TABER'S
Condensed Medical Dictionary

by

CLARENCE WILBUR TABER

Author, Taber's Cyclopedic Medical Dictionary, Taber's Dictionary
of Gynecology and Obstetrics, and Dictionary of
Food and Nutrition, etc., etc.

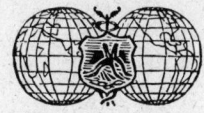

F. A. DAVIS COMPANY, PUBLISHERS
PHILADELPHIA

Preface

This dictionary is an abridgement of *Taber's Cyclopedic Medical Dictionary*. It has been prepared to meet the requirements of those who feel the need of a more adequate type of medical word book than heretofore obtainable; one that has not been abbreviated by clipping definitions found in the large and more exhaustive medical dictionaries. This process often distorts the meaning of the words included.

The majority of medical students and nurses will undoubtedly continue to use the Cyclopedic edition. Those who want a more elementary type of dictionary will find in this work a better presentation of subject material than may be found elsewhere in a concise form.

Vocabulary: With the exception of the names of foods, the vocabulary in this dictionary is exactly the same as that in the Cyclopedic edition. Medical synonyms are also included.

Pronunciations: Over 99% of the vocabulary words have been respelled for pronunciation and marked with diacritical symbols.

Definitions: They are exactly the same as those in the larger work, written especially for the purpose and not abbreviated from other sources.

The abridgement has been made by eliminating supplementary material, illustrations, and tabulated matter in the appendix of the *Cyclopedic Medical Dictionary*.

* * *

Abbreviations Used in the Text

abbr.	abbreviation	inf.	inferior
adm.	administration	int.	interior, internal
anat.	anatomy	K	potassium, kalium
ant.	anterior	L.	Latin
anti.	antidote	lat.	lateral
app.	appendix	LL.	Late Latin
art.	artery	m.	male
AS.	Anglo-Saxon	ME.	Middle English
at. wt.	atomic weight	med.	medical
bact.	bacteriology	mg.	milligram
bet.	between	Mg	magnesium
biol.	biology	N	nitrogen
BNA	Basle nomina anatomica or Basle anatomical nomenclature	Na	sodium, natrium
		neur.	neurology
		NP.	nursing procedure
br.	branch, branches	NNR.	new and nonofficial remedy
C.	Centigrade	nut.	nutrients
C	carbon	O	oxygen
Ca	calcium	OB.	obstetrics
Cal.	large Calorie or Calories	O. Fr.	Old French
cal.	small calorie or calories	OPHTH.	ophthalmology
carbo.	carbohydrates	opp.	opposite
cc.	cubic centimeter	orig.	origin
cf.	compare	ORTH.	orthopedics
chem.	chemistry	OTO.	otology
Cl	chlorine	ONP	operating nursing procedure
comp.	composition	p	page
contra.	contraindication	P	phosphorus
Cu	copper, cuprum	PATH.	pathology
der.	derivative	pert.	pertaining
dis.	distribution	PHARM.	pharmacy
E.	English	PHYS.	physiology
(e	indicates the word may also be terminated with "e"	pl.	plural
		post.	posterior
e. g.	for example	pre.	prefix
elect.	electricity	pro.	protein
esp.	especially	prog.	prognosis
etiol.	etiology	PSY.	psychiatry, psychoanalysis, psychology
ex.	example		
ext.	exterior, external	PT.	physical therapy
F.	Fahrenheit	q.v.	which see
Fr.	French	rel.	relating
Fe	iron, ferrum	RS.	related subjects
fem.	female, feminine	S	sulfur
ff. ind.	fact finding index	sing.	singular
funct.	function	sp. gr.	specific gravity
G.	Greek	sup.	superior
Ger.	German	SYM.	symptoms
Gm.	gram or grams	SYMB.	symbol
gr.	grain or grains	SYN.	synonym
gyn.	gynecology	USP	United States Pharmacopeia
H	hydrogen	viz.	namely
I	iodine	*	denotes more information may be found under the word indicated
i. e.	that is		
ind.	indication		

A

a. Abbr. for *accommodation, anode, anterior,* and *total acidity.*

A. Symb. for *argon.*

A. or **A. u.** Abbr. for *Angström unit.*

A₂. Abbr. for *aortic second sound.*

A. A. Abbr. for *achievement age.*

āā, āā. Prescription sign denoting the stated amount of each of the substances is to be taken.

a-, an-. Prefix meaning *without, away from, not,* as *atypical.*

Aaron's sign. Distress in region of heart or stomach upon pressure over Mc-Burney's point* as in *appendicitis.*

ab-. Prefix meaning *from, away from, negative,* as *abnormal.*

abacte′rial. Without bacteria.

abactio (ab-ak′shĭ-o). Induced abortion.*

abactus venter. Nonspontaneous abortion.

Abadie's sign (ă-bă-dēz′). 1. In exophthalmic goiter, spasm of the *levator palpebrae superioris.* 2. In tabes dorsalis, insensibility to pressure over *tendo Achillis.*

abaissement (a-bās′mon). 1. Depression. 2. Couching. 3. Falling.

abalienated (ab-āl′yen-ā-ted). Deranged.

abalienatio mentis (ab-al-yen-a′shĭ-o men′tis). Insanity.

abalienation (ab-āl-yen-ā′shun). Physical or mental decay; lunacy or derangement.

abanet (ab′an-et). Girdle or girdlelike bandage. SYN: *abnet.**

abarognosis (ă-bar-og-no′sis). Without sense of weight.

abarthrosis (ab-ar-thro′sis). A movable joint or point upon which bones move freely upon each other; diarthrosis.*

abartic′ular. At a distance from a joint.

abarticula′tion. Dislocation of a joint.

abasia (a-ba′zĭ-ă). Motor incoördination in walking; astasia. Inability to stand or walk due to loss of coördination; organic disease in such cases usually easily recognized; if not, hysteria is probable.

    a. astasia. Inability to stand or walk.

    a. atactia. Uncertain movements.

    a., choreic. That due to cramps in the limbs similar to movements of chorea.

    a., paralytic. That in which the legs give way from body weight.

    a., paroxysmal trepidant. That caused by trepidation, stiffening legs and making walking impossible.

    a., spastic. Paroxysmal trepidantia.

    a. statica. Uncertainty of movement.

    a., trembling, a. trepidans. That due to trembling of the legs.

abasic (ă-ba′sik). Pert. to abasia.

abate (a-bāt′). 1. To lessen or decrease. 2. To cease or cause to cease.

abate′ment. Decrease in severity of pain or symptoms.

abatic (ab-at′ik). Pert. to abasia. SYN: *abasic.**

abaxial (ab-ak′si-al), **abaxile.** 1. Without the axis of the body. 2. At the opp. end of the axis of a part.

Abbé's catgut ring (ab′bā′s). A ring of catgut to reinforce the suture in intestinal anastomosis.

    A.'s condenser. Several nonachromatic lenses to increase illumination under lens of a microscope.

    A.'s operation. 1. For relief of the tic douloureux by resection of the 5th c. nerve. 2. Lateral anastomosis of the intestine.

Abbé-Zeiss apparatus. An instrument for estimating number of blood corpuscles.

Abb′ot's paste. A paste for killing a nerve of a tooth.

Abbott's method. Treatment of lateral curvature of the spine by a series of plaster jackets.

A. B. C. lin′iment. Liniment composed of aconite 40, belladonna 40, chloroform 20.

a.b.c. process. The use of alum, blood, and charcoal in purification of water or sewage or deodorization.

Abderhalden's reaction or test (äb′der-hāl-denz). Creation of ferments in circulation as result of injection of foreign protein, fat, or carbohydrate. Used in testing for pregnancy, acute infections, malignancies, goiter, dementia precox.

abdomen (ab-do′men). Cavity in body between diaphragm and pelvis.

    a., accordion. Nervous pseudotympany.

    a., acute. Any acute abdominal condition demanding prompt operation.

    a., boat-shaped. SEE: *a., scaphoid.*

    a., carinate. SEE: *a., scaphoid.*

    a., navicular. SEE: *a., scaphoid.*

    a. obstipum. Congenital shortness of the rectus abdominus muscle.

    a., pendulous. A relaxed condition of the abdominal wall.

    a., scaphoid. Sunken as in emaciation and in meningitis. One whose ant. wall is hollowed.

abdominal (ab-dom′i-nal). Pert. to the abdomen, its function and disorders.

    a. cavity. Cavity within the peritoneum.

    a. gestation. Abdominal pregnancy. Extrauterine fetation in belly cavity.

    a. reflexes. These consist of muscular contraction of either side of the abdomen, being induced by friction on that part. [dominal wall.

    a. rings. The apertures in the ab-

    a. section. Abdominal incision for any operation on internal organs. SEE: *laparotomy.*

abdominoanterior (ab-dom″ĭ-no-an-te′rĭ-or). Position of fetus in utero with belly facing ant. abdominal wall of mother.

abdom″inocar′diac re′flex. Increased heart consciousness when abdominal sympathetics are stimulated.

abdominocentesis (ab-dom″ĭ-nō-sen-te′sĭs). Abdominal puncture by tapping. SYN: *paracentesis abdominis.*

abdominocys′tic. Pert. to abdomen and bladder.

abdominogen′ital. Pert. to abdomen and genital organs.

abdom″inohysterec′tomy. Removal of uterus through abdominal wall.

abdom″inohysterot′omy. Incision into the uterus through an abdominal opening.

abdom″inoposte′rior. Position of fetus in utero with abdomen toward mother's back.

abdom″inos′copy. Examination of abdomen or its viscera.

abdom″inoscro′tal. Pert. to abdomen and scrotum.

   a. muscle. Cremaster m.

abdominothoracic (ab-dom″ĭ-no-tho-ras′-ik), Pert. to abdomen and thorax.

   a. arch. Pert. to both abdomen and thorax.

abdom′inous. Having a prominent abdomen.

abdom″inouterot′omy. Cesarean section. SYN: *abdominohysterotomy.*

abdom″inovag′inal. Pert. to abdomen and vagina.

abdom″inoves′ical. Pert. to abdomen, urinary system, or gallbladder.

   a. pouch. Peritoneal fold which includes urachal folds.

abduce (ab-dūs′). To draw away.

abducens (ab-dū′senz). 1. The 6th cranial nerve. 2. The external rectus muscle of the eye, which moves the eyeball outward. 3. Pert. to certain muscles or their nerves drawing from the median line of the body.

   a. labiorum. Abducens oris, *q.v.*

   a. nerve. Sixth cranial nerve.* Motor nerve supplying lateral rectus muscle of eye. ORIG: *Fasciculus teres.*

   a. oculi. BNA. *Musculus rectus lateralis.* Muscle of eye.

   a. oris. Muscle of mouth. BNA. *Musculus caninus.*

abdu′cent. Abducting, leading away from.

abduct′. To draw away from axis of body or one of its parts.

abduc′tion. Movement away from midline of body, turning outward.

abduc′tor. A muscle which draws certain parts away from a common center.

Abel's bacillus. One found in nasal secretion in ozena; *Klebsiella ozaenae.*

abenteric (ab-en-ter′ĭk). Located in a part outside the intestines, as *abenteric typhoid.*

abepithymia (ab-ep-ĭ-thī′mĭ-ă). 1. Perverted desire or longing. 2. Solar plexus paralysis.

Abernethy's fascia (ab′er-nĕ-thēz). Superperitoneal areolar tissue separating *ext.*

iliac art. from iliac fascia over the psoas.

   A.'s sarcoma. A circumscribed fatty tumor occurring principally on the trunk.

aber′rant. Wandering from the normal or usual course.

   a. pyramidal tract. Several groups of fibers from motor cortex to the cranial nerve nuclei, running apart from the rest of the pyramidal system.

aberratio (ab-er-a′shĭ-o). Aberration.

   a. humorum. Abnormal flow of blood to another tract, as in vicarious menstruation (*aberratio mensium*).

aberra′tion. 1. Deviation from a normal course. 2. Mental unsoundness, but not insanity. 3. Imperfect refraction.

   a., chromatic. Unequal refraction of different wave lengths of the spectrum producing a blurred image.

   a., diopteric. Spherical aberration.

   a., distantial. Blurring of a distant object.

   a., mental. Mental unsoundness that may or may not amount to insanity.

   a., spherical. Imperfect focus produced by a convex lens.

aberrom′eter. An instrument for measuring optical error.

abevacuation (ab-ē-vak-u-a′shun). Abnormal evacuation either in excess or in deficiency.

abeyance (a-bā′ăns). A temporary suspension of activity, sensation, or pain.

abiochemistry (ab-i-o-kem′ĭs-trĭ). Inorganic chemistry.

abiogenesis (ab-i-o-jen′e-sĭs). Spontaneous generation.

abiogenet′ic, abio′genous. Pert. to spontaneous generation.

abiological (ab-ĭ-o-loj′ĭ-kal). Not related to biology or the science of life.

abiology (a-bi-ol′o-jĭ). The study of inanimate things.

abionergy (ab-ĭ-on′ur-jĭ). Premature degeneration. SYN: *abiotrophy.*

abiosis (ab-i-ō′sĭs). Absence of life.

abiot′ic. Incompatible with life; not viable.

abiotro′phia. Abiotrophy.

abiotrophy (ab-i-ot′ro-fĭ). Premature loss of vitality or degeneration of tissues and cells.

abirritant (ab-ir′it-ant). Relieving irritation; soothing.

abirrita′tion. 1. Asthenia, or atony. 2. Lowered tissue irritability.

abiuret (a-bi′ū-ret). Nonbiuret. Not giving the biuret reaction.

ablactation (ab-lak-ta′shun). Free of, or cessation of milk secretion; weaning.

ablastem′ic. Not germinal.

ablate′. To remove, especially by excision.

ablatio (ab-la′shĭ-o). Ablation, removal, detachment.

   a. placentae. Premature detachment of a normally situated placenta.

   a. retinae. Detachment of retina.

ablation (ab-la′shun). Removal of a part, as by cutting. SEE: *ablatio.*

-able; -ible; -ble. Suffixes: Capable of being; power to be, as *audible.*

ablepsia (ă-blep'sĭ-ă). 1. Blindness. 2. Dulled perception.

ab'luent. An agent possessing cleansing qualities, as a detergent.

ablu'tion. A cleansing or washing. PT: Pouring water out of bucket over body or part. Mechanical effect mild; action depends mainly on temperature.

abmor'tal. Passing from dead or dying to living muscular fiber, as an electric current.

abner'val. Passing from a nerve to a muscular fiber.

ab'net. A girdle or girdlelike bandage.

abneural (ab-nu'ral). Ventral. Remote from neural or dorsal aspect.

abnor'mal. Not normal. SEE: *chondral-loplasia, chondrodysplasia*.

ab"normal'ity. That which is not normal.

abnormity (ab-norm'ĭ-tĭ). 1. Deformity; abnormality. 2. A monstrosity.

aboiment (ăbwa-mon'). The making of barking sounds.

aboli'tion. Doing away with anything.

aborad (ab-o'rad). Away from the mouth.

abo'ral. Opposite to, or away from, the mouth.

abort'. 1. To cause expulsion of an embryo or of the fetus before time of viability. 2. To arrest progress of disease. 3. To arrest growth or development; rudimentary.

aborticide (a-bor'tĭ-sĭd). A term etymologically incorrect for an agent causing death of fetus and expulsion from uterus.

abortient (ab-or'shent). 1. Producing abortion. 2. Abortifacient. 3. Sterile.

abortifacient (a-bor-tĭ-fā'shent). A drug which causes an abortion.

abortion (ab-or'shun). 1. The arrest of any physical action or disease. 2. The termination of pregnancy before the term of viability, *i. e.*, before the 28th week, the fetus measuring 35 cm. or less, and weighing less than 3¼ lb. (1500 Gm.). The term *miscarriage* is sometimes applied when occurring after 4th mo. and before 7th mo.; *premature delivery* after 7th mo. and before full term.

   a., accidental. That which occurs spontaneously and accidentally without criminal intent.

   a., artificial. When induced or performed purposely, as by a surgeon.

   a., criminal. When produced for other than medical purposes.

   a., embryonic. Before 4th month.

   a., fetal. After 4th month.

   a., habitual. When in course of repeated pregnancies with no apparent cause.

   a., incomplete. When some of products of conception are retained with continuation of symptoms.

   a., induced. When brought on intentionally, criminally or therapeutically.

   a., inevitable. That which cannot be stopped or when occurring after the embryo is dead.

   a., infected. When accompanied by infection of retained material with resultant febrile reaction.

   a., justifiable. When done to save the mother's life.

   a., missed. That in which the fetus died with products of conception retained in uterus.

   a., ovular. That which occurs within first three weeks after conception.

   a., partial. In multiple pregnancy, aborting of only 1 fetus, or less than the entire number. [terference.

   a., spontaneous. Occurring without in-

   a., therapeutic. One done when life of mother is endangered by continuation of the pregnancy.

   a., threatened. When only earliest signs of abortion are present.

   a., tubal. An ectopic (abnormally placed) pregnancy in which the ovum has been expelled through the fimbriated end of tube.

abortionist (a-bor'shun-ist). One who performs a criminal abortion.

abortive (a-bor'tiv). 1. Preventing the completion of. 2. Abortifacient; that which prevents a natural or regular course. 3. Rudimentary.

abortus (a-bor'tus). An abortion.

aboulia (ă-boo'lĭ-ă). Inability to exercise will power. SYN: *abulia, q.v.*

aboulomania (ă-boo'lo-ma'nĭ-ă). Mental disorder with loss of will power. SYN: *abulomania.*

abrade'. 1. To chafe. 2. To roughen or remove by friction.

Abrams' heart reflex. Reduction of area of cardiac dullness resulting from manual friction of precordial and epigastric areas.

   A. lung reflex. Following irritation of the skin over the thorax or upper abdominal region, there is an increase in pulmonary area.

abra'sio cor'neae. Removal of corneal excrescences by scraping.

abrasion (ab-ra'shun). An injury resulting from scraping away of a portion of skin or of a mucous membrane. A brush burn.

abra'sive. 1. Producing abrasion. 2. That which abrades.

abreaction (ab-re-ak'shun). PSY: Reevaluation of an emotion-laden experience during its free discussion with an understanding psychotherapist. Freud calls the process *catharsis.**

abrosia (ab-rō'zĭ-ă). 1. Fasting; the need for food. 2. A wasting away.

abruptio (ab-rup'shĭ-o). A tearing away from.

   a. placentae. Premature detachment of normally situated placenta. SEE: *ablatio placentae.*

abscess (ab'ses). A localized collection of pus in a cavity; the pus formed by disintegration of tissue.

   a., acute. One which runs a short course with fever and inflammation.

   a., alveolar. One of the gum or alveolus.

   a., amebic. One containing amebae.

   a., anorectal. One in the tissue near the rectum.

a., apical. One at the apex of lung or at extremity of root of a tooth.

a., appendiceal, appendicular. Pus formation about vermiform appendix.

a., arthrifluent. A wandering abscess having origin in a diseased joint.

a., atheromatous. Atheromatous softening in wall of an artery.

a., Bezold's. A deep abscess in the neck.

a., blind. A dental granuloma.

a., Brodie's. Tuberculosis with suppuration of articular end of a bone.

a., bursal. One in a bursa.

a., canalic'ular. An abscess of breast discharging into the milk ducts.

a., caseous. One in which the pus has a cheesy appearance.

a., cheesy. Caseous abscess.

a., chronic. One of slow development.

a., circumscribed. An abscess limited by exudation of lymph.

a., circumtonsillar. Quinsy.

a., cold. Usually a chronic one in bones, joints, or tuberculous glands. It has little surrounding inflammation.

a., congestive. One that shows pus at a point distant from where formed.

a., diffuse. A collection of pus not circumscribed by a well-defined capsule.

a., dry. One that disappears without pointing or breaking.

a., embolic. One formed in the clot of an embolism.

a., fe'cal. A stercoral abscess.

a., fixation. One produced artificially by subcutaneous injection of an irritant.

a., gas. An abscess containing gas due to *B. aerogenes* or other gas-forming microörganism.

a., gravitation. An abscess in which the pus migrates, sinking to lower depths.

a., hypostatic. A gravitation abscess.

a., ischiorectal. One in the ischiorectal fossa.

a., lacrimal. Suppuration of a lacrimal gland.

a., lacunar. One in the urethral lacunae.

a., lumbar. One in the lumbar region.

a., lung. Abscess occurring in the lung.

a., mammary. One in the female breast.

a., metastatic. A secondary one at a distance from focus of infection.

a., miliary. A small embolic abscess. One discharging numerous small collections of pus.

a., milk. A mammary abscess during lactation.

a., mural. One in tissues of the abdominal wall following celiotomy.

a., peribronchitic. Abscess in inflamed tissue around the bronchi. SYN: *Faubel's granule.*

a., pericemental. An alveolar abscess not involving apex of a tooth.

a., peridental. Periodontal abscess.

a., perinephric. One in tissue about the kidney.

a., periodontal. An alveolar abscess.

a., phlegmonous. An acute abscess.

a., primary. One originating at point of infection.

a., psoas. One with pus descending in sheath of psoas muscle due to vertebral disease.

a., rectal. One in the rectum.

a., residual. One occurring in old inflammatory products.

a., retropharyngeal. One in post. wall of the oropharynx.

a., root. Dental granuloma. Granulations at root of a tooth.

a., scrofulous. One due to tuberculous degeneration of bone, or lymph glands.

a., secondary. Embolic abscess.

a's., shirt-stud. Two abscesses communicating by a sinus.

a., stercoral. One containing pus and fecal matter.

a., stitch. One formed about a stitch or suture.

a., strumous. A cold abscess of tuberculous causation.

a., subphrenic. One beneath the diaphragm.

a., thecal. One in sheath of a tendon.

a., wandering. One at a distance from focus of disease with pus along fascial sheaths of muscles.

a., warm. An acute abscess.

abscession (ab-sesh'un). 1. Metastasis. 2. A critical discharge. 3. An abscess.*

abscission (ab-sī'shun). The removal of a part by excision.

absentia epilep'tica (ab-sen'shĭ-ă). The loss of consciousness in the mild form of epilepsy.

ab'solute al'cohol. Alcohol with no more than 1% of water.

   a. temperature. Temperature reckoned from the absolute zero.

   a. zero. 273.7° below zero Cent. The lowest possible temperature.

absorb'. To suck up as through pores. SEE: *absorbent.*

absorbefacient (ab-sor-be-fā'shent). Causing or that which causes absorption.

absorb'ent. 1. A substance that causes absorption of diseased tissue. 2. Taking up by suction.

   a. cotton. Cotton prepared to absorb moisture.

   a. glands. Lymph glands.

absorptiometer (ab-sorp-shĭ-om'e-ter). An instrument for measuring thickness of liquid drawn by capillary attraction between glass plates.

absorption (ab-sorp'shun). 1. The taking up of liquids by solids, or of gases by solids or liquids. 2. The taking up of light or of its rays by black or colored rays. 3. The taking up by the body of radiant heat, causing a rise in body temperature. 4. PHYS: The passage of a substance through some surface of the body into body fluids and tissues, as the passage of ether through the respiratory epithelium of lungs into the blood during anesthesia, or passage of oil of wintergreen through the skin, the result of several processes.

a. lines. Dark lines of solar spectrum. SYN: *Fraunhofer's lines.**

a., pathological. Absorption of contents of an excretion or an abnormal product into blood stream.

a. of radiation. Grotthuss' law states only rays which are absorbed are physiologically active.

a. spectrum. A spectrum showing absorption lines.

absorp'tion co''effi'cient. PT: The ratio of the linear rate of change of intensity of roentgen rays in a given homogeneous material to the intensity at a given point within the same mass.

absorp'tive. Absorbent.

abstergent (ab-stur'jent). 1. A cleansing agent. 2. Having cleansing properties. 3. A purgative.

abstersion (ab-ster'shun). Cleansing.

abster'sive. Abstergent. Cleansing.

abstinence (ab'stĭ-nens). Going without voluntarily.

a. symptoms. Partial collapse resulting from withdrawal of alcohol, stimulants, and some opiates.

ab'stract. 1. A preparation containing the soluble principles of a drug evaporated and mixed with sugar of milk. 2. *v.* **abstract'.** To remove from. 3. To condense or abbreviate.

abstraction (ab-strak'shun). Bloodletting.

abter'minal. Away from an end toward the center, noting course of.

abulia (a-boo'lĭ-ă). Absence of or inability to exercise "will power"; hesitation; indecision. Seen in dementia precox.

abulic (ab-u'lik). Pert. to abulia.

abulomania (a-boo'lo-ma'nĭ-ă). A mental disorder accompanied by impaired (or loss of) will power. These are obsolete terms. [anchored.

abut'ment. The tooth to which a bridge is A. C. Abbr. for anodal closure.

a. c. Abbr. for L. *ante cibos*, before meals.

a. c. interval. One bet. beginning of auricular and carotid wave; intersystolic period.

acacia (ak-ka'shĭ-a). USP. A dried, gummy exudation from the tree *Acacia senegal.*

acalcerosis (ă-kal-ser-o'sis). Lack of calcium in the body.

acalculia (a-kal-kŭ'lĭ-ă). Inability to solve mathematical problems.

acampsia (a-kamp'sĭ-ă). Inflexibility of a limb; rigidity, ankylosis.

acan'tha. 1. The spine. 2. A vertebral spinous process.

acanthesthesia (a-kan-thes-the'zĭ-ă). A sensation as of a prick; a form of paresthesia, *q.v.*

Acan'thia lectula'ria. The common bedbug, *Cimex lectularius.*

acan'thion. Tip of ant. nasal spine.

Acanthocephala (ă-kan-tho-sef'ăl-ă). An order of nematodelike entozoa, including Echinorhynchus. Parasitic in man.

acanthocephaliasis (ă-kan''tho-sef-ăl-ĭ'ă-sis). Infestation with Acanthocephala.

acan'thoid. Thorny; spiny; of a spinous nature.

acanthokeratodermia (ă-kan''tho-ker''ă-to-der'mĭ-ă). Hypertrophy of hands and feet.

a. adenoides cysticum. Sweat gland edema.

a. alveolaris. Tumor of epithelium. SYN: *epithelioma.*

a. verrucosa seborrhoica. Warty growths in the senile.

acantholysis (a-kan-thol'is-is). Any disease of the skin accompanied by atrophy of the prickle layer.

a. bullosa. A skin condition of large bullae produced by irritation. SYN: *Epidermolysis bullosa.**

acanthoma (a-kan-tho'ma). 1. Papilloma. 2. Cancer of skin.

a. adenoides cysticum. Eruption arising in the rete spinosum of the skin and resembling spiradenoma.

acanthopel'vis. A prominent and sharp pubic spine on a rachitic pelvis.

acanthosis (a-kan-tho'sis). Disease of prickle cell layer of skin.

a. nigricans. Chronic inflammatory disease of skin in adult life generally associated with cancer of some internal organ.

acanthot'ic. Pert. to acanthosis.

acanthulus (a-kan'thu-lus). An instrument for removing thorns or splinters from wounds.

acap'nia. The presence of less than normal amount of carbon dioxide in blood and tissues, *e. g.*, after voluntary overbreathing and the condition resulting therefrom.

acap'nial. Showing or pert. to acapnia.

acar'bia. Diminution of carbonate of the blood due to asphyxia.

acariasis (ak-ă-rĭ'a-sis). Any disease caused by a mite or *acarus* (*Acaridae*).

acaricide (a-kar'ĭ-sĭd). 1. An agent that destroys acarids. 2. Destroying a member of order *Acarina.*

ac'arid, acar'idan. A tick or mite; member of order *Acarina.*

acaridi'asis. Disease caused by a mite. SYN: *acariasis.*

acarinosis (ă-kar-ĭ-no'sis). Disease caused by a mite. SYN: *acariasis.*

acarodermatitis (ak-a-ro-der-mă-tī'tis). The itch. Inflammation of skin caused by a mite.

ac'aroid. A mite, or resembling one.

acarophobia (a-kar-o-fo'bĭ-ă). PSY: Delusion that the skin is infested with mites or worms.

acarpia (a-karp'ĭ-a). Barrenness; sterility.

ac'arus. A mite or tick.

acaryote (ă-kar'ĭ-ōt). Without a nucleus.

acatalepsia (a-kat-a-lep'sĭ-ă). 1. Dementia. Impairment of mind. 2. Diagnostic uncertainty.

acat'alepsy. 1. Dementia or impairment of mind. 2. Uncertainty. SYN: *acatalepsia.**

acatalep'tic. 1. Deficient mentally. 2. Uncertain or doubtful.

acatamathesia (a-kat-a-ma-the'zĭ-ă). PSY: 1. Psychic blindness or deafness, or blunting of sensation. 2. Inability to comprehend words, conversation, or signs, due to a brain lesion.

acataphasia (a-kat-a-fa'zĭ-ă). Inability to formulate a sentence.

acataposis (ă-kă-tap'o-sis). Dysphagia. Difficulty in swallowing.

acatastasia (ă-kat-as-ta'zĭ-ă). Irregularity or fixed characteristics in the course of a disease or in excretion.

acatharsia (a-ka-thar'sĭ-ă). Foulness; impurity; lack of purging.

acathectic (ă-ka-thek'tĭk). Inability to retain. Lack of retention.

    a. jaundice. That due to inability of liver cells to prevent bile from passing into lymph and blood.

acathexia (a-ka-theks'ĭ-ă). An inability to retain excretions or secretions.

acathisia (a-ka-thĭz'ĭ-ă). Inability to remain seated.

acaulino'sis. A disease due to a fungus, causing eczematous eruption.

ACC. Abbr. for *anodal closure contraction.*

accelerans (ak-sel'er-ans). The acceleration heart rate.

accelera'tion. Increasing the motion of, as pulse or respiration.

accelerator (ak-sel'er-a-tor). Anything that increases action or function.

    a. nerve. Nerve increasing heart rate and action. SEE: *accelerans.*

    a. urinae. Bulbocavernosus muscle.

accentua'tion. Marked with a special stress; emphasis.

accept'or. A substance absorbing nascent hydrogen freed by a reducing enzyme.

    a., hydrogen. Substance which receives hydrogen from a hydrogen donator.

accesso'rius. Accessory, supplementary, as certain muscles, glands, nerves.

    a. nerve. 11th cranial nerve. Motor nerve made up of a cranial and a spinal part which supplies the trapezius and sternomastoid muscles and pharynx. Accessory portion joins the vagus, to which it supplies its motor and some of its cardio-inhibitory fibers.

    a. Willis'ii. Spinal accessory nerve.

acces'sory. Auxiliary; assisting, as accessory glands of the pancreas or Brunner's glands.*

    a. articles of diet. Condiments,* flavors, and stimulants.

ac'cident. 1. An unexpected event. 2. An unforeseen occurrence of an unfortunate nature, a mishap.

accipiter (ak-sip'it-er). A bandage for the face with clawlike tails.

acclima'tion. To become accustomed to a climate.

acclimatization (a-kli-ma-ti-za'shun). Becoming accustomed to a new climate.

acclimatize (ak-klī'mă-tīz). To make accustomed to a new climate.

accommoda'tion. 1. Adjustment. 2. Adaption.

    a., absolute. Accommodation of either eye separately.   [*commodation.*

    a., amplitude of. SEE: *range of ac-*

    a., binocular. Meeting of both eyes at a point in order to carry the object's image to the retina of both.

    a., histologic. Change in cell form and function due to change in surrounding conditions.

    a., mechanism. Method by which curvature of eye lens is changed in order to focus close objects on the retina.

    a., negative. Relaxation by the eye to adjust itself for long distances.

    a., positive. Contraction by the eye to adjust itself for short distances.

    a., range of. Space of vision between its closest and most remote points.

    a., reflex. The normal dilation and contraction of pupil as eye focuses for near and far objects. SEE: *Argyll-Robertson pupil.*

    a., relative. Accommodation produced by the two eyes acting together.

accom'modative iridoplegia. Noncontraction of pupils during accommodation.

accouchée (ak-koo-shay'). One who has been delivered of a child.

accouchement (a-koosh-mon'). The act of delivery in childbirth; parturition.

    a. forcé. Forcible hand delivery.

accoucheur, accoucheuse (ak-koosh-er', a-koo-shŭz') (*Fem.*). One who practices obstetrics.

accrementition (a-kre-men-tish'un). Increase of growth by interstitial development from blastemia and by reproduction by cellular fission. Gemmation, *q.v.*

accretion (ak-re'shun). 1. Adherence of parts. 2. Accumulation.

accubation (ak-u-ba'shun). 1. Act of taking to one's bed or assuming a reclining posture. 2. Lying in bed with another person.

accum'ulator or storage battery. PT: A vessel containing sulfuric acid diluted until its sp. gr. is 1.200. In this are immersed lead plates.

a.c.e. mixture. An anesthetic for general inhalation made up of one part of *alcohol,* two parts of *chloroform,* and three parts of *ether.* Now seldom used.

acedia (a-sē'dĭ-ă). Indifference. Insensibility. Lack of emotion. SYN: *apathy.*

acenesthesia (a-sen-es-the'zĭ-ă). Absence of a feeling of well-being, present in such disorders as hypochondriasis and neurasthenia.

acen'tric. Not central; peripheral.

aceph'alocyst, acephalocys'tis. An echinococcus cyst; hydatid.

    a. racemo'sa. A hydatid uterine mole.

acephalous (ă-sef'al-us). Without a head.

acerbity (a-serb'ĭ-tĭ). Astringency combined with acidity.

acervuline (ă-ser'vu-līn). Aggregated, occurring in clusters.

acervuloma (ă-ser-vu-lo'ma). Intracranial tumor containing brain sand.

acer'vulus. Sandy, sabulous.

    a. cer'ebri. Sabulous matter filling the follicle of the pineal gland; brain sand.

acescence (a-ses'ens). 1. Slight acidity. 2. Process of souring.

acesent (a-ses'ent). Slightly acid.

acestoma (a-ses-to'mă). The fresh granulations which later form a cicatrix.

acetabular (as-et-ab'u-lar). Pert. to the acetabulum.

acetabulum (as-et-ab'u-lum). The rounded (cotyloid) cavity on the external surface of the innominate bone (*os coxae* or *os innominatum*) which receives head of femur.

acetanilid (as-et-an'il-id) (antifebrin). USP. A white powder or crystalline substance obtained by interaction of glacial acetic acid and aniline.

DOSAGE: 3 gr. (0.2 Gm.).

acetarsone (as-et-ar'sŏn). An organic arsenical compound originally introduced as "stovarsol" containing 27.1 to 27.4% arsenic.

DOSAGE: Orally: 4 gr. (0.25 Gm.).

acetate (as'e-tāt). A salt of acetic acid.

acetbroman'ilid. Antisepsin, asepsin, an analgesic and hypnotic.

acetic (a-se'tĭk). Pert. to vinegar; sour.

a. acid. Gives vinegar sour taste.

a. a. test for albumen. Acetic acid is added to heated urine. If cloudy, albumen present. SEE: *albumen.*

a. fermentation. A continuation of alcoholic fermentation.

aceticoceptor (ă-se"tik-o-sep'tor). One of the side chains which have an affinity for the acetic acid radical.

acet'idin. Ethyl acetate.

acetify (a-se'tĭ-fĭ). To produce acetic fermentation or vinegar.

acetimeter (ă-se-tĭm'e-ter). An apparatus which determines the acetic acid in fluid.

Acetobac'ter. A genus of *nitrobacteriaceae.*

A. ace'ti. A form of Acetobacter producing vinegar from wine or cider.

acetone (as'e-tōn). Dimethyl ketone ($CH_3)_2CO$, a colorless, volatile, inflammable liquid, miscible with water, useful as a solvent, and having a characteristic irritating odor.

DOSAGE: 5-15 gr. (0.3-1.0 Gm.).

a. bodies. Certain substances related to acetone. An example is *acetoacetic acid, q.v.* under *acid.*

acetonemia (as-e-to-nē'mĭ-ă). Large amounts of acetone in blood. SYM: *erethism, gradual depression, acidosis.*

acetonuria (as-e-to-nu'rĭ-ă). The occurrence of acetone and diacetic bodies in the urine, as in the *ketosis* of diabetes, starvation, etc., which may be due to incomplete oxidation of albuminous substances.

acetophenetidin (as-ĕ-to-fe-net'id-in) (phenacetin) USP. A crystalline substance manufactured from coal tar.

DOSAGE: 5 to 15 gr. (0.32-1.0 Gm.).

acetous (as'e-tus). 1. Pert. to vinegar. 2. Sour in taste.

acetum (pl. *aceta*) (a-se'tum). Vinegar.

acetylcholine (ă-sĕt-ĭl-kō'lēn). An alkaloid from ergot.

It causes a lowering of blood pressure.

a. chloride. It is dissolved in glucose and given in daily doses of 0.5-1.0 Gm., intramuscularly.

acetylsalicylic acid (as'ĕt-il-sal-ĭ-sil'ik)

(aspirin) USP. A white powder or crystalline substance obtained by action of acetic anhydride on salicylic acid.

DOSAGE: 5 to 15 gr. (0.3-1.0 Gm.).

achalasia (ă-kal-a'zĭ-ă). Failure to relax; said of muscles, such as sphincters, the normal function of which is a persistent contraction with periods of relaxation.

achieve'ment age. Determined by test for proficiency in a subject measured by what average child of that chronological age can do. SEE: *age.*

a. quo'tient (A.Q.). A state of progress in learning ascertained by dividing the achievement age by the mental age.

Achil'les jerk. The motor response to striking tendon of gastrocnemius muscle.

Achilles tendon (a-kil'ēz) (*tendo achillis* or *tendo calcaneus*). The tendon of the soleus and gastrocnemius muscles, at the back of the heel.

A. t. reflex. Plantar flexion of foot and contraction of calf muscles following blow upon tendon of Achilles. Absent in sciatica.

achillobursitis (a-kil-o-bur-si'tis). Inflammation of the bursa lying over the Achilles tendon.

achillodynia (a-kil-o-din'i-ă). Pain caused by inflammation bet. the *tendo calcaneus* and the bursa.

achillorrhaphy (a-kil-or'raf-ĭ). Suture of *tendo achillis.*

achillotomy (a-kil-ot'o-mĭ). A division of *tendo achillis.*

achi'lous. Without lips.

achiria (a-ki'rĭ-ă). 1. Congenital lack of hands. 2. Loss of sense of possession of one or both hands. 3. Inability to tell on which side of body a stimulus is applied.

achlorhydria (a-klor-hi'drĭ-ă). Absence of free hydrochloric acid in the gastric juice.

achloride (ă-klo'rĭd). A salt other than a chloride; nonchloride.

achloropsia (ă-klo-rop'se-ă). Color blindness as regards green. [of bile.

acholia (ak-o'lĭ-ă). An absence or want

acholic (ak-o'lĭk). Pert. to acholia.

acholuria (a-kol-u'rĭ-ă). In some forms of jaundice, absence of bile pigments in the urine.

achondroplasia (ă-kon-dro-pla'sĭ-ă). Defect in the formation of cartilage at the epiphyses of long bones, producing a form of dwarfism; sometimes seen in rickets.

achor (a'kor). 1. Small pustules on hairy parts of body. 2. Pointed pustules. 3. Scabby eruption on scalp and face of infants.

achoresis (ă-ko-re'sis). Contraction of the bladder, stomach, or other hollow viscus, reducing its capacity.

Achorion (ă-ko'rĭ-on). A genus of fungous organisms found in the skin, esp. in hair follicles.

A. schoenleinii. A species of Achorion in ringworm.

achreocythemia (a-kre-o-sĭ-the'mĭ-ă). Absence of coloring in the blood.

achroacyte (a-krō'a-sīt). A lymphocyte; a colorless cell.

achroacytosis (a-kro-ă-si-to'sis). Many lymphocytes in the peripheral circulation.

achroiocythemia (ă-kroy"o-sĭ-the'mĭ-ă). Deficiency of hemoglobin in red blood cells.

achroma (a-kro'ma). 1. A form of macula.* 2. An absence of color. Leukoderma. Hereditary, circumscribed skin areas deficient in pigmentation.

achromacyte (ak-ro'mă-sīt). A decolorized erythrocyte.*

achromasia (ak-ro-ma'zi-ă). 1. Albinism, vitiligo, or leukoderma. 2. Lack of pigment in the skin. 3. Pallor due to poor nutrition.

achromate (ak'rō-māt). One who is color blind.

achromatic (ak"rō-mat'ĭk). Colorless.
    a. lens. One correcting chromatic aberration.
    a. sensation. A descriptive name for visual sensation in white, black, and gray, contrasted with the chromatic or colored sensations.

achromatin (ă-krō'mat-ĭn). The basis of a cell nucleus, so-called because it is not readily colored by basic stains.

achro'matism. Colorlessness.

achromat'ocyte. A decolorized red blood cell.

achromatolysis (ă-kro-mă-tol'is-is). Dissolution of cell achromatin.

achromatophil (ă-kro-mat'o-fĭl). A cell not stainable the usual way.

achromatopsia (ă-kro-mă-top'sĭ-ă). Color blindness; partial or total.

achromatop'sy. Color blindness. SYN: *achromatopsia.*

achromatosis (a-chro"ma-tō'sis). Condition of being without natural pigmentation. SEE: *achroma.*

achromatous (a-krō'mă-tus). Without color.

achromaturia (ă-krō"mă-tu'rĭ-ă). Colorless or nearly colorless urine.

achrom'ia. Absence of color. SYN: *achroma.* SEE: *chloranemia.*
    a. parasitica. Skin disease causing spotted appearance.

achromic (ă-kro'mĭk). Lacking color.

achromoder'mia. Lack of color in skin.

achro'mophil. Not staining easily.

achromotrich'ia. Lack of color in the hair.

achroödextrin (ak"ro-o-deks'trĭn). One of the varieties of dextrin resulting from the first splitting of a polysaccharide molecule, the other being *erythrodextrin.*

achylia (a-ki'lĭ-ă). Absence of chyle.
    a. gas'trica. Hypoacidity; a deficiency of hydrochloric acid and of gastric enzymes.
    a. pancreat'ica. Absence or deficiency of pancreatic secretion.
    SYM: Emaciation, fatty stools, impaired nutrition, etc. [SYN: *achylia.*

achylosis (ă-kĭ-lo'sis). Absence of chyle.

achylous (ak-i'lus). 1. Lacking in any digestive secretion. 2. Without chyle.

achymia, achymosis (a-ki'mĭ-ă, a-ki-mo'sis). Deficiency or absence of chyme.

acicular (a-sĭk'u-lar). Needle-shaped.

a'cid. 1. Any substance containing hydrogen replaceable by metals, yielding hydrogen ions as the only positive ions, when dissolved in water, and affecting indicators in certain ways. SEE: *indicator.* 2. Sour. [taste to vinegar.
    a., acetic, CH_3COOH. It gives the sour
    a., a., glacial. A pure anhydrous preparation which melts at 16.7° C. and is consequently crystalline in a cold room.
    a., acetoacetic, $CH_3CO.CH_2COOH$. SYN: *Diacetic acid;* occurs in diabetic urine.
    a., amino. A series of compounds that can be prepared from proteins or made synthetically and which have the general formula $NH_2R.COOH$. Ex: *acid, aminoacetic, histidine,* and *tryptophan.*
    a., aminoacetic, NH_2CH_2COOH. The same as glycerine, one of the simplest examples of an amino acid.
    a., ascorbic. Synthetic vitamin C ($C_6H_8O_6$). Similar to natural vitamin in citrus, etc., in comp. and therapeutic value.
    DOSAGE: Infants and children: *prophylactic,* ⅙-¾ gr. (0.01-0.05 Gm.); *curative,* ½ gr. (0.03 Gm.). Adults: *prophylactic,* ¾ gr. (0.05 Gm.); *curative,* ¾-1½ gr. (0.05-0.1 Gm.).
    a., barbituric, $C_4H_4O_3N_2$. Malonyl urea. A heterocyclic compound from which veronal and other hypnotics are derived.
    a., benzoic, C_6H_5COOH. A white crystalline material prepared from coal tar; used in keratolytic ointments.
    a., betaoxybutyric. SYN: for: *acid, acetoacetic.*
    a., bile. Any substance occuring in the form of salt in the bile. Ex: *glycocholic, acetic, taurocholic acids.*
    a., boric, H_3BO_3, **a., boracic.** A white crystalline substance giving very weakly acid solutions, poisonous to plants and animals, and useful as a bacteriostatic.
    a., butyric, C_3H_7COOH. A liquid having odor of vomitus and rancid butter.
    a., carbolic. Obsolescent name for phenol.
    a., carbonic, H_2CO_3. A weak acid from carbon dioxide dissolved in water.
    a., carboxylic. Any one containing the group COOH. The simplest examples are *formic* and *acetic.*
    a., citric, $C_6H_8O_7.H_2O$. USP. Prepared from lemon or lime juice in form of large white or transparent crystals.
    DOSAGE: 8 gr. (0.5 Gm.).
    a., diacetic. Same as acetoacetic.
    a., fatty. One of a series of carboxylic acids which can be combined with *glycerol* to form fats; the simplest members of the series are *formic* and *acetic;* most typical: *stearic* and *oleic.*
    a., formic, HCOOH. The simplest member of the series of fatty acids; a liquid heavier than water and 12 times as strong as acetic acid.

a., gallic, $C_6H_2(OH)_3COOH$. A crystalline acid that can be prepared from tanbark and plant galls.

a., glutamic, $COOH.CH_2.CH_2.CHNH_2-COOH$. An important amino acid.

a., glycocholic, $C_{26}H_{43}NO_6$. Occurs as a sodium salt in bile and can be decomposed into aminoacetic and cholic acids.

a., glycuronic, $CHO.(CHOH)_4COOH$. Related to the carbohydrates; is found in small quantities in the urine, and occurs among the decomposition products of mucoids.

a., hydriodic, HI. Used in medicine for its iodine content; its salts are called iodides.

a., hydrochlor'ic (HCl) (Muriatic acid), USP. An aqueous solution of a gas produced by the interaction of sulfuric acid and sodium chloride.

DOSAGE: Diluted (10%) : 15 ♏ (1 cc.). Taken through a glass tube.

a., hydrocyanic, HCN. A weak, unstable, poisonous volatile acid which forms salts called cyanides; has a characteristic odor suggesting almonds, and in minute doses stimulates respiration.

DOSAGE: (Dil.) 1½ gr. (0.1 Gm.).

a., lactic, $C_3H_6O_3$. Results in nature from the fermentation of lactose (as in sour milk) and when pure is a clear syrupy liquid.

a., linoleic, $C_{18}H_{32}O_2$. May be prepared from linseed and cottonseed oils and is an example of unsaturated fatty acid.

a., malic, $C_4H_6O_5$. Found in certain sour fruits as apples and apricots.

a., mineral. Acids prepared from nonorganic materials, as sulfuric, hydrochloric, nitric, and phosphoric.

a., muriatic. Obsolescent name for *acid, hydrochloric.*

a., nitric, HNO_3. A strong corrosive acid prepared from sulfuric acid and a nitrate.

a., oleic, $C_{18}H_{34}O_2$. An unsaturated fatty acid that can be prepared from various fats and oils.

a., oxalic, $C_2H_2O_4$. A white crystalline solid found in cranberries, rhubarb, and other plants; is poisonous in large quantities, and occurs (as calcium oxalate) in urinary calculi.

a., palmitic, $C_{16}H_{32}O_2$. A fatty acid prepared from palm oil.

a., pectic, $C_{16}H_{22}O_{15}$. An acid derived from pectin.

a., phosphoric, H_3PO_4. Gives rise to salts called phosphates and related compounds widely distributed in nature.

DOSAGE: (10%) 15 gr. (1.0 Gm.).

a., phosphorous, H_3PO_3. A dibasic oxyacid of phosphorus. It has 1 atom less of oxygen than phosphoric acid.

a., phosphotungstic, $P_2O_5.12WO_342H_2O$. Used in chemical and histologic technic. Precipitates proteins and alkaloids.

a., picric, $C_6H_2(NO_2)_3OH$. An explosive poisonous crystalline substance which reacts with proteins and alkaloids and leaves bright yellow stains.

a., prussic. Obsolescent name for *acid, hydrocyanic.*

a., pyrogallic. Same as pyrogallol, $C_6H_3(OH)_3$. A white crystalline substance which absorbs oxygen rapidly in alkaline solution and is used in gas analysis and photography.

a., pyruvic, $CH_3CO.COOH$. The simplest of the ketonic acids, important in metabolism because of its close relation to *acid, lactic.*

a., salicylic, $C_6H_4(OH)COOH$. A white, crystalline powder used for its antiseptic and keratolytic actions; its derivatives, the salicylates, are much used as analgesics.

DOSAGE: 5-20 gr. (0.3-1.3 Gm.).

a., stearic, $C_{17}H_{35}COOH$. A fatty acid prepared from animal fats, esp. beef.

a., sulfonic. Any organic compound of the general formula $R.SO_3H$ generally prepared by the action of strong sulfuric acid on benzene or its derivatives.

a., sulfuric, H_2SO_4. A corrosive, heavy liquid prepared from sulfur and indispensable in the industries.

a., sulfurous, H_2SO_3. An acid existing in solutions of sulfur dioxide in water and giving rise to salts called sulfites.

DOSAGE: (6%) 15-60 gr. (1.0-4.0 Gm.).

a., tannic. A glucoside prepared from oak galls and sumac and yielding gallic acid and glucose on hydrolysis.

a., tartaric. USP. $C_4H_6O_6$. Occurs free or as tartrates in fruit juices. A light yellow powder, from nut galls, freely soluble in water and glycerin.

DOSAGE: 8 gr. (0.5 Gm.).

a., taurocholic. A substance occuring in bile and yielding cholic acid and taurine on hydrolysis.

a., unsaturated. Organic acid containing less than the maximum possible number of hydrogen atoms. For example, compare unsaturated *oleic* and *linoleic* acids with the saturated *acid, stearic.*

a., uric. A crystalline solid (formula $C_5H_4N_4O_3$) prepared from urine.

a., valeric, $C_5H_{10}O_2$. Same as valerianic acid an oily liquid of the fatty acid series, existing in 4 isomeric forms, having a disgusting odor, and prepared from valerian root. ADM: Dilute well with water. Protect teeth by giving through straw or glass tube.

DOSAGE: 1-8 gr. (0.06-0.5 Gm.).

acidaminuria (as″id-am″in-ū′rĭ-ă). Excess of amino acids in voided urine.

acid-ash diet. Decrease or omit fruits, vegetables, milk. Adjust cals. by increasing neutral or acid-ash foods.

acid-base balance. In metabolism, the balance of acid to base (alkaline ash) necessary to keep the blood neutral (slightly alkaline), between pH 7.35 and pH 7.43.

acidemia (as-i-de′mĭ-ă). A condition in which uncompensated reduction in alkaline reserve or uncompensated increase in circulating acid substances results in increased acidity of the blood.

so that the *p*H drops from a normal range of 7.72–7.64 to lower, more acid values, *e. g.*, 7.36, as measured by the indicator method. SEE: *acid-base balance, acidity, acidosis.*

acid-fast. Not decolorized easily when stained by acids. Ex: *smegma, tubercle,* and *hay-bacilli.*

acid″ifica′tion. Becoming sour; conversion into an acid.

acidifiable (a-sid-ĭ-fī′ă-bl). Capable of transformation into an acid.

acidimeter (as-ĭ-dim′ĕ-ter). Instrument for testing purity of acids.

acidimetry (as-ĭ-dim′ĭ-trĭ). Determination of an acid's strength, or of the acidity of a fluid.

ac′idism, acidis′mus. Poisoning due to acids introduced from outside.

acidity (a-sid′ĭ-tĭ). Quality of being acid; having an excess of acid; sourness.

   a. **of stomach.** Sourness due to fermentation of food in the stomach, or oversecretion of acid. It does not necessarily indicate acidosis.

acidophil(e (as-sid′o-fil or fīl). Capable of being stained by acid stains such as eosin. Said of cells or parts of cells prepared for microscopic study.

acidophilic (a-sid″o-fil′ik). Having affinity for acid or pert. to certain tissues and cell granules. SYN: *acidophilous.*

acidophilism (ă-sĭd-of′il-izm). State due to acidophil adenoma of the hypophysis, causing acromegaly.

acidophilous (as-ĭ-dof′ĭ-lus). Capable of being stained by acid stains, said of cells. SYN: *acidophil, q.v.*

   a. **milk.** Milk fermented by *Lactobacillus acidophilus* cultures.

acidoresis′tant. Acid resisting; said about bacteria.

acido′sic. Having acidosis.

acidosis (as-i-do′sis). A disturbance of the acid-base balance of the body.

acidotic (as-id-ot′ik). Pert. to acidosis.

a′cid pois′oning. Acids have a sour taste and many of them are corrosive or poisonous.

acid-proof. Acid-fast.

acid-salt. A compound formed when only a part of the hydrogen of an acid is replaced by a metal.

acid′ulate. To make somewhat sour or acid.

acidulous (a-sid′u-lus). Slightly sour or acid.

acidum (as′i-dum). Acid.

acidu′ric. Capable of growing in an acid medium, but prefering a slightly alkaline medium, as certain bacteria.

acinesia (as-in-e′sĭ-a). Akinesia. 1. Loss of voluntary motion. 2. Immobility. 3. Interval following the systolic heartbeat.

acinesic (as-in-e′sĭk). Acinetic, akinetic.

acinetic (as-in-et′ĭk). 1. One afflicted with akinesia. 2. That which lessens muscular action.

acini. Pl. of acinus.

aciniform (as-in′ĭ-form). Resembling grapes.   [glandular acini.

acinitis (as-in-i′tis). Inflammation of

acinous (as′ĭn-us). Pert. to certain glands resembling a bunch of grapes, such as *acini* and *alveolar* glands.

ac′inus (pl. *acini*). 1. Smallest division of a gland; a group of cells surrounding a saccular or tubular cavity. 2. A liver lobule. 3. An air cell of the lung.

acladio′sis. An ulcerative dermatitis due to the fungus *Acladium castellanii.*

aclasia (ă-kla′sĭ-ă). Pathologic continuity of structure: chondrodystrophy.

   a., **diaphyseal.** Imperfect formation of cancellous bone in cartilage bet. diaphysis and epiphysis.

aclasis (ak′lă-sis). Pathological continuity of structure. SYN: *aclasia.*

aclas′tic. Not refracting light rays.

acleistocardia (ă-klīs-to-kar′dĭ-ă). Patent foramen ovale.

aclu′sion. Imperfect adjustment of opposing tooth surfaces.

acmastic (ak-mas′tik). Pert. to disease with regular increase of symptoms (*epacmastic*) and decrease (*paracmastic*), or period of decline.

acme (ak′me). 1. The time of greatest intensity of a symptom. 2. Acne.

acne (ak′ne). Any inflammatory disease of the sebaceous glands.

   SEE: *bacchia, bottle nose, stictacne.*

   a. **albida.** Whitish nodules on face. SEE: *milium.*

   a. **artificialis.** Acne caused by external disturbance or irritation.

   a. **atrophica.** SEE: *acne varioliformis.*

   a. **ciliaris.** That which affects the edges of the eyelids.

   a. **decalvans.** Quinquad's disease; a purulent folliculitis of the scalp resulting in irregular bald patches.

   a. **disseminata.** SEE: *acne vulgaris.*

   a. **generalis.** Acne spread over the entire body.

   a. **hypertrophica.** Thickening of the lips and sides of the nose accompanying *acne rosacea.*

   a. **indurata.** Form of *acne vulgaris* with chronic discolored indurated surfaces.

   a. **keratosa.** Acne in which a horny plug takes the place of the comedo.

   a. **papulosa.** Common acne in which the lesions are papular.

   a. **punctata.** A form with pointed papular lesions, the centers of which are black-tipped comedones.

   a. **rosacea.** Called also brandy nose, toper's nose, brandy face, rosy drop; characterized by congestion and telangiectasis and frequently accompanied by acne and seborrhea, usually of angioneurotic origin.

   a. **simplex.** SEE: *acne vulgaris.*

   a. **tarsi.** Acne affecting the sebaceous glands of the eyelids.

   a. **urticaria** (kaposi). A form with itching patches.

   a. **varioliformis.** Variety with pustular eruptions. Contagious. SEE: *molluscum contagiosum.*

   a. **vulgaris.** Common acne, *acne simplex.*

acneform (ak'ne-form). Resembling acne.

acneiform (ak-ne'ĭ-form). Acneform.

acnemia (ak-ne'mĭ-ă). Wasting of the calves of the legs.

acnitis (ak-ni'tis). A papular eruption which becomes pustular, leaving slight scars.

acoin (ak'o-in). A white crystalline powder; bactericide and local anesthetic.

acolasia (ak″o-la'zĭ-ă). 1. Lust. 2. Unrestrained self-indulgence. Intemperance.

acom'atol. Pancreatic hormone.

aco'mia. Baldness. SYN: *alopecia*.

aconite (ak'o-nīt). USP. A poisonous and very powerful alkaloid.
   DOSAGE: Of tincture (10%) 5 to 15 ℳ (0.3-1 cc.).

ac'tol. Silver lactate, containing 50% silver. Usually employed in solutions from 1: 5000 to 1: 1000 in dentistry as an antiseptic.

aconuresis (a-kon″u-re'sis). An involuntary voiding of urine.

acoprosis (ă-kop-ro'sis). Imperfect formation of feces.

acoprous (ă-kop'rus). Absence of feces in the intestines.

acor (a'kor). Acidity.

acoria (a-ko'rĭ-ă). 1. Lacking in satisfaction after eating but not from hunger. 2. Gluttony. SEE: *bulimia, hyperorexia, pica, parorexia, polyphagia*.

acouesthe'sia. Sense of hearing.

acoumeter (a-kōō'me-ter). An instrument for determining acuteness of hearing.

acouophonia (ă-koo-o-fo'nĭ-ă). Auscultatory percussion.

acouphone (a'koo-fōn). An electric appliance to aid the deaf to hear.

acousia (a-kōō'zĭ-ă). The hearing faculty.

acousma (a-kooz'mă). Nonverbal auditory hallucination.

acousmatagnosis (ă-koos-mă-tag-no'sis). Inability to understand what is said, due to mental disorder.

acousmatamnesia (ă-koos-mă-tam-ne'zĭ-ă). Loss of memory for sounds.

acoustic (a-koos'tik). Pert. to sound or to the sense of hearing.
   a. **center.** In the temporal lobe of the cerebrum.   [canal.
   a. **meatus.** The external auditory
   a. **nerve** (*nervus acusticus*). 8th cranial nerve. FUNCT: Special sense of hearing and equilibrium. ORIG: Two roots, cochlear and vestibular. DIS: Cochlea, vestibule body canals. BR: Cochlear, vestibular. SEE: *cranial nerves*.

acous'ticon. A type of hearing aid.

acoustics (a-koo'stiks). The science of sounds and their perception.

acquired'. Not congenital; gotten after birth.

acraconitine (ak-ra-kon'ĭ-tin). An alkaloid derived from *Aconitum ferox*. SYN: *pseudaconitine*.

acragnosis (ak-rag-no'sis). Absence of sensibility in limbs.

a'cral. Pert. to extremities.

acraldehyde (ak-ral'de-hīd). Volatile liquid produced by dry distillation of glycerin. SYN: *acrolein*.

acra'nia. Congenital absence of the cranium, either partial or complete.

acrasia (a-kra'zĭ-ă). Without self-control; intemperate.

acratia (a-kra'shĭ-ă). 1. Loss of strength; impotence. 2. Incontinence, or loss of control.

acraturesis (a-krat-u-re'sis). 1. Urinary incontinence. 2. Vesicle atony causing feeble urination.

acremonio'sis. A condition marked by fever and development of swellings, due to *Acremonium potronii*.

acribom'eter. Instrument which measures minute objects.

acrid (ak'rid). Burning, bitter, irritating.

acriflavine (ak'rĭ-fla-vene) USP. A dye manufactured from coal tar.
   DOSAGE: For irrigations and treatment of wounds, 1: 4000 to 1: 1000 solutions in normal saline.
   a. **neutral.** Same as acriflavine but less acid and less irritant.
   DOSAGE: Orally, ½ to 1½ gr. (0.3-0.1 Gm.).

acrimony (ak'rĭ-mō″nĭ). Quality of being pungent, acrid, irritating.

acrinia (a-krin'ĭ-ă). Suppression or diminution of an excretion or secretion.

acrisia (a-kris'ĭ-ă). Condition of uncertainty in diagnosis and prognosis.

acritical (ak-rit'ik-al). Not marked by a crisis.

acritochro'macy. Color blindness.

acroagnosis (ak-ro-ag-no'sis). Absence of feeling in a limb.

acroanesthesia (ak″ro-an-es-the'zĭ-ă). 1. Absence of sensation. 2. Lack of sensation in one or more of the extremities.

acroarthritis (ă-kro-ar-thri'tis). Arthritis of the hands or feet.

acroasphyx'ia. Cold, pale condition of hands and feet; sym. of Raynaud's disease.

acroataxia (a″kro-ă-taks'ĭ-ă). Ataxia involving, or limited to, the fingers and toes.   [blast.*

ac'roblast. The outer layer of the meso-

acrobystiolith (ă-kro-bis'tĭ-o-lith). A calculus of the prepuce.

acrobystitis (ă-kro-bis-ti'tis). Preputial inflammation.

acrocepha'lia. Pointed condition of the top of the cranium.

acrocephalic (ak″ro-se-fal'ik). A skull with a vertical index above 77; pert. to one with a peaked head.

acrocephaly (ak″ro-sef'ă-lĭ). A malformed cranial vault having a high or peaked appearance due to premature closure of the coronal, sagittal, and lambdoid sutures.

acrocinesia, acrocinesis (ă-kro-sin-e'sĭ-ă, -sis). Excessive motion.

acrocinetic (a-kro-sin-et'ik). Showing acrocinesis.

acrocontrac'ture. Contracture of the hands or feet.

acrocordon (a-kro-kor'dŏn). A soft, pedunculated growth.

acrocyanosis (ak-ro-si-a-no'sis). Cyanosis of finger tips, and other extremities.

acrodermatitis (ak″ro-der-ma-ti′tis). Dermatitis of the extremities.

a., continuous. An obstinate eczematous eruption confined to the extremities.

a. hiemalis. A form occurring in winter, affecting the extremities and tending to spontaneous disappearance.

acrodynia (ak-ro-din′ĭ-ă). 1. Disorder of skin and limbs in children. 2. Multiple neuritis of digits.

acroesthesia (ak-ro-es-the′zĭ-ă). 1. Marked hyperesthesia. 2. Pain in the extremities.

acrogno′sis. Sensory perception of limbs.

acrohy′pothermy. Abnormal coldness of extremities.

acrokinesia (ak-ro-kin-e′sĭ-ă). Excessive motion. SYN: *acrocinesia*.

acrolein (ak-ro′le-ĭn). A volatile liquid produced by dry distillation of glycerin.

acromac′ria. Spider-fingers. SYN: *arachnodactyly*.

acromania (ak-ro-ma′nĭ-ă). Mania accompanied by great motor activity and sometimes by muteness.

acromasti′tis. Inflammation of the nipple; thelitis.

acromegaly (ak-ro-meg′ă-lĭ), **acromegalia** (ac-ro-me-ga′lĭ-ă). A chronic disease (Marie's disease), characterized by progressive enlargement of the bones of the head, and soft parts of the hands, feet, thorax, and face; often associated with hypertrophy of the pituitary body or with diseases of thyroid gland.

acromelalgia (ak-ro-mel-al′jĭ-ă). A disease of the extremities, esp. the feet, with pain upon walking.

acrometagenesis (ă-kro-mĕt-ă-jen′ĕ-sis). Abnormal growth of extremities leading to deformity.

acromial (ak-ro′mĭ-al). Rel. to the acromion.*

a. angle. The angle at edge of spine of the *scapula* where it ascends to become the *acromion, q.v.*

a. process. The acromion.

a. reflex. Flexion of forearm with internal rotation of hand resulting from quick blow upon acromion. Elicited in hyperkinetic states.

acromicria (ak-ro-mik′rĭ-ă). Congenital shortness or smallness of the extremities.

acromioclavicular joint (a-kro″mĭ-o-klă-vik′u-lar). Joint between the acromion (outward extension of spine of the *scapula*, forming part of shoulder) and *clavicle*.

acromiocoracoid (a-kro″mi-o-kor′ă-koid). Rel. to the acromion and coracoid process.

acro′miohu′meral. Pert. to acromion and humerus.

a. muscle. Deltoid muscle.

acromion (a-kro′mĭ-on). The lateral, triangular projection of spine of scapula, forming point of the shoulder, and articulating with the clavicle. SEE: *acromiohumeral, acromiothoracic.*

acromiothoracic (a-kro″mĭ-ō-thō-ras′ĭk). Pert. to acromion and thorax.

acromphalus (ak-rom′fal-us). 1. Center of navel. 2. Beginning of umbilical hernia, marked by abnormal projection of umbilicus.

acromyle (ak-rŏm′ĭl-e). The patella.*

acromyotonia (ak″ro-mĭ-ō-to′nĭ-ă). Myotonia of extremities causing spasmodic deformity.

acronarcotic (a-kro-nar-kot′ĭk). Having the property of a narcotic and yet irritant in local effects.

acro″neuro′sis. Any neurosis, usually vasomotor, in extremities.

acronyx (ak′ro-nĭks). Ingrowing of a nail.

acropachy (ak′ro-pak-ĭ). Thickening of fingers or toes.

acroparal′ysis. Paralysis of one or more extremities.

acroparesthesia (ak″ro-par-es-the′zĭ-ă). Extreme paresthesia or morbid sensation of the extremities.

acro″pathol′ogy. Pathology of extremities.

acropathy (ak-rop′ath-ĭ). Any disease of extremities .

acrophobia (ak-ro-fo′bĭ-ă). Morbid fear of high places.

acroposthitis (ak-ro-pos-thi′tis). Inflammation of prepuce.

acroscleroderma (ak″ro-skler-o-der′mă). Hard, thickened skin condition. SYN: *scleroderma.*

ac′rose. A substance forming starting point for synthesis of fruit sugars.

acrosinosis (ăk″rō-sĭ-nō′sĭs). Condition of having pointed or malformed sinuses.

ac′rosome. The ant. end of head of the spermatozoon.

acrosphacelus (ak-ro-sfas′el-us). Gangrene of digits. SYN: *Raynaud's disease.*

acroteria (ak-ro-te′rĭ-ă). The extremities.

acrotic (a-krot′ĭk). 1. Pert. to failure of or defective beating of the heart. 2. Pert. to the surface or glands of the skin.

acrotism (ak′ro-tizm). Apparent absence of the pulse.

acrotrophoneurosis (ak-ro-tro″fo-nu-ro′sis). Trophoneurosis of extremities.

acrylaldehyde (ak-ril-al′de-hĭd). A volatile liquid from glycerin. SYN: *acrolein.*

act re′flex. Involuntary reflex act immediately following any stimulus.

actinic (ak-tin′ĭk). Pert. to the chemical action of the sun's rays.

a. burns. Those caused by ultraviolet or sun rays. F. A. TREATMENT: As for dry heat burns. SEE: *burns.*

actinism (ak′tin-izm). That property of radiant energy which produces chemical changes, as in photography or heliotherapy.

ac″tinochem′istry. Action of rays from a luminous source.

actinocutitis (ak″tin-o-ku-ti′tis). Cutaneous inflammation. SYN: *actinodermatitis.*

actinodermatitis (ak″tin-o-der-ma-ti′tis). Actinoneuritis. Cutaneous inflammation, acute or chronic, caused by roentgen rays or radium. [element.

actinogen (ak-tin′o-jen). Any radioactive

actinogenesis (ak″tin-o-jen′es-is). The source or production of actinic rays.

actinogenic (ak″tin-o-jen′ik). Producing rays; radiogenic.

actin′ogram. Roentgen ray photograph.

actin′ograph. A skiagraph. An x-ray picture.

actinol′ogy. Radiology; science of the chemical effects of light.

actinometer (ak″tin-om′e-ter). PT: An instrument to measure the intensity of an actinic effect.

Actinomyces (ak-tin-o-mi′sēz). A vegetable parasite (*Actinomycetaceae*), causing actinomycosis.

actino″myce′tic. Pert. to Actinomyces.

actino″myco′ma. A tumor produced by actinomycosis.

actinomycosis (ak-tin-o-mi-ko′sis). A ray fungus disease in animals, sometimes communicated to man, invading the brain, lungs, gastroenteric tract, or jaw (lumpy jaw).

actino″mycot′ic. Pert. to actinomycosis.

actinon (ak′tin-on). Emanation from actinium, which is one of the radium, actinium, and thorium series.

actino″neuri′tis. Neuritis due to exposure to radium or x-rays.

actino″prax′is. Employment of radioactive rays in diagnosis and treatment.

actinos′copy. Examination of deep structures by x-rays.

actinostereos′copy. Examination by x-ray. SYN: *actinoscopy*.

ac′tinother′apy. PT: Treatment of disease by rays of light, esp. actinic or chemical light.

ac′tinotoxe′mia. Blood poisoning produced by x-ray or radioactivity.

ac′tion. Performance of a function, or process; in pathology, a morbid process.

    a., *antagonistic.* The ability of one drug to antagonize the effect of another.

    a., *astringent.* One in which the tissue cells are contracted by a chemical combination of drug and tissues, forming an albuminate. If this is not dissolved in fluids surrounding tissues, they are not acted upon further by the drug.

    a. *current.* PT: Same as *action potential.*

    a. *of arrest.* Inhibition.

    a., *poisonous.* SEE: *toxicological action.*

    a. *potential.* The momentary difference in electrical potential between active and resting parts of a nerve fiber found when the two parts are connected with a sensitive galvanometer.

    a., *reflex.* Involuntary movement produced by a sensory nerve and carried to a center and returned by an efferent nerve to its origin or source of stimulus.

    a., *synergistic.* The ability of one drug to aid the effect of another.

    a., *toxicological.* The effect resulting from an overdose of a drug.

ac′tivate. 1. To make active. 2. To make radioactive.

ac′tivator. A substance in the body that activates glandular or chemical function, such as cholesterol and cod-liver oil, which stimulate the parathyroid glands, or enterokinase* which activates the trypsinogen* of the pancreatic juice. Sunlight and ultraviolet light are also activators. SEE: *antibody.*

ac′tive prin′ciples. The action of chemical substances in drugs which cause changes in activity of the body.

actual (ak′chu-al). Real, existent.

    a. *cautery.* Cautery acting by virtue of its heat and not chemically.

acufilopressure (ak-u-fi′lo-presh-ŭr). Acupressure increased by a ligature.

acu′ity. Clearness, sharpness.

acu′minate. Conical or pointed.

acupressure (ak′u-presh″ur). Compression of arteries by means of needles.

    a. *forceps.* Spring-handled forceps for compressing blood vessels.

    a. *needles.* Elastic needles for same purpose.

ac′upuncture. Puncture with needles for diagnostic and therapeutic purposes; also in treatment of edemas of lower limbs.

acus (a′kus). A surgical needle.

acusection (ak-u-sek′shun). Section by an electrosurgical needle.

acus′ticus. The auditory or 8th cranial nerve.

acute′. 1. Sharp, severe. 2. Having rapid onset, severe symptoms and a short course; not chronic.

acutenaculum (ak″u-ten-ak′u-lum). A needle holder.

acutor′sion. Twisting of an artery with a needle to control hemorrhage.

acyanoblepsia (a″si-an-o-blep′si-ă). Inability to discern blue colors. SYN: *acyanopsia.*

acyanopsia (a-si-an-op′si-ă). Inability to discern blue colors.

acyesis (ă-si-e′sis). 1. Absence of pregnancy. 2. Sterility of the female. 3. Incapability of natural delivery.

acystineuria (ă-sis-tin-u′rĭ-ă). Inability to control nervous mechanism of the bladder.

ad-. Prefix. Adherence, increase, toward, as *adduct.*

-ad. Suffix. Toward; in direction of.

a. d. Abbr. *right ear.*

A. D. A. American Dental Association or American Dietetic Association.

ad′alin (Carbromal). USP. A white crystalline powder containing 36% bromine in combination with urea.

    DOSAGE: As a sedative, 5 to 10 gr. (0.3-0.6 Gm.) in cold water. As hypnotic, from 10 to 15 gr. (0.6-1 Gm.).

adamantine (ad-ă-măn′tin). Very hard. Pert. to enamel of teeth.

ad″amantino′ma. A tumor of the jaw, esp. the lower one, arising from the enamel organs.

    It may be partly cystic, partly solid, and may reach a large size; sometimes malignant.

adamantoblast (ad-a-măn′to-blast). An enamel cell from which tooth enamel is formed.

adamantoblastoma (a-dă-man-to-blas-to'-mă). Overgrowth of an enamel cell.

adamanto'ma. An enamel tissue tumor.

Adam's apple. The laryngeal prominence formed by the union of the thyroid, cricoid, and epiglottic cartilages. SEE: *prominentia laryngea*.

Adams' operation. Subcutaneous palmar aponeurotomy for Dupuytren's contraction.

    A.'s saw. A saw used in osteotomy.

Adams-Stokes syn'drome. Slow, perhaps irregular pulse, vertigo, syncope, and occasional pseudoepileptic convulsions and Cheyne-Stokes breathing.

adapta'tion. The adjustment of the pupil of the eye to light variations.

adap'ter. A device for joining one part of an apparatus to another part.

adaptom'eter. Device for measuring time required for ocular adaptation. [ger.

addephagia (ad-ef-a'jĭ-ă). Insatiable hunger.

ad'dict. 1. To form a habit for the use of a drug. 2. One habituated to the use of a drug.

addiction (ă-dĭk'shun). Enslavement to some habit, esp. the drug habit.

    a. state. A condition in which cessation of narcotic or other drug produces definite "symptoms of abstinence." SEE: *alcoholism, narcotism.*

addiment (ad'im-ent). A substance described by Ehrlich, which resembles a ferment in its action and is present in normal serum.

add'isin. A substance supposed to be present in gastric juice which tends to keep red blood cells and hemoglobin at a normal level through stimulation of bone marrow; named after Thomas Addison, who described pernicious anemia during first half of 19th century.

addisonism (ad'ĭ-sŭn-izm). Symptom complex not due to disease of suprarenal glands, resembling that of Addison's disease.

Addison's disease. One due to deficiency of the suprarenal capsule, or to tuberculous wasting of the adrenals causing hypofunction of the adrenal medulla; *melasma suprarenale.*

    A.'s keloid. Firm, round, discolored patches on skin. SYN: *morphea.* SEE: *scleroderma.*

ad'duct. To draw toward a center.

adduc'tion. 1. Movement of a limb toward the body's center or beyond it. 2. Position assumed by such a movement.

    a. of the foot. Its movement about its own axis, or inward rotation around the leg's axis.

adduc'tor. A muscle which draws toward the medial line of the body or to a common center.

    a. reflex. Contraction of adductors of right thigh, indicative of appendicitis, elicited with patient lying completely relaxed and with thighs half flexed. Pressure is exerted outward by a finger on inner side of each knee.

adelomorphous (ad''el-ō-mor'fus). Having undefined form, as the pepsin glands.

adelphotaxis (ă-del'fō-tăk"sis). Grouping of cells in mutual relationships.

adenalgia (ad-en-al'jĭ-ă). Adenodynia.* Pain in a gland.

ad'enase. Enzyme secreted by the pancreas, spleen, and liver, and which converts *adenine** into *hypoxanthine.** SEE: *enzymes.*

adenasthenia (ad''en-ăs-the'nĭ-ă). Deficient glandular functional activity.

adendrit'ic. Without dendrites, as certain cells in spinal ganglia.

adenectomy (ad-en-ek'to-mĭ). Excision of a gland.

ad''enecto'pia. A gland out of its normal place.

ad''enemphrax'is. Obstruction to discharge from a gland.

adenia (ad-e'nĭ-ă). Hypertrophy of lymphatic glands with hyperleukocytosis absent.

aden'iform. Like a gland in form.

adenin(e (ad'en-in). 6-amino purine, $C_5H_5N_5$, a solid substance of the uric acid group, and derivable from the nucleic acids; *e. g.*, of ox pancreas.

adeni'tis. Inflammation of lymph nodes or a gland.

adeniza'tion. Abnormal change into a glandlike structure.

ad'enoblast. 1. Any active gland cell. 2. Embryonic cell which forms a gland.

adenocarcinoma (ad-en-o-kar-sin-o'mă). Adenoma* combined with carcinoma.

adenocele (ad'ĕ-no-sēl). A cystic tumor arising from a gland. A tumor of glandular structure.

adenocellulitis (ad''en-o-sel-u-li'tis). Inflammation of a gland and adjacent cellular tissue.

adenochondroma (ad''ĕ-no-kon-dro'mă). Adenoma with added characteristics of chondroma.

adenocyst (ad'e-no-sist). A cystic tumor arising from a gland.

adenocystoma (ad''en-o-sis-to'mă). Cystic adenoma.

adenodynia (ad-en-o-din'ĭ-ă). Pain in a gland. SYN: *adenalgia.*

adenofibro'ma. Fibrous and glandular tissue tumor frequently found in the uterus.

adenogenous (ad-en-oj'en-us). Having origin in glandular tissue.

adenog'raphy. Study of or treatise on glands.

adenohypersthenia (ad''e-no-hi"pers-the'-nĭ-ă). Excessive glandular activity.

adenoid (ad'en-oid). A lobulated, lymphoid mass composed of lymphoid tissue similar to the tonsils, and containing masses of lymphocytes* found in tonsils, lymph nodes, spleen, and in the nodules of the intestines. SYN: *pharyngeal tonsil.*

    a. tissue. Reticular tissue with lymph cells in the meshes of the network; also called lymphoid tissue.

adenoidectomy (ad-en-oid-ek'to-mĭ). Excision of adenoids.

adenoiditis (ad''ĕ-noi-di'tis). Inflammation of an adenoidal growth.

ad''enolipo'ma. A tumor with characteristics of adenoma and lipoma.

adenol'ogy. Science of the glands.

adenolymphitis (ad-ĕ-no-lim-fi'tis). Inflammation of a lymphatic gland. SYN: *lymphadenitis*.

adenolymphocele (ad″en-o-lim'fo-sēl). Cystic dilatation of a lymph node from obstruction.

adenolymphoma (ad″cn-o-lim-fo'mă). A lymph gland adenoma.

adenoma (ad-en-o'mă) (pl. *adenomata*). A neoplasm of glandular epithelium.

  a., acinous. Form with glands having acinous structure.

  a., chromophobe. Tumor of pituitary gland composed of cells that do not stain readily.

  a., malignant. Adenoma combined with carcinoma. SYN: *adenocarcinoma*.

  a., multiglandular. Adenoma containing many small changed glands.

  a. sebaceum. Steatadenoma; acanthoma of sebaceous glands. Benign tumorlike growths developing from epithelium of sebaceous glands which undergo fatty but never colloid metamorphosis.

  a. simplex. Form with hyperplastic condition of the glands.

adenomalacia (ad″ĕ-no-mal-a'sĭ-ă). Glandular softening.

adenomatome (a-dĕ-no'mă-tōm). Instrument for removing adenoids.

ad″enomato'sis. Multiple glandular tissue overgrowths. [adenomas.

adenomatous (ad-ĕ-no'mă-tus). Pert. to

adenomere (ad'en-o-mēr). The functional part of a gland.

adenomycosis (ad″dĕ-nō-mī-ko'sis). Disease of the lymph nodes. SYN: *Hodgkin's disease*.

adenomyoma (ad-ĕ-no-mĭ-o'mă). A tumor containing glandular and smooth muscular tissue.

adenomyometritis (ad-en-o-mi-o-me-tri'tis). GYN: A hyperplastic condition of the uterus which is the result of pelvic inflammation and grossly resembles an adenomyoma.

adenomyosis (ăd-ĕ-no-mi-o'sis). Ectopic adenomatous growths.

ad″enomyxo'ma. A tumor with adenoma and myxoma characteristics.

ad″enomyx″osarco'ma. A tumor with adenoma, myxoma, and sarcoma characteristics.

adenoncus (ad-en-on'kus). A tumor of a gland or its enlargement.

adenopathy (ad-en-op'ă-thī). Swelling and morbid change in lymph nodes; glandular disease.

ad″enopharyngi'tis. Inflammation of tonsils and pharyngeal mucous membrane.

adenophlegmon (ad-ĕ-no-fleg'mon). Inflammation (acute) of a gland and its adjacent tissue.

ad″enophthal'mia. Inflammation of the meibomian glands.

ad″enosarco'ma. A tumor with characteristics of adenoma and sarcoma.

adenosclerosis (ad-ĕ-no-skle-ro'sis). Glandular induration.

adenosis (ad-en-o'sis). Any disease of a gland, esp. of a lymphatic gland.

adenotome (ad'en-o-tom). An instrument for incision of a gland.

ad″enot'omy. 1. Glandular anatomy. 2. Excision or incision of a gland.

adenotyphus (ad″en-o-ti'fus). Abdominal typhus fever.

adeps (ad'eps). Lard; omental hog fat.

  a. anseri'nus. Goose grease.

  a. benzoina'tus. Benzoinated lard.

  a. la'nae. Wool fat.

  a. ovil'lus, a. ovis. Mutton suet or tallow.

ader'mia. Lack of skin, congenital or acquired.

ader″mogen'esis. Imperfect growth or repair of skin.

adherent (ad-he'rent). 1. Attached to, as of two surfaces. 2. OB: A placenta that remains attached to the uterine wall after delivery.

adhe'sion. Abnormal joining of parts to each other.

  a., primary. Healing by first intention.

  a., secondary. Healing by second intention.

adhesive (ad-he'siv). 1. Causing adhesion. 2. Sticky; adhering. 3. That which causes 2 bodies to adhere.

  a. inflammation. A serous membrane inflammation exudating fibrinous matter making adhesions possible.

  a. plaster [*emplastrum adhaesivum*]. A heavy material, as cloth, coated with gummy sticky materials to remain in place after application.

adiadochokinesis (a-dĭ-ad″o-ko-kin-e'sis). 1. Inability to make rapid alternating movements. 2. Incessant movement. 3. NEUR: Rapid antagonistic movements which cannot be carried out with accuracy. Seen in cerebellar disease.

adiaphoresis (ă-di-af-o-re'sis). Deficiency or absence of sweat.

adiapneustia (ad-ĭ-ap-nŭ'stĭ-ă). Absence of perspiration. SYN: *adiaphoresis*.

adiastole (ă-di-as'to-le). Imperceptibility of diastole.

adiathermancy (ă-dĭ-ă-thur'măn-sĭ). State of being impervious to heat.

adiemorrhysis (ad″i-em-or'i-sis). Arrest of capillary circulation.

adip'ic. Relating to fat; fatty.

adipocele (ad'ĭ-pō-sēl). Fat in a hernial sac. Lipocele.

adipocel'lular. Made up of or pert. to fat and connective tissue.

adipocere (ad'ĭ-pō-sēr). A waxy substance converted from dead tissue.

ad″ipofibro'ma. A fibroma and adipoma.

adipogenous (ad-ĭ-poj'en-us). Inducing the formation of fat.

adipolysis (ad-ĭ-pol'ĭ-sis). The hydrolysis of fat.

adipolytic (ad″ip-o-lit'ik). Pert. to adipolysis.

adipoma (ad-ip-o'mă). Fatty tissue tumor. SYN: *lipoma*.

a″dipopex'is. The storing of fat.

a'dipose. Fatty, pert. to fat.

  a. capsule. Renal fat.

  a. fossae. Fatty accumulations on outer mammary surface.

a. tissue. Connective or areolar tissue containing masses of fat cells.

adiposis (ad-ĭ-po'sis). Abnormal accumulation of fat in the body. SYN: *corpulence, liposis.*

a. doloro'sa. A neurosis, the symptoms of which are nodular formations, chronic bronchitis, and pain.

a. hepat'ica. Fatty degeneration or infiltration of the liver.

a. tuberosa simplex. A disease resembling adiposis dolorosa in which the fat occurs in small circumscribed nodules sensitive or painful to touch. SYN: *Anders' disease.*

adipositis (ad-ĭ-po-si'tis). Infiltration of an inflammatory nature in and beneath subcutaneous adipose tissue.

adipos'ity. Excessive fat in the body. SYN: *adiposis.*

adipo"sogen'ital syndrome. Combination of adiposity, impaired development of genital organs, and change in secondary sex characteristics. SEE: *Fröhlich's syndrome.*

adiposuria (ad-ĭ-pō-su'rĭ-ă). Fat in the urine. SYN: *lipuria.*

adip'sia, ad'ipsy. Absence of thirst.

adipsous (ă-dĭp'sus). Quenching thirst.

ad'itus. An approach; an entrance.

a. ad antrum. The recess of the tympanic cavity, which lodges head of malleus and greater part of incus.

a. ad aquaeductum Sylvii. The entrance to the sylvian aqueduct, situated at lower posterior angle of third ventricle of brain.

a. ad infundibulum. A small canal leading from the third ventricle into the infundibulum.

a. ad laryngem, a. laryngis. Upper aperture of larynx.

adjuster (ad-jus'ter). Device for holding together the ends of the wire forming a suture.

ad'juvant. 1. That which assists. 2. MAT. MED: A drug added to a prescription to hasten or increase the action of a principal ingredient; synergist.

Adler's organ-inferiority. A theory that ascribes psychic compensations to structural defects, tending to minimize the importance of psychosexual and other functional inadequacies.

ad lib. Abbr. L. *ad lib'itum,* at pleasure.

admax'illary. Accessory to the jaw.

a. gland. An occasional accessory salivary gland located near the angle of the jaw excreting through the parotid duct.

adnata (ad-na'tă). Layer of conjunctiva touching the eyeball. SEE: *tunica adnata.*

adner'val. Near a nerve.

adneu'ral. Adnerval.

adnex'a. Accessory parts as *adnexa u'teri,* the oviducts, and ovaries.

a. oculi. Lacrimal glands.

a. uteri. Ovaries and oviducts.

adnex'al. Adjacent or appending.

adnexi'tis. Inflammation of the *adnexa uteri.*

adnexopexy (ad-neks'ō-peks-ē). Fixing the fallopian tube and ovary to the abdominal wall.

adolescence (ad-o-les'ens). Period from beginning of puberty until adult life. In temperate climates 15 yr. for boys and 13-14 yr. for girls. Recent research proves adolescence is earlier in temperate climates and later in hot and cold regions.

ad"oles'cent. 1. Pert. to adolescence.* 2. Young man or woman not fully grown.

adoral (ad-o'ral). Toward or near the mouth.

adosculation (ad-ŏs-kū-la'shun). 1. Impregnation without intromission of the penis. 2. Insertion of one part into the cavity of another.

adre'nal. 1. Near the kidney. 2. Pert. to an artificial preparation made from the adrenal gland, known as *adrenalin, epinephrine,* and other trade names. 3. A suprarenal body or capsule over each kidney (SEE: *capsule*) necessary to life and containing a secretion that regulates blood pressure and which affects the muscular layer of the arteries, the muscular tissue of the heart, and the skeletal muscles.

adrenalectomy (ad-ṉē-năl-ek'tō-mĭ). Excision of an adrenal body.

adren'alin (epinephrin(e). USP. ($C_9H_{13}O_3N$). An internal secretion derived from the adrenal glands (suprarenal capsules) and commercially prepared from the adrenal glands of the sheep; a hormone of the medulla of the suprarenals.

ADM: (a) Locally; (b) hypodermically. DOSAGE: *Internally,* 5 to 15 ㎖ (0.3-1.0 cc.) of the 1: 1000 solution. *Subcut.,* $\frac{1}{120}$ ㎖ (0.005 cc.). *Locally,* 1:·10,000 to 1: 1000 solutions. In recent years a solution of 1: 100 has been marketed, and recommended for use by inhalation in allergic conditions, particularly asthma.

adrenaline'mia. Adrenalin in the blood.

adrenalinu'ria. Adrenalin in the urine.

adren'alism. Illness due to overactivity of suprarenal glands.

adrenalitis (ad-re"nal-i'tis). Inflammation of the suprarenal gland; adrenitis.

adrener'gic. Stimulated by adrenalin; applied to agents stimulating sympathetic nervous system.

adrenin(e (ad-ren'ĭn). A preparation made from the medulla of the suprarenal gland; the adrenal hormone.

adreni'tis. Inflammation of the suprarenal gland. SYN: *adrenalitis.**

adrenop'athy. Suprarenopathy. Any disease of the suprarenal glands.

adren"oster'one. Male sex hormone obtained from urine.

adren'otrope, adrenotrop'ic. One of adrenal type. Pert. to adrenotropism.

adren"otrop'in. Hormone obtained from male urine, controlling islands of Langerhans.

adrenotropism (ad-rĕn-ōt'ro-pizm). A type dominated by adrenal influence.

adrenotropism (ad-rĕn-ōt'ro-pizm). A type dominated by adrenal influence.

adsorp'tion. 1. A process whereby a gas or a dissolved substance becomes concentrated at the surface of a solid or at the interfaces of a colloid system. Ex: removal of dyes from solutions by filtration through charcoal. 2. Attachment of one substance to the surface of another.

adter'minal. Toward extremity of any structure.

adul'terant. That which adulterates or weakens a substance.

adultera'tion. The addition of an impure or weaker substance to another one.

adus'tion. 1. Being scorched, parched, dry. 2. Application of cauterization.

advancement (ad-vans'ment). Operation to remedy strabismus, by which the insertion of an ocular muscle is attached at a point further removed from its origin.

    a., capsular. Attachment of capsule of Tenon in front of its normal position.

adventitia (ad-ven-tish'yä). The outermost covering of a structure or organ, such as the *tunica adventitia,* or outer coats of an artery.

adventitious (ad-ven-tish'us). 1. Acquired; accidental. 2. Arising sporadically. 3. Pert. to adventitia.

ad'vitant. A vitamin.

adynamia, adynamy (a-din-am'ĭ-ă, -dĭn'-a-mĭ). Asthenia,* debility.

adynamic (ad-ĭ-nam'ĭk). Weak, feeble, asthenic. Pert. to adynamia.

aegophony (e-gof'o-nĭ). A goatlike bleating sound heard on auscultation of the chest.

aerated (a'er-a-ted). Containing air or gas.

aeration (a-er-a'shun). 1. Act of airing. 2. Change of venous into arterial blood in the lungs. 3. Saturating a fluid with gases.

aerendocardia (a-er-en-do-kar'dĭ-ă). Bubble of air in the blood within the heart.

aerenterectasia (a″er-en-ter-ek-ta'zĭ-ă). Distention of intestine with gas.

aerial (a-e'rĭ-al). Pert. to the air.

aeriferous (a-er-if'er-us). Carrying air.

aeriform (a-er'ĭ-form). Airlike; gaseous.

a'erobe. A microörganism which can live and grow only in the presence of free oxygen.

aerobian (a-er-o'bi-an). Aerobiotic; living only in the presence of oxygen.

aerobic (a-er-o'bik). 1. Living only in presence of oxygen. 2. Concerning an organism living only in oxygen.

aero'bion (pl. *aerobia*). An organism which lives only in presence of oxygen.

    a., facultative. One able to live without oxygen under some conditions, but which normally requires it.

    a., obligate. One which cannot live without air.

aerobiosis (a-er-o-bi-o'sis). Living in an atmosphere containing oxygen.

aerobiotic (a-er-o-bĭ-ot'ĭk). Pert. to aerobiosis.

aerocele (a'er-o-sēl). Gas within and distending a cavity.

aerocolpos (a″er-o-kol'pos). Distention of the vagina with air.

aerocoly (ă-ĕ-rok'ō-lĭ). Distention of colon with gas.

aerocystoscopy (a-ĕr-ō-sis-tos'kō-pĭ). Examination of the bladder, when distended by air, with a cystoscope.

aerodermectasia (a-er-ō-der-mek-ta'zĭ-ă). Subcutaneous emphysema.

aerodynam'ics. Science of air or gases in motion.

aeroembolism (a-er-ō″em'bō-lizm). A condition in which nitrogen bubbles form in blood and tissues during rapid ascent to high altitudes.

aerogen (a'er-o-jen). A gas-forming microörganism.

aerogenesis (a-er-o-jen'e-sis). Formation of gas.

aerogenic (a-er-o-jen'ik). Gas-forming.

aerogenous (a-er-oj'en-us). Gas-forming.

aerogoniscope (a-er-og-on'is-kōp). Device for collecting organic dust from the air.

aerohydrop'athy, aerohydrother'apy. Treatment by application of air and water.

aerometer (a-er-om'e-ter). Device for measuring density of gases.

aeromicrobe (a-er-o-mi'krōb). Any aerobic organism.

aeroneurosis (a-er-o-nu-ro'sis). A chronic functional nervous disorder affecting aeroplane flyers.

aeropathy (a-er-op'ath-ĭ). Morbid condition caused by atmospheric pressure, such as *mountain sickness,* and caisson disease.

aeroperito'nia. Distention of peritoneal cavity with gas.

aerophagy (a-er-of'aj-ĭ). Swallowing of air.

aerophilous (a-ĕr-of'ĭ-lŭs). Requiring air for development. SYN: *aerobic.*

aerophobia (a-er-o-fo'bĭ-ă). Morbid fear of a draft or of fresh air.

aerophore (a'er-o-fōr). 1. Conducting air. 2. Apparatus for introducing air into lungs of stillborn child.

a'erophyte. An organism or plant that lives upon air.

aeroplethysmograph (a-er-o-ple-thiz'mo-graf). Instrument for recording air respired.

aeropleura (a″er-o-plu'ră). Pneumothorax; air in pleural cavity.

aeroporotomy (a″er-o-po-rot'o-mĭ). Operation for admitting air into the air passages.

aeroscope (a'er-o-skōp). Device for examining air dust.

aerotaxis (a″er-o-tak'sis). Movement of organisms away from or toward air, said of aerobic and anaerobic bacteria.

aerotherapy (a-er-o-ther'a-pĭ). PT: Air-bath therapy.

aerothermotherapy (a″er-o-ther″mo-ther'-ă-pĭ). Applications of hot air.

aerotonometer (a-er-o-to-nom'e-ter). Apparatus for measuring tension of gases of the blood.

aerotympanal (a″er-o-tĭm'pă-năl). Pert. to air in tympanum.

aerourethroscope (a″er-o-u-rēth′ro-skōp). An apparatus for making urethral examination by electric light, after dilatation by air.

aerourethroscopy (a″er-ō-ū-rē-thros′kō-pĭ). Examination of the urethra when distended with air.

aer″teriver′sion. Eversion of artery ends to stop hemorrhage. SYN: *arterioversion.*

aer″teriver′ter. Instrument for use in aerteriversion. SYN: *arterioverter.*

aesthet′ic moral′ity. Right conduct as an expression of the ego ideal apart from any consideration of prudence or fear of wrongdoing.

afeb′rile. Without fever.

afen′il. Compound of calcium chloride and urea in aqueous solution.

ACTION AND USES: For calcium deficiency; coagulative.

DOSAGE: 10% solution, 10 cc. intravenously every 2nd or 3rd day.

af′fect. PSY: The emotional reactions associated with an experience. SYN: *psychic trauma.*

affec′tive. Stimulating emotion.

a. insanity. Impulsive or emotional insanity.

a. memory. Memory of a psychic trauma causing recurrence of emotion.

a. psycho′sis. PSY: An emotional one as manic-depressive psychosis.

a. spasms. Attacks of laughing, screaming, or weeping in hysteria.

af′ferent. Carrying impulses toward a center, as when a sensory nerve carries a message toward the brain; also said of certain veins and lymphatics. Opp. of efferent.*

affinity (ă-fĭn′ĭt-ĭ). 1. Common relationship; attraction. 2. Chemical attraction bet. two substances, *i. e.,* oxygen and hemoglobin. SEE: *chemoreceptor.*

a., chemical. Force combining atoms of various substances.

a. of composition. Tendency to form a compound without destroying any previously formed compound.

a., elective. Force causing a substance to elect 1 substance rather than another with which to unite.

af′flux. Rush of blood to a part.

affluxion. Affiux; congestion.

affu′sion. The pouring of water upon, as on the body, for cooling, cleansing, or therapeutic purposes.

NP: Patient may lay on a rubber sheet arranged to direct the water into a pail at bedside. A thin sheet may cover patient. Water can be poured on body through a watering can.

af′ter-action. A term used particularly in connection with nerve centers to designate the fact that they continue to react for some time after the stimulus ceases. In the sensory centers this action gives rise to after-sensations.

af′terbirth. Placenta and membranes expelled after birth of child.

af′terbrain. Section of embryonic brain which develops subsequently into oblon-

gata, auditory nerve and 4th ventricle. SYN: *metencephalon.*

af′tercat″aract [*cataracta secundaria*]. Retained portion of lens substance bet. agglutinated layers of capsule; seen after extracapsular cataract extraction.

af′terimage. One that persists subjectively after disappearance of object seen.

af′terpains. Uterine cramps due to contraction of uterus, occuring during first few days after confinement (*puerperium*); commonly seen in multiparae.* Pains more severe during nursing.

af′tersensa′tion. Sensation persisting after stimulus causing it has ceased.

Ag. Chem. symb. of silver.

agalactia (ă-găl-ak′tĭ-ă). Absence of milk

agalorrhea (ă-gal-ō-re′ă). Arrest of milk flow.

agalorrhea. Arrest of milk flow.

agamogen′esis. Asexual reproduction.

agar (ag′ar) (Agar-Agar). The dried mucilaginous substance, or gelatin, extracted from algae.*

DOSAGE: 60-240 gr. (4.0-15.0 Gm.).

AgCl. Silver chloride.

age. The time of existence of anything.

a., achievement. One determined by a proficiency test in any schoolroom study, measured by the mental ability of the average child of chronological age.

a., chronolog′ical. The years of one's life. SEE: *chronological.*

a., marriageable. One at which the individual is physically suited for marriage. SYN: *nubility.*

a., mental. The age of a person with regard to his mental development; this is determined by a series of mental tests as devised by Binet. Thus, if a woman of 30 can pass only the tests of a child of 12, she is said to have a mental age of 12. SEE: *Binet.*

a. of consent. An arbitrary age fixed by state statutes when a girl is supposed to be responsible for giving her consent to coitus.* It ranges from 10 to 18 years of age. Under that age the act is legally *rape* even though consented to. In England the age of consent is 13, but between that age and 16, sexual intercourse* is a misdemeanor.

-age. Suffix: put in motion; to do; to move, as *manage.*

agenesia, agenesis (ă-jen-e′sĭ-ă, ă-jen′es-is). 1. Sterility; impotence. 2. Incomplete development.

agenitalism (a-gen′i-tal-ism). Symptoms resulting from absence of the testicles or ovaries.

agenosomia (ah-jen-o-so′mĭ-ă). Imperfect development of genitals.

ageusia (ă-gŭ′sĭ-ă). Absence of the sense of taste; a partial loss or an impairment of the sense of taste.

a., gustatory. This is caused by a disordered condition of the taste buds* or of the lingual mucous membrane, or from contact with an irritating substance.

agger (aj′er). ANAT: A mound or pile.

a. na'si (BNA). *Crista ethmoidalis.* Ridge of nose.

agglomerate (ag-lom'er-āt). To congregate; to form into a mass.

agglu'tinable. Capable of agglutination.

agglutinant (a-glu'tin-ant). 1. Anything causing adhesion. 2. Causing to unite or adhere, as healing of a wound.

agglutination (ag-glu-tin-a'shun). 1. Clumping of microörganisms when a specific immune serum is added to a culture. 2. Adhesion of surfaces of a wound.

  SEE: *antiagglutinin, autoagglutination.*

  a., immediate. Healing by first intention.

  a., mediate. Healing by second intention.

agglu'tinative. Causing or capable of causing agglutination.

agglutinin (ag-lu'tin-in). A specific principle or antibody in blood serum of an animal affected with a microbic disease which is capable of causing the clumping of bacteria peculiar to that disease so that they are more easily engulfed by the white cells.

  a., chief. Agglutinin causing immunity in the blood, which has been immunized.

  a., group. Agglutinin acting as a specific on 1 species, but which will act on others.

  a., haupt-. SEE: *chief agglutinin.*

  a., immune. Agglutinin causing immunity, found in the blood either because of recovery from the disease or of having been inoculated with the microörganism.

  a., major. SEE: *chief agglutinin.*

  a., minor. Agglutinin acting on another organism than the 1 utilized for serum production, in lower dilution.

  a., partial. SEE: *minor agglutinin.*

agglutinogen (ag-gloo-tin'o-jen). 1. A substance inherited which agglutinates only the blood of parent and child. 2. A substance causing the formation of agglutinin when introduced into the body.

agglutinoid (ă-glu'tin-oid). One with the zymotoxic group deficient or absent.

agglutinophilic (a-glu-tin-o-fil'ik). Contributing to agglutination.

agglu'tinophore. The active agent producing agglutination.

agglutogenic (ag-gloo-to-jen'ik). 1. Pert. to substances from which agglutinins originate. 2. Causing agglutinins.

agglutom'eter. Device to simplify the agglutination or Widal test.

ag'gregate, ag'gregated. 1. Total substances making up a mass. 2. To cluster or come together.

  a. glands. Lymphoid follicles found mainly in the ileum. SYN: *Peyer's patches.*

aggres'sin. A supposed substance which renders the action of bacteria more aggressive by lowering the activity of the phagocytes and weakening resisting power.

a'gitated depres'sion. PSY: A psychiatric phase differing from the manic or depressive phases; involution melancholia or a rel. condition.

aglaukopsia (a-glaw-kop'sĭ-ă). Green blindness.

aglobu'lia. Marked decrease of red blood cells.

aglutition (ag-lu-tish'un). Difficulty in swallowing or inability to swallow.

aglycosu'ric. Free from glycosuria.

agmatol'ogy. The study of fractures.

agminate(d (ag'min-āt). Aggregate; grouped in clusters.

  a. glands. Lymphoid follicles found mainly in the ileum. SYN: *Peyer's patches.*

ag'nail. 1. Hangnail. 2. Whitlow.*

agne'a. A condition in which objects are not recognized; agnosis, *q.v.*

agno'sia. Loss of comprehension of auditory, visual, or other sensations although the sensory sphere is intact; inability to recognize an object.

  a., auditory. Deafness of mind.

  a., optic. Blindness of the mind.

  a., tactile. Inability to distinguish objects by sense of touch.

agomphiasis (ag-ŏm-fi'as-is). 1. Looseness of the teeth. 2. Without teeth.

agonad (ă-go'nad). One without gonads.

agon'adal. Having no gonads.

ag'onal. Rel. to the moment of death, or to agony.

agonia (ag-o'nĭ-ă). 1. Extreme anguish; mental distress. 2. The death struggle.

ag'onist. The muscle directly engaged in contraction as distinguished from muscles which have to relax at the same time.

agony (ag'o-nĭ). 1. Extreme suffering, mental or physical. 2. Death struggle.

  a. clot, a. thrombus. Clot formed in the heart after long heart failure and when dying.

agoraphobia (ag-o-ra-fo'bĭ-ă). 1. Morbid dread of open spaces. 2. Dread of crowds of people.

-agra. Suffix: pert. to gout or a gouty affection; loosely, a severe pain; seizure.

agraffe (ă-graf'). An appliance for clamping together edges of a wound.

agrammat'ica. Agrammatism.

agram'matism. Inability to form a grammatical or intelligible sentence or to arrange words in grammatical sequence. ETIOL: Cerebral disease.

agranulocyte (ă-gran'u-lō-sīt). A nongranular leukocyte.

agranulocytic (a-gran-ū-lō-sīt'ik). Pert. to agranulocytosis.

agranulocytosis (a-gran''u-lō-sī-tō'sĭs). 1. Condition marked by destructive ulcerative lesions of the throat, *leukopenia.** 2. Marked reduction of polymorphonuclear leukocytes in the blood and bone marrow.

  a., Ludwig's. Purulent inflammation about the flor ɔ of the mouth, submaxillary glands and beneath the jaw.

  a., Plaut-Vincent's. An infectious ulceromembranous disease of the mucosa caused by *B. fusiformis* associated with a spirillum (*Spironema vincentii*).

agranuloplas'tic. Capable of forming nongranular cells.

agranulo'sis. Marked reduction of granular leukocytes in blood and bone marrow. SYN: *agranulocytosis.*

agraphia (ah-graf'ĭ-ă). A loss of ability to express oneself in writing due to a central lesion, or to muscular incoordination.

agraph'ic. Pert. to agraphia.

agre'mia. Blood condition in gout.

agria (ag'rĭ-ă). Herpes; malignant pustules or pustular eruption.

agroma'nia. Unreasonable desire for solitude or solitudinous wandering. Morbid desire to live in solitude or in the country.

agrypnia (a-grip'nĭ-ă). Inability to sleep. SYN: *insomnia;* * *ahypnia.* *

agrypnot'ic. 1. Afflicted with insomnia. 2. That which causes wakefulness.

ague (a'gu). 1. Intermittent or malarial fever; typified by chills, fever, and sweating. 2. A chill. SEE: *malaria.*

ah. Abbr. for *hypermetropic astigmatism.*

Ahlfeld's sign (ahl'felt). OB: Uterine irregular contractions after the 3rd month of pregnancy.

ahypnia (ah-hip'nĭ-ă). Insomnia or sleeplessness; agrypnia. *

aichmophobia (ăk-mō-fo'bĭ-ă). Morbid fear of pointed instruments or of being touched by them or with a finger.

ailurophobia (i'lu-ro-fo'bĭ-ă). PSY: Morbid fear of cats.

A symbolism of psychoneurotic origin.

air (ār). The invisible, tasteless, odorless mixture of gases surrounding the earth.

   a., alveolar. Air in the alveoli.

   a., complemental. The amount that may be breathed in over and above the tidal air by deepest possible inspiration.

   a., minimal. The small amount of air left in the alveoli by collapse of small bronchi when the supplemental and residual air is driven out when the lungs collapse with the thorax open. This makes it possible for the excised lungs of animals to float, hence the term "lights."

   a., reserve. Residual air plus supplementary air in the chest after normal expiration. About 5 pt. (2600 cc.).

   a., residual. The amount remaining in the lungs after the fullest possible expiration. About 1500 cc.

   a., supplemental. Amount that may be forcibly expired after a quiet expiration. About 1600 cc.

   a., tidal. The amount that flows in and out of the lungs with each quiet respiration; average of adult male about one pint (500 cc.).

air bed. Large inflated air cushion used as a mattress. SEE: *air cushion.*

air cell. An air vesicle.*

air conditioning. Adjustment of normal temperature and humidity while insuring adequate ventilation.

air cushion. An airtight inflatable cushion. To inflate, a pump like a bicycle pump may be used.

   NP: When inflating orally, place layer of gauze over opening and between lips.

air em'bolism. Obstruction of a blood vessel brought about by entrance of air into the blood stream.

air hun'ger. Shortness of breath marked by rapid, labored breathing. SYN: *dyspnea.* *

air sac. An air vesicle.*

airsickness. Condition similar to seasickness occurring during airplane flight.

air swal'lowing. Oral intake of air either voluntarily or involuntarily.

air vesicle. Pulmonary tissue saccule filling with air during breathing.

air'way. A metallic or rubber instrument inserted into the mouth to keep the air passages of a postanesthetic patient clear until he is conscious.

Aix-Les-Bains (eks-la-băn) **douche massage.** * Water up to 115° F. flowing from a tube on a certain part of body while operator massages that part.

akatamathesia (ah-kăt-ăm-ath-e'zĭ-ă). Inability to understand.

akathisia (ah-kath-iz'ĭ-ă). PSY: Inability to remain seated.

   Seen in catatonia,* in agitated melancholia, and in some compulsive conditions.

akinesia (ah-kin-e'sĭ-ă). Loss of movement for any reason. Acinesia, *q.v.*

   a. algera. Form with intense pain caused by any movement.

   a. amnestica. Form marked by failure of muscular power due to lack of use.

akos'ma. Auditory hallucination, consisting of tinnituslike sounds of buzzing, whistling, etc., but also much more complex noises of groans, screams, etc.

akutomy (a-koo'to-mĭ). PT: The electrical cutting current; acusection.

Al. Chemical symbol for aluminum.

-al. Suffix: Pert. to, as *abdominal.*

ala (a'la) (pl. *alae*). 1. An expanded or winglike structure or appendage. 2. Axilla.*

a'lae na'si. The cartilaginous flap on the outer side of each nostril.

ala'lia. Loss of ability to speak due to defect or paralysis of the vocal organs. Aphasia.

alar (a'lar). 1. Pert. to or like a wing. 2. Axillary.

   a. artery. Small br. of axillary. Supplies tissues of axilla.

   a. cartilage. Lower lateral; one on each side of nose.

   a. vein. One accompanying the alar artery.

alas'trim. A modified smallpox with pustules not umbilicated and with no secondary rise of temperature.

alate (al'āt). Winged.

al'ba. 1. White. 2. White substance of the brain.

albar'as. A disease of the skin, forming white anesthetic patches on which the hair turns white.

albedo (al-be′do). Whiteness. Reflection of light from a surface.

    a. ret′inae. Retinal edema.

    a. unguium. White semilunar area at nail root. SEE: *lunula.*

Albee's operation (awl′bez). Removal of upper end of head of femur and corresponding edges of the acetabulum with approximation; artificial ankylosis of the hip.

Albers-Schönberg disease (ăl-bărs-shĕn′bărg). Abnormal bone calcification giving bones spotted, marblelike appearance and causing them to fracture spontaneously. SYN: *osteosclerosis fragilis; marble bones.*

Al′bert's disease. Achillodynia. Inflammation of the retrocalcanean bursa.

al′bicans (pl. *albicantia*). 1. White or whitish. 2. One of the *corpora albicantia*.

    a., corpus. Whitish body in ovarian cortex.

albidum (ăl′bĭ-dŭm). White.

albidu′ria. 1. Passing of white or colorless urine and of low specific gravity. 2. Chyluria.*

Albini's nodules (ăl-bĭ′nĭ). Minute nodules on margins of mitral and tricuspid valves of the heart; sometimes seen in newly born.

albinism (al′bin-ism). 1. Abnormal, nonpathological absence of pigment in skin, hair, and eyes, partial or total, frequently accompanied by astigmatism, photophobia, and nystagmus, because the choroid is not sufficiently protected from light because of lack of pigment. 2. A form of macula.* Permanent.

    TREATMENT: None.

albino (al-bi′no). A person deficient in pigment; one afflicted with albinism.

albinu′ria. Passing of white or colorless urine of low specific gravity. SYN: *albiduria.*

albocinereous (al-bō-sĭn-e′rē-ŭs). Pert. to both white and gray matter of brain and spinal cord.

albuginea (al-bu-jĭn′ĭ-ă). A layer of firm, white, fibrous tissue forming the investment of an organ or part.

    a. epididymidos. The fibrous coat of the epididymis, resembling the *albuginea testis,* but with less firmness and strength.

    a. lienis. The white, highly elastic fibrous coat, lying directly beneath the serous investment of the spleen. SYN: *tunica propria of the spleen.*

    a. ovaril. The layer of firm fibrous tissue lying beneath the epithelial ovarian covering.

    a. penis. A strong, very elastic white fibrous coat, forming a sheath common to both corpora cavernosa of the penis.

    a. renis. The fibrous renal capsule.

    a. testiculi, a. testis. The thick, unyielding layer of white fibrous tissue lying under the tunica vaginalis.

albugineotomy (al-bu-jĭn-e-ot′o-mĭ). Incision of tunica albuginea of the testis.

albuginitis (al-bu-jĭn-i′tĭs). Inflammation of any tunica albuginea.

albu′go. White opacity of the cornea.

albu′kalin. A substance in leukemic blood.

albu′men. Any simple protein soluble in water and dilute salt solutions, and coagulable by heat, as *e. g.,* the protein of egg white; albumins, *q.v.*

    a. water. After removing the specks from 2 eggs, separate the white from the yolk, and then cut the whites across several times, but do not beat. Add ½ pt. of cold boiled water. Stir lightly and add a pinch of salt or a few drops of lemon. For infants the lemon is omitted, and the albumen water must be strained through gauze.

albumimeter (al-bu-mim′et-er). An instrument for quantitative estimation of albumin in urine.

albu′min. A protein substance found in nearly every animal or plant tissue and fluid.

    a., acid. Compound resulting from action of acid on albumin.

    a., alkali. Compound resulting from action of weak alkalies on albumin.

    a., blood. Body albumin found in blood serum, said to be very similar to that present in albuminous urine.

    a., circulating. Albumin present in the liquids of the body.

    a., derived. Albumin changed by chemical action.

    a., egg. Form in egg white.

    a., floating. SEE: *circulating albumin.*

    a., incipient. Imperfect form of albumin found in chyle.

    a., muscle. Form found in muscular tissue.

    a., myosin. Albumin of meat.

    a., native. Any albumin present in an organism normally.

    a., serum. SEE: *blood albumin.*

    a., soluble. One that has not been altered by chemical action so that it is insoluble in water.

    a., vegetable. Albumin seen in vegetable tissue. [whey.

    a., whey. Albumin obtained from

albu′minate. Metaprotein, a product of hydrolysis of albumen and globulin.

albuminatu′ria. Albuminates in voided urine.

albuminiferous (al-bu-min-if′er-us). Producing albumin.

albuminimeter (al-bu-min-im′e-ter). Instrument for measuring amount of albumin in urine. SEE: *albumimeter.*

albuminiparous (al-bu-min-ip′ar-us). Yielding albumin.

albuminogenous (al″bu-min-oj′en-us). Producing albumin.

albu′minoid. 1. Resembling albumin. 2. Any one of a large class of proteins, such as (a) *collagen** in white fibers of connective tissue, which produces gelatin on boiling; (b) *elastin,* in yellow fibers of connective tissue, and (c) *keratin,** found in hair, skin, and finger nails; *osseins* in osseous tissue, and *chondrigen* in cartilage.

    They resemble *proteids** in origin and composition of which *albumin* is a type.

albuminolysis (al-bu-min-ol'ĭ-sis). Proteolysis; decomposition of protein.

albu'minone. Noncoagulable protein in blood serum.

albuminoptysis (al-bŭ-mĭn-op'tĭ-sis). Albumin in sputum.

albuminoreac'tion. The presence or absence of albumin in the sputum.

Positive reaction indicates inflammatory condition of lungs.

albuminorrhe'a. Albumin in urine.

albuminose (al-bu'min-oz). 1. Albumose. 2. Albuminous.

albumino'sis. Abnormal increase of albuminous constituents in blood plasma.

albu'minous. Having the nature of albumen.

albu"minuret'ic. Pert. to albuminuria.

albuminuria (al-bu-min-u'rĭ-ă). The presence of albumin in the urine, indicating either a simple mixture of albuminous matters with the urine, or a pathological state of the kidneys.

a., cardiac. Caused by disease of the heart valves.

a., cyclic. Deposit at regular diurnal intervals of small amounts of albumen in the urine, esp. in childhood and youth.

a., extrarenal or accidental. Due to contamination of urine with pus, chyle, or blood.

a., functional or transient. One in which the only finding is occasional presence of albuminuria, associated with physical or mental distress or slight emotional excitement. Occurs in some after taking certain foods.

a. gravidarum. Albuminuria developing in pregnant women.

a., pathological. Albuminuria caused by a disease.

a., physiological. Albuminuria in a temporary form, existing without evidence of pathology.

a., renal. Due to changes in epithelial cells of kidneys, making them pervious to proteins of the blood as in all forms of nephritis.

a., toxic. Due to toxins generated within the body or by poison from outside source.

albuminu'ric retini'tis. Inflammation of retina characterized by hazy retina, blurred disc margin, distention of retinal arteries, retinal hemorrhages, and white patches in the fundus, esp. the stellate figure at the macula.* SEE: *retinitis.*

albu'moscope. An instrument for determining the presence of albumen in the urine.

al'bumose. The intermediate product produced by enzymes in the splitting of proteins which in the course of digestion becomes peptones.

albumosemia (al-bu-mo-se'mĭ-ă). Albumose in the blood.

albumosuria (al-bū-mō-sū'rĭ-ă). Albumose in the urine.

Alcock's canal. A space in the external fascia of the *ischiorectal fossa,* above the tuberosity of the ischium.*

It contains the internal pudendal artery, veins, and nerve.

al'cohol. One of many carbon compounds of the general formula

R^1, R^2—COH, where R^1 R^2 and R^3 may be R^3 hydrogen atoms or any organic radicals.

a., absolute. Contains 99% alcohol or not more than 1% by weight of water.

a., denatured. Alcohol rendered unfit for use as a beverage or medicine.

a., ethyl. Ordinary or grain alcohol.

a., methyl. Wood spirit.

alcoholase (al'ko-hŏl-āz). A ferment converting lactic acid into alcohol.

alcohol'ic. Pert. to alcohol.

a. fermentation. That which is produced by yeast in bread. RS: *Fermentation, acetic* and *lactic.*

alcoholism (ăl'kō-hŏl-izm). Diseased condition due to acute or chronic excessive indulgence in alcoholic liquors.

a., acute. Excessive indulgence in alcohol.

a., chronic. Continued use of alcohol.

a. psychoses. These include (a) pathological intoxication, (b) delirium tremens,* (c) Korsakoff's psychosis.* (d) acute hallucinosis,* and (e) other types.

alcoholize (al'ko-hol-īz). 1. To impregnate with alcohol. 2. To make into alcohol.

alcoholomania (al-ko-hol-o-ma'nĭ-ă). Abnormal craving for intoxicants.

alcoholometer (al-ko-hol-om'et-er). An instrument for measuring quantity of alcohol in a fluid.

alcoholophilia (al"ko-hol-o-fil'ĭ-ă). Morbid craving for alcohol.

alcoholu'ria. Alcohol in the urine.

alcosol (al'kō-sŏl). A sol using alcohol as the solvent instead of water.

aldehyde (al'de-hīd). 1. Oxidation product of a primary alcohol. 2. A hydrocarbon wherein hydrogen has been replaced by the —CHO group. 3. Carbon compounds of the general formula $\frac{H}{R}>CO$; formaldehyde H_2CO, acetaldehyde CH_3CHO, and benzaldehyde C_6H_5CHO are members of this group. Formaldehyde is a combustible gas but soluble in water; its 40% solution is called formalin. Acetaldehyde and benzaldehyde are liquids.

alembic (al-em'bik). Utensil used for distillation.

alemmal (ă-lĕm'al). Without a neurilemma, as a nerve fiber.

Alep'po boil, button, evil, or sore. Oriental boil.

aleuco-. For words beginning thus, see *aleuko-* words.

aleukemia (ă-lū-kē'mĭ-ă). 1. Deficiency of white blood corpuscles. The existence of leukopenia or aleukocytosis. 2. Pseudoleukemia.

aleukemic (a-lu-ke'mik). 1. Marked by aleukemia. 2. Pert. to an early stage of Hodgkin's disease, before blood changes occur.

a. leukemia. Leukemia in which the total count of white blood corpuscles is normal, regardless of quantitative changes of the blood or leukemic changes in tissues.

aleukia (ă-lu′kĭ-ă). 1. Leukopenia. 2. Absence of blood plates.

aleukocytosis (a-lu-ko-si-to′sis). A diminished production of white corpuscles in the blood.

aleuron (al-u′ron). The protein granules of seeds in which the vitamins* are supposed to be stored.

aleuronat (al-ū′ro-năt). Vegetable albumin used for bread for diabetics.

ale′wife. Shadlike fish eaten salted in West Indies. Average serving, 230 grams. Pro. 44.6, Fat 11.3.

Alexand′er-Adam's operation. Shortening the round ligaments, suturing their ends to the ext. abdominal ring, for uterine displacements.

alexeteric (ăl-eks-ĕ-ter′ik). Protective against infection, venom, and poison.

alex′ia. Inability to read, due to a central lesion; word-blindness. A form of aphasia.

a., musical. Inability to read music. It may be sensory, optical or visual, but not motor. SEE: *anarthria, aphemia.*

alexic (al-ek′sik). Defensive, as an alexin.*

alexin (al-ek′sin). Defensive substance in normal serum which, in presence of a sensitizer, destroys bacteria and exerts a lytic action on cells. SYN: *complement, q.v.*

alexin′ic un′it. The lowest amount of alexinic serum required to dissolve a measured quantity of red blood corpuscles in the presence of an excessive amount of hemolytic serum.

alexipharmic (ă-leks-ĭ-far′mik). 1. An antidote. 2. Antidotal. Warding off the ill effects of a poison.

alexipyretic (ă-lĕk″sĭ-pĭ-ret′ĭk). That which lessens fever. SYN: *febrifuge.*

alexocyte (ă-lĕks′o-sit). A leukocyte supposed to secrete alexin.

alexofixagen (al-ĕks-o-fĭk′sa-jĕn). An antigen stimulating production of complement-fixing antibodies.

aleze (ă-lĕz′). A folded cloth to protect the bed from discharges.

algae (al′je). Seaweed; aquatic cryptograms.*

a., Hawaiian. Edible variety. Average serving 25 grams. Pro. 0.7. Contains Vit. A and B.

alganesthesia (al-gan-ĕs-the′zĭ-ă). Absence of normal sense of pain. SYN: *analgesia.*   [refrigerant.

algefacient (al-je-fa′shent). Cooling, or

algesia (al-je′zĭ-ă). Supersensitiveness to pain, hyperesthesia.

algesic (al-je′sik). Hyperesthesic; painful.

algesichronometer (al-je″sĭ-kro-nom′et-er) An instrument for measuring time taken to feel pain.

algesimeter (al-jes-im′et-er). An instrument for measuring sensitiveness of cutaneous surfaces.

algesthesia (al-jes-the′zĭ-ă). Unusual sensitivity to sensory stimuli, as pain or touch. SYN: *hyperesthesia.*

algetic (al-jet′ik). Painful.

-algia. Suffix signifying *pain*, as in neur-*algia*.

algicide (al′jis-id). That which destroys algae.

algid (al′jid). Cold, chilly.

a. pernicious fever. A form of malaria with symptoms of collapse.

a. stage. Cold and cyanotic skin occurring in cholera and some other diseases.

algiomotor (al″jĭ-o-mo′tor). Causing painful contraction of muscles.

algiomus′cular. Causing painful contraction of muscles. SYN: *algiomotor.*

algogenic (al-go-jen′ik). 1. Causing neuralgic pain. 2. Lowering body temperature below normal.

algolagnia (al-go-lag′nĭ-ă). A sex perversion on part of one who cannot enjoy love or sex when dissociated from some form of pain to the sexual partner, male or female. The subject may be a sadist or a masochist. SEE: *masochism, sadism.*

algolagnist (al-go-lag′nist). One who practices algolagnia.*

algom′eter. Instrument for testing the sensitiveness to pain.

algophily (al-gŏf′ĭ-lĭ). Sexual pleasure in experiencing bodily pain or inflicting it upon others. Algolagnia.*

algophobia (al-go-fo′bĭ-ă). Morbid aversion to witnessing or experiencing pain.

algopsychalia (al-go-sĭ-ka′lĭ-ă). Hallucinatory depression in which the dread and suicidal trends are ascribed to the hallucinations.

al′gor. 1. A chill. 2. The sensation of cold; cold.

algos (al′gos). Pain.

alible (al′ĭ-bl). Absorbable; nutritive; assimilable.

alices (al′ĭs-ēz). The red spots appearing before pustulation in smallpox.*

alienation (al-yen-a′shun). Mental disorder, including every form of deviation from the physiological mental activities in conduct. In law, a psychosis varying according to situation involved.

a′lienism. Science of mental diseases.

a′lienist. One who studies disease from an antisocial standpoint.

aliform (al′ĭ-form). Having form of a wing.

a. process. Wing of the sphenoid.

al′iment. Nutriment, food.

alimen′tary. Possessing the qualities of nourishing.

a. canal or tract. The digestive tube from the beginning of the esophagus to the rectum, and accessory glands.

a. duct. The thoracic duct.

alimenta′tion. The general process of nourishing the body; it includes mastication, swallowing, digestion, absorption, and assimilation.

a., artificial. Feeding of patient unable to take nourishment normally.

a., forced. 1. Feeding of a patient

unwilling to eat. 2. Therapeutic feeding of more nourishment than necessary.

a., rectal. Injection of food through the rectum. However, little if any nutrients are absorbed through the colon.

alimentotherapy (al-im-en-to-ther'ap-ĭ). Treatment employing dietetics.

alina'sal. Pert. to the *alae nasi* or wings of the nose.

alinement (al-īn-ment). The line along which adjustment of the teeth is made.

aliphatic (al-ĭ-fat'ĭk). 1. Belonging to that series of carbon compounds characterized by straight or branching chains of carbon atoms, related to methane and ethane, and including the fats and fatty acids; opposite of *aromatic.* 2. Fatty.

aliquot (al'ĭ-kwot). A fractional part divisible into the whole without a remainder.

alisphenoid (al-ĭ-sfe'noyd). Pert. to the greater wing of the sphenoid bone.

alkalemia (al-kal-e'mĭ-ă). An excessive alkalinity of the blood due to a decrease in the *hydrogen ion* concentration of the blood, which normally is balanced with the *hydroxyl ions,* thus giving the blood a neutral reaction.

alkales'cence. 1. Slight alkalinity. 2. Process of becoming alkaline.

alkales'cent. Alkaline or becoming alkaline.

al'kali. 1. A metallic oxide (except ammonia) that has the property of combining with an acid to form a salt, or with an oil to form soap. Ex: *caustic soda, caustic potash.* 2. Any caustic substance which can neutralize acids and affect indicators in certain ways. Ex: *sodium hydroxide,* which turns litmus blue.

alkalimeter (al-kal-im'et-er). Device for measuring strength of alkalies.

alkalim'etry. Measurement of degree of alkalinity in a mixture.

al'kaline. Pert. to an alkali or having the reactions of one.

al'kaline ash diet. One consisting of normal amount of protein with moderate salt restriction, adequate in all known essentials.

al'kaline reserve. The amount of material in the blood available for neutralizing the acids produced in the course of metabolism,* particularly carbonic acid.

al'kaline tide. The increase in *alkaline reserve* and occasional occurrence of alkaline urine during gastric digestion, compensating for the simultaneous secretion of acid in the stomach.

alkalin'ity. State of being alkaline. SEE: *antalkaline, hydrogen ion.*

al'kalinize. To make alkaline.

alkalinu'ria. An alkaline urine.

alkalipe'nia. Low alkali reserve of the body.

alkalitherapy (al-kal-i-ther'ap-ĭ). Alkali therapy.

alkaliza'tion. Process of making alkaline.

al'kaloid. 1. An active bitter principle that reacts with an acid to form a salt, the latter being used because of its solu-

bility, rather than the alkaloid. 2. An alkaline principle of organic origin; any nitrogenous base, esp. one of vegetable origin having a toxic effect.

alkalom'etry. Dosimetry. Administration of alkaloids.

alkalo'sis. A condition in which the alkalinity of the body tends to increase beyond normal, due to excess of alkalies or withdrawal of acid or chlorides from the blood.

alkalot'ic. Pert. to alkalosis.

alkaluretic (al-ka-lu-ret'ĭk). Causing or that which causes an alkaline urine.

alkap'ton(e. A yellowish-red substance sometimes occurring in urine, the possible result of incomplete oxidation of tyrosin.

alkaptonuria (al-kap-ton-u'rĭ-ă). The presence of a yellowish nitrogenous substance in the urine not esp. indicative of disease or a local lesion although found in pulmonary tuberculosis. It turns the urine dark or black.

alkyl (al'kil). Any univalent alcohol radical.

allachesthesia (al-ă-kes-the'zĭ-ă). Tactile sensation remote from point of stimulation.

allantiasis (al-an-tī'ă-sis). 1. Sausage-poisoning. 2. Botulism.*

allantochorion (al-lăn-tō-ko'rĭ-ŏn). Fusion of the allantois and chorion into one structure.

allanto'ic. Pert. to the allantois.

allan'toid. 1. Sausage-shaped. 2. Allantois. 3. Pert. to the allantois.

allan'toin (chemical name, glyoxyldiuride). A white crystalline powder, considered to be secreted by maggots.

   DOSAGE: ½-2 gr. (0.03-0.12 Gm.). In 0.4% solutions or as an ointment.

allantoinu'ria. Allantoin in the urine.

allantois (al-an'tois). A diverticulum (cul-de-sac) of the hind gut in the embryo, which later surrounds the entire embryo, internally forming into the bladder and externally into the umbilical cord and placenta.

allantox'icon. A ptomaine generated in decomposing sausage.

allelocatalysis (al-le-lo-kat-ăl'ĭ-sis). Stimulation of a bacterial culture by the addition of cells of same type.

allelomorph (al-le'lo-morf). One of a pair of character units, the descendants not showing a mixture of the pair, but one or the other of the unit characters.

allel'otaxis. Development of a part from different embryonic structures.

Allen-Doisy unit. Injection in a spayed mouse of the smallest amount of estrus-producing hormone secreted during pregnancy, producing desquamation of vaginal epithelium in the mouse.

   A test for female sex hormone in women.

Allen's law. The more carbohydrate taken by a diabetic, the less he utilizes.

A.'s treatment. Certain days (7 to 10) of absolute fasting followed by a spare diet with little carbohydrate;

starvation treatment for diabetics preceding treatment by insulin. Water and a little alcohol permitted, followed by increasingly small amounts of carbohydrates, until sugar appears in urine, then fats until acetonuria* is produced, then protein until 1500 to 2000 calories are reached.

allen′thesis. Introduction of a foreign substance into the body.

allergen (al′er-jen). A hypothetic substance supposed to produce allergy.*

allergia (al-er′jǐ-ǎ). Hypersensitivity to a specific substance. SYN: *allergy.**

aller′gic. Pert. to or sensitive to an allergen.

   a. extracts. Made from protein of various substances believed to have specific action in producing morbid conditions.

al′lergin. A substance supposed to produce allergy. SYN: *allergen.*

allergiza′tion. Sensitization.

al′lergy. 1. Hypersensitivity to a specific substance. 2. A clinical change in the capacity of an organism to react to an infection following a primary one, as in increased susceptibility, or immunity.

allesthesia (al-es-the′sǐ-ǎ). A sensation in one limb which is referred to the other one; allochiria.

alliaceous (al-ǐ-a′se-us). Tasting like garlic or onions.

allitera′tion. Dysphrasia, in which words are spoken according to sound.

allo-. 1. A prefix meaning differentiation from the normal. 2. Indicating a body made stable by heat. 3. CHEM: An isomer, close relative or variety of a compound. Isomerism when there is relative asymmetry.

allochesthe′sia. Tactile sensation remote from point of stimulation. SYN: *allochiria, allesthesia.*

allochezia, allochetia (al-o-ke′zǐ-ǎ, al-o-ke′shǐ-ǎ). 1. Excretion of nonfecal matter from the bowels. 2. Excretion of feces through an abnormal opening.

allochiria (al-o-ki′rǐ-ǎ), **allocheiria.** Sensation referred to side of body opposite its origin; allesthesia.
   Observed in locomotor ataxia and in hysteria.

allochroism (al-ŏk′rō-izm). Change in color.

allochromasia (al-ō-krō-mā′sǐ-ǎ). Change in color of hair or skin.

allocinesia (al-o-sin-e′sǐ-ǎ). Movement on side of body opposite to the one directed. SEE: *allokinesis.*

alloerotism (al-lo-er′ot-ism). Gratification of the sexual instinct directed to an external object. Cf. *autoerotism.*

allokinesis (al-o-kin-e′sis). Movement on side of body opposite to the one directed.

allokinetic (al-o-kin-et′ik). Movement caused by external forces.

allola′lia. Speech defect, esp. if due to disease of speech center.

allonal (ǎl′o-nol). A derivative of barbituric acid. A trade name.

USES: Hypnotic, sedative, and analgesic.
   DOSAGE: Average 2 2/3 gr. (0.170 Gm.).

all′opath. A misnomer for a regular medical practitioner.

allopathy (al-lop′a-thǐ). A misnomer for a system of therapeutics administering medicines which produce effects different from those of the disease treated; in principle, the opp. of homeopathy. A term erroneously used for the regular practice of medicine.

allophasis (al-off′as-is). Incoherency; delirium.

alloplasia (al-o-pla′zǐ-ǎ). *Heteroplasia.** Replacement of normal cell forms by other cell forms latent in the tissue.

al′loplasty. Plastic surgery with nonhuman tissue.

allopsychic (al-lo-si′kik). Ideas not related to the patient's personality, but to the external environment.

allopsycho′sis. Derangement of perceptive powers.

allorhythmia (al-o-rith′mǐ-ǎ). Irregular cardiac rhythm.

allosome (al′o-sōm). A chromosome differing in appearance and behavior from an ordinary one.

allotherm (al′o-therm). An organism whose temperature is directly dependent on its culture medium.

allotox′in. A substance within the body which protects by destroying toxins inimical to it.

allotriogeustia (al-ot-rǐ-o-just′ǐ-ǎ). Perverted taste.

allotriophagy (al-o-trǐ-of′ǎ-jǐ). The habit of eating injurious, unusual, and nonedible substances.   [urine.

allotriuria (al-ot-rǐ-u′rǐ-ǎ). Abnormal

allotropic (al-lo-trop′ik). 1. CHEM: Pert. to different forms of the same element without change of chemical composition. 2. Possessing an altered nutritive value.

   a. type. One much concerned with what others think, say, or do.

allot′ropism, allot′ropy. Presence of an element in two or more distinct forms with unlike properties.

allox′an. A substance obtained by the action of nitric acid or of nascent chlorine upon uric acid.

$$C(OH)_2 \begin{matrix} > \end{matrix} \begin{matrix} CO—NH \\ CO—NH \end{matrix} \begin{matrix} > \end{matrix} CO.$$

allox′in. Any one of a series of *xanthin* bases derived from the splitting of *chromatin*, which on oxidation produces uric acid.

allox′ur bases or bodies. Xanthine bases. Nitrogenous substances formed by splitting of nucleins.

alloxuremia (al-oks-u-re′mǐ-ǎ). Xanthine* bases in the blood.

alloxu′ria. Xanthine bases in the urine.

al′lyl. A univalent radical. It is present in garlic and mustard.

Almén′s tests (ǎl-māns′). Three tests of urine for blood, albumin, and sugar.

alochia (ǎ-lo′kǐ-ǎ). Absence of puerperal* vaginal discharge following childbirth.

aloe (al'o). USP. The inspissated juice of several species of aloe.

DOSAGE: As a purgative: 2 to 5 gr. (0.125 to 0.3 Gm.).

alo'gia. Inability to express oneself through speech. SYN: *aphasia.*

alopecia (al-o-pe'shĭ-ă). Natural or abnormal baldness or deficiency of hair, partial or complete, localized or generalized.

a. adnati. Congenital baldness.

a. areata, a. Celsi, a. circumscripta. Baldness is sharply defined; circumscribed patches which leave the scalp smooth and white, and which are probably due to nervous disturbances or parasites.

a., congenital. Form with absence of hair bulbs at birth.

a. follicularis. Inflammation of the hair follicles of the scalp causing loss of hair from affected areas.

a. furfuracea. Called also *alopecia capillitii, pityriasis capitis, seborrhea capillitii,* and *dandruff.* Chronic in course and marked by hyperemia, dandruff and itching, and falling out of hair (exfoliation of scales), which becomes harsh, dry, and lusterless.

a. localis, a. neuritica. Falling of hair in circumscribed spots in area of distribution of scalp nerves.

a. neurotica. Baldness following a nervous disease or injury to nervous system, and occurring at site of injury.

a. pityroides. Falling of both scalp and body hair, together with abundant branlike desquamation.

a. senilis. Baldness of old age.

a. simplex. Baldness prematurely.

a. symptomatica. Loss of hair after prolonged fevers or during course of some disease; also may result from changes in internal secretions.

a. toxica. Loss of hair thought to be due to toxins of infectious disease.

a. universalis. General loss of hair from all parts of body.

al'pha. First letter of Greek alphabet. CHEM: Denotes first in a series of isomeric compounds.

a. leukocyte. One that disintegrates during blood coagulation.

a. test. A U. S. army test for recruits capable of reading English.

alphus (al'fus), **al'phos.** 1. Psoriasis. 2. A pustular, scrofulous affection of the skin accompanied by white crusts.

al'terant. An alterative. That which brings about a favorable change in the body functions.

alterative (awl'ter-a-tiv). A medicine that alters the processes of nutrition and excretion, restoring the normal functions of the system.

al'ternate host. A carrier of disease germs, such as the louse, and other insects.

al'ternating cur'rent. PT: An electrical current the direction of which reverses constantly.

al'ternator. PT: So-called sinusoidal alternator: an electromagnetic device consisting of a revolving armature which cuts the lines of force in a magnetic field and which delivers a sinusoidal current from secondary coil of the apparatus.

al'therm, altherm pad. A device containing chemicals applying heat to the eye or a sinus.

altricious (al-trish'us). Slow in developing; requiring long nursing.

al'um (ammonium alum, or potassium alum). USP. Large, colorless crystals, or white powder, with sweetish, strongly astringent taste.

DOSAGE: As an astringent, 5 to 15 gr. (0.3-1 Gm.). As an emetic, 1 drachm (4 Gm.).

alu'men. Alum.

a. exsiccatum. Alum that has been dried or burnt.

aluminosis (al-ū-min-o'sis). Chronic catarrhal inflammation of the lungs in alum workers.

alu'minum. A silver-whitish metal. SYMB: *Al.* Atomic weight 26.97.

aluminum acetate (as'et-āt). A salt formed by the reaction between aluminum sulfate and lead acetate. Its aqueous solution, containing 4 to 5%, is known as Burow's Solution.

alumnol (a-lum'nol). A fine, white, nonhygroscopic powder.

DOSAGE: As surgical antiseptic, in from ½ to 3% solutions; in gynecology, in from 2 to 5%.

alusia (al-u'sĭ-ă). Morbidity; hallucination.

alvajel (al-vă-jel'). An ointment made from a tropical plant, of the cactus family, and recommended in x-ray burns.

Alvegniat's pump (al-văn-yats'). Mercurial vacuum pump for removing gases from the blood.

alveobronchi'tis. Inflammation of the bronchioles, and pulmonary alveoli; bronchopneumonia.*

alve'olar. A small depression or pert. to an alveolus.

SEE: *chilognathopalatoschisis.*

a. air. The mixture of gases collected by having the subject first execute a normal expiration and then exhale as much additional air (which comes from the alveoli of the lungs) into the collecting device as possible.

a. process. One of four processes which make up each maxillary bone.

alve'olate. Honeycombed; pitted.

alveoli (al-ve'o-li). Pl. of alveolus.

a. dentales (BNA). Tooth sockets.

alveoli'tis. Inflammation of the alveolar processes; pyorrhea.*

alveoloclasia (al-ve-o-lo-kla'zĭ-ă). Absorption of any part of the alveolar process.

alveolus (al-ve'o-lus) (*pl. alve'oli*). 1. A little hollow. 2. The socket of a tooth. 3. Air cell of the lungs. 4. A small depression such as those contained in the honeycomb cells of the gastric mucous membrane. 5. A follicle of a racemose gland.

a., mucous, of the salivary glands.

Those that secrete the ropy material of the saliva, containing mucin.

a., parietal. An air space in the wall of an alveolar passage in the lung.

a. pulmoneus. A pulmonary air space.

a., serous, of the salivary glands. Those that secrete thec serous albumin of the saliva, which coagulates when heated.

a., terminal. An air space connected with a pulmonary infundibulum.

alveus (al′ve-us). A canal, tube, duct, or cavity.

a. ampullascens. Dilation at the receptaculum chyli.

a. hippocampi. Medullary layer investing the hippocampus major.

alvine (al′vīn). Pert. to the intestines or abdomen.

a. concretion. Intestinal stone.

a. discharge. Stools.

a. flux. Watery feces.

alvi′nolith. An intestinal mass formed from calcareous salts and other matter.

al′vus. Abdomen and viscera.

alycin (a-li′sin). A combination of natural salicylates with an alkaline base. Given usually as a powder, or an elixir.

DOSAGE: Average, 1 teaspoonful.

alymphopotent (a-lĭm′fō-pō″tĕnt). Unable to develop lymphocytes or lymphoid cells.

Alzheimer's disease (ahlts′hi-mer). PSY: Presenile dementia with hyaline degeneration of the smaller blood vessels of the brain.

Am. Symbol for *mixed astigmatism*, or for *ametropic*.

ama (a′mă). Enlargement of a bony canal of labyrinth of the internal ear at the end opposite the ampulla.

A. M. A. Abbr. for American Medical Association.

amaas (ä′mähs). A mild form of smallpox, milk-pox.

am′acrine cell. Nerve cell without any axis cylinder process.

amal′gam. Any alloy containing mercury.

amal′gamate. To make an amalgam.

amara (am-a′ră). Bitters.

amarthritis (am-ar-thri′tis). Polyarthritis. Inflammation of more than one joint at the same time.

amasesis (ă-mas-ē′sis). Inability to masticate.

amas′tia. Failure of breast development.

am′ative. 1. Expressing sexual desire. 2. Propensity to love.

Amat′o bod′ies. Those seen in leukocytes in scarlet fever.

amaurosis (am-aw-ro′sus). Blindness, partial or total, without known lesions of optic nerve or of the eye. It may occur as result of hysteria.

a., albuminuric. Amaurosis caused by kidney affection.

a., amaurotic. Amaurosis caused by the atrophying of optic nerve or vision centers.

a., cerebral. Amaurosis caused by brain malady.   [on.

a., congenital. Amaurosis from birth

a., diabetic. Amaurosis in connection with diabetes.

a., epileptoid. Sudden seizure of blindness, considered to be similar to epilepsy.

a., lead. Amaurosis caused by lead poisoning.

a., reflex. Amaurosis due to reflex action caused by irritation of a remote part.

a., saburral. Amaurosis in conjunction with acute gastritis.

a., tobacco. Amaurosis caused by tobacco poisoning.

a., toxic. Blindness from optic neuritis caused by poison.

a., uremic. Amaurosis caused by uremic condition.

amaurotic (am-ă-rot′ik). Pert. to one afflicted with amaurosis.

a. family idiocy. Form of idiocy in which the vision is imperfect. SEE: *idiocy, idiot.*

amaxophobia (ă-maks-o-fo′bĭ-ă). Morbid dread of carriages and wagons or riding in them.

ambi-. Prefix: both or both sides; around; about, as *ambidextrous.*

ambidex′trous. Ability to work effectively with either hand.

ambilat′eral. Pert. to both sides.

ambile′vous. Awkward in use of both hands.

ambio′pia. Double vision. SYN: *diplopia.**

ambisinis′ter. Awkward in use of both hands. SYN: *ambilevous.*

ambiten′dency. PSY: The association of diverging impulses to action and opposite trends of thought or emotion with a central idea—an essential mechanism in conflict.

ambivalence (am-biv′ă-lens). 1. Possessing ability of equal power or value in two directions. 2. PSY: Linking of opposite or contrary emotional values (love and hate) to the same idea, or toward the same person. The fluctuation from strong like to dislike found in schizophrenia.

ambiv′alency. The condition of being ambivalent.

ambiv′alent. Have equal power or value in both directions.

a. feelings. Two opposite emotions, such as love and hate, for the same person at same time.

ambloma (amblo′mă). An aborted fetus.

amblosis (am-blo′sis). An abortion.

amblyacusia (am″blĭ-ă-koo′sĭ-ă). Dullness of hearing.   [touch.

amblyaphia (am-ble-af′ĭ-ă). Dull sense of

amblychromasia (am″blĭ-kro-ma′sĭ-ă). The state in which the cell nucleus stains faintly.

amblychromat′ic. Staining faintly.

amblygeustia (am-blĭ-jus′tĭ-ă). Defective or blunted taste.

amblyopia (ăm-blĭ-o′pĭ-ă). Reduced or dimness of vision, not dependent upon visible changes in the eye and not refractive (alcoholic, astigmatic, diabetic, *ex anopsia*, malarial, methyl alcohol, quinine, tobacco, toxic, uremic).

a. exanopsia. Dimness of vision resulting from inaccurate focusing on retina due to refractive errors, cataract, etc.

a., postmarital. Amblyopia caused by excessive sexual activity.

a. reflex. Amblyopia due to irritation of peripheral area.

amblyoscope (am'blĭ-os-kōp). Instrument for training an amblyopic eye for better vision.

am'bo. Annular fibrocartilage producing an elevation about a joint cavity, and the elevation itself.

amboceptor (am-bo-sep'tor). So called by Ehrlich. An immune substance or antibody forming a union between an antigen and complement (agent that completes lytic action), as it is assumed it has one affinity for the antigen and one for the complement.

a. unit. Smallest amount of amboceptor required in the presence of which a given quantity of red blood corpuscles will be dissolved by an excess of complement.

ambon (am'bon). The ring which surrounds the sockets in which the heads of long bones are received, as the *glenoid cavity*.

am'bos. Incus or anvil bone.

ambrine (am'brĭn). A preparation of paraffin used in treating extensive burns.

am'bulance. Wagon for transportation of the sick and wounded.

am'bulant, ambulatory. Able to walk, not confined to bed.

a. typhoid fever. A mild attack of typhoid fever, in which the patient is not confined to bed. SEE: *typhoid*.

ambustial (am-bus'shal). Pert. to a burn or scald.

ambustion (am-bus'shun). A burn or scald.

ame'ba. A one-celled protozoan minute animal form of life that constantly changes its shape by sending out processes of its protoplasm, by which it moves about and obtains its nourishment.

a. bucca'lis. Ameba found in dental infections.

a. coli. Those which frequent the upper part of the large intestine.

a. dysenteriae. Those appearing in the intestines and which are responsible for amebic dysentery.

a. movements. Those possessed by leukocytes which "wander" through capillary walls into surrounding tissues; a process known as "migration."

amebiasis (am-e-bi'as-is). Infection with amebas, of which *amebic enteritis** is one form. Many forms are not recognized as being due to parasitic infection.

ame'bic. Pert. to or caused by amebas.

a. carrier state. That in which an individual harbors a form of pathogenic ameba. At least one per cent of the population harbor *E. histolytica*. Often a subacute or chronic form will follow an attack.

a. dysentery. SEE: *amebic enteritis*.

a. enteritis. Intestinal amebic infection.

a. hepatitis. Abscess of the liver of amebic origin.

a. proctitis. Infection with amebas affecting the anus and rectum.

ame'bicide. Destructive to or any agent that kills amebas.

ame'biform. Formed like an ameba.

amebocyte (a-me'bo-sīt). A cell showing ameboid movements.

ame'boid. Having the appearance and characteristics of an ameba.

ame'boidism. Amebalike movements, noting a condition shown by certain nerve cells.

amebula (am-e'bū-lă). The amebalike spore of the malarial parasite.

amebu'ria. Amebas in the urine.

amelioration (ă-me-lĭ-or-a'shun). Improvement; moderation of a condition.

ame'loblast. A cell from which tooth enamel is formed.

ameloden'tinal. Pert. to both enamel and dentine.

Amend's solution (a'mends). An organic iodine preparation, stable, and causing less gastric disturbances than Lugol's solution.

DOSAGE: From 10 to 20 drops in glassful of water, ½ to 1 hour before meals.

ame'nia. Absence of the menses; amenorrhea.*

amenomania (a-me-no-ma'nĭ-ă). Insanity characterized by happiness.

amenorrhea (a-men-o-rē'a). Absence or suppression of menstruation; normal before puberty, after the menopause, during pregnancy and lactation.

a., partial. Appearing occasionally and at irregular intervals.

a., physiological. Periods when normally free from menstruation; pre-puberty, pregnancy, lactation, postmenopause periods.

a., primary. *Emansio mensium.* That in which menses have never made their appearance.

a., secondary. *Suppressio mensium.* That in which, having appeared, they subsequently cease.

amenorrhe'al. Pert. to, caused or accompanied by amenorrhea.

amenorrhe'ic. Pert. to amenorrhea.

ament (ă'ment). An idiot; one without evidence of mind.

amentia (am-en'shĭ-a). PSY: Intellectual defect of varying degrees.

ameristic (a-mer-is'tik). Not segmented.

ametrohemia (ah-mĕt-rō-he'mĭ-ă). Lack of uterine blood supply.

ametrom'eter. Instrument for measuring ametropia.

ametropia (a-me-tro'pĭ-ă). Imperfect refractive powers of eye (hyperopia, myopia, astigmatism), in which the principal focus does not lie on the retina.

ametrop'ic. Pert. to ametropia.

amianthinopsy (ăm-ĭ-an'thin-op"sĭ). Violet blindness.

amicro'bic. Not due to microbes.

am'icron(e. A colloid particle unrecognizable through the ultramicroscope.

amicroscop'ic. Too small to be detected through the ultramicroscope.

am'ide. A chemical compound produced by the substitution of an acid radical for one of the hydrogen atoms of ammonia.

am'idin. 1. The part of starch soluble in water. 2. A monacid base. The group $C.NH.NH_2$.

amido-. A prefix signifying amine, *q.v.*

amid'ulin. Soluble starch.

amimia (a-mim'ĭ-ă). Loss of power to express ideas by signs or gestures; inability to comprehend gestures.

amine (am'in). One of a group of organic compounds containing the amine (NH_2) group, substituted for ammonias, and possessing the general formula RNH_2, characterized by strong pharmacologic activity, and including the ptomaines and alkaloids.

amino- (a-mē'no, am'in-o). Prefix denoting compound containing amine.

amino acid. One of the compounds, of which about 22 different ones are known, derived from the fatty acids by the exchange of a hydrogen atom of the hydrocarbon radical for an amino group. Intermediary products in the catabolism and anabolism of protein. Organic acids in which NH_2 has replaced one of the hydrogen atoms.

amino compound. Substance containing the group NH_2; same as amines, *q.v.*

amino group. The NH_2 group which characterizes the amines.

aminoacetic acid (am-in'o-ă-sē'tik) (glycocoll, glycine). One of the normal constituents of the bile.
DOSAGE: Average, 1½ drams (5 grams) *t.i.d.*

amino acide'mia. Amino acids in the blood.

aminol'ysis. Splitting of amines.

aminophyllin(e (a-min''ō-fil'in). Mixture of theophylline inducing diuretic action and acting as a myocardial stimulant. SEE: *theophylline.*
DOSAGE: 1½ gr. (0.1 Gm.).

aminopyrine (am''in-o-pi'rēn) (Pyramidon) USP.
DOSAGE: 0.3 to 0.4 Gm. (5 to 6 gr.).

aminosis (am-in-o'sis). Production or presence of amino acids in the blood.

aminosuria, aminuria (am-in-o-su'rĭ-ă, -u'rĭ-ă). Amines in voided urine.

amito'sis. Multiplication by division or cleavage of cells. Cell and nucleus division without changes in the nucleus, occurring during regular processes of cell reproduction.

amitotic (ah-mĭt-ot'ik). Characterized by amitosis.

am'meter. PT: An instrument calibrated to read in amperes the strength of a current flowing in a circuit.

ammone'mia. Ammonia in the blood due to urea decomposition. SYN: *ammoniemia.*

ammon'ia. 1. A gas formed by decomposition of nitrogen-containing substances.

2. Water charged with the same is called *ammonia water.*
    a., **aromatic spirit of.** A stimulant or an inhalant.
DOSAGE: ½ to 2 drams by mouth.
    a. **water.** Solution of ammonia in water.
DOSAGE: (10%) 15 ㎜ (1.0 cc.).

ammo'niac. Ammoniacal.

ammoni'acal. Having the characteristics of or pert. to ammonia.

ammo'niated. Containing ammonia.

ammoniemia (am-mō-nĭ-e'mĭ-ă). Ammonia in the blood due to decomposition of urea.

ammonium car'bonate (am-o'nĭ-um). Occurs as hard mass with strong odor of ammonia. On exposure to air loses CO_2 and ammonia.
DOSAGE: 0.3 Gm. (5 gr.).
    a. **chlor'ide.** White crystalline powder without odor.
DOSAGE: 0.3 Gm. (5 gr.). As a diuretic: 1¼ to 4 drams (5 to 15 Gm.).
    a. **hydrox'ide.** This is a solution of ammonia gas in water, used about the house for cleaning purposes, used in artificial ice, and electric refrigerators.

ammoniuria (am-o-nĭ-u'rĭ-ă). An over amount of ammonia in the urine.

amnesia (am-ne'zĭ-ă). A loss of memory.
    a., **auditory.** Loss of memory as to word meanings.
    a., **periodic.** Amnesia occurring in a period of double consciousness.
    a. **traumatica.** Amnesia caused by injuries.
    a., **visual.** Inability to remember the appearance of objects that have been seen or to be cognizant of printed words.

amnesic (am-ne'sik). Pert. to amnesia.
    a. **aphasia.** Loss of memory. SYN: *amnesia.*

amnestic (am-nes'tik). Amnesic, or causing amnesia.

amniochorial (am''nĭ-o-ko'rĭ-ăl). Rel. to both amnion and chorion.

am''niochorion'ic. Rel. to both amnion and chorion. SYN: *amniochorial.*

am''nioclep'sis. Gradual unperceived loss of amniotic fluid.

amniog'raphy. Radiography of amniotic sac.

am'nion. Bag of waters. The inner of the fetal membranes, a thin, transparent sac which holds the fetus suspended in the *liquor amnii,* or amniotic fluid, *q.v.*

amniorrhea (am-nĭ-or-re'ă). Premature escape of the *liquor amnii.*

amniorrhexis (am-nĭ-o-rek'sis). Rupture of the bag of waters, or amnion.

amnios (am'nĭ-os). The amnion, or the *liquor amnii.*

amniotic (am-ne-ot'ik). Pert. to the amnion.
    a. **fluid.** *Liquor amnii.* The liquid or albuminous fluid contained in the amniotic sac, *q.v.*
    a. **sac.** The bag or sac formed by the amnion.*

am'niotin. Commercial estrogenic hormone product.

amniotitis (am-nĭ-o-ti′tis). Inflammation of the amnion.

amniotome (am′ni-o-tōm). Instrument for puncturing fetal membranes.

amnitis (am-ni′tis). Inflammation of the amnion. Syn: *amniotitis*.

amok (am-ok′). A state of murderous frenzy.

amor (am′or). Love.

> **a. insanus.** Unrestrained libido in the insane. Syn: *erotomania.**
> **a. lesbicus.** Urningism* as practiced by the female sex. Saphism*; Lesbianism.*
> **a. sui.** Vanity; love of self.
> **a. veneris.** The clitoris.

amoralia (a-mŏ-ra′lĭ-ă). Moral imbecility.

amoralis (a-mo-ra′lis). A moral imbecile.

amorphia (a-mor′fĭ-a). Without form. Syn: *amorphism.*

amorphism (a-mor′fĭzm). State of being without definite form. Syn: *amorphia.*

amorphous (a-mor′fus). Without crystalline form, as *gelatin.*

amotio (am-o′shĭ-o). A detachment.

am″pelother′apy. Grape cure.

amperage (ăm-per′āj). PT: Strength of the electrical current expressed in amperes or milliamperes.

ampere (ăm′pēr). PT: Practical unit of intensity of electric current, being that which is produced by 1 volt acting through resistance of 1 ohm.

> **a. meter.** Instrument denoting in amperes the strength of a current. See: *ammeter.*

amperemeter (am′per-me″ter). Apparatus for measuring amperage of an electric current.

amphet′amine sul′fate. Synthetic white powder employed as a vasomotor stimulant. Syn: *benzedrine sulfate.*

amphi-. Prefix. On both sides, as *amphibious.* Chem: Denotes certain positions or configurations.

amphiarthrosis (am-fi-ar-thro′sis). A form of articulation intermediate between diarthrosis and synarthrosis, in which the articulating bony surfaces are separated by an elastic substance to which both are attached, so that the mobility is slight, but may be exerted in all directions. The articulations of the bodies of the vertebrae are examples.

amphiaster (am′fĭ-ăs″ter). Double star found during mitosis.*

Amphib′ia. A class of animals which live on land and in water.

amphiblas′tula. A morula formed by unequal segmentation.

amphiblestri′tis. Inflammation of retina. Syn: *retinitis.*

amphibo′lia. The uncertain period of a fever, or disease.

amphibolic (am-fi-bol′ik). Uncertain; ambiguous.

> **a. period, or stage.** The critical period of a disease when the outcome cannot be certain.

amphib′olous. Changeable; amphibolic.

amphicelous (am-fĭ-se′lus). Concave on each end.

amphicentric (am-fĭ-sen′trik). Centering at both ends.

amphichroic, amphichromatic (am-fĭ-kro′-ik, -kro-mat′ik). 1. Turning red litmus paper blue, and blue, red. 2. Reacting both as an acid and an alkali.

amphicra′nia. Pain on both sides of head.

am″phicreat′ine, amphicreat′inine. A leukomaine formed in muscles.

amphicyte (am′fĭ-sīt). One of the capsule cells enveloping the body of ganglionic neurons.

amphicyt′ula. Impregnated ovum having unequal segmentation of the vitellus.

amphidiarthrosis (am-fĭ-di-ar-thro′sis). An articulation with amphiarthrosis and diarthrosis, such as that of the lower jaw.

amphigas′trula. The human ovum in advanced gastrula stage.

amphigony (am-fĭg′o-nĭ). The sexual process.

amphimixis (am-fĭ-miks′is). 1. Sexual reproduction. 2. Psy: Pregenital energies and mechanisms diverted to the genitals during psychosexual maturity.

am″phimor′ula. The morula in ovum with unequal composing cells.

amphipyrenin (am′fĭ-pi′ren-in). The basophile substance of the nuclear membrane of a cell.

amphithe′atre. An operating room with seats arranged around it for students and others.

amphitrichate, amphitrichous (am-fit′rĭ-kāt, -kus). Pert. to certain organisms having flagella, or a flagellum at both ends.

ampho-. Prefix: both, as *amphodiplopia.*

am″phodiplo′pia. Double vision in each eye.

amphojel (am′fō-jĕl) [Alumina gel]. A colloidal suspension of hydrated alumina, capable of neutralizing the free hydrochloric acid in not less than 12 volumes of gastric juice of average strength.

> Dosage: Average, 1 teaspoonful.

am″phopep′tone. First peptone formed by tryptic digestion of protein.

amphophil, amphophilous (am′fo-fil, am-fof′il-us). Having affinity for either acid or basic dyes.

amphor′ic. Pert. to a sound as that caused by blowing across the mouth of a bottle; a resonance; a cavernous sound heard on percussion of a pulmonary cavity.

amphoric′ity. Producing amphoric sounds.

amphoriloquy (am-fo-ril′ok-wĭ). Having amphoric sounds in speaking.

amphoroph′ony. Amphoric voice sound.

amphoter′ic, amphot′erous. Affecting both red and blue litmus.

> **a. compounds.** Those which may act as a base or an acid, *i. e., protein.*

amphoterism (am-fo′ter-izm). Having both acid and basic properties.

amphot″erodiplo′pia. Double vision in each eye. Syn: *amphodiplopia.*

amphoton′ic. Pert. to both vagotony and sympathicotony.

amphot'ony. Tonicity of the sympathetic and parasympathetic systems.

amplexatio (am-pleks-a'shĭ-o). Sexual intercourse, coitus.

ampliation (am-plĭ-a'shun). Distention of a part or cavity.

amplifica'tion. 1. Enlargement of visual area in microscopy. 2. Magnification of sound in telephony.

am'plifier. That which increases magnification of vision or sound.

am'plitude. 1. In physics, the distance between extreme limits of an oscillation or vibration. Thus, the amplitude of vibration of a pendulum is the chord of the arc through which it oscillates; the amplitude of vibration of a wave is the distance from the crest to the trough of the wave. 2. Of the pulse, its fullness, *i. e.*, the extent of dilatation of the artery at each impulse of the heart.

    a. **of accommodation.** Total range of eye's accommodative power.

amuck'. State of murderous frenzy. SYN: *amok.*

ampoule, ampule (am'pōōl). A small glass that can be sealed and its contents sterilized. This is a French invention for containing hypodermic solutions. SEE: *sterule, ampulla.*

ampul'la. 1. Sacklike dilatation of a canal, as the mammary lactiferous ducts, or semicircular canals of the ear. 2. A small, hermetically sealed flask containing a solution for parenteral use; an ampoule.

    a., **Lieberkuhn's.** Lacteal's blind end in intestinal villi.

    a. **of rectum.** Portion situated above the perineal flexure.

    a. **of vagina.** Upper vaginal area.

    a. **of vas deferens.** Ampulla underneath bladder near the termination of the vas.

    a. **of Vater.** Enlargement at gateway of common bile duct and pancreatic duct into the duodenum.

ampulli'tis. Inflammation of any ampulla, esp. dilated extremity of *vas deferens.*

amputation (am-pu-ta'shun). Surgical removal of a part.   [in.

    a., **primary.** Before inflammation sets

    a., **secondary.** During period of suppuration.

amusia (a-mu'sĭ-ă). Music-deafness; inability to produce or comprehend music, as loss of the ability to play a musical instrument. ETIOL: Brain lesion, but cause not clearly understood.

Amussat's operation (am-ū-sä's). One for formation of an artificial anus, by lumbar colotomy in ascending colon.

amychophobia (ă-mĭ-ko-fo'bĭ-ă). PSY: Morbid fear of being scratched; fear of the claws of any animal.

amyctic (am-ik'tĭk). 1. Irritating, caustic. 2. A caustic or corrosive agent.

amyeloneuria (ă-mi-el-o-nu'rĭ-ă). Spinal cord paresis.

amyelotrophy (ă-mi-el-ot'ro-fĭ). Spinal cord atrophy.

amygdala (a-mig'da-lă). 1. Tonsil. 2. A mass of gray matter in the ant. portion of the temporal lobe.

amygdalectomy (a-mig-dal-ek'to-mĭ). Excision of a tonsil.

amygdaline (a-mig'dal-ĭn). 1. Pert. to a tonsil. 2. A bitter tasting glucoside in bitter almonds and cherry laurel leaves.

    a. **fissure.** One on ventral side of temporal lobe, *incisura temporalis.*

amygdalitis (a-mig-dal-i'tis). Inflammation of a tonsil; tonsillitis.

amygdaloid (a-mig'da-loid). Resembling a tonsil or an almond.

    a. **fossa.** A depression for the tonsil.

    a. **tubercle.** A projection from the middle cornu of the lateral ventricle, marking the location of amygdaloid nucleus.

amygdalolith (a-mig'da-lo-lith). Stone in a distended crypt of a tonsil.

amygdalop'athy. Any disease of a tonsil.

amygdalothrypsis (a-mig''dal-o-thrip'sis). Crushing of a tonsil followed by excision.

amygdalotome (a-mig-dal'o-tom). Instrument for excision of a tonsil.

amygdalotomy (a-mig-da-lot'o-mĭ). Removal of a portion of the tonsils.

amyl (am'ĭl). A hypothetical univalent radical, C_5H_{11}, nonexistent in a free state.

amyla'ceous. Starchy.

amylase (am'ĭl-laz). A ferment or amylolytic enzyme of the saliva, pancreatic juice and intestinal juice that hydrolyzes starch, producing achroödextrin and maltose.

amyle'mia. Hypothetical presence of starch in the blood.

amylin(e (am'ĭl-in). 1. Part of starch soluble in water. 2. A monacid base. The group $C.NH.NH_2$. SYN: *amidin.*

amyl nitrite (am'ĭl ni'trite). A clear yellowish liquid. Ethereal odor.

    DOSAGE: 3 ℳ (0.2 cc.) by inhalation.

amylodex'trin. Soluble substance produced during the change of starch into sugar.

amylodyspep'sia. Inability to digest starchy foods.

amylogen (am-il'o-jen). Soluble starch.

amylogenesis (am-i-lo-jen'es-is). The production of starch.   [ducing.

amylogenic (am-il-o-jen'ik). Starch-pro-

am'yloid. Starchlike, somewhat resembling hyalin. SEE: *chitinous.*

    a. **kidney.** Enlarged, firm, smooth kidney usually associated with amyloid diseases of spleen or liver.

amyloido'sis. Amyloid deposit in tissues and organs.

amylolysis (am-il-ol'is-is). Changing of starch into sugar in the process of digestion.

amylolytic (am-il-o-lit'ik). 1. Having the qualities of a hydrolytic enzyme. 2. Pert. to a starch-splitting enzyme converting polysaccharides* into disaccharides* such as ptyalin, *q.v.*

    a. **enzyme.** A ferment that hydrolyzes starch, producing achroödextrin and maltose. SYN: *amylase.*

amylop'sin. Diastatic enzyme in pancreatic juice which changes starch into achroödextrin and maltose. SEE: *digestion; duodenum; enzymes.*

amylose (am'ĭ-lōz). A group of carbohydrates containing starch, cellulose, and dextrin. SEE: *glycose, saccharose.*

amylosis (am-il-o'sis). Albuminoid degeneration of the cells.

amylosu'ria. Amylose in the urine.

amylum (am-i'lum). Starch.

amylu'ria. Starch in the urine.

amyocardia (ă-mi-o-kar'dĭ-ă). Weakness of the heart muscle. SYN: *Myasthenia cordis.*

a'myon. Absence of muscular tissue.

amyostasia (am-i-o-sta'sĭ-ă). Difficulty in standing because of lack of coördination or because of muscular tremors. SEE: *tremor.*

amyosthenia (am-i-os-the'nĭ-ă). Lack of muscular tone or power.

amyosthen'ic. Pert. to muscular weakness.

amyotaxy (am-i'o-taks-ĭ). Muscular ataxia.

amyotonia (am-i-o-to'nĭ-ă). Failure of muscular tone.
  a. congenita. Thomsen's disease, a disease, usually congenital and hereditary, characterized by tonic spasm and rigidity of certain muscles when an attempt is made to move them after a period of rest or when mechanically stimulated. The stiffness disappears as the muscles are used.

amyotrophia (am-ĭ-o-tro'fĭ-a). Muscular wasting.
  a., progressive spinal. Progressive muscular atrophy.

amyotrophic (am-i-o-trof'ik). Pert. to muscular atrophy.
  a. lateral sclerosis. A progressive muscular atrophy. SYN: Spastic irritability of muscles; increased reflexes.

amyotrophy (am-i-ot'ro-fĭ). Muscular wasting. SYN: *amyotrophia.**

amyous (am'ĭ-us). Weak. Deficient in muscular strength.

amytal (am'it-al). A derivative of barbital.
  DOSAGE: As sedative: 1/3 to 3/4 gr. (0.2 to 0.4 Gm.). Hypnotic: 1½ to 5 gr. (0.1 to 0.3 Gm.).

amyxia (ă-miks'ĭ-a). Deficient mucous secretion.

amyxorrhea (ă-miks-or-ri'ă). Lack of normal secretion of mucus.

an-. Prefix: negative; without or not, as *anemia.*

An. SYMB: Actinon.   [*ciation.*

A. N. A. Abbr. *American Nurses Asso-*

ana (an'ă). Meaning "one of each" used in writing prescriptions as āā. SEE: *prescription.*

anab'asis. Period of increase in a disease.

anabatic (an-ă-bat'ik). Increased severity; pert. to anabasis.

anabio'sis. Revival of a body which seemed lifeless. SYN: *resuscitation.*

anabiotic (an-ă-bi-ot'ik). Restorative. Any agent that resuscitates or restores.

anabole (an-ab'o-le). Vomiting; regurgitation; expectoration.

anabol'ic. Promoting or pert. to anabolism.
  a. nerve. Nerve controlling building processes.

anab'olin. A product of anabolism.

anabolism (an-ab'o-lizm). The building up of the body substance; the constructive or synthetic chemical reactions included in metabolism.

anabrosis (an-ab-ro'sis). Superficial ulceration.

anacampsis (an-ă-kamp'sis). A flexure.

anacamp'tics. Study of reflection of light or sound.

anacamptometer (an-a-camp-tom'et-er) Device for measuring reflexes.

anacatharsis (an-ak-ath-ar'sis). Vomiting; expectoration.

anacathar'tic. That which causes vomiting.

anachlorhydria (an-ă-klor-hīd'rĭ-ă). Absence of free hydrochloric acid in the gastric juice. SYN: *achlorhydria.**

anacid (an-as'id). Subacid, slightly acid; lacking in acidity.

anacidity (an-as-id'it-ĭ). Abnormal lack or deficiency of acidity.

anaclasim'eter. Instrument for measuring refraction of eyes.

anaclisis (an-ak'lis-is). Reclining.

anaclit'ic choice. An early expression of psychosexual development, the opposite of narcissism,* in which the object of one's love is influenced by dependence upon the mother or whoever is responsible for the child's early care, more or less inhibiting other expressions of the sex instinct.

anacroasia (an-ă-kro-a'sĭ-ă). Inability to understand spoken words.

anacrotic (an-a-krot'ik). 1. Pert. to a pulse with more than one expansion of the artery. 2. Pert. to two heartbeats traced on the ascending line of a sphygmogram. SEE: *pulse.*
  a. limb. Up-stroke of a pulse wave.
  a. wave. A wave on the up-stroke of a pulse wave.

anac'rotism. Existence of a double beat on ascending line of sphygmogram. SYN: *anadicrotism.**

anacusia, anacu'sis (an-ak-oo'sĭ-ă, -sis). Complete deafness.

anadenia (an-ad-e'nĭ-ă). 1. Lowered glandular function. 2. Chronic lack of gastric secretion.

anadicrot'ic. 1. Pert. to a pulse with more than one artery expansion. 2. Pert. to two heartbeats traced on the ascending line of a sphygmogram. SYN: *anacrotic, q.v.*

anadicrotism (an-ă-dik'ro-tizm). Existence of a double beat on ascending line of the sphygmogram.

anadipsia (an-a″dip'se-ă). Intense thirst.

anadrome (an-ad'ro-me). 1. Ascending pain. 2. Globus hystericus. 3. Upward determination of the blood.

anaerobe (an-a'er-ōb). A microörganism which thrives best or lives only without oxygen.

anaerob'ic. Having the power to use oxygen for metabolism from oxygen compounds; having the ability to live without air as some microbes.

anaerobiosis (an-a-er-o-bi-o'sis). Life in an oxygen-free atmosphere.

anaerobiotic (an-a-er-o-bi-ot'ik). Able to exist without free oxygen.

anagnosasthenia (an"ag-no-sas-the'nĭ-ă). Distressing symptoms when trying to read.

anagoge, anagogia (an-ă-go'je, -jĭ-ă). Vomiting.

anakatesthe'sia. A sensation as of hovering or bearing down upon one.

anaku'sis. Complete deafness. SYN: *anacusia.**

anal (a'nal). Rel. to the anus or outer rectal opening.

  a. canal. The terminal portion of the colon, its external aperture being the anus. This is protected by an internal and external sphincter muscle, and remains closed except during defecation. It is about 2.5 to 3.8 cm. (1½ inches) long.

  a. erotic (e-rot'ik). PSY: One who indulges in anal erotism,* or that which pertains to it.

  a. e. character. One who has persisted in anal erotism after childhood. SYM: Orderliness in all habits, obstinacy, sometimes the manifestation of revenge, spite, and miserliness. SEE: *erotism.*

  a. reflex. Contraction of anal sphincter following irritation of skin about anus. Reflex is lost in lesions of posterior columns of cord and is exaggerated in anal fissures.

analepsis (an-al-ep'sis). Gaining strength after an illness. Restoration to health. 2. Epilepsy accompanied by gastric aura. 3. Suspension as in a swing.

analeptic (an-a-lep'tik). 1. Invigorating. 2. A restorative. 3. That which restores health.

analgesia (an-al-je'zĭ-ă). Absence of normal sense of pain.

  a. algera, a. dolorosa. Severe pain with loss of sensitivity in a part.

  a., paretic. Complete analgesia of upper limb, in conjunction with partial paralysis.

analgesic (an-al-je'sik). A medicine which relieves pain when given by mouth.

analgetic (an-al-jet'ik). Analgesic; producing freedom from pain, or an agent that lessens pain.

analgia (an-al'jĭ-ă). State of being without pain.

analgic (an-al'jik). Without pain.

analogue (an'al-og). An organ or part similar in function, but differing in structure.

analosis (an-al-o'sis). Wasting away; atrophy.

analysand (an-al'ĭ-zand). PSY: A patient who is being psychoanalyzed.

analysis (ă-năl'ĭ-sĭs). 1. Separation of anything into its constituent parts. 2. CHEM: Determination of, or separation into, its constituent parts of a substance

or compound. 3. PSY: Diagnosis and treatment.

  a., qual'itative. Determining the nature of the elements in a substance.

  a., quantita'tive. Determining the nature and the quantity of elements in a substance.

  a., spectrum. Determining the nature of a gas by use of the spectroscope.

analyst (an'ă-list). One who analyzes.

analytic (an-ă-lit'ik). Pert. to any analysis.

analyze (an'al-īz). To make an analysis.

anamnesis (an-am-ne'sis). 1. Recollection; faculty of remembering. 2. That which is remembered. 3. The personal and case history of a patient and his family history. SEE: *catamnesis.*

anamnes'tic. 1. Pert. to previous medical history of patient. 2. Assisting the memory.

anamniot'ic. Without an amnion.

ananabasia (an-an-ab-a'zĭ-ă). An abulia in which the person seems unable to ascend heights.

ananaphylaxis (an-an-ă-fi-lak'sis). That which neutralizes anaphylaxis.*

ananastasia (an-an-as-ta'zĭ-ă). An abulia in which the person is unable to rise from a sitting position.

anandria (an-an'drĭ-ă). Impotence; lack in virility.

anangiopla'sia. Imperfect vascularization of a part.

anangioplas'tic. Pert. to imperfect development of the vascular system.

anapeiratic (an-ă-pi-rat'ik). Pert. to a nervous affection arising from excessive muscular activity, as an occupational neurosis.

  a. cramp. One arising from excessive muscular activity.

  a. c., cyclists. Pain in scrotum, perineum, and thighs from excessive riding.

  a. c., occupational. Writer's cramp.

  a. c., professional. Spasmodic disorder affecting groups of muscles used in special work or movements.

anaphase (an'a-fāz). A stage in mitosis when the newly divided chromosomes move towards the opposite poles of the chromatic spindle to form the *diaster.*

anaphia (an-ă'fĭ-ă). 1. Abnormal sensitiveness to touch. 2. Defective sense of touch. 3. Palpation that reveals no diagnosis.

anaphoresis (an-ă-for-e'sis). 1. Insufficient activity of the sweat glands. 2. Transmission of electropositive bodies into tissues by passage of electric current, the flow toward the positive pole.

anaphoria (an-ă-for'ĭ-ă). Tendency of eyeballs to turn upward. SYN: *anatropia.*

anaphrodisia (an-af-ro-diz'ĭ-ă). Diminished or absent sex desire.

anaphrodis'iac. An agent that will depress the sexual function.

anaphrodite (an-af'ro-dīt). One with an impairment of sexual desire or with an absence of it. [tion.

anaphylac'tia. Any anaphylactic condi-

anaphylactic (an-ă-fi-lak'tĭk). Pert. to increasing susceptibility to an infection.

   a. shock. Intense symptoms often accompanied by a rash, as the result of a foreign protein injection. SEE: *shock.*

anaphylactin (an-ă-fi-lak'tin). The substances supposed to produce hypersusceptibility following injection of a foreign protein.

anaphylac'togen. That which produces anaphylaxis or anaphylactin.

anaphylactogen'esis. The process of producing anaphylaxis.

anaphylactogenic (an-ă-fi-lak-to-jen'ik). Producing anaphylaxis or the agent producing anaphylactic reactions.

anaphylatox'in. The poisonous element in anaphylaxis.

anaphylatox'is. Anaphylatoxic reaction.

anaphylaxis (an-a-fil-aks'is). The opposite of *prophylaxis.** A condition produced artifically and experimentally in lower animals and dependent upon well defined antigen-antibody reaction. A hypersensitive state of the body to a foreign protein or a drug, so that the injection of a second dose brings about an acute reaction; known also as *protein sensitization* and *serum sickness.* The term implies symptoms severe enough to produce serious shock.

anapla'sia. 1. Reversion of cells to a more embryonic type. 2. Alteration in cells which produces malignancy.

anaplas'tic. Pert. to anaplasia or restoration of lost part.

anaplasty (an'a-plas-tĭ). Grafting or restoring lost parts.

anaplero'sis. Transplantation of tissue.

anapnea (an-ap-ne'ă). 1. Respiration. 2. Regaining the breath.

anapneic (an-ap-ne'ik). Pert. to anapnea or relieving dyspnea.

anapnograph (an-ap'no-graf). An instrument for measuring pressure and speed of respiration.

anapnoic (an-ap-no'ik). 1. Pert. to anapnea. 2. Relieving dyspnea.

anapnom'eter. Instrument for measuring respiratory movements.

anapnother'apy. Any gas treatment.

anapophysis (an-ă-pof'ĭ-sis). An accessory spinal process of a vertebra.

anap'tic. Pert. to anaphia or diminished or lost tactile sense.

anarithmia (an-ă-rith'mĭ-ă). Inability to count or to use numbers. ETIOL: Brain lesion.

anarthria (an-ar'thrĭ-ă). 1. Loss of motor power to speak. 2. State of being without vigor. 3. Condition of being without joints.

   a. centralis. A central lesion causing partial aphasia.

   a. literalis. Stammering.

anasarca (an-ă-sar'kă). A general dropsical condition.

   a. acute. With natural color of skin.

anasarcous (an-ă-sar'kus). Dropsical.

anaspadias (an-ă-spa'dĭ-ăs). Urethral opening upon upper surface of penis.

anastal'tic. 1. Very astringent. 2. Afferent.

anastasis (an-as'tas-ĭs). 1. Convalescence. 2. Resuscitation. 3. An upward flow of body fluids.

anastate (an'as-tāt). Anything characteristic of an anabolic process.

anastole (an-as'to-le). Shrinking away or retraction of the lips of a wound.

anastomose (an-as'to-mōs). 1. To make an opening of one vessel into another, or the passage of nerve fibers into each other. 2. To make such a connection, surgically.

anastomosis (an-as-to-mo'sis). 1. A communication between two vessels. 2. The surgical or pathologic formation of a passage between any two normally distinct spaces or organs. 3. An end-to-end union.

   SEE: *circle of Willis, inosculation.*

   a., antiperistaltic. Enterostomy in which the two parts are so joined that the peristaltic wave in each part is in opposite directions.

   a., arteriovenous. Anastomosis between an artery and a vein.

   a., collateral. A natural one, as that of the arteries at knee joint.

   a., crucial. An arterial anastomosis in the proximal part of the thigh, formed by the anastomotic branch of the sciatic, and internal circumflex, the first perforating, and the transverse portion of the external circumflex.

   a., Galen's. The anastomosis between the sup. and inf. laryngeal nerves.

   a., heterocladic. Anastomosis between branches of different arteries.

   a., homocladic. Anastomosis between branches of the same artery.

   a., Hyrtl's. An occasional looplike anastomosis between the right and left hypoglossal nerves in the geniohyoid muscle.

   a., intestinal. The establishment of a communication between two portions of the intestines.

   a., isoperistaltic. Intestinal anastomosis in which the two parts are so joined that the peristaltic wave in each part is in the same direction.

   a., Jacobson's. The anastomosing part of the tympanic plexus.

   a., precapillary. Anastomosis between small arteries just before they become capillaries.

   a., Schmidel's. Abnormal communications between the vena cava and the portal system.

   a., terminoterminal. Anastomosis between the peripheral end of an artery and the central end of the corresponding vein, and between the central end of the artery and terminal end of the vein.

   a., unreterotubal. An anastomosis between the ureter and the fallopian tube.

anastomot'ic. Pert. to, or marked by, anastomosis.

anastomot'ica mag'na. 1. *Arteria genu suprema.* 2. *Arteria collateralis ulnaris inferior.*

anatherapeusis (an-ă-ther″ă-pū′sis). Treatment by steadily increasing doses.

anathrepsis (an-ath-rep′sis). The regaining of flesh after an illness.

anatomic (an-ă-tom′ik). Of or rel. to the anatomy or structure of an organism.

anatomist (an-at′o-mist). A skilled student of anatomy.

anatomy (an-at′o-mĭ). The structure or study of structure of organs or a treatise on same.

    a., applied. That applied to diagnosis and treatment, esp. surgical treatment.

    a., comparative. Comparison of structure of different animals.

    a., descriptive. Study of physical structure.

    a., gross. Study of structures seen with the naked eye.

    a., morbid or pathological. That of abnormal structure.

anat′opism. Inability to conform to social usage.

anatoxic (an-a-toks′ik). 1. Pert. to anatoxin. 2. Anaphylactic.

anatoxin (an-a-toks′in). A modified toxin retaining the antigenic properties with lessened toxic properties.

anatricrotic pulse (an-a-tri-krot′ik). Three beats on the ascending curve of a pulse wave.

anatripsis (an-at-rip′sis). 1. A centripetal, or upward movement in massage. 2. Inunction. Rubbing or removing by scraping. 3. Crushing as of a stone.

anatriptic (an-at-rip′tik). An agent to be rubbed in.

anatro′pia. Tendency of eyeballs to turn upward; anaphoria.

anaxon(e (an-aks′on). A nerve cell having no neuraxon as those of the retina.

anazoturia (an-az-o-tu′rĭ-ă). Without urea or nitrogenous substances in the urine.

anchone (ang-ko′nĕ). Spasm of the throat in hysteria.

anchorage (ang′ko-rāj). 1. Operative fixation of displaced viscus. 2. The part to which anything is fixed, as a tooth to which a bridge is fastened.

ancipital (an-sip′it-al). Two-edged.

anconad (ang′ko-nad). Toward the elbow.

anconagra (ang-ko-nag′ră). Gout of the elbow.

anconal, anconeal (ang′ko-nal, -ne-al). Pert. to the elbow.

    a. fossa. Fossa olecrani.

anconeus (ang-ko′ne-us). Short muscle with origin in external condyle of humerus and inserted with shaft and olecranon of ulna.

anconitis (ang-ko-ni′tis). Inflammation of the elbow joint.

ancyroid (an′sir-oid). Shaped like fluke of an anchor.

Andernach's ossicles (ăn′der-năkh). Small bones found in cranial sutures. SYN: *wormian bones.*

Anders' disease. One in which fat occurs in painful nodules. SYN: *adiposis tuberosa simplex.*

An′dersch's ganglion. Ganglion petrosum.

    A.'s nerve. Nervus tympanicus.

An′dral's decu′bitus. Lying on sound side during beginning of pleurisy.

andrase (an′drāz). The hypothetical substance determining male sex. Opp. of *gynase.*

andriat′rics. Study of diseases of male genitals.

andro- (an′drō). A prefix signifying man.

androgalactozemia (an-dro-gal-ak-to-ze′-mĭ-ă). Oozing of milk from male breast.

androgen (ăn′drō-jĕn). Substance producing or stimulating male characteristics, as the male hormone.

androgyne (an′dro-jĭn). One possessing genital and sexual characteristics of both sexes. SYN: *hermaphrodite.*

androgynoid (an-droj′ĭ-noyd). A male of hermaphroditic sexual characteristics and tendencies mistaken for a woman.

androgynous (an-droj′in-us). 1. Resembling or possessing characteristics of both sexes; hermaphroditic. 2. Without definite sexual characteristics.

androg′ynus. A hermaphrodite.

android (ăn′droyd). Shaped like that of a man, as a female pelvis.

andrology (an-drol′o-jĭ). Study of diseases of the male.

andromania (an-dro-ma′nĭ-ă). Abnormal sexual desire in the female. SYN: *nymphomania.*

andromimetic (ăn″drō-mĭm-ĕt′ĭk). Simulating human processes, as certain types of protozoa.

androp′athy. Any disease peculiar to the male, as *prostatitis.*

an′drophile. Preferring man, as parasitic organisms.

androphobia (an-dro-fo′bĭ-ă). Abnormal fear of the male sex.

androphonomania (an-dro-fo-no-ma′nĭ-ă). Psychotic homicidal trends, esp. when violent.

androsterone (an-dro-ster′ōn). Testicular hormone of male sex, found in urine, which regulates changes taking place at puberty.

-ane. Indicating a saturated hydrocarbon.

anebous (an-e′bous). Immature.

aneilema (an-i-le′mă). 1. Flatulence. 2. Colic.

anelectrotonus (an-el-ek-trot′o-nus). The state of diminished irritability of a nerve or muscle produced in region near the anode during the passage of an electric current.

Anel's operation (ah-nelz′). Ligation of an artery immediately above and on proximal side of an aneurysm.

    A.'s probe. A probe for the lacrimal and nasal ducts.

anemato′sis. 1. General anemia. 2. Pernicious anemia.

anemia (an-e′mĭ-ă). A deficiency of red blood corpuscles, hemoglobin, or both. The total volume of the blood may or may not change.

    a., aplastic. This is a form of primary anemia in which bone marrow does not supply new red blood corpuscles.

    a., chlorosis (green sickness). Form

of anemia in adolescent girls, perhaps due to faulty diet during puberty. SEE: *chlorosis.*

a., drepanocytic. Anemia in which red blood cells of person assume a sickle shape, legs ulcerate.

a., essential, a., idiopathic. Anemia caused by pathology of the blood or blood-building organs. SYN: *pernicious anemia.*

a., lymphatica. Anemia in conjunction with tumors of the lymph glands. SEE: *Hodgkin's disease.*

a., macrocytic. Anemia marked by abnormally large erythrocytes.

a., microcytic. Anemia with abnormally small erythrocytes.

a., myelopathic. Anemia caused by disruption in bone marrow function.

a., myelophthisic. Anemia in which blood-building tissues are mechanically displaced.

a., normocytic. Anemia in which the hemoglobin content remains normal.

a., primary or pernicious. Disease of the blood characterized by severe progressive anemia and achlorhydria.

NP: Guard against decubitus. Rest in bed and keep warm. Keep mouth clean. Relieve headache.

a., secondary. Anemia which results from an injury or disease.

a., sickle-cell. SEE: *drepanocytic anemia.*

a., septic. Anemia due to septic condition in the body.

a., splenic. Anemia accompanied by an enlarged spleen.

anemia, words pert. to: anematosis, anemotrophy, anencephalohemia, antianemic, chloranemia, chloremia, chlorosis, ischemia, sickle cell, sura.

anemic (an-e′mik). Pert. to anemia; deficient in red blood cells, or in hemoglobin, or in amount of blood.

anemop′athy. Treatment by inhalation.

anemophobia (an-em-o-fo′bĭ-ă). Abnormal fear of drafts, or of the wind.

anemot′rophy. Anemia from deficient formation of blood; atrophy of blood.

anencephalohe′mia. Anemia of the brain.

anepia (an-ep′ĭ-ă). Inability to speak.

anergasia (an-er-ga′sĭ-ă). Anergia; functional inactivity.

anergastic reaction (an-er-gas′tik). Disorders involving cerebral lesions, or organic psychoses.

anergia (an-er′jĭ-ă). Inactivity; sluggishness.

anergic (an-er′jik). Sluggish; inactive. Deficient in energy; listless.

a. stupor. Acute phase of dementia.

aneroid (an′er-oid). Operating without a fluid, as air. Ex: *aneroid barometer.*

aneroplasty (an-er′o-plas-tĭ). Immersion of a wound to exclude air.

anerythrocyte (an-er-ĭ′thrō-sīt). A red blood cell without hemoglobin.

anerythroplasia (an-er″ĭ-thrō-plā′zĭ-ă). Without formation of red blood cells.

anerythroplastic (an-er″ĭ-thrō-plas′tik). Marked by anerythroplasia.

anerythropsia (an-er-ith-rop′sĭ-ă). Inability to distinguish red clearly.

anesis (an-e′sis). A lessening of symptoms or of their severity.

anesthecinesia (an″es-the″sĭn-e′sĭ-ă). Combined sensory and motor paralysis.

anesthesia (an-es-the′zĭ-ă). Partial or complete loss of sensation, as result of disease, injury, or administration of a drug or gas.

a., block. That resulting from nerve blocking by injection of alcohol or other substance into or very near to a nerve trunk.

a., bulbar. Pons lesion causing central anesthesia.

a., caudal. Spinal anesthesia induced by injection in region of cauda.

a., dolorosa. Painfulness of a part with anesthesia of that part, as in thalamic lesions.

a., general. One that is complete and affecting the entire body, with loss of consciousness, when the anesthetic acts upon the brain.

a., Gwathmey's. Anesthesia induced by injecting an olive oil and ether solution into the rectum.

a., infiltration. Local anesthesia achieved by injecting water or a weak cocaine solution.

a., inhalation. General anesthesia achieved by inhaling ether or chloroform vapors, or the like, or nitrous oxide gas.

a., local. One affecting a local area only, the anesthetic acting upon nerves or nerve tracts. SEE: *block anesthesia, infiltration anesthesia.*

a., mental. Failure to recognize sensory stimulations.

a., mixed. Production of general anesthesia by more than one drug, as nitrous oxide gas continued by ether.

a., neural. Injection of an anesthetic into a nerve or immediately around it (*intraneural* and *paraneural*).

a., primary. First stage of anesthesia, *q.v.*

a., rectal. General anesthesia produced by introduction of anesthetic agent into rectum.

a., regional. Nerve or field blocking causing insensibility over a particular area.   [of sexual desire.

a., sexualis. Anaphrodisia or absence

a., spinal or spinal* puncture. When the injection into the theca is up to level at which nerves of the area enter the spinal cord.

a., surgical. When depth of anesthesia produces relaxation of muscles and loss of sensation and/or consciousness.

a., twilight. State of light anesthesia induced to alleviate sharp pains. SEE: *twilight sleep.*

anesthesimeter (an-es-thes-im′et-er). For measuring anesthetic administered.

anesthesin (ăn-es′thē-sĭn). Proprietary local anesthetic.

DOSAGE: 0.2 to 0.5 Gm. (3 to 8 gr.).

anesthesiology (an-es-thē-zē-ol'ō-jĭ). Science of anesthesia and anesthetics.

anesthesiophore (an-es-the'zĭ-ō-fōr). Carrying anesthetic action, as *cocaine*.

anesthetic (an-es-thet'ĭk). An agent that produces insensibility to pain or touch. According to action, they are subdivided into general and local. SEE: *anesthesia*.

anesthetist (an-es'thē-tist). One who administers anesthetics, esp. for general anesthesia.

anesthetiza'tion. Induction of anesthesia.

anesthetize (an-es'thē-tīz). To place under an anesthetic.

anes'thetizer. One who administers an anesthetic.

anetic (a-net'ĭk). 1. Relaxing, soothing. 2. Anodyne.

anetodermia (an-et-ō-der'mĭ-ă). Relaxation of the skin.

an'etus. Any intermittent fever.

aneuria (a-nu'rĭ-ă). Defect in or deficiency of nervous energy.

aneur'ic. Pert. to aneuria.

aneurosis (ä-nū-ro'sĭs). Lacking in nervous susceptibility.

aneurysm (an'u-rizm). Arterial dilatation due to pressure of blood on weakened tissues, forming sac of clotted blood.

   a., **aortic.** Affecting any part of the aorta.

   a. **of arch of aorta.** ETIOL: Pressure on trachea, esophagus, veins, or nerves. SYM: Dyspnea, cough, sputum, dysphagia, congestion of head and neck. Inequality in the two radial pulses.

   a., **arteriovenous.** One in which artery and vein become connected by a saccule. ETIOL: Trauma. Weak point, in walls of an artery, due to syphilis, sudden strain, or injury. SYM: Pain, expansile pulsation, bruit. NP: Avoid increasing heart action or raising blood pressure.

   a., **dissecting.** One in which the blood makes its way between the layers of a blood vessel wall, separating them.

   a., **fusiform.** All the walls of the blood vessels dilate more or less equally, creating a tubular swelling.

   a., **sacculated.** One due to the yielding of a weak patch on one side of the vessel and which does not involve the entire circumference; usually due to an injury.

   a., **varicose.** Aneurysm forming a blood-filled sac bet. an artery and a vein.

aneurysmal (an-ū-riz'măl). Pert. to aneurysm.

aneurysmectomy (an-u-riz-mek'to-mĭ). Extirpation of an aneurysm by removal of its sac.

aneurysmotomy (an-u-riz-mot'o-mĭ). Incision of the sac of an aneurysm, allowing it to heal by granulation.

anfractuosity (an-frak-tu-os'ĭ-tĭ). A cerebral sulcus.

anfractuous (an-frak-tu'us). Bending; sinuous.

angeitis (an-ge-i'tĭs). Inflammation of a blood vessel or a lymphatic. SYN: *angiitis.**

an'gel's wing. A very prominent scapula, due to deformity.

Angelucci's syndrome (ăn-jĕ-loot'che). Great excitability, palpitation, and vasomotor disturbance associated with venal conjunctivitis.

angi (an'gĭ). Inguinal buboes.

angiasthe'nia. Loss of vascular tone.

angiectasia, -sis (an-jĭ-ek-ta'zĭ-ă, -tas-is). Enlarged capillaries or abnormal dilation of a vessel.

angiec'tomy. Excision of section of a blood vessel.

angiectopia (an-jĭ-ek-to'pĭ-ă). Displacement of a vessel.

angiemphraxis (an-je-em-fraks'ĭs). Obstruction of any vessel.

angiitis (an-jĭ-i'tĭs). Inflammation of a blood vessel or of a lymphatic.

angina (ăn-jĭ'na, L. an-jĭ'na). 1. A sense of suffocation. 2. Disease of the pharynx or fauces.

   a., **acute.** Simple sore throat.

   a. **cruris.** Angina due to obstruction of an artery, causing pain and cyanosis of the affected part, with periodic lameness.

   a., **follicular.** Angina of the larynx and pharynx from public speaking, excessive drinking of alcoholic liquors.

   a. **laryngea.** Inflammation of the larynx.

   a. **ludovici, a. ludwigii.** Purulent inflammation in the submaxillary region.

   a., **Ludwig's.** Phlegmonous cellulitis of the neck.

   a. **maligna.** Diphtheria.

   a., **necrotic.** Form with gangrenous patches in the mucosa of the air passages, seen in scarlet fever and occasionally in diphtheria.

   a. **parotidea.** Inflammation of the parotid glands. SYN: *mumps.*

   a. **pectoris.** Pain and oppression about the heart; a paroxysmal affection characterized by severe pain radiating from the heart to the shoulder, thence down the left arm, or, rarely, from the heart to the abdomen; apparently dependent upon some lesion of the coronary arteries of the heart, its walls, or valves. Attacks may occur in lesions of the aortic valves. Generally afflicts males of middle age.

   a. **simplex.** Sore throat. SEE: *acute angina.*

   a. **streptococcus.** Angina caused by the streptococcus.

   a. **tonsillans.** Quinsy.

   a. **trachealis.** Croup.

   a., **Vincent's.** Ulceration and inflammation of floor of mouth. SEE: *trench mouth.*

anginal (an'jĭ-nal). Pert. to angina.

anginoid (an'jĭ-noid). Resembling angina pectoris, or any angina.

anginophobia (an-jĭ-no-fo'bĭ-ă). Intense fear of an attack of angina pectoris.

anginose (an'jĭ-nōs). Pert. to or resembling angina.

an'ginous. Resembling angina. SYN: *anginose.*

angio- (an-gĭ-o). A prefix pert. to a vessel.

an'gioatax'ia. Variability in arterial tonus.

angioblast (an'jĭ-o-blast). Embryonic cells from which blood vessels develop.

angiocardiokinet'ic. Stimulating or that which affects movements of heart and blood vessels.

angiocarditis (an-ji-o-kar'di-tis). Inflammation of the heart and large blood vessels. SEE: *carditis.*

angiocav'ernous. Rel. to conditions present in angioma cavernosum.

angiocholecystitis (an"jĭ-ō-kō-lē-sis-ti'tis). Inflammation of gallbladder and bile vessels.

angiocholitis (an-jĭ-ō-kō-li'tis). Inflammation of biliary vessels; cholangitis.

angiocrine (an'jĭ-ō-krin). Marked by vasomotor disorders resulting from disturbances of the endocrine glands.

angiodermatitis (an"jĭ-ō-der-mă-ti'tis). Inflammation of cutaneous vessels.

angiodystrophia (an-jĭ-ō-dis-tro'fĭ-ă). Faulty nutrition of vessels.

angiofibro'ma (pl. *-fibromata*). An angioma having connective tissue overgrowth.

angiogenesis (an"jĭ-ō-jen'es-is). Development of blood vessels.

angiogenic (an"jĭ-ō-jen'ik). Pert. to angiogenesis; of vascular origin.

an'gioglio'ma. A mixed angioma and glioma.

angiograph (an'jĭ-o-graf). A variety of sphygmograph.

angiography (an-jĭ-og'ră-fĭ). A description of blood vessels and lymphatics.

angiohyalinosis (an"jĭ-ō-hi"al-in-o'sis). Hyaline or glassy degeneration of the muscular coat of blood vessels.

an'giohyperto'nia. Angiospasm; spasmodic contraction of arteries.

an'giohypoto'nia. Angioparalysis; angioparesis; vascular relaxation.

angioid (an'jĭ-oyd). Resembling a blood vessel.

　　a. streaks. Dark, wavy, anastomosing striae lying beneath retinal vessels.

angiokeratoma (an"jĭ-o-ker-ă-to'mă). A skin disease occurring chiefly on feet and legs.

angiokinet'ic. Pert. to action of blood vessels.

angioleukasia (an-gĭ-o-lū-ka'sĭ-ă). Dilatation of lymphatics.

angioleukitis (an-jĭ-o-lu-ki'tis). Inflammation of lymphatics.

angiolipo'ma. A mixed angioma and lipoma.

angiolith (an'jĭ-o-lith). 1. A venous calculus. 2. Calcareous deposit in wall of a blood vessel.

angiology (an-jĭ-ol'o-jĭ). The science of the blood vessels and lymphatics.

angiolymphitis (an"jĭ-ō-lim-fi'tis). Inflammation of the lymphatics. SYN: *lymphangitis.*

an'giolympho'ma. Tumor of dilated lymphatics.

angiolysis (an-jĭ-ol'ĭ-sis). Obliteration of blood vessels in newly born infants after tying of the cord.

angioma (an-ji-o'mă). A growth made up of dilated blood vessels.

　　a. cavernosum. Is congenital and appears as an elevated dark red tumor, ranging in size from a pea to that of the hand. It frequently has pulsation; commonly involves the subcutaneous or submucous tissue.

　　a. simplex (port wine mark). One that is congenital, made up of capillaries, nonelevated, bright red or purple-red in color; may cover a large surface; usually found on the face, commonly called "Mother's mark."

　　a., telangiectatic. Is acquired. Appears as bright spot composed of dilated capillaries. Is associated with acne rosacea, gouty predispositions, and exposure to weather.

angiomalacia (an-jĭ-o-ma-la'sĭ-ă). Softening of blood vessel walls.

angiomatosis (an-jĭ-o-ma-to'sis). Condition of multiple angiomata.

　　a. retinae. Primary angioma of retina.

angiomatous (an-jĭ-om'ă-tus). Like an angioma.

angiomeg'aly. Enlargement of blood vessels, esp. in the eyelid.

angiometer (an-jĭ-om'et-er). Instrument for measuring tension and diameter of vessels.

angiomyocardiac (an-jĭ-o-mi-o-kar'dĭ-ak). Pert. to blood vessels and cardiac muscle.

angiomyoma (an"jĭ-o-mĭ-o'mă). An angioma mixed with a myoma.

angiomyosarco'ma. Tumor containing elements of angioma, myoma, and sarcoma.

angioneurectomy (an-jĭ-o-nu-rek'to-mĭ). Excision of vessels and nerves.

angioneuroedema (an"jĭ-o-nu-ro-ē-de'mă). Acute swelling of subcutaneous or submucous tissue due to vasomotor lesion.

angioneurosis (an-jĭ-o-nŭ-rō'sis). Spasm or paralysis of blood vessels.

angioneurotic (an-ge-o-nŭ-rot'ik). Pert. to angioneurosis.

　　a. edema. Swelling of submucous or subcutaneous tissues. Sometimes periodic with gastric disturbances. ETIOL: Probably a toxemia.

angioneurotomy (an-jĭ-o-nu-rot'o-mĭ). Cutting of vessels and nerves.

angionoma (an-jĭ-on-o'mă). Ulceration of a vessel.

angioparal'ysis. Vasomotor relaxation of blood vessel tone.

angioparesis (an-jĭ-ō-pă'rē-sis). Partial paralysis of the vasomotor system.

angiopathol'ogy. Morbid changes of the blood vessels.

angiopathy (an-jĭ-op'a-thĭ). Any disease of blood vessels or lymphatics.

angioplania (an"jĭ-o-plan'ĭ-ă). Abnormality or irregularity in course of a blood vessel.

angioplas'ty. Plastic surgery upon blood vessels.

angiopoietic (an"jĭ-ō-poy-et'ik). Causing the formation of blood vessels, pert. to certain cells. [pressure.

angiopres'sure. Control of hemorrhage by

angiorhigosis (an-jĭ-ō-rĭ-go'sis). Rigidity of vessels.

angiorrhaphy (an-jĭ-or'af-ĭ). Suture of a vessel or vessels.

angiorrhexis (an-jĭ-or-eks'is). Rupture of a blood vessel.

angiosarco'ma. Mixed sarcoma and angioma.

angiosclero'sis. Hardening of the walls of the vascular system.

angioscope (an'jĭ-o-skōp). A microscope for studying capillary vessels.

angiosialitis (an"jĭ-o-si-al-i'tis). Inflammation of a salivary duct.

angiosis (an-jĭ-o'sis). Any disease of the lymphatics or blood vessels.

an'giospasm. Excessive blood vessel tone.

angiospas'tic. Pert. to angiospasm.

angiostaxis (an"jĭ-o-stax'is). 1. Hemophilia. 2. Oozing of blood.

angiosteno'sis. Contraction of caliber of blood vessels.

angiosteosis (an"jĭ-os-te-o'sis). Calcareous degeneration of arteries.

angios'tomy. Artificial fistulous opening into a blood vessel for an implantation.

angiostrophy (an-jĭ-os'tro-fĭ). Twisting cut end of a vessel for the arrest of bleeding.

angiosynizesis (an"jĭ-ō-sin-ĭ-ze'sis). Collapse of walls of a vessel and their subsequent adhesion.

angiotelectasis (an"jĭ-ō-tel-ek'ta-sis). Dilatation of terminal arterioles.

angiotitis (an-jĭ-ō-ti'tis). Inflammation of blood vessels of the ear.

angiotome (an'jĭ-o-tōm). One of the segments of the vascular tissues of the embryo.

angiotomy (an-ji-ot'o-mi). Dissection of blood vessels.

angioton'ic. Pert. to increase of arterial tension.

angiotribe (an'jĭ-ō-trīb). Instrument for crushing the end of an artery to check hemorrhage.

angiotripsy (an'jĭ-ō-trip-sĭ). The use of an angiotribe.

angiotroph'ic. Pert. to nutrition of blood vessels.

angi'tis. Inflammation of the blood vessels or lymphatics. SYN: *angiitis*.

angle (ang'gl). A point or corner where two lines meet.

    a., alpha. One found by intersection of visual line with optic axis.

    a., alveolar. Meeting point of the base of the nasal spine and the middle point of the alveolus of the upper jaw.

    a., basilar. Formed by the intersection of a projection line from the nasal point to a line drawn at the base of the nasal spine.

    a., biorbital. Formed by the meeting of the axes of the orbits.

    a., cerebellopontine. Junction of the cerebellum and pons.

    a., costal. Meeting point of the lower border of the false ribs with the axis of the sternum.

    a., craniofacial. The angle formed at the point where the basifacial and basi-

cranial axes join at the midpoint of the sphenoethmoidal sutures.

    a., facial. The angle made by lines from the nasal spine and external auditory meatus meeting between the upper middle incisor teeth.

    a., gamma. Angle formed by line of fixation with optic axis.

    a. of incidence. The angle between a ray incident on a surface and a line drawn perpendicular to the surface at the point of incidence.

    a. of iris. Angle between the cornea and iris at the periphery of the ant. chamber of the eye.

    a. of jaw. The angle at the point where the post. edge of the ramus of the mandible and the lower surface of the body of the mandible join.

    a. of mandible. Angle of the jaw.

    a., metafacial. Angle between the base of the skull and the pterygoid process.

    a., occipital. Formed by the intersection of lines from the basion and from the lower border of the orbit at the opisthion.

    a., ophryospinal. Angle formed by the joining of lines drawn from the auricular point and the glabella at the ant. nasal spine.

    a., parietal. Formed by the meeting of the prolongation of the two lines tangent to the prominent portion of the zygomatic arch and the parietofrontal suture.

    a., pontine. Same as cerebellopontine angle.

    a., pubic. Junction of the rami of the pubes.

    a., sphenoid. Formed by the intersection of lines coming from the nasal point and the tip of the rostrum of the sphenoid, at top of the sella turcica.

    a., sternal. Angle between the manubrium and body of the sternum.

    a., venous. Angle of the internal jugular and subclavian vein.

angophrasia (an-go-fra'zĭ-ă). Drawling, choking speech in paralytic dementia.

angor (ang'gor). Violent distress as in angina* pectoris.

Angström's unit (öng'strum). PT: An internationally adopted unit of measurement of wave length, one ten-millionth of a millimeter, or one two hundred and fifty-four millionth inch.

Anguil'lula. Genus of nematode worms.

    A. aceti. Vinegar eel.

    A. intestinalis. Parasitic form of nematode infesting intestine in tropics and near tropics.

    A. stercoralis. Free stage of *Anguillula intestinalis.*

anguilluli'asis. Infestation with *Anguillula intestinalis.*

angular. Having corners or angles.

    a. artery. The artery at the inner canthus of the eye; facial artery.

angulation (ang-gu-la'shun). Formation of angular loops in the intestine.

anhaphia (an-ha'fĭ-ă). Abnormal or defective sense of touch. SYN: *anaphia.*

anhedonia (an-hed-o'nĭ-ă). Psy: Lacking in interest or pleasure; apathy.

anhedonic (an-he-don'ik). Pert. to anhedonia.

anhelation (an-hel-a'shun). Dyspnea, shortness of breath.

anhelitus (an-hel-it'us). Asthma; difficult breathing.

anhelose, anhelous (an'hel-ōs, -us). Panting.

anhemato'sis. Defective or insufficient blood formation.

anhemolytic (an-hem-o-lit'ik). Not destructive to the blood cells.

anhepatia (an-he-pa'shĭ-ă). Failure or lack of liver function.

anhepat'ic. Not produced by the liver.

anhepatogenic (an-hep-at-o-jen'ik). Not produced by the liver. SYN: *anhepatic.*

anhidrosis (an-hi-dro'sis). Abnormal deficiency of sweat, general or localized, temporary or permanent, accompanying disease conditions.

anhidrotic (an-hi-drot'ik). Checking or anything that checks or prevents perspiration.

anhis'tic, anhis'tous. Seemingly without structure.

anhydra'tion. The state of not being hydrated.

anhydremia (an-hi-dre'mĭ-ă). A lessening of the normal quantity of fluids in the blood.

anhydride (an-hi'drīd). A substance from which the hydrogen and oxygen in the ratio in which they exist in water have been removed.   [acid.

anhydrochlo'ric. Lacking in hydrochloric

anhydromyelia (an-hi-dro-mi-e'lĭ-ă). Deficiency in spinal fluid.

anhy'drous. Containing no water.

anhypnia (an-hip'nĭ-ă). Insomnia; sleeplessness; anhypnosis.

anhypno'sis.

anianthinopsy (an-ĭ-an'thin-op"sĭ). Inability to recognize violet tints.

anidros (an-id'ros). Exhibiting no perspiration.

anidrosis (an-id-ro'sis). Abnormal deficiency of sweat. SYN: *anhidrosis.*

anidrotic (an-i-drot'ik). Pert. to anidrosis. SYN: *anhidrotic.*

anid'rus. Showing no perspiration. SYN: *anidros.*

anile (an'īl). Infirm; like an old woman.

aniline (an'i-lin). The simplest aromatic amine, $C_6H_5NH_2$, an oily liquid derived from benzene.

DOSAGE: 1 gr. (0.06 Gm.).

anilinophil, anilinophilous (an"ĭ-lin'o-fil, -fil-us). A structure staining readily with aniline dyes.

anilism (an'il-izm). Chronic aniline poisoning.

SYM: Cardiac and gastric weakness, intermittent pulse, vertigo, muscular depression, cyanosis.

anil'ity. Old age in females.

anima (an'im-ă). The vital principle; breath; air; mind; consciousness.

animalcule (an-i-mal'kule). Unicellular animal organism; protozoan.

anincretinosis (an-ĭn-krĕ-tĭn-o'sis). A disorder due to failure of some organ of internal secretion.

anion (an'i-on). PT: An ion carrying a negative charge. Since unlike forms of electricity attract each other, the ion is attracted by, and travels to, the positive anode. Examples are acid radicals and corresponding radicals of their salts. SEE: *ion.*

anirid'ia. Congenital absence, complete or partial, of iris; irideremia.*

anischuria (an-is-ku'rĭ-ă). Incontinence of urine.

aniseikonia (an-is-ĭ-ko'nĭ-ă). A condition in which the size and shape of the ocular image of one eye differs from that of the other.

anis'ergy. Varying degrees of blood pressure in different parts of the system.

aniso (an'is-o). Prefix. Unequal, unsymmetrical in combination.

anisochromatic (an-i-so-kro-mat'ik). Not of uniform color.

anisocoria (an-is-o-ko'rĭ-ă). Inequality of the diameter of the pupil; may be normal or congenital.

anisocytosis (an-ĭ-so-si-to'sis). Inequality in size of cells, esp. erythrocytes. An abnormal condition.

anisog'amy. Sexual fusion of two gametes of different form and size.

anisognathous (an-ĭ-sog'na-thus). Having upper jaw wider than lower one.

anisohypercytosis (an-is-o-hi-per-si-to'-sis). Increase in number of leukocytes with altered proportion of the different varieties. Opposite of *anisohypocytosis.*

anisohypocyto'sis. Decrease in number of leukocytes with altered proportion of different varieties. OPP: *anisohypercytosis.**

anisoiconia (an-ĭ-so-ĭ-ko'nĭ-ă). Failure of retinal images to coalesce.

an"isomas'tia. Breasts unequal in size.

an"isome'lia. Inequality between two paired limbs.

anisometrope (an"ĭ-so-me'trŏp). One afflicted with anisometropia.

anisometropia (an-i-so-me-tro'pĭ-ă). Inequality in refractive power of the two eyes.

anisometrop'ic. Having unequal refractive power.

anisonormocyto'sis. Abnormal relation in numbers of different forms of leukocytes but with normal number of total leukocytes.

aniso'pia. Inequality of visual power of both eyes.

anisopiesis (an-ĭ-so-pi-e'sis). Apparent inequality of blood pressure in different parts of the body.

anisorhythmia (an-ĭ-sŏ-rith'mĭ-ă). Absence of synchronism in rate of the auricles and ventricles or irregular heart action.

anisospore (an'ĭ-so-spōr). A sexual cell. Opp. of *isospore.*

an"isosthen'ic. Not of equal muscle strength.

anisotropal (an-is-ot'ro-pal). 1. Not equal

in every direction. 2. Unequal in power of refraction.

anisotrop'ic. Having different optical properties in different directions, as have certain crystals; double polarizing.

anisotropous (an-ĭ-sot'ro-pus). 1. Not equal in every direction. 2. Unequal in refractive power. SYN: *anisotropal*.

anisuria (an-is-u'rĭ-ă). Alternate polyuria and oliguria, *q.v.*

ankle (ăng'kl). The part between the foot and lower end of leg.
   SEE: *astragalus, malleolus.*
   a. **bone.** The astragalus.
   a. **clonus.** A rhythmic extension-flexion of the ankle induced by its sudden dorsiflexion, evidencing upper motor neuron* disease, such as spastic paraplegia, hemiplegia, etc.
   a. c. reflex. Succession of rapid contractions and relaxations when foot is pressed dorsally. Occurs in lateral tract disease and disseminated sclerosis.
   a. joint. A hinge joint. Lower part of *tibia*, its *medial malleolus* and *lateral malleolus* of *fibula* forming socket for the *astragalus.*
   a., tailor's. An abnormal bursa over the head of the fibula in tailors from pressure caused by sitting cross-legged on the floor.

ankyloblepharon (ang-ki-lo-blef'ar-on). Adhesion of ciliary edges of lids to each other.   [of lips to each other.

ankylochilia (ang-kĭ-lo-ki'lĭ-ă). Adhesion

ankyloglos'sia. Tongue-tie.

ankyloproctia (ang-ki-lo-prok'shĭ-ă). Stricture or imperforation of the anus.

ankylosed (ang'ki-lozd). Denoting fixation of a joint. Stiffened; held by adhesions.

ankylosis (an-kyl-o'sis). Abnormal immobility and consolidation of a joint.
   a., artificial. The surgical fixation of a joint.
   a., bony. The abnormal union of the bones of a joint, also called true ankylosis.
   a., extracapsular. That caused by rigidity of parts outside a joint.
   a., false. Spurious ankylosis; that due to rigidity of the surrounding parts.
   a., fibrous. That due to the formation of fibrous bands within a joint only.
   a., intracapsular. That due to the undue rigidity of structure within a joint.
   a., ligamentous. Ankylosis by ligaments or fibrous structures.
   a., true. Same as bony ankylosis.

Ankylos'toma. Old world hookworm, a genus of nematode parasites.
   A. americanum. American hookworm.
   A. duodenale. The hookworm.

ankylos'toma. Trismus, lockjaw.

ankylostomiasis (ang-kil-o-sto-mi'as-is). Disease caused by hookworms in the intestine; hence commonly called "hookworm."

ankylotia (ang-kĭ-lo'shĭ-ă). Closure or imperforation of external auditory meatus of ear.

ankylotome (ang'kil-o-tōm). An instrument for cutting *fraenum linguae.*

ankylurethria (ang-kĭl-ŭ-re'thrĭ-ă). Stricture or imperforation of the urethra.

ankyroid (ang'kĭ-royd). Hook-shaped.
   a. cavity. The posterior or descending cornu of lateral ventricle.

anlage (ahn'lăg-ĕ). 1. Rudiments in a developing embryo. 2. The embryonic part in which differentiation first appears.

annatto (an-at'o). Reddish coloring matter obtained from the pulp of *Bixa orellana,* a tropical tree. SYN: *annotto, arnotto.*

annec'tent. Linking together.

annex'a. Accessory parts. SYN: *adnexa.*

annexi'tis. Inflammation of *adnexa uteri.* SYN: *adnexitis.*

annex'opexy. Fixation of fallopian tubes and ovary to abdominal wall. SYN: *adnexopexy.*

annot'to. Reddish coloring matter obtained from pulp of *Bixa orellana,* a tropical tree. SYN: *annatto, arnotta.*

annuens (an'u-enz). *Musculus rectus capitis anticus minor.*

ann'ular. Circular; ring-shaped.

annulorrhaphy (an-u-lor'ă-fĭ). Closure of a hernial ring by suture.

ann'ulus. A ring-shaped structure; a ring.
   a. ciliaris. Boundary between choroid and iris.
   a. tympanicus. The tympanic ring.
   a. umbilicus. Umbilical ring. SEE: *abdominal.*

anoci-association (a-no'sĭ-as-o-sĭ-a'shun). The blocking or exclusion of neuroses, fear, pain, and harmful influences or associations to prevent shock, by injection of narcotics hypodermically.

anococcygeal (a-no-kok-sij'e-al). Rel. to both anus and coccyx.
   a. body. The muscle and fibrous tissue lying between the coccyx and anus.
   a. ligament. A band of fibrous tissue joining the tip of the coccyx with the external sphincter ani.

anod'al. Pert. to the anode.
   a. closure contraction. Contraction of muscles at anode on closure of circuit.

anode (an'ōd). The positive pole of an electrical source. Only galvanic (direct current) and static electricity have distinct polarity.

anodinia (an-o-din'ĭ-ă). Absence of vertigo.

anodmia (an-od'mĭ-ă). The want or absence of the sense of smell; anosmia, *q.v.*

an'odyne. An agent that will relieve pain; milder in form than an analgesic, *q.v.*

anodyn'ia. 1. Cessation or absence of pain. 2. Loss of sensation.

anoesia (an-o-e'sĭ-ă). Without power of comprehension; anoia,* imbecility, idiocy.

anoetic (an-o-et'ik). Rel. to the borderline of consciousness; not fully conscious.

anoia (an-oy'ă). Anoesia, *q.v.* Idiocy.

anomalous (an-om'al-us). Irregular. Contrary to the normal.

anom'aly. Anything contrary to general rule.

anomia (an-o′mĭ-ă). Inability to remember names of persons and objects.

anonychia (an-o-nik′ĭ-ă). Absence of the nails.

anonymous (an-on′im-us). Nameless.
  a. artery. *Arteria anonyma.*
  a. veins. *Venae anonymae.*

anoopsia (an-o-o-op′sĭ-ă). Tendency of one eye to turn upward. SYN: *hyperphoria.* *

Anopheles (an-of′el-ēz). The mosquito whose bite is responsible for the malaria parasite in man.

anopho′ria. Tendency of one eye to turn upward. SYN: *hyperphoria,* * *anopia.* *

anophthal′mia. Congenital absence of eyes.

ano′pia. Tendency of 1 eye to turn upward. SYN: *anopsia, hyperphoria.* *

anop′sia. 1. Hyperphoria. 2. Inability to use the vision as in those confined in the dark, or from disuse of an eye in strabismus, or resulting from cataract, or in refractive errors.

anorectal (an-o-rek′tal). Pert. to the anus and rectum.

anorectic, anorectous (an-o-rek′tic, -tus). Having no appetite.

anorexia (an-or-eks′ĭ-ă). Loss of appetite.
  a. nervo′sa. Loss of appetite for food not explainable by local disease. It may be a part of a psychosis.*

anoria (an-or′ĭ-ă). Immaturity.

anor′mal. Abnormal.

anorrhorrhea (an-or-or-e′ă). Diminished or imperfect secretion of serous fluid.

anorthography (an-or-thog′ră-fĭ). Agraphia,* esp. motor agraphia; loss of power to express oneself in writing. SEE: *agraphia.*

anorthopia (an-or-tho′pĭ-ă). 1. Vision in which straight lines do not appear straight; symmetry and parallelism not properly perceived. 2. Squinting.

anorthosis (an-or-tho′sis). Absence of or diminished erectility.

anosia (an-o′sĭ-ă). Normal; without disease.

anosmatic (an-oz-mat′ik). Deficient sense of smell.

anosmia (an-oz′mĭ-ă). Absence of the sense of smell; anodmia,* anosphrasia.* Frequent in neurasthenia, hysteria, and sometimes in ataxia.

anosmic (an-oz′mik). Lacking in sense of smell.

anos′mous. Anosmic. Pert. to anosmia.

anosodiaphoria (an-o-so-di-af-or′ĭ-ă). Real or pretended indifference to presence of disease, esp. paralysis.

anosognosia (an-o-sog-no′zĭ-ă). Real or pretended ignorance of the presence of disease, esp. paralysis. Opp. of *pathodixia, q.v.*

anosphrasia (an-os-fra′zĭ-ă). Absence or imperfect sense of smell.

anospi′nal. Pert. to center in the spinal cord which controls the contraction of the anal sphincter.

anostosis (an-os-to′sis). A defective formation or development of bone; failure to ossify.

anotro′pia. Farsightedness. SYN: *hyperopia.* *

anoves′ical. Rel. in any way to both anus and urinary bladder.

anov′ular, anov′ulatory. Not pert. to ovulation.

anoxemia (an-oks-e′mĭ-ă). Lack of oxygen in the blood.

anoxia (an-ox′ĭ-ă). Deficiency of oxygen.
  a., anemic. Deficiency in the oxygen carrying power of the blood.
  a., anoxic. Lessened oxygen tension in arterial blood, but with normal oxygen capacity.
  a., stagnant. Increase in oxygen removed from the blood due to insufficiency of circulation.

anox′ic. Pert. to or caused by a general lack of oxygen, and characterized by a generally subnormal oxygen tension of the blood.

anoxybiosis (an-oks′ĭ-bĭ-o′sis). Life in an oxygen-free atmosphere. SYN: *anaerobiosis.*

an′sa. Any anatomical structure in the form of a loop.
  a. capitis. The zygomatic arch.
  a. hypoglos′si. Loop of the hypoglossal nerve.
  a. lenticular. Fibers entering the lenticular nucleus from the thalamus by way of the thalamic radiation.
  a. of the spinal nerves. Connecting loops of fibers between the ant. spinal nerves.
  a. peduncularis. Fibers passing from the thalamus through the thalamic radiation, under the lenticular nucleus to the cortex of the temporal lobe and insula.
  a. sacralis. Nerve cord connecting the sympathetic trunk with the ganglion impar.
  a. subclavia. Loop of nerve fibers winding around the ant. aspect of the subclavian artery.

anselaphesia (an-sel-af-e′zĭ-ă). Absence of sense of touch or feeling or sensation, esp. of tactile sensibility.

anserine (an′ser-in). Pert. to a goose.

ant-, anti-. Prefixes: Opposed to; counteracting; against, as *antifebrile.*

antacid (ant-as′id). An agent that will neutralize acidity, esp. in digestive tract.

antag′onism. Opposition or contrary action, as bet. muscles or medicines.

antag′onist. That which counteracts the action of anything, as a muscle or drug.

antalge′sic. Pain-relieving agent. SYN: *anodyne.*

antalgic (ant-al′jik). An anodyne or analgesic.

antalkaline (ant-al′kal-in). Neutralizing or reducing alkalinity.

antaphrodis′iac. Lessening sexual desire.

antarthritic (ant″ar-thrit′ik). Remedy for gout.

antasthenic (ant-as-then′ik). 1. Strengthening, invigorating. 2. Agent which invigorates.

antasthmat′ic. 1. An agent that prevents an asthmatic attack. 2. Relieving asthma.   [curing atrophy.

antatrophic (ant-ă-trof′ik). Preventing or

ante-. Prefix: Before, as *antenatal.*

antebrachium (an-te-bra'ke-um). The forearm.

antecurvature (an-te-ker'va-tūr). Bending forward abnormally. SYN: *anteflexion.*

an'tedating. The theory that hereditary defects manifest themselves earlier with each successive generation and often more severely though the clinical picture may change.

antefebrile (an-te-feb'ril). Pert. to the period before a fever.

anteflex'ion. Abnormal bending forward, *i. e., uterus,* bending forward at its body and cervix.

anteloca'tion. Forward displacement of an organ or part of the human body.

antemetic (an-tem-et'ik). 1. Arresting vomiting. 2. Remedy that controls vomiting and nausea.

ante mor'tem. Before death.

   a.-m. statement. One made immediately preceding death.

an'te par'tum. The time before the onset of labor.

antephialtic (ant-ef-ĭ-al'tik). Preventing nightmare.

anteposition. Anterior displacement of the uterus.

anteprostati'tis. Inflammation of glands of Cowper.

antepyret'ic. Before the development of fever; antefebrile. SEE: *antipyretic.*

anteresis (ant-er'e-sis). Resistance during reduction of a dislocation.

anterethic (an-ter-eth'ik). Soothing.

ante'rior. Before, or in front of.

   a. chamber. Aqueous chamber. Bounded in front by cornea, behind by iris and lens.

antero-. Prefix: Anterior; front; before, as *anterosuperior.*

anterograde (an'ter-o-grād). Extending backward.

antero-infe'rior. In front and below.

anterolat'eral. In front and to one side.

anterome'dian. In front and toward the central line.

anteroposter'ior. Passing from front to rear.

anterosuper'ior. In front and above.

antever'sion. 1. A tipping or bending forward of an organ. 2. A forward placement of the uterus, the normal position of the healthy uterus.

   a. uteri. A forward tipping of the uterus.

antever'ted. Inclined or bent forward; said of uterus.

anthelix (an'the-liks). External ear's inner curved ridge. SYN: *antihelix.*

anthelmintic (an-thel-min'tik). An agent used to expel intestinal worms. Ex: *santonin, phenyl salicylate, thymol.*

   a. enema. One given to expel worms. SEE: *enema.*

Anthemis (an'them-is). Chamomile.

anthemorrha'gic. Agent for preventing or arresting hemorrhage.

anthocy'anin. Pigment of red beet root.

anthocyanine'mia. Anthocyanin in the blood.

anthocyaninu'ria. Anthocyanin in urine.

Anthomy'ia canicula'ris. A small black horse fly, whose larvae may infest the human intestine, often resulting in alarming gastrointestinal symptoms.

Anthony's fire, St. Name given to erysipelas.

anthopho'bia. Morbid dislike of flowers.

anthorism, anthorisma (an'thor-izm, -iz'mă). A diffuse swelling.

anthracemia (an"thra-se'mĭ-ă). Presence in the blood of *B. anthracis.*

anthracia (an-thra'sĭ-ă). Presence of carbuncles.

anthracoid (an'thra-koid). Like or pert. to anthrax.

anthracoma (an-thra-ko'mă). Carbuncle.

anthracometer (an-thra-kom'e-ter). An instrument for measuring the carbon dioxide in the air.

an"thraconecro'sis. Necrosis of tissue into dry, black gangrene.

anthraco'sis. 1. Miner's phthisis. A condition of the pulmonary organs due to coal dust inhalation; a pneumonoconiosis. 2. A carbuncle, or a corroding ulcer.

anthrax (ăn'thrăks). 1. A carbuncle. 2. Acute, infectious disease caused by *Bacillus anthracis,* usually attacking cattle and sheep.

anthropo- (an'thro-pō). Prefix: Pert. to man.

anthropogeny (an-thro-po'je-nĭ). Origin and development of man.

anthropoid (an'thro-poid). 1. Resembling a man. 2. An ape.

anthropol'ogy. The science which treats of man.

anthropometry (an-thro-pom'et-rĭ). Science of measuring the human body and its parts and functional capacities.

anthropoph'agy. The eating of human flesh.

an"thropopho'bia. A morbid fear of society or of a particular man.

anthroposomatology (an"thro-po-so-ma-tol'o-jĭ). Branch of anthropology dealing with human body.

an"thropotox'in. Supposed poison exhaled by human lungs.

anthydropic (ant-hi-drop'ik). 1. Correcting dropsy. 2. Agent for relieving dropsy.

anthypnotic (ant-hip-not'ik). 1. Preventing sleep. 2. Agent hindering sleep.

anthysteric (ant-his-ter'ik). 1. Relieving hysteria. 2. Agent soothing hysteria.

anti-. Prefix: Against, as *antibody.*

antiagglu'tinin. A specific antibody opposing action of agglutinin.

antial'bumate, antial'buminate. A product resulting from incomplete proteolysis of albumin; parapeptone.

antialbu'min. An albumin constituent; supposed to be source of antialbumose.

antial'bumose. A product formed by peptic digestion of albumin; becomes antipeptone by further hydrolysis.

antialex'in. Anticomplement.

antiam'boceptor. Substance inhibiting action of an amboceptor.

antiam'ylase. Substance neutralizing action of amylase.

antianaphylac'tin. An antibody specific to anaphylactin.

antianaphylax'is. A state of immunity.

antiane'mic. Curing or preventing anemia.

antian'tibody. An antibody counteracting effect of antitoxin which produced it.

antiapoplec'tic. Relieving or preventing apoplexy.

antiarthritic (an-tĭ-ar-thrĭt'ĭk). Medicine given to relieve gout.

antibacte'rial. Destroying or stopping the growth of bacteria.

antibacterin (an-tĭ-bak'ter-in). An antibody injected to prevent further germ growth in the body. SEE: *germ theory.*

antibechic (an-tĭ-bek'ĭk). 1. Relieving cough. 2. A cough remedy.

antibilious (an-tĭ-bil'yus). Relieving bilious conditions.

antibio'sis. An association of two organisms detrimental to one of them.

antibiotic (an-tĭ-bi-ot'ĭk). Tending to destroy life.

antiblennorrhagic (an-tĭ-blen-o-raj'ĭk). 1. Preventing or curing gonorrhea or catarrh. 2. Remedy for these diseases.

an'tibody. A substance in the body which incites immunity (antagonistic to invading bodies) such as the reacting agents in the serum.

antibrachium (an-te-bra'kĭ-um) (BNA). The forearm.

antibro'mic. 1. Deodorizing. 2. A deodorant.

antical'culous. Antilithic.

antican'crin. Cancroin. Supposed cancer antibody.

anticar'dium. Precordial depression.

anticarious (an-tĭ-ka're-us). Preventing decay of teeth.

anticathode (an-tĭ-kath'ōd). Portion of vacuum tube opposite cathode. SYN: *target.*

anticheirotonus (an-tĭ-ki-rot'o-nus). Spasmodic bending inward of thumb in epilepsy or before attack.

anticholagogue (an-tĭ-ko'la-gog). Depressing hepatic function.

anticholerin (an-tĭ-kol'er-in). Substance from cultures of *Spirillum cholerae asiaticae:* employed against cholera.

antic'ipating intermittent. Intermittent with paroxysms recurring earlier each day before the regular time.

an"ticipa'tion. Theory that hereditary defects manifest themselves earlier in each successive generation and often more severely. SYN: *antedating.*

anticli'nal. Leaning in opp. directions.

    a. vertebra. Tenth thoracic vertebra.

anticomplement (an-tĭ-kom'ple-ment). A substance combining with and thus neutralizing a complement.

anticonvul'sive. 1. Relieving convulsions. 2. Agent preventing convulsions.

anticreatinin (an-tĭ-kre-at'ĭn-in). A leukomaine from creatinine.

anti'cus (BNA). Anterior. That part nearest the ventral or front surface.

anticu'tin. An antibody neutralizing tuberculin to prevent cutaneous tuberculin reaction.

anticyclic acid (an-tĭ-sik'lik). An antipyretic drug.

anticytol'ysin. Antibody inhibiting cytotoxin. SYN: *anticytotoxin.*

anticy'tost. An antibody which gives immunity to cytost; named by Turck.

anticytotox'in. An antibody specifically inhibiting cytotoxin.

antidiabe'tin. A preparation of saccharine and mannite (a sweetish substance taken from the flowering ash) used as substitute for sugar in diabetes.*

antidiarrhe'ic en'emas. These include the demulcents, astringents, antiseptics, carminative, or sedative enemas, *q.v.*

antidinic (an-tĭ-din'ĭk). 1. Relieving giddiness. 2. Agent preventing vertigo.

antidiphtherin (an-ti-dif'ther-in). A substance taken from the culture of diphtheria bacillus and used to prevent the disease.

antidiuretic (an"tĭ-di-u-ret'ĭk). 1. Lessening urine secretion. 2. A drug having such an action.

antido'tal. Acting as or pert. to an antidote.

antidote (an'tĭ-dōt). A substance which neutralizes poisons or their effects.

antido'tum. An antidote.

antidromic (an-tĭ-drom'ĭk). Running in a direction opposite the usual stream, as when a nervous impulse runs along a sensory fiber in the direction of the sense-organ.

antidyscratic (an-tĭ-dis-krat'ĭk). Relieving dyscrasia.

antidysenter'ic. 1. Relieving or preventing dysentery. 2. An agent curing dysentery.

antiemet'ic. An agent that will prevent or arrest vomiting.

antienzyme (an-tĭ-en'zĭm). 1. Enzyme neutralizer. 2. An enzyme retarding the activity of another.

antiephial'tic. Hindering nightmare. SYN: *antephialtic.*

an'tifat. An agent which lessens accumulation of fat.

antifeb'rile. 1. A medium reducing fever. 2. Reducing or relieving fever.

antifebrin (an-tĭ-feb'rin). Acetanilid.

    DOSAGE: 3 gr. (0.2 Gm.).

    a. salicylate. Salifebrin.

antifer'ment. Hindering, or an agent which hinders, the action of an enzyme. SYN: *antienzyme.*

antifermen'tative. Preventing the fermentation process. SYN: *antizymotic.*

antigalactagogue (an-ti-gal-ak'tă-gog). An agent that lessens the secretion of milk. Ex: *belladonna,* probably all *hydragogue purgatives.*

antigalactic (an-tĭ-gal-ak'tic). Diminishing or retarding the secretion of milk.

an'tigen. Any immunizing agent which, when inoculated into the body of a susceptible person, may produce antibodies.*

    a. unit. Smallest quantity of antigen required to fix 1 unit of complement, preventing hemolysis.

antigenic (an-tĭ-jen'ĭk). Capable of causing the production of an antibody.

antigenophil (an-tǐ-jen'o-fĭl). Having an attraction for the antigen. SYN: *antigentophil*.

antigentophil (an-tǐ-jen'to-fĭl). Having affinity for antigen.

antigentother'apy. Stimulating antibody formation by injecting antigens.

antiglob'ulin. A precipitin which precipitates globulin.

an"tigonorrhe'ic. 1. Curing gonorrhea. 2. An agent relieving gonorrhea.

antihe'lix. Inner curved ridge of external ear.

antihemicra'nin. A proprietary drug for headache. SYN: *antimigraine*.

antihemol'ysin. A substance which neutralizes hemolysin.

antihidrot'ic. Preventing or checking perspiration. SYN: *anhidrotic*.

antihormone (an-tǐ-hor'mōn). An inhibitory autacoid opposing hormone action.

antihydrop'ic. 1. Relieving dropsy. 2. Agent causing disappearance of dropsy.

anti-icter'ic. 1. Relieving icterus. 2. Agent for curing jaundice.

an"ti-immune'. Preventing immunity.

an"ti-isoly'sin. A substance inhibiting action of an isolysin.

antikenotox'in. A substance counteracting fatigue toxins.

antiketogen'esis. Lowering of acidosis through body oxidation of sugar, alcohol, glycerin, and allied substances.

antiketogenet'ic, antiketogen'ic. Pert. to antiketogenesis.

an'tikol. Proprietary antifebrile medicine.

antilac'tase. An antibody counteracting lactase.

antilemic (an-tǐ-le'mǐk). 1. Preventing plague. 2. An agent curing the plague.

antilepsis (an-tǐ-lep'sis). 1. Application of a remedy to a healthy part. 2. An attack or seizure. 3. Taking effect or root. 4. Support of a bandage.

antileptic (an-tǐ-lep'tǐk). 1. Assisting, supporting. 2. Revulsive.

antilethargic (an-tǐ-leth-ar'jĭk). Preventing sleep.

antilith'ic. An agent that prevents the formation of, or favors the removal of, stones or calculi in the urinary or biliary tracts.

antilo'bium. The tragus.

antilogia (an-tǐ-lo'jǐ-ä). Contradictory symptoms which render diagnosis uncertain.

antiluetic (an-tǐ-lu-et'ĭk). Antisyphilitic.

antilysin (an-tǐ-li'sin). A substance neutralizing the lysins of a disease against which an animal has been immunized.

antilysis (an-tǐl'is-is). The result of the action of antilysin.

antilys'sic. Preventing or checking rabies. SYN: *antirabic*.

antimalar'ial. An agent that will prevent or relieve malaria. Ex: *quinine*.

antimere (an'tǐ-mēr). Any body segment bounded by planes at right angles to the long axis of the body.

antimetro'pia. An ocular disorder in which one eye is hypermetropic, the other myopic.

antimiasmat'ic. Preventing or checking malaria. SYN: *antimalarial*.

antimicro'bic. 1. Not believing in the pathogenicity of microörganisms. 2. Preventing the development or pathogenic action of microbes.

antimicro'bin. Antibody used to prevent further germ growth in the body. SEE: *germ theory*.

antimo'nial. Pert. to or containing antimony.

antimony (an'tǐ-mo"nǐ). SYMB: *Sb*. An element of metallic appearance and crystalline structure. Atomic weight 121.77. Its salts form various poisons and medicinal drugs.

antimycotic (an-tǐ-mi-kot'ĭk). Checking or destroying bacteria. SYN: *antibacterial*.

antinarcot'ic. Relieving stupor caused by a narcotic.

antinephritic (an-tǐ-nef-rit'ĭk). Serviceable in renal inflammation.

antiner'vin. Bromacetanilid and salicylanilid used as an antineuralgic.

antineuralgic (an-tǐ-nu-ral'jĭk). 1. Relieving neuralgic pain. 2. Agent curing neuralgia.

antineurit'ic. Counteracting nerve inflammation.

antineu'ritin. Antineuritic vitamin or Vitamin B_1.

antin'ion. Frontal pole of the skull.

antiop'sonin. A substance that retards opsonin action.

antioxida'tion. Prevention of oxidation.

antiox'ygen. A substance hindering oxidation.

antiparalyt'ic. Reputedly relieving paralysis.

antiparasit'ic. 1. Destructive to parasites. 2. Insecticide.*

antiparastati'tis. Inflammation of Cowper's glands.

antipathic (an-tǐ-path'ĭk). Opposite; unlike.

antip'athy. 1. Aversion; disgust; or that which excites repugnance. 2. Chemical incompatibility.

antipepsin (an-tǐ-pep'sin). An antibody counteracting pepsin.

antipeptone (an-tǐ-pep'tōn). Peptone derived from antialbumose through hydrolysis.

antiperiod'ic. Antimalarial; preventing regular recurrences.

antiperistal'sis. A wave of contraction in the gastrointestinal tract moving towards the oral end.

antiperistal'tic. 1. Pert. to antiperistalsis.* 2. Impeding peristalsis.*

antiphlogistic (an-ti-phlo-jis'tik). An agent that tends to relieve inflammation.

antiphthisic (an-tǐ-tiz'ĭk). Checking or relieving phthisis.

antiphthi'sin. Modified tuberculin.

antiplas'tic. 1. An agent preventing granulation of tissue. 2. One which thins the blood.

antipneumotox'in. An antitoxin opposing pneumotoxin.

antip'odal cell. One of two nuclear cells at the base of embryo sac in a seed.

antipraxia (an-tĭ-praks' ĭ-ă). Functions or symptoms antagonistic to each other.

antiprostate (an-tĭ-pros'tāt). Cowper's glands.*

antiprostati'tis. Inflammation of Cowper's glands.

antiprothrom'bin. Agent preventing formation of thrombin; anticoagulant. SEE: *clotting.*

antiprotozo'al. Destructive to protozoa.

antipruritic (an-tĭ-pru-rit'ĭk). That which relieves itching.

antipsoric (an-tip-so'rĭk). An agent used to prevent or arrest itching. It may be local or general.

antiputrefac'tive. Preventive of putrefaction.

antipyic (an-tĭ-pi'ĭk). Checking suppuration; antipyogenic.

antipyogenic (an"tĭ-pi-o-jen'ik). Preventing or checking pus formation.

antipyre'sis. Use of antipyretics in fever.

antipyret'ic. An agent that reduces febrile temperatures.

antipyrine (ăn"tĭ-pi'rĭn). White crystalline powder, odorless and having a slightly bitter taste.
  DOSAGE: 5 gr. (0.3 Gm.).

antipyrotic (an-tĭ-pi-rot'ĭk). That which allays the pain from burns.

antirab'ic. Preventive of, or curing, hydrophobia; antilyssic.

antirachit'ic. 1. Helping to cure rickets. 2. Agent for treating rickets.
  a. vitamin. Vitamin D. SEE: *vitamins.*

antirheumat'ic. An agent that will prevent or relieve rheumatism. Ex: *sodium salicylate, acetylsalicylic acid, colchicum.*

antiricin (an-tĭ-ri'sin). An antibody to ricin.

antiscabious (an-tĭ-ska'bĭ-us). Preventing or relieving scabies.

antiscorbutic (an-ti-skor-bu'tik). An agent effective against or a remedy for scurvy. Vitamin C is antiscorbutic.

antisep'sin. Monobromacetanilide. An analgesic, antipyretic and antiseptic drug. SYN: *asepsin.* [germs.

antisep'sis. The exclusion of putrefactive

antiseptic (an-tĭ-sep'tĭk). An agent that will prevent the growth or arrest the development of microörganisms.

antisep'ticism. Therapeutic employment of antiseptic measures.

antiserum (an-tĭ-se'rum). A serum containing an antibody specific in relation to the substance which has produced it through repeated injections.

antisialic (an-tĭ-si-al'ĭk). Checking or that which checks the secretion of saliva.

antisialogogue (an-tĭ-si-al'o-gog). An agent that lessens or checks the flow of saliva.

antispasmod'ic. An agent that will relieve muscular spasm.

antispas'tic. Agent relieving muscular spasm. SYN: *antispasmodic.*

antistal'sis. Backward movement of bowel contents. Opp. peristalsis, *q.v.*

antistaphylococ'cic. Destructive to staphylococcus.

antistaphylol'ysin. Blood serum substance counteracting staphylolysin.

antistat'ic. Counteracting; hostile. SYN: *antagonistic.*

antistreptococ'cic. Destructive to streptococcus.

antistreptococ'cin. The antitoxin of any type streptococcus.

antisu'doral. Checking perspiration. SYN: *antihidrotic.*

antisu'dorin. Commercial name of remedy to correct sweating.

antisyphilit'ic. An agent that will prevent or relieve syphilis. Ex: *mercury, arsenic, bismuth.*

antitabetic (an-tĭ-ta-bet'ĭk). 1. Preventing tabes dorsalis. 2. Agent which mitigates tabetic symptoms.

antith'enar. Placed opposite to the thenar.

antither'mic. 1. Reducing temperature. 2. Agent lowering temperature. SYN: *antifebrile, antipyretic.*

antithrombin (an-tĭ-throm'bin). A substance in the blood which prevents or retards coagulation.

antithyroi'din. A serum from sheep's blood after thyroid has been removed.
  DOSAGE: 0.5 to 1 cc.

antiton'ic. Diminishing tone or tonicity.

antitoxic (an-tĭ-tok'sĭk). Neutralizing a poison, specifically an antitoxin.
  a. unit. Sufficient quantity of antitoxin to neutralize 100 toxic units. SYN: *immunizing unit.*

antitox'igen. An antigen stimulating antitoxin production in the blood.

antitox'in. A protein that defends the body against *toxins*. It may be in the tissues, or produced in the body by introduction of some toxic substance.
  a. serum. A serum taken from the blood of an animal, principally the horse, cow, or goat, that has been immunized against poisonous toxins, by repeated injections of the toxins required (*antitoxin diphtheria, tetanus**), beginning with small doses (causing a temperature reaction) and increasing according to tolerance, until no reaction is present.

antitox'inogen. An antigen promoting production of antitoxin in the blood. SYN: *antitoxigen.*

antitragicus (an-tĭ-traj'ik-us). A small muscle in the pinna of the ear.

antitragus (an-tit-ra'gus). A projection on the ear of the cartilage of the auricle in front of the tail of the helix, post. to the tragus.

antitrismus (an-tĭ-trĭs'mus). A condition in which the mouth cannot close because of tonic spasm.

antitrope (an'tĭ-trōp). 1. A symmetrical pair of organs. 2. Antibody.

antitro'pin. An antibody.*

antitryp'sin. An antibody or antiferment inhibiting tryptic action.

antitryp'tic. Opposed to fermentation.

antituberculot'ic. Inhibiting the advance of tuberculosis.

antitu'lase. A serum used in treating for tuberculosis.

antiuratic (an-tĭ-u-rat'ĭk). Preventing the precipitation of urates.

antivaccina'tion. Opposition to vaccination. [to vaccination.

antivaccina'tionist. One who is opposed

antiven'ene. Blood serum of an animal rendered immune to snake bite.
USES: A specific in treating certain poisonous snake bites.

antivene'real. Preventing or curing venereal diseases.

antivenin (an-tǐ-ven'in). An antigenic substance prepared from immunized animal sera used by injection to overcome the effects of snake bite.

antiven'om. A snake venom antitoxin.

antiven'omous. Inhibiting venom.

antivi'ral. Inhibiting a virus.

antivi'rus. A bacterial filtrate from a broth medium heated to reduce toxicity; used in the Besredka local immunity method.

antixe'nic. Pert. to living tissue reaction to any foreign substance.

antizymot'ic. An agent that will prevent or arrest fermentation. Ex: *salicylic acid, alcohol.*

antlia (ant'lǐ-ă). A pump or syringe.

antodontalgic (ant-o-don-tal'jik). 1. Relieving toothache. 2. Remedy for toothache.

an'tozone. Hydrogen peroxide.

an'tra. Pl. of antrum.

antracele (an'tra-sēl). Accumulation of fluid in Highmore's antrum.

antral (an'tral). Pert. to an antrum.

antrec'tomy. Excision of the walls of an antrum.

antritis (an-tri'tis). Inflammation of an antrum, esp. that of the antritis of Highmore.

antroatticotomy (an-tro-at-ǐ-kot'o-mǐ). Operation to open and remove contents of the antrum and the attic of the tympanum.

antrocele (an'tro-sēl). Fluid accumulation in Highmore's antrum. SYN: *antracele.*

antrona'sal. Rel. to the maxillary sinus and nasal fossa.

antrophore (an'tro-fōr). A medicated bougie for local treatment of any accessible cavity or canal.

antroscope (an'tro-skop). An instrument for examining the maxillary sinus.

antros'copy. Examination of any cavity by the antroscope.

antros'tomy. Operation to open an antrum for drainage.

antrotome (an'tro-tōm). An instrument for cutting open a cavity, esp. in bone.

antrot'omy. Opening an antral wall.

an''trotympan'ic. Rel. to the mastoid sinus and the tympanic cavity.

an''trotympani'tis. Chronic inflammation of middle ear and mastoid antrum.

an'trum (pl. *antra*). Any nearly closed cavity or chamber in a bone.
    a. auris. External acoustic meatus.
    a. cardiacum. Cardiac portion of the stomach, proximal or superior portion.
    a. mastoideum. Tympanic antrum.
    a., maxillary. The maxillary sinus. SEE: *sinus.*
    a. of Highmore. The air sinus in the maxillary bone.

    a. puncture. Made near floor of nose 1½ inches from external opening. Pus is then drained.
    a. pyloricum. Bulge in the pyloric portion of the stomach along the greater curvature on distention.
    a. tympanicum. The mastoid antrum.

antu'itrin. Extract of anterior lobe of pituitary body.
    a. G, a. growth. Commercial product derived from the ant. pituitary, containing the growth stimulating element.
    a. gonadotropic. Commercial product derived from the ant. pituitary, containing the gonadotropic hormone.
    a. S. A gonadotropic hormone extracted from the urine of pregnant women.
    a. T, a. thyrotropic. Commercial product derived from the ant. pituitary, containing the thyrotropic element.

anure'sis. Failure of kidney to secrete sufficient urine, suppression or failure to reach bladder if secreted; found in nephritis (if acute), or congestion, renal abscess, and last stages of chronic nephritis.

anuret'ic. Pert. to anuresis, *q.v.*

anu'ria. Failure of kidney function. SYN: *anuresis.*

a'nus. The outlet of the rectum lying in the fold bet. the nates.
    The end of the anal* canal (2.5 to 3 cm.). Fissures of anus in newly born indicative of congenital syphilis.
    a., artificial. Opening of the bowel (usually surgical).
    a., fissure in. A crack in mucosa of rectum.
    a., fistula in. A fistulous connection bet. lumen of rectum and perianal skin.
    a., imperforated. Where the natural opening is closed.
    a., vulvovaginal. An opening into the vulva from the anus.

anvil (an'vil). Middle ossicle of ear. SYN: *incus.*

anxietas (ang-zi'et-ăs). Anxiety, apprehension, restlessness.
    a. tibia'rum. Tiredness, twitching, and unrest in legs when in bed. ETIOL: Increase of the muscular sense.

anxiety neuro'sis. A functional disease in which fear (or the somatic evidences of fear) is the essential part of the picture.

anxious agitated depression. PSY: Depression accompanied by worry, uneasiness, and agitation, esp. rel. to poverty and want, or ruin.

anydremia (an-ǐ-dre'mǐ-ă). Decrease in normal fluid content of the blood. SYN: *anhydremia.*

anypnia (an-ip'nǐ-ă). Condition of sleeplessness.

A. O. C. Abbr. for Anodal Opening Contraction. [catalepsy.

aochlesia (a-ok-le'zǐ-ă). Tranquillity; rest;

aolan (ā'o-lan). A sterile solution of lactalbumin in colloidal form.
USES: In nonspecific protein therapy, to relieve pain in gonorrheal complications.

DOSAGE: From 5 to 10 cc., at intervals of 5 to 6 days, intramuscularly.

aor'ta. The main artery of the trunk.

aor'tal. Pert. to the aorta.

aortalgia (a-or-tal'jĭ-ă). Pain due to pathological aortic conditions.

aortarctia (a-or-tark'shĭ-ă). Aortic narrowing.

aortectasia (a-ort-ek-ta'zĭ-ă). Dilatation of the aorta.

aor'tic. Pert. to aorta or its orifice in the left ventricle of the heart.

   a. murmur. Symptom of aortic valvular disease.

   a. opening. 1. Path through diaphragm for aorta. 2. Post. opening in the diaphragm.

   a. regurgita'tion.* Leakage of the blood from the aorta back into the left ventricle at the recoil of the aorta's elastic walls. ETIOL: Diseases of the heart or blood vessels, or weakness of the same.

   a. valves. Three valves in left ventricle at the aortic opening.

aortitis (a-or-ti'tis). Inflammation of the aorta.

aortocla'sia. Aortic rupture.

aortog'raphy. Examination of abdominal aorta by x-ray after injection of contrast fluid.

aortolith (a-or'to-lith). Calcareous deposit in the aortic wall.

aortomalacia (a-or-to-mal-a'sĭ-ă). Softening of the aorta's walls.

aortop'athy. Any aortic disease.

aortopto'sia, aortopto'sis. Sinking down of abdominal aorta.

aortorrhaphy (a-or-tor'af-ĭ). Suture of the aorta.

aortosclero'sis. Aortic sclerosis.

aortostenosis (a-or-to-sten-o'sis). Narrowing of the aorta.

aortot'omy. Incision of the aorta.

aos'mic. Without odor.

A. O. T. A. Abbr. *American Occupational Therapy Association.*

apallesthesia (ă-pal"es-the'zĭ-ă). Inability to detect vibrations of a tuning fork placed against the body.

apan'dria. Aversion to males.

apanthropia, apanthropy (a-pan-thro'pi-ă, -ĭ). Morbid aversion to society or to man.

aparalyt'ic. Marked by lack of paralysis.

aparathyrosis (ă-par-ă-thī-ro'sis). Parathyroid deficiency.

apareunia (a-pa-ru'nĭ-ă). Impossibility or absence of coitus.

aparthrosis (ap-ar-thro'sis). 1. Diarthrosis. 2. Dislocation.

apastia (ap-as'tĭ-ă). Abnormal refusal to eat.

apathetic (ap-ă-thet'ik). Indifferent; without interest. SYN: *apathic.*

apath'ic. Indifferent. SYN: *apathetic.*

apathism (ap'ath-izm). Slow to react; opp. to erethism.*

ap'athy. Indifference; insensibility; without emotion, sluggish, opp. of erethism.*

apectomy (a-pek'to-mĭ). Eradication of apex of a tooth root. SYN: *apicoectomy.*

ape-hand. Nerve lesion in which the thumb remains at right angle from hand.

apeidosis (ap-e-i-do'sis). Slow disappearance of characteristic form in a disease.

apella (ap-el'ă). 1. A circumcised male. 2. One with a short prepuce.

apellous (ă-pel'us). 1. Without skin. 2. Circumcised.

apenteric (ap-en-ter'ik). Away from the bowels.

apep'sia. 1. Absence of pepsin in the gastric juice. 2. Imperfect digestion or its cessation.

apepsin'ia. Absence of pepsin in the gastric juice.

apeptous (ä-pep'tus). 1. Indigestible; crude. 2. Apeptic.

ape'rient. A very mild purgative, particularly applied to mild purgative waters.

aperistal'sis. Absence of peristalsis.

aper'itive. 1. An appetizer. 2. Mild purgative. SYN: *aperient, q.v.*

apertura (ap-er-tu'ră). An opening.

aperture (ap'er-chure). An orifice or opening.

a'pex (*pl. apices*). The summit or extremity of anything.

   a. beat. The point of maximum impulse of the heart against the chest wall felt in the 5th left intercostal space, 3½ inches from middle of sternum about an inch within a line drawn from middle of clavicle parallel with sternum (the mammary line).

   a. murmur. One over the apex of the heart.   [tooth.

   a. root. The end of the root of a

apex'ograph. An instrument for determining apex of a tooth root.

A. P. H. A. 1. Abbr. *American Public Health Association.* 2. *American Protestant Hospital Association.*

aphacia (a-fa'sĭ-ă). Lack of eye lens.

apha'cic. Pert. to aphacia.

aphagia (a-fa'jĭ-ă). Inability to swallow.

aphakia (a-fa'kĭ-ă). Absence of eye's crystalline lens. SYN: *aphacia.*

apha'kik. Pert. to aphakia.

aphasia (a-fa'zĭ-ă). Inability to express oneself properly through speech, or loss of verbal comprehension.

   a., amnesic. Loss of memory for words.

   a., ataxic. Inability to articulate. Similar to *aphasia, motor.*

   a., auditory. Aphasia due to pathology of center of hearing.

   a., conduction. ETIOL: Due to lesion of conduction path bet. motor and speech centers.

   a. gibberish. Utterance of meaningless phrases.

   a., motor. Patient knows what he wants to say but cannot say it. Muscles coördinating speech unable to coordinate. May be complete or partial. Broca's area is disordered or diseased.

   a., optic. Inability to call name of an object recognized by sight without the aid of sound, taste, or touch; a form of *agnosia.*

a., sensory. Inability to understand spoken words, if word center is involved (auditory aphasia) or the written word if visual word center is affected (visual aphasia). If both centers are involved, will not understand spoken or written word.

a., traumatic. Aphasia caused by head injury.

apha'sic, apha'siac. Pert. to aphasia.

aphelotic (af-el-ot'ĭk). Absent minded; given to reverie.

aphelxia (af-elks'ĭ-ă). Absent minded; oblivious of external conditions.

aphemesthesia (ă-fem-es-the'zĭ-ă). Word deafness, or word blindness.

aphemia (a-fe'mĭ-ă). Loss of speech due to impairment of the word memory center; amnesic aphasia.* SEE: *alexia, amnesia, anarthria.*

aphephobia (af-e-fo'bĭ-ă). Abnormal aversion to being touched by anyone.

aphlogistic (ă-flo-jist'ĭk). 1. Not inflammable. 2. Burning without flame.

aphonia (a-fon'ĭ-ă). Loss of voice with intact inner speech and not due to central lesion. May obtain in chronic laryngitis.

a. clericorum. Clergyman's sore throat.

a. paranoica. The silence of the insane.

aphoresis (ă-for-e'sis). 1. Lack of endurance, esp. of pain. 2. Any separation of a part.

aphoria (ă-fo'rĭ-ă). Sterility in the female.

aphose (ă'fōz). A subjective perception of darkness, or of a shadow.

aphrasia (a-fra'zĭ-ă). Morbid refusal to speak; seen in dementia precox, *q.v.*

a., paralytic. Due to paralysis of the faculty of ideation.

a., superstitious. Avoidance of certain words because of scruples or aversion to their use.

aphrenia (a-fre'nĭ-ă). An apparent lack of intellect seen in some forms of dementia.

a. apoplexy. Unconsciousness.

aphrenic, aphrenous (ă-fren'ĭk, 'us). Insane.

aphrodisia (af-ro-dis'ĭ-ă). Sexual desire, esp. when morbid, or sexual congress.

aphrodisiac (af-ro-diz'ĭ-ak). An agent which stimulates sexual desire.

aphronesia (ă-fro-ne'sĭ-ă). 1. Silliness. 2. Dementia.

aphronia (ă-fro'nĭ-ă). Mental deficiency; defective functional activity of cerebrum.

aphtha (af'thă). 1. Very small ulcer on a mucous membrane. 2. Thrush.

aphthenxia (af-thengks'ĭ-ă). An aphasia with articulate sounds imperfectly expressed.

aphthongia (af-thon'gĭ-ă). Aphasia due to spasm of muscles controlled by the hypoglossal nerve.

aphthous (af'thus). Pert. to, or characterized by, ulcers.

aphylac'tic. Having no immune power.

aphylaxis (ă-fĭ-laks'ĭs). Without immunity against disease.

apical. Pert. to the apex.

apices (a'pis-ez). Pl. of apex.

apiceotomy (ap'ĭs-e-ot'o-mĭ). Eradication of apex of a tooth root. SYN: *apicoectomy.*

apicitis (ap-ĭ-sī'tis). Inflammation of any apical structure, esp. apex of lung or tooth root.

apicoectomy (ap-ĭ-ko-ek'to-mĭ). Amputation of apex of a tooth root.

apicoloca'tor. Instrument for locating apex of a tooth root. SYN: *apexograph.*

apicolysis (ap-ĭ-kol'ĭs-is). Artificial collapse of the apex of a lung by making an opening through the anterior chest wall.

apicotomy (ap-ĭ-kot'o-mĭ). Removal of apex of a tooth root. SYN: *apicoectomy.*

apiectomy (ap-ĭ-ek'to-mĭ). Eradication of apex of a tooth root. SYN: *apicoectomy.*

apinealism (ă-pin'e-al-izm). Syndrome due to absence of pineal gland.

ap'inoid. Free from dirt; clean.

a. cancer. Hard cancer.

apiphobia (ă-pĭ-fo'bĭ-ă). Abnormal fear of bees or of insects which buzz like a bee.

apisination (ap-ĭs-in-a'shun). Poisoning from bee stings.

apituitarism (ă-pit-u'ĭt-ar-izm). Condition due to total abeyance of function or removal of pituitary body. Leads to cachexia thyreopriva.*

aplanat'ic lens. Free from spherical or chromatic aberration. Not wandering.

aplasia (a-pla'zĭ-ă). Failure of an organ or part of the body to develop naturally.

aplas'tic. Having deficient or arrested development.

apnea (ap-ne'a). 1. Temporary absence of respiration following a period of overbreathing or overabundance of oxygen and a decrease of carbon dioxide, a feature of some types of dyspnea.* 2. Asphyxia. 3. Temporary cessation of breathing seen in the Cheyne-Stokes breathing, named after the first two physicians who noticed this type of breathing.

apneumato'sis. Noninflation of air cells.

apo- (ap'o). Gr. prefix: From, away, separation, as *apophysis.*

ap'ocain. Local anesthetic, mildly toxic, employed for surface anesthesia and infiltration. SYN: *tutocain.*

apocamnosis (ap-o-kam-no'sis). Weariness, easily induced fatigue.

apocenosis (ap-o-sen-o'sis). 1. Increased flow of blood or body fluids. 2. Partial evacuation. [*matic.*

apochromat'ic. Without color. SYN: *achro-*

apocope (ă-pok'o-pe). Amputation.

apocopous (a-pok'o-pus). Castrated.

apocoptic (ap-o-kop'tic). The effect resulting from the removal of a part.

apocrine (ap'o-krin). Pert. to cells which lose part of their protoplasm while functioning.

apocrustic (ap-o-krus'tĭk). 1. Astringent. 2. Repellent. 3. Defensive.

apodemialgia (ap-o-de-mĭ-al′gĭ-ă). 1. An abnormal desire to wander from one's abode or environment; wanderlust. 2. Morbid dislike of a home.

apogee (ap′o-gē). Highest stage of a disease.

apokamnosis (ap″o-kam-no′sis). Abnormal tendency to fatigue, as in neurasthenia.

apolarthron (ap-o-lar′thrŏn). A natural fish liver oil, of great concentration, each capsule containing 25,000 USP units of Vitamin D, and 30,000 units of Vitamin A.

   DOSAGE: From 2 to not more than 6 capsules per day.

apolepsis (ap-o-lep′sis). 1. Cessation of a function. 2. Retention or suppression of an excretion or secretion.

apolexis (ap-o-leks′is). 1. The catabolic condition or process. 2. Decline of life.

apomorphine (ap-o-mor′fēn). A morphine derivative prepared from the alkaloid by extraction of one molecule of water.

   a. **hydrochloride.** A grayish white powder; should not be used if it at once imparts a greenish color when dissolved in 100 parts distilled water.

   DOSAGE: $\frac{1}{12}$ gr. (0.005 Gm.) *hypodermically;* as *expectorant,* $\frac{1}{60}$ gr. (0.001 Gm.).

apomyelin (ap-o-mi′el-ĭn). A brain substance containing no glycerol.

apone (a′pōn). An anodyne.

aponeurosis (ap-o-nu-ro′sis). Extension of connective tissue beyond a muscle in round or flattened tendons, or expanded sheets for the attachment of muscular fibers, or means of insertion or origin of a flat muscle, or as a fascia for other muscles.

ap″oneurol′ogy. The science of aponeuroses.

ap″oneuror′rhaphy. Aponeurotic suture.

aponeurositis (ap-on-ū-ro-si′tis). Aponeurotic inflammation.

aponeurot′ic. Pert. to, or rel. to, an aponeurosis.

aponeurotome (ap-on-ū′ro-tōm). Knife for dividing an aponeurosis.

aponeurotomy (ap-on-u-rot′om-ĭ). Surgical cutting of an aponeurosis.

aponia (a-pon′ĭ-ă). 1. Abstaining from labor. 2. Absence of pain.

aponic (ap-on′ĭk). Rel. to aponia.

aponoia, aponoea (a-pon-oy′ă, ă-pon-e′ă). Amentia.

apophlegmatic (ap-o-fleg-mat′ik). Producing a mucous discharge; expectorant.

apophyseal (ap-o-fĭz′e-al). Rel. or pert. to an apophysis.

apoph′ysis. 1. A projection, esp. from a bone; an outgrowth without an independent center of ossification. 2. The pineal gland.

   a. **of Ingrassias.** Smaller wing of sphenoid bone.

   a. **lenticularis.** Temporal bone's orbicular process.

   a. **of Rau.** Long process of malleus.

   a. **raviana.** Gracile process of malleus.

apophysitis (a-pof-i-si′tis). Inflammation of a bony process which has never been entirely separated from the bone of which it forms a part.

apoplasmia (ap-o-plaz′mĭ-ă). Deficiency of blood plasma.

apoplectic (ap-o-plek′tĭk). Pert. to apoplexy.

apoplec′tiform. Like apoplexy.

apoplectig′enous. Causing apoplexy.

apoplec′toid. Like apoplexy. SYN: *apoplectiform.*

apoplexy (ăp′ō-plĕk-sĭ). 1. Sudden diminution of, or loss of, consciousness and paralysis, due to hemorrhage into brain or spinal cord, or formation of an embolus or thrombus, which occludes an artery. SYN: *stroke.* 2. Condition of an organ marked by a hemorrhage into its substance, as apoplexy of the lung.

apopsychia (ap-op-sik′ĭ-ă). Fainting; syncope.

apoptosis (ap-op-to′sis). Falling off or out, as a scab or hair.

aporioneurosis (ap-or-ĭ-o-nu-ro′sis). Anxiety neurosis.

aporrhegma (ap-o-reg′mă). 1. A biological separation of one substance from another. 2. Any nitrogen-containing substance formed by the removal of carbon dioxide from protein-derivatives, as when histamine, $C_3H_5N_2(CH_2)_2NH_2$, is formed by putrefaction from histidine, $C_3H_5N_2CH(NH_2)COOH$.

aporrhinosis (ap-or-in-o′sis). Nasal discharge.

aporrhipsis (ap-or-ip′sis). Removal of clothing or bedclothes; seen in some psychotic conditions or in delirium.

aposia (a-po′zĭ-ă). Absence of thirst.

apositia (ap-o-sit′ĭ-ă). Anorexia* associated with disgust for food.

apos′pory. Absence of spore-producing ability.

apostasis (ap-os′tă-sis). 1. The crisis or end of a disease. Termination by crisis. 2. An abscess. 3. An exfoliation.

apostaxis (ap-o-staks′ĭs). 1. Epistaxis. 2. Discharge by drops.

apostem (ap′o-stem). An abscess.

apostema (ap-os-te′mă). An abscess.

aposthia (ah-pos′thĭ-ă). Congenital absence of the prepuce.

apothanasia (ă-poth-ă-na′zĭ-ă). Prolongation of life.

apoth′ecaries' meas′ure. A system of measuring drugs in English speaking countries rapidly being displaced by the metric system, *q.v.*

   The scruple and the pound are now seldom used. A portion of a grain is expressed fractionally, as gr. ½, not decimally. The quantity is written in Roman numerals, *q.v.*, with the symbol before it, as gr. v.

Weight

20 grains (gr.)	= 1 scruple (℈)
60 grains (gr.) (3℈)	= 1 dram (3)
8 drams (3)	= 1 ounce (℥)
12 oz. (℥) (5760 gr.)	= 1 pound (lb.)

Volume

60 minims	$(\mathfrak{m}) = 1$ fluidram	(f ʒ)
8 fluidrams	(f ʒ) = 1 fluidounce	(f ʒ)
16 fluidounces	(f ʒ) = 1 pint	(pt.)
2 pints	(pt.) = 1 quart	(qt.)
4 quarts	(qt.) = 1 gallon	(C)

Some Points to Remember Are: The character ʒ represents 60 grains, while f ʒ represents 60 minims. ʒ represents 480 grains only, while f ʒ is necessary to express 480 minims. A minim is not the equivalent of a grain. 480 minims (1 f ʒ) of water weighed at the standard temperature weighs 456.37 grains. This should be remembered for percentage solutions. Specific gravities of liquids vary; a pint of a liquid is not necessarily a pound.

apoth′ecary. A druggist or pharmacist. In England and Ireland one licensed by the Society of Apothecaries as an authorized physician and dispenser of drugs.

ap′othem, ap′otheme. The brown precipitate which appears when vegetable decoctions or infusions are exposed to the air, or are boiled a long time.

apothesine (ap-oth′es-in). A local anesthetic of the procaine type (in that it is relatively ineffective when applied to the mucous membrane), but slower in action than procaine. Its toxicity is about equal to that of cocaine, but twice that of procaine.

DOSAGE: 0.08 Gm. (1½ grains).

apothesis (ap-oth′es-is). Reduction of a fracture or dislocation.

apotheter (a-poth′e-ter). Navel string repositor.

apotox′in. The anaphylactic substance due to action of toxogenin on injected toxin.

apotrip′sis. Removal of opacity in cornea.

apozem(e (ap′o-zēm). A decoction.

appara′tus. 1. A number of parts acting together in the performance of some special function. 2. A mechanical appliance or appliances, used in operations and experiments.

    a., acoustic. Auditory apparatus, the assemblage of parts essential for hearing.

    a., Clover's. A device used in administering ether or chloroform.

    a., Desault's. Desault's bandage.

    a., Fell-O'Dwyer's. An instrument for performing artificial respiration, and for preventing collapse of the lung in chest operations.

    a. ligamentosus colli. The occipito-axoid ligament.

    a. major. Median lithotomy.

    a. minor. Lateral lithotomy.

    a., sound conducting. Those parts of the acoustic apparatus that transmit sound.

    a., sound perceiving. Those central parts of the acoustic apparatus that are essential for the perception of sounds.

    a., vocal. The various organs collectively that subserve phonation.

appendal′gia. Pain in lower right quadrant in region of vermiform appendix.

appendectomy (ap-en-dek′to-mi). Surgical removal of the vermiform appendix.

appen′dical, appendi′ceal. Pert. to an appendix.

    a. reflex. Tenderness at McBurney's point accompanied by rigidity considered a reflex expression by way of sympathetic cerebrospinal arc.

appendicectasis (ap-pen-dis-ek′tă-sis). Appendical dilatation.

appendicectomy (ap-en-dis-ek′to-mi). Surgical removal of the appendix.

appendices epiploicae (ap-pen′dī-sēz ep-ip-lo′is-e). Pouches of peritoneum, filled with fat and attached to the colon.

appendicial (ap-pen-dis′ī-al). Pert. to the appendix. SYN: *appendical.*

appendicitis (ap-pen-di-si′tis). Inflammation of the vermiform appendix.

    a. obliterans, a., protective. Appendicitis with adhesions closing the appendical cavity.

appendico-enterostomy (ap-pen-dik-o-enter-os′to-mi). 1. Appendicostomy. 2. The establishment of an anastomosis bet. appendix and intestine.

appendicolithi′asis. Formation of calculi in the vermiform appendix.

appendicolysis (ap-pen-di-kol′ī-sis). Operation which frees appendix from adhesions by a slit in the serosa at its base.

appendicopathy (ap-pen-di-ko′path-ī). Any disease of the vermiform appendix.

    a. oxyurica. Lesion of the appendical mucosa supposedly due to oxyurids.*

appendico′sis. Noninflammatory state of the appendix. SYM: Dull pain, local soreness, afebrile, but continual discomfort.

appendicostomy (ap-pen-dik-os′to-mi). Operation for irrigating cecum and colon.

appendic′ular. 1. Appendical. 2. Pert. to limbs or that appended to another part.

appen′dix. An appendage.

    a., auricular. A forward prolongation of the heart-auricle.

    a., ensiform. The third or lowest portion of the sternum.

    a., gangrenous. When inflammation is extreme, blood vessels are blocked in the mesentery, circulation to appendix cut off, and diffuse peritonitis ensues.

    a. vermiformis (*appendix, vermiform* or *processus vermiformis*). A worm-shaped process projecting from the cecum, whose mucous membrane also lines the appendix, which contains many solitary glands. Its average length is 7.5 cm., and its position is variable. It secretes 1 to 2 cc. of fluid per day.

appen′dotome. An instrument for excision of appendix.

apperception (ap-per-sep′shun). The mental process whereby new knowledge is organized and interpreted in the light of past knowledge and experiences.

appercep′tive. Pert. to apperception.

ap′petence(y. An appetite or desire.

ap′petite. Desire, esp. for food; not necessarily hunger.

a. juice. Gastric secretion brought about by psychic causes such as sight or odor of food, and by tasting and chewing. It ceases 15 to 20 minutes after mastication is completed.

appeti′zer. That which promotes appetite.

applanatio (ap-plan-a′shĭ-o). A flattening, as the corneal surface.

a. cornea. Flattened cornea.

ap′ple-head. Dwarf's broad, thick skull.

applicator (ăp′lĭ-kā-tēr). Device, usually a slender rod of glass or wood, used with a pledget of cotton on the end, to apply medicine to the nose, throat, uterus, or any other body cavity.

apposi′tion. 1. Development by accretion. 2. Addition of parts. 3. Fitting together, as the edges of two surfaces.

approximal (a-proks′im-ăl). Contiguous; next to.

apraxia (a-praks′ĭ-ă). 1. Inability to perform certain purposive movements without loss of motor power, sensation, or coördination. 2. Ridiculous and out of the ordinary acts performed by the insane. Inability to understand the meaning of things.

a. algera. Induction of severe headache by a hysterical attack, thus preventing motion.

a., ideational. Misuse of objects due to failure to identify them.

a., motor. Inability to willfully perform acts.

aprication (ap-rĭ-ka′shun). 1. Sunstroke. 2. Sunbath. Basking in the sun.

aproctia (ă-prok′shĭ-ă). Imperforation or absence of anus.

aproctous (ă-prok′tus). Having an imperforate anus.

a′pron. Garment to cover front of the body, for protection of clothing during surgical operations, etc.

a., Hottentot. Hypertrophy of labia minora.

aprosex′ia. Unintentional inattention, esp. from defective hearing, sight, or mental weakness. Inability to concentrate on anything.

apselaphesia (ap-sel-af-e′zĭ-ă). Absence of tactile sense.

apsithyria, apsithurea (ăp-sith-ĭ′rĭ-ă, -u′re-ă). Hysterical loss of voice with inability to whisper.

apsychia (ăp-si′kĭ-ă). Unconsciousness; a faint.

apsychosis (ăp-si-ko′sis). Inability to think.

aptyalia, aptyalism (ap-ti-ă′lĭ-ă, -ti′al-izm). 1. Absence or deficiency of saliva. 2. A condition due to excessive expectoration through loss of oxydases.

apulosis (ap-u-lo′sis). A cicatrix.

apyetous (ă-pi′et-us). Nonsuppurative, nonpurulent.

apyknomorphous (ă-pik″no-mor′fus). Pert. to a cell which stains lightly as its stainable material is scattered.

apyogenous (ă-pi-oj′en-us). Not due to pus.

apyous (ă-pi′us). Without pus.

apyretic (ă-pi-ret′ik). Without fever. SYN: *afebrile.*

apyrexia (ă-pi-reks′ĭ-ă). 1. Absence of or intermission of fever. 2. Nonfebrile period of an intermittent fever.

apyrogenetic, apyrogenic (a-pi-ro-jĕ-net′-ĭk, -jen′ĭk). Not causing fever.

aqua (ak′wă) (pl. *aquae*). Water.

a. ammoniae. Water charged with ammonia and stimulants.

a. chlori. Water charged with chlorine for antisepsis and cleaning.

a. communis. Faucet water.

a. destillata. A water obtained by distillation.

a. fortis. Nitric acid.

a. labyrinthi. The fluid in the labyrinth of the ear.

a., medicated (water). An aqueous solution of a volatile substance. Usually contains only a comparatively small percentage of the active drug. Many of them are merely water saturated with a volatile oil. They are used more as vehicles and to give odor and taste to solutions. There are 14 official waters.

a. menthae piperitae. Peppermint water.

a. oculi. The fluid (aqueous humor) of the eye.

a. pura. Purified water.

a. re′gia. Nitrohydrochloric acid, nitromuriatic acid, *q.v.*, for F. A. Treatment.

a. rosae. Rosewater, used mainly as a flavor.

a. sedativa. Sedative lotion containing ammonia water and spirit of camphor.

a. vitae. Brandy.

aquacapsuli′tis. Serous iritis. SYN: *aquocapsulitis.*

aquaeductus (ak-we-duk′tus). A channel or canal to convey fluids.

a. cerebri. Canal lined with ciliated epithelium and going from the third ventricle through the mesencephalon to the fourth ventricle.

a. cochleae. Canal connecting subarachnoid space and the perilymphatic space of the cochlea.

a. Fallopii. Canal for facial nerve in petrous part of temporal bone.

a. Sylvii. Aquaeductus cerebri.

aquamedin (ak-wa-med′ĭn). A preparation from the isolation of a hormone from the ant. lobe of the pituitary gland which seems to control the water balance in the tissues as insulin controls the balance of sugar in the body.

aquapuncture (ak′wă-pungh′chur). 1. Injection of water hypodermically as a placebo. 2. A fine jet of water sprayed on the skin as a counterirritant.

aqueduct (ak′we-dukt). Canal or passage. SYN: *aquaeductus.*

a. vestibuli. Small passage reaching from the vestibule to the post. surface of the temporal bone's petrous section.

aqueous (ăk′wē-ŭs). Of the nature of water; watery.

a. chamber. Ant. chamber of the eye.

a. humor. Watery liquid, transparent, containing trace of albumin and small amount of salts. Produced by iris and ciliary body. Passes into post. chamber, then through *ligamentum pectinatum* (Fontana's spaces) and Schlemm's canal and passes into ant. ciliary veins.

aquiferous (ak-wif'er-us). Carrying water or lymph.

aquocapsuli'tis. Serous iritis.

arabinose (ar'ab-in-ōs). Gum sugar, a pentose, obtained from boiling gum arabic and 0.5 per cent sulfuric acid.

arabinosu'ria. Arabinose in the urine.

arachnidism (ar-ak'nid-izm). Systemic poisoning from spider bite.

arachnitis (ar-ak-ni'tis). Inflammation of the arachnoid membrane. SYN: *arach-noiditis, q.v.*

arachnodactyly (ar-ak-no-dak'til-ĭ). Spider fingers; a state in which fingers and sometimes toes are abnormally long, slender, and curved.

arachnoid (ar-ak'noid). Resembling a web.

a. cavity. (a) The space between the arachnoid membrane and the dura mater (*cavum subdurale*); (b) the space between the arachnoid membrane and the pia mater (*cavum subarachnoidale* or *subarachnoid space*). The latter contains the cerebrospinal fluid.

a. membrane (*arachnoidea encephali*). The middle (bet. the dura and pia mater) or serous membrane of the brain and spinal cord. SEE: *basiarachnitis.*

arachnoidea (ar-ak-noid'e-ă). A thin, fibrous, middle membrane covering the brain and spinal cord; *arachnoidea enceph'ali* and *arachnoidea spina'lis.*

arachnoiditis (ar-ak-noid-i'tis). Arachnitis; inflammation of the arachnoid membrane.

arachnopia (ar-ak-no'pĭ-ă). Pia and arachnoid considered as one membrane.

Aran-Duchenne's disease (ar-ahn-du-shens'). Muscular atrophy beginning in the upper extremities and progressing to other parts of the body.

araneous (ă-ra'ne-us). Arachnoid; resembling a cobweb.

Arantius's body, A.'s nodule (ar-an'shĭ-us). Nodule at center of free border of each of the six semilunar valves.

A.'s ventricle. Small sac on floor of fourth ventricle.

ar'bor vi'tae. ANAT: 1. A treelike structure; a treelike outline seen in a section of the cerebellum and the interior fold of the cervix. 2. A series of branching ridges within the cervix of the uterus.

arborescent (ar-bor-es'ent). Branching; treelike.

arborization (ar-bor-i-za'shun). Interlacing; ramification; applied to nerve process terminations, fibers, and arterioles. SEE: *nerve.*

arc re'flex. The arc or path of a reflex. Reflex resulting from impulse passing from point of stimulus along afferent nerve to spinal center and out along efferent nerve to point of activation.

arcade', Flint's. Vascular arch at base of renal pyramids.

arca'num. Secret remedy or nostrum.

arcate (ar'kăt). Arched, bow-shaped.

arch-, archi-. Prefix: First, principal, or chief. Beginning, as *archetype.*

arch, arches. Any structure or structures of a curved or bowlike outline.

a., abdominothoracic. The lower boundary of the front of the thorax.

a., alveolar. The arch of the alveolar process of either jaw.

a., ant. metatarsal. Formed by the inferior surfaces of the heads of the metatarsal bones of the foot.

a. of the aorta. Proximal curved part of aorta extending to 3rd dorsal vein.

a.'s, aortic. 1. Same as arch of the aorta. 2. Four pairs of cartilaginous arches of the fetus in the region of the neck.

a.'s of Corti. A series of arches made up of the rods of Corti.   [ligament.

a., crural. Femoral arch. Poupart's

a., deep crural. A band of fibers arching in front of the sheath of the femoral vessels.

a., dental. An arch formed by the alveolar process on either jaw, containing teeth and covered by the gums.

a.'s, embryonic. Fetal arches, the aortic, branchial, mandibular, hyoid, pulmonary, and thyrohyoid arches.

a., femoral. Poupart's ligament.

a., hemal. Arch formed by the body and processes of a vertebra, a pair of ribs and the sternum, or other like parts; also the sum of all such arches.

a., hyoid. The second fetal arch which persists in the styloid process, the stylohyoid ligament, and lesser cornu of the hyoid bone.

a., Langer's axillary. A thickened border of fascia forming a bridge across the occipital groove.

a., longitudinal. Formed by the bones, ligaments, and soft tissues of the medial aspect of the sole of the foot.

a., mandibular. The fetal arch whence are developed the jawbones, with the malleus and incus.

a., nasal. The arch formed by the nasal bones and by the nasal processes of the superior maxilla.

a., neural. The arch of a vertebra formed by its pedicles and laminae; also the sum of all such arches.

a., palmar. BNA. *arcus volaris. Deep,* an arch formed in the palm by the communicating branch of the ulnar and the radial artery. *Superficial,* an arch in the palm forming the termination of the ulnar artery.

a.'s, pharyngeal. The branchial arches of the fetus.

a., plantar. BNA. *arcus plantaris.* The arch formed by the external plantar artery and the dorsalis pedis.

a.'s, postaural. The branchial arches.

a., pubic. The portion of the pelvis formed by the rami of the ischia and the ossa pubis on either side.

a., pulmonary. The fifth of the aortic arches on the left side. It becomes the pulmonary artery.

a., stylohyoid. One of the embryonic arches made up of four segments, *viz.*: the pharyngobranchial, which develops into the styloid process, the epibranchial, developing into the stylohyoid ligament, the ceratobranchial and hypobranchial which together develop into the lesser cornu of the hyoid bone.

a., supraorbital. A bony arch formed by the prominent margin of the orbit.

a., thyroid. The third fetal arch; its cartilage is represented by the greater cornu of the hyoid bone.

a., transverse. Articulations (meta-tarsophalangeal) at ball of foot.

a. of a vertebra. The arching portion of a vertebra enclosing the spinal foramen.

a.'s, visceral. The fetal arches.

a., zygomatic. The arch formed by the malar and temporal bones.

archaic type of reaction. An inadequate immature reaction to reality; a reversion to a type once acceptable as normal (*e. g.*, in infancy).

archamphiaster (ark-am'fĭ-as″ter). Amphiaster formed when polar globules are extruded.

archebiosis (ar-ke-bi-o'sis). Spontaneous generation.

archegenesis (ar-ke-jen'e-sis). Generation spontaneously. SYN: *archebiosis.*

archenteron (ark-en'ter-on). Cavity formed by invagination of the blastodermic vesicle.

archeocyte (ar'ke-o-sīt). A wandering cell.

ar″cheokinet'ic. Pert. to a low and primitive type of motor nerve mechanism as found in the peripheral and ganglionic nervous systems. SEE: *neokinetic, paleokinetic.*

archepyon (ar-ke-pi'on). Unusually thick pus.

ar″chespore, ar″chespo'rium. Cells giving rise to mother cells of spores.

archetype (ar'ke-tip). Primitive type, from which other forms have developed by differentiation.

archiblast (ar'kĭ-blast). The outer layer which surrounds the germinal vesicle.

archiblas'tic. Derived from, or pert. to, the archiblast.   [sue.

archiblasto'ma. Tumor of archiblastic tis-

archigaster (ar-kĭ-gas'ter). The primitive embryonic alimentary canal.

archinephron (ar-kĭ-nef'ron). Primordial kidney, an organ of the embryo. SYN: *mesonephros, wolffian body.*

archineu'ron. The central cell of the cerebral cortex, and all its processes.

archipal'lium. Olfactory cortex, older than neopallium.

ar'chiplasm. The substance of the attraction sphere.

archistome (ar'kis-tōm). Invagination of blastula making little opening into archenteron. SYN: *blastopore.*

architis (ar-ki'tis). Inflammation of the anus; proctitis.

archocele (ar'ko-sēl). Hernia of the rectum.

archocystocolposyrinx (ar-ko-sis-to-kol-po-sir'inks). Fistula of rectum, vagina, and bladder.

archocystosyrinx (ar-ko-sis-to-sir'inks). Anovesical fistula.

ar'chon. Poisonous radical of all proteins.

archoptoma (ar-kop-to'mă). Prolapse of the rectum.

archoptosia (ar-kop-to'sĭ-ă). Prolapse of rectum. SYN: *archoptosis.*

arehoptosis (ar-kop-to'sis). Prolapse of rectum.

archorrhagia (ar-ko-ra'jĭ-ă). Hemorrhage from the rectum; archorrhea.

archorrhea (ar-kor-re'ă). Rectal hemorrhage.

archos (ar'kos). The anus.

archostenosis (ar-ko-sten-o'sis). Stricture of the rectum.

arc lamp. Source of light consisting of gaseous particles from the electrodes of an electric arc which are raised to a temperature of incandescence by an electric current.

arciform (ar'sif-orm). Bow-shaped.

arctation (ark-ta'shun). Stricture of any canal opening.

arcuate (ar'ku-āt). Bowed.

arcuation (ar-ku-a'shun). A bending.

arculus (ar'kū-lŭs). Support, in the form of an arch for bedclothes, to protect a part.

ar'cus. An arc or arch.

a. denta'lis. Dental arch.

a. plantaris. The plantar arch.

a. seni'lis. Opaque white ring about corneal periphery, seen in aged persons. Due to deposit of fat granules.

a. senilis, false. Has no diagnostic significance. Marked by a sharply delineated ring, yellow or yellowish white. Due to deposit of fat. Keratitis, ulcer, *q.v.*

ardanesthe'sia. Inability to feel heat.

ardent (ar'dent). Burning; feverish.

a. spirits. Distilled alcoholic liquors.

ar'dor. Burning; great heat.

a. urinae. A burning sensation during urination.

a. veneris. Sexual desire.

a. ventriculi. Heart burn; pyrosis.

area (a're-ă). A circumscribed space; one having definite boundaries. SEE: *McBurney's point, mesal, mesial.*

a., Broca's. Area in the left hemisphere in post. portion of inferior frontal convolution. Controls speech. In left-handed persons it is in the right hemisphere.

a. germinativa. Area of germination of the ovum.   [the occipital bone.

a., occipital. Portion of brain below

a. pellucida. Clear central portion of *area germinativa.*

a., rolandic. Area situated in ant. central convolution in front of fissure of Rolando in each hemisphere. Governs motor acts of the body.

areatus (a-re-a'tus). Occurring in circumscribed areas or patches.

arec'oline. Oily anthelmintic and miotic alkaloid derived from betel nut. DOSAGE: 0.05-0.1 gr. (0.003-0.006 Gm.).

areflex'ia. State without reflexes.

arenaceous (ar-ě-na'se-us). Resembling sand or gravel.

arenation (ar-ě-na'shun). A sand bath or application of hot sand.

arenoid (ar'e-noid). Like sand.

are'ola. 1. A cellular, highly fleecy connective tissue, with meshes capable of distention; a tissue occupying the interspaces of the body. 2. A form of macula* showing a hyperemic area about a skin lesion such as that about a boil. 3. A ringlike discoloration as that about the nipple.

    a. papilla'ris. The darkened ring about the female nipple.

    a., secondary. An additional ring surrounding the areola during pregnancy.

areolar (ar-e'o-lar). Rel. to the areola.

    a. tissue. Connective tissue which occupies the interspaces of the body.

areoli'tis. Inflammation of mammary areola.

areometer (a-re-om'e-ter). Instrument for measuring sp. gr. of fluids. [pact.

areosis (ar-e-o'sis). Dilution; less common.

arevareva (ar-e''va-ra'va). Severe skin disease accompanied by decay of vital powers.

argamblyopia (ar-gam-bli-o'pi-a). Amblyopia due to not using the eye.

Ar'gand burner. Gas or oil lamp having an inner tube by which air is supplied to the flame to increase combustion.

Argas (ar'gas). Genus of ticks usually infecting birds, but may attack man, causing severe pain, also fever.

ar'gema. White corneal ulcer.

argentaffine (ar-jent'af-fin). Taking a silver stain.

argentaffino'ma. Growth containing argentaffine elastic fibers.

    May be benign or malignant. Practically without symptoms unless pressing on neighboring structures.

argen'tum. SYMB: Ag. Silver; atomic weight 107.12.

argil'la. Clay.

argillaceous (ar-jĭl-a'shus). Resembling or composed of clay.

ar'ginase. Enzyme of the liver that splits up arginine and forms urea.

arginine (ar'jĭ-nēn). Crystalline amino acid, $C_6H_{14}N_4O_2$, obtained from decomposition of vegetable tissues, protamines, proteins and also prepared synthetically.

ar'gol, ar'gols. Impure cream of tartar formed in wine casks.

ar'gon. An inert gas in the atmosphere.

Argyll-Robertson pupil. More properly the name of a symptom often present in paralysis and locomotor ataxia, in which the light reflex is absent but there is no change in the power of contraction during accommodation.

argyria (ar-ji'rĭ-ă). Bluish discoloration of skin and mucous membranes as a result of the administration of silver.

argyri'asis. Bluish discoloration of skin due to use of silver. SYN: *argyria.*

argyric (ar-jir'ik). Pert. to silver.

argyrism (ar'jir-izm). Blush discoloration of skin due to use of silver. SYN: *argyria.*

argyrol (ar'jĭ-rol) (silver vitellin). A dark brown, crystalline, protein substance, containing 20% silver.

    DOSAGE: In strengths of 5% to 50% depending upon the condition.

argyrophil (ar-ji'ro-fĭl). Staining readily or easily impregnated with silver.

argyrosis (ar-ji-ro'sis). Bluish discoloration of skin due to use of silver. SYN: *argyria,* q.v.

arhyth'mia. Irregular heart action. SYN: *arrhythmia.*

    a., continuous. Permanent arhythmia.

    a., inotropic. Arhythmia caused by disorder of heart muscle's contraction.

    a., perpetual. SEE: *continuous arhythmia.*

    a., respiratory. Increase of heart action due to disorder of respiratory movements.

    a., sinus. Disorder of the impulses arising at the sinoauricular node causing heart action to be irregular.

arhythmic (ah-rith'mik). Pert. to arhythmia. SYN: *arrhythmic.**

ariboflavinosis (ă-ri-bō-flā''vĭn-ō'sĭs). Condition arising from a deficiency of riboflavin in the diet.

aridura (ar-ĭd-u'ră). Dryness, wasting, withering.

aristocar'dia. Cardiac deviation to the right.

aristogen'ics. Control of factors tending to improve the race. SYN: *eugenics.*

aristol (ă-ris'tol) (thymol-iodide). A reddish brown powder, with faint odor of iodine.

arithmomania (ar-ĭth-mo-ma'nĭ-ă). Repetition of consecutive numbers, unnecessary counting, and insane interest in numbers.

arkyochrome (ar'kĭ-o-krōm). A nerve cell in which the stainable substance is arranged in a network.

arkyostichochrome (ar''kĭ-o-stik'o-krōm). A nerve cell in which the stainable material is arranged both as a network and in parallel lines.

arm. The upper extremity from the shoulder to the elbow, which includes the *humerus,* the *ulna,* and the *radius.*

    a. center. Center in rolandic area controlling arm motion.

    a., golf. A form of neurosis seen in golf players after excessive exercise.

    a. hole. Armpit. SYN: *axilla.*

    a., Saturday-night. A form of paralysis of the brachial plexus, usually seen in drunkards. ETIOL: Sleeping in a chair, with the arm hanging over the back of the chair while the head rests on the shoulder or arm.

armamentarium (ar-mă-men-ta'rĭ-um). All that a physician or surgeon uses in his practice.

arm'ature. A part of a dynamo consisting of a coil of insulated wire mounted around a soft iron core.

armil′la. The annular ligament of the wrist.

arm′pit. Axilla. SEE: *hemorrhages, etc.*

arm-to-arm vaccination. Transferring vaccine virus from one patient to another.

ar′my itch. Chronic itch prevalent during U. S. Civil War.

Arneth's classification of neutrophiles (ar′neth). Based on the number of nuclear lobes which polynuclear neutrophiles contain. The normal are:

Lobes	1	2	3	4	5
%	5	35	41	17	2

A.'s formula. Method of procedure for elaborate differential blood count to estimate number of immature leukocytes. SEE: *formula.*

Ar′nold's canal. Passage in the temporal bone for small superficial petrosal nerve.

A.'s ganglion. Otic ganglion.

A.'s nerve. Auricular branch of vagus nerve.

aro′ma. An agreeable odor.

aromat′ic. 1. Having an agreeable odor. 2. Belonging to that series of carbon compounds in which the carbon atoms form closed rings (as in *benzene*) as distinguished from the *aliphatic* series in which the atoms form straight or branched chains.

a. compounds. Ring or cyclic compounds related to benzene, many having a fragrant odor.

a. spirits of ammonia. Contains about 35% ammonium carbonate in aromatic dilute alcohol.
DOSAGE: 2 cc. (30 ♏) freely diluted with water.

arrachment (ă-răsh-mon′). Pulling out the capsule in a membranous cataract, through a corneal incision.

arrec′tor muscles. Involuntary muscle fibers inserted in the hair follicles on the side toward which the hair slopes. Under the influence of cold or terror they contract, straighten the follicles, and raise the hairs, resulting in "gooseflesh," or *cutis anserina.*

arrecto′res pilo′rum. Muscles whose contractions cause "gooseflesh." SEE: *arrector muscles.*

arrhea (ar-re′ă). Suppression or cessation of a discharge.

arrhenoblastoma (a-re-no-blas-to′mă). An ovarian tumor made up of masculine sex cells and producing virile sex characteristics.

arrhythmia (ar-ith′mǐ-ă). Irregular heart action causing absence of rhythm.

arrhyth′mic. Signifying loss of rhythm.

arrosion (ar-o′shun). Ulcerous destruction of vessel walls.

ar′senfast. Resistant to the poisonous action of arsenic, esp. the spirochetes which acquire immunity after repeated arsenic administration.

arseni′asis. Chronic arsenical poisoning.

arsenic (ar′sen-ik). SYMB: As. Atomic weight, 74.93; atomic no., 33. A metal

of grayish white color, very poisonous, used in the manufacture of dyes and in medicine.

a. triox′ide. Used internally in form of Fowler's solution (Solution of Potassium Arsenite) 1%.
DOSAGE: 0.2 cc. (3 ♏) increased to 1.0 (15 ♏).

arsenic-fast. Resistant to toxic action of arsenic. SYN: *arsenfast.*

arsen′ical. Pert. to or of nature of arsenic or its compounds.

arsenicism (ar-sen′is-izm). Chronic arsenic poisoning. SYN: *arseniasis.*

arsenicophagy (ar-sen-ĭ-kof′ă-jĭ). Habitual eating of arsenic.

arsenioniza′tion. Electrolytic diffusion of arsenic ions in tissues.

arse′nium. Arsenic.

arsen′oblast. Male element in nucleus of impregnated ovum; a masculonucleus.

arsenoph′agy. Habitual eating of arsenic. SYN: *arsenicophagy.**

arsenorelap′sing. Pert. to syphilitic case which relapses after apparent cure by arsenic.

arsenoresis′tant. Resistant to arsenic compounds.

arsenother′apy. Treatment with arsenic and its compounds.

ar′senous. Of the nature of, or pert. to arsenic or its compounds. SYN: *arsenical.*

ar′sin. A very poisonous gas.

arsonvaliza′tion. Application of high frequency current.

arsphenamine (ars-fen-am′ĭn) (salvarsan). A light yellow powder containing about 30% arsenic.
DOSAGE: Intravenously, in 0.2 to 0.6 Gm. (3 to 9 gr.) doses.

ar′tefact. An unnatural structure or change due to manipulation, death, or reagents.

arterec′tomy. Excising an artery or arteries.

arte′ria (pl. *arteriae*). Artery.*

arteriag′ra. Pain in an artery.

arte′rial. Pert. to one or more arteries.

a. bleeding. Blood is bright red and pumped out. Arrest by pressure on proximal side of vessel (nearest heart).

a. circulation. It is maintained by the pumping of the heart; elasticity and extensibility of arterial walls; peripheral resistance in the areas of small arteries. and by the quantity of blood in the body. SEE: *circulation.*

a. varix. An enlarged and tortuous artery.

arterializa′tion. Aeration of the blood, changing it from venous into arterial.

arteriarctia (ar-te-rĭ-ark′tĭ-ă). Stenosis or constriction of an artery.

arteriasis (ar-te-rĭ′ăs-is). Degeneration of an artery.

arteriectasis, arteriectasia (ar-te-rĭ-ek′-tas-is, -tă′zĭ-ă). Arterial dilatation.

ar′terin. Coloring matter of arterial blood.

arterio-at′ony. Lack of tone in arterial walls.   [capillaries.

arteriocap′illary. Pert. to arteries and

a. fibrosis. Arteriosclerosis of capillaries and arterioles.

arteriofibro'sis. Arteriocapillary fibrosis.

arte'riogram. Recording of arterial pulse. SYN: *sphygmogram.*

arteriog'raphy. Description of arteries.

arterio'la. Small artery.

a. rec'ta. One of the small renal arteries going to the medullary pyramids.

arterioles (ar-te'ri-ole). The smallest arteries leading at their distal ends into the capillaries.

arte'riolith. An arterial calculus.

arteriol'ogy. Science of arteries, usually combined with study of other vessels, as in angiology.*

arterioisclero'sis. Thickening of the arterial walls with loss of elasticity and contractility.

arterioisclerot'ic. Rel. to arterioisclerosis.

arteriomala'cia. Softening of the arteries.

arteriom'eter. Instrument measuring variations in the size of a beating artery.

arteriomo'tor. Causing changes in size of arteries by dilatation and constriction.

arteriomyomatosis (ar-te'ri-o-mi-o-mă-to'sis). Thickening of arterial walls due to overgrowth of muscular fibers.

arterio"necro'sis. Arterial necrosis.

arter"iop'athy. Any disease of the arteries.

arterio"pla'nia. The presence of an anomalous course in an artery.

arterioplasty (ar-te'ri-o-plăs-tĭ). Repair of an aneurysm, restoring continuity of channel of the artery.

arteriopres'sor. Causing increased arterial blood pressure.

arteriorrhaphy (ar-te-rĭ-or'af-ĭ). Arterial suture.

arteriorrhexis (ar-te-rĭ-or-eks'ĭs). Rupture of an artery.

arterioisclero'sis. A degeneration and hardening of the walls of arteries, capillaries, or veins, due to chronic inflammation and resulting in fibrous tissue formation.

arterioisclerot'ic. Pert. to arterioisclerosis.*

arte'riospasm. Arterial spasm.

arteriosteno'sis. Contraction of the lumen of an artery, either temporary or permanent.

arteriosto'sis. Calcification of an artery.

arteriostrep'sis. Twisting of divided end of an artery to arrest hemorrhage.

arteriosympathec'tomy. Removal of arterial sheath containing fibers of sympathetic nerve.

arteriotome (ar-te'rĭ-o-tōm). Knife for opening an artery.

arteriotomy (ar-te-rĭ-ot'o-mĭ). Surgical division or opening of an artery.

arteriotony (ar-te-rĭ-ot'o-nĭ). 1. Blood pressure. 2. Intraärterial blood tension.

arteriove'nous. Rel. to both arteries and veins.

arteriover'sion. Everting wall of artery to arrest hemorrhage from open end.

arterioverter (ar-te-ri-ov'er-ter). An instrument for everting cut end of an artery for arresting hemorrhage.

arteri'tis. Inflammation of an artery.

a. defor'mans. Inflammation of inner coat of an artery. SYN: *chronic endarteritis.**

a. oblit'erans. Inflammation of intima of artery causing closure of vessel's lumen. SYN: *endarteritis obliterans.**

ar'tery. One of the vessels carrying blood from the heart to the tissues.

arthragra (ar-thra'gră). Seizure in the joints. SYN: *gout.*

ar'thral. Pert. to a joint.

arthralgia (ar-thral'jĭ-ă). Articular neuralgia. Pain in the joints.

arthrectomy (ar-threk'to-mĭ). 1. The operation of opening into a joint cavity with the object of removing dead or diseased tissue. 2. Excision of a joint.

arthredema (ar-thred-e'mă). Edema of a joint.

arthrempyesis (ar-threm-pĭ-ē'sis). Suppuration in a joint.

arthresthesia (ar-thres-the'zĭ-ă). Joint sensibility; the perception of articular motions.

arthric (ar'thrik). Pert. to a joint.

arthrifuge (ar'thrĭ-fūg). A remedy for gout.

arthritic (ar-thrit'ik). 1. Gouty. 2. Pert. to arthritis.   [aid arthritics.

arthriticin (ar-thrit'is-in). Preparation to

arthritide (ar'thrit-īd). A skin eruption assumed to be of gouty origin.

arthritis (ar-thri'tis). A joint affection characterized by inflammation and probably due to focal infection.

a., acute secondary. One caused by osteitis. SYM: Severe pain, redness, and swelling.

a., acute suppurative. Purulent distention of synovial sac; a serious form.

a., atrophic. One followed by atrophy.

a. deformans. One with deformity. SYM: Begins in fingers; develops progressively. Deformity due to ankylosis, exostosis, and atrophy of soft parts.

a. fungosa. Tuberculosis of a joint.

a., gonorrheal. One due to gonorrheal infection. SYM: Usually attacks knee joint; during acute stage several joints may be affected.

a., hypertrophic. Deformed enlargement of the cartilage at the edge of a joint.

a., pneumococcic. One sometimes appearing as a sequel to lobar pneumonia, affecting one or more joints, and the middle ear.

a., rheumatoid. A chronic joint disease, with enlarged cartilage and synovial membrane.

a., syphilitic. One due to acquired or hereditary syphilis. SYM: Enlarged, but not very painful joint.

a., tubercular. Arthritis involving epiphyseal cartilage, synovial membrane, and joint.

arthritism (ar'thrĭ-tizm). A condition or tendency to inflammation and gouty conditions of the joints and their processes. SEE: *oxypathia.*

arthro-. Prefix: Pert. to joints.

arthrobacte′rium. A bacterium which reproduces by segmentation or fission.

arthrocace (ar-throk′ă-se). Caries of a joint.

arthrocele (ar′thro-sēl). 1. Hernia of a synovial membrane, penetrating the capsule of a joint. 2. Any joint swelling.

arthrochondri′tis. Inflammation of an articular cartilage.

arthroclasia (ar-thro-kla′sĭ-ă). Breaking an ankylosed joint.

arthrodesis (ar-throd′es-is). The surgical fixation of a joint; artificial ankylosis.

arthrodia (ar-thro′dĭ-ă). Gliding joints articulating by surfaces which glide upon each other.

arthrodyn′ia. Pain in a joint.

arthroempye′sis. Suppuration in a joint. SYN: *arthrempyesis.**

arthroendos′copy. Inspection of interior of a joint by endoscope.

arthrog′raphy. A description of the joints.

arthrogryposis (ar″thro-gri-po′sis). 1. Persistent contracture of a joint. 2. Tetany.

arthrokleisis (ar-thro-kli′sis). Ankylosis,* both natural and surgical.

ar′throlith. Calculous deposit in a joint.

arthrology (ar-throl′o-jĭ). The science of joints.

arthrol′ysis. The operation of restoring mobility to an ankylosed joint.

arthromeningi′tis. Inflammation of a synovial membrane. SYN: *synovitis.*

arthrom′eter. Instrument for measuring the degree of movement of a joint.

ar′thron. An articulation or joint.

arthron′cus. 1. Tumor of a joint. 2. Swelling of a joint.

arthroneural′gia. Pain in a joint.

arthrono′sos. Joint disease.

a. defor′mans. Arthritis causing deformity. SYN: *arthritis deformans.**

arthropathol′ogy. Joint disease pathology.

arthropathy (ar-throp′ă-thĭ). Any joint disease.

a., Charcot′s. A trophic joint disease with effusion of fluids into a joint, seen in locomotor ataxia and in syringomyelia and sometimes in general paresis.

a., inflammatory. An inflammatory joint disease; arthritis.

a., osteopulmonary. Enlargement and swelling of the ends of the long bones following pulmonary disease.

a., static. A disturbance in a joint of a given extremity secondary to a disturbance in some other joint of the same extremity, as one in the right knee joint secondary to one in the right hip joint.

a., tabetic. Same as Charcot's arthropathy.

arthrophlysis (ar-throf′lis-is). An eczematous eruption occurring in rheumatic subjects.

arthrophyma (ar-thro-fi′mă). An articular swelling.

ar′throphyte. Abnormal growth in joint cavity.

arthroplasty (ar′thro-plas-tĭ). Surgical formation or reformation of a joint.

arthropyosis (ar-thro-pi-o′sis). Suppuration of a joint.

arthrorheu′matism. Rheumatism of the joints.

arthrosclero′sis. Stiffening or hardening of the joints, esp. in the aged.

arthro′sis. 1. Joint. 2. Joint affection due to trophic degeneration.

ar′throscope. An endoscope for examining interior of a joint.

arthros′copy. Direct point visualization by means of an arthroscope.

ar′throspore. A bacterial spore formed by segmentation; has greater resistance than an endospore.

arthrosteitis (ar-thros-te-i′tis). Inflammation of the bony structures of a joint.

arthros′tomy. The formation of a temporary opening into a joint for drainage purposes.

arthrosynovi′tis. Inflammation of synovial membrane of a joint.

arthrous (ar′thrus). Jointed or pert. to a joint.

arthrotome (ar′thro-tōm). Knife for making incisions into a joint.

arthrotomy (arth-rot′o-mĭ). Cutting into a joint.

arthroxesis (ar-throx-e′sis). Scraping a joint.

ar′tiad. CHEM: An element of an even numbered valence. SEE: *perissad.*

artic′ular. Pert. to articulation.

artic′ulate. 1. To join together as a joint. 2. To adjust artificial teeth properly. 3. Clearly spoken. 4. To speak clearly.

artic′ulated. State of articulation or of being jointed.

articula′tion. The connection of bones; joints.

a., confluent. Speech in which syllables are not clearly enunciated.

artic′ulatory. Rel. to articulation (3.), *q.v.*

artic′ulo mor′tis. At the time of death.

articulus (ar-tik′u-lus). 1. A knuckle or a joint. 2. A segment.

artifi′cial. Not natural; formed in imitation of nature. SEE: *feeding.*

a. hyperemia. A method to bring blood to the superficial tissues by means of "cups," and elastic bandage, or unctions.

a. pneumothorax (nu-mo-thor′aks). Artificial introduction of air into pleural cavity. Oxygen or nitrogen, or filtered atmospheric air is used. SEE: *pneumothorax.*

artifi′cial respira′tion. Maintenance of respiratory movements by artificial means in cases of suspended breathing; resuscitation.

ar′tisan's cramp. A spasmodic affection of the muscles induced by prolonged work requiring delicate coördination and occurring only in performance of that particular work.

artus (ar′tus). A joint or joints; a limb.

aryepiglottic (ar-ĭ-ep-ĭ-glot′ĭk). Pert. to the arytenoid cartilage and epiglottis.

ar′yl. A prefix denoting a radical of the aromatic series.

a. group. In chemistry, a radical

group of the aromatic or benzene series.

arylarsonate (ar-ĭ-lar'so-nāt). Salt of arylarsonic acid.

arytenoid (ar-it'en-oid). 1. Pert. to *arytenoid cartilages* (two), which regulates tension of vocal bands. 2. Funnel or pitcher-shaped.

arytenoidectomy (ar-it″e-noy-dek'to-mĭ). Excision of arytenoid cartilage.

arytenoid'itis. Inflammation of arytenoid cartilage.

As. 1. Abbr. for *astigmatism*. 2. Symb: *arsenic*.

a. s. Abbr. *left ear*.

asafetida (as-e-fet'id-a). USP. A gum resinous substance with characteristic odor and taste.

Dosage: 0.4 Gm. (6 gr.) in pill form or an emulsion as an enema of 1 dram to 100 cc. water.

asaphia (as-af'ĭ-ă). Inability to articulate properly due to cleft palate.

asarcia (ă-sar'sĭ-ă). Leanness; emaciation.

asbes'tiform. Having structure similar to asbestos.

asbes'tos. Fibrous form of magnesium and calcium silicate.

asbesto'sis. Lung disease due to protracted inhalation of asbestos particles.

ascariasis (as-kar-ĭ'as-is). Symptoms produced by gastrointestinal worms (*ascarides*, round and thread worms).

ascar'ides. Pl. of *Ascaris.**

ascaridiasis (as-kar-ĭ-dĭ'ă-sis). Ascarides in intestine and symptoms they cause.

Ascaris (as'kar-is). [Pl. *ascarides*]. A nematode worm belonging to the family Ascaridae, and commonly infesting the intestinal canal. See: *ascariasis*.

    A. lumbricoides. The round worm.

    A. vermicularis. The thread worm.

Aschheim-Zondek test (ash'him-tson'dĕk). A test for pregnancy. See: *test*.

Asch'ner's phenomenon. Slowing of the pulse caused by eyeball pressure.

Aschoff's bodies (ahsh'of). Rheumatic nodules in the myocardium; also in lungs in rheumatic fever complicated by pneumonia.

    A.'s node. Atrioventricular node.

ascia (a'sĭ-ă, as'kĭ-ă). Spinal bandage without reverse, each turn overlapping the previous one for a third of its width.

ascites (ă-si'tez). A collection of serous fluid in the peritoneal cavity.

    a. chylosus. Chyle in the ascitic fluid.

ascit'ic. Pert. to ascites.

    a. fluid. Sp. gr. 1.005-1.015, clear and pale, straw color with greenish tinge in some cases.

Ascoli's reaction (ahs-ko'lĭs). 1. Precipitation test for anthrax. 2. Miostagmin reaction.*

as'cospore. Spores within an *ascus,** or sac.

as'cus. A spore case; a sac containing spores.

-ase. A suffix to the name of a substance upon which an enzyme acts, as *lipase* (from lipoid), a fat-splitting enzyme, or when added to a word to indicate its

action upon some other substance, as *oxidase*, indicating a catalytic ferment.

ase'mia, asema'sia. Inability to comprehend any type of symbol. See: *asymbolia*.

asepsin (ă-sep'sin). An antiseptic analgesia, antipyretic drug. Syn: *antisepsin*.

asep'sis. A condition free from germs; free from infection; sterile, free from any form of life. See: *antisepsis, antiseptics, sterile, sterilization.*

asep'tic. Rel. to asepsis; free from septic matter.

asep'tic-antisep'tic. Both aseptic and antiseptic.

asep'ticize. To make sterile; to free from pathogenic matter.

asex'ual. Without sex; nonsexual See: *parthenogenesis.*

asexualization (ah-seks-u-al-iz-a'shun). Ablation of the ovaries or testes and in this manner desexing the individual.

ash (ăsh). Incombustible, powdery residue of an organic substance that has been burned.

    Residue from food digested in the body is either alkaline or acid.

asialia (as-ĭ-a'lĭ-ă). Failure to secrete saliva or deficiency of it.

Asiat'ic cholera. An epidemic, acute infectious disease. See: *cholera.*

asidero'sis. Deficiency of iron in the circulating blood.

asitia (a-sish'ĭ-ă). 1. Aversion to food. Syn: *anorexia.** 2. The want of food.

asonia (ă-so'nĭ-ă). Tone deafness.

aspastic (ă-spas'tik). Nonspastic.

as'pect. 1. That part of a surface looking in any designated direction. 2. Appearance, looks.

aspermat'ic. Pert. to aspermatism.

aspermatism (a-sper'mă-tizm). Lack of formation of spermatozoa due to defective secretion of semen; aspermia.

asper'mia. Lack of or failure to ejaculate semen.

asper'mous. Pert. to aspermia. Syn: *aspermatic.*

as'perous. Uneven; having minute elevations.

asper'sion. Sprinkling an affected part with water; a form of hydrotherapy.*

asphalgesia (as-fal-je'zĭ-ă). A burning sensation and convulsions sometimes felt during hypnosis on touching certain articles.

asphyctic, asphyctous (as-fik'tik, -tus). 1. Asphyxiated. 2. Without pulse.

asphyxia (ăs-fĭk'sĭ-ă). 1. Suspended animation in living organisms due to interference with the oxygen supply of the blood. 2. Suspension of the pulse beat. 3. Cyanosis due to interference with circulation. May be general or local.

    a. carbonica. Suffocation from inhalation of coal or water gas.

    a. livida. When there is difficulty in breathing, but the superficial reflexes are present.

    a., local. The congested stage of Raynaud's disease.

    a. neonatorum. Imperfect breathing in the new born child.

a. pallida. When difficulty in breathing is accompanied by weak and thready pulse, pale skin, and absence of superficial reflexes. This is the most serious type.

a., traumatic. Discoloration of the head and neck due to compression of the trunk.

asphyx′ial. Pert. to asphyxia; asphyctic.

asphyx′iant. An agent, especially any gas that will produce asphyxia. [asphyxia.

asphyx′iate. To cause asphyxiation, or

asphyx′ia″tion. A state of asphyxia or suffocation. Act of producing asphyxia. SEE: *asphyxia.*

aspidium (as-pid′i-um) (Male fern) USP. The dried root of *filix-mas*, used only in form of oleo-resin.
    DOSAGE: 4 Gm. once daily according to condition of patient.

as′pirate. 1. Aspiration; to remove by suction. 2. A sound like that of the letter *h*.

aspiration (as-pir-a′shun). 1. To draw in or out as by suction. Foreign bodies may be aspirated into the nose, throat, or lungs on inspiration. 2. The withdrawing of a fluid from a cavity by means of suction with an instrument called an aspirator.

aspirator (as′pir-a-tor). 1. Apparatus for evacuating fluid contents of a cavity. 2. Instrument used in chemical analysis of gases.

aspirin (as′pir-ĭn). Commercial name of acetylsalicylic acid. POISONING: Due to hypersusceptibility, or to large doses.
    DOSAGE: 5 gr. (0.3 Gm.).

asporogen′ic. Not reproducing by spores.

asporous (ă-spor′us). Having no spores.

assafet′ida, assafoet′ida. A resinous substance used as a carminative and antispasmodic in hysteria. SEE: *asafetida.*

assana′tion. Improvement of sanitary conditions.

assault′, crim′inal. Cohabitation without consent is always legal rape, but even with consent, if the victim is insane, it is legally considered rape.

asses′ milk. Average serving, 245 grams. Pro. 4.9, Fat 3.7, Carbo. 14.9.

assident (as′ĭd-ent). Usually associated with a disease, as *assident* symptoms.

assimilable (as-sim′il-a-bl). Capable of assimilation.

assim′ilate. To absorb digested food.

assimila′tion. The processes whereby the products of digestion are changed to resemble the chemical substances of the body tissues, first passing through the lacteals and blood vessels; transformation of food into living tissue.

assisting patient to walk. Aiding an injured or convalescent patient to walk by means of support. SEE: *transportation.*

asso′ciated movements. Synchronous correlation of 2 or more muscles (or muscle groups) which, though apparently not essential for the performance of some function, nevertheless, normally accompany it, as the swinging of arms accompanies normal walking.

asso′ciation ar′eas. Small islands in the brain surrounded by cerebral tissue known as motor and sense areas or association areas, as association fibers connect the motor and sense areas.

a. center. One controlling associated movements.

a., controlled. An idea suggested by a word uttered by the physician.

a. of ideas. The linking together in a memory chain of two or more ideas associated by some similiarity, relationship, or by both having been experienced at the same time.

a. neuron. A neuron which transmits impulses from afferent to efferent neurons.

assonance (as′o-nans). Abnormal impulse to use alliteration.

assuetude (as′wē-tūd). 1. Becoming habituated to conditions. 2. Acquiring tolerance of a drug until it loses its effect.

as′surin. Complex substance occurring in brain tissue.

astasia (as-ta′sĭ-ă). Motor incoördination instanding.

a. abasia. Combined incoördination for standing or walking. PSY: A mental conflict making it difficult to stand or walk without swerving or swaying.

asteatosis (as′te-ă-to′sis). Any disease condition in which there is scantiness or absence of the sebaceous secretion.

a. cutis. A dry, fissured condition of the skin together with deficient secretion.

as′ter. The stellate rays forming round the dividing centrosome* during mitosis.*

astereognosis (a-ster-e-og-no′sis). Inability to recognize objects or forms by touch.

aste′rion. A craniometric point at occipital, parietal, and temporal bones.

aster′nal. Not connected with the sternum

asteroid (as′ter-oid). Star-shaped.

asthenia (as-the′nĭ-ă). Lack or loss of strength; debility. Any weakness, but one esp. originating in muscular or cerebellar disease.

a., neurocirculatory. A condition due to excessive stimulation of the adrenal-sympathetic system frequently seen in soldiers.

asthenic (as-then′ik). Weak; pert. to asthenia.

a. body type. A thin, more or less tall person with flat chest, accompanied by inferior muscular development, who centers his interest in his inner self Usually an introvert.* SEE: *pyknic type*

asthenometer (as-the-nom′ĕ-ter). An instrument for determining loss of strength.

as′thenope. One affected with weak sight

astheno′pia. Weakness or tiring of eyes due to fatigue of ciliary muscle or extraocular muscles. Painful vision.

a., accommodative. Refractive errors such as hyperopia and astigmatism.

a., muscular. Anomalies of external muscles.

a., nervous. Hysteria and neurasthenia.

a., photogenous. Excessive or improper illumination.

a., reflex. Disease in other organs, as nose, sinuses, teeth.

asthenop'ic. Rel. to asthenopia.

asthenox'ia. Deficient oxygenation of waste products.

asthma (az'mä). Paroxysmal dyspnea accompanied by the adventitious sounds caused by a spasm of the bronchial tubes or due to swelling of their mucous membrane.

a., cardiac. Dyspnea due to heart disease.

a. convulsivum, a., bronchial, a., dyspeptic. Asthma due to a nervous reflex.

a., hay. Hay fever, *q.v.*

a., renal. Occurring in Bright's disease.

a., thymic. Due to enlargement of the thymus. The attacks are sudden and may prove fatal (status lymphaticus).

asthmat'ic. Pert. to or of the nature of asthma.

astigmatic (as-tig-mat'ik). Pert. to or afflicted with astigmatism.

astig'matism. Form of ametropia in which refraction of several meridians of eyeball is different, usually due to change in curvature of cornea and lens.

astigmat'oscope. Instrument which detects and measures astigmatism.

astigmatos'copy. Use of the astigmatoscope.

astigmometer (ah-stig-mom'ĕ-ter). An instrument for measuring astigmatism.

asto'matous, as'tomous. Without mouth or oral aperture.

astragalar (as-trag'ă-lar). Pert. to the astragalus.

astragalectomy (as-trag-al-ek'to-mĭ). Excision of astragalus.

astragalus (as-trag'al-us). BNA *Talus.* A bone of the foot which articulates with the tibia and fibula above, and with the calcaneum (os calcis) below. The ankle bone. SEE: *sustentaculum.*

astraphobia (as-tra-fo'bĭ-ă). Anxiety and terror of thunderstorms.

astrict'. 1. To contract or *constrict*, as the action of an astringent. To *compress*, as an artery in a hemorrhage. 2. To constipate.

astriction (a-strik'shun). Contraction; compression; constriction.

astring'ent. 1. Styptic. 2. Agent checking secretion of mucous membranes and which contracts and hardens tissues, limiting secretion of glands.

a. enema. One given to contract intestinal tissue and to provoke subsequent evacuation of worms. SEE: *enema.*

a., mineral. They coagulate the albumins when applied to wounds or mucous surfaces, protecting them and making healing possible. They also stop bleeding. In the digestive tract they check secretions and lessen peristalsis, creating constipation.

astro-. Prefix: A star or star-shaped.

as'troblast. Primitive cell which develops into an astrocyte.

astroblasto'ma. Tumor composed of astroblasts.

as'trocyte. 1. Star-shaped cell forming the neuroglia fibers. 2. Star-shaped bone corpuscle.

astrocyto'ma. Tumor formed from astrocytes.

astrog'lia. Astrocytes making up neuroglia tissue.

astrokinet'ic motions. Movements of centrosome.*

astropho'bia. Morbid fear of stars and celestial space.

astrosphere (as'tro-sfēr). Small body in the nucleus considered an independent and indispensable cell constituent.

astrostat'ic. Pert. to astrosphere in its resting condition.

Astu'rian rose. Pellagra; a disease characterized by a rosy rash on the body. SEE: *pellagra.*

astysia (ă-stiz'ĭ-ă). An inability to fully (normally) erect the penis.

asurre'nalism. Deficient suprarenal function.

asyllabia (ă-sil-a'bĭ-ă). Recognition of letters but not syllables or words.

asy'lum. An institution for the care of those unable to care for themselves, as the infirm, the aged, the insane, the blind.

a. ear. Bloody tumor of ear found in the insane. SYN: *hematoma auris.**

asymbo'lia. Inability to comprehend words, gestures, or any type of symbol; asemia. Sensory aphasia.

asymmetry (ă-sim'et-rĭ). Lack of symmetry of parts or organs on opp. sides of body.

asymphytous (ă-sim'fĭt-us). Not grown together.

asymptomat'ic. Without symptoms.

asyn'chronism (ah-sin'klit-ism). Lack of concurrence in time.

asynclitism (ah-sin'klit-ism). GYN: An oblique presentation of the fetal head.

a., Litzmann's. Where the post. parietal bone of the fetal head presents.

a., Naegele's. Where the ant. parietal bone of the fetal head presents.

asynergia, asynergy (a-sin-er'jĭ-ă, -jĭ). Lack of coördination between muscle groups. Movements are in serial order instead of being made together. Seen in cerebellar diseases.

asynesia (a-sĭn-e'zĭ-a). Stupidity.

asyn'dia. Sexual impotence.

asynovia (ă-sin-o'vĭ-ă). Lack of or insufficient secretion of synovial fluid of a joint.

asystemat'ic. Diffuse; not limited to one system or set of organs.

asystole, asystolia (ă-sis'to-le, -to'lĭ-ă). Faulty contraction of ventricles of the heart.

asystolism (ă-sis'tol-izm). Retention of contents of the right ventricle of the heart seen in last stages of mitral incompetence.

atabrin(e (at′ă-brin). Commercial preparation used in treatment of malaria.
DOSAGE: 1½ gr. (0.1 Gm.) three times a day for 3 days. SYN: *atebrin.*

atactic (at-ak′tik). Incoördinate, irregular, as muscular incoördination, esp. in aphasia.   [ataxia.

atactiform (ă-tak′tĭ-form). Similar to

atactilia (ă-tak-til′ĭ-ă). Inability to recognize tactile impressions.

atarax′ia, a′taraxy. Imperturbability.

atavico′sis. Intestinal degeneration from eating highly concentrated foods.

atavism (ăt′ă-vĭzm). 1. Recurrence of characteristics of a remote ancestor, after remaining latent for 1 or more generations. 2. Reappearance, in a descendant, of a disease or abnormality experienced by a remote ancestor. A reversion to an original type.

atavis′tic. Pert. to atavism.*

ataxaphasia (at-aks-ă-fa′zĭ-ă). Inability to arrange words in sentences.

ataxaphemia (at-aks-a-fe′mĭ-ă). Lacking in lingual coördination.

ataxia (a-taks′i-a). Motor incoördination manifest during a purposive movement by irregularity and lack of precision.

　　a., alcohol. Ataxia seen in drinkers, caused by peripheral neuritis.

　　a., autonomic. Incoördination bet. sympathetic and parasympathetic nervous systems.

　　a., Briquet's. Hysteria with skin and leg muscle anesthesia.

　　a., cerebellar. Muscular incoördination due to cerebellar disease.

　　a., choreic. Lack of muscular coördination seen in persons with chorea.

　　a., hereditary cerebellar. Disease of late adolescence. ETIOL: Atrophy of cerebellum. SYN: Ataxia gait, hesitating and explosive speech, nystagmus, and sometimes optic neuritis.

　　a., hereditary spinal. Friedreich's disease.* Sclerosis of the post. and lateral columns of spinal cord; occurs in children. SYN: Ataxia in lower extremities, extending to upper; paralysis and contractures follow.

　　a., hysterical. Ataxia of leg muscles due to hysteria.

　　a., intrapsychic. A state in which emotional expressions appear to have no logical bases or relationship, other than those found in the Unconscious.

　　a., locomotor. A sclerosis affecting the post. columns of spinal cord, most commonly due to syphilis.

　　a., Marie's. Hereditary cerebellar ataxia.*

　　a., motor. Lack of ability for proper coördination of muscles.

　　a., spinal. Due to spinal cord disease, as in locomotor ataxia.*

　　a., static. Loss of deep sensibility causing inability to preserve equilibrium in standing.

　　a., thermal. Condition in which body temperature changes irregularly.

　　a., vasomotor. Form of autonomic ataxia.*

ataxiadynamia (ă-taks″ĭ-ad-ĭ-nam′ĭ-ă). Muscular weakness in combination with incoördination.

atax′iagram. Ataxiagraph record or tracing.

ataxiagraph (ă-taks′ĭ-a-graf). Instrument measuring swaying in ataxia.

ataxiam′eter. Apparatus measuring ataxia.

ataxiamnesia (at-aks′ĭ-am-ne′zĭ-ă). Suffering from muscular ataxia and amnesia.

atax′ic, atax′ial. Pert. to, or marked by, ataxia.

ataxoadynamia (at-aks-o-ă-dĭ-nam′ĭ-ă). Ataxia associated with muscular weakness.   [muscles.

ataxophe′mia. Incoördination of speech

ataxopho′bia. Morbid dread of ataxia.

a′taxy. Lack of muscular coördination. SYN: *ataxia.*

-ate. CHEM: Ternary acids, the names of which end in ic, take the ending *ate* to indicate salts formed from them. SEE: *-ide, -ite.*

atebrin(e (at′ĕ-brin). Proprietary drug used to treat malaria.
DOSAGE: 1½ gr. (0.1 Gm.) three times a day for 3 days. SYN: *atabrin.*

atelectasis (at-e-lek′tă-sis). Lack of air in the lungs as in a fetus, or in a portion of an adult lung due to pleural effusion exerting pressure, and blocking the small bronchial tubes.

atelia (at-e′lĭ-ă). The retention of childish characteristics in the adult.

atelic (at′el-ik). Without function.

ateliosis (ă-tĕ-lĭ-o′sis). A form of infantilism due to pituitary causes in which growth may be arrested without deformity. The voice and face may resemble those of a child.

ateliot′ic. Infantile.

atelo-. Prefix: Imperfect development.

athermic, athermous (ă-ther′mĭk, -mus). Without fever.

athermosystaltic (ath-er-mo-sis-tal′tĭk). Not contracting under ordinary temperature variations, said of striated muscle.

atheroma (ath-e-ro′mă). 1. A sebaceous cyst. 2. Fatty degeneration or thickening of the wall of the larger arteries. SEE: *arteriosclerosis.*

atheromasia (ath-er-o-ma′zĭ-ă). Atheromatous degeneration.

atheromatosis (ath-er-o-mă-to′sis). Generalized atheromatous condition.

atheromatous (ath-er-o′mă-tus). Pert. to atheroma.

atheronecro′sis. Necrosis or degeneration accompanying arteriosclerosis.

atherosclero′sis. Senile type of arteriosclerosis characterized by atheromatous degeneration of walls of arteries.

athero′sis. Fatty degeneration of arterial walls.

athetoid (ath′e-toid). 1. Similar to athetosis. 2. Affected with athetosis.

athetosis (ath-ĕ-to′sis). Slow, repeated, involuntary, purposeless, vermicular, muscular distortion involving part of a limb, toes, and fingers or almost the entire body.

ath′lete's foot. Infection of skin of foot by *Tinea microsporon* or *T. megalosporon.*

ath′lete's heart. Incompetence of the aortic valves.

athlet′ic in′juries. SEE: *Under nature of injury, as abrasion, burn, Charley horse, contusion, fracture, golf arm, sprain, strain, tennis elbow, etc.*

athrepsia, athrepsy (a-threp′sĭ-ă, -ĭ). Malnutrition, marasmus.*

athreptic (ath-rep′tĭk). Marasmic; pert. to or afflicted with athrepsia.

athrom′bia. Defective blood clotting.

athymia (ă-thi′mĭ-ă). 1. Confusional insanity; amentia. 2. Without emotion. 3. Lack of thymus gland or its secretion.

athymic (ath-i′mĭk). Pert. to athymia.

athy′mism. Absence of thymus gland or its secretions. SYN: *athymia* (3).

athyrea (a-thi′re-ă). A condition due to the absence of the thyroid gland or insufficiency, or suppression of its function resulting in imperfect development of the physical and mental tissues of the body.

athyreo′sis. Condition due to absence of thyroid gland or its secretions, causing imperfect development. SYN: *athyria.**

athyria (a-thi′rĭ-ă). Absence of thyroid gland or its secretions, causing imperfect development. SYN: *athyrea.*

athy″roide′mia. Morbid condition of blood due to absence of thyroid gland or its secretions.

athyroidism (ă-thi′roy-dĭzm). Suppression of thyroid secretions, or absence of the thyroid gland; athyrea.

atlan′tad. Toward the atlas.

atlan′tal. Pert. to the atlas.

at′las. The first cervical vertebra by which the head articulates with the occipital bone, so called because of Atlas who was supposed to support the world on his shoulders. SEE: *atlantal, atloaxoid.*

atloaxoid (at-lo-aks′oid). Pert. to atlas and axis.

atmiat′rics, atmi′atry. Treatment of respiratory disease by medicated vapors.

atmic (at′mik). Consisting of or pert. to vapor.

atmo-. Prefix: Breath, vapor, steam.

atmocau′sis. Application of superheated steam; substitute for uterine curettage.

atmocautery (at-mo-kaw′ter-ĭ). Device for cauterization with steam.

atmograph (at′mo-graf). A spirograph. Device for tracing respiratory movements.

atmometer (at-mom′e-ter). Instrument for measuring exhalations.

at′mos. A unit of air pressure; one dyne per one sq. cc.

at′mosphere. 1. The gases surrounding the earth to the height of 200 miles. 2. Climatic condition of a locality. 3. PHYSICS: Pressure at sea level of the atmosphere—14.7 lbs. to the sq. in. 4. CHEM: Any gaseous medium around a body.

atmospher′ic. Pert. to the atmosphere.

atmospheriza′tion. Process of transforming venous into arterial blood.

atmother′apy. 1. Treatment of disease by medicated vapors. SYN: *atmiatrics.** 2. Treatment by some method of condensing air.

atocia (at-o′sĭ-ă). Female sterility.

at′om. The smallest particle of an element that can exist and take part in a chemical change, retaining its identity, and which cannot further be divided without change of its structure.

atom′ic. Pert. to an atom or atoms.

atom′ic the′ory. Formulated by Dalton, who taught that all matter is composed ultimately of atoms.

atom′ic weight. The weight of different atoms as compared with that of *hydrogen*, which is the lightest, and is represented as 1. The heaviest known is that of *uranium. Oxygen* is 16.

atomicity (at-om-is′ĭ-tĭ). 1. Chemical valence or combining power. 2. Number of hydroxyl groups in an alcohol, or in a base.

atomiza′tion. Converting a fluid into form of a spray.

a′tomize. To reduce a liquid to the form of a spray or a vapor.

atomizer (at′om-i-zer). Apparatus for changing jet of liquid to a spray.

atonic (a-ton′ik). Without tension or tone; relaxed.

atonicity (at-ŏ-ne′ĭ-tĭ). State of being atonic, or without tone.

atony (at′o-nĭ). Debility; or lack of normal tone.

   a., gastric. Lack of muscle tone in stomach and failure to contract normally, causing slow movement of food out of stomach. Secondary to certain diseases.

at′open. An allergen, exciting cause of any form of idiosyncrasy or hypersensitiveness.

atophan (a′to-fan). Analgesic and antipyretic drug. SEE: *cinchophen.*

   DOSAGE: 8 gr. (0.5 Gm.).

atop′ic. Pert. to atopy.* Displaced; misplaced.

atopognosis (at-o-pog-nō′sis). An inhibited sense of touch or feeling, the victim not being able to know where one has touched his skin.

atopomenorrhea (at-op-o-men-or-e′ă). Periodic hemorrhage from any part of the female body other than the uterus; vicarious menstruation.

at′opy. 1. Hereditary allergic disease. 2. The many forms of hypersensitivity or idiosyncrasies.

atox′ic. Nonpoisonous.

atrabil′iary. Melancholic.

   a. capsules. Suprarenal capsules.

atremia (at-re′mĭ-ă). Absence of trembling or tremor.   [cells.

atrepsy (ă′trep-sĭ). Immunity to tumor

atre′sia. Pathological closure of a normal anatomical opening or congenital absence of the same, esp. that of the esophagus. SEE: *gynatresia.*

atre'sic. Imperforate; pert. to atresia.

atretic (a-trĕt'ĭk). Imperforate, closed. SYN: *atresic.*

atreto-. Prefix: Imperforate.

atretogastria (ă-tret-o-gas'trĭ-a). Gastric imperforation.

atreturethria (ă-tret-u-re'thrĭ-ă). Urethral imperforation.

a'tria. Pl. of atrium.

atrial (a'trĭ-al). Pert. to an atrium.

atrichia (ă-trik'ĭ-ă). Absence of hair.

atrichosis (ă-tri-ko'sis). Having no hair, atrichia.*

atri'chous. Being without flagella.

atrionector (a'trĭ-o-nek'tor). Sinoauricular node of Keith.*

at'riotome. Instrument which cuts connections between the cardiac auricle and ventricle.

atrioventric'ular. Pert. to both auricle and ventricle.

atriplicism (ă-trip'lĭ-sizm). Poisoning due to eating one form of spinach, *At'riplex littora'lis.* SEE: *allantiasis.*

a'trium (pl. *a'tria*). 1. A cavity or sinus. 2. BNA: Cardiac auricle, the upper chamber of each half of the heart. 3. Portion of tympanic cavity lying below the malleus. 4. Site of entrance of bacteria causing an infectious disease. SEE: *auricle, heart.*

   a. of lungs. The place of entry and termination of a bronchiole, each atrium having a series of alveoli or air cells, thus increasing surface exposed to air.

   a. of ventricle. That part of a lateral ventricle connected with temporal and occipital cornua. SEE: *atria, atrial.*

atro'phia. Wasting of a part from lack of nutrition. SYN: *atrophy.*

atrophic (a-tro'fĭk). Pert. to, or marked by, atrophy.

atrophied (ă'tro-fēd). Wasted. Afflicted with atrophy.

atrophoderma (ăt-rō-fō-der'mă). Cutaneous atrophy.

   a. pigmentosum. Rare skin disease characterized by ulcers, disseminated pigment discolorations, etc. SYN: *xeroderma pigmentosum, q.v.*

atrophodermato'sis. Any skin disease which has atrophied skin as a sym.

at'rophy. A wasting due to lack of nutrition of any part.

   a., acute yellow. Extensive degeneration of liver cells with jaundice, mental disturbances, and cutaneous hemorrhages.

   a., Buchwald's. Progressive wasting of the skin.

   a., compression. Compression of a part causing atrophy.

   a., correlated. Wasting of a part following destruction of another part.

   a., Cruveilhier's. Progressive wasting of the muscles.

   a. of disuse. Atrophy from failure to normally use a part.

   a., Hoffman's. Progressive muscular wasting, in the legs, hands, and forearms.

   a., idiopathic muscular. Progressive

atrophy affecting muscle groups and due to muscular changes, developing in early life.

   a., Landouzy-Dejerine. Muscular wasting in face and scapulohumeral area.

   a., muscular. Muscular wasting.

   a., progressive muscular. Chronic disease marked by progressive wasting of the muscles and paralysis, beginning with the extremities and ultimately causing death from paralysis of muscles of respiration. SYN: *poliomyelitis, chronic anterior; palsy, wasting.*

   a., trophoneurotic. Wasting due to disease of the nerves or nerve centers.

   a., unilateral facial. Progressive atrophy of the facial tissues on one side only.

   a., white. Wasting of nerve, leaving only white connective tissue.

atrophy, words pert. to: antatrophic, atrophic, auantic, cataplasia, claw-foot, claw-hand, macies, trophoneurosis, wasting palsy.

atrop'ic. Displaced.

a'tropine sul'fate. USP. The salt of an alkaloid obtained from belladonna.

   DOSAGE: $1/120$ gr. (0.0005 Gm.).

at'ropinism, at'ropism. Atropine poisoning.

atropiniza'tion. Production of physiologic effect of atropine.

at'ropinize. To bring under the influence of atropine.

atten'tion. Power to focus on some phase of consciousness including some aspect of the world of reality.

   a. reflex. Change in size of pupil when attention is suddenly fixed. SYN: *Piltz's reflex.*

atten'uant. 1. Diluting, making thin or weak. 2. An agent that thins the blood.

atten'uated. 1. Diluted. 2. Pert. to reduced virulence of pathogenic microorganism.

   a. virus. One made less virulent.

attenua'tion. 1. Dilution. 2. Dynamization. 3. Lessening of virulence.

at'tic. Upper portion of tympanic cavity above tympanic membrane.

   a. disease. Chronic suppurative inflammation of attic.

attici'tis. Inflammation of tympanic attic.

atticoantrot'omy. Operation to remove contents of the attic and mastoid antrum.   [attic.

atticot'omy. Surgical opening of tympanic

at'titude(s. Bodily posture(s), esp. the stereotype seen in catatonia* and the theatric expression often seen in hysteria.

   a. of combat. The rigid, defensile attitude of the corpse, due to contractions caused by fear, fire, etc.

   a., crucifixion. Body rigid with arms at right angles, seen in conditions of hysteroepilepsy.

   a., defense. Position automatically assumed to avert pain.

   a., forced. Abnormal position due to disease or contractures.

   a., frozen. Stiffness of gait, seen in amyotrophic lateral sclerosis.

a., illogical. Peculiar attitudes caused by disease, esp. hysteroepilepsy.

a., passional, a., passionate. Theatric or dramatic gestures and expressions of face and figure assumed by hysteric patients.

a., stereotyped. Position taken and held for a long period, seen frequently in mental diseases.

attol′lens. Raising or lifting up.

attrac′tion. Tendency of particles to approach each other.

a., capillary. The force by which liquids rise in fine tubes, or through pores of loose material.

attrahens (at-ra′hens). Drawing forward, as a muscle.

attrax′in. Hypothetical substance in solutions supposed to exert chemotactic influence on certain body cells.

attrition (at-rish′un). 1. A chafing or abrasion. 2. Any friction that breaks the skin.

atylosis (at-I-lo′sĭs). Nontypical tuberculosis.

atyp′ical. Deviating from the normal.

Au. Symb. for gold (aurum).

A. u. or Å. Abbr. for Angström's unit.

auantic (aw-an′tik). Wasted away. SYN: atrophic.

au′digram. Chart of variations of acuteness of hearing.

audile (aw′dil). 1. Pert. to hearing. 2. Ear-minded. 3. PSY: One whose mental images are auditory. SEE: visile and motile.

audiogram (aw′dĭ-o-gram). Record of the audiometer.

audiom′eter. A delicate instrument for testing hearing; consists of a thermoionic tube circuit in which the tube is placed into oscillation. By varying the electrical constants of the circuit, one may make the emitted tone assume various pitches.

audiom′etry. Testing of the hearing sense.

audiphone (aw′dĭ-fon). Instrument for conveying sound to auditory nerve through the teeth or a bone.

audi′tion. Hearing.

a., colored. Color sensation is perceived when certain sounds reach the ear.

a., mental. The recollection of a sound based on previous auditory impressions.

a., m. verbal. Mental audition, the sounds being words.

auditive (aw′di-tiv). One who is auditory minded, depending upon hearing in learning, or recall.

au″ditogno′sis. 1. Understanding and interpretation of sounds. 2. Diagnosis by percussion and auscultation.

aud″itoŏc″ulogy′ric reflex. The sudden turning of the head and eyes in direction of an alarming sound.

aud′itory. Pert. to the sense of hearing. SEE: deafness, hearing.

a., canal (meatus acusticus externus). The external canal, about 2.5 cm. from the concha to the tympanic membrane.

a., nerve (n. acusticus). A part of the 8th pair of cranial nerves; it is a sensory nerve with two sets of fibers: (a) cochlear n. (of hearing), and (b) vestibular n. (of equilibrium), the latter having three branches, the sup., inf., and middle br.

a., reflex. Blinking of the eyes upon the sudden, unexpected production of a sound.

a., m. verbal. Mental auditory, the sounds being words.

a. teeth. Toothlike projections in the cochlea.

a. tube. Eustachian tube, q.v.

aud′itus. The power or the sense of hearing.

Auenbrugger's sign (ow′en-broog-er's). Epigastric prominence due to marked pericardial effusion.

Auerbach's plexus. A plexus of sympathetic nerve fibers situated bet. the longitudinal and circular fibers of the muscular coat of the stomach and intestines. Also called the plexus myentericus.

Auer's bodies. Rodlike bodies in lymphocytes in leukemia.

Aufrecht's sign (owf′rekht's). Diminished breathing sound heard above the jugular notch in tracheal stenosis.

augment (aug′ment). 1. To add to or increase. 2. The increasing stage of a fever, or of an acute disease.

augmen′tor. Increasing.

a. nerves. Those increasing force and rapidity of the heartbeat.

aula (aw′lä). Ant. part of third ventricle.

aulatela (aw-lä′tĕ-lä). Membrane covering the aula.

auliplex′us. Aulic part of choroid plexus.

aulix (aw′liks). Monro's sulcus.

au′ra. The preëpileptic phenomenon.

aural (aw′ral). 1. Pert. to the ear. 2. Pert. to an aura.

auranti′asis. Yellowish skin color due to eating large quantities of oranges.

auran′tium. Orange.

auric (aw′rik). Pert. to gold (aurum).

auricle, auricula (aw′rik-1, -u-la). BNA. 1. The external ear; pinna or flap. 2. (atrium, BNA). One of the two smaller and upper chambers of the heart.

auric′ular. 1. Rel. to the auricle of the ear. 2. Pert. to the auricles of the heart and its nerves and arteries. SEE: polyotia.

a. fibrillation. Irregular and rapid contractions of the auricles which work independently of the ventricles.

a. ventricular tract. A neuromuscular bundle of nerve fibers which pass as the bundle of His* from the right auricle into the ventricle. SEE: pulse and heart.

auricula′re (pl. auricula′ria). A craniometric point at center of opening of external auditory canal.

auric″ulocer′vical nerve re′flex. Congestion of ear on same side resulting from stimulation of distal end of divided auriculocervical nerve.

auric″ulopalpe′bral re′flex. Closure of an

eye resulting from stimulation by heat or some tactile irritant on the ext. auditory meatus or deeper portions of canal up to the tympanum. SYN: *Kisch's reflex.*

auriculoventric'ular. Pert. to both auricle and ventricle. SYN: *atrioventricular.*

a. bundle. A fascicular bundle which forms part of the myocardium, and is made up of the bundle of His,* Tawara's node,* and the Purkinje network.*

auriform (aw'rĭ-form). Ear shaped.

auriginous (aw-rij'in-us). Pert. to jaundice.

aurilave (au'rĭ-lāv). An apparatus for cleansing the ear.

auripuncture (aw'rĭ-punk-tur). Puncture of tympanic membrane.

auris (aw'ris). The ear.

au'riscalp, auriscal'pium. 1. Scraping instrument to remove foreign matter from ear. 2. Earpick.

auriscope (aw'ris-kop). Instrument for making an aural examination.

aurist (aw'rist). Ear specialist. SYN: *otologist.*

auris'tics. Art of treating ear diseases.

auristil'lae. Ear drops.

aurococcus (aw'ro-kok'us). Pyogenic microbe forming golden cultures found in boils, abscesses, carbuncles, pyemia, etc. SYN: *Staphylococcus pyogenes aureus.*

aurometer (aw-rom'et-er). Instrument which measures hearing of each ear.

aurother'apy. Treatment of disease by adm. of gold salts.

aurum (aw'rum). Gold.

auscult', aus'cultate. To examine by auscultation.

auscultation (aws-kul-ta'shun). Process of listening for sounds produced in some of the body cavities, esp. chest and abdomen, in order to detect or judge some abnormal condition.

a., immediate. When ear is applied directly to bared or thinly covered surface.

a., mediate. When sounds are conducted from the surface to ear through an instrument.

ausculta'tory. Pert. to auscultation.

a. percussion. Auscultation at the same time percussion is made.

auscultoplec'trum. Instrument used for both auscultation and percussion.

autacoid (aw'ta-koyd). Any chemical substance which is produced normally by chemical reactions within a given tissue, is released into the blood, and affects the activity of some remote tissue whither it is carried.

autarcesiology (aw-tar-sĕ-sĭ-ol'o-jĭ). Branch of immunology pert. to autarcesis.

autarcesis (aw-tar'sĕ-sis). Resistance to infection through natural immunity.

autarcetic (aw-tar-set'ik). Pert. to autarcesis.

autechoscope (aw-teck'os-kop). Instrument for auto-auscultation.

autemesia (aw-tem-e'sĭ-ă). Vomiting without apparent cause.

autism (aw'tizm). PSY: Mental introversion in which the attention or interest is fastened upon the victim's own ego. A self-centered mental state from which reality tends to be excluded.

autistic thinking (aw-tis'tik). Daydreaming; phantasy of wish fulfillment.

auto-. Prefix: Self, as *autoinfection.*

autoactiva'tion. Gland activation by its own secretion.

autoagglutina'tion. Blood corpuscle agglutination of an individual by his own serum.

autoanal'ysis. Patient's own analysis of mental state underlying his mental disorder.

autoan'tibody. Antibody acting against products of individual in whom it is formed.

autoantitox'in. Antitoxin produced by body itself.

autoau'dible. Audible to oneself; pert. to sounds produced in one's own body.

au'toblast. Independent cell, as a bacterium.

autocatalysis (aw-to-kat-al'ĭs-ĭs). Production of substances by enzymes which increase their activity.

autocath'eterism. Passage of the catheter upon oneself.

autochthonous (aw-tok'tho-nus). Found where it is developed.

autochthonous ideas (aw-tok'tho-nus). Ideas which compel attention and which are not in harmony with one's character, and which arise spontaneously, including auditory hallucinations.

autocinesia, autocinesis (aw-to-sin-e'sĭ-ă, -e'sis). Voluntary movement.

autoclasis (aw'tok'lă-sis). Destruction of a part from internal causes.

autoclave (aw'to-klave). An apparatus for sterilization by steam under high pressure of 20 lb. per sq. in. at 260° F.

autocondensa'tion. A method of applying high frequency currents for therapeutic purposes.

autoconduc'tion. A method, formerly much in vogue in France, of administering high frequency currents.

autocys'toplasty. Plastic repair of bladder with grafts from patient's own body.

autocytolysin (aw-to-sĭ-tol'ĭ-sin). Agent in serum destroying erythrocytes. SYN: *autolysin.*

autocytolysis (aw-to-sĭ-tol'ĭ-sis). Self-digestion or self-destruction of cells.

autoder'mic. Pert. to one's own skin, esp. rel. to dermatoplasty,* with patient's own skin.

autodiagno'sis. Diagnosis of one's own disease.

autodiges'tion. Self digestion. SYN: *autopepsia.*

autodrain'age. Drainage of a cavity by sending the fluid through a channel made in patient's own tissues.

autoecholalia (aw"to-ek-o-la'lĭ-ă). Repetition of words of one's own statements.

autoecic (aw-te'sik). Pert. to parasite always infesting the same organism.

autoerot'ic. Attracted sexually to oneself.

autoerot′icism. Self-love sexually, apart from masturbation. SYN: *autoerotism*.

autoerotism (aw″tō-ĕr-ŏt′izm). The spontaneous generation of sexual emotion in the absence of an external stimulus, normally or abnormally, and apart from masturbation. SEE: *eroticism*.

autofundoscope (aw-to-fun′do-skōp). Apparatus for autoexamination of the eye vessels about the macular region.

autogenesis (aw-to-jen′ĕ-sis). Abiogenesis; self-production; spontaneous generation.

autogenetic (aw-to-jen-et′ik). Pert. to self-production or autogenesis.

autogenic (aw-to-jen′ik). Rel. to self-production. SYN: *autogenetic*.

autogenous (aw-toj′en-us). 1. Self-producing. 2. Originating within the body. 3. Denoting a vaccine from a culture of bacteria from the patient who is to be inoculated with it.

au′tograft. A graft taken from one part of a person's body to fill in another part.

autog′raphism. Nervous state in which tracings made upon the skin leave wheals.

autohem′ic. Done with one's own blood.

autohemol′ysin. Antibody acting on corpuscles of individual in whose blood it is formed.

autohemol′ysis. Hemolysis of a person's blood corpuscles by his own serum.

autohemother′apy. Treatment by withdrawal and injection of patient's own blood.

autohypno′sis, autohyp′notism. Self-induced hypnosis, usually in a very susceptible person.

autoimmuniza′tion. Immunization produced by an attack of the disease.

autoinfec′tion. Infection by toxins produced within the organism.

autoinfu′sion. Forcing blood from extremities to body by applying Esmarch bandages.

autoinocula′tion Secondary infection from disease focus already present in body.

au″tointoxica′tion. A condition produced by poisonous products set free within the body. SEE: *autotyphization*.

autokinesis (aw-to-kĭn-ē′sis). Voluntary action.

autokinet′ic. Being able to move voluntarily.

autolesion (aw-to-le′shun). Injury self-inflicted.

autolysate (aw-tŏl′ĭ-sāt). Specific product of autolysis.

autolysin (aw-tŏl′ĭ-sin). Agent in serum destroying erythrocytes. SYN: *hemolysin*.

autol′ysis. The self-solution or self-digestion which occurs in tissues or cells by ferment in the cells themselves, even after death and in the absence of putrefactive bacteria. SEE: *autolysate, autolysin*.

autolyt′ic. Rel. to autolysis. SEE: *enzymes*.

automat′ic. Spontaneous; involuntary.

autom′atin. Hypothetical heart substance which is supposed to be the natural excitant of the heartbeat.

automatin′ogen. Heart substance which is activated into automatin.

automatism (aw-tom′ă-tizm). Automatic actions or behavior without conscious purpose or knowledge.

automat′ograph. Instrument which records automatic movements.

automysopho′bia. Morbid dread of personal uncleanliness.

autonephrec′tomy. Ureteral stricture, completely closing it.

autonomic (aw-to-nom′ik). Spontaneous, self-controlling.

　a. nervous system. A part of the nervous system which is concerned with reflex control of bodily functions.

auton′omin. A hormone supposed to correlate endocrine gland activity, inhibiting or stimulating secretions of each according to systemic need.

autonomotrop′ic. Drawn to the autonomic nervous system.

auton′omous. Independent of external influences.

auton′omy. Functional independence.

autop′athy. A disease originating without apparent external cause.

autopep′sia. Digestion by self, as of gastric wall by its own secretion.

autopha′gia, autoph′agy. Biting oneself.

autophil (aw′to-fil). Person having sensitive autonomic nervous system.

autophilia (aw-to-fil′ĭ-ă). Narcissism, *q.v.* Self-love.

autophobia (aw-to-fo′bĭ-ă). 1. A psychoneurotic fear of being alone. 2. Abnormal fear of being egotistical.

autophonia (aw-to-fo′nĭ-ă). Suicide.

autophony (aw-tof′on-ĭ). The vibration and echolike reproduction of the patient's own voice, breath sounds, and murmurs.

autoplas′tic. PSY: Rel. to psychic modifications in adapting oneself to reality.

autoplasmother′apy. Treatment through injecting patient's own blood plasma.

autoplasty (aw′to-plas-tĭ). A grafting of fresh parts taken from the patient's body for the repair of wounds.

autoprecipitin (aw-to-pre-sip′ĭ-tĭn). Precipitin active against serum of animal that developed it.

autopsia (aw-top′sĭ-ă). 1. An exploratory incision to determine cause of a disorder or nature of a disease. 2. Autopsy.

autopsy (aw′top-sĭ). Examination of the organs of a dead body to determine cause of death, or pathological conditions.

autopsycho′sis. Mental disease in which patient's ideas about himself are disordered.

autopyother′apy. 1. Treatment of disease by adm. of patient's own pathological excretions. 2. Self-treatment.

autoreinfu′sion. Intravenous injection of patient's own blood which has been effused in his body cavities.

autor′rhaphy. Wound closure by tissue taken from edges of the wound.

autoseptice′mia. Septicemia from poisons existing within the organism.

autoserodiagno'sis. Diagnosis through serum from patient's blood.

aut″o-ser″o-sal′var-san. Blood serum from patient after salvarsan injection used on the patient himself.

autoserother′apy. Treatment by hypodermic injection of patient's own blood serum.

autose′rous. Pert. to autoserum.

autose′rum. Serum obtained from patient's own blood or cerebrospinal fluid.

autosuggestibil′ity. Peculiar lack of resistance to any suggestion that may be offered.

autosugges′tion. Acceptance of an idea uninfluenced by others that induces mental or physical action or change.

PSY: 1. Hysteroid aggravation of actual injury. 2. Persistence into normal consciousness of impressions occurring during secondary states. SEE: *hypnotism*.

autosynnoia (aw-to-sĭn-noy′ă). PSY: Intense concentration to the extent of loss of interest in the outside world; a state of introversion.

autotem′nous. Pert. to cells propagating by spontaneous division.

autother′apy. 1. Spontaneous cure. 2. Treatment of disease by administering patient's own pathological secretions.

autotomy (aw-tot′o-mĭ). A surgical operation performed by oneself.

autotopnosia (aw-to-top-no′zĭ-ă). Inability to orient various parts of body correctly.

autotoxe′mia, autotoxico′sis. Self-poisoning due to absorption of ferment or poison generated within the body.

autotox′in. Poison generated within the body upon which it acts.

autotransform′er. A transformer that has part of its turns common to both primary and secondary circuits. SEE: *transformer*.

autotransfusion (aw-to-trans-fu′shun). 1. Bandaging the limbs to force the blood to the vital centers. 2. A method of treating internal hemorrhage by returning the patient's own extravasated blood to the circulation.

autotransplanta′tion. Transferring a piece of tissue from one part to another in same person.

autotrophic (aw-to-trof′ik). Self nourishing; pert. to green plants and bacteria which form pro. and carbo. from inorganic salts and carbon dioxide.

autotuber′culin. Tuberculin prepared from cultures of patient's own sputum.

autotyphization (aw-to-ti-fiz-a′shun). Production of state resembling typhoid fever; due to autointoxication.

autourother′apy. Treatment of various allergic diseases by injections of the patient's own urine.

autovaccina′tion. Vaccination with autovaccine.*

autovac′cine. Vaccine prepared from virus developed in patient's own body.

autoxida′tion. Spontaneous combining with oxygen.

au′tumn catarrh. Type of hay fever.

auxanography (awks-an-og′ră-fĭ). Determination of most suitable medium for bacterial cultivation.

auxanology (awks-an-ol′o-jĭ). Scientific study of growth.

auxesis (awks-e′sis). Enlarged in bulk, or size.

auxet′ic. Promoting proliferation in leukocytes and other cells.

auxilytic (awks-ĭ-lit′ik). Favoring lysis (2), *q.v.*

auximone (awks′im-ōn). Vitaminlike substance favoring growth in plants.

aux′in. Plant-sprout and human urine hormone promoting growth in plant cells and tissues.

auxocyte (awks′o-sīt). Cell taking part in growth.

auxogluc (awks′ō-glŭk). A group of tasteless atoms which combine with gluciphores to form sweet-tasting compounds. SEE: *gluciphore*.

auxol′ogy. Scientific study of growth of organisms.

a′va, a′va-ka′va. 1. Intoxicating beverage. 2. Drug used in cystitis, gout, and wasting illnesses. SYN: *kava*.

av′alanche theory. Theory that nervous impulses increase in intensity in passing along efferent nerves.

avasculariza′tion. Expulsion of blood, as by use of Esmarch bandage.

Avel′lis′ syndrome. Paralysis of one-half of soft palate, the pharynx, larynx, and loss of pain and heat and cold sensation on opp. side.

averse′ depres′sion. Depression accompanied by defective judgment and rutformation, esp. in the presenile period.

evertin (a-ver′tin). A tribromethanol; is a white, crystalline substance with a melting point at 79° to 80° C. (174° to 176° F.), and which is 3½% soluble in water at a temperature of 40° C. Its use is that of a basal narcotic.

a′viator's disease. Vasomotor disturbances, headache, and drowsiness seen in aviators.

avidin (av-id′in). A proteinlike substance isolated from eggwhite. Said to be an inhibitor of biotin,* a B vitamin named Vit. H.

avirulent (ă-vir′u-lent). Without virulence.

avitaminosis (a-vi-tă-mĭ-no′sis). Disease due to lack of vitamins in the diet; a deficiency disease. SEE: *avitaminotic, vitamin*.

avitaminotic (ă-vi-tam-in-ot′ĭk). Pert. to or affected with avitaminosis.*

avivement (a-vēv-mon′). Refreshing of edges of a wound by operation to hasten healing.

Avogad′ro's law. Equal volumes of gases contain equal numbers of molecules, pressure and temperature being same.

A.'s number. Number of molecules in one gram-molecular weight of a compound.

avoirdupois′ meas′ure. A system of weighing or measuring all coarse and heavy articles. 7000 grains equal one pound. Some medicines are bought and sold by avoirdupois weight.

Dry Measure

16 drams (dr.) equal... 1 ounce (oz.)
16 ounces equal .... 1 pound (lb.)
25 pounds equal .... 1 quarter (qr.)
4 quarters equal ......100 weight (cwt.)
20 cwts. equal .... 1 ton (T.)

Liquid Measure

2 pints equal .....1 quart equals 57¾ cubic inches.
4 quarts equal ....1 gallon equals 231 cubic inches.

avulsion (a-vul'shun). 1. A turning away from as in disgust. 2. A tearing away forcibly of a part or structure. If surgical repair is necessary, merely apply a sterile dressing.

axanthopsia (aks-an-thop'sĭ-ă). Yellow blindness.

axial (aks'ĭ-al). Situated in or pert. to an axis.

   a. skeleton. Head and trunk.

axifugal (aks-if'u-gal). Receding from the center. SYN: *centrifugal.**

axilem'ma. Sheath of an axis cylinder.

axil'la (pl. *axil'lae*). The armpit.

axillar (aks'ĭ-lar). Pert. to axilla. SYN: *axillary.*

axillary (aks'ĭ-lar-ĭ). Pert. to the axilla.

ax'ion. Brain and spinal cord. The cerebrospinal axis.

axioplasm (aks'ĭ-o-plazm). Neuroplasm of an axis-cylinder.

ax''ip'etal. Directed toward the axis. SYN: *axopetal.*

ax'is. The second cervical vertebra* or backbone.

   a., basicranial. Axis connecting basion and gonion.

   a., basifacial. Axis from subnasal point to gonion.

   a., binauricular. Axis bet. the 2 auricular points.

   a., celiac. Celiac artery from abdominal aorta.

   a., cerebrospinal. Central nervous system.

   a. cylinder. Nerve fiber core. SYN: *axon, neuraxon.*

   a., frontal. Imaginary line running transversely through the center of the eyeball.

   a., neural. SEE: *cerebrospinal axis.*

   a., optic. Line of vision.

   a., sagittal. Imaginary line running through the eyeball anteroposteriorly.

axis cylinder process. Axon, *q.v.*, or neuraxon. The conducting portion of a nerve fiber. SEE: *axilemma, axioplasm, axite, axofugal, axopetal, axoplasm, axospongium.*

axis traction (ak'sis trak'shun). Traction made on the fetus in the direction of the birth canal.

   a. t. forceps. Device used to aid in traction made on the fetus.

axite (aks'īt). Any terminal filament of an axis cylinder.

axo- (aks'o). Prefix: Axis.

axodendrite (aks-o-den'drīt). Process given off from a nerve cell axon (not an axis cylinder).

axofugal (aks-of'u-gal). Extending from an axis cylinder process.

axolem'ma. Axis cylinder sheath. SYN: *axilemma.*

axolysis (aks-ol'ĭ-sis). Destruction of the axis cylinder of a nerve.

ax'on, ax'one. 1. The neuraxon or axis cylinder process, the conducting part of a nerve cell. 2. The cerebrospinal axis. 3. The body axis. SEE: *nerve.*

axoneme (aks'o-nēm). Axial thread of a chromosome.

axoneuron (aks-o-nu'ron). A nerve cell of the cerebrospinal system.

axonometer (aks-o-nom'e-ter). Device for determining the axis of astigmatism.

axopetal (aks-op'et-al). Directed toward an axis cylinder process.

axophage (aks'o-fāj). Glia cell found in myelin excavations in myelitis.

ax'oplasm. Material surrounding fibrils of axis cylinder.

axospongium (aks-o-spon'jĭ-um). The fine fibrillar network of axis cylinder of a nerve cell.   [body fat.

axungia (aks-un'jĭ-ă). 1. Lard. 2. Internal

Ayerza's disease (ă-yer'să). One characterized by dyspnea, chronic cyanosis, erythemia, enlargement of spleen and liver, and hyperplasia of bone.

Az. Abbr. for *azote.*

aza'lein. A red dye. SYN: *fuchsin.*

azo-. Prefix indicating substance from a hydrocarbon by replacement by nitrogen of a part of the hydrogen.

azoamyly (az-o-am'ĭ-lĭ). Diminution of amount of glycogen stored up in the liver.

azochloramid (ă-zo-klor'ă-mid). A stable, chlorine substance, crystalline and yellow in appearance, soluble in water or triacetin, etc.
   DOSAGE: Used in solutions of 1: 500.

azo-compounds. Organic substances of which an example is azobenzene, $C_6H_5N: NC_6H_5$.
   They are related to aniline, and include important dyes and indicators.

azoic (az-o'ĭk). Containing no living organisms.

azoospermia (ah-zo-o-sper'mĭ-ă). Deficient vitality of the spermatozoa or their absence.

azopro'tein. A horse serum protein.

azoru'bin S. A dark red dye excreted in the bile after intravenous injection. Test of hepatic function.

azotation (az-o-ta'shun). Nitrogen absorption from the air.

az'ote. Nitrogen.

azotemia (az-o-te'mĭ-ă). Presence of nitrogenous bodies in the blood. SYN: *uremia.**

azotene'sis. Disease due to excess of nitrogen in system. Ex: *scurvy, gangrene.*

azotifica'tion. Atmospheric nitrogen fixation.

azotized (az'ot-īzd). Containing nitrogen.

azotom'eter. Instrument measuring amount of uric acid and urea in urine.

azotorrhea (az-o-to-re′ă). Excess of nitrogenous matter in the feces or urine.

azotu′ria. Increase of urea in the urine.

Az′tec type. Microcephalic idiocy.*

azurophil(e (azh-u′ro-fil). Staining readily with azure dye.

azurophil′ia. Condition in which some blood cells have azurophil granules.

azygos (az′ĭ-gos). Occurring singly, not in pairs.

    a. veins. Three unpaired veins of the abdomen and thorax. Azygos major arises from *vena cava inferior* through the aortic orifice of the diaphragm and the post. mediastinum, ending in the *vena cava superior*.

azygous (az′ĭg-us). Single, not paired.

azymia (a-zi′mĭ-ă). State of being without a ferment.

azymic, azymous (ă-zi′mik, -mus). 1. Unfermented or unleavened. 2. Denoting the absence of a ferment.

B

Ba. Symb. barium.

Bab'bitt metal. Antifriction alloy used occasionally in dentistry.

Babcock's test. Psy: The difference between a vocabulary and a nonvocabulary test indicating the degree of mental deterioration.

Ba'bes-Ernst bodies. Metachromatic* bodies seen in bacterial protoplasm.

Babe'sia. Genus of protozoans thought to be always transmitted by ticks.

 B. bovis. Found in blood cells of cattle, causing hemoglobinuria.

 B. hominis. Believed by some to be pathogenic organism of Rocky Mountain tick fever.

 B. ovis. Causes hemoglobinuria and jaundice in sheep.

babesi'asis. Infection caused by a species of *Babesia*.

Babinski's reflex. Extension of the great toe (extensor plantar) on stroking sole of foot; sometimes a flexion of the other toes when irritation is applied to the sole of the foot. It indicates a lesion of the pyramidal tract and is found in organic hemiplegia,* diseases of nervous system, but not in hysteria.

 B.'s ear-reflex. Inclination of head to diseased side, in middle and internal ear diseases, when galvanic electrode is placed near the ear and when galvanic current is closed.

 B.'s method. Producing reflex contraction of Achilles tendon by tapping it with patient kneeling on a chair.

 B.'s sign. A loss or diminished reflex produced by the Achilles tendon. It is found in sciatica, not in hysteric sciatica.

bacca (bak'ă). A berry.

Baccelli's sign (băt-chel'ēz). Good conduction of a whisper through nonpurulent effusions. Shows a serous pleuritic exudate.

bacchia (bak'e-ă). Acne rosacea.*

bacciform (bak'sĭ-form). Berry-shaped; coccal.

bacillac (bas'il-ăk). Milk preparation soured by *Lactobacillus acidophilus.*

bacillae'mia. Bacillemia.*

bacillar, bacillary (bas'il-ar, bas'il-ar-ĭ). Pert. to or caused by bacilli or rodlike forms.

 b. layer. Rod-and-cone retinal layer.

bacille'mia. Presence of bacilli in the blood.

bacil'licidal, bacillicid'ic. Destructive to bacilli.

bacillicide (bas-il'is-īd). An agent destructive to bacilli.

bacil'liculture. 1. Propagation of bacilli. 2. Culture containing bacilli.

bacil'liform. Resembling a bacillus in shape.

bacilliparous (ba-sĭl-ip'ar-us). Producing bacilli.

bacillogen'ic, bacillogenous (ba-sil-oj'e-nus). 1. Producing bacilli. 2. Originating in bacilli.

bacillopho'bia. Morbid fear of bacilli.

bacillo'sis. Condition due to infection by bacilli.

bacillum (bas-il'um). 1. Sponge holder. 2. A stick.

bacilluria (bas-il-u'rĭ-ă). Bacilli in the urine, though *B. coli* is normally in the bowels.

bacil'lus (pl. *bacilli*). 1. Spore bearing, nonmotile, microscopic, rod-shaped organism of the Bacillaceae family found in soil, in milk, and in the contents of the intestines, most of them not being pathogenic.

 2. Anat: A rod-shaped structure, as in the layer of cones and rods of the retina.

 B. abortus. Organism causing infectious abortion in cattle.

 b., acid-fast. One very resistant to decoloring effect of acids after staining.

 B. acidi lactici. One causing lactic acid fermentation; *Lactobacillus acidophilus.*

 B. acidophilus. Acid producing microorganism.

 B. actinobacter. Nonpathogenic bacillus causing butyric acid fermentation, found in milk, water, old cheese, dust, earth, etc. Syn: *B. butyricus.*

 B. aerogenes. Normal inhabitant of the intestines; pathogenic only under unusual conditions.

 B. aerogenes capsulatus. Causative agent of gas gangrene; of variable virulence.

 B. aertrycke. One of the paratyphoid group; pathogenic for man, sometimes by infection, sometimes by intoxication.

 B., Afanassiew's. Bacillus seen in whooping cough sputum.

 B. albicans pateriformis. Bacillus found in skin in seborrhea.

 B. albuminis. Nonpathogenic species seen in feces.

 B. albus cadaveris. Pathogenic species in blood of a cadaver.

 B. amylobacter. See: *B. butyricus.*

 B. alcaligines. Characterized by its failure to ferment any carbohydrate; rarely pathogenic.

 B. anthracis. Causative agent of anthrax, both as "malignant pustule" and as "wool-sorter's disease."

 B. asiaticus. Bacillus causing a fever, found in India.

 B. aureus. One found in the skin in seborrheic cases.

 b., Bang's. *Bacillus abortus.*

 B. beribericus. Bacillus seen in persons with beriberi.

B-1

B. bienstockii. Pathogenic species found in human feces.

B. bipolaris septicus. Bacillus of the hemorrhagic septicemia group.

B., Boas-Oppler. Species seen in stomach in cancer.

b., Bordet-Gengou. Bacillus pertussis.

B. botulinus. Causative agent of food poisoning with neuroparalytic symptoms due to toxin formed during the growth of this bacillus in foods.

B. bronchitidis putridae. Species of putrid bronchitis.

B. butylicus, butyricus. Nonpathogenic bacillus causing butyric acid fermentation, found in water, milk, old cheese, dust, and earth.

B. capsulatus mucosus. Pathogenic species in nasal secretions of influenza patients.

B. cavicidus. Pathogenic species in human feces.

B. cholerae asiaticae. Asiatic cholera spirillum.

B. chovaei. Anthrax bacillus.

B. coli. Normal inhabitant of intestines; pathogenic only under unusual conditions.

B. coprogenes parvus. Pathogenic fecal bacillus of man.

B. crassus. Broadest species of bacillus known.

B. c. sputigenus. Pathogenic species found in human sputum.

B. cystiformis. Nonpathogenic species found in urine of patient with cystitis.

B. dentalis viridans. Pathogenic bacillus causing dental caries.

B. diphtheriae. Diphtheria bacillus.

b., Ducrey's. Chancroid bacillus.

B. dysenteriae. Organism producing dysentery and summer diarrhea in infants.

B. endocarditidis capsulatus. Pathogenic species found in viscera of endocarditic cadavers.

B. e. griseus. Pathogenic species from heart in patient with ulcerative endocarditis.

B. enteridis. One pathogenic for man, through either infection or intoxication.

B. fusiformis. One causing Vincent's angina.

B. geniculatus. Nonpathogenic species found in stomach.

B. gingivae pyogenes. One from decaying dental pulp; pathogenic.

B. influenzae. One specific for influenza.

B. leprae. Causative agent of leprosy.

B. malariae. One from the blood of patients having malaria.

B. mallei. Bacillus causing glanders.

B. mucosus capsulatus. One of the pneumonia bacilli.

B. murisepticus pleomorphus. Pathogenic bacillus found in uterine discharges of pyemia.

B. oedematis maligni. Gram-positive, motile, fairly large, rod-shaped organism with rounded ends. Infectious to man only through wounds.

B. ozaenae. One always present in ozena or fetid rhinitis.

b., paracolon. One present in paratyphoid fever.

B. paradoxus. One found in tropical dysentery.

B. paradysenteriae. One present in paradysentery.

B. perfringens. Bacillus aerogenes capsulatus.

B. pertussis. Believed to be causative agent of whooping cough.

B. pestis. One causing bubonic and sylvatic plague.

B. pneumoniae. One causing pneumonia.

B. pseudopneumonicus. Pathogenic variety found in blue pus.

B. pyocyaneus. Bacillus of blue and green pus.

B. pyogenes. Pus bacillus.

B. rhinoscleromatis. One present in rhinoscleroma, but not yet proved to be its causative agent.

B. salivarius septicus. Pneumonia diplococcus.

B. saprogenes. One from putrefying pus and gangrenous tissue.

B. of Scheurlen. Nonpathogenic bacillus found in cancer and healthy breasts.

B. septicaemiae. A saprophyte from the blood.

B. septicus acuminatus. Pathogenic variety found in blood and organs of child dead from septicemia.

B. s. sputigenus. Pneumonia diplococcus.

b., Shiga's. Bacillus dysenteriae.

B. smegmatis. Acid fast, nonpathogenic organism found in smegma, q.v.

B. suipestifer. One of the paratyphoid group.

B. tetani. One found in tetanic pus.

B. tuberculosis. Causative agent of tuberculosis.

B. tussis convulsivae. Pathogenic species in whooping cough sputum.

B. typhosus. Pathogenic for man, causing typhoid fever.

B. utpadel. Pathogenic bacillus in human small intestine.

B. welchii. Bacillus aerogenes capsulatus.

bacte′ria (pl. for bacterium). Unicellular, vegetable microörganisms, concerned with fermentation and putrefaction.

Bacteriaceae (băk-te-rĭ-a′se-e). Family of Eubacteriales with rod-shaped cells without endospores.

bactericide (bak-ter′ĭ-sid). That which destroys bacteria.

bacteriemia (bak-ter-ĭ-e′mĭ-ă). Living bacteria in the blood.

bacterine (bak′ter-en). A bacterial vaccine.

bacterio-. Prefix: Pert. to bacteria.

bacteriogenic (bak-tē-re-ō-jen′ik). Caused by bacteria.

bacteriolog′ic, bacteriolog′ical. Pert. to bacteriology.

bacteriol′ogist. One versed in bacteriology.

bacteriol'ogy. Science of microörganisms.

bacteriolysin (bak-te-rǐ-ol'is-in). A substance (antibody) developed as the result of infection of the white blood cells by a bacterium that destroys the same kind of a bacterium.

bacteriolysis (bak-tē-rē-ŏl'is-is). The disintegration of bacteria generally by a specific antibody.

bacteriolytic (bak-te"rǐ-o-lit'ik). Pert. to bacteriolysis.

bacterioöpso'nin. An opsonin acting on bacteria.

bacteriopathol'ogy. Pathology as it relates to bacteria or their toxins.

bacteriophage (băk-tē'rǐ-ō-fāj). Nonspecific agent destructive to bacteria, normally present in the intestinal tract, esp. of those recovering from a bacterial disease; also found in urine, pus, blood, etc.

bacteriopha'gia. Destruction of bacteria by lytic agents.

bacteriopha'gic. Pert. to bacteriophage.

bacteriopho'bia. Abnormal dread of bacteria.

bacterioprecip'itin. Precipitin occurring in bacteria-treated serum.

bacteriopro'tein. One of the proteins in bacteria bodies.

bacterioscop'ic. Rel. to bacterioscopy.

bacterios'copy. Microscopic examination of bacteria.

bacteriosis (bak-tē-rǐ-o'sis). 1. Infection by bacteria. 2. The action of bacteria in the system.

bacteriosol'vent. Agent causing lysis or solution of bacteria.

bacteriostasis (bak-tē-rǐ-os'tās-is). The arrest of bacterial growth.

bacte'riostat. An agent inhibiting bacterial growth.

bacteriostat'ic. Retarding or inhibiting growth of bacteria.

bacteriotherapeu'tic. Pert. to bacteriotherapy.

bacteriother'apy. Treatment of infectious disease through introduction of bacteria into system.

bacteriotox'ic. 1. Toxic to bacteria. 2. Due to bacterial toxins.

bacteriotox'in. Toxin specifically destructive to bacteria.

bacteriotrop'ic. Attracted toward or causing to be attracted to bacteria.

bacteriotryp'sin. A ferment formed by *S. cholerae asiaticae.*

bacterit'ic. Due to or characterized by bacteria.

bacter'ium (pl. *bacteria*). Unicellular vegetable microörganism causing putrefaction and fermentation.

bacteriu'ria. Passage of bacteria in the urine.

bacteroid (bak'ter-oid). Like a bacterium.

bacteru'ria. Bacteriuria.

baculiform (bak-u'li-form). Rod-shaped.

Baer's vesicle (bārz). The ovule.

bag-of-waters. The amnion.* The membrane enclosing the *liquor amnii* and the fetus.

bag, hydrostatic. OB: Rubber or silk bag which is inserted into the uterine cavity and then distended with fluid in order to initiate labor and aid in dilatation of cervix.

　　b., Pol'itzer's. Soft rubber bag for middle ear inflation.

baker. Two or more electric lamps mounted in semicircular containers, called electric light bakers

baker leg. Knock knee; genu valgum.

Baker's cyst. One containing synovial fluid communicating with synovial fluid of a joint.

baker's dermatitis. Eczematous affection of hand caused by yeast. SEE: *baker's itch.*

baker's itch. Manual eczema from irritation of yeast. SEE: *baker's dermatitis.*

baker's salt. Ammonium carbonate.

baker's stigmata. Manual callosities from kneading dough.

bal"aneu'tics. The study of giving baths for therapeutic purposes.

balanic (ba-lan'ik). Pert. to the *glans clitoris** or *glans penis.**

balanism (bal'an-ism). Gynecological treatment by use of pessaries or suppositories.

balanitis (bal-an-i'tis). Inflammation of the glans penis, infectional or gonococcal, and of mucous membrane beneath it with purulent discharge. The prepuce is often affected. 　　[glans penis.

balano- (bal-an-o). Prefix: Pert. to the

bal"anoblennorrhe'a. Gonorrheal inflammation of the external glans penis.

balanoplasty (bal-an-o-plas'tǐ). Plastic surgery of glans penis.

balanoposthitis (bal-an-o-pos-thi'tic). Inflammation of the glans penis and prepuce; balanitis.*

balanoprepu'tial. Pert. to glans penis and prepuce.

balanorrhagia (bal"an-ŏ-ra'jǐ-ă). Hemorrhage from glans penis.

balanorrhea (bal-an-o-re'a). Balanitis with purulent discharge.

balbuties (bal-bu'shǐ-ēz). Stuttering.

baldness. Lack of hair on head. RS: *acomia, alopecia, atrichia, atrichous, hair.*

Bal'four's disease. Chloroma.*

Balkan frame. A framework (usually wood) to fit over a bed so that weights may be suspended from it to produce the desired continuous traction and yet permit freedom of motion while maintaining immobilization of the desired part being treated.

ball-and-socket joint. Joint in which one rounded bone head fits into cavity of another bone. SYN: *enarthrosis.**

ballism (bal'izm). 1. Condition characterized by jerking, twisting movements. 2. Paralysis agitans.*

ballis'tics. Science of curves of projectiles.

ballistopho'bia. Morbid fear of missiles.

balloon'ing. The distention of a cavity, as vagina, by air or otherwise for examination.

ballot'table. Capable of showing the ballottement* phenomenon.

ballottement (bal-ot-mon'). The rebound of a fetal extremity when displaced by the examining finger either through abdominal wall or vagina.

ball thrombus. Clot in the ante mortem heart. SEE: *thrombus*.

balm. 1. A balsam. 2. A soothing or healing ointment.

    b. of Gilead. 1. Mecca balsam from *Commiphora opobalsamum*, probably Biblical myrrh. 2. Balsam fir, source of Canadian balsam. 3. Poplar bud resin.

balneary (bal'ne-ă-rĭ). Institution for adm. of balneotherapy.   [and baths.

balneography. Treatise on mineral springs

balneology (bal-ne-ol'o-jĭ). The science of treating disease by baths.

balneotherapeutics (bal''ne-o-ther-ă-pu'-tiks). Treatment of disease by baths. SYN: *balneotherapy.**

balneotherapy (bal-ne-o-ther'a-pĭ). The treatment of disease by baths.

bal'neum (pl. *bal'nea*). A bath.

    b. are'nae. A sand bath.

    b. lu'teum. A mud bath.

balop'ticon. Apparatus for projecting image of an opaque object on a screen.

bal'sam. Oleoresin or resin containing benzoic acid or cinnamic acid.

balsam of Peru. USP. A dark-brown, viscid, resinous liquid. ACTION AND USES: Locally same as benzoin. May be used full strength or in ointment.

    DOSAGE: 15 gr. (1.0 Gm.).

balsam'ic. 1. Pert. to balsam. 2. Aromatic.

    b. tincture. Compound tincture of benzoin

Bal'ser's fatty necrosis. Pancreatitis with gangrenous and fatty necrotic areas in interlobular tissue, and sometimes in pericardial fat and bone marrow.

banana oil, poisoning. Resulting from amyl acetate used as a vehicle for suspending metals for the purpose of painting with metals, as gilding.

band'age. Piece of gauze or other material for application to a limb or other portion of the body.

band forms. Neutrophil granular leukocytes with bandlike or horseshoe-shaped nuclei. Constitute about 4 per cent of total leukocytes.

Bandl's ring. Line of depression corresponding to site of internal os uteri, sometimes felt just above pubis during labor pains.

ban'dy leg. Bowleg. SYN: *genu varum*.

Banti's disease. A syndrome combining anemia, splenic enlargement, hemorrhages, and ultimately cirrhosis of liver.

baptorrhea (bap-tor-e'ă). An infectious discharge from a mucous membrane.

baragnosis (bar-ag-no'sis). Inability to estimate weights.

Barba'does leg. Disease marked by hypertrophy of skin and subcutaneous tissue, due to obstruction of circulation in lymphatic or blood vessels. SYN: *elephantiasis, pachydermia*.

barber's itch. Fungous affection of the bearded portions of face and neck. SYN: *Tinea sycosis*.

    b. rash. Barber's itch. SEE: *sycosis*.

barbital (bar'bit-al) (veronal). USP. USES: As sedative and hypnotic in simple insomnia, neurasthenia, and sleeplessness of hysteria.

    DOSAGE: 5 to 10 gr. (0.32-0.65 Gm.). in hot water or milk.

    b. sodium (soluble barbital, medicinal). USP. Has same properties as barbital but because of greater solubility, more rapidly absorbed. DOSAGE: 8 gr. (0.5 Gm.).

bar'bitalism. Acute or chronic poisoning from use of barbital or its derivatives. SYN: *barbituism, q.v.*

barbituism (bar-bit'u-izm). Poisoning from use of barbital or its derivatives. SYN: *barbitalism, barbiturism*.

barbit'urate. Barbituric acid salt.

    Picrotoxin is the best antidote at present.

barbitu'rics. Derivatives of barbituric acid such as *luminal* (phenobarbital), *barbital* (veronal), *dial, amytal, allonal*, and many others.

barbiturism (bar'bĭ-tu-rizm). Acute or chronic poisoning from use of veronal, luminal, or any barbituric acid derivatives. SYN: *barbituism*.

barbotage (bar-bo-tăzh'). Spinal anesthesia by withdrawal of spinal fluid to which the drug is added before reinjection.

baresthesia (bar-es-the'zĭ-ă). The pressure sense.

baresthesiometer (bar-es-the-si-om'ĕ-ter). Instrument for determining sensibility to pressure in different parts of body.

ba'ric. Pert. to barium.

barium (ba'rĭ-um). SYMB: Ba. A metallic element of the alkaline group. Atomic weight 136.4. Barium sulfate is used for taking x-ray pictures of the abdominal tract.

bark. The outer cover of the woody parts of a plant. Ex: *cascara sagrada, cinchona, wild cherry*.

Barkow's ligaments (bar'kŏvs). Ant. and post. ligaments of elbow.

Barlow's disease. Infantile scurvy;* a deficiency disease; occurs in bottle-fed babies who lack other foods.

barm. Yeast.

Barnes' bag or **dilator.** Rubber bag used to induce premature labor by dilating uterine cervix.

    B.'s curve. The segment of a circle whose center is the sacral promontory.

baro-. Prefix: Weight, heaviness.

barognosis (bar-og-no'sis). The ability to estimate weights. OPP: *baragnosis*.

barograph (bar'o-graf). Self-registering barometer.

baromachrometer (bar-o-ma-krom'et-er). Instrument for measuring and weighing infants at time of birth.

bar'oscope. Instrument noting atmospheric pressure variations, without accurately weighing them.

bar'ospirator. Apparatus producing artificial respiration by means of air pressure variations in a closed chamber

barotax'is. Protoplastic reaction to any form of pressure.

barot'ropism. Protoplasmic reaction to any form of pressure. SYN: *barotaxis.*

bar'rel chest. A form of thorax resembling a cylinder.

bar'ren. Sterile; incapable of producing offspring.

Bartholin's abscess (bar'to-linz). This develops when Bartholin's glands* are affected in gonorrhea and when they become occluded in an acute inflammatory process.

    B.'s cyst. In chronic inflammation of Bartholin's glands* cysts are commonly formed. Carcinoma is rare.

    B.'s ducts. Large ducts of the sublingual salivary gland. They parallel Wharton's duct* and open with it.

    B.'s glands. Two small compound, racemose, mucous glands, pea to bean size, situated beneath the vestibule, one on each side of the vaginal opening and at the base of the labia majora.

bartholinitis (bar-to-lin-i'tis). Inflammation of a vulvovaginal gland.

Baruch's law. Water has a sedative effect when its temperature is the same as that of the skin, and a stimulating effect when it is below or above the skin temperature.

    B.'s sign. When rectal temperature remains high after a 15-minute bath in water at 75° F. it points to typhoid fever.

baruria (bar-u'rĭ-ă). Urine having a high specific gravity.

bary-. Prefix: Heavy, dull, hard.

baryecoia (bar"ĭ-e-koy'ă). Hardness of hearing; deafness.

baryesthesia (bar-ĭ-es-the'zĭ-ă). The pressure sense. SYN: *baresthesia.*

baryglossia (bar-ĭ-glos'ĭ-ă). Having a slow, thick utterance.

barylalia (bar-ĭ-la'lĭ-ă). Indistinct, husky speech.

baryodmia (bar-ĭ-od'mĭ-ă). Disagreeable, heavy odor.

baryodynia (bar-ĭ-ō-din'ĭ-ă). Severe pain.

baryphonia (bar-ĭ-fo'nĭ-ă). Difficulty in speaking words.

bary'ta, bary'tes. Barium oxide, BaO; caustic and poisonous.

barythymia (bar-ĭ-thi'mĭ-ă). Sullen, gloomy, or melancholy state of mind.

ba'sad. Denoting the direction toward the base of anything.

ba'sal. 1. Pert. to the base of anything; the base. 2. Of primary importance.

    b. ganglia. The *optic thalamus* and *corpus striatum* located in the floor of the lateral ventricles of the brain.

basal metab'olism. The minimal amount of energy or number of calories sufficient to support the basic metabolic processes of a resting individual in the postabsorptive state.

bascula'tion. 1. Replacement of a retroverted uterus by swinging it into place. 2. Systolic recoil of the heart.

base. 1. The lower part of anything. 2. The principal substance in a mixture.

3. In chemistry, a substance which is able to neutralize an acid and to form a salt.

    b. of heart. Heart surface back and upward, containing pulmonary vein and vena cavae openings.

base or basic substance. A compound usually composed of a metal with oxygen, or oxygen and hydrogen, and possessing the following properties: with an acid it forms a salt; it has (when soluble in water) an alkaline taste.

    b., animal. A leukomaine or ptomaine.

    b.'s, hexone. The amino acids, *lysin, arginin,* and *histidine.*

baseball finger. Results from violent backward dislocation of the terminal phalanx onto the dorsum of the middle phalanx, as when a finger is struck on its tip when extended.

Basedow's disease (baz'e-do). Grave's disease; exophthalmic goiter.

    B.'s syndrome. Flashes of heat, sweating crisis, tachycardia.

basement membrane. A thin layer of flattened cells underlying the epithelium of mucous surfaces; a part of the corium.* SEE: *membranes.*

base'plate. Plastic material for making dental trial plates.

bas-fond (bah-fawn'). A fundus.

basi-, basio-. Prefixes: base.

ba'sial. Pert. to the basion.

basiarachnitis (ba-sĭ-ar-ak-ni'tis). Inflammation of the arachnoid membrane at base of brain.

basiarachnoiditis (ba-sĭ-ar-ak-noy-di'tis). Inflammation of the arachnoid membrane at base of brain. SYN: *basiarachnitis.*

basibregmat'ic axis. Vertical line from the basion to junction of coronal and sagittal sutures.

ba'sic. 1. Possessing properties opposite to those of an acid. 2. Fundamental.

    b. diet. Protein 1 Gm. per Kg. ideal body weight. Emphasize milk, all vegetables, all fruits except prunes, plums, cranberries, and possibly grapes. Limit meat, cereals, eggs.

    b. salt. A compound formed when only part of the hydroxide radicals of a base are replaced by the acid radical of an acid.

basicity (ba-sis'ĭ-tĭ). 1. Basic in character. 2. The combining power of an acid; the valence. It is expressed by a number indicating number of hydrogen atoms replaceable by a base.

basicra'nial axis. Straight line from the basion to point of angle of mandible.

basifa'cial axis. Straight line from the point of angle of mandible to the subnasal point.

basihyal, basihyoid (ba-sĭ-hi'al, -oyd). The body of the hyoid arch or either of the two bones forming it.

bas'ilar. Basal; pert. to a base.

basilat'eral. Both lateral and basilar.

basilem'ma. 1. Basement membrane. 2. Basis supporting framework of nervous tissue of cerebrospinal axis.

basil'ic. Prominent, important.

    b., vein. Large vein on inner side of biceps. Usually chosen for intravenous injection or for withdrawal of blood.

basilysis (bas-il'i-sis). Crushing the fetal head in labor.

basilyst tractor (ba'sil-ist). Instrument devised by Sir A. R. Simpson consisting of three blades for perforating the fetal head and obtaining a substantial grasp to facilitate delivery of the child.

basioccipital bone (bas-ĭ-ok-sip'it-al). Basilar process of occipital bone.

basioglossus (bas-ĭ-o-glos'us). Part of hyoglossus muscle attached to base of hyoid bone.

ba'sion. Point at middle border of the foramen magnum.

basiot'ic. Pert. to base of ear.

basiotribe (ba'si-o-trīb). Instrument for crushing the fetal head.

basiotripsy (ba-sĭ-o-trip'sĭ). Crushing fetal head.   [ing.

basiphobia (bas-ĭ-fo'bĭ-ă). Fear of walk-

basirrhinal fissure (bas-ĭ-ri'nal). 1. Pert. to base of brain and to the nose. 2. A cerebral fissure at base of olfactory lobe.

basis (ba'sis). Base.

    b. cranii. Base of skull.

basisphenoid (bas-ĭ-sfe'noid). Lower portion of sphenoid bone.

basisyl'vian fissure. Transverse basilar portion or stem of sylvian fissure.

basket cell. A multipolar ganglion cell in outermost gray layer of cerebellum.

ba'sograph. Device for registering abnormalities of gait.

basophil(e (bas'o-fĭl or fīl). In histology, applied to cells or parts of cells which are readily stained with basic dyes like methylene blue; esp. a class of white corpuscles (mast cells or basophilic leukocytes). Function unknown.

basophilia (bas-o-fĭl'ĭ-ă). 1. A pathological condition of the blood in which the erythrocytes develop basophile granules. 2. A condition in which many mast cells are present.

basophilic (ba-so-fĭl'ik). Pert. to method of staining various cells.

basophobia (bas-ō-fo'bĭ-ă). 1. Emotional inability to stand or walk without muscle impairment. 2. Abnormal fear of walking.

bass deaf'ness. Deafness to bass notes, the higher ones being heard.

Bassini's operation (bah-sĭ'nĭz). One for inguinal hernia.

bas'tard. 1. One born out of wedlock. 2. Not legitimate.

bath. The medium and method of cleansing the body or any part of it, or to treat it therapeutically, as with air, light, steam, vapor, water, etc.

    b., acid. 5 oz. hydrochloric acid or 1 gal. vinegar to 30 gal. water.

    b., air. Therapeutic use of air, warmed or vaporized, on the nude body.

    b., alcohol. Use of alcohol on patient, as a stimulant and defervescent, in dilute form.

    b., alkaline. For chronic rheumatism. 1 lb. sodium bicarbonate or washing soda to 30 gal. water.

    b., alum. Use of alum in washing solution, as an astringent.

    b., animal. Therapeutic use of a recently killed animal or its pelt on a patient.

    b., antipyretic. SEE: *Brand bath.*

    b., antiseptic. For irritating, offensive, and parasitic skin diseases. SEE: *carbolic, creosote, sulfur baths.*

    b., aromatic. One to which some volatile oil or perfume is added, or some herb.

    b., arthritic. Alum, ½ lb., to 30 gal. water, or boric acid solution, 2½%, made by adding 2-3 lb. boric acid to 30 gal. water. Tannic acid only as ordered. Amount of any of these baths must be specified by physician and amount checked.   [bath.

    b., arsenical. Weak solution in tepid

    b., astringent. Bathing in liquid containing an astringent.

    b., blanket. One in which wet pack and blankets are used.

    b., blood. One using fresh animal blood.

    b., bog. Peaty mud bath, for therapeutic purposes.

    b., borax. Glycerin and borax solution for bathing.

    b., box. One in which patient is completely enclosed in box except for his head.

    b., bran. 2-3 lb. bran to 30 gal. water, or 3-5 lb. malt or starch to 1 gal. water added to full bath at 95° F. to 96° F., may be used to stop itching.

    b., Brand. Full bath of 65° F. combined with strong friction in the water, used in typhoid fever.

    b., brine. 7 lb. sea salt to 30 gal. water.

    b., bubble. Mechanical production in a bathtub of water of tiny air bubbles by (1) an air distributor which consists of a number of metal tubes through which the air passes to the water, (2) an air pump, and (3) an electric motor that drives the pump.

    b., cabinet. Exposure of the skin of the body except the head, to heat from electric lamps, live steam, steam radiators, or electric heaters. Bath cabinets are constructed of wood, marble, or steel.

    b., camphor. Bath in air charged with camphor.

    b., carbolic. Strength 1-100. Mix 48 oz. pure carbolic in 5 pt. boiling water, putting it into bath before 30 gal. water are added, to make sure of mixing.

    b., carbon dioxide. An effervescent saline bath consisting of water, salts, and CO_2. The natural CO_2 baths are known as Nauheim baths, and approach closely CO_2 baths in their therapeutic effects.

    b., cold. One used for stimulation, being followed by brisk rub.

b., cold plunge. Tub bath with water at 85-79° F., duration ½ to 3 minutes, with bather using friction while in water.

b., colloid. One containing bran, gelatin, starch, etc., for treatment of dermatitis.

b., continuous. One that is administered for hours, days, weeks, or months. It is a continuous, flowing bath if the prescribed temperature is maintained by keeping a stream of water flowing through the tub.

b., contrasted. Used for hands or feet. Two large basins or pails of sufficient depth, filled with water, one as hot as can be borne, the other as cold as can be borne. Change or add hot and cold water frequently to keep temperatures same as in beginning. Put part to be treated in hot water for 1 minute, then into cold for ½ minute, then again into hot water. Repeat for prescribed length of time, ending with cold water.

b., cresote. 1-2 drams cresote to 30 gal. water, to which 10 oz. glycerine are sometimes added.

b., douche. Large jets of water sprayed on the body.

b., drip sheet. Modified sheet bath.

b., earth. Bathing in warmed earth or sand.

b., electric light. Exposure of the nude body, except the head, to rays from a large number of electric lights placed on the inside walls of a cabinet.

b., electrotherapeutic. An electric current sent through water in which the patient lies, or in which a limb is immersed. Only a faradic current is used for a faradic bath.

b., emollient. Used for irritation and inflammation of skin, and after erysipelas. SEE: *glycerine, linseed, oatmeal, powdered borax, starch baths.*

b., foam. Tub bath to which has been added an extract of a saponin containing vegetable fiber, and through this mixture, O or CO_2 is driven through porous wood or the foam is produced mechanically.

b., foot. Immersion of feet and legs to a depth of 4 inches above ankles in water at 98° F. The temperature of the water is increased.

b., full. Bath in which the whole body except the head is immersed in water.

b., galvanic. Entire body or one or more limbs immersed in large tub or several smaller basins made of insulating material (porcelain or wood), with electrodes consisting of metal plates in wooden frame to prevent direct contact with patient's body.

b., glycerine. 10 oz. to 30 gal. water.

b., half. Tub bath with about 18 inches of water; the temperature depends on the case and the desired action.

b., Heller. A form of hydroelectric bath.

b., herb. One to 2 pounds of herbs, such as chamomile, wild thyme, or spearmint, are tied in bag, boiled with 1 gal. of water, and the decoction added to the full bath.

b., hip. SEE: *sitz bath.*

b., hot. Tub bath with the water covering the body to a little above the nipples and temperature gradually raised from 98° F. to desired degree (to 108° F.).

b., hot air. Exposure of entire body except head to hot air contained in a bath cabinet.

b., hydroelectric. Application of faradic, galvanic, or sinusoidal current conducted to the patient through water.

b., hyperthermal. One in which the body except head is immersed in water from 105-120° F. for 1 to 2 minutes.

b., immersion. Free tub bath.

b., incandescent light. SEE: *electric light bath.*

b., internal. Introduction of large amounts of water into rectum and stomach.

b., kinetotherapeutic. Bath given for underwater exercises of weak or partially paralyzed muscles.

b., linseed. 1-2 lb. to 30 gal. water. Boil emollient in a tied muslin bag, and add the mucilage to the 30 gal. water.

b., lukewarm. Bath in which patient's whole body except head is submerged in water, temperature, 94-96° F., duration 15-60 minutes.

b., medicated. Bath to which bran, oatmeal, starch, sodium bicarbonate, epsom salts, pine products, tar, sulfur, potassium permanganate, or salt is added.

b., milk. Bath taken in milk, as an emollient or cosmetic.

b., mud. Old form of applying moist heat which depends on availability of certain soils heated by thermal springs or artificially.

b., mustard. For irritant effect, and to draw blood from deeper parts, as in a febrile cold, infantile convulsions, infantile diarrhea, and for shock. A heaping tablespoonful of fresh mustard for each gallon of water. In adults it is used as a hot foot bath.

b., Nauheim (naw'hĭm). A bath in which the human body is immersed in warm water and subjected to the action of carbon dioxide gas.

b., neutral. One in which no circulatory or thermic reaction occurs, temperature 92-97° F.

b., neutral sitz. Same as hot sitz bath, except temperature between 92-97° F., and foot bath, 104-110° F., duration 15-60 minutes.

b., oatmeal. 2-3 lb. to 30 gal. water.

b., oxygen. Given by introducing O into the bath through a special device consisting of a metal plate provided with bamboo reeds which are connected to an oxygen tank or by generating the O by chemicals.

b., paraffin. Member is immersed in warm paraffin, 140-150° F., withdrawn, immersed again, withdrawn repeatedly until it is encased.

b., Peng. A form of foam bath, *q.v.*

b., pine needle. One-half to 1 lb. extract pine needles added to a bath covering the whole body to the chin, temperature 93-98° F., duration 20 minutes.

b., powdered borax. One-half lb. to 30 gal. water; 5 oz. glycerine may be added.

b., reducing. One given to reduce patient's temperature.

b., Russian. Warm vapor bath followed by rubbing and cold plunge.

b., saline. Given in artificial sea water made by dissolving 8 lbs. of sea salt, or a mixture of 7 lb. of sodium chloride and ½ lb. of magnesium sulfate in 30 gal. of water.

b., Sandor. A form of foam bath, *q.v.*

b., Schnee. Four cell hydroelectric bath.*

b., seawater or salt. Antipruritic.

b., sedative. A prolonged warm bath. Continuous flow of water may be used. Use air cushion and back rest.

b., sheet. Given by wrapping the patient in a sheet previously dipped in water 80-90° F., and rubbing the whole body with vigorous strokes on the sheet, until all parts of the sheet feel warm.

b., sitz. Immersion of thighs, buttocks, and abdomen below the umbilicus in water. In a hot sitz bath the water is first 92° F. and elevated to 106° F., duration 3 to 10 minutes.

b., sponge. One in which patient's body is moistened with washcloth or sponge.

b., starch. 1 lb. mixed in cold water, pouring boiling water to make starch mucilage, which add to 30 gal. water.

b., steam. Given in a chamber into which steam under low pressure is allowed to escape.

b., stimulating. One which increases cutaneous effect; used for tonic purposes. [water.

b., sulfur. 2 or 3 oz. sulfur to 30 gal.

b., sweat. One given to induce perspiration, as in temperature reduction.

b., tonic. One which, through its stimulation of the cutaneous nerves and the response of the autonomic nervous system, quickens the circulation of the blood throughout the body.

b., towel. Given by applying towels dipped in water 70-60° F. to arms, legs, ant. and post. surfaces of trunk successively, removing the towel and drying the part.

b., vapor. Exposure of skin of body except head to vapor.

b., whirlpool. Continuous localized douches for the arm and leg.

b., Ziemssen (tsĕm'sen). Tub bath at 88° F., cold water added slowly until temperature reaches 65° F., patient is rubbed vigorously; duration 20-30 minutes or until chilled.

bathesthe′sia. Consciousness of joints, muscles, and organs beneath the skin. Syn: *bathyesthesia.*

bath′mic. Pert. to the vital force controlling nutritional function.

bath′mism. The force that regulates nutrition and growth.

bathmotrop′ic. Promoting excitability of tissues in response to stimuli.

bathopho′bia. A fear of high objects.

bath″yanesthe′sia. Loss of deep sensibility.

bathycar′dia. A fixed abnormally low position of the heart.

bathyesthesia (bath-ĭ-es-the′zĭ-ä). A consciousness of muscles, joints, and organs beneath the skin.

bathygastry (bath′ĭ-gas-trĭ). Abnormally low stomach. Syn: *Gastroptosis.*

bathyhyperesthesia (bath-ĭ-hi″per-es-the′-zĭ-ä). Sensitiveness of muscular tissues and deep structures.

batono′ma. A tumor supposed to be caused by vegetable organisms of higher grade than bacteria.

batophobia (bat-ō-fo′bĭ-ä). 1. Acrophobia; fear of heights. 2. Dread of anything high.

batrachoplasty (bat′rak-o-plăs-tĭ). Plastic operation for ranula.

battarism (bat′ä-rizm). Stuttering.

bat′tery. Device for generating galvanic currents by chemical action.

Bat′tey's operation. Excision of healthy ovaries to induce menopause or for other therapeutic purposes.

bauchstiel (bowch′shteel). The abdominal pedicle by which the embryo is attached to the chorionic membrane.

Baudelocque's diameter (bō-dloks′). Distance bet. the depression just beneath the spine of the last lumbar vertebra and the ant. and upper margin of the *symphysis pubis.* The ext. conjugate diameter.

B.'s method. Manipulation to convert a face presentation into one of the vertex.

Bauer qual′imeter. Instrument for measuring intensity and penetrating power of roentgen rays through various metals. See: *penetrometer.*

Bauhin's valve (bo-anz′). The ileocecal valve; *valvula coli.*

baunscheidtism (bown′shĭd-izm). Acupuncture for producing counterirritation.

Bava′rian splint. A splint of plaster of Paris between two flannel cloths.

Bayle's disease. A general paresis described in 1822 by Antoine Bayle.

bay′onet leg. Backward dislocation at knee joint of tibia and fibula.

Bazin's disease (bah-zanz′). 1. Buccal psoriasis. Purple or reddish nodules on legs which may ulcerate. 2. Erythema induratum.

B. C. G. Abbr. *Calmette-Guérin bacillus.*

b. d. Abbr. L. *bis die,* twice a day.

bdellometer (del-lom′et-er). Artificial substitute for a leech consisting of a scarificator, cupping glass, and exhausting syringe.

beaded. Referring to disjointed colonies

along the inoculation line in a streak or stab.

beads, rachitic. Visible swelling where the ribs join their cartilages, seen in rickets. "Rachitic rosary."

beaker (bē′ker). Glass vessel with wide mouth for mixing or holding liquids.

bear′ing down. The expulsive effort of a parturient woman, in second stage of labor.

beat. Pulsation of blood in the heart and blood vessels.

　　b., apex. Stroke of the heartbeat felt by the hand when held over the fifth intercostal space on left of chest wall.

　　b., ectopic. One beginning at a place other than sinoauricular node.

　　b., forced. Extrasystole brought on by artificial heart stimulation.

　　b., premature. An extrasystole.

beat knee. A subcutaneous connective tissue inflammation over the patella.

Beccaria's sign (bek-kā′rĭ-ă′s). Occipital pulsation in pregnancy.

bechesthesis (bek-es′thes-is). A feeling in the throat causing one to cough.

bech′ic. 1. Controlling a cough. 2. A cough medicine.

Bechterew-Mendel reflex (bekh′te-rev). A reflex indicating a lesion of the pyramidal tract, and manifested when the cuboid bone is tapped, causing a flexion of the 4 outer toes.

Bechterew's reflex (běk′těr-ěv). 1. Contraction of facial muscles due to irritation of nasal mucosa. 2. Dilatation of pupil on exposure to light. 3. Plantar flexion of foot. 4. Flexion of foot in dorsal direction and flexive movement of knee and hip following passive flexion of toes and plantar extension of foot. 5. Contraction of lower abdominal muscles when skin of inner surface of thigh is stroked.

Béclard's hernia (bā-klärs′). Hernia through opening for the saphenous vein.

bed. A piece of furniture for rest of body or during sleep or illness.

　　b., air. One inflatable with air.

　　b. blocking. Placing bedblocks under bed to raise it at head or foot.

　　b. case. Hysteria with refusal to leave the bed.

　　b. fast, b. ridden. Unable or unwilling to leave the bed.

　　b., fracture. One for patients with fracture.

　　b., Gatch. One with a jointed bed rest that can be raised into a half-sitting position.

　　b., hydrostatic. A water bed.

　　b., metabolic. One arranged to catch the feces and urine.

　　b. rest. A device for propping up patients in bed.

　　b., water. A rubber mattress filled with water. Uses: Prevention of bed sores.

bedbug (*Cimex lectularius*). An insect which injects an irritating substance causing a purpuric* reaction, or an urticarial* wheal.

Bed′nar's aph′thae. Minute yellowish patches on either side of the palate of the newly born.

bedpan. Device for receiving fecal and urinal discharges from patient confined to the bed.

bedsore. Pressure sore. Syn: *decubitus.* Decubitus consists of ulceration and gangrene of a localized area, usually over the sacrum, due to pressure which limits the nutrition of the affected area.

bed′wetting. Name for habit of young children of wetting bed at night. Syn: *enuresis, q.v.*

Beer's operation. Flap operation for cataract or artificial pupil.

beestings (best′ings). Colostrum*; first milk after parturition.

beg′ma. 1. A cough. 2. Expectorated matter.

behav′iorism. A theory of conduct which regards normal and abnormal behavior as the result of conditioned reflexes quite apart from the concept of will. It does not apply to conditions resulting from structural disease.

behavior reflex. One acquired as result of training and repetition.

Beh′ring's law. Serum of an immunized person confers immunity on another into whom diphtheria antitoxin is injected.

belch. Escape of gas from the stomach through the mouth; to eructate.

belching. Raising of gas from the stomach.

belem′noid. Dart shaped; styloid.

belladonna (bel-a-don′a) (Deadly Nightshade). USP. The dried leaves and roots of *Atropa belladonna*, the active principle of which is atropine.*

　　Dosage: Tr. belladonna. USP. 10 ♏ (0.6 cc.). Fluid extract. USP. 1 ♏ (0.06 cc.).

Bellini's ducts (bel-lǐ′nǐ). The excretory tubules of the kidneys.

　　B.'s ligament. A fasciculus of capsular ligament of the hip reaching the great trochanter.

Bell-Magendie's law. That ant. spinal nerve roots only contain motor fibers and post. roots sensory fibers.

bell′-metal resonance. A metal-like sound heard in pneumothorax.

Belloc's cannula or **sound** (bel-loks′). An instrument for drawing in a plug through nostril and mouth in epistaxis.

bell sound. Bell metal resonance.

Bell's disease. Acute delirious mania; acute periencephalitis.

　　B.'s law. Post. spinal nerve roots are sensory and ant. ones motor.

　　B.'s nerves. Internal and external respiratory nerves.

　　B.'s paralysis. Facial motor lower neuron paralysis affecting 7th cranial nerve.

　　B.'s spasm. Convulsive facial tic.

belly. Abdomen; stomach.

　　b. ache. Colic gastralgia.

　　b. button. Umbilicus.

　　b. of muscle. Nontendinous thick central part of a muscle.

belonepho'bia. Morbid fear of sharp-pointed objects.

belonoid (bel'o-noid). Needle shaped.

belonoskiascopy (bel-o-no-ski-as'ko-pĭ). Subjective retinoscopy by means of shadows and movements to determine refraction.

Bence-Jones' albumose. Protein bodies appearing in the urine of persons suffering from disease of the bone marrow.

bends [caisson disease]. Pain and weakness caused by increased atmospheric pressure.

beneceptor (be'ne-sep-tor). A nerve organ for the reception and transmission of beneficial stimuli.

Ben'edikt's syndrome. Hemiplegia with oculomotor paralysis and clonic spasm on opp. side.

benign (be-nin'). 1. Not recurrent. SYN: *benignant.* 2. Not malignant. 3. Mild.
    b. stupor. A stupor sometimes seen in the depression of manic-depressive psychosis.

benig'nant. 1. Not malignant. 2. Not recurrent. SYN: *benign.*

benzedrine (ben-ze-drēn'). A colorless mobile liquid, producing local effects similar to those of ephedrine.
    DOSAGE: As a spray, 1% solution in liquid petrolatum, as an inhalant, one or two inhalations through each nostril at hourly intervals. Continued use should be guarded against, sleeplessness and restlessness may be the result.
    b. sulfate. A white, odorless powder, a cerebral stimulant, similar in its action to caffeine.
    DOSAGE: Average, 10 mg.

benzene, or benzol. C_6H_6. A volatile liquid, immiscible with water, able to dissolve fats.
    DOSAGE: 2-10 ℳ (0.12-0.6 cc.).

benzidin test diet. This consists of milk, crackers and rice.

ben'zoate. Any salt of benzoic acid.

benzocaine (benz-o-kain'). Nontoxic local anesthetic. SEE: *anesthesin.*
    DOSAGE: 5 gr. (0.3 Gm.).

benzo'ic acid, USP. May be obtained by sublimation from gum benzoin.
    DOSAGE: 5-15 gr. (0.3-1.0 Gm.).

benzoin (ben'zoin, -zo-in). USP. A balsamic resin from styrax benzoin.

ben'zol. Same as benzene. Widely used in industry as from coal tar distillation, manufacture of motor fuels, rubber industry, manufacture of cans, lacquer and paint trades.

Bérard's aneurysm (bā-rars'). An arteriovenous aneurysm in the tissues surrounding the injured vein.

Béraud's ligament (ba-rōz'). Pericardial suspensory ligament.
    B.'s valve. Krause's* valve. Fold of mucous membrane at beginning of nasal duct.

Ber'covitz test. For pregnancy: Several drops of patient's citrated blood instilled into one eye; if contraction or dilatation of the pupil occurs, sometimes the two eyes alternately, pregnancy is assumed.

Bergeron's chorea (bair-zhĕ-rawn'). A hysterical type of chorea.

Bergmann's incision. One in flank for exposing the kidney.

Bergonie's chair (bair-go-nyas'). A specially designed chair, the back and seat of which take the form of four large electrodes. Other electrodes are applied to the abdomen, forearms, and thighs. The muscles are stimulated with a specially constructed instrument giving a faradic current. Used in obesity and constipation.

beriberi (ber'ĭ ber'ĭ). An Oriental disease; an endemic and infective form of *polyneuritis.**

Bernard's canal or duct (ber-nar'). An accessory pancreatic duct. *Ductus pancreaticus accessorius.* BNA.
    B.'s granular layer. Inner layer of cells lining acini of pancreas.

Bernreuter test (bern'rū-ter). A "yes" and "no" test of 125 questions, used to ascertain the attitudes and interest of a patient.

bertillonage (ber'tē-yon-äj). Physical measurement for identification of criminals.

Bertin, Bertini, columns of (ber'tan). Renal cortical columns supporting the blood vessels in the kidneys. The part that separates the medullary pyramids.
    B.'s ligament. Iliofemoral ligament.

besoin de respirer (ba-zwan de res-pĭ-ra'). Sensation inducing act of breathing.

bestiality (bes-tĭ-alʹĭ-tĭ). Coition with an animal.

beta. Second letter of Greek alphabet. Used as a prefix to chemical words to note isomeric variety or position in compounds of substituted groups.

betanaphthol (be-tă-naf'thol). Occurs as a colorless or buff colored crystalline powder, with faint odor of phenol.
    DOSAGE: 4 gr. (0.25 Gm.).

Beta rays. Negatively charged particles emitted by radium; more penetrating than alpha rays. Absorbed by 1 mm. lead or 0.6 mm. platinum.

beta test (ba'ta). An army group intelligence test used with those unable to read English.   [to other consonants.

be'tacism. Speech defect giving *b* sound

betaine hydrochloride (bē-tain'). A colorless crystalline substance, containing 23% hydrochloric acid, and obtained from an alkaloid found in the beet, and other plants.
    DOSAGE: 8 gr. (0.5 Gm.), dissolved in water, which corresponds to about 18 ℳ dilute hydrochloric acid USP.

betalin S (bā'ta-lin). Synthetic vitamin B_1. 1 mg. contains 400 Sherman units.

betaxin (be-taks'in). Synthetic crystalline vitamin B_1 hydrochloride.
    DOSAGE: Orally, from 1 to 5 mg. daily. Intramuscularly, from 1 to 10 mg.

Betz cell. A form of giant pyramidal cell in the cortical motor area.

bex (bĕks). A cough or condition characterized by a cough.
    b. convulsiva. Whooping cough.

Bezold's abscess (be′zolt's). Mastoiditis which involves the tip cell, causing abscess underneath insertion of sterno-cleidomastoid muscle.

Bi. CHEM: Symb. for bismuth.

bi-. Prefix: Two, double, twice, as *biceps*.

biartic′ular. Pert. to two joints; diarthric.

bibasic (bī-ba′sik). Pert. to an acid with two hydrogen atoms replaceable by bases to form salts.

bibulous (bib′u-lus). Absorbent.

bicam′eral. Having two cavities or hollows; esp. an abscess divided by a septum.

bicap′sular. Having a double capsule.

bicar′bonate. A salt resulting from the incomplete neutralization of carbonic *acid*, or from the passing of an excess of carbon dioxide into a solution of a *base*.

bicar′diogram. A cardiogram curve representing the combined effects of the right and left ventricles.

bicellular (bi-sel′u-lar). 1. Composed of two cells. 2. Having two chambers or compartments.

bi′ceps. Two-headed; in front of humerus and behind femur.

   b. brachii. Muscle of the upper arm, having two heads. Flexes and supinates forearm.

   b. femoris. Muscle of the thigh.

   b. reflex. Biceps muscle contraction when tendon is percussed.

bicep′tor. A receptor having two complementophil groups.

Bichat's canal (bī-shäs′). The subarachnoid canal extending from third ventricle to middle of Bichat's fissure carrying the veins of Galen.

   B.'s fat ball or **pad.** Mass of fat behind the buccinator muscle.

   B.'s fissure. The horseshoe fissure separating cerebrum from cerebellum.

   B.'s foramen. Same as Bichat's canal.

   B.'s ligament. Lower fasciculus of post. sacroiliac ligament.

   B.'s membrane. *Lamina basalis.*

   B.'s tunic. The tunica intima of the blood vessels.

bichloride of mercury (bī-klo′rīd) (corrosive mercuric chloride). A crystalline salt, $HgCl_2$.

   DOSAGE: Internally, 0.16-0.5 gr. (0.001-0.003 Gm.).

bicho (bē′chō). Epidemic gangrenous proctitis.

biciliate (bi-sil′ī-āt). Having two cilia.

bicip′ital. 1. Pert. to a biceps muscle. 2. Having two heads.

Bi₃(CO₃)₃. Bismuth carbonate.

bicon′cave. Concave on each side, as a lens.

bicon′vex. Convex on two sides, as a lens.

bicor′nuate, bicornuous. Having two processes or hornlike projections.

   b. uterus. Anomalous uterus resulting from incomplete union of the mullerian ducts. May be double or single organ with two horns.

bicoro′nial. Pert. to the two coronas.

bicor′porate. Having two bodies.

bicus′pid. Having two cusps or prongs.

   b. valves. Valves bet. the left ventricle and left auricle (atrium). SEE: *heart.*

bicuspid (bī-kus′pĭd). One of 2 teeth above and below on each side between the molars and canines.

b. i. d. Abbr. for *bis in die,* twice daily.

Bidder's gang′lion. One of two ganglia or cardiac nerves.

bidermo′ma. A teratoid growth having two germ layers; didermoma.

bidet (bī-det′). A receptacle with attachments for giving injections, for a hip bath or sitz bath, or for washing the genitals or for douching.

biduous (bid′u-us). Continuing for two days.

Biederman's sign (be′der-mans). Dusky redness of the lower ant. pillars of fauces in certain cases of syphilis.

bier′merin. Hormone in gastric juice. SYN: *addisin.*

Bier's cup (beers). A clear glass cup provided with a pump and bulb named after the inventor.

bifa′cial. Having similar opposite surfaces.

bi′fid. Cleft or split into two parts.

   b. spine. Congenital fissure of vertebral column.

   b. tongue. Cleft tongue.

bifo′cal. Having two foci, as *bifocal eyeglasses.*

bifo′rate. With two openings.

bifurcate (bi-fur′kate). Having two branches or divisions; forked.

bifur′cated. Having two branches; forked.

bifurcation (bī-fûr-kā′shŭn). A separation into 2 branches; the point of forking.

Big′elow's ligament. The iliofemoral ligament; Y-ligament.

   B.'s septum. Bony tissue layer under neck of femur. SYN: *calcar femorale.*

bigem′inal. Double, paired.

   b. bodies. Small portion of brain lying behind third ventricle. The corpora quadrigemina.

   b. pulse. Pulse in which beats are in groups of two with pause in between groups. SEE: *pulse, bigeminal.*

bigem′inum. A bigeminal body.

bigeminy (bī-jĕm′ĭn-ĭ). Pulse marked by occurrence of 2 beats close together followed by a pause before next pair of beats. SYN: *pulse, bigeminal.*

bilabe (bi′lăb). Device used for urethral extraction of vesical calculi.

bilat′eral. Pert. to, affecting, or rel. to two sides of the body.

   b. symmetry. Symmetry of paired organs. SYN: *bilateralism.*

bilateralism (bī-lat′ĕr-ăl-ĭzm). Arrangement on 2 sides; symmetry.

bile (bīl). A secretion of the liver. SYN: *gall.*

   b. acids. Complex acids, of which cholic, choleic, glycocholic, and taurocholic acids are examples, and which occur as salts (*e. g.,* sodium taurocholate) in bile.

   b. ducts. Intercellular biliary passages conveying the bile from the liver to the hepatic duct which joins the duct from the gallbladder (cystic duct), to form the common bile duct (ductus choledochus), and which enters the duodenum about 3 inches (7.5 cm.) below the pylorus. SEE: *hepatic duct, cystic duct, common bile duct, gallbladder.*

   b. pigments. Complex, highly colored substances found in bile, derived from the red pigment (hemoglobin) of the blood, and imparting the brown color to intestinal contents and feces. Ex: *bilirubin, biliverdin.*

   b. salts. Alkali salts of bile.

bilharzia (bil-har′zĭ-ă). A parasitic fluke in blood supply of the liver. The eggs are found in great numbers in bladder or rectum.

bili-. Prefix: Pert. to bile.

biliary (bil′ĭ-ar-ĭ). Pert. to or conveying bile.

   b. calculus. Cholelithiasis. Formation of stone in any of the biliary passages.

   b. colic. Pain caused by the pressure or passing of gallstones.

   b. ducts. Passages conveying bile from liver to hepatic duct. SEE: *bile ducts.*

biliation (bil-ĭ-a′shun). Excretion or secretion of bile.

bilifecia (bil-if-e′sĭ-ă). Presence of bile in the feces.

bilifica′tion. The formation of bile.

bilifla′vin. A yellow pigment derived from biliverdin.

biliful′vin. Biliverdin mixed with other substances.

bilifuscin (bil-ĭ-fus′ĭn). A dark green pigment in gallstones.

biligenesis (bil-ĭ-jen′ĕ-sis). The formation of bile.

biligenet′ic. Forming bile.

biligenic (bil-ĭ-jen′ik). Forming bile. SYN: *biligenetic.**

bilihu′min. A dark residue after applying solvents to bile or gallstones.

bi′lin. Mixture of sodium glycocholate and sodium taurocholate extracted from bile.

bilineurin (bil′′ĭ-nū′rin). $C_6H_{15}NO_2$. A toxic ptomaine from organic substances; choline.

bil′ious. 1. Pert. to bile. 2. Afflicted with biliousness.

   b. fever. Fever with vomiting of bile.

   b. remittent. SEE: *bilious fever.*

biliousness (bil′yus-nes). 1. A symptom due to disordered condition of the liver causing constipation, headache, loss of appetite, and vomiting of bile. 2. Excess of bile; bilious fever. Fever with vomiting of bile.

biliphein (bil-ĭ-fe′ĭn). An impure bilirubin.

bilipra′sin. Green pigment similar to bilirubin.

bilipur′pin, bilipurpu′rin. A purple pigment derived from biliverdin.

bilirachia (bil-ĭ-ra′kĭ-ă). Bile in the spinal fluid.

bilirubin (bil-ĭ-ru′bin) ($C_{16}H_{18}N_2O_3$). The orange-colored or yellowish pigment in bile.

bilirubinemia (bil-ĭ-roo-bin-e′mĭ-ă). Bilirubin in blood.

bilirubinu′ria. Bilirubin in urine.

bil′is. Bile.

   b. bovina, b. bulbata. Oxgall, used as laxative, cholagogue, and intestinal antiseptic. SYN: *fel bovis.*

bilither′apy. Treatment with bile salts.

biliuria (bil-ĭ-u′rĭ-ă). Bile in the urine.

biliverdin (bil-ĭ-ver′dĭn). A greenish pigment in bile formed in oxidation of bilirubin. RS: *bilifulvin, bilipurpin, choleverdin.*

biloc′ular. 1. Having two cells. 2. Divided into compartments.

bilron (bil-ron′). Iron bile salts.

   DOSAGE: 15 to 60 gr. daily (0.97-3.9 Gm.).

biman′ual. With both hands; with two hands, as *bimanual palpation.*

binary (bi′nar-ĭ). 1. Compounded of two elements. 2. Separating into two branches.

   b. acid. One containing hydrogen and one other element.

binau′ral. Pert. to or having two ears.

   b. arc. The arc from one aural point to another across top of cranium.

binauric′ular. Pert. to or having two ears. SYN: *binaural.**

binder. A broad bandage, most commonly used as an encircling support of abdomen or chest.

   b., abdominal. A wide band fastened snugly about the abdomen for support.

   b., chest. A broad band used for encircling the chest to apply heat, dressings, or pressure, and supporting the breasts. Improved by using shoulder straps to keep from slipping.

   b., double T. A horizontal band about the waist to which two vertical bands are attached in back; each brought around leg and again fastened to horizontal band. As means of holding dressings about the perineum or genitalia (esp. in the male).

   b., obstetrical. A broad bandage encircling entire abdomen from ribs to pelvis, affording support—usually after childbirth.

   b., T. Two strips of material fastened together, resembling a T, used as a bandage to hold a dressing on perineum of women; or vertex of head, etc.

   b., towel. A towel encircling abdomen or chest with ends pinned or sewed together for support.

bind′web. 1. Connective tissue. 2. Tissue forming framework of brain and spinal cord. SYN: *neuroglia.*

Binet age (bĭ-na′). Intellect as measured by the Binet-Simon tests as compared with the age of a normal child. The Binet age of an idiot is 1-2 yr.; the imbecile, 3-9 yr.; the moron, 8-12 yr.

binoc′ular. Pert. to both eyes.

   b. vision. Normal vision and use of both eyes.

binot′ic. Pert. to or having two ears. SYN: *binaural.**   [ova.

binov′ular. Derived from or pert. to two

binu'clear, binu'cleate. Having two nuclei.

binucleolate (bi-nū-kle'o-lāt). Having two nucleoli.

bio-. Prefix: Life.

bio-assay'. Estimation of strength of a drug.

bi'oblast. A corpuscle that has not yet become a cell; micella.

biocatalyst (bi-o-kat'al-ist). An enzyme; a biochemical catalyzer.

biochem'istry. The chemistry of living things; the science of the chemical changes accompanying the vital functions of plants and animals.

biochemorphic (bi"o-kem-or'fik). Pert. to the relation bet. biologic action of drugs and foods and their chemical constitution.

biochemorphology (bi"o-kĕ-mor-fol'o-jĭ). Science of chemical structure of substances as related to their action on the body.

bioclimatology (bi"o-kli-ma-tol'o-jĭ). Relations of climate to life.

biocolloid (bi-o-kol'oyd). A colloid in animal or vegetable organism.

biocy'toculture. A culture made from live leukocyte bearing pus.

biocytoneurology (bi-o-cī-to-nu-rol'o-jĭ). The science of living nerve cells.

biodynam'ics. The doctrine or science of living force or energy.

biogen (bi'o-jen). 1. Protoplasm. 2. Assumed substance of a spiritual body.

biogen'esis. Begetting living things from living things opp. to spontaneous generation or abiogenesis,* *q.v.*

biogenet'ic. Pert. to biogenesis.

biokinet'ics. The science of changes in developing organisms.

biolog'ic, biolog'ical. Pert. to biology.

biolog'icals. 1. Complex substances of organic origin, depending for their action on the processes effecting immunity, used esp. in diagnosis and treatment of disease, as vaccines, serums, or antigens. 2. Complex products, of organic or synthetic origin, obtained or standardized by biological methods, as pituitary extract or insulin.

biol'ogist. A professional student of or a specialist in biology.

biology (bi-ol'o-jĭ). Science of life and living things.

   b., dynamic. Science of activities of living organisms.

   b., static. Science of structures and potentialities of living organisms.

biolysis (bi-ol'ĭs-ĭs). Devitalization or destruction of living tissue by action of living organisms.

biolytic (bi-o-lit'ik). Capable of destroying life.

biomax'illary. Pert. to or afflicting both jaws.

biometer (bi-om'et-er). Instrument for measuring life sounds.

biomet'rics. Biometry.

biom'etry. 1. Application of statistics to biological facts. 2. Computation of life expectancy.

bion (bi'on). Any living organism.

bionergy (bi-on'er-jĭ). Vital energy or force.

bionomics (bi"ō-nŏm'ĭks). Branch of science dealing with the relations of organisms to their environment. SYN: *ecology.*

bion'omy. The science pert. to vital functions and their laws.

biono'sis. Any disease due to pathogenic organisms.

biophagism, biophagy (bi-of'ă-jizm, -ă-jĭ). Absorbing nourishment from living matter.

bioph'agous. Feeding on nonparasitic matter.

biophilia (bi-o-fil'ĭ-ă). Instinct of self-preservation.

biophore (bi'o-fōr). The ultimate unit having vital energy.

biophylac'tic. Tending to preserve life.

biophysics (bi-o-fiz'ĭks). Vital process phenomena.

biophysiol'ogy. Study of morphology and physiology.

bi'oplasm. Protoplasm. Living substance. SEE: *biogen.*

bioplas'mic. Pert. to bioplasm.

bioplas'min. A hypothetical substance contained in every living cell, essential to its life.

bioplast (bi'o-plast). The cellular unit.

bioplas'tic. Pert. to a bioplast.

bi'opsy. Excision of a small piece of tissue for microscopic examination.

bios (bi'os). Life.

bios'copy. Examination to determine life.

biose (bi'ōs). A saccharide.

biospectrom'etry. Clinical spectrometry to determine presence of foreign matter.

biospectros'copy. The clinical spectroscopy of living tissue.

biostat'ics. Science of metabolism.

biotax'is, bi'otaxy. 1. The selecting and arranging activity of living cells. 2. Systematic classification of living organisms. [ganisms.

biot'ics. Pert. to the laws of living or-

biotin (bi-ot'in). A B vitamin named Vit. H. The most powerful life substance known and a great stimulator. It is active in concentrations of one part to four hundred billion parts. It, with avidin,* seems to maintain an equilibrium of vital forces. Lack of this equilibrium may be the cause of disease.

biotomy (bi-ot'o-mĭ). Operation on living animals for pathological or physiological study. SYN: *vivisection.*

biotox'in. A toxin from living tissues and juices.

biotrip'sis. A condition of the skin seen in old people in which skin wears away.

biotropism (bi-ot'ro-pizm). Increased virulence resulting from therapeutic procedures.

Biot's breathing or respiration (bĭ-ōs'). Rapid breathing with rhythmical pauses. Unfavorable in meningitis.

bio'type. Fundamental constitution of an organism or those possessing it.

biov'ular twins. Twins from two separate ova.

bip'ara. Woman who has had two labors.

bip'arous. Giving birth to two at a time.

biparasit'ic. Pert. to parasite living upon another parasite.

biparen'tal. Derived from both parents.

biramous (bi-ra'mus). Possessing two branches.

bipol'ar. 1. Having 2 poles or processes. 2. Pert. to the use of 2 poles in electrotherapeutic treatments.

    b. nerve cell. Cell with 2 processes.

    b. version. Braxton Hicks version; a combined one. Changing a *cephalic* position into a *podalic* one, or *vice versa,* by placing 1 hand on fundus of uterus and 2 fingers of other hand in cervix.

B. I. P. P. The letters stand for *bismuth, iodoform, paraffin paste.* A paste used during the first World War.

Birdsall punch. Modification of the caulk punch for using the cutting current for excision of the prostatic median bar.

birefrac'tive, birefrin'gent. Splitting a ray of light in two.

birth. Act of being born. Passage of a child from uterus.

    b., complete. The instant of complete separation of the body of the infant from that of the mother, regardless of cord or placenta detached.

    b. control. Any method used to prevent conception, such as artificial devices used by the male or the female.

    b., cross. With fetus across the uterus.

    b., live. An infant showing one of the three evidences of life (breathing, heart action, movements of a voluntary muscle) after complete birth.

    b. mark. Nevus; mark from birth injury.

    b. palsy. Paraplegia or hemiplegia caused by birth injury. Injury to some shoulder muscles may cause Erb's palsy.

    b., still. An infant not exhibiting evidence of life after complete birth. SEE: *live birth.*

bisacro'mial. Pert. to both acromial processes.

bisection (bi-sek'shun). Division into 2 parts. SYN: *hemisection.*

bisex'ual. Hermaphroditic; having imperfect genitalia of both sexes in one person.

bisferious (bis-fer'i-us). Having two beats; dicrotic.

bisiliac (bis-il'i-ăk). Pert. to the two most distant points of the two iliac crests.

bis in d., bis in die. Twice a day.

bismarsen (bis-mar'sen). A bismuth derivative of arsphenamine containing approximately 13% arsenic and 24% bismuth.

    DOSAGE: Initial, 0.1 Gm. intramuscularly, succeeding doses, 0.2 Gm. at weekly intervals; a few drops of a 2% solution of butyn should be added to lessen the pain on administration.

bismosol (biz'mo-sol). A solution of potassium sodium bismuthotartrate (containing 35% bismuth).

    DOSAGE: Intramuscularly in 1 cc. doses every 2 to 7 days for 20 doses; after interval of 1 month a second course may be given.

bismuth (biz'muth). A drug used as a protective for inflamed surfaces, and as an opaque medium for x-ray visualization.

    b. sodium tartrate. Contains 72.7 to 73.9% bismuth. USES: In treatment of syphilis. DOSAGE: ½ gr. (0.03 Gm.) intramuscularly.

    b. subcarbonate. USP. USES: As an antacid. SEE: *bismuth subnitrate.* DOSAGE: 15 gr. (1 Gm.).

    b. subgallate (Dermatol). USP. A bright yellow powder without odor or taste. DOSAGE: 15 gr. (1 Gm.).

    b. subnitrate. USP. Occurs as heavy white odorless powder. DOSAGE: 15 gr. (1 Gm.).

bistoury (bis'to-rĭ). Small surgical knife used in minor operations; special varieties are tenotomes, gum lancets, hernia knives, and lithotomy bistouries.

bite (bīt). 1. To cut with the teeth. 2. A puncture by an insect. 3. Occlusion of the teeth.

    b., close, closed. One in which lower incisors lie behind upper incisors.

    b., end-to-end. One in which incisors of both jaws meet along cutting edge when jaw is closed.

    b., open. One in which labial teeth cannot come together.

    b., over. One in which upper incisors overlap lower ones when jaws are closed.

bitelock. Device for retaining position biterims outside the mouth.

bitem'poral. Pert. to both temples or temporal bones.

bite plate. A plate to support a biterim.

biterim. A rim of wax placed on base plate as a guide for inserting artificial teeth.

biter'minal. Using an alternating current and two poles in electrotherapeutic treatment. SEE: *bipolar.*

bites. Injuries in which body surfaces are torn by insects or animals, resulting in abrasions, punctured, or lacerated wounds.

    b., insect. They contain an acid substance resembling formic acid and consequently are relieved by alkalies, as ammonia water, baking soda paste or even soap paste rubbed on.

bitter (bĭt'er). 1. Having a disagreeable taste. 2. Sensation of taste stimulated by strong, disagreeable flavor.

bit'ters. Herb tonic for stimulating the tone of gastrointestinal mucous membrane.   [matic properties.

    b., aromatic. Substances having aro-

    b., simple. Those which stimulate the digestive mucosa.

    b., styptic. Those with styptic and astringent properties.

bi'uret''. A crystalline decomposition derivative of urea.

    b. reaction. Rose to violet coloring in an aqueous solution of protein, when dilute solution of copper sulfate and sodium hydroxide are added to it.

b. test. Use of above reaction to detect presence of urea or any soluble protein. SEE: *test, biuret.*

bivalent (bī-vā'lĕnt). 1. Having a valence of 2. 2. BIOL: Double, as a chromosome consisting of 2 joined chromosomes. 3. A bivalent chromosome.

biven'ter. A muscle with two bellies; pert. to several muscles.

biven'tral. Digastric; with two bellies.

Bizzozero's corpuscles (bit-sot'ser-os). Nucleated red blood cells, round or elliptical.

Bjerrum screen. Tangent plane for mapping field of vision, esp. central and paracentral scotomata.

B. sign. One seen in glaucoma, a sickle-shaped blind spot usually found in central zone of the visual field. SEE: *sign.*

black (blăk). 1. Devoid of color; reflecting no light. 2. Marked by dark pigmentation.

b. blood. Impure or venous blood.

b. body. PHYS: A body that absorbs all radiation falling upon it.

b. cancer. An abnormal deposit of black matter in various parts of the body in melanosis.

b. death. A contagious, malignant disease, as the bubonic plague.

b. eye. Subcutaneous extravasation of blood into the eye or orbit, usually the result of injury.

b. head. Comedo.*

b. measles. A severe type of measles in which the eruption is very dark due to hemorrhage under the skin.

b. tongue. Presence of dark patch on back of tongue caused by microphytes. SYN: *glossophytia.*

b. vomit. The vomiting of black matter as in yellow fever.

blackwater fever. Hemoglobinuria.* A pernicious, fatal, infectious malarial fever due to the destruction of the red blood cells by the malarial organism.

black widow. *Lactrodec'tus mac'tans.* A poisonous spider.*

bladder. 1. A membranous sac or receptacle for a secretion, as the *gallbladder, q.v.* 2. The vesicle which acts as a reservoir for urine. SEE: *urinary bladder.* [to lack of muscular tone.

b., atony of. Inability to urinate, due

b., catarrh of. Cystitis.

b., exstrophy of. Turning inside out of the bladder.

b., irritable. Marked by a constant desire to urinate.

b., nervous. Irritable bladder with incomplete urination.

b., stammering of. Interruption of urination.*

b., urinary (*vesica urinarius*). The muscular, membranous, distensible reservoir for the urine, which it receives from the kidneys through the ureters, and which it discharges from the body through the urethra.* It has no function other than that of a reservoir.

b.-worm. Larval type of tapeworm.

bland. Soothing, mild.

b. diet. One soothing in flavor and texture; all food which causes chemical, mechanical, or thermal irritation is avoided.

Blandin's glands (blan-dăns'). Glandula lingualis ant. or Nuhn's glands. Glands near tip of tongue.

blast. A nucleated erythrocyte; also called an *erythroblast.*

blaste'ma. Protoplasm from which cells and tissues are formed.

blas'tid, blas'tide. Marking site of the nucleus in the impregnated ovum.

blas'tin. That which stimulates growth of cells.

blasto-. Prefix: Germ or bud.

blastocele (blas'to-sēl). The cavity in morula of a blastosphere.

blastoce'lic. Pert. to a blastocele.

blastochyle (blas'to-kīl). Blastocelic fluid.

blastocyst (blas'to-sist). The germinal vesicle, or blastodermic vesicle.

blas'tocyte. The morula after change into a cyst.

blastocyto'ma. A tumor composed of blastocytes.

blas'toderm. The germinal vesicle of an ovum or egg made up of several cell layers, the *ectoderm** or *epiblast** or outer layer; the *entoderm** or *hypoblast** or inner layer; and the *mesoderm** or *mesoblast** or middle layer.

blastoderm'ic vesicle. A vesicular structure or sphere consisting of one layer of cells which surround a cavity filled with fluid in which the impregnated ovum expands.

blastogen'esis. 1. Multiplication by budding. 2. Transmission of characteristics from parents to offspring by the germ plasma.

blastol'ysis. Lysis or destruction of a germ cell.

blasto'ma (pl. *blastomata*). A granular tumor formed by a single type of tissue, including *fibromas* and *chondromas.*

blastomere (blas'to-mere). A nucleated cell into which the fecundated vitellus divides, forming a fluid-filled ball of cells, a modified *blastula* known as the *blastocyst, q.v.*

blastomerot'omy. Destruction of blastomeres.

blastomycetes (blas-to-mĭ-sē'tēs). Saccharomycetes; budding fungi; yeast fungi.

blastomyco'sis. A disease caused by budding yeast fungi in the tissues.

blastoneuropore (blas''to-nu'ro-pōr). Opening formed by the union of the blastopore and neuropore.

blastophyllum (blas''to-fil'ŭm). A blastodermal layer.

blastopore (blas'to-pōr). The small opening into the archenteron made by invagination of the blastula.

blas'tosphere. Blastula or germinal vesicle.

blas'tospore. A thallospore formed by budding from a hypha.

blastula (blas'tu-lă). A blastocyst; the

blastodermic vesicle. The fecundated ovum when it is a hollow sphere filled with a gelatinous substance.

blas'tular. Pert. to a blastula.

blastulation (blas-tu-la'shun). The formation of the blastula or blastosphere.

Blat'ta orienta'lis. The common cockroach.

Blaud's pills. Named after a French physician. Contents are sulfate of iron and carbonate of potash. Their use is indicated in anemia,* amenorrhea,* etc.

bleaching powder (blēsh'ing). Chlorinated lime.

blear-eye. Marginal blepharitis. Chronic inflammation of margins of eyelids.

bleb. Elevation of the epidermis, irregularly shaped.

bleeder. One who bleeds an abnormal amount. SEE: hemophilia.

blee'der's disease. Congenital blood condition marked by inability of blood to coagulate. SYN: hemophilia.*

bleeding (blēd'ing). 1. Emitting blood. 2. Process of emitting blood, as a hemorrhage or operation of letting blood.

   b., arterial. This is indicated by bleeding in spurts. Color, bright red.

   b., venous. Flow continuous. Color of blood, dark red.

   TREATMENT: Patient recumbent. Pressure below wound with wound bet. heart and hand. Bandage over wound above and below.

blena'na. Mucus.

blennadenitis (blen-ad-en-i'tis). Inflammation of mucous glands.

blennelytria (blen-el-it'rĭ-ă). An abnormal white mucous discharge from vagina or cervical canal. SYN: leukorrhea.

blennemesis (blen-em'es-is). Vomiting of mucus.

blennenteritis (blen-en-ter-i'tis). Enteritis accompanied by a flow of mucus.

blennisthmia (blen-isth'mĭ-ă). Catarrh of the pharynx.

blenno-. Prefix: Pert. to mucus.

blennocystitis (blen-o-sis-ti'tis). Inflammation of the urinary bladder.

blennogenic, or **blennogenous** (blen-o-jen'ik, or blen-oj'en-us). Secreting mucus.

blennoid (blen'oid). Like mucus; mucoid.

blennometritis (blen-o-me-tri'tis). Inflammation of the uterus.

blennophlogisma, blennophlogosis (blen-o-flo-jis'mă, blen-o-flo-jo'sis). Inflammation of a mucous membrane.

blennophthalmia (blen-off-thal'mĭ-ă). Catarrhal conjunctivitis.

blennoptysis (blen-op'tis-is). Expectoration of mucus from the bronchi.

blennorrhagia (blen-o-a'jĭ-ă). 1. A discharge from mucous membranes, esp. gonorrheal discharges from the genital or urinary tract. 2. Gonorrhea.

   b. of conjunctiva. OPHTH: Adult form: gonorrheal ophthalmia.

   b. of lacrimal sac. A chronic catarrhal inflammation of the mucous membrane lining the lacrimal sac, resulting in retention of the mucous secretion and tears.

blennorrhagic (blen-o-raj'ik). Pert. to blennorrhea; blennorrheal.

blennorrhea (blen-or-ē'ă). Discharge from mucous membranes, esp. gonorrheal discharge from genital or urinary tract. SYN: blennorrhagia.*

blennorrheal (blen-o-re'ăl). Blennorrhagic; pert. to blennorrhea.

blennorrhinia (blen-or-in'ĭ-ă). Coryza. Catarrh of the nasal passages.

blennosis (blen-o'sis). Any disease of a mucous membrane.

blennostasis (blen-os'tas-ĭs). The checking of any mucous discharge.

blennostat'ic. Diminishing mucous secretion.

blennostrumous (blen-o-stru'mus). Pert. to gonorrhea and scrofula.

blennothorax (blen-o-tho'raks). Pulmonary catarrh.

blennotorrhea (blen-ot-or-ē'ă). A discharge of mucus from the ear.

blennurethria (blen-u-rē'thrĭ-ă). Gonorrhea of the urethra.

blennuria (blen-nu'rĭ-ă). Excess of mucus in the urine.

blepharadenitis (blef-ar-ad-en-i'tis). Inflammation of the meibomian glands. SYN: blepharoadenitis.

blepharal (blef'ar-al). Pert. to an eyelid.

blepharedema (blef-ar-ĕ-de'mă). Swelling of the eyelids.

blepharelosis (blef″ar-el-o'sis). Ingrowing eyelashes.

bleph'arism. Twitching of the eyelids.

blepharitis (blef-ar-i'tis). Inflammation of the edges of the eyelids involving hair follicles and glands opening on surface; ulcerative and nonulcerative.

   NP: Bathe lids with borax and warm water to remove crusts. Ointment to edges. Good food, cod-liver oil.

   b. ciliaris, b. marginalis. Inflammation affecting the ciliary margins of the eyelids.

   b. squamosa. Blepharitis with scaling.

   b. ulcerosa. Blepharitis with ulceration.

blepharo- (blef-ar-o). Prefix: Pert. to the eyelid.

blepharoadenitis (blef-ar-o-ad-en-i'tis). Inflammation of meibomian glands.

blepharoadenoma (blef-ar-o-ad-e-no'mă). Adenoma or glandular tumor of eyelid.

blepharoatheroma (blef″ar-o-ath-ĕ-ro'mă). Sebaceous cyst of an eyelid.

blepharochalasis (blef-ar-o-kal'as-is). Relaxation of skin of eyelid due to loss of elasticity following edematous swellings, such as in recurrent angioneurotic edema of lids.

bleph'arochromidro'sis. Discolored sweat of the eyelid.

bleph'aroc'lonus. Clonic spasm of muscles of the eye.

blepharoconjunctivitis (blef-ar-o-con-junc-tī-vi'tis). Inflammation of eyelids and conjunctiva.

blepharodiastasis (blef-ar-o-di-as'tas-is). Excessive separation of eyelids.

blepharolithiasis (blef-ar-o-lith-i'ăs-ĭs). Concretions within the eyelid.

blepharoncus (blef-ar-on′kus). Tumor of the eyelid.

blepharon (blef′ar-on). The eyelid; palpebra.

blepharopachynsis (blef″ar-o-pă-kin′sis). Thickening of the eyelid.

blepharophimosis (blef-ar-o-fī-mo′sis). Narrowing of slit between eyelids at external angle of eye due to angle being covered by vertical fold of skin.

blepharophryplasty (blef″ă-rof′rĭ-plas-tĭ). Plastic operation for restoration of eyelid and eyebrow.

bleph′aroplast. A minute mass of chromatin in a cell forming the base of a flagellum.

blepharoplasty (blef′ar-o-plas-tĭ). Plastic operation upon the eyelid.

blepharoplegia (blef-ar-o-ple′jĭ-ă). Paralysis of an eyelid.

blepharoptosis (blef-ar-op-to′sis). Dropping of the upper eyelid.

blepharopyorrhea (blef-ăr-o-pī-or-ē′ă). Pus flowing from the eyelid.

blepharorrhea (blef-ăr-or-e′ă). Discharge from the eyelid.

blepharorrhaphy (blef″ă-ror′răf-ĭ). Reducing length of palpebral fissure by stitching margins of eyelids at outer canthus.

blepharospasm (blef′ar-o-spazm). A twitching or spasmodic contraction of the orbicularis palpebrarum muscle due to habit spasm, eyestrain, or nervous irritability.

blepharosphincterectomy (blef″ar-o-sfinkter-ĕk′to-mĭ). Excision of part of the orbicularis palpebrarum to relieve pressure of eyelid on cornea.

blepharostat (blef′ar-o-stat). Device for separating the eyelids during an operation.

blepharostenosis (blef″ar-o-sten-o′sis). Narrowing of the palpebral slit through inability to open the eye normally.

blepharosynechia (blef″ar-o-si-nek′ĭ-ă). Permanent adhesion of the eyelids.

blepharotomy (blef-ar-ot′o-mĭ). Cutting of eyelid.

blepsopathia (blep-so-path′ĭ-ă). Eyestrain.

Blessig's groove. A mark in the embryonic eye indicating the *ora serrata*, or retinal anterior edge. SEE: *groove.*

blind. Without sight.

blindness. Amaurosis; loss of sight.

 b., color. Inability to distinguish one or more primary colors.

 b., day. Inability to see in daylight; hemeralopia.

 b., letter. Inability to understand the meaning of letters; a form of aphasia.

 b., night. Nyctalopia; inability to see at night.

 b., psychic. Sight without recognition due to brain lesion.

 b., snow. ETIOL: Glare of sunlight upon the snow; temporary.

 b., word. Inability to understand written or printed words.

blind spot. Physiological scotoma situated 15° to outside of fixation point; corresponds to entrance of optic nerve in eye. SYN: *optic disc.*

blister. 1. A bleb or vesicle containing serum, sometimes caused by a pressure. 2. A collection of fluid below the epidermis, usually the result of a burn.

 b., blood. Small subcutaneous or intracutaneous extravasation of blood due to rupture of blood vessels.

 b., fly. Known as *cantharides* and Spanish fly blister, the therapeutic value of which consists in the irritation which it produces, drawing a large amount of blood to an area, thereby relieving the congestion, and improving the circulation.   [than 1 place.

 b., flying. One to be used in more

 b., water. One containing water.

bloated (blōt′ĕd). Swollen or distended beyond normal size, as by serum, water, gas, etc.

block. 1. To deaden all sensory impressions in a nerve, or in the nerve trunk and roots of the spinal cord through the use of an anesthetic for operative purposes. 2. To obstruct. 3. An obstruction or stoppage.

 b., heart. Interferences with the heart's contraction, causing disassociation of the auricular and ventricular rhythms.

blocking. 1. Interruption in free association during psychoanalysis as a defense against unpleasant ideas.

 2. PSY: A sudden, unaccountable stoppage of speech or thought. May be due to a conflict or painful thought, and exhibited in dementia precox.

 3. Process of obstructing or deadening, as a nerve.

Blondlot rays (blon-lo′). Rays of shorter wave length but which resemble light, making certain bodies luminous; also called *n*-rays.

blood. The fluid that circulates through the heart, arteries, veins, and capillaries carrying nourishment and oxygen to the tissues and taking away waste matter and carbon dioxide.

 b., clotting of. The process whereby blood changes into a jellylike, nonfluid mass.

 b. constituents. The preceding tables give pertinent data on this subject.

 b., defibrinated. If whole blood is stirred in a dish, *e. g.*, with a stick of wood, the stringy, elastic *fibrin* comes out on the stirrer; it can be washed until white. The remaining thick, red blood can no longer clot, and is called defibrinated blood.

blood bank. Storing place for reserve blood kept for emergency transfusions.

blood cell. Minute body in the blood of 2 types: erythrocyte,* or red cell, and leukocyte,* or white cell.

 b. c. casts. Masses of red cells molded by the renal tubules, the blood originating from the glomeruli. Abnormal microscopic body in the urine composed of coagulated serum covered with red blood cells.

blood clot. Coagulated mass of blood. SYN: *coagulum.*

blood corpuscles. The solid or cellular elements in the blood. SEE: *erythrocytes, leukocytes.*

blood count. Enumeration of the red corpuscles and the leukocytes per cubic millimeter.

blood dust. Minute colorless bodies in the blood, particles of the blood corpuscle. SYN: *hemoconia.*

blood examinations. They may be (a) morphological,* (b) chemical, (c) physical, (d) bacteriological, and (e) serological.*

bloodless. Without blood.

    b. operation. One by which the blood is expelled by compresses from the part which is to be operated upon, or by electrocautery.

blood motes. Minute colorless particles in the blood, bits of blood corpuscles. SYN: *blood dust, hemoconia.*

blood platelets. Derived from giant bone marrow cells. They are pale discs found in normal blood, and they aid in coagulation.

blood poisoning. The entrance of noxious materials, such as bacteria and their toxic products, into the blood stream.

blood pressure. As popularly used, the pressure existing in the large arteries at the height of the pulse wave; the systolic intraärterial pressure.

    More generally, the pressure exerted by the blood on the wall of any vessel.

    b. p., diastolic. Lowest point to which it drops between beats.

    b. p., hypertonic. Same as the highest osmotic pressure of blood serum.

    b. p., hypotonic. Same as the lowest osmotic pressure of blood serum. SEE: *hypertension, hypotension.*

    b. p., isotonic. The same as the osmotic pressure of blood serum.

    b. p., normal. Should show a high systolic pressure of about 145 mm. with 10 mm. less for women. Normal diastolic pressure, 60 mm. to 90 mm.; 120 mm. average systolic pressure at the age of 20, and ½ mm. for each year above that age, which would give 135 mm. as normal systolic pressure for a man about 50. Arterial pressure is not uniform.

    b. p., systolic. The highest point caused by the contraction of the heart. 120 to 145 mm.

blood'shot. Locally congested with blood.

blood smear. Drop of blood spread on a slide for purpose of examination.

blood sugar. Sugar in the form of about 0.08 to 0.12% dextrose in the blood or about 80-120 mg. per 100 cc. of blood.

    b. s. test. Increased sugar content of the blood, or presence of sugar in the urine indicates faulty metabolism and diabetes. The urine may be free of sugar but the blood sugar may have increased, which necessitates a test being made.

blood test. To ascertain contents of the blood.

blood transfusion. Transferring of blood from blood vessels of one person directly into those of another.

blood urea. Normally it is about 12 mg. per 100 cc. It rises with increasing age. An abnormal amt. indicates deficient kidney action.

blood vessel. A canal carrying blood. RS: *artery, capillary, sinus, vein.*

bloody flux. Dysentery.

bloody sweat. Excretion of blood or blood pigment through the sweat glands. SYN: *hemathidrosis.*

bloody vomit. A result of rupture of the blood vessels of the upper alimentary tract due to injury, disease, or swallowing of blood.

bloody weeping. Hemorrhage from conjunctiva.

Blot's perforator (blos). Instrument used to perforate the fetal skull to facilitate its delivery.

blow'fly. Flesh fly that deposits its eggs in flesh; *Musca vomitoria.*

blow'ing respiration. Bellows murmur; bruit de soufflet.

blue. 1. A primary color of the spectrum; sky color; azure. 2. Cyanotic.

    b. baby. A child born with a very blue color due to mixture of the venous and arterial blood through a defect in the heart.

    b. mass. A compound pill of mercury.

    b. ointment. Mercurial ointment. SEE: *mercury.*

    b. stone. POISONING: (copper sulfate). SYM: Vomiting which is bluish and which turns darker on addition of ammonia. Pain and cramps in upper part of the abdomen. Convulsions. Pulse first strong and rapid, and later feeble. TREATMENT: Empty stomach by means of a stomach tube or an emetic. Give large quantities of milk or the white of eggs in water. Follow with barley water or gruel or similar demulcent.

    b. vitriol. SEE: *copper sulfate.*

bluefish. NUTRIENTS: A. P. Prot. 19.4, Fat 1.2. FUEL VALUE: 100 Gm.—88 cal.

Blumenau's nucleus (bloo'men-ows). Outer part of the cuneate fasciculus.

Blu'menbach's clivus. Sloping part of sphenoid bone behind post. clinoid processes.

blush'ing. Rush of blood to the face caused by embarrassment or other emotion. SEE: *rubedo.*

B. M. A. Abbr. for *British Medical Association.*

B. M. R. Abbr. for *basal metabolism rate.*

B. M. S. Abbr. for *Bachelor of Medical Science.*

BNA. Abbr. for *Basle nomina anatomica,* an anatomical nomenclature adopted by the German Anatomical Society in 1895, at Basle, Switzerland. It includes some 4500 terms.

Boas motor meal. Test for tonicity of bowels.

    B. point. A tender spot left of the 12th dorsal vertebra in cases of gastric ulcer.

    B. reagent. Formula for testing hydrochloric acid in gastric juice.

B. sign. The presence of lactic acid in the gastric contents.

B. test meal. This is a nonlactic-acid-containing meal.

Bochdalek's ganglion (bok'dal-ek). Ganglion of plexus of dental nerve in the maxilla above the canine tooth.

Bo'do. A genus of protozoan organisms. Some are parasitic in man's intestines.

body. Soma; corpus. 1. The physical man. 2. The trunk without the head and extremities. 3. The principal part of anything.

b. cavities. The thorax, abdomen and pelvis.

b., chromophilic. One of the granular bodies in cytoplasm of a nerve cell which stain readily with basic dyes.

b., ciliary. The ciliary processes and muscles.

b., Donovan. Organism supposedly causing granuloma inguinale.

b., Negri. One of rounded particles in protoplasm of nerve cells of animals or persons dead from rabies.

b., Nissl's. SEE: *chromophilic body.*

b., perineal. Tissues bet. the vagina and rectum.

b., tigroid. SEE: *chromophilic body.*

body mechanics. Mechanical correlation of the various systems of the body. SEE: *posture.*

boil. A furuncle. An acute circumscribed inflammation of the subcutaneous layers of the skin, gland, or hair follicle. SYN: *furunculus.*

boiling. Vaporization of a liquid.

1. Boiling water destroys organic impurities. 2. Boiling toughens and hardens albumin in eggs. 3. Boiling toughens fibrin and dissolves tissues in meat. 4. Boiling bursts starch granules. 5. Boiling softens cellulose in cereals and vegetables.

b. point. The degree of heat required to bring a liquid to a boil. It depends upon the liquid. Water boils at 212° F. (100° C.) under ordinary conditions. To kill microörganisms water should be boiled 3-15 minutes. Aeration (pouring from one vessel to another) will overcome the flat taste of boiled water.

bolom'eter. 1. Device for measuring the force of the heartbeat apart from blood pressure. 2. An instrument for gauging minute degrees of radiant heat.

bo'lus. A pill-shaped mass.

b., alimentary. A mass of masticated food ready to swallow.

bond. A mark or short line bet. atoms to indicate the number and attachments of the valencies of an atom giving a graphic representation of arrangement of the atoms of elements in the molecules of compounds; as, H-Cl.

bone. Osseous tissue. The hardest connective tissue that forms the framework of the body.

b., ankle. The astragalus or talus.

b., breast. The sternum.

b., cartilage. A bone developed from cartilage.

b., cavalry. Rider's bone or bony formation in adductor magnus femoris.

b., collar. Clavicle.

b. conduction. Sound perception through skull bones.

b. cyst. Bone tumor of cystic variety.

b., dermal. A bone formed by the ossification of the cutis.

b., epactal, epipteric. A wormian bone, occasionally present at the pterion or junction of the parietal, frontal, great wing of the sphenoid, and squamous portion of the temporal bones.

b., haunch. Hip bone, os coxae.

b., Inca's Os interparietal, os incae.

b., jugal. Os zygomaticum.

b., lenticular. Processus lenticularis.

b., lentiform. Os pisiforme.

b., lingual. Os hyoideum.

b., membrane. A bone developed from membrane.

b., penis. A more or less extensive area of ossification of the cavernous body of the penis in certain lower animals, a vestige of which is occasionally found in man.

b., ping pong. The thin shell of osseous tissue covering a giant cell sarcoma in a bone.

b., pneumatic. Hollow bone, one containing many air cells.

NAMES OF PRINCIPAL BONES:

b., carpal. Situated in the wrist, consisting of the navicular, lunate, triangular, pisiform, greater multangular, lesser multangular, capitate, hamate. SEE: *skeleton.*

b., clavicle. Forms the ant. portion of the shoulder girdle.

b., ethmoid. Light bone at the ant. part of the base of the skull.

b., femur. Longest, or thigh, bone of the lower extremity.

b., fibula. Bone on outer side of leg (shin bone).

b., frontal. Forms the forehead and aids in the formation of the roofs of the orbital and nasal cavities.

b., humerus. The longest, or arm bone of the upper extremity.

b., hyoid. A horseshoe shaped bone suspended from the tips of the styloid processes of the temporal bone.

b., incisive. Fetal bone behind forepart of sup. maxilla, with which it fuses in the adult.

b., inferior nasal concha. Extends along the lateral wall of the nasal cavity.

b., innominate. Hip bone, composed of the ilium, ischium, and pubis.

b., lacrimal. Bone aiding in the formation of the orbit.

b., mandible. Forms the lower jaw.

b., maxilla. One of two bones forming the upper jaw.

b., metacarpal. The bones of the palm.

b., metatarsal. The bones forming the ant. portion of the foot.

b., nasal. Two small, oblong bones that form the bridge of the nose.

b., palatine. Bone situated at th'

back part of the nasal cavity bet. the maxilla and pterygoid process of the sphenoid.

    b., phalanges. Bones of the digits.

    b., rib. One of 12 sets of arched bones, which form a large part of the thoracic skeleton.

    b., tarsal. Bones of the ankle and proximal part of the foot.

    b., vertebra. One of 33 bones forming the spinal column. It is made up of 7 cervical, 12 thoracic, 5 lumbar, 5 sacral, and 4 coccygeal bones.

    b., zygomatic. Bone situated at the upper and lateral side of the face. SEE: *skeleton.*

bone cell. Bone corpuscle. Osteoblast.

bone graft. A piece of bone taken either from some animal (foreign) or the body of the patient in which it is to be used (autogenous) and placed so as to encourage its growth and union with the bone it is being placed in contact with.

bone grafting. Transplanting a healthy bone to replace missing or defective bone.

bone'let. A small bone.

bone marrow. Medulla or soft tissues in the hollow of long bones and in the extremities of long bones. SEE: *marrow.*

bone reflex. Any result of bone percussion.

Bonnet's capsule (bon-nā'). Tenon's capsule.

bo'ny. Resembling or of the nature of bone. SYN: *osseous.*

boopia (bo-op'ĭ-ă). Ox-eyes observed in hysteria.

booster. A device, consisting essentially of a small induction coil with adjustable core, for increasing the electromotive force of an alternating current circuit, or a device, such as a dynamo, in series to increase the voltage of a direct current circuit.

boracic acid (boric acid, *acidium boricum*). An odorless, white, crystalline powder obtained by condensation and evaporation from certain mineral salts.

    TREATMENT: Wash out stomach. Give saline cathartic and large volumes of water. Stimulants as necessary.

bo'rate. A basic salt of boric acid.

bo'rated. That to which borax has been added.

borax. A sodium salt of a form of boric acid.

    It is found in some arid regions, and is made by combining a complex boric acid with sodium diborate. Its chief use is as a detergent and water softener; also a weak antiseptic.

borborygmus (bor-bor-ig'mus). (pl. *borborygmi*). A gurgling, splashing sound heard over the large intestine; intestinal flatus.

border cells. Those in the stomach from which the secretion of acid takes place. They are fewer in number at the cardiac and pyloric ends of the stomach.

Bordet's theory (bor'das). That bacteriolytic sera owe their action to (a) an *antibody* and (b) *alexin.*

boric acid (bo'ric). White crystalline powder of which boron forms base.

    DOSAGE: 8 gr. (0.5 Gm.).

bo'rism. Symptoms caused by internal use of borax or boron compounds.

boroglycerol (bo-ro-glis'er-ōl). A liquid made by heating boroglycerid and glycerin.

borolyptol (bo-ro-lip'tōl). An antiseptic compound of formaldehyde, eucalyptus, myrrh, storax, etc.

bo'ron. SYMB: B. At. weight, 11. A nonmetallic element; with oxygen it forms boric acid.

Borrelia (bor-rel'ĭ-ă). A genus of spirochetes including organisms responsible for relapsing fever.

    B. vincen'ti. A species found in Vincent's angina.

Borsieri's line (bor-sĭ-a'rĭ's). In the early stage of scarlet fever, a line drawn on the skin with the finger nail leaves a white mark which quickly turns red and becomes smaller in size. SEE: *scarlatina.*

boss. A circumscribed roundish protuberance, as that of a humpback.

bos'selated. Marked by numerous bosses.

bossela'tion. One or more small bosses.

Bossi's dilator (bos'sĭ). Metal instrument used to dilate the cervix by means of force.

Botal's (Botal'lo's) duct. The ductus arteriosus.

    B.'s foramen. Orifice bet. the two atria of the fetal heart.

    B.'s ligament. Relic of the ductus arteriosus.

bot flies. Genus *Oestrus.* They lay eggs under the skin of their victim which cause swellings simulating a boil. Multiple furuncles appear with hatching of larva.

bothrenchyma (both-ren'kĭ-mă). Tissue that is pitted.

botryoid (bot'rĭ-oid). Resembling a bunch of grapes.

Botryomyces (bot"rĭ-o-mi'sēz). A genus of fission fungi or bacteria.

botryotherapeutics, botryotherapy (bot"rĭ-o-ther-ă-pu'tiks, -ther'a-pĭ). The grape cure.

bot'tle nose. Acne rosacea of the nose.

botuliform (bot-u'lif-orm). Shaped like a sausage.

botulin (bot'u-lin). A toxin sometimes found in sausages and imperfectly canned meats and vegetables.

botulin'ic acid. A toxin found in putrid sausage.

botulism (bot'u-lizm). Poisoning due to *Botulism botulinus* in food ingested.

Bouchard's nodules (boo-shars'). Thickening of first interphalangeal joints, seen in dilatation of stomach.

    B.'s coefficient. Proportion of fluid to solids in urine.

Bouchut's method (boo-shus'). Intubation of larynx.

    B.'s respiration. Expiration longer than inspiration in children with bronchopneumonia.

    B.'s tube. One used for intubation.

bougie (boo-zhē'). Instrument for exploring and dilating canals, esp. the male urethra.

   b., armed. One with caustic attached.

   b., filiform. One of very small size.

   b., obstetrical. GYN: Rubber catheter inserted bet. the fetal membranes and the uterine wall for instituting labor.

bouillon (boo-yawn'). Clear beef broth.

   b. culture. Bouillon used as a basis for a bacteriological culture.

boulimia (boo-lim'ĭ-ă). Abnormal hunger sensation a short time after a meal. SYN: *bulimia, q.v.*

bouquet (boo-kā'). 1. The aroma of a wine. 2. A cluster of blood vessels.

Bourdin's paste (boor-dans'). A caustic mixture of nitric acid and sublimed sulfur.

Bourdon's test (boor-don'). One administered to determine the alertness of attention, time and accuracy being requisite.

bourdonnement (boor-dŏn-mon'). A humming sound.

boutonnière operation (boo-tŏn-yār'). 1. Incision through perineum behind an impervious stricture. 2. A buttonhole-like opening in a membrane.

bo'vine. Pert. to cattle.

   b. lymph. Vaccine virus from a heifer.

bo'vinoid. Like that of cattle.

bow'el. The intestine.

   b. movement. Evacuation of feces. SYN: *stool.*

bowleg. A bending outward of the lower limb. Bandyleg, genu* varum.

Bowman's capsules. Malpighian capsules of the kidneys.

   B. membrane. Thin homogeneous membrane separating corneal epithelium from corneal substance. SEE: *membrane.*

boxnote. A hollow sound heard on percussion in emphysema.

box splint. One for fractures below the knee.

Boyer's bursa (bwă-yas'). One ant. to the thyrohyoid membrane.

   B.'s cyst. A subhyoid cyst.

Boyle's law. The volume of a given mass of gas, at any given temperature, varies inversely as the pressure it bears.

Boze'man-Fritsch catheter. Double-current uterine catheter with several openings at tip.

B. P., B. Ph. Abbr. for *British Pharmacopeia.*

Br. CHEM: SYMB: *bromine.* BACT: Abbr. for *Brucella.*

bra'chia. Pl. of *brachium,* arm.

brachial (bra'kĭ-al). Pert. to the arm.

   b. artery. Main artery of arm. Continuation of the axillary artery on the inside of the arm.

   b. glands. Lymphatic glands of the arm.

   b. plexus. Network of lower cervical and upper dorsal spinal nerves supplying arm, forearm and hand. SEE: *nerve plexuses.*

   b. veins. Those accompanying the brachial artery.

brachialgia (bra-kĭ-al'jĭ-ă). Intense pain in the arm.

brachio-. Prefix: Pert. to the brachium

brachiocephalic (bra-kĭ-ō-sef-al'ĭk). Pert. to arm and head.

brachiocrural (bra-kĭ-o-kru'ral). Pert. to arm and leg.

brachiocu'bital. Pert. to the arm and forearm.

brachiocyllosis (bra-kĭ-o-sil-o'sis). Curvature of the arm.

brachiofa'cial. Pert. to arm and face.

brachioncus (bra-kĭ-on'kus). A chronic. hard swelling of the arm.

brachiotomy (bra-kĭ-ot'o-mĭ). Surgical removal or cutting of an arm of the fetus to facilitate delivery.

bra'chium. 1. The upper arm from shoulder to elbow. 2. One of the white tracts of the brain.

brachy-. Prefix: short.

brachybasia (bră-kĭ-ba'sĭ-ă. A slow, shuffling gait seen in partial paraplegia. SEE: *gait.*

brachycardia (brak-ĭ-kar'dĭ-ă). Slowness of heart action. SYN: *bradycardia, q.v.*

brachycephalic, brachycephalous (brak-ĭ-sef-al'ik, -al-us). Having a head disproportionately short.

brachyceph'alism, brachyceph'aly. Shortness of the head.

brachydactylia (brak-ĭ-dak-til'ĭ-ă). Shortness of the fingers.

brachygnathia (brak-ĭg-na'thĭ-ă). Abnormal shortness or recession of under jaw.

brachymetropia (brak-ĭ-me-trop'ĭ-ă). Myopia; nearsightedness.

brachymetropic (brak-ĭ-me-trop'ik). Nearsighted; myopic.

brachyphalan'gia. Shortness of phalanges.

brachypnea (brak-ĭp-ne'ă). Shortness of breath.

brachyuran'ic. Having a short palate, or a palatomaxillary index over 115.

bradesthesia (brad-es-the'zĭ-ă). Blunted perception. SYN: *bradyesthesia, q.v.*

Bradford frame. An oblong frame, about 7 x 3, made of 1 in. pipe, covered with canvas strips which run from one side of the frame to the other and which are movable, thus permitting the patient to urinate and defecate without moving the spine or changing position.

brady-. Prefix: Slow, as *bradycardia.*

bradyacusia (brad-ĭ-ak-oo'sĭ-ă). Hardness of hearing.

bradyarthria (brad-ĭ-ar'thrĭ-ă). Bradylalia; unusual slowness of articulation of words.

bradycardia (brad-ĭ-kar'dĭ-ă). Slow heart action. SEE: *arrhythmia, tachycardia.*

   b., sinus. A sinus rhythm with a rate below 60 in an adult, or below 70 in a child.

bradycar'dic. Pert. to bradycardia.

bradycinesia (brad-ĭ-sĭn-e'sĭ-ă). Extreme slowness of movement. SEE: *bradykinesia.*

bradycrote (brad'ĭ-krōt). Slowness of pulse.

bradycrotic (brad-ĭ-krot'ĭk). Pert. to slowness of pulse.

bradydiastole (brad-ĭ-di-as'to-le). Prolongation of the diastolic pause, as in myocardial lesions.

bradyecoia (brad-ĭ-ek-oi'ă). Hardness of hearing.

bradyesthesia (brad-ĭ-es-the'zĭ-ă). Blunted perception.

bradyglossia (brad-ĭ-glos'ĭ-ă). Unusual slowness of speech. SYN: *bradylalia, bradyarthria, bradylogia, bradyphasia, bradyphemia.*

bradykinesia (brad-ĭ-kin-e'sĭ-ă). Extreme slowness of movement.

bradykinetic (brad-ĭ-kin-et'ik). Relating to slow movements.
    A slow motion picture exhibiting details very plainly is used for analysis of the patient.

bradylalia (brad-ĭ-la'lĭ-ă). Slowness of utterance.

bradylexia (brad-ĭ-lex'ĭ-ă). Slowness in reading due to a brain disorder.

bradylogia (brad-ĭ-lo'jĭ-ă). Unusual slowness of speech. SYN: *bradylalia, bradyphasia, bradyphemia.*

bradypepsia (brad-ĭ-pep'sĭ-ă). Slow digestion.

bradyphagia (brad-ĭ-fa'jĭ-ă). Slowness in eating.

bradyphasia (brad-ĭ-fa'zĭ-ă). Extreme slowness of speech. SYN: *bradylalia, bradylogia, bradyphemia.*

bradyphemia (brad-ĭ-fe'mĭ-ă). Unusual slowness of utterance of words. SYN: *bradylalia.*

bradyphrasia (brad-ĭ-fra'zĭ-ă). Slowness of speech; seen in some types of mental disease.

bradyphre'nia. Extreme fatigue as a result of epidemic encephalitis.

bradypnea (brad-ip-ne'ă). Abnormally slow breathing.

bradyspermatism (brad-ĭ-sper'mat-izm). Abnormally slow emission of semen.

bradysphygmia (brad-ĭ-sfĭg'mĭ-ă). Abnormally slow pulse.

bradystal'sis. Slow peristalsis.

bradytocia (brad-ĭ-to'sĭ-ă). Slow parturition.   [passing urine.

bradyuria (brad-ĭ-u'rĭ-ă). Slowness in

braidism (bra'dizm). Hypnotism.

brain. A large, soft mass of nerve tissue contained within the cranium.
    b., abdominal. The solar plexus.
    b. fever. Meningitis.
    b. mantle. Cerebral cortex. SYN: *pallium.*
    b. tumor. Usually used inexactly to describe any intracranial mass, neoplastic, cystic, inflammatory (abscess), or gummatous.

brain storm. Temporary outburst of mental excitement; often maniacal, esp. in paranoia.

Brain's reflex. Extension of flexed arm on assuming quadripedal posture.

branchial (brang'kĭ-al). Pert. to gills.
    b. arches. Four pairs of curved cartilages separating the branchial cleft near upper pole of the embryo.
    b. clefts. A series of openings bet. the branchial arches.

branchiogenous (brang-kĭ-oj'en-us). Having origin in a branchial cleft.

branchiomerism (brang-kĭ-om'er-izm). Segmental division of the entoderm.

brandy. Spiritous liquor distilled from wine and containing about 50% alcohol by volume.

branks (brangks). Mumps.

Brasdor's operation (brah-dors'). Ligation of an artery below an aneurysm.

brash. 1. A cutaneous eruption. 2. Pyrosis.
    b., water. Acidity of the mouth.

brass founders' a'gue. Tremors due to zinc poison from inhalation.

brass poisoning. Due to the inhalation of fumes of zinc and zinc oxide with destruction of tissue in respiratory passage.

Brauch-Romberg symptom (browkh-rom'berg). A sign of ataxia; swaying of body when eyes are closed and feet held together.

Braun's hook (browns). Instrument for fracturing clavicle or to assist in decapitation of the fetal head.

Braune's canal (brow'nehs). The parturient canal formed by the uterus, dilated cervix and vulva.
    B.'s ring. A point, supposedly 10 cm. above the margins of the dilated external os.

braw'ny induration. Pathological hardening and thickening of tissues.

Braxton Hicks sign. Intermittent painless uterine contractions observed every 5-15 minutes throughout pregnancy, after uterine body becomes palpable.

breakbone fever. Acute epidemic febrile disease. SEE: *dengue.*

breast. 1. The upper ant. aspect of the chest. 2. One of the mammary glands
    b., chicken; b., pigeon. Deformity in which chest is protruding, caused by rickets or obstructed respiration in infancy.
    b. milk. Mother's milk. SEE: *colostrum.*
    b. pump. One to draw milk from the female breast.

breath (brĕth). The air inhaled and exhaled in act of respiration.
    b., rattling and shortness of. Edema; presence of fluids in the air passages.
    b., sighing. Air hunger. Occurs in internal hemorrhage.

breathe (brĕth). 1. To inhale and exhale air; to respire. 2. To inject by breathing.

breathing (brĕth'ing). Act of inhaling and exhaling air. SYN: *respiration.*
    b., asthmatic. Harsh breathing with a prolonged wheezing expiration. Is heard all over the chest.
    b., bronchial or tubular. Harsh breathing with a prolonged high, pitched expiration which has sometimes a tubular quality.
    b., cogged wheel or jerky. Respiratory murmur not continuous, but broken into waves, not indicative of any special disease, but frequently observed in bronchitis and in incipient phthisis.

b. of emphysema. Weak with prolonged, low pitched or inaudible expiration.

b., exaggerated. Almost same peculiarity as puerile breathing. Heard over lung that is doing extra work necessitated by some impairment of its fellow.

b., odorous. Due to drugs, alcohol, tobacco, diabetes, kidney disease.

b., puerile. Type heard normally over lungs of children, loud, expiration, higher pitched than in vesicular breathing and almost as long as inspiration.

b., rapid. In pneumonia, high fevers, or interference with oxygenation.

b., slow. Found in narcotic poisoning, sleep, or rest, and in cases of brain compression.

b., stertorous. Due to a relaxation of the palate and is characterized by a deep snoring on inspiration.

b., weak or shallow. Noted: (a) When chest walls are thick; (b) in the old and feeble; (c) in emphysema; (d) in pleural effusion; (e) in incipient phthisis; (f) in painful affections of the chest, like pleurodynia and beginning pleurisy; (g) in pulmonary edema.

bredouillement (bra-dwē-mon'). Pronunciation of only part of a word due to rapid utterance.

breech. The nates, or buttocks.

b. presentation. The presentation of the buttocks instead of the head in childbirth. Occurs in 1/60 of all full-time labors.

breeze. A movement of air.

b., static. If a dry stick is brought near a patient on an insulated platform receiving a charge from a static machine, the charge will pass gradually to the conductor from the patient in the form of a bluish brush.

bregma (breg'mă). That point on the skull where the coronal and sagittal sutures join. The ant. fontanelle in the fetus and young infant.

bregmat'ic. Pert. to the bregma.

breg″mocard′iac reflex. Reduced heart rate following pressure on post. fontanel.

Breisky's disease (bri'skĭs). Atrophy of the vulva. Kraurosis vulvae.

Brenner tumor. A benign fibroepithelioma of the ovary.

brenzkatechinuria (brents″kat′ek-in-u′-rĭ-ă). Alkaptonuria. Condition in which alkapton is present in urine, causing it to darken on standing.

breviduc′tor. Adductor brevis muscle.

breviflex′or. A flexor brevis muscle.

brick dust. A red deposit of urates in the urine.

bricklayers' cramp. A neurosis with incoordination of muscles of the hand when using the trowel.

b. itch. Eczema from lime mortar.

brickmakers' disease. Hookworm disease. Ankylostomiasis; uncinariasis.

bridge. 1. Narrow band of tissue. 2. Dental plate fastened to a tooth at each end.

b. of nose. The ridge formed by the nasal bones.

bridgework (brij-werk). A partial plate held in place by permanent attachments to other teeth.

b., fixed. Partial plates held by crowns or inlays fastened to the natural teeth.

b., removable. Partial plates held by clasps which permit their removal.

brightic (brīt′ik). Pert. to Bright's disease.

brightism. Chronic Bright's disease.

Bright's disease. A generic term for acute and chronic disease of the kidneys. It is usually associated with dropsy and albuminuria. Known also as *nephritis*.

brim. 1. An edge or margin. 2. Brim of pelvis. The boundary of the superior strait of the pelvis.

brim′stone. Sulfur.

brisement forcé (brēz-mon′). Breaking, by forcible means, of adhesions.

Brissaud's reflex (brĭs-sos′). Contraction of fascial femoris muscle following tickling of sole of foot.

British thermal unit. Amount of heat necessary to raise the temperature of one pound of water 1 degree F. SEE: *calorie*.

broach. A dental instrument for enlarging a tooth canal or for removing the pulp.

broad ligaments. These are massive tissues covered internally by peritoneum which spread in all directions from the uterus to the pelvic brim.

Broadbent's sign. A visible retraction of the left side and back in region of 11th and 12th ribs synchronous with the cardiac systole, in adherent pericardium.

Bro′ca's area. On left side of brain, controlling movements of tongue, lips, vocal cords, or motor speech area. Loss of speech due to hemorrhage from here.

B.'s convolution. Third left frontal convolution.

B.'s fissure. One surrounding Broca's convolution.

Brodie's abscess. An abscess of the head of the tibia, or it may be an abscess of any bone.

brokaw ring. Rubber tubing ring threaded with catgut for intestinal anastomosis.

brom-, bromo-. Prefixes: Presence of bromine. [foods.

bromatology (bro″mă-tol′o-jĭ). Science of

bro″matother′apy. Diet in treatment of disease.

bro″matox′ism. Poisoning by infected food.

bro′melin. Ferment allied to trypsin; found in pineapple juice.

It digests 1500 times its weight of proteins.

bromides (bro′mīds). Salts of bromine.

bromidrosiphobia (bro-mid-ros-ĭ-fo′bĭ-ă). Abnormal fear of personal odors, accompanied by hallucinations.

bromidrosis (brom-ĭ-dro′sis). Fetid or offensive sweat. It occurs mostly on *feet, groins*, and *axillae*.

bromine (bro′mēn). SYMB: Br. A liquid element, reddish brown in color, which gives off stifling odors.

bromism, brominism (bro′mizm, bro′min-izm). The results of prolonged use of bromides.*

bromoa′cetone. A lethal war gas causing lacrimation.

bro″moder′ma. Acnelike eruption due to chronic bromide poisoning.

bromo″hyperhidro′sis. Fetid and excessive sweat. SEE: *bromidrosis.* [dides.

bromo″i′odism. Poisoning from bromoio-

bromomania (bro-mo-ma′nĭ-ă). Insanity caused by use of bromides.

bromomenorrhea (bro-mo-men-or-e′ă). Offensive and disordered menstruation.

bromopnea (brom-op-ne′ă). Offensive breath.

bromo seltzer (bro′mo selt′zer). A proprietary headache powder.

bromural (brō″mur′al). A white, crystalline substance, α-monobromisovaleryl-urea derived from bromine.

DOSAGE: As nerve sedative, 5 gr. (0.3 Gm.) 3 times a day. As hypnotic, 10 gr. 0.6 Gm.).

bronchadenitis (bronk″ad-en-i′tis). Inflammation of bronchial glands.

bronchi (bron′ki) (sing. *bronchus*). The tubes into which the trachea divides opp. 3rd dorsal vertebra. The right bronchus is shorter and more vertical than the left one.

bronchia (bron′kĭ-ă). The bronchial tubes.

bronchial (bron′ke-al). Pert. to the bronchial tubes.

 b. crises. Paroxysm of coughing in locomotor ataxia.

 b. glands. Glands surrounding the bronchi at lung root.

 b. tree. Bronchi and bronchial tubes.

 b. tubes. The smaller divisions of the bronchi.

bronchiarctia (bron-kĭ-ark′shĭ-ă). Bronchial tube stenosis.

bronchiectasis (bron-kĭ-ek′tas-is). Dilatation of a bronchus or bronchi, secreting large amounts of offensive pus.

bronchiectatic (bron-kĭ-ĕk-tăt′ĭk). Pert. to bronchiectasis.

bronchiloquy (bron-kil′o-kwĭ). Unusual vocal resonance over a bronchus covered with consolidated lung tissue.

bronchiocele (bron′kĭ-o-sēl). Circumscribed dilatation of a bronchus.

bronchiocrisis (bron-kĭ-o-kri′sis). Bronchial crisis.

bronchiogenic (bron-kĭ-o-jen′ĭk). Having origin in the bronchi.

bronchiolectasis (bron″kĭ-o-lek′ta-sis). Dilatation of the bronchioles; capillary bronchiectasis.

bronchioles, bronchioli (bron′kĭ-ols, -o′li). The very minute bronchial tubes formed by the subdivision of the bronchi.*

bronchiolitis (bron-kĭ-o-li′tis). Inflammation of the bronchioles.

 b., exudativa. A form with fibrinous exudation.

 b., vesicular. Bronchopneumonia.

bron′chiospasm. Spasmodic narrowing of the lumen of the bronchial tubes.

bronchiosteno′sis. Narrowing of the bronchial tubes. SYN: *bronchiarctia.*

bronchis′mus. Spasmodic narrowing of the lumen of the bronchial tubes. SYN: *bronchiospasm.*

bronchit′ic. Pert. to bronchitis.

bronchitis (bron-ki′tis). Inflammation of bronchial mucous membrane.

 b., acute catarrhal. Chilliness, malaise. Soreness and constriction behind sternum, increased by coughing; slight fever, 100°-102° F. Cough at first dry and painful, later mucopurulent expectoration which becomes free as inflammation subsides.

 b., capillary. An inflammation of the smaller bronchi, generally secondary to simple bronchitis.

 b., chronic. Persistent cough, mucopurulent expectoration. Soreness behind sternum. Fever absent unless disease is severe—dyspnea on exertion.

 b., fetid. Bronchitis with foul-smelling expectoration.

 b., fibrinous. A primary inflammatory disease of the bronchi associated with formation of false membrane.

 b., putrid. Chronic form with foul-smelling sputum.

 b., rheumatic. Severe cough in paroxysms, expectoration of scanty, tenacious mucus; aching pains in chest, does not yield to ordinary treatment for bronchitis.

bronchium (brong′kĭ-um) (pl. *bronchia*). A bronchial tube.

broncho-. Prefix: Rel. to the bronchi.

bronchoadeni′tis. Inflammation of bronchial glands. SYN: *bronchadenitis.*

broncho″blennorrhe′a. Copious, thick sputum accompanying chronic bronchitis.

bronchocele (bron′ko-sēl). Goiter.

bronchoclysis (bron-kok′lĭ-sis). Introduction of a medicated solution into the bronchi.

bron″choconstric′tion. Constriction of the lumen of the bronchi. [chus.

bron″chodilata′tion. Dilatation of a bron-

bronchoegophony (bron-ko-ĕ-gof′o-nĭ). Egobronchophony; a goatlike sound.

bronchogenic (bron-ko-jen′ĭk). Having origin in the bronchi.

bron′chogram. A roentgenogram of the lungs and bronchi.

bronchog′raphy. Radiography of the bronchi; making a bronchogram.

broncholith (bron′ko-lith). Calculus in the bronchus or bronchial tube.

broncholithiasis (bron-ko-lith-i′ă-sis). Calculi in the bronchi.

bronchomoniliasis (bron-ko-mon-il-i′ă-sis). Infection of the bronchial membrane with a species of Monilia.

bronchomo′tor. 1. Causing change of caliber of the bronchi. 2. An agent causing such a change.

bronchomycosis (bron-ko-mi-ko′sis). Any bronchial disease due to microbes or fungus.

bronchopathy (bron-kop′ath-ĭ). Any disease of the air passages.

bronchophony (bron-kof′o-nĭ). The voice as heard over a normal bronchus.

 b., whispered. Bronchophony when patient whispers.

bronchoplasty (bron′ko-plas-tĭ). Operation of closing tracheal fistula.

bronchoplegia (bron-ko-ple'jĭ-ă). Paralysis of the bronchial tubes.

bronchopneumonia (bron-ko-nu-mo'ne-a). Inflammation of the terminal bronchioles and alveoli.

bron"chopul'monary. Pert. to bronchi and lungs.

bronchorrhagia (bron-kor-a'jĭ-ă). Bronchial hemorrhage.

bron"chor'rhaphy. Suturing of a wound of the bronchus.

bronchorrhea (bron-ko-re'ă). Abnormal secretion from the bronchial mucous membrane, sometimes very offensive (fetid bronchitis*).

bronchorrhoncus (bron-kor-on'kus). A bronchial râle.

bronchoscope (bron'ko-skōp). An instrument for examining the interior of a bronchus.

bronchoscopy (bron-kos'kō-pĭ). Examination of the bronchi through a bronchoscope.

bronchosinusi'tis. Infection of bronchi and sinuses at the same time.

bron'chospasm. Spasm of the bronchus.

bronchospirochetosis (bron-ko-spī-rō-kē-to'sis). Hemorrhagic bronchitis; bronchopulmonary spirochetosis resulting from *Spirochaeta bronchialis.*

bronchostenosis (bron-ko-sten-o'sis). Narrowing of a bronchus.

bronchos'tomy. Formation from without of an opening into a bronchus.

bron"chotet'any. Extreme dyspnea due to spasm in the bronchi preventing access of air.

bronchotome (bron'ko-tom). Instrument for making an incision of the trachea.

bronchotomy (bron-kot'o-mĭ). Incision of a bronchus, the larynx, or trachea.

bron"chotra'cheal. Pert. to both bronchi and trachea.

bron"choty'phoid. Typhoid fever marked by severe bronchitis in initial stage.

bron"choty'phus. Typhus fever accompanied by bronchial catarrh.

bron"chovesic'ular. Pert. to bronchial tubes and air passages of the lungs.

bronchus (bron'kus) (pl. *bronchi*). 1. One of the 2 large branches of the trachea. 2. The trachea including the bronchi.

bronzed skin. A characteristic symptom of Addison's disease which is due to inflammation of the suprarenal capsules.

brood cells. The mother cells surrounding the daughter cells.

brossage (brōs-sazh'). Brushing the averted eyelids with stiff brush to remove granulations, as in trachoma.

Brouha's test (broo'ăs). A test for pregnancy.

brow'ache. Supraorbital neuralgia; migraine.

Brownian movement. BACT: Oscillatory movement distinguished from self motility of living microörganisms.

Brown-Se'quard's paralysis (sa-kars'). Reflex flaccid paraplegia occurring during some urinary tract affections.

B.-S.'s syndrome. Anesthesia of one side of the body and paralysis and hy-peresthesia of the other side; found in unilateral compression of the spinal cord.

brow presentation. When the brow or face of the infant comes first on presentation in labor; makes birth almost impossible. Cesarean section indicated.

Brucella (bru-sel'ă). A genus of bacteria, nonmotile, nonsporing, aerobic, gram negative, and pathogenic. Genus *Alcaligenes*, except for *Brucella tularensis.*

brucel'lar. Pert. to Brucella.

brucelliasis (broo-sel-li'a-sis). Infection with Brucella; undulant fever.

brucel'lin. A vaccine made from several species of Brucella.

bruce'losis (bru-sel-o'sis). Infection with Brucella. SYN: *brucelliasis.*

Bruce's septicemia. Malta fever.

Bruch's glands (brooks). Lymphoid glands in the palpebral conjunctiva.

B.'s membrane. The vitreous lamina.

brucine (bru'sin). A poisonous alkaloid from *Strychnos nux vomica* and other *Strychnos* species. Similiar to but less powerful than strychnine, *q.v.*

Bruenning electric head-cabinet (bru'ning). Apparatus to apply infrared radiation over face and sinus areas.

bruise. An injury with diffuse effusion into subcutaneous tissue, and in which skin is discolored but not broken.

b. of head, chest, and abdomen. May be associated with internal injuries.

b. of or contusion of breast. SYM: Pain, swelling, discoloration.

bruissement (bru-ēs-mon'). A purring sound heard in auscultation.

bruit (broo'ē). An adventitious sound of venous or arterial origin heard on auscultation.

b. de craquement. Crackling.

b. de diable. 1. The venous hum of anemia. 2. Subjective tinnitus of chlorotic patients and a humming hallucination of hearing in the insane.

b. de frottement. Frictionlike sound.

b., placental. A purring or blowing noise heard in the pregnant uterus due to fetal circulation of blood, and synchronous with the maternal pulse.

b. de pot fêlé. Cracked pot sound.

b. de râpe. Rasping.

b. de soufflet. Bellows sound.

Brunner's glands. Compound glands of the duodenum and upper jejunum. Also known as duodenal glands.

brush discharge. In electrotherapeutics, the discharge from a static machine (less commonly from a high frequency apparatus), having a disruptoconvective character and peculiarities that can be produced by the passage of an electrical current through a resistance such as a tube containing glycerine or a damp (or "green") wooden wand. SEE: *static breeze.*

Bryce's test. A second vaccination after 5th or 6th day from appearance of vesicles of previous vaccination as a test of latter. [liferation.

bryocytic (brī-o-si'tic). Having cell pro-

bubo (bu'bo). Suppuration of a lymphatic gland, particularly in the axilla or groin, of chanchroidal, tuberculous, gonorrheal, or syphilitic origin

bubonadenitis (bu-bon-ad-en-i'tis). Inflammation of an inguinal gland.

bubonal'gia. Pain in the groin.

bubon d'emblée (bu-boh" dähm-blä'). Venereal bubo appearing without previous lesion.

bubon'ic plague. A very fatal, acute, infectious disease, common in the Orient, esp. India.

bubonocele (bu-bon'o-sēl). Inguinal hernia.

bubononcus (bu-bon-on'kus). A swelling in the inguinal region.

bubonopanus (bu-bon-o-pa'nus). An inguinal bubo.

bucar'dia. Severe hypertrophy of the heart.

bucca (buk'a). 1. The mouth. 2. Hollow part of the cheek.

    buc'cal. Pert. to the cheek or mouth.

    b. cavity. The mouth.

    b. glands. Small glands situated in the mucous membranes of the mouth which secrete saliva.

buccella'tion. Hemostasis by use of a lint pad or compress.

buccinatolabialis (buk-sin-at-o-lä-bĭ-a'lis). The buccinator and orbicularis oris as one.

buccinator (buk'sin-a-tor). The muscle of the cheek. SEE: *muscles.*

buccoversion (buk-o-ver'shun). Position of part buccal to line of occlusion; said of a tooth.

buccula (buk'ŭ-lă). A double chin.

Buck's extension. An apparatus consisting of a weight and pulley for applying extension to a limb.

bucnemia (buk-ne'mĭ-ă). Inflammation of the leg; elephantiasis.

budding. A form of fission in which the mother cell puts out budlike processes containing their proportion of chromatin, which then separate and become individual cells. SEE: *gemmation.*

Buerger's disease (bur'gers). A disorder affecting the muscles and blood vessels of the legs.

buffer (bŭf'ĕr). 1. A substance, esp. a salt of the blood, tending to preserve original hydrogen-ion concentration of its solution, upon adding an acid or base. 2. A substance tending to offset reaction of an agent administered in conjunction with it.

    b. action. Buffer salts absorb an excess of either acid or alkali without upsetting the hydrogen ion concentration.

    b. food values. The ability of foods to combine with base or acid without changing their reaction.

    b. salts. Substances in the blood which act as a buffer.

buf'fy coat. Light stratum of a blood clot when coagulation is delayed.

buggery (bug'er-ĭ). Unnatural sexual relations through the anus. SYN: *sodomy.*

bugs. Insects, some of which bite or sting, causing punctures or abrasions on body surfaces. SEE: *bites.*

Buhl's disease (bools). Epidemic hemoglobinuria if associated with acute fatty degeneration. SEE: *Winckel's disease.*

bulb. An expansion of a canal, vessel, or organ.

    b. of the aorta. The dilatation of the aorta at its beginning.

    b., duodenal. Upper duodenal area just beyond pylorus.

    b. of the eye. The eyeball.

    b., hair. The expanded portion at the lower end of the hair root.

    b., olfactory. The ant. enlargement of the olfactory tract.

    b. of the urethra. The post. portion of the spongy body.

bul'bar. 1. Pert. to a bulb. 2. Shaped like a bulb. 3. Pert. to the medulla oblongata.

    b. paralysis. Paralysis due to changes in motor centers of the oblongata. SEE *paralysis.*

bul'biform. Shaped like a bulb.

bulbitis (bul-bi'tis). Inflammation of the urethra in its bulbous portion.

bul'bi vestib'uli (pl.). The glands of Bartholin.

bulbocaverno'sus. Ejaculator seminis; accelerator urinae, sphincter vaginae muscle.

bulbocav'ernous reflex. Contraction of bulbocavernous muscle on percussing dorsum of penis.

bulbomim'ic reflex. Contraction of facial muscles following pressure on eyeball.

bulbonu'clear. Pert. to the nuclei in the medulla oblongata.

bulbourethral glands (bul"bo-u-re'thral). Cowper's glands. Two small glands about the size of a pea, one on each side of the prostate gland, each with a duct about 1 inch (2.5 cm.) long, terminating in the wall of the urethra. They secrete a viscid fluid forming part of the seminal fluid.

bul'bus. Bulb.

    b. aortae. The bulb or beginning of the aorta and pulmonary artery.

    b. vestib'uli. Erectile tissue on both sides of the vagina.   [will.

bulesis (bu-le'sis). An act of the will; the

bulimia (bu-lim'ĭ-ă). Hunger experienced a short time after a meal; morbid hunger.

bulim'ic. Pert. to bulimia.

bulla (bul'la) (pl. *bullae*). A large blister or skin vesicle filled with fluid; a bleb, *q.v.*

    b. ethmoidal'is. A rounded projection into the middle meatus of the nose underneath the middle turbinated bone, formed by an ant. ethmoid cell.

    b. ossea. The dilated portion of the bony external meatus of the ear. SEE: *pompholyx.*

bullate (bul'āt). Said of a surface growth which appears blistered because of convex prominences.

bullation (bul-a'shun). 1. Division into small compartments. 2. Inflation.

Buller's shield. Watch glass securely held in place by adhesive plaster, or junction of skin and plaster sealed with collodion.

bullet wound. Puncture wound from a bullet. SEE: *wounds*.

bullous (bul'us). Having the nature of a bulla.

bun'dle. A group of fibers; a fasciculus.

   b., Arnold's. The frontal tract of the crusta cerebri.

   b., atrioventricular, auriculoventricular. Bundle of His.

   b., Gratiolet's. Fibers from optic thalamus to optic center.

   b. of His. Small bundle of fibers passing from auricle to ventricular musculature and septum.

   b., Keith's. Fibers in wall of auricle bet. the *venae cavae.*

   b., respiratory. The solitary fasciculus.*

   b., Schultze's. Comma-shaped path of fibers in middle of spinal cord's fasciculus cuneatus.

   b., sino-atrial. Bundle of muscular fibers bet. *venae cavae* in wall of atrium of heart.

   b., solitary. Tractus solitarius.

   b. of Vicq d'Azyr. Fasciculus thalamomillaris. White fibers around base of optic thalamus.

bundle-branch block. A form of heart block in which the two ventricles contract independently of each other.

bunioid (bun'ĭ-oid). Round, as a tumor.

bunion (bun'yun) (*Hallux valgus*). Inflammation and thickening of the bursa of the joint of the big toe.

bunogaster (bu-no-gas'ter). Protrusion of the abdomen.

Bunsen burner. A burner named after its inventor.

buphthalmia, buphthalmos (buf-thal'mĭ-ă, -mos). Condition of infantile glaucoma resulting in uniform enlargement of eye.

Burdach's tracts. Continuation of dorsolateral column of spinal cord into medulla oblongata. SYN: *cuneate fasciculus.*

buret, burette. A graduated tube for measuring a reagent.

burn (burn). The effect of exposure to heat, chemicals, *q.v.*, sunshine, electricity, *q.v.*, etc., classified simply into 3 degrees.

   b., acid. Due to exposure to corrosive acids, as sulfuric, hydrochloric, nitric, etc.

   b., alkali. Due to caustic alkalies, as lye, caustic potash (potassium hydroxide), caustic soda (sodium hydroxide), etc.

   b., brush. A combined burn and abrasion resulting from friction. TREATMENT: Like abrasion, *q.v.*

   b., chemical. Injuries due to the action of corrosive or irritating chemicals, as acid burns, *q.v.*, alkali burns, *q.v.*

   b., electric. A result of exposure to electricity. The extent of destruction is much greater than that evidenced by initial inspection.

   b. of eye. F. A. TREATMENT: Wash well with warm water and instill bland oil, as sweet oil or paraffin oil.

   b., fireworks, from. Such injuries are usually burns, *q.v.*, often with imbedded foreign bodies and a high incidence of infection and tetanus which should be prevented by meticulous care of injury and the administration of antitetanic serum.

   b., flash. Lesion from electric arc.

   b., gunpowder, from. Often followed by tetanus which should be prevented by administration of antitetanic serum and meticulous care of injury.

   b., heat. From exposure to heat, steam, electric arc, or spark.

Burns' amauro'sis. Dimness of sight or blindness following sexual excesses.

bur'rowing. The formation of: (1) A subcutaneous tunnel made by a parasite, or (2) a fistula or sinus containing pus.

bur'sa. A sac or pouch in connective tissue chiefly about joints.

bur'sal. Pert. to a bursa.

bursa'lis. Obturator internus muscle.

bursalogy (ber-sal'o-jĭ). Anatomy, pathology, and physiology of bursae.

bursectomy (ber-sek'to-mĭ). Excision of a bursa.

bursi'tis. Inflammation of a bursa.

   NP: Painting skin with iodine. Application of figure-of-eight bandage. Post. leg splint may be necessary; otherwise surgery.

bur'solith. A calculus formed in a bursa.

bursop'athy. Any pathological condition of a bursa.

bursula (bur'sū-la). A small bursa.

   b. testium. The scrotum.

Burton's line. A blue line along the margin of the gums visible in chronic lead poisoning.

butane (bu'tan). C_4H_{10}. An anesthetic from petroleum.

butesin (bu'tes-in). A white, crystalline powder derived from aminobenzoic acid, and having an action similar to anesthesin.

   DOSAGE: As a dusting powder, pure or diluted; may also be used in form of troches, ointment, or suppository; internally, from 1½ to 3 gr. (0.1-0.2 Gm.).

   b. picrate (pik'rat). A yellow powder combining anesthetic action of butesin and antiseptic effect of picric acid.

   USES: As 1% ointment in treatment of burns and ulcers.

buttocks (but'uks). The gluteal prominence, commonly called the "seat" or "rump."

button anastomosis. One made to unite severed portions of the hollow viscera without suture. Devised by Murphy.

button forceps. Those for holding parts of an anastomosis button while it is being adjusted and placed.

buttonhole. A straight cut through the wall of a cavity.

   b. fracture. Perforation of a bone by a missile.

   b., mitral. Contraction of any orifice to a slit, as that of the heart.

b. operation. Boutonnière's operation. An artificial slit in a membrane.

button suture. One for preventing a suture from cutting through or into underlying tissue.

butylchloral hydrate (bu'til-klo'ral hi'-drāt). A preparation similar in action to chloral, but said to be less depressant and more analgesic.

DOSAGE: 5 to 20 gr. (0.3 to 1.3 Gm.).

butyn (bu'tin). A colorless, odorless, solid substance derived from coal tar.

DOSAGE: For its anesthetic action in eye, nose, or throat, 1 to 2%.

butyraceous (bu-tir-a'shus). Containing or resembling butter.

butyrate (bu'tir-āt). A salt of butyric acid.

butyr'ic acid. A rancid, viscid acid found in butter and animal excretions.

butyrin (bu'tir-in). A soft, yellowish, semiliquid fat which gives butter its flavor. It represents 5% of butter fat.

butyroid (bu'tir-oid). Having the appearance or consistency of butter.

butyrometer (bu-tir-om'e-ter). Device for estimating amt. of butter fat of milk.

butyrous (but'ir-us). Of butterlike consistency.

Byrd-Dew method. One for resuscitating newborn child suffering from asphyxia.

bys'ma. A plug or tampon.

byssa'ceous. Resembling flaxlike threads.

byssino'sis. Pulmonary condition from inhalation of cotton dust.

byssocausis (bis-o-kaw'sis). Cauterization by moxa; moxibustion.

bys'soid. Consisting of a filamentous fringe, the filaments being of unequal length.

byssophthisis (bis-o-this'is). Pulmonary condition caused by inhalation of cotton dust. SYN: *byssinosis.**

byssus (bis'us). The growth of hair on the pubic region.

byth'us. The lower abdominal region.

C

C. SYMB: Carbon. Abbr. for congius (gallon), compound, centigrade, Celsius, clonus, closure, etc.

C. Abbr. L. *centum*, one hundred.

C₃ population. Those who are the products of imperfect development, mentally or physically.

Ca. SYMB: Calcium; abbr. for cathode.

Cabot's ring bodies. Ring-shaped bodies sometimes seen in red blood cells in pernicious anemia, lymphatic leukemia, and lead poisoning.

cac-. Prefix: Bad, as *cachexia*.

CaC₂. Calcium carbide.

cacaerometer (kak-ă-er-om'ĕ-ter). Instrument for testing impurity of air.

cacan'thrax. Malignant anthrax.

cacao (kă-kā'o). Theobroma. Seed used to prepare cacao butter, chocolate, and cocoa. SEE: *cocoa*.

cacation (kak'at-or-ī). Defecation; going to stool.

cacatory (kak'at-or-ī). Accompanied by diarrhea or excessive bowel movements.

cacemia (kas-e'mĭ-a). A poor condition of the blood.

cacergasia (kas-er-ga'sĭ-ă). Defective functioning, mentally or physically.

cacesthesia (kak-es-the'zĭ-ă). 1. Disorder of sensibility, morbid or otherwise. 2. Malaise.

caché (kash-a'). A lead cone covered with paper layers, with mica bottom, used for applying radiotherapy, radium, or any radioactive substance.

cachectic (kă-kek'tĭk). Pert. to cachexia.

cachet (kă-sha'). Two concave pieces of wafer (rice paper) bet. which is placed medicine to be administered, the margins being pressed together so they will adhere.

cachexia (ka-keks'ĭ-ă). A state of ill health, malnutrition, and wasting.

  c., cancerous. Cachexia caused by cancerous condition.

  c., lymphatic. Cachexia caused by Hodgkin's disease of the lymph nodes.

  c., malarial. Cachexia due to chronic malaria.

  c., pachydermic. Cachexia due to myxedemic condition.

  c., pituitary. Group of symptoms caused by atrophy of pituitary gland. SYN: *Simmond's disease*.

  c. splenectica. Cachexia caused by disease of the spleen. SYN: *pseudoleukocythemia*.

  c. strumipri'va or **c. thyreopriva.** Adult type of thyroid activity due to surgical removal of the thyroid gland.

  c., thyroid. Goiter.

cachinna'tion (kak-in-a'shun). Hysteric laughter.

CaCl₂. Calcium chloride; a bleaching powder.

Ca(ClO)₂. Calcium chlorate.

CaCO₃. Calcium carbonate; chalk.

CaC₂O₄. Calcium oxalate.

cacocholia (kak-o-ko'lĭ-ă). Abnormal condition of bile.

cacochylia (kak-o-ki'lĭ-ă). Impaired digestion.

cacochy'mia. 1. Disordered metabolism. 2. Cacochylia.

cacocolpia (kak-o-kol'pĭ-ă). 1. Diseased condition of the vagina. 2. Gangrene of the vulva.

cacodontia (kak-o-don'tĭ-ă). Bad teeth.

cacoethes (kak-o-e'thes). 1. Any bad habit, propensity, or disorder. 2. A malignant ulcer.

cacoethic (kak-o-eth'ĭk). Malignant.

cacogenesis (kak-o-jen'ĕ-sis). Any abnormal development or growth.

cacogen'ic. Pert. to race degeneration.

cacogen'ics. Race degeneration.

cacogeusia (kak-o-gū'sĭ-ă). A bad taste.

cacoglossia (kak-o-glos'ĭ-ă). Gangrene of tongue.

cacomorphia (kak-o-mor'fĭ-ă). Malformation; deformity.

caconychia (kak-o-nik'ĭ-ă). Disease of the nails.

cacop'athy. Malignant disease; a severe disorder.

cacophonia (kak-o-fo'nĭ-ă). An altered, or abnormal voice.

cacoplasia (kak-o-pla'zĭ-ă). The formation of diseased structures.

cacoplas'tic. 1. Pert. to or causing morbid growth. 2. Incapable of normal development or formation.

cacorhythmic (kak-o-rith'mik). Showing irregularity of rhythm.

cacorrhinia (kak-or-in'ĭ-ă). Any disease of the nose.

cacosmia (kă-kos'mĭ-ă). A form of parosmia.* Imaginary foul odors which do not exist.

cacosphyxia (kak-os-fiks'ĭ-ă). A disordered pulse.

cacothenics (kă-ko-then'ĭks). Racial degeneration from bad environment.

cacothymia (kak-o-thi'mĭ-ă). A disorder of the mind; moral depravity; insane morbidity of temper.

cacotrichia (kak-o-trik'ĭ-ă). A diseased state of the hair.

cacot'rophy. Malnutrition.

cacozyme (kak'o-zīm). A ferment capable of inducing a disease.

cacumen (kak-u'men). Part of cerebellum below the declivis.

cadaver (kăd-av'er). A dead body; a corpse. SEE: *cleavage lines*.

cadaveric (kă-dav'er-ĭk). Pert. to a dead body.   [corpse.

cadaverous (kă-dav'er-us). Resembling a

caduca (kad-dū'kă). Thickened membrane of the uterus.

cadu'ceus. The wand of Hermes or Mercury; used as a symbol of the medical profession.

caducity (kad-u'sĭ-tĭ). Feebleness or senility of old age.

cadu'cous membrane. Mucous membrane which develops at conception and envelops the impregnated ovum. SYN: *decidua.*

caffeine, caffeina (kaf'e-in, -ă). USP. $C_5H_{10}N_4O_2$. An alkaloid of coffee and tea that is a stimulant and a diuretic.
DOSAGE: 1-5 gr. (0.065-0.32 Gm.).
 c. citrate. USP. A mixture of caffeine and citric acid, containing about 52% caffeine.
 DOSAGE: From 3-8 gr. (0.2-0.5 Gm.).
 c. with sodium benzoate. USP. A mixture of equal parts of caffeine and sodium benzoate.
 DOSAGE: 5 gr. (0.3 Gm.). *Hypoderm.*, 3-7½ gr. (0.2-0.5 cc.).
 c. s. salicylate. NF. A mixture of caffeine with sodium salicylate, containing about 52% caffeine.
 DOSAGE: 3 gr. (0.2 Gm.).

caffeinism (kaf'e-in-ĭzm). Chronic effects of excessive use of coffee.

CaH₂O₂. Calcium hydroxide; slaked lime.

cainotophobia (ki-no-to-fo'bĭ-ă). Inability to adapt oneself to a new environment or to anything new. SEE: *nostomania.*

caisson disease (ka'son). A disease due to rapid fluctuations of atmospheric pressure occurring among those who work in caissons at great depths under water; diver's paralysis.

caked breast. A stagnation of milk in the secreting ducts.

Cal. Abbr. of large calory.

cal. Abbr. of small calory.

calage (kal-azh'). Fixation of body in a berth by means of pillows to prevent movement and so to relieve seasickness.

calamine, prepared (kal'a-mĭn). A pink powder, containing zinc oxide with small amt. of ferric oxide.

calca'neal, calca'nean. Pert. to the calcaneum. [in the heel.

calcaneodynia (kal-ka-ne-o-din'ĭ-ă). Pain

calcaneum, calcaneus (kal-ka'ne-um, -us). 1. The heel bone, or *os calcis.* It articulates anteriorly with the cuboid bone, and with the astragalus above. 2. Talipes calcaneus, *q.v.*

calcanodynia (kal-kan-o-din'ĭ-ă). Pain in the heel when standing or walking.

cal'car. A spurlike process.
 c. avis. Hippocampus minor, lower of two elevations on inner wall of post. horn of lateral ventricle of brain.
 c. femorale. A bony spur that strengthens the femoral neck.

calca'rea. Lime.

calcareous (kal-ka're-us). Of the nature of lime; chalky.

calcarine (kal'kar-ĭn). Spur shaped.

calcariuria (kal-kar-ĭ-u'rĭ-ă). Calcium salts in the urine.

calcaroid (kal'kar-oid). Calciumlike deposit in brain tissue.

calcemia (kal-se'mĭ-ă). Excess of calcium in the blood. [bile.

calcibilia (kal-si-bil'ĭ-ă). Calcium in the

calcic (kal'sĭk). Pert. to calcium or lime.

calcicosis (kal-si-ko'sis). Pneumonoconiosis caused by inhaling dust from limestone, esp. by marblecutters.

calcidin (kal'si-dĭn). A combination of calcium and iodine, containing 15% of the latter.
 DOSAGE: From 1-3 gr. (0.065-0.2 Gm.) in hot water every 15 or 30 minutes to be effective; larger doses for iodine effect.

calciferous (kal-sif'er-us). Containing calcium, chalk, or lime.

calcific (kal-sif'ĭk). Forming lime.

calcification. Deposit of lime salts in the tissues; normally in bone.

calcigerous (kal-sij'er-us). Containing lime or 'ime salts.
 c. tubes. Dentinal tubules of dentin.

calcigrade (kal'sig-rād). Walking on the heels.

calcim'eter. Device for measuring the calcium in the blood.

calcina'tion. Expulsion of water and animal matter by heat.

calcine (kal'sĭn). To cause calcination.

calcinorrhachia (kal-sin-or-ra'kĭ-ă). Calcium in the spinal fluid.

calcino'sis. Deposit of lime salts in tissues.

calcipectic (kal-sĭ-pek'tik). Pert. to calcipexis.*

calcipenia (kal-sĭ-pe'nĭ-ă). Calcium deficiency in body tissues and fluids.

calcipexis, calcipexy (kal-sĭ-pēk'sis, -pēks'ĭ). The fixation of calcium in body tissues.

calciphilia (kal-sĭ-fĭl'ĭ-ă). Tendency to calcification.

calciprivia (kal-sĭ-priv'ĭ-ă). Deficiency or absence of calcium.

calciprivic (kal-sĭ-priv'ĭk). Pert. to deficiency or absence of calcium in the body.

calcis, os. Heel bone.

cal'cium. SYMB: Ca. Atomic weight, 40.09. Silver-white metallic element, the basis of limestone.
 c. carbonate. $CaCO_3$ (precipitated chalk). USP. A fine, white, tasteless and odorless powder.
 DOSAGE: 15 gr. (1 Gm.).
 c. chloride ($CaCl_2$). USP. A very deliquescent salt occurring as translucent crystals having a sharp saline taste.
 DOSAGE: 15 gr. (1 Gm.).
 c. deficiency. SYM: Brittle bones and their poor development, including the teeth, dental caries, rickets, tetany, heart atony, hyperirritability, excessive bleeding.
 c. gluconate. A granular or white powder without odor or taste, containing an equivalent of 8-9% calcium.
 DOSAGE: Orally, 75 gr. (5 Gm.); intramuscularly or intravenously, 15 gr. (1 Gm.).
 c., high diet. A normal adequate diet including 1½ qt. milk and all other foods high in calcium. Cheese is used frequently instead of meat.

c. lactate. USP. A white, odorless and nearly tasteless powder, less irritating than the chloride.
DOSAGE: 15 gr. (1 Gm.).

c., low diet. Milk, cheese, and other foods high in calcium are avoided.

c. oxide. USP. Occurs as white or grayish-white hard mass.

calcium phosphate precipitated. A white, amorphous powder.
DOSAGE: From 15-60 gr. (1-4 Gm.).

cal'coid. Neoplasm of the tooth pulp.

calcopherous (kal-kof'er-us). Containing or producing lime or any salts of calcium.

calcospherite (kal-kos-fe'rīt). One of many small calcareous bodies found in tumors, nervous tissue, the thyroid, and prostate.

calcreose (kal'kre-oze). A chemical combination of creosote and lime containing approximately 50% creosote.
DOSAGE: 4-16 gr. (0.25-1 Gm.).

calculary (kal'ku-la-rĭ). Pert. to calculus.

cal'culi. Pl. of calculus, q.v.

calculif'ragous. Breaking or reducing a stone in the bladder.

calculo'sis. Having a calculus.

calculous (kal'ku-lus). Like a calculus.

calculus (kal'ku-lus) (pl. calculi). Commonly called "stone"; any abnormal concretion within the animal body, and usually composed of mineral salts.

c., biliary. Cholelithiasis*; gallstones.
SEE: gallbladder.

c., hemic. One formed of coagulated blood.

c., pancreatic. Stone in the pancreas, q.v.

c., renal. Stone in the kidney.

c., salivary. Stone in salivary duct. Usually affects duct of submaxillary gland.

c., urinary. Stone in the urethra.

c., vesical. Stone in the bladder.

calefacient (kal-ĕ-fa'shent). Conveying or that which conveys a sense of warmth when applied to a part of the body.

calf. The swelling on back part of the leg below the knee formed by the gastrocnemius and soleus muscles.

cal'iber. The diameter of any orifice or opening.

calibra'tion. Estimation of the caliber of an opening.

calibrator (kal'ib-ra-tor). Instrument for measuring openings.

c., anastomosis. One for determining size of opening to be united by anastomosis.

c., vaginal. One for determining degree of vaginal relaxation.

calic'ulus. A cup-shaped structure.

c. gustato'rius. A taste bud.

c. ophthal'micus. (BNA). The optic cup.

caliectasis (kal-ĭ-ek'tas-is). Dilatation of the renal calyx.

caliga'tion. Dimness of vision; caligo.

cali'go. Dimness of vision. SYN: caligation.*

caliper(s (kal'ip-er). 1. Instrument for

measuring diameters, as those of chest or pelvis. 2. A mechanical apparatus to aid patients who are suffering from fractures of the legs to walk.

Calliphoria vomitoria. Common blowfly causing intestinal disorders.

callisec'tion. Vivisection under anesthesia.

Cal'lisen's operation. Lumbar colotomy for an artificial anus.

callomania (kal-lo-ma'nĭ-ă). Belief in one's own beauty; a delusion of the insane.

callo'sal. Pert. to the corpus callosum.

callosity, callositas (kal-os'it-ĭ, -as). Circumscribed thickening and hypertrophy of the horny layer of the skin.

callosomar'ginal. Pert. to the corpus callosum and marginal gyrus, marking sulcus bet. them.

callosum (kal-o'sum). The great commissure of the brain bet. the cerebral hemispheres. SYN: corpus callosum.

callous (kal'us). Hard; like a callus.

cal'lus. Hypertrophied thickening of circumscribed area of horny layer of skin: callosity.* 2. The osseous material thrown out bet. ends of a fractured bone.

c., definitive. Cartilage found bet. 2 ends of a fractured bone.

c., provisional. Temporary deposit bet. ends of a fractured bone.

cal'mant. 1. A soothing or calming medicine; sedative. 2. Of a soothing nature.

calm'ative. 1. Sedative; soothing. 2. An agent that acts as a sedative.

Calmette's reaction (kal-mets'). Slight injection of conjunctiva in one with an infective disease upon introduction of toxins of same disease. SYN: ophthalmic reaction, q.v.

calomel (kal'o-mel). Mercurous chloride, q.v.
DOSAGE: Laxative (fractional), 2½ gr. (0.15 Gm.).

calor (ka'lor). 1. Heat. 2. Moderate heat of fever; with rubor, tumor, dolor, it represents the 4 classical signs of inflammation.

c. anima'lis. Normal heat of the body.

calora'diance. Giving out heat rays.

calorescence (kal-or-es'ens). Producing by means of a lens incandescence of a body.

caloric (kal-or'ĭk). 1. Heat. 2. Relating to heat,* or to a calory.*

caloricity (kal-or-is'it-ĭ). Heating power of the body.

calorie (kăl'or-ē). A unit of heat. SYN: calory, q.v.

calorifacient (kal-or-ĭ-fa'shent). Producing heat.

calorific (kal-or-if'ĭk). Producing heat; calorifacient.*

calorigenet'ic. Pert. to heat production or its increase. SYN: calorigenic.

calorigen'ic. Pert. to heat production or its increase.

calorimeter (kal-or-ĭm'e-ter). Instrument for determining heat of bodies.

calorimetry (kal-or-im'e-trĭ). A calory measure of heat thrown off by the body under different conditions.

caloripuncture (kal-o″rĭ-punk′tur). Use of heated needles in cauterization by puncture. SYN: *ignipuncture.*

Calori's bursa (kal-o′rĕz). One bet. arch of aorta and trachea.

cal′ory, or gram-cal′ory. The amount of heat necessary to raise the temperature of one kilogram of water from zero to 1° C.

In dietetics and metabolimetry a unit 1000 times as large is used; it is called the kilogram-calory, large calory, or simply Calory (capitalized). By the law of conservation of energy, a calory can be converted, under certain conditions, into other forms of energy in definite proportions; the conversion factors for various energy units are given in the above table. SEE: *therm, thermal.*

Calot's solution. Solution of creosote, iodoform, ether, olive oil, and guaiacol, used externally on painless granulations of fistulas and in chronic otorrhea. SEE: *solution.*

calva′ria. Skull cap; cranium, skull.

calvities (kal-vish′ĭ-ēz). Baldness, alopecia.*

calx (kalks). 1. Lime. 2. The heel.

  c. chlorinata. Chlorinated lime. Used as a deodorant and disinfectant.

  c. sulfurata. Sulfurated lime. Used as a depilatory.

  c. usta, c. viva. Burnt lime, quicklime.

calyciform (ka-lis′ĭ-form). Cup-shaped.

calyculus (kal-ik′u-lus) (pl. *calyculi*). In anat. a cup- or bud-shaped structure.

  c. gustatoril. Taste bud.

calyx (ka′lix). Any cuplike division of the kidney pelvis.

  c. ovum. Wall of graafian follicle from which the ovum has escaped.

cam′era. Any body cavity.

  c. aquosa. Ant. aqueous chamber of eye.

  c. cordis. Interior or enveloping membrane of pericardium.

  c. oculi. Chamber of eye.

  c. o. ant. (major). Same as *camera aquosa.*

  c. o. post. (minor). Post. chamber of eye.

Camerer's law. Two children of same weight but different ages require same amt. of food.

camisole (kam′ĭ-sōl). A straitjacket used for restraining violent mental patients.

Cammidge reaction (kam′ij). Urinal reaction in pancreatic disease.

The result is a light yellow flocculent precipitation in a few hours following test.

cam′phor. USP. A gum obtained from an evergreen tree native to China and Japan.

  DOSAGE: 8-15 ℳ (0.5-1 cc.) hypodermically of a 10% sterile solution in olive oil.

  c. ice. Cosmetic preparation used for mild eruptions and for toilet.

cam′phorated. Combined with or containing camphor.

  c. oil. Liniment containing camphor.

camphoromania (kam-for-o-ma′nĭ-ă). Abnormal craving for camphor.

campimeter (kamp-im′e-ter). Device for measuring field of vision.

campimetry (kam-pim′et-rĭ). Measurement of field of vision. SYN: *perimetry.*

cam′pospasm. 1. Abnormal flexing of the body. 2. Static deformity produced in war.

camptocor′mia. Abnormal flexing of body. SYN: *campospasm.*

camptodactylia (kamp-to-dak-tĭl′ĭ-ă). Permanent flexion of fingers or toes.

camp′tospasm. Camptocormia; forward trunk flexion seen in soldiers.

canal (kă-năl). A narrow tube, channel, or duct.

  c., alimentary. The mouth, pharynx, esophagus, stomach, and intestines.

  c., Bartholin's. Duct of Bartholin's gland.

  c., birth. Canal through which the child must pass during its delivery, namely, uterus, vagina, and vulva.

  c., Braune's. Uterine cavity and vagina after complete effacement and dilatation of the cervix.

  c., cervical. Canal of the cervix uteri which communicates with the vaginal canal.

  c., genital. Canal for the passage of the ovum and for coitus.

  c.'s Ha′vers (Haversian). A system of longitudinal canals in bone, with their transverse and oblique branches, all containing lymphatics and blood vessels.

  c., Nuck. Tubule of peritoneum descending from the uterus into the inguinal canal.

  c., parturient. Space from the fundus uteri to the exterior, the birth canal.

  c. of Petit. Space which encircles the periphery of lens.

  c., Schlemm's. Plexus of veins at sclerocorneal junction to outer side of spaces of Fontana. Aqueous humor leaves the eye through spaces of ligamentum pectinatum and Schlemm's canal, passing into anterior ciliary veins.

  c., semicircular. OTOL: The long canals of the labyrinth bony and membranous, horizontal, anterior vertical, posterior vertical. Part of apparatus for maintaining equilibrium.

  c., urogenital. The structures formed from the lower buds of the Wolffian and Mullerian ducts after their junction.

  c., uterocervical. The canal of the uterus and cervix.

  c., vaginal. Space within the vagina.

  c.'s Volkmann's. Small canals found in long bones through which blood vessels proceed from the periosteum to join the Haver's or Haversian canals.

  c., vulvar. Vestibule of the vagina.

  c., vulvouterine. The vaginal tube. SEE: *uterus; vagina.*   [canaliculus.

canalicular (kan-al-ik′u-lar). Pert. to a **canaliculi** (kan-al-ik′u-lī) (sing. *canaliculus*). Small canals, esp. those opening into the *lacunae* of bones.

canaliculus (kă-nal-ĭk'u-lŭs). A small channel or canal.

  c. lacrimalis. Lacrimal canal carrying tears from eyes to nose. Extends from puncta to lacrimal sac.

canal'is. A canal or channel.

  c. arteriosus. Blood vessel connecting pulmonary artery and the aorta in the fetus.

  c. venosus. Duct connecting the umbilical vein in hepatic region to the ascending vena cava.

canalization (ka-nal-ĭ-za'shun). Formation of channels in tissue.

can'cellated. Reticulated; latticelike.

cancelli (kan-sel'lī). Reticulations forming spongy tissue of bones.

can'cellous. Having a reticular or latticework structure, as the spongy tissue of bone.

  c. tissue. Reticular or spongy tissue of bone.

cancellus (kăn-sĕl'ŭs). An osseous plate of which cancellous bone is composed.

cancer (kan'ser). 1. A malignant tumor. 2. Specifically, hyperplasia of epithelial or gland cell with infiltration and destruction of tissue.

  c., adenoid. Malignant variety with tubular cylinders with a lining of epithelium.   [tion.

  c., black. Cancer with dark pigmenta-

  c., breast. Scirrhous, hard, and medullary soft.

  c. cell. Cell composing cancerous epithelium.

  c., cervix uteri. Scirrhous, encephaloid, and epitheliomatous.

  c., hard. Cancer composed of fibrous tissue.

  c., lips. Epithelioma, usually in men, smokers, and on lower lip.

  c., scirrhous. SEE: *hard cancer.*

  c., stomach. Colloid, epithelial, hard or soft. Usually at pyloric end and lesser curvature. SYM: Pain, dyspepsia; emaciation. Constipation and vomiting.

cancerate (kan'ser-āt). Cancerous; developing into cancer.

cancerigenic (kan-ser-ĭ-jen'ĭk). Causing or capable of producing cancer.

cancerine (kan'ser-ēn). A ptomaine obtained from urine in uterine carcinoma.

cancerism (kan'ser-izm). Tendency to cancerous formation; cancerous diathesis.

cancerocidal (kan″ser-o-si'dal). Destructive to cancer cells.

canceroderm (kan″ser-o-derm). Telangiectasis of skin on chest and abdomen sometimes seen in cancer.

cancerogenic (kan″ser-o-jen'ik). Cancerigenic.* Causing or producing cancer.

cancerology (kan-ser-ol'o-jĭ). The science of cancer. SYN: *cancrology.*

canceromyces (kan-ser-o-mi'sēz). An organism bet. a mycete and a mold considered by Niessen as a cause of cancer.

cancerophо'bia. Morbid fear of cancer.

can'cerous. Pert. to malignant growth.

cancriform (kang'krĭ-form). Having the appearance of cancer.

cancroid (kan'kroid). 1. Like a cancer. 2. A type of keloid.* 3. Epithelioma.*

cancrology (kang-krol'o-jĭ). The study of cancer. SYN: *cancrology.*

cancrum (kang'krum). A rapidly spreading ulcer.

  c. na'si. Gangrenous inflammation of nasal membranes.

  c. o'ris Gangrenous stomatitis, noma. NP: Cleanse mouth not less than every 2 hours, the oftener the better. Fluids by mouth, nasal feeding.

  c. puden'di. Ulceration of vulva.

candle, international. A unit of luminosity.

  c. power. Amt. of light thrown out by a lighted candle, measured in international candles. SEE: *unit, light unit.*

canescent (kan-es'ent). Grayish in color.

cane sugar. Table sugar obtained from sugar cane. SYN: *saccharose.*

ca'nine. 1. Pert. to a dog. 2. Pert. to the canine teeth or the 4 teeth known as the eyeteeth (upper and lower) bet. the incisors and molars.

  c. appetite. Abnormal hunger a short time after eating. SYN: *bulimia.*

  c. eminence. Ridge on ant. surface of sup. maxilla.

  c. fossa. Depression on sup. maxilla external to the canine eminence.

  c. tooth. Tooth situated bet. incisors and 1st premolar tooth. SEE: *dentition, tooth.*

canities (kan-ish'ĭ-ez). Congenital (rare) or acquired whiteness of the hair.

canker (kang'ker). Thrush; white spots on mucous membrane of the mouth, aphthae, noma, gangrenous stomatitis.

cannula (kan'u-lă). A tube or sheath enclosing a trocar, the tube allowing the escape of fluid after withdrawal of the trocar.

Cantani's diet (kăn-tä'nēz). Exclusive meat diet in diabetes mellitus.

can'thal. Pert. to a canthus.

canthar'idal. Pert. to or containing cantharides.

cantharides (kan-thar'id-ēz). USP. Dried insects obtained from Spain or Russia. SYN: *Spanish fly.*

  ACTION AND USES: Locally, an irritant; as a vesicant in the form of a plaster. Its use has been almost entirely discontinued.

canthectomy (kan-thek'to-mĭ). Excision of a canthus.

canthitis (kan-thi'tis). Inflammation of a canthus.

cantholysis (kan-thol'ĭs-is). Incision of a canthus to widen palpebral slit.

canthoplasty (kan'tho-plas-tĭ). Plastic surgery of canthus of the eye. Enlargement of palpebral fissure by division of the external canthus.

canthorraphy (kan-thor'ă-fĭ). Suturing of canthus.

canthotomy (kan-thot'o-mĭ). Division of canthus.

can'thus. The angle at either end of the slit bet. the eyelids; *external, internal.* BNA. *Commissura palpebrarum.*

can'tus gal'li. Children's disease marked

by spasm of the larynx followed by noisy inspiration. SYN: *laryngismus stridulus.*

CaO. Calcium oxide, quicklime, calx.

CaOC. Abbr. for cathodal or negative opening contracture.

cap (kăp). 1. A covering. SYN: *tegmentum.* 2. Tissue over the end of a lymph follicle. 3. First part of the duodenum. SYN: *pyloric cap.*

    c., knee-. Bone in front of the knee. SYN: *patella, q.v.*

capac'itance. That property of a system of conductors and dielectrics which permits the storage of electric charges. For units of capacitance. SEE: *farad.*

capac'itor. A device used primarily because it possesses the property of capacitance.

    It consists of two conducting surfaces separated by a nonconductor or dielectric.

capac'ity. 1. Capability. 2. Cubic content. 3. Holding power. SEE: *capacitance.*

    c., unit of. Unit of electrical capacity. Capacity of a condenser which, charged with 1 coulomb, gives a potential of 1 volt. SYN: *farad.*

capeline (kap'e-lĭn). A bandage used for the head, or the stump of an amputated limb.

capiat (ka'pĭ-at). An instrument for removing placental remnants, etc., from the uterus.

capillarectasia (kap'ĭ-lar-ek-ta'sĭ-ā). Dilatation of capillary vessels.

capillaries (kap'il-lā-rēs). 1. Minute blood vessels. 2. Small lymphatic ducts. SEE: *capillary.*

cap'illariomo'tor. Vasomotor, esp. pert. to the capillaries.

capillari'tis. Inflammation of the capillaries; telangiitis.

capillar'ity. Process by which a liquid's surface, at the point of contact with a solid, is elevated or lowered. SYN: *capillary attraction.*

capillarop'athy. Capillary disorders or disease.

capillaros'copy. Examination of capillaries for diagnostic purposes.

cap'illary. 1. Minute blood vessel, 0.008 mm. in diameter, finer than a hair, carrying blood and forming the capillary system. Capillaries connect the smallest arteries (arterioles) with the smallest veins (venules). 2. One of the small lymphatic ducts which allow passage of nutrient matter and oxygen from the blood to the tissues, and of waste matter from the tissues into the blood. 3. Pert. to a hair; hairlike.

    c. attraction. The relative results attending the mutual attraction (cohesion) bet. the molecules of a liquid, and their attraction by a touching solid (adhesion), according to which the fluids rise above or sink away from their level about the sides of the containing vessel, or of capillary tubes or rods or plates immersed in them. When the fluid rises, the phenomenon is known as *attraction,* and cohesion dominates; when it sinks,

the phenomenon is styled *repulsion,* and adhesion dominates. (*The Practical Standard Dictionary.*)

capilliculture (kap-il'ĭ-kul-chur). Systematic treatment for improvement of the hair.

capillose (kap'ĭl-os). Hairy.

capillus (kap-il'us). 1. A hair, esp. of the head. 2. A filament. 3. A hair's breadth; 1/10-1/12 of a line.

capistration (kap-is-tra'shun). 1. Narrowing of opening of prepuce, so that it cannot be retracted behind the glans penis. SYN: *phimosis.* 2. Lockjaw. SYN: *trismus.*

cap'ital. 1. Pert. to the head. 2. Of great importance to life.

cap'itate. Head-shaped; having a rounded extremity.

    c. bone. Third bone in distal row of carpus. SYN: *os capitatum.*

capitatum (kap-ĭ-ta'tum). Third bone in distal row of carpus. SYN: *os magnum.*

capitel'lum. BNA. *Capitulum humeri.* The round eminence at lower end of the humerus articulating with radius; its radial head.

capitones (kap'it-ōn-ēz). Fetuses with heads too large for normal delivery.

capitular (kă-pit'u-lar). Pert. to a capitulum.

capit'ulum. A small, rounded articular end of a bone.

capotement (kă-pōt-mon'). A sound like splashing in the stomach.

cappa (kap'ă). A layer of gray matter, *ectocinereal lamina,* of the mesencephal.

cap'reolate, cap'reolary. Spiral or tendril shaped.

    c. vessels. Spermatic vessels.

capric (kap'rik). 1. Pert. to a goat. 2. Having the odor of a goat.

caprizant (kap'rĭ-zant). Leaping or irregular pulse.

caprokol (cap'ro-kol). A resorcin compound relatively nontoxic, and having a phenol coefficient of over 70.

    c. solution (S. T. 37). A 1:1000 solution of caprokol.

    DOSAGE: 2½-10 ♏ (0.15-0.6 Gm.).

capsicum (kap'si-kum). USP. Cayenne pepper; dried, ripe fruit of capsicum.

    DOSAGE: Tincture: 8 ♏ (0.5 cc.).

capsitis (kap-si'tis). Capsulitis of crystalline lens.

capsot'omy. Incision through Tenon's capsule.

cap'sula. Any capsule, esp. the internal capsule of the brain.

    c. articula'ris. Capsule of a joint.

    c. bul'bi. Tenon's capsule.

    c. fibro'sa hep'atis. Glisson's capsule.

    c. glomer'uli. Bowman's capsule; malpighian capsule.

    c. len'tis. Crystalline lens.

cap'sular. Pert. to a capsule.

    c. ligament. A ligament which surrounds a movable joint.

capsula'tion. Enclosure in a capsule.

cap'sule. 1. A membranous bag or a covering enveloping a part. 2. A gela-

tinous shell for administering medicine.
3. **Lens capsule.** Capsule enclosing the lens of the eye.

c., atrabiliary. SEE: *suprarenal capsule.*

c., auditory. Embryonic cartilaginous capsule which becomes ext. ear.

c. of Bowman. The glomerular capsule of the kidneys.

c. of the brain. Two divisions of cerebral substance, int. and ext.

c., cartilage. Cartilage cell lining in cartilage cavity.

c., Glisson's. An outer capsule of fibrous tissue in which is invested the liver, its ducts and vessels.

c., nasal; c., optic. Embryonic cartilage developing into nose and eyes.

c., suprarenal or **adrenal.** A glandular body at the apex of each kidney, size about 2x1¼x¼ inches, weight 1 dram. Left one is larger.

c. of Tenon. The *fascia bulbi,* a serous sac enveloping the eyeball, forming a socket in which it rotates.

capsulec'tomy. Excision of a capsule.

capsuli'tis. Inflammation of a capsule.

capsulocil'iary. Pert. to capsule of lens and ciliary structures.

cap"suloplas'ty. Plastic surgery of a capsule, esp. one of a joint.

capsulorrhaphy (kap-su-lor'ă-fĭ). Suture of a joint capsule or of a tear in a capsule.

capsulotome (kap'su-lo-tōm). Instrument for making incision into capsule of crystalline lens.

capsulotomy (kap-su-lot'o-mĭ). Cutting of capsule of crystalline lens.

captation (kap-ta'shun). The first stage of hypnosis.

caput (ka'put) (pl. *cap'ita*). 1. The head. 2. The upper part of an organ.

c. coli. Cecum; colonic head.

c. cornu. Enlarged portion of post. horn of spinal cord's gray matter.

c. gallinaginis. Round protuberance on urethral floor. SYN: *verumontanum.*

c. Medusae. Plexus of veins about the umbilicus in 1 form of cirrhosis of the liver indicating obstruction.

c. obstipum. Wryneck.

c. succedaneum. Swelling produced on the presenting part of the fetal head during labor. It may be mistaken for the bag-of-waters.

carbarsone (kar'bar-sōn). A white, crystalline, odorless solid, derived from arsenilic acid; contains about 28% arsenic, having a chemical structure resembling tryparsamide.

DOSAGE: *Orally* for adults, 3¾ gr. (0.25 Gm.) twice a day for 10 days.

As a retention enema for adults, 30 gr. (2 Gm.) dissolved in 200 cc. of warm 2% sodium bicarbonate solution, every other night, for a maximum of 5 doses, if necessary. Oral administration should be interrupted during this interval.

carbohemia (kar-bo-he'mĭ-ă). Incomplete carbon dioxide elimination from blood.

carbohyd'rates. The monosaccharoses, disaccharoses, and polysaccharoses. A class of organic compounds so called because in them the hydrogen and oxygen are in the same ratio as they are in water, so that the group can be represented by the formula CxH_2yOy.

c. high diet. Large amounts of carbohydrate. 0.65 Gm. pro. per Kg. ideal body weight. Bet. meal nourishments.

carbohydratu'ria. Sugar in the urine. SYN: *glycosuria.*

carbolic acid. Colorless crystalline coal tar derivative which is a poisonous antiseptic and disinfectant.

DOSAGE: 1 gr. (0.06 Gm.).

carbolism (kar'bo-lizm). Poisoning by carbolic acid.

car'bolize. To add or mix with carbolic acid.

carbolu'ria. Phenol in the urine.

car'bon. SYMB: C. This nonmetallic element is the characteristic constituent of organic compounds.

car'bonate. A salt of carbonic acid.

c. of soda. Sodium carbonate commercially in crude form, as washing soda. The free alkali present is irritating and in larger concentrations has the effect of sodium hydroxide, *q.v.*

car'bon diox'ide. A colorless, pungent, and acid-tasting gas (CO_2), heavier than air, generally produced in the combustion, decomposition, or fermentation of carbon or its compounds, and found in the air and exhaled by all animals.

c. d. combining power test. This test, done on blood serum, is a determination of the amount of carbon dioxide which the blood serum can hold in chemical combination.

c. d. inhalation. Carbon dioxide mixed with oxygen for inhalation stimulates breathing the same way as increased carbon dioxide production from exercise. Inhalation of oxygen and carbon dioxide is used as an accessory during artificial respiration and as a continuation of resuscitation after spontaneous breathing has returned.

c. d. (solid) therapy. Solid carbon dioxide (CO_2 snow) is used for therapeutic refrigeration. Solid CO_2 has a temperature below 0° F. Application to skin 1-2 seconds causes superficial frostbite, 4-5 seconds a blister, 10-15 seconds superficial necrosis, 15-45 seconds ulceration. Now used mostly for certain nevi and warts, occasionally for telangiectasia* and lupus erythematosus.

carbonemia (kar-bo-ne'mĭ-ă). Excess accumulation of carbonic acid in the blood.

carbon'ic. Pert. to carbon.

c. acid. Acid resulting from mixture of carbon dioxide and water.

c. a. gas. A colorless, pungent, acid-tasting gas, heavier than air, produced in the combustion of carbon or its compounds, and found in the air exhaled by all animals. SEE: *carbon dioxide.*

car'bonize. To char.

car'bon monox'ide. An insidious poisonous

gas. It is a colorless, tasteless, odorless gas, gives no warning of its presence, and it is widely distributed as the result of imperfect combustion and oxidation.

carbonom'etry. Determination of presence and amt. of carbon dioxide exhaled.

car'bon tetrachloride (tet-ra-chlo'rīd). USP. A clear, colorless liquid, with ethereal odor resembling chloroform; not inflammable.

DOSAGE: Adult, from 30-45 ♏ (2-3 cc.), best given in capsule on empty stomach, and followed by a saline purge within 3 hours, or may be given in magnesium sulfate solution. Precaution should be taken in not administering to alcoholics nor to patients low in calcium reserve.

carbonu'ria. The presence or excretion of carbon dioxide or its compounds in the urine.

carbonyl (kar'bon-ĭl). A characteristic group of aldehydes and ketones:

$$R-C=O.$$
$$\underset{R}{|}$$

carboxyl (kar-box'ĭl). The characteristic group of an organic acid: $R-C\underset{OH}{\overset{O}{<}}$

carboxyhemoglobin (kar-bok''sĭ-hem-o-glo'bin). Compound formed by carbon monoxide and hemoglobin in poisoning by carbon monoxide.

carbuncle, carbunculus (kar'bung-kl, -ku-lus). A circumscribed inflammation of the skin and deeper tissues which terminates in a slough and suppuration and is accompanied by marked constitutional symptoms.

carbun'cular. Pert. to a carbuncle.

carbunculosis (kar-bun-ku-lo'sis). Appearance of several carbuncles in succession.

Carcasonne's ligament (kar-kă-suns'). The deep perineal fascia. Colles's fascia.

carcinectomy (kar-sin-ek'to-mĭ). The excision of a cancerous growth.

carcinelcosis (kar-sin-ĕl-ko'sis). An ulcer of a cancerous nature.

carcinogenesis (kar''sin-o-jen'e-sis). The production or origin of cancer.

carcinogenic (kar''sin-o-jen'ik). Causing cancer.

car'cinoid. An epithelial growth resembling a cancer, but having a benign course.

carcinolysis (kar-sin-ol'is-is). Destruction of carcinoma cells.

carcinolytic (kar-sin-o-lit'ik). Destructive to cancer cells.

carcinoma (kar-sin-o'mă). An epithelial cell new growth or malignant tumor, enclosed in connective tissue, and tending to infiltrate and give rise to metastases.

  c., epithelial. Epithelial cell cancer.

  c., glandular. Carcinoma with cells of the secreting variety. SEE: adenocarcinoma.

  c., lipomatous. Carcinoma with fatty tissue.

  c., melanotic. Carcinoma containing melanin.

  c., ossificans, c. osteoid. Carcinoma with bony deposit.

  c. sarcomatodes. Carcinoma showing transition to sarcomatous type.

  c., scirrhous. Carcinoma with firm structural form.

  c., squamous. Carcinoma arising from the squamous epithelium.

carcinomatophobia (kar-sin-no''mă-to-fo'-bī-ă). Morbid fear of carcinoma.

carcinomatosis (kar-si-no-ma-to'sis). The condition giving rise to carcinomata.

carcinomatous (kar-sin-o'mă-tus). Pert. to or affected with cancer.

carcinomec'tomy. Excision of a cancer.

carcinomelcosis (kar''sin-o-mel-ko'sis). An ulcerating cancer.

carcinophobia. Morbid fear of cancer.

carcinosarco'ma. A mixed tumor of carcinoma and sarcoma.

carcinosectomy (kar-sin-o-sek'to-mĭ). Excision of a cancer.

carcinosis (kar-sin-o'sis). 1. Tendency to the development of malignant disease. 2. A form of carcinoma, beginning generally in the uterus, or the stomach, and spreading to the peritoneum.

carcinous (kar'sin-us). Pert. to or of the nature of carcinoma. SYN: cancerous.

car'damom, car'damon. Dried ripe fruit of Elettaria repens, used as an aromatic and carminative.

Cardarelli's sign (kar-dă-rel'lĭs). Tracheal tugging significant of aneurysm of aorta.

cardia (kar'di-a). 1. The heart. 2. Upper orifice (esophageal) of stomach connecting with the esophagus. SEE: heart.

car'diac. 1. Pert. to the heart or esophageal orifice of the stomach. 2. One afflicted with heart disease. 3. A heart tonic.

  c. atrophy. Fatty degeneration of the heart.

  c. cycle. The period from the beginning of one beat of the heart to the beginning of the next succeeding beat, including the systole, or contraction of the auricles and ventricles propelling the blood onward, and the diastole, the period during which the cavities are being refilled with blood.

  c. diet, Smith. A variation of the Karrell diet. Maintenance protein (2/3 to 1 Gm. per Kg.) mostly milk or eggs. The calories made adequate by addition of some cream by the liberal use of carbohydrates. Fluids limited, salt restricted in cases complicated with edema. For the first few days diet is liquid, milk and cream, orange juice and added sugars. After that soft foods are added, pureed vegetables, fruits, toast, cereal, carbohydrate pushed by use of sugars, jelly, honey or sugar candy.

  c. movements. Those caused by the movement of the air in the lungs from the pulsation of the heart.

  c. plexus. Plexus cardiacus.

  c. reflex. Reduction of area of cardiac dullness resulting from manual friction of precordial and epigastric areas.

cardiactia (kar-dĭ-ak'tĭ-ă). Cardiac stenosis.

cardiagra (kar-dĭ-a'gră). Serious pains in the chest of a constricting nature. SEE: *angina pectoris.*

cardialgia (kar-dĭ-al'jĭ-ă). Pain at the pit of the stomach or region of the heart, usually occurring in paroxysms.

cardiam'eter. Device for marking position of the cardia.

cardiamor'phia. Malformation of the heart.

cardianastrophe (kar-dĭ-an-as'tro-fĭ). Congenital transposition of the heart to the right side. SYN: *dextrocardia.*

cardianesthe'sia. Lack of sensation in the heart.

cardianeuria (kar-dĭ-ă-nu'rĭ-ă). Lack of nerve stimulus to the heart.

cardianeurysma (kar-dĭ-an-u-riz'mă). Aneurysm of the heart.

cardiant (kar'dĭ-ant). 1. Affecting, or that which affects the heart. 2. A cardiac stimulant.

cardiaortic (kar-dĭ-a-or'tĭk). Pert. to the heart and the aorta.

cardiasthenia (kar-dĭ-as-the'nĭ-ă). Type of neurasthenia with predominance of cardiac symptoms.

cardiasthma (kar-dĭ-az'mă). Dyspnea due to heart disease.

cardiataxia (kar-dĭ-ă-taks'ĭ-ă). Incoördination of the heart contractions; very irregular heart action.

cardiatrophia (kar-dĭ-at-ro'fĭ-ă). Atrophy of the heart.

cardiechema (kar-dĭ-ek-e'mă). A heart sound.

cardiectasia, cardiectasis (kar-dĭ-ek-ta'-sĭ-ă, -sis). Dilatation of the heart.

cardiectomy (kar-dĭ-ek'to-mĭ). Excision of the cardiac end of the stomach.

cardielcosis (kar-dĭ-el-ko'sis). Ulceration of the heart.

cardiemphraxia (kar-dĭ-em-fraks'ĭ-ă). Obstruction of the blood flow in the heart.

cardiethmoliposis (kar-dĭ-eth-mo-lip-o'sis). Fat in connective tissue of the heart.

cardieurysma (kar-dĭ-u-riz'mă). Dilatation of the heart.

cardinal. Principal, as the cardinal symptoms, temperature, pulse, respiration.

cardio-. Prefix: Pert. to the cardia or heart.

cardioaccel'erator. That which increases the rate of the heartbeat.

cardioangiology (kar"dĭ-o-an-jĭ-ol'o-jĭ). The science of the heart and blood vessels.

cardioaortic (kar"dĭ-o-ă-or'tĭk). Pert. to the heart and the aortic artery.

cardiocele (kar'dĭ-o-sēl). Hernia of the heart.

cardiocentesis (kar-dĭ-o-sen-te'sis). Surgical puncture of the heart to relieve engorgement of one of its chambers.

cardiocinetic (kar"dĭ-o-sin-et'ĭk). Influencing heart action.

cardioclasia (kar-dĭ-o-kla'zĭ-ă). Rupture of the heart.

cardiodemia (kar-dĭ-o-dē'mĭ-ă). Fatty degeneration of the heart.

cardiodi'lator. Device for dilating the cardia.

cardiodio'sis. Dilating the cardiac end of the stomach.

cardiodynia (kar-dĭ-o-din'ĭ-ă). Pain in the region of the heart.

cardiogen'ic. Having origin in the heart itself.

car'diogram. A tracing of movements of the heart.

cardiograph (kar'dĭ-o-graf). A device for registering heart pulsations in graphic form.

cardiograph'ic. Pert. to cardiography.

cardiog'raphy. Recording the heart movements.

cardiohepat'ic. Pert. to heart and liver.

car"dioinhib'itory. Slowing action of the heart. [heart.

cardiokinet'ic. Influencing action of the

car'diolith. A concretion or calculus in the heart.

cardiol'ogist. A specialist in treatment of heart disease.

cardiol'ogy. The science of the heart.

cardiol'ysin. A lysin acting on heart muscle.

cardiolysis (kar-dĭ-ol'is-is). Freeing pericardial adhesions to surrounding tissues, involving resection of the ribs and sternum.

cardiomalacia (kar-dĭ-o-mal-a'sĭ-ă). Softening of the heart walls

cardiomegaly (kar-dĭ-o-meg'a-lĭ). Hypertrophy of the heart.

cardiometer (kar-dĭ-om'ĕ-ter). Device for locating impulse or apex of the heart's beat.

cardiomotil'ity. The ability of the heart to function.

cardiomyoliposis (kar"dĭ-o-mi"o-lip-o'sis). Fatty degeneration of the heart.

cardiomyot'omy. Severing the constricting muscle of the heart to relieve cardiospasm.

cardioncus (kar-dĭ-on'kus). Heart aneu, rysm or aneurysm of the aorta near the heart.

cardionecro'sis. Necrosis of the heart.

cardionephric (kar-dĭ-o-nef'rĭk). Pert. to heart and kidney.

cardioneu'ral. Pert. to nervous control of the heart.

cardioneuro'sis. Functional neurosis with cardiac symptoms.

cardiopalmus (kar-dĭ-o-păl'mus). Palpitation of the heart.

cardiopal'udism. Irregularity of heart action resulting from malaria.

car'diopath. One with heart disease.

cardiopathy (kar-dĭ-op'ath-ĭ). Any disease of the heart.

cardiopericardi'tis. Inflammation of myocardium and pericardium.

cardiophobia (kar"dĭ-o-fo'bĭ-ă). Morbid fear of heart disease.

cardiophone (kar'dĭ-o-fōn). Device for listening to sound of the heart.

cardiophtharsis (kar-dĭ-of-thar'sis). Destruction of the heart's substance.

cardioplasty (kar-dĭ-o-plas'tĭ). Operation of the stomach to relieve cardiospasm.

cardioplegia (kar-dĭ-o-ple'gĭ-ă). Paralysis of the heart.

cardiopneumat'ic. Pert. to the heart and the lungs.

cardiopneumograph (kar-dĭ-o-nu'mo-graf). Device for recording motion of heart and lungs.

cardioptosis (kar-dĭ-op-to'sis). Prolapsus of the heart.

cardiopul'monary. Pert. to both heart and lungs.

car'diopuncture. Surgical puncture of the heart. SYN: *cardiocentesis.*

cardiopylor'ic. Pert. to the cardiac and pyloric ends of the stomach.

cardiore'nal. Pert. to both heart and kidneys.

cardiorrhaphy (kar-dĭ-or'af-ĭ). Suturing of the heart muscle.

cardiorrhexis (kar-dĭ-or-reks'is). Heart rupture.

cardiosclerosis (kar-dĭ-o-sklĕ-ro'sis). Hardening of the cardiac tissues and arteries.

car'dioscope. Istrument for listening to heart sounds. SYN: *cardiophone.*

cardiospasm (kar'dĭ-ō-spazm). 1. Heart spasm. 2. Spasm of the cardiac sphincter of the stomach.

cardiosphyg'mograph. Instrument for graphically recording movements of the heart and pulse.

cardiostenosis (kar-dĭ-o-sten-o'sis). Heart constriction and its development.

cardiosym'physis. Destruction of pericardial sac by adhesions.

cardiotachometer (kar″dĭ-o-tak-om'et-er). An instrument for determining rapidity of heartbeat.

cardiother'apy. The treatment of cardiac diseases.

cardiotomy (kar-dĭ-ot'o-mĭ). Incision of the heart.

cardioton'ic. Increasing tonicity of the heart.

cardiotoxic (kar-dĭ-ō-toks'ik). Exercising a poisonous effect upon or through the heart.

cardiotromus (kar-dĭ-ot'ro-mŭs). Heart flutterings.

cardiotrophother'apy. Nutritional treatment of heart disorders.

cardiovalvuli'tis. Inflammation of valves of the heart. Valvular endocarditis.

cardiovalvulotome (kar-dĭ-o-val'vū-lo-tōm). An instrument for excising part of a valve, esp. the mitral valve.

cardiovas'cular. Pert. to the heart and blood vessels.

   c. reflex. Sympathetic increase in heart rate when increased pressure in or distention of great veins occurs.

cardiovasology (kar″dĭ-o-vas-ol'o-jĭ). Science of the heart and blood vessels. SYN: *cardioangiology.*

cardi'tis. Inflammation of the heart muscles.

cargile membrane (kar'gĭl). One made from the ox's peritoneum to prevent surgical adhesions.

caribi (kar-ĭ'bĭ). Epidemic gangrenous proctitis.

caricous (kar'ĭk-us). Fig-shaped.

caries (ka'rez). Decay and death of a bone or tooth associated with inflammation and the formation of abscesses in the periosteum and surrounding tissues.

   c. fungo'sa. A tuberculosis of bone.

   c., necrotic. Caries with pieces of bone in a suppurative cavity.

   c. sic'ca. Dry tuberculosis of ends of bones and joints unaccompanied by fluid or swelling.

carina (kar-i'nă). A keel-like structure.

carinate (kar'in-ăt). Keel-shaped; resembling the bottom of a boat.

carious (ka'rĭ-us). 1. Affected with or relating to caries. 2. Having pits or perforations. SEE: *caries.*

carmin'ative. An agent that will remove gases from the gastrointestinal tract. Ex: *asafetida, peppermint, cardamon.*

   c. enema. Given to relieve distention caused by flatulence and also to stimulate peristalsis. SEE: *enema.*

carnal (kar'nal). Rel. to the flesh.

   c. knowledge. Having awareness or sexual practices.

carneous (kar'ne-us). Fleshy.

   c. columns. *Columnae carneae.* Muscular projections from inner coat of the heart ventricles.

carnification (kar-nĭf-ĭk-a'shun). Denoting alteration of tissues, esp. pulmonary tissue.

carniformis (kar-nĭ-form'is). Fleshlike in appearance.

carnivorous (kar-niv'or-us). Flesh eating.

carnopho'bia. Abnormal aversion to meat.

carnose (kar'nos). Having the consistency of or resembling flesh.

carnosity (kar-nos'it-ĭ). An excrescence resembling flesh; a fleshy growth.

caro (ka'ro). Flesh.

   c. luxurians. Excessive spongy granulations.

carot'enase. An enzyme that converts carotene into vitamin A.

carotene (car'o-tēn') (pro-vitamin A). This is a reddish, crystalline pigment found in many vegetables, such as carrots, tomatoes, pumpkins, etc.

carotene'mia. Carotene in the blood.

caroteno'sis. Pigmentation of tissues caused by carotene in the blood.

carotic (kar-ot'ik). 1. Carotid. 2. Resembling stupor; stupefying. 3. A sleep-producing drug.

carot'id. The principal artery of the neck. It divides into the right and left branches. SEE: *aorta.*

   c. gland. A ductless gland at the bifurcation of the common carotid artery.

carotidynia (kar-ot-ĭ-din'ĭ-ă). Pain elicited by pressure on the common carotid artery.

caro'tin. A coloring matter in carrots; a lipochrome.

car'otinase. A ferment converting carotin into vitamin A. SYN: *carotenase.**

carotinemia (kă-ro-tĭn-e'mĭ-ă). Carotin in

circulating blood, causing yellowish skin if in excess.

caro′tinoid. Having the qualities of carotin, esp. the yellow color of carotin.

carpagra (kar-pag′rä). Sudden pain in the wrist.

   c. articulation. Wrist joint.

carpale (kar-pa′lē). Any wrist bone.

carpec′tomy. Excision of the carpus or portion of it.

carphologia, carphology (kar-fo-lo′jĭ-ă, -fŏl′ō-gĭ). Involuntary picking at bedclothes, seen esp. in febrile or exhaustive delirium, of the low muttering type.

carpi′tis. Inflammation of a carpal joint or joints.

carpo-. Prefix: Pert. to the carpus.

car′pometacar′pal. Pert. to both carpus and metacarpus.

carpope′dal. Pert. to wrist, foot, feet, or hands.

   c. spasm. Spasm of the hands and feet, sometimes seen in laryngismus stridulus, *q.v.*

carpoptosis (kar-pop-to′sis). Wrist drop.

carpus (kar′pus). The 8 bones of the wrist.

carreau (kar-ō). Tuberculosis and scrofulosis of organs of digestion.

Carrel-Dakin treatment. A method of wound irrigation first utilized by Dr. Alexis Carrel and Dr. Henry Dakin in 1915.

car′rier. 1. One who or that which carries disease germs. 2. That which carries anything.

   c., acute. Patient who is a carrier only during and just subsequent to the convalescent period.

   c., chain saw. Instrument for carrying one end of a thread around a bone to be cut.

   c., chronic. Individual carrying the disease-producing organism for a long period of time or permanently.

   c., drainage tube. Instrument for placing drainage tubes in narrow or deep seated tracts.

   c., ligament. Flat, needlelike instrument for drawing ligament through perforations made in the fascia.

   c., ligature. Instrument for carrying ligatures.

   c., renal. Instrument for introduction into kidneys. Flexible ones, about 20 in. long.

   c., suppository bladder. Instrument for depositing suppositories, etc., in the bladder.

   c., temporary. Healthy individual who has not had the disease, but nevertheless carries the organism in his body.

   c., urethral. Instrument for introductions into ureters. Flexible ones, about 12 in. long.

Carron oil (kar′on). A mixture of linseed oil and lime water used as a dressing in treatment of burns.

car sickness. Sickness induced by riding in cars. SYM: Similar to seasickness.

cartilage (kar′til-äj). Gristle. A strong, tough, elastic substance or nonvascular tissue forming part of the skeleton, as the costal cartilages, the larynx, ears, and nostrils.

   c., articular. Cartilage lining osseous articular surfaces.

   c., hyaline. Articular cartilage. It covers the ends of the bones in the joints. As costal cartilage, it forms the cartilage of the ribs and they are known also as skeletal cartilage.

   c., white fibro. Bundles of white fibers pervading the intercellular substance and containing bet. them the cartilage cells. This cartilage joins bones together.

   c., yellow or elastic. A network of yellow elastic fibers, holding cartilage cells, and pervading intercellular substance. Found in the epiglottis, the external ear, the auditory tube, strengthening them and maintaining their shape.

cartilagin (kar-til′aj-ĭn). A characteristic principle of hyaline cartilage.

cartilaginification (kar-til-aj-in-if-ik-a′shun). Formation of, or conversion into, cartilage.

cartilaginoid (kar-til-aj′in-oid). Resembling cartilage.

cartilaginous (kar-til-aj′in-us). Pert. to or consisting of cartilage.

cartila′go. Cartilage.

car′uncle. A small, fleshy growth.

   c., lacrimal. *Caruncula lacrimalis.* One found on the conjunctiva near the inner canthus. A small, reddish elevation of modified skin.

   c., urethral. *Carunculae myrtiformes.* A small, red, papillary growth, highly vascular, sometimes found at the urinary meatus in females.

caruncula (kar-ung′ku-lä) (pl. *carunculae*). A tiny, fleshy protuberance. SYN: *caruncle.*

   c. myrtiformes. Shreds of the ruptured hymen. SEE: *caruncle.*

carus (ka′rus). A lethargic, deep sleep.

   c. catalep′tica. Catalepsy.

   c. ecsta′sis. A trance, or catalepsy.

   c. lethar′gus. Lethargy.

caryenchyma (kar-ĭ-en′kĭ-mä). The fluid portion of the protoplasm of a nucleus.

caryocinesia, caryocinesis (kar′ĭ-o-sin-e′sĭ-ä, -e′sis). Nuclear changes in cell division. SYN: *karyokinesis.*

caryogenesis (kar-ĭ-o-jen′es-is). The development of a cell nucleus.

caryogenic (kar-ĭ-o-jen′ik). Pert. to the cell nucleus.   [shaped nucleus.

caryolobic (kar-ĭ-o-lo′bik). Having a lobe-

caryolymph (kar′ĭ-o-limf). The nuclear fluidlike substance.

caryolysis (kar-ĭ-ol′is-is). Nuclear changes in cell division. SYN: *caryocinesis.* *

caryom′itome. Chromatin threads and membranes of the cell nucleus. SYN: *nuclear fibril.*

caryomito′sis. Nuclear changes in cell division. SYN: *caryocinesis.* *

caryorrhexis (kar-ĭ-or-ek′sis). Splitting of a nucleus into chromatin particles. SYN: *karyorrhexis.*

cascara sagrada (kas-kar'ă sag-rä'dă). USP. The dried bark of *Rhamnus purshiana*, a small tree grown on western U. S. coast, and in parts of South America. The bark is seldom used, either extract or fluid extract being preferable.
DOSAGE: From 10 to 30 gr. (0.6-2.0 Gm.).

c. s., aromatic fluid extract. USP. DOSAGE: From 20 to 60 ♏ (1.2-4.0 cc.).

c. s., extract. USP. DOSAGE: From 2 to 8 gr. (0.13-0.5 Gm.).

c. s., fluid extract. USP. USES: Mild laxative, less pleasant, but more efficient than the aromatic fluid extract. DOSAGE: From 10 to 30 ♏ (0.6-2 cc.).

case. A particular example of a disease; incorrectly a patient.

c. brain. The calvaria; cranium, skull cap.

c. fatality rate. Number per thousand of fatal terminations from a disease or operation.

c. taking. A record of symptoms and history pert. to a patient. SEE: *casuistics*.

casease (ka'se-as). A casein digesting enzyme, produced by bacteria, *i. e., Tyrothrix tenuis*.

caseate (ka'se-at). 1. To undergo cheesy degeneration. 2. A lactate.

caseation (ka-se-a'shun). 1. Process of converting necrotic tissue into a granular amorphous mass resembling cheese. 2. Precipitation of casein during coagulation of milk.

casein (ka'se-in). The principal protein in milk, seen in milk curds.

c., vegetable. A protein in beans, peas, and other legumes. SYN: *legumin*.

caseinogen (ka-se-in'o-jen). The principal protein in milk from which casein is derived.

caseose (ka'se-os). The product of gastric digestion of casein.

caseous (ka'se-us). Resembling cheese; pert. to transformation of tissues into a cheesy mass.

CaSO₄. Calcium sulfate.

casoid (ka'soyd). Bread made of a meal prepared from casein for diabetics.

Casoni's reaction (kă-so'nĭz). Appearance of a white papule on skin at site of an injection of fluid from a hydatid cyst; if it remains and increases after operation, another cyst remains.

cassava (kas-äh'vă). 1. Tapioca. 2. The manioc plant.

casse'rian ganglion. Ganglion of sensory root of 5th cranial nerve. Term used erroneously for gasserian ganglion. SEE: *gasserian ganglion*.

cast. 1. A solid mold of a part, usually applied *in situ* for immobilization, as in fractures, dislocations, and other severe injuries.
2. Plastic or fibrous material thrown off in various pathological conditions, the product of effusion. It is molded to the shape of the part in which it has been accumulated.

c., bacterial. Formed from a hyaline matrix filled with these elements. Their

presence indicates their origin, the kidneys.   [*q.v.*]

c., bloody. Same as bacterial casts.

c., broad. Same as "renal failure" casts, *q.v.*

c., bronchial. Seen in sputum of cases with asthma and some cases of bronchitis.

c., epithelial. Contain cells from inner lining of uriniferous tubules. Seen in acute nephritis.

c., fatty. Those containing epithelium that has undergone degenerative changes, found in very advanced cases of renal degeneration.

c., fibrinous. Yellowish-brown, sometimes with ragged fractures, and highly refractile.

c., granular. Of varying sizes and made up of albumin and white blood cells, and of serious import in nephritis in its acute and chronic forms.

c., hyaline. Pale cylinders with rounded edges and variable size. Found in irritating conditions of the kidneys, nephritis, and its varying forms.

c., pseudo-. These are epithelial cells swollen and held in groups resembling casts. Alkaline urine has a tendency to dissolve casts.

c., pus. Found in urine in suppuration of kidney.

c., "renal failure." Those occurring only in last stages of severe renal disease.

c., urinary. Those found in the urine. They may be *hyaline casts*.

c., uterine. Those from the uterus passed in exfoliative endometritis or membranous dysmenorrhea.

c., waxy. Light yellowish, well defined, with tendency to split transversely, found in some cases of amyloid degeneration, and advanced nephritis.

cas'tor oil. A fixed oil expressed from the seed of the plant.
DOSAGE: 4 drams (15 cc.) for adults; 1 dram (4 cc.) for children.
ADM: Give cold with fruit juices, brandy, whiskey, or sodium carbonate.

cas'trate. 1. To remove the testicles or ovaries. 2. One who has been castrated. SEE: *spay*.

cas'trated. Desexed; emasculated.

castration (kas-tra'shun). Emasculation; excision of the testicles or ovaries; the analogy of spay.*

c. complex. Morbid fear of castration.

casualty (kaz'u-al-tĭ). 1. Accident causing injury or death. 2. One so disabled, as a soldier.

casuistics (kaz-ū-is'tiks). Study of pathological cases.

cata-. Prefix: Down or downward; against, or according to, as *catabolism*.

catabasis (kat-ab'as-is). The decline of a disease.

catabat'ic. Pert. to catabasis.*

catabiotic (kat″ă-bī-ot'ĭk). Used up in the performance of the vital processes

catabol'ergy. The energy expended by catabolic processes.

catabolic (kat-a-bol'ik). Pert. to catabolism.

catab'olin. Any product of catabolism.

catabolism (ca-tab'o-lizm). Catabolism is the disintegration of living cells into simpler substances, most of which are excreted.

catabolite (kat-ab'o-līt). Any catabolism product. SYN: *catabolin.*

cataclasis (kat-ă-clas'is). A fracture.

catacleisis (kat-ak-li'sis). Closure of eyelids by spasm or adhesion.

catacrot'ic. Manifesting the downstroke of a pulse tracing interrupted by an upstroke.

catacrotism (kat-ak'ro-tizm). A pulse with one or more secondary expansions of artery following main beat.

catadicrotic (kat-a-di-krot'ik). Manifesting 1 or more secondary expansions of a pulse.

catadi'crotism. Two minor expansions following the main beat of an artery.

catadioptric (kat'ă-dī-op'trik). Pert. to refraction and reflection of light.

catadrome (kat'ad-rōm). The onset or the decline of a disease.

catagenesis (kat-ă-jen'es-is). Retrogression or involution.

catagma (kat-ag'mă). A fracture; a broken bone.

catalase (kat'a-lās). An assumed ferment capable of decomposing hydrogen peroxide.

catalepsy (kat'al-ep-sĭ). 1. A neurosis characterized by a loss of sensibility and voluntary movements without any perceptible alteration in circulation. 2. Abnormal condition of muscular rigidity and loss of will, accompanied by hysterical coma. 3. Muscular rigidity occurring under hypnosis.*

catalep'tic. Pert. to catalepsy.

cataleptiform (kat-al-ep'tĭ-form). Having the form of catalepsy.

catalep'toid. Resembling or simulating catalepsy.

catalysis (kat-al'is-is). Decomposition produced chemically by a substance not affected by the reaction.

catalyst (kat'al-ist). 1. An agent producing catalysis. 2. An agent employed to speed or maintain a reaction in which it does not participate. SEE: *catalytic agent.*

catalytic (kat-al-it'ik). Pert. to catalysis.*
   c. agent. A material or substance that, without itself reacting or undergoing change, induces a reaction that cannot take place without its presence.

catalyzer (kat'al-i-zer). An agent which speeds or maintains a reaction in which it does not take part; a catalyst.

catamenia (kat-a-me'nĭ-ă). The menses. Periodic menstrual discharge of blood from the uterus.

catame'nial. Pert. to the menses or catamenia.

catamnesis (kat-am-ne'sis). A patient's history, after first being seen by physician, including all subsequent examinations.

cataphasia (kat-a-fa'zĭ-ă). A speech disorder causing an involuntary repetition of the same word.

cataphora (kat-af'o-ră). Lethargy with short remissions.

cataphoresis (kat-a-for-e'sis). The transmission of electronegative ions or drugs into the body tissues or through a membrane by use of an electric current.

cataphoria (kat-af-o'rĭ-ă). Tendency of visual axes to incline below the horizontal plane.

cataphor'ic. Pert. to cataphora or cataphoresis.

cataphre'nia. A dementia type tending to recovery but which shows mental debility.

cataphylaxis (kat-ă-fĭ-laks'is). The process of carrying antibodies, leukocytes, etc., to the site of an infection.

cataplasia (kat-ă-pla'zĭ-ă). Degenerative change in tissues or cells.

cataplasis (kat-ap'las-is). 1. The period of decline in life. 2. Application of a coating or a plaster.

cat'aplasm. A poultice, *q.v.* The most commonly used are flaxseed, onion, bread and milk, and bran. They are used as counterirritants, drawing the blood to the surface of the body, thereby removing deep-seated inflammation.

cataplectic (kat-ă-plek'tĭk). Pert. to cataplexy.

cataplexy, cataplexia (kat'a-pleks-ĭ,-pleks'ĭ-a). A form of sudden shock, accompanied by loss of muscular tone, without loss of consciousness, the patient falling to the floor.

cataptosis (kat-ap-to'sis). Ptosis; apoplexy, epilepsy, paralysis.

cat'aract. Opacity of lens of eye or its capsule or both.

cataractous (kat-ar-ak'tus). Affected with or of the nature of a cataract.

catarrh (ka-tar'). Inflammation of mucous membrane.
   c., dry. Severe spells of coughing with little or no expectoration. Generally seen in the old in association with emphysema or asthma.
   c., epidemic. Influenza.
   c., gastric. Gastritis.
   c., intestinal. Enteritis.
   c., nasal. Coryza.
   c., pulmonary. Bronchitis.
   c., uterine. Endometritis.
   c., vernal. A chronic form of conjunctivitis occurring usually in spring and summer. Must be differentiated from trachoma and follicular conjunctivitis.
   c., vesical. Cystitis.

catarrhal (kat-ă'ral). Of the nature of or pert. to catarrh.

catastalsis (kat-as-tal'sis). Downward contraction of stomach during digestion; not preceded by a wave of inhibition.

catastaltic (kat-as-tal'tik). 1. A nerve impulse passing from above downward. 2. An astringent. 3. A sedative or inhibitory agent. 4. Inhibiting, restraining.

catastasis (kat-as'tas-is). Decline or quieting of symptoms. Restitution of a part.

catastate (kat'as-tāt). One of a succession of catabolic conditions or substances, each being less complex, more stable, and exhibiting less functional activity than its predecessor. 2. Stupor.

catastat'ic. Pert. to catastasis or a catastate.

catato'nia. 1. Intervention of maniacal, melancholic, or stuporous intervals in the progressive dementia of a form of dementia precox accompanied by muscular tension. 2. Stupor.

caton'ic. Stuporous; pert. to catatonia.

catatricrotic (kat-ă-tri-krot'ĭk). Manifesting a third impulse in the descending stroke of the sphygmogram.

catatricrotism (kat-a-tri'kro-tĭzm). State in which the pulse is catatricrotic.

catatropia (kat-ă-tro'pĭ-ă). Having both eyes turned downward.

cataxia (kă-taks'ĭ-ă). The breaking up of pathogenic microörganisms.

cat bite. Usually a punctured or lacerated wound, potentially infected with bacteria. Frequently infected wounds follow even under careful management. If animals are rabid, may lead to hydrophobia.

cat'electrot'onus. The state of increased excitability produced in a nerve or muscle in the region near the cathode during the passage of an electric current.

catenating (kat'en-āt"ing). Linking or connecting, as one disease associated with another.

catenoid (kat'en-oid). Chainlike; pert. to protozoan colonies whose individuals are joined end-to-end.

cat'gut. Sheep's intestine twisted for use as an absorbable ligature.

catharma (kath-ar'mă). Product or result of purging.

cathar'sis. 1. Purgative action of the bowels. 2. The freudian method of freeing the mind by recalling the patient's memory of an event or experience that was the exciting cause of a psychoneurosis; abreaction, q.v.

cathar'tic. An active purgative, usually producing several evacuations which may or may not be accompanied by pain or tenesmus.

cathedral glass. Window glass substitute for transmitting antirachitic rays of sunlight.

catheresis (kath-er'e-sis). 1. Weakness resulting from medication. 2. Caustic or feebly caustic action.

catheretic (kath-e-re'tik). 1. Weakening. 2. Slightly caustic.

catherization (kath"e-ri-za'shun). Act of weakening by medication.

catheter (kath'et-er). A tube for evacuating or injecting fluids through a natural passage.

   c., double channel. One providing for inflow and outflow.

   c., elbowed. One which has an acute bend near the beak. USES: Cases of enlarged prostate.

   c., eustachian. One for injection into eustachian tube through nasal passages.

   c., female. One about 5 inches long.

   c., ndwelling. One which keeps its position in the ureter.

   c., male. One for bladder evacuation. 12-13 inches long.

   c., prostatic. One designed to pass prostatic obstruction. 15-16 inches long.

   c., self-retaining. One which can be retained at will, effecting bladder drainage.

   c., vertebrated. One in sections to be fitted together, so that it is flexible.

   c., winged. One with little flaps at each side of beak to aid in retaining it in the bladder.

catheter fever. Reactionary rise in temperature from passing of a catheter or urethral bougie.

catheterization (kath"et-er-i-za'shun). Introduction of a catheter through the urethra into the bladder for withdrawal of urine.

catheterize (kath'e-ter-īz). To draw the urine through a catheter.

cathetom'eter. Device to aid in the reading of thermometers.

cathexis (kath-eks'is). The emotional or mental energy imparted to an idea.

cath'odal. Pert. to the cathode.

cath'ode. The negative pole, as opposed to the anode, or positive pole.

   c. dark space. The nonluminous region which envelops and follows the outline of the cathode in a discharge tube at moderately low pressures.

   c. stream. Negatively charged electrons, sent out as particles from the cathode in discharges through the vacuum. SEE: *cathode rays.**

cathod'ic. Pert. to a cathode.

cathod'ograph. An x-ray picture; skiagram.

catholicon (ka-thol'ĭ-kŏn). A remedy for all diseases; a panacea.

cation (kat'ĭ-on). The name given by Faraday to the element or elements of an electrolyte in electrochemical decomposition appearing at the negative pole, or cathode.   [ble edges.

catlin (kat'lin). Surgical knife with doucatochus (kat'o-kus). 1. Coma vigil; catalepsy. 2. A trance; deathlike.

catoptric (kat-op'trik). Pert. to reflected light or mirrors.

catoptrophobia (kat-op-trō-fo'bĭ-ă). Morbid fear of mirrors or of breaking them.

catoteric (kat-o-ter'ĭk). A cathartic or purgative.

cat's ear. An ear resembling that of a cat.

cat's-eye pupil. A slitlike pupil.

cat's purr. A purring bruit due to defect of the mitral valve heard on auscultation.

catulotic (kat-ul-ot'ĭk). Tending to cause cicatrization.

cat unit. Amount of a drug, per Kg. of animal's weight, required to kill it, when injected intravenously.

cau'da. Tail. The lower part of an anatomical structure.

c. cerebelli. Cerebellar tail-like process.

c. equi'na. Termination of spinal cord.

c. stria'ti. Tail-like post. extremity of corpus striatum.

caudad (kaw'dad). Toward the tail; in a post. direction.

caudal (kawd'al). 1. Pert. to any tail-like structure. 2. Inferior in position.

caudate (kaw'dāt). Possessing a tail.

caudation (kaw-da'shun). A lengthened or elongated clitoris.

caudle (kawd'l). A nutritious food made of egg, gruel, sherry, and flavoring.

caul (kawl). 1. The great omentum. 2. Membranes or portions of the amnion covering head of fetus at birth.

cauli'flower ear. Malformation of auricle due to injury, as seen in boxers.

c. excrescence. Condyloma of the cervix uteri.

cauloplegia (kaw-lo-ple'jĭ-ă). Paralysis of the penis.

cauma (kaw'mă). An inflammatory fever; pyrexia, heat, fever.

c. enteritis. An acute intestinal catarrh.

caumesthesia (kaw-mes-the'zĭ-ă). A sense of heat without cause of same.

causalgia (kaw-sal'jĭ-ă). Intense burning pain with a glossy skin.

causoma (kaw-so'mă). A burning; an inflammation of a burning nature.

caustic (kaw'stik). 1. Corrosive and burning. 2. An agent that will destroy living tissue. SEE: escharotic.

c. potash. Potassium hydroxide, q.v.

c. soda. Sodium hydroxide, q.v.

cauterant (kaw'ter-ant). 1. Escharotic; caustic. 2. A caustic agent.

cauterization (kaw-ter-i-za'shun). Burning a part; cautery.

c., actual. By hot iron. Atmocausis. By steam.

c., chemical. Cautery by electrolysis. By chemical means.

c., electrical. By platinum wires heated to incandescence by an electric current; galvanocautery.

c., potential. By applying a corrosive substance.

cauterize (kaw'ter-iz). To burn with a cautery, or to apply one.

caut'erodyne. A radio knife for bloodless surgery.

It is a small pencil-like tube with a wire coil in place of a blade. It seals minor blood vessels. Used for cancer and goiter operations.

cautery (kaw'ter-ĭ). A means of destroying tissue by electricity, heat, or corrosive chemicals.

cava (ka'vah). Vena cava.

ca'val. Pert. to the vena cava.

cav'alry bone. Rider's bone; bony deposit in the adductor muscles of the thigh.

cavascope (kav'ă-skōp). Instrument for examining cavities.

cavernil'oquy. Low pitched sound over pulmonary structures.

caverni'tis. Inflammation of the corpus cavernosum penis.

caverno'ma. A cavernous angioma.

cavernosi'tis. Inflammation of the corpora cavernosa.

cavernosum (kăv-ĕr-nō'sŭm). One of 2 erectile columns of the dorsum of the penis or clitoris. SYN: corpus cavernosum.

cavernous (kăv'ĕr-nŭs). Containing hollow spaces.

c. angioma. A vascular tumor with many large spaces.

c. body. Corpus cavernosum.

c. râle. Bubbling hollow sound.

c. resonance. Amphoric resonance.

c. respiration. Hollow sound heard when there is a lung cavity.

c. rhoncus. A cavernous râle.

c. sinus. Blood sinus on body of sphenoid bone.

c. tumor. An angioma.

cav'itary. 1. Hollow; having or forming cavities. 2. Any nematode worm.

cavita'tion. Formation of a cavity. Ex: Formation of lung cavity in tuberculosis.

cavitis (ka-vi'tis). Inflammation of a vena cava.

cavity (kav'it-ĭ). A hollow space, such as a body organ or the hole in a carious tooth.

c., abdominal. The cavity of the peritoneum bet. the diaphragm and pelvis.

c., amniotic. That within the amnion.

c., buccal. The mouth.

c., cotyloid. The acetabulum.

c., glenoid. Cavity in head of scapula, which holds the humerus.

c., pelvic. One containing the bladder and rectum and the uterus in the female.

c., pulp. One in a tooth containing the dental pulp and nerve termination.

c., Rosenmüller's. One on either side of openings of eustachian tube.

c., splanchnic. One of three, the cranial, thoracic, and abdominal, including the pelvic cavity.

c., visceral. The splanchnic cavity.

ca'vum. A cavity or a hole.

c. septi pellucidi. BNA. Cavity of the 5th ventricle of the brain.

c. tympani. Middle ear cavity.

ca'vus. Condition of exaggerated height of arch of foot. SYN: talipes cavus.

Cayenne pepper (kī-ĕn', kā-ĕn'). Capsicum, q.v.

Cazenave's lupus (kahz-nāv'). 1. Lupus erythematosus. 2. Pemphigus foliaceus.

cc. Abbr: Cubic centimeter; about 16 minims.

CCl₃CHO. Chloral.

c.cm. Abbr. for cubic centimeter.

Cd. Symb. of cadmium.

Ce. Symb. of cerium.

ceasmic (se-as'mĭk). Pert. to an abnormal cleavage of parts or to a fissure.

cebione (sē'bĭ-ōn). SEE: cevitamic acid.

cecal (se'kal). 1. Pert. to cecum. 2. Blind, terminating in a closed extremity.

cecectomy (se-sek'to-mĭ). Removing part of or incision into the cecum.

cecitis (se-si'tis). Inflammation of the cecum.

cecoileostomy (se-ko-il-e-os'to-mĭ). Making an opening through the abdominal wall into the ileum at the ileocecal valve.

cecopexy (se'ko-peks-ĭ). Surgical fixation of the cecum to the abdominal wall.

cecoplica'tion. Reduction of a dilated cecum by making a fold in its wall.

cecoptosis (se-kop-to'sis). Falling displacement of the cecum.

cecosigmoidostomy (se-ko-sig-moid-os'to-mĭ). Formation of a communication bet. the cecum and sigmoid.

cecos'tomy. Surgical formation of a cecal fistula or artificial anus.

cecot'omy. Cutting into the cecum.

cecum (se'kum). A blind pouch at the junction of the small intestines with the ascending colon, and to which the ileum is attached.

celarium (se-la'rĭ-um). The epithelium of the celom.

-cele. Suffix: A swelling.

celectome (se-lek'tōm). Instrument for obtaining a piece of tissue from a tumor for examination.

celiac (se'lĭ-ak). Rel. to the abdominal regions.

 c. artery. Artery running through abdomen. See: *aorta, artery.*

 c. axis. A branch of the abdominal aorta.

 c. disease. Dilatation of the small and large intestines causing intestinal indigestion, and occurring in children and infants, usually bet. the 9th and 18th months; sometimes bet. the 3rd and 6th years.

 c. plexus. Sympathetic plexus lying near the origin of celiac artery. See: *plexuses.*

celiagra (se-lĭ-ag'ră). Gouty affection of any abdominal organ.

celial'gia. Abdominal pain.

celiectasia (se-lĭ-ek-ta'sĭ-ă). Distention of the abdomen.

celiectomy (se-lĭ-ek'to-mĭ). Removal of an abdominal organ.

celiocentesis (se-lĭ-o-sen-te'sis). Puncture of the abdomen. Syn: *paracentesis.*

celiocolpotomy (se''lĭ-o-kol-pot'o-mĭ). Vaginal opening into the abdomen for removing the products of ectopic pregnancy.

celioelytrotomy (se-lĭ-o-el-ĭ-trot'o-mĭ). Opening through the vagina into the abdomen.

celioenterotomy (se-lĭ-ō-en-ter-ot'o-mĭ). Incision in the abdominal wall to gain access to the abdomen.

celiogastrostomy (se-lĭ-ō-gas-tros'to-mĭ). Incision in the abdominal wall for making a gastric fistula.

celiogastrotomy (sel-ĭ-o-gas-trot'o-mĭ). Incision of stomach with abdominal section.

celiohysterectomy (se''lĭ-o-his-ter-ek'to-mĭ). Removal of uterus through an abdominal incision.

celiohystero-oöthecectomy (se-lĭ-o-his-ter--o-o-ō-the-sek'to-mĭ). Removal of the uterus and the ovaries through an abdominal incision.

celiohystero-salpingo-oöthecectomy (se-lĭ-o-his-ter-o-sal-pin-go-o-ō-the-sek'to-mĭ). Removal of the uterus, fallopian tubes and ovaries through an abdominal incision.

ce''liohysterot'omy. Opening into the uterus through an abdominal incision.

celioma (se-lĭ-o'mă). An abdominal tumor.

celiomyal'gia. Rheumatic pain in muscles of the abdomen.

celiomyomectomy (se-lĭ-o-mĭ-o-mek'to-mĭ). Removal of fibroid tumors through an abdominal incision.

celiomyomotomy (se-lĭ-o-mĭ-o-mot'o-mĭ). Incision of muscles of abdomen.

celiomyositis (se-lĭ-o-mi-o-si'tis). Inflammation of muscles of the abdomen.

celioncus (se-lĭ-on'kus). An abdominal tumor.

celioparacentesis (se-lĭ-o-par-ă-sen-te'sis). Puncture of the abdomen.

celiopathy (se-lĭ-op'ath-ĭ). Any disease of the abdomen.

celiopyosis (se-lĭ-o-pī-o'sis). Purulent peritonitis.

celiorrhaphy (se-lĭ-or'af-ĭ). Suture of wound in the abdominal wall.

celiosalpingectomy (se-lĭ-o-sal-pin-jek'to-mĭ). Removal of the fallopian tubes through an abdominal incision.

celiosalpingotomy (se-lĭ-o-sal-pin-got'o-mĭ). Opening of the fallopian tube through an abdominal incision.

celioscope (se'lĭ-o-skōp). Device for illumination of abdominal cavity.

celioscopy (se-lĭ-os'ko-pĭ). Use of the celioscope.

celiotomy (se-lĭ-ot'o-mĭ). Surgical incision into the abdominal cavity.

 c., vaginal. Entering the abdomen through the vagina.

celitis (se-li'tis). Peritonitis; abdominal inflammation.

cell. 1. A small, enclosed or partly enclosed cavity, such as an air cell. 2. Protoplasmic body which constitutes the unit of all life in itself, a complete organism.

 c., adipose. A fat cell.

 c., blood. An erythrocyte or a leukocyte.

 c. body. Part of the nerve cell or neuron which contains the cell nucleus and cytoplasm. See: *nerve.*

 c., brood. A mother cell.

 c. carrier. Phagocyte.

 c., daughter. One from a parent cell.

 c., endothelial. A flat cell making up the lining membranes of vessels.

 c., epithelial. One forming epithelial surfaces of membranes and skin.

 c., giant. Osteoclast. Found in marrow, esp. red marrow.

 c., glia. Spider or mossy cell in neuroglia tissue. See: *neuroglia cell.*

 c., goblet. Epithelial cell distended with mucus.

 c., interstitial, c., Leydig's. One of many found in connective tissue of the seminiferous tubules of the testes, and such tissues of the ovary which account for their internal secretion.

 c., irritation. See: *plasma cell.*

c., mossy. Neurogliar tissue cell with many short processes and large body. SEE: *spider cell.*

c., mother. One which gives rise to 2 or more daughter cells.

c., mucous. A goblet cell.

c., neuroglia. Spider cells and mossy cells.

c., plasma. Phagocytic leukocyte whose protoplasm is not granular and is densest in periphery and with chromatin arranged in a wheel-like shape. SYN: *plasmacyte.*

c., prickle. One of the cells of the stratum germinatorum of the skin.

c., pus. Pyocyte, pus corpuscle.

c., pyramidal. A nerve cell of the cerebral cortex.

c., sickle. An abnormal erythrocyte in anemia.

c., spider. Star-shaped cell in neuroglia tissue.

c., squamous. Flat, scalelike, epithelial cell.

c., stimulation. SEE: *plasma cell.*

cellase (sel'as). A ferment acting upon cellose.*

cell-color ratio. The product of dividing the percentage of hemoglobin into the number of red blood cells in a cc.

cellophane (sĕl'ō-fān). Thin, transparent, waterproof sheet of viscose.

cell-organ. A part of certain cells which may perform digestive functions. Ex: *cytosome, plastic.*

cel'lose. The product of hydrolysis of cellulose. SEE: *cellase.*

cel'lula (pl. *cellulae*). 1. A minute cell. 2. A small compartment.

cel'lular. 1. Pert. to, composed of, or derived from cells. 2. Areolar; having interstices.

c. tissue. Loose connective tissue.

cellule (sel'ul). A minute cell; cellula.*

cellulicidal (sel-ū-lĭ-sī'dal). Destructive to cells.

cellulif'ugal. Extending or moving away from a cell.

cellulin (sel'ū-lin). A carbohydrate forming the basis of vegetable fiber. SYN: *cellulose.*

cellulipetal (sel-ū-lip'et-al). Extending or moving toward a cell.

cellulitis (sel-u-lī'tis). Inflammation of cellular or connective tissue, spreading as in erysipelas.

c., diffuse. That accompanied with pus.

c., pelvic. Parametritis; inflammation of the parametrium.* Occurs in puerperal fever, or septic conditions of the uterus and appendages.

cellulocutaneous (sel-ū-lō-kū-ta'nē-us). Pert. to subcutaneous connective tissue and the skin.

cellulofi'brous. Both cellular and fibrous.

celluloneuritis (sel''u-lo-nū-ri'tis). Inflammation of nerve cells.

c., acute anterior. Polyneuritis and Landry's paralysis.

cellulose (sel'u-los). A fibrous form of carbohydrate constituting the supporting framework of plants; plant fiber.

c. high diet. High residue diet, *q.v.*

cellulotox'ic. 1. Poisonous to cells. 2. Caused by cell toxins.

cel'oglass. Window glass substitute for transmitting antirachitic rays of sunlight.

celol'ogy. The surgical study of hernias.

celom, celoma (se'lom, se-lo'mă). The body cavity, esp. of the embryo.

celonychia (se-lo-nik'ĭ-ă). Fingernails with concave outer surface.

celoschisis (se-los'kĭ-sis). Congenital fissure of the abdominal wall.

celoscope (se'los-kōp). Device for throwing light into a cavity.

celosomia (se-lo-so'mĭ-ă). Congenital protrusion of viscera.

celotomy (se-lot'o-mĭ). A cutting operation for strangulated hernia.

celozo'ic. Inhabiting any cavity of the body, such as parasitic protozoa.

Cel'sius scale. The reverse of the centigrade scale; a degree Celsius being 1.8 degree Fahrenheit; the boiling point; F. 212°, being zero C., the freezing point, F. 32°, being 100° C.

cementi'tis. Inflammation of the dental cementum.

cementoblast (se-men'to-blast). A dental cell developing into the substantia ossea.

cementocla'sia. Decay of the cementum of a tooth root.

cemento'ma. A tumor having its origin in the substantia ossea.

cenesthesia, cenesthesis (sen-es-the'zĭ-ă, -sis). 1. A hysterical condition resulting in loss of the consciousness of identity. 2. The sense of pleasurable or painful existence in states of exaltation or depression. 3. The sensing of the normal functioning of the body organs.

cenesthe'sic, cenesthet'ic. Pert. to cenesthesia.

cenesthopathia (sen-es-tho-path'ĭ-ă). Any abnormal perversion of consciousness.

cenopho'bia. Morbid fear of open spaces and of crowds. SYN: *agoraphobia.*

cenopsychic (sen-o-si'kik). Only recently appearing in mental development.

cenosis (se-no'sis). 1. Evacuation. 2. Inanition.

cenosite (se'no-sīt). A microörganism not depending for life upon its host, but parasitic in character.

cenotic (se-not'ik). 1. Purgative; drastic. 2. Pert. to cenosis.

cenotophobia (se-no-to-fo'bĭ-ă). Morbid aversion to new things and new ideas.

cenotype (sen'o-tīp). An original type.

cen'sor. PSY: A psychic inhibition that prevents abhorrent unconscious thoughts or impulses from seeking objective expression unless in a form unrecognized by consciousness.

center (sen'ter). 1. Middle point of a body. 2. Nerve cells governing a function.

c., accelerating. One in the medulla accelerating to the heart.

c., arm. One in cerebral cortex controlling arm movements.

c., association. Center controlling associated movements.

c., auditory. One for hearing, in the gyri in sylvian fissure.

c., cardioinhibitory. Medullary center which slows heart action.

c., ciliospinal. One which dilates the pupils.

c., deglutition. One which controls swallowing.

c., diabetic. One in ant. half of floor of fourth ventricle, post. part; glycosuria excited by its puncture.

c., epiotic. Ossification center of mastoid process.

c., erection. Found in lumbar region of spinal cord; controlled from oblongata.

c., gustatory. One in cerebrum which controls taste.

c., leg. One controlling leg movements; located in ascending frontal convolution.

c., motor cortical. Nerve center controlling voluntary movement.

c., nerve. One of many in cerebrospinal or ganglionic nervous systems originating or controlling vital function.

c., ossification. Spot where ossification begins in bones.

c., reflex. Cerebral center transforming sensory impressions into efferent motor ones.

c., respiratory. Medullary center in fourth ventricle controlling breathing.

c., spasm. At junction of medulla and pons; injury causes convulsions.

c., speech. One for articulate speech memories; located in post. part of third left frontal convolution.

c., sweat. Medullary center, subsidiary centers in spinal cord. Controls sweating.   [temperature.

c., temperature. One controlling body

c., trophic. One of many located in cerebrospinal and sympathetic systems presiding over nutrition.

c., visual. In occipital lobe. Controls sight.

c., word. Cerebral center controlling perception of word meanings.

centesimal (sen-tes'im-al). Divided into or rel. to hundredths.

centesis (sen-te'sis). Puncture of a cavity.

centigrade (sen'ti-grād). A thermometer divided into 100° bet. the boiling and freezing point, which is 0 degree. SEE: *thermometer.*

cen'tigram. A measure of weight; the hundredth part of a gram; 0.15432 gr. SEE: *metric measure.*

centiliter (sen'ti-le-ter). One-hundredth part of a liter; 10 cc.

centimeter (sen'ti-me-ter). One-hundredth part of a meter; 2/5 of a linear inch (0.3937).

centinormal (sen-ti-nor'măl). One-hundredth part of the normal, as the strength of a solution.

centrad (sen'trad). Toward the center.

central (sen'tral). Situated at, or rel. to, a center.

c. nervous system. Brain and spinal cord, including their nerves and end organs, controlling voluntary acts. Also called cerebrospinal system, and voluntary nervous system.

centraphose (sen'tra-fōz). A subjective sensation of a dark spot originating in the optic brain centers. SEE: *centrophose, chromophose.*

c. bodies. Attraction center of a cell. SYN: *centrosome.*

cen'tre. Center.

centric (sen'trik). Pert. to a center.

centriciput (sen-tris'ĭ-put). The central part of upper surface of skull, bet. the occiput and sinciput.

centrifugal (sen-trif'u-gal). Receding from the center.

SEE: *axifugal, centrifuge.*

c. force. The force which impels a thing, or parts of it, outward from the center of rotation.

centrifuge (sen'trĭ-fūj). A machine for the separation of heavier materials from lighter ones, through the employment of centrifugal force.* Used in testing for solids, in urine, corpuscles in blood, etc.

centriole (sĕn'trĭ-ōl). Minute granule which is focus of an attraction sphere. SEE: *metaphase, prophase, telephase.*

centripetal (sen-trip'e-tal). Toward the center.

centrocinesia (sen"tro-sĭn-e'zĭ-ă). Movement excited from central stimulation.

centrocinetic (sen"tro-sin-et'ĭk). Exciting motor action; pert. to centrocinesia.

centrocyte (sen'tro-sĭt). A cell having single and double, hematoxylin stainable, granules of varying size in its protoplasm.

centrodesmus (sen-tro-dez'mus). The matter connecting the 2 centrosomes in a nucleus during mitosis.

centrolecithal (sen-tro-les'ith-al). With the yoke in the center.

centrophose (sĕn'trŏ-fōz). A subjective sensation of a light spot having its origin in the optic brain centers. SEE: *centraphose.*

centrosclero'sis. Ossification filling a bone cavity.

cen'trosome. The attraction center from which springs the reproductivity of a cell; central body.

centrosphere (sen'tro-sfēr). The envelope encasing 2 centrosomes.

centrostaltic (sen-tro-stal'tĭk). Pert. to a center of motion.

centrother'apy. Any local application that acts upon nerve centers.

centrum (sen'trum). Any center, esp. an anatomical one.

c. commu'ne. The solar plexus.

c. semiova'le. A mass of white matter at center of each cerebral hemisphere.   [diaphragm.

c. tendin'eum. Central tendon of the

cephalad (sef'al-ad). Toward the head.

cephalalgia (sef-ă-lal'jĭ-ă). Headache, pain in the head.

cephalalgic (sef-al-al'jik). Of the nature of cephalalgia.

cephalea (sef-al-e'ă). Pain in the head; headache. SYN: *cephalalgia.**

cephaledema (sef-ăl-ē-de'mă). Edema of the head.

cephalemometer (sef-ă-lĕ-mom'et-er). Apparatus for determining blood pressure in the head.

cephalhematocele (sef"ăl-hem-at'o-sēl). A bloody tumor communicating with the dural sinuses under the pericardium.

cephalhematoma (sef-al-he-mă-to'mă). A subcutaneous swelling containing blood, often found on the head of a baby several days after birth, when delivery was accompanied by use of forceps. SYN: *caput succedaneum.*

cephal'ic. 1. Cranial; pert. to the head. 2. Superior in position.

    c. version. Turning the fetus during labor so head will present.

cephalin (sef'al-in). A substance resembling lecithin derived from brain substance of an animal. USES: Locally, to arrest hemorrhage.

cephalitis (sef-al-i'tis). Inflammation of the brain and membranes.

cephalocele (sef-al'o-sēl). Brain hernia.

cephalocentesis (sef-ă-lo-sen-te'sis). Surgical puncture of cranium.

cephalodynia (sef-al-o-din'ĭ-ă). Pain in the head; headache, cephalalgia.

cephalogas'ter. Embryonic enteron nearest the ant. pole.

cephalohemometer (sef-al-o-hem-om'et-er). Instrument for determining changes in intracranial blood pressure.

cephalo'ma. A soft carcinoma.

cephalomenia (sef-ă-lo-me'nĭ-ă). Vicarious menstruation from the nose or head.

cephalomeningitis (sef-ă-lo-men-in-ji'tis). Inflammation of the cerebral meninges.

cephalometer (sef-al-om'et-er). Device for measuring the head.

cephalometry (sef-al-om'e-trĭ). Measurement of the head.

cephalomo'tor. Pert. to movements of the head.

cephalone (sef'al-ōn). An idiot with a large head and sclerotic hyperplasia of the brain.

cephalonia (sef-a-lo'ni-a). Macrocephaly with hypertrophy.

cephalopathy (sef-al-op'ath-ĭ). Any disease of the head or brain.

cephaloplegia (sef-al-o-ple'gĭ-ă). Paralysis of muscles about head, or—less accurately—face.

cephalorhachidian (sef"al-o-ră-kid'ĭ-an). Pert. to the head and spine.

cephaloscope (sef'al-o-skōp). Device for auscultation of the head.

ceph'alostat. Device for holding the head.

cephalotome (sef'al-o-tōm). Instrument for cutting the head of the fetus.

cephalotomy (sef-ăl-ot'o-mĭ). Cutting the fetal head to facilitate delivery.

cephalotractor (sef'al-o-trak'tor). Obstetrical forceps.

cephalotribe (sef'al-o-trĭb). Instrument for crushing head of fetus.

cephalotripsy (sef'al-o-trip-sĭ). Crushing of fetal head in dystocia.

cephalotrypesis (sef'al-o-trip-e'sis). Removing a bone disk from the skull. SYN: *trephination.*

ceptor (sep'tor). 1. A receptor. 2. A nervous mechanism for receiving and transmitting sensations.

    c., chemical. One which initiates chemical reactions in the body.

    c., contact. One which apprehends stimuli contributed by direct physical contact.

    c., distance. One which perceives stimuli at a distance, by aerial or ethereal forces.

cera (se'ra). Wax.

    c. alba. White wax.

    c. flava. Yellow wax.

ceram'ics, dental. The use of porcelain in dental work.

ceramodon'tia. Dental ceramics.

ceramuria (ser-am-u'rĭ-ă). Excessive phosphate excretion in urine. SYN: *phosphaturia.*

cerate (se'rat). Unctuous substance of such consistency that it may be spread easily, at ordinary temperature, upon muslin or similar material with a spatula, and yet not so soft as to liquefy and run when applied to the skin; not often prescribed. Three cerates are official.

ceratocele (ser'ă-to-sēl). Hernia of Descemet's membrane through outer layer of the cornea.

ceratonosus (ser-ă-ton'o-sus). A disease of the cornea.

ceratotome (se-rat'o-tōm). A knife for division of the cornea.

ceratum (se-ra'tum). An unctuous solid for application to the skin. SYN: *cerate.*

cercaria (ser-ka'rĭ-ă). The final larval stage of trematode worms.

cerclage (sair-klazh'). Binding with metal wire of the ends of a fractured bone.

Cercomonas. A genus of flagellate infusoria.

    C. intestinal'is. A species in the human intestine in certain cases of diarrhea.

cercomoni'asis. Infestation with *Cercomonas intestinalis.*

cercus (ser'kus). A hairlike structure.

cerea flexibilitas (sē're-ă fleks-ĭ-bil'ĭ-tas). PSY: A condition in which the limbs can be molded into any desired position.

cerebellar (ser-e-bel'lar). Pert. to the cerebellum.

cerebellif'ugal. Extending or proceeding from the cerebellum.

cerebellip'etal. Extending toward the cerebellum.

cerebellitis (ser-ĕ-bel-li'tis). Inflammation of the cerebellum.

cerebellospinal (ser-ĕ-bel-lo-spi'nal). Pert. to cerebellum and spinal cord.

cerebellum (ser-ĕ-bel'um). Lower or back brain, bet. the pons and medulla oblongata, and below the post. portion of the cerebrum.

cerebral (ser'ĕ-bral, ser-e'bral). Pert. to the cerebrum.

    c. hemorrhage. The result of rupture

of a sclerosed or diseased blood vessel in brain. Often associated with high blood pressure. RS: *apoplexy, hemiplegia.*

cerebral cortex reflex (ser-ĕ-bral kor'tĕks). Pupillary contraction of both eyes, when a bright object is brought within field of vision.   [headache.

cerebralgia (ser-ĕ-bral'jĭ-ă). Cephalalgia,

cerebrasthenia (ser''ĕ-bras-the'nĭ-ă). Neurasthenia characterized by feelings of unreality, doubt and anxiety. SYN: *psychasthenia.*

cerebration (ser-ĕ-bra'shun). Mental action of the brain.

cerebriform (sĕr-ĕ-brĭ-form). Resembling the brain in form or structure.

cerebrifugal (ser-ĕ-brif'ŭ-gal). Away from the brain; pert. to efferent nerve fibers.

cerebrin (ser'ĕ-brin). One of a number of fatty nitrogenous principles from nerve tissue, containing phosphorus.

cerebripetal. Proceeding toward the cerebrum, as nerve fibers or impulses.

cerebritis. Inflammation of the brain, esp. the cerebrum.

cerebroid (ser'ĕ-broid). Cerebriform; resembling the brain substance.

cerebrology (ser-ĕ-brol'o-jĭ). Science of the brain.

cerebroma (ser-ĕ-bro'mă). Brain hernia; any mass in the brain.

cerebromalacia (ser-ĕ-bro-mal-a'sĭ-ă). Softening of the brain, esp. of the cerebrum.

cerebromeningitis (ser-e-bro''men-in-ji'tis). Inflammation of the cerebrum and its membranes.

cerebrometer (ser-e-brom'et-er). Device for registering cerebral impulses.

cerebropathy (ser-e-brop'ath-ĭ). Any disease of the brain, esp. cerebrum.

cerebrophysiology (ser''e-bro-fiz-ĭ-ol'o-jĭ). Physiology of the brain.

cerebropontile (ser-e-bro-pon'tĭl). Pert. to the brain and pons Varolii.

cerebropsychosis (ser-e-bro-sĭ-ko'sis). Any mental disorder due to cerebral lesion.

cer''ebrosclero'sis. Hardening of the brain, esp. of the cerebrum.

cerebroscope (ser-e'bro-skōp). Instrument for brain diagnosis.

cerebroscopic (ser-e-bro-skop'ĭk). Pert. to cerebroscopy.

cerebroscopy (ser-e-bros'ko-pĭ). Diagnostic use of the ophthalmoscope as applied to the brain.

cerebrose (ser'e-brōs). $C_6H_{12}O_6$, a compound (brain sugar) derived from brain tissue.

cerebroside (ser'e-bro-sīd). A phosphorous-free class of compounds existing in the brain.

cerebrosis (ser-e-bro'sis). Any brain disease. SYN: *encephalosis.*

cerebrospinal (ser''e-bro-spi'nal). Referring to the brain and spinal cord, as the cerebrospinal axis.

    c. fever. Cerebrospinal meningitis. Inflammation of the brain and spinal cord; sometimes called "spotted fever" because of rash on the body.

    c. fluid. A water cushion protecting the brain and spinal cord from shock.

    c. nervous system. Nervous system of brain and spinal cord. SYN: *central nervous system, q.v.*

    c. puncture. Surgical puncture, usually at the fourth lumbar interspace, to remove a specimen of the fluid for clinical examination.

cerebrospi'nant. 1. Any agent affecting the brain and spinal cord. 2. Affecting the brain and spinal cord.

cerebrosuria (ser''e-bro-su'rĭ-ă). Cerebrose in the urine.

cer''ebrot'omy. 1. Incision of the brain to evacuate an abscess. 2. Dissection of the brain.

cerebrum (ser'e-brum, ser-e'brum). The forebrain. The larger part of the brain consisting of two hemispheres where the sensory stimuli are received and the motor impulses originate. The supposed center of the intellect, the emotions, and the will.

ceroma (se-ro'mă). A waxy tumor that has undergone amyloid degeneration.

ce'roplasty. The manufacture of anatomical models and pathological specimens in wax.

cerosis (se-ro'sis). Morbid condition of membranes resembling waxlike scales.

cer'tifiable. Pert. to infectious diseases which must be reported to the health authorities.

cerumen (se-rŭ'men). The waxlike, soft brown secretion found in the external canal of the ear; inspissated, dried earwax.

ceru'minal. Pert. to the cerumen.

cerumino'sis. Excessive wax formation.

ceru'minous. Pert. to cerumen.

    c. glands. Modified sweat glands in the skin lining the external auditory canal, which secrete a yellowish brown substance, cerumen.

ceruse (se'rŭs). White lead.

cervical (ser'vik-al). 1. Pert. to the neck or to any cervix. 2. GYN: Pert. to the cervix uteri.

    c. plexus. That formed by loops joining the ant. rami of first 4 cervical nerves; it receives communicating rami from the sympathetic ganglia. SEE: *plexus.*

    c. region. That of neck in relation to position of cervical vertebrae.

    c. vertebrae. First 7 bones of the spinal column. SEE: *skeleton.*

cervicectomy (ser-vĭ-sek'to-mĭ). Removal of the cervix uteri.

cerviplex (ser-vis'ĭ-pleks). The cervical plexus.*

cervicit'is. Inflammation of the cervix uteri.

    May be induced by invasion of the gonococcus.

cervico-. Prefix: Pert. to the neck.

cervicobra'chial. Pert. to the neck and arm.

cervicobuc'cal. Pert. to the buccal surface of neck of a molar or premolar tooth.

cervicofa'cial. Pert. to the neck and face.

ce. vicoves'ical. Pert. to the cervix uteri and bladder.

cervimeter (ser'vĭ-me-ter). Instrument for measurement of cervix uteri.

cervix (sĕr'vĭks). The neck or a part of an organ resembling a neck. SEE: "cervico-" words.

    c. uteri. Neck of the uterus. The lower part from the internal os, outward to the external os.

    c. vesicae, c., vesical. Neck of the bladder.

cesarean section (sē-zar'ē-ăn). Removal of the fetus by means of an incision into uterus, usually by way of abdominal wall.

    c. s., absolute. Where the child cannot be delivered through the natural passages under any circumstances.

    c. s., relative. Where the child could be delivered through the natural passages, but where such a delivery might jeopardize the life of the mother or the child. [section.

cesarotomy (sez-ă-rot'o-mĭ). Cesarean*

Cestoda (ses-tōd'ă). *Taenia.* Tapeworms.

cestode (ses'tōd). A tapeworm; one of the Cestoda.

ces'toid. Like a tapeworm.

Cestoidea (ses-toi'de-ă). An order of *Platyhelmintha,* including the flatworms and tapeworms.

Cetraria (sē-trā'rĭ-ă). 1. A genus of lichens, chiefly found in northern latitudes. 2. *Cetraria islandica,* or Iceland moss, a lichen used in treating lung and bowel disorders.

cevitamic acid (sev-i-tam'ĭk). Crystalline vitamin C. This acid was first introduced as ascorbic acid, and is found in abundance in citrus fruits, many vegetables, such as cabbages, tomatoes, paprika, spinach, etc.

    DOSAGE: As a protective in infants, 1/6 gr. (0.01 Gm.), corresponding to about 1 oz. fresh orange juice; adult, 5/6 gr. (0.05 Gm.). Intravenously, 1 1/2 gr. (0.1 Gm.) to 15 gr. (1 Gm.).

C. G. S. Abbr. for *centimeter-gram-second,* a name given to a system of units for distance, weight and time.

C₂H₄. Ethylene.

CH₄. Methane; marsh gas.

C₂H₂. Acetylene.

C₆H₆. Benzene.

Chaddock's reflexes (chad'dok). 1. Extension of great toe resulting from irritation around ext. malleolus. 2. Flexion of wrist and fanning of fingers when forearm is irritated above and near wrist.

chaeromania (ke-ro-ma'nĭ-ă). Mania characterized by exaltation and cheerfulness. SYN: *amenomania.*

chain. In bacteriology, 3 or more cells attached end to end. In chemistry, atoms held together by one affinity.

    c. reflex. One in a consecutive series.

chalarosis (kal-ar-o'sis). Infection with *Chalara,* a fungus producing subcutaneous nodules which break down, forming ulcers.

chalaza (kal-a'ză). Inflammation of a meibomian gland causing small tumor of eyelid border. SYN: *chalazion.*

chalazion (ka-la'zĭ-on). Small, hard tumor analogous to sebaceous cyst developing on the eyelids, formed by distention of a meibomian gland with secretion. A meibomian cyst. SEE: *chalaza, steatoma.*

chalcosis (kal-ko'sis). 1. Chronic poisoning from copper. 2. Copper deposits in lungs and tissues.

chalice cell (tshal'is). Crateriform shell remaining after mucus has been discharged from an epithelial cell. SYN: *goblet cells.*

chalicosis (kal-ĭ-ko'sis). Lung disorder due to inhalation of stone particles. SYN: *pneumoconiosis, q.v.*

chalinoplasty (kal-in'o-plas-tĭ). Plastic surgery of the mouth and lips, esp. of corners of mouth.

chalone (kal'on). An autacoid that inhibits the action of a hormone* or which diminishes cellular activity. SEE: *autacoid.*

chalybeate (kal-ib'e-ăt). 1. Pert. to or composed of iron; ferruginous. 2. Agent containing iron.

Chamberland filter (sham-ber-län). An unglazed porcelain filter through which water can be forced under pressure. Intercepts all but ultramicroscopic microorganisms.

chamber (chām'ber). Compartment or closed space.

    c., anterior. The space bet. the cornea and iris.

    c., aqueous. Ant. and post. chambers of the eye, containing the aqueous humor.

    c., posterior. Space behind the iris, ant. to the lens.

    c., vitreous. Cavity behind the lens in the eye containing the vitreous humor.

chamomile (kam'o-mīl). Flowers of the *Anthemis* yielding a bluish volatile oil and a bitter infusion.

chancre (shang'ker). A hard, syphilitic, primary ulcer. The first sign of syphilis.

    c., hard; c., hunterian. Primary lesion of syphilis. SEE: *chancre.*

    c., simple; c., soft. A nonsyphilitic venereal ulcer. SYN: *chancroid.*

    c., true. SEE: *hard chancre.*

chancroid (shang'kroyd). A nonsyphilitic venereal ulcer, highly infectious; a simple or soft chancre.

chancrous (shang'krus). Pert. to or of the nature of chancre. [teric.*

change of life. The menopause;* climac-

charbon (shar-bon'). Infection with *B. anthracis.* SYN: *anthrax.*

charcoal (shär'kōl). Wood charcoal. USP. Very fine powder prepared from soft charred wood.

    DOSAGE: 5 to 20 gr. (0.32-1.3 Gm.).

    c. fumes. SEE: *carbon monoxide.*

Charcot-Leyden crystals (shar-ko'-li'den). Elongated, double pyramid-shaped crystals made up of spermine and found in the sputum of bronchial asthma.

Charcot-Robin crystals (shar-co'-ro-ban') Tiny crystals found in blood in leukemia.

Charcot's arthropathy (shar-ko'). Joint effusion seen in locomotor ataxia.

C.'s disease. Multiple cerebrospinal sclerosis with locomotor ataxia.

C.'s joint. Result of disease of the sympathetic innervation, producing atrophic disorder of a joint.

charlatan (shar'lă-tăn). A boasting pretender to special knowledge or ability, as in medicine. SYN: *quack.*

charlatanry (shar'lă-tăn-rĭ). Undue pretension to knowledge or skill or an instance of it. SYN: *quackery.*

Charles' law. All gases on heating expand equally, and on cooling contract equally, according to temperature relation. Same as Gay-Lussac's law.

charley horse [slang]. An athletic injury, usually a bruised or a torn muscle associated with cramping in the muscles. F. A. TREATMENT: Cold applications.

charpie (shar'pĭ). Shreds of linen for dressing wounds.

charta (kar'ta). Preparation intended mainly for external application made by saturating paper with medicinal substances or by applying the latter to the surface of paper by addition of adhesive liquid.   [medicinal powder.

chartula (kar'tu-lă). A paper containing a

chaude-pisse (shōd-pēs'). The burning sensation during urination in acute gonorrhea.

chauffage (sho-fazh'). A heated cautery at low temperature applied over a part about ¼ in. from it.

Charting, Latin Abbr. Which May Be Used in, and Their Meanings

Abbr.	Phrase	Meaning
a or āā	ana	of each
abs. feb.	absente febre	when there is no fever
a.c.	ante cibos	before eating
ad	ad	to, up to
ad effect.	ad effectum	until effectual
ad gr. acid	ad gratam aciditatem	to an agreeable acidity
ad gr. gust	ad gratum gustum	to an agreeable taste
ad lib.	ad libitum	at pleasure; as much as is needed
ad neut.	ad neutralizandum	to neutralization
ad sat.	ad saturandum	to saturation
adst. feb.	adstante febre	when fever is present
ad us.	ad usum	according to custom
ad us. ext.	ad usum externum	for external use
aeq.	aequales	equal
ag. feb.	aggrediente febre	when the fever increases
agit. ante sum.	agita ante sumendum	shake before taking
alt. dieb.	alternis diebus	every other day
alt. hor.	alternis horis	alternate hours
alt. noc.	alternis nocta	every other night
aq.	aqua	water
aq. bull.	aqua bulliens	boiling water
aq. cal.	aqua calida	warm water
aq. dest.	aqua destillata	distilled water
aq. ferv.	aqua fervens	hot water
aq. frig.	aqua frigida	cold water
aq. menth. pip.	aqua menthae piperitae	peppermint water
aq. pur.	aqua pura	pure water
arg.	argentum	silver
bal.	balneum	bath
bal. sin.	balneum sinapis	mustard bath
bib.	bibe	drink
b. i. d.	bis in die	twice daily
bis.	bis	twice
bis in 7d.	bis in septem diebus	twice a week
b.p.		blood pressure; boiling point
bull.	bulliat	let it boil
C.		Centigrade
		carbon
		calory
c.	cum	with
cap.	capsula	a capsule
cat.	cataplasma	a poultice
cc.		cubic centimeter
chart.	charta	paper
cito disp.	cito dispensetur	let it be dispensed quickly
c.m.	cras mane	tomorrow morning
c.m.s.	cras mane sumendus	to be taken tomorrow morning
c.n.	cras nocte	tomorrow night

Charting, Latin Abbr. Which May Be Used in, and Their Meanings *(Continued)*

Abbr.	Phrase	Meaning
cochl. amp.	cochleare amplum	tablespoonful
cochl. infant.	cochleare infantis	teaspoonful
coch. mag.	cochleare magnum	a tablespoonful
coch. med.	cochleare medium	a dessertspoonful
coch. parv.	cochleare parvum	a teaspoonful
comp.	compositus	compounded of
cong.	congius	a gallon
contra	contra	against
cont. rem.	continuantur remedia	let the medicines be continued
c.v.	cras vespere	tomorrow night
cyath.	cyathus	glassful
cyath. vinos.	cyathus vinosus	wineglassful
D.	dosis	dose
d.	da	give
d. d. in d.	de die in diem	from day to day
decub.	decubitus	lying down
det.	detur	let it be given
dieb. alt.	diebus alternis	on alternate days
dil.	dilue	dilute
dim.	dimidius	half
div.	divide	divide
div. in p. aeq.	divide in partes aequales	divide into equal parts
don.	donec	until
emp.	emplastrum	a plaster
en.		enema
exhib.	exhibeatur	let it be given
ext.	extractum	extract
ext. liq.	extractum liquidum	liquid extract
Fahr.		Fahrenheit (temperature scale)
Fe.	ferrum	iron
f.h.	fiat haustus	make a draught
f.m.	fiat mistura	make a mixture
f.p.	fiat pilula	make a pill
ft.	fiat	let it be made
Gm.		gram
gr.	granum	grain
gtt.	gutta	a drop
h. n.	hac noc'te	tonight
hor. som. or h. s.	hora somni	at bedtime
ind.	indies	daily
inf.	infusum	an infusion
inj.	injectio	an injection
liq.	liquor, oris	a liquor
m.	misce	mix
mod. praes.	modo praescripto	as prescribed
mor. dict.	more dicto	in the manner directed
mor. sol.	more solito	in the usual manner
n. b.	no'ta be'ne	note well
noct.	noc'te	night
non rep.	non repetatur	do not repeat
O.	octarius	a pint
o. d.	oculus dexter	right eye
ol.	oleum	oil
o.m.	omni mane	every morning
omn. bid.	omnibus bidendis	every 2 days
omn. bih.	omni bihoris	every 2 hours
omn. hor.	omni hora	every hour
omn. noct.	omni nocte	every night
o. s.	oculus sinister	left eye
p.a.a.	parti affectae applicetur	let it be applied to the affected region
part aeq.	partes aequales	equal parts
post. cib. or p. c.	post cibos	after eating
p.r.	per rectum	by the rectum
p. r. n.	pro re nata	as needed
pulv.	pulvis	a powder
p.v.	per vaginam	by the vagina
q. i. d.	qua'ter in di'e	four times a day

Charting, Latin Abbr. Which May Be Used in, and Their Meanings (Continued)

Abbr.	Phrase	Meaning
q.l.	quantum libet	as much as is wanted
q. s.	quantum sufficiat	a sufficient quantity
q.v.	quantum volueris	at will
℞	recipe	take (thou)
rep.	repetatur	let it be repeated
rep. sem.	repetatur semel	let it be repeated once only
s.a.	secundum artem	by skill
sig.	signetur	let it be labeled
sing.	singulorum	of each
s. o. s.	si o'pus sit	if necessary
ss.	semi	one-half
stat.	statim	at once
sum.	sumat or sumendum	let him take, or let it be taken
s.v.	spiritus vini	spirits of wine
s. v. gall.	spiritus vini gallici	brandy
T.		temperature
tab.	tabella, tabellae	a tablet, tablets
t. i. d.	ter in die	thrice daily
tinct. or tr.	tinctura	tincture
ung.	unguentum	ointment
ur.		urine

Chauffard's syndrome (sho-fars'). Peculiar symptoms of polyarticular joint disease with splenic and glandular enlargement in young children.

Chaussier's areola (sho-sī-ās'). Indurated tissue around the lesion of a malignant pustule.

check. 1. To slow down or arrest the course of. 2. To verify.

    c. bite. Impression of teeth on plastic material to check articulation.

    c. experiment. Control experiment, or one checked against another.

cheek. Side of face forming lateral wall of mouth below the eye.

    SEE: *bucca, buccal, buccinator, gena, malar bone, melitis, meloncus.*

    c. bone. The malar bone, *os zygomaticum.*

    c. muscle. Buccinator.

    c. retractor. Device for enclosing cheek at the mouth's angle for properly exposing operating field.

cheilitis (ki-li'tis). Inflammation of the lip.

    c. exfoliativa. Seborrheic dermatitis of the lips.

cheilognathopalatoschisis (kī-lŏg''năth-ō-păl-ā-tŏs'kĭ-sĭs). Malformation in which there is a cleft in the hard and soft palate, upper jaw, and in the lip.

cheiloplasty (kil'o-plas-tĭ). Plastic operation upon the lips.

cheilosis (kī-lō'sĭs). Morbid condition of lips with reddened appearance and fissures at the angles, seen frequently in vitamin B deficiency, ariboflavinosis.*

cheilostomatoplasty (kil-os-to'mat-o-plas-tĭ). Plastic building up of mouth.

cheilotomy, chilotomy (ki-lot'o-mĭ). Excision of part of the lip.

cheloid (ke'loid). Keloid skin disease with fibrous growths at site of a scar.

chem'ic, chem'ical. Pert. to chemistry. SEE: *base, bond, "chem-" words.*

    c. balance of the body. Foods burned within the body may produce either an alkaline or an acid ash.

    c. compound. A compound formed of 2 or more substances which cannot be separated by mechanical means.

    c. reflex. Any physiologic response to action of a hormone.

chemicocautery (kem-ik-o-kaw'ter-ĭ). Cauterization by chemical agents.

chemicogen'esis. Chemical fertilization of an ovum.

cheminosis (kem-in-o'sis). Any disease caused by chemical agents.

chemiotaxis (kem-ĭ-o-taks'ĭs). Cellular repulsion and attraction.

chemise (she-mēz'). Surgical dressing to prevent hemorrhage after surgery upon bladder or rectum.

chem'ism. Chemical energy.

chemist (kem'ist). One trained in chemistry.

chem'istry. The science that treats of the molecular and atomic structure of bodies.

chemokine'sis. Increased energy incited by a chemical substance.

chemolysis (kem-ol'is-is). Chemical decomposition or decay.

chemomorphosis (kem-o-mor-fo'sis). Change of form as the result of chemical action.

chemophysiol'ogy. Physiologic chemistry.

chemorecep'tor. Side chain in a living cell having an affinity for chemical substances and fixing them.

chemore'flex. Reflex resulting from chemical action.

chemosis (ke-mo'sis). Swelling of conjunctiva about the cornea.

chemotactic (kem-o-tak'tĭk). Pert. to chemotaxis.

chemotaxis (kem-o-tak'sis). Attraction and repulsion of living protoplasm to a chemical stimulus.

chemotherapy (kem-o-ther'a-pĭ). Application of chemical reagents in treatment of disease, that have a specific and toxic effect on microörganism causing the disease, without harming the patient.

chemotic (ke-mot′ĭk). Pert. to chemosis.

chemotropism (kem-ot′ro-pizm). Ability or impulse to progress or turn in a certain direction due to the influence of certain chemical stimuli. SYN: *chemotaxis.*

chenopodium oil (ken-o-po′dĭ-um). USP. Oil of American wormseed. Colorless, a pale yellow volatile oil with pungent, irritating odor.

  DOSAGE: From 5 to 15 ℳ (0.3-1 cc.).

cherophobia (ker-o-fo′bĭ-ă). Morbid fear of and aversion to gaiety.

chest. The thorax.

Cheyne-Stokes reflex (chān-stōks). Rhythmic acceleration, deepening, and stopping of breathing movements.

Cheyne-Stokes respiration. An irregular type of arrhythmic breathing occurring in certain acute diseases of the central nervous system, heart, lungs, and in intoxications.

chiasm, chiasma (ki′azm, ki-az′ma). 1. A crossing. 2. An incomplete crossing of the optic fibers (the outer fibers not crossing each other); the point of crossing of the fibers of the optic nerves.

chiastometer (ki-as-tom′et-er). Instrument for measurement of deviation of optic axes.

chicken breast. Abnormal prominence of the sternum. SYN: *pectus carinatum.*

  c. fat clot. A yellowish blood clot.

chickenpox. A mild, contagious, infectious disease, marked by an eruption of vesicles on skin and mucous membranes. SEE: *varicella.*

chiq′gers. A tick or mite (*acarina* of the order *Arachnida*) which gets under the skin and causes acarodermatitis.

  TREATMENT: Extraction of the flea with a flat needle, followed by a bichloride of mercury dressing. As a preventive, pyrethrum powder may be sprinkled on walls, floors, or furniture.

chignon fungoid (shĕn-yon′). A bacterial invasion of the hair.

chigo, chigre (chĕ′go, chĕ′grā). A jigger or sand flea.

chilblains (chil′blāns). Inflammation and swelling of the feet, toes, or fingers caused by cold.

child′bed. Puerperium. Period during and immediately subsequent to parturition.

  c. b. fever. Puerperal fever.

childbirth. The process of bringing forth a child; parturition. SEE: *labor.*

child crowing. Spasmodic closure of glottis, of brief duration, and succeeded by noisy inspiration. SYN: *laryngismus stridulus.*

chilectro′pion. Eversion of the lip.

chilitis (ki-li′tis). Inflammation of the lips. SEE: *cheilitis.*

chill (chĭl). A disturbance of the heat regulating mechanism of the body, accompanied by shivering and fall of temperature.

  c., nervous. Accompanied by a chilly sensation but not with fever.

chiloangioscopy (ki-lo-an-jĭ-os′ko-pĭ). Microscopical examination of the circulation in the lip.

chilognathopalatoschisis (kĭ-log″nath-o-pal-at-os′kis-is). Fissure of the lip, palate, and alveolar process.

Chilomas′tix mesnil′i. A species of Mastigophora that is parasitic in the intestines.

chiloschisis (ki-los′kis-is). Harelip.

chilostomatoplasty (kĭ-los-to′mă-to-plas″-tĭ). Plastic operation for harelip.

chilot′omy. 1. Surgical removal of a portion of the lip for excision of a growth. 2. Cutting of an overgrowth at the articular end of a long bone to free its movement.

chim′ney-sweeps′ cancer. Epithelioma of the scrotum.

chiniofon (kin′ĭ-o-fŏn). USP. A derivative of sulfonic acid, containing approximately 27% iodine.

  DOSAGE: Orally, for adults, from 4-15 gr. (0.25-1 Gm.) 3 times a day; rectally, 15-75 gr. (1-5 Gm.) dissolved in 200 cc. water. Treatment combining both has been used in acute cases, and serious chronic ones, and course of treatment requiring from 7 to 14 days.

chin cough. Whooping cough, *q.v.*

  c. jerk. Reflex contraction of muscles of mastication on suddenly depressing the jaw.

  c. reflex. Clonic movement resulting from percussing or stroking lower jaw.

chionablepsia (kĭ-on-ab-lep′sĭ-ă). Snow blindness.

chirapsia (kĭ-răp′sĭ-ă). Friction; massage.

chirognostic (kĭ-rog-nos′tĭk). Having the ability to distinguish the right from the left.

chirokinesthesia (kĭ-ro-kin-es-the′sĭ-ă). Subjective perception of motions of the hand.

chiromeg′aly. Enlargement of the hands, wrists, or ankles. [hand.

chi′roplasty. A plastic operation on the

chiropodalgia (kĭ-ro-pod-al′jĭ-ă). Pain in hands and feet. SYN: *acrodynia.*

chiropodist (ki-rop′o-dist). One who practices chiropody.

chiropody (ki-rop′od-ĭ). Treatment of disorders of hands and esp. feet.

chiropompholyx (ki-ro-pom′fo-liks). Inflammatory disease of skin confined to hands and feet. SYN: *pompholyx, q.v.*

chiropractic (ki-ro-prak′tik). A system of correction, teaching health from anatomic relationship; that disease results from anatomic distortion, which must be removed by hand correction.

chiropractor (ki-ro-prak′tor). One who practices chiropractic methods.

chirospasm (ki′ro-spazm). Spasmodic affection of muscles of hand, or writers′ cramp.

chirurgery (ki-rur′je-rĭ). Surgery.

chirurgia (ki-rur′jĭ-ă). Surgery.

chirurgical (ki-rur′jĭk-al). Surgical.

chitinous (ki′tin-us). Pert. to a keratoid substance.

c. degeneration. Amyloid degeneration.

chloasma (klo-az'mă). Pigmentary skin discolorations, usually those occurring in yellowish brown patches or spots.

c. gravida'rum. Same as chloasma uterinum, q.v.

c. hepaticum. So-called "liver spot" following dyspepsia.

c., idiopathic. Chloasma caused by external agents, such as sun, heat, mechanical means, x-rays, etc.

c., symptomatic. Chloasma caused by various diseases, as syphilis or cancer.

c. traumaticum. Skin discolorations from traumatic agencies.

c. uteri'num. Brown discolorations of skin in pregnancy.

chloracetization (klo-ras-ĕt-iz-a'shun). Production of local anesthesia by chloroform and glacial acetic acid.

chloralamide (klo'răl-ăm'id). A hypnotic safer than chloral.

DOSAGE: 15-45 gr. (1.0-3.0 Gm.).

chloral hydrate (klo'ral). USP. Colorless, transparent crystals having aromatic, slightly acrid odor, and caustic, faintly bitter taste; soluble in alcohol and water.

DOSAGE: From 10-30 gr. (0.65-2.0 Gm.).

chloranemia (klor-an-e'mĭ-ă). An anemia resembling that of chlorosis occurring in some diseases, such as cancer and tuberculosis.

chlorate (klo'rāt). A salt of chloric acid. SEE: *potassium chlorate.*

chlorbu'tanol. Colorless crystals, with taste and odor resembling camphor.

chlorbu'tol. Colorless crystals, with odor and taste resembling camphor. SEE: *chlorobutanol.*

chlorcosane (klor-co-sān') (chlorinated paraffin). Used as a solvent for dichloramine T, *q.v.*

chloremia (klo-re'mĭ-ă). Anemia with diminution of hemoglobin and decrease in number of red corpuscles.

chlorephidrosis (klor-ef-ĭ-dro'sis). Greenish perspiration.

chloretone (klō'rĕ-tōn). Colorless crystals, resembling camphor in odor and taste. SEE: *chlorobutanol.*

chlorhydria (klor-hi'drĭ-ă). Excess of hydrochloric acid in stomach.

chloride (klō'rīd). Any binary compound of chlorine.

chloridemia (klor-ĭ-de'mĭ-ă). Chlorides in the blood.

chloridim'eter. An instrument for estimating amt. of chlorides in a fluid.

chloridimetry (klor-ĭ-dim'e-trĭ). Determination of amt. of chlorides in the body fluids.

chloridrom'eter. Device for estimating amt. of chlorides in urine.

chloriduria (klor-id-u'rĭ-ă). Presence or excess of chlorides in urine.

chlorinated (klor'in-ă-ted). Impregnated with chlorine.

c. lime. Calcium hypochlorite widely used in solution as a bleach, as an antiseptic, and as a ringworm preventive.

chlorina'tion. Treatment of water by addition of chlorine and its compounds for the killing of bacteria. 0.15 to 0.7 parts are used for million gallons of water.

chlorine (klo'rēn). SYMB: Cl. A nonmetal element of a gaseous nature not found in a free state, but usually combined in chlorides with alkaline earths. With sodium it forms sodium chloride, or salt.

c. preparations. Those used for disinfecting.

chlorite (klo'rit). A salt of chlorous acid; used as a disinfectant and bleaching agent.

chloroanemia (klor-o-a-ne'mĭ-ă). Anemia occurring in cachectic conditions. SYN: *chlorosis.*

chloroblast (klō'rō-blăst). A rudimentary red blood corpuscle. SYN: *erythroblast.*

chlorobutanol (klō-ro-bū'tan-ol). USP. (Chlorbutol, chloretone.) Colorless crystals, with odor and taste resembling camphor.

DOSAGE: From 5-20 gr. (0.3-1.3 Gm.), preferably in capsule.

chlor'oform. CHCl₃. USP. A heavy, clear, colorless liquid with strong ethereal odor, formed by the action of chlorinated lime on methyl alcohol.

DOSAGE: 5 ℳ (0.3 cc.).

c. anesthesia. For some time chloroform anesthesia was more popular than ether. It is 6 times as strong, but it was found to be more harmful.

chlorofor'min. A toxin extracted by chloroform from the tubercle bacilli.

chloroformism (klo'ro-form-izm). The habit of inhaling chloroform and the resulting symptoms.

chloroleukemia (klo-ro-lŭ-ke'mĭ-ă). Leukemia combined with chlorosis.

chloroma (klo-ro'mă). A greenish sarcoma of the periosteum of cranial bones; "green cancer."

chloromyeloma (klo-ro-mĭ-el-o'mă). Chloroma accompanied by multiple growths in bone marrow.

chloropenia (klo-ro-pe'nĭ-ă). Deficiency in chlorine; hypochloremia. [chlorine.

chloropenic (klo-ro-pen'ik). Deficient in

chlorophane (klo'ro-fān). A green-yellow pigment in the retina.

chlorophyl, chlorophyll (klo'ro-fĭl). The green coloring matter in plants.

chloro'pia. Vision in which all things appear green.

chloroplas'tid. A chlorophyl granule.

chloroprivic (klor-o-priv'ĭk). Lack of, or due to loss of, chlorides.

chlorop'sia. Vision in which all things seem green. SYN: *chloropia.*

chlorosarco'ma. Sarcomatous form of chloroma.

chloro'sis. A form of anemia* in adolescent girls, perhaps due to faulty diet during puberty.

chlorotic (klo-rot'ĭk). Of the nature of or afflicted with chlorosis.

chloroxyl (klō-roks'ĭl). Cinchophen hydrochloride.

USES AND DOSAGE: Same as cinchophen.

chlorum (klo'rum). Official name of chlorine.

chloruremia (klor-u-re'mĭ-ă). Urinary chlorides retained in the blood.

chloru'ria. Chlorides in the urine.

chlo'ryl. Anesthetic mixture of ethyl and methyl chlorides.

Ch.M. Abbr. for *Chirur'giae magis'ter*, Master of Surgery.

choana na'rium (ko-a'na). Post. nares or opening into the nasopharynx of the nasal fossa on both sides.

choanoid (ko'an-oyd). Shaped like a funnel.

chocolate. 1. Preparation made by grinding roasted cacao or theobroma seeds. 2. Beverage prepared by dissolving in water or milk. SEE: *cocoa*.

choked disk. Inflammation of the optic disk. SEE: *disk*.

choking. Obstruction within respiratory passage or constriction about the neck, interfering with breathing and circulation of brain.

cholago'gia. Excretion of bile from gallbladder.

cholagogue (ko'lă-gog). A purgative that stimulates the flow of bile.

cholangiogastrostomy (ko-lan″jĭ-o-gas-tros'to-mĭ). Formation of a communication bet. a bile duct and the stomach.

cholangiography (ko-lan-jĭ-og'ră-fĭ). X-ray or skiagraphic examination of the bile ducts.

cholangioma (ko-lan-jĭ-o'mă). A tumor of the biliary ducts.

cholangiostomy (kol-an-jĭ-os'to-mĭ). The surgical formation of a fistula into the gallbladder.

cholangiotomy (kol-an-jĭ-ot'o-mĭ). Incision of an intrahepatic bile duct for removal of gallstones.

cholangitis (ko-lan-jī'tis). Inflammation of the gall or bile duct. May be obstructive or catarrhal.

cholascos (ko-las'kos). Escape of bile into the peritoneal cavity.

cholecyst (kol'e-sist). A pear-shaped sac on the undersurface of the right lobe of the liver, the reservoir for the bile. SYN: *gallbladder, vesica fellea.*

cholecystalgia (ko-lē-sis-tal'jĭ-ă). Biliary colic.

cholecystectasia (ko-le-sis-tek-ta'zĭ-ă). Dilatation of the gallbladder.

cholecystectomy (ko-le-sis-tekt'o-mĭ). Excision of a gallbladder.

cholecystendysis (ko-le-sis-ten'dĭ-sis). Removal of a gallstone by incision, suturing wound in gallbladder and abdominal wall.

cholecystenterorrhaphy (ko-le-sist-en-ter-or'ă-fĭ). Suture of gallbladder to intestinal wall.

cholecystenterostomy (ko-le-sist-en-ter-os'to-mĭ). Suturing of gallbladder to intestine.   [gallbladder.

cholecystic (ko-le-sis'tĭk). Pert. to the

cholecystitis (ko-lē-sis-ti'tis). Inflammation of the gallbladder. It may be acute or chronic.

cholecystnephrostomy (ko″le-sist-nef-ros'to-mĭ). Making an anastomosis of gallbladder into renal pelvis.

cholecystocolostomy (ko-le-sis-to-ko-los'-to-mĭ). Making a passage from gallbladder to colon.

cholecystocolotomy (ko-le-sis-to-ko-lot'o-mĭ). Incision into gallbladder and colon.

cholecystoduodenostomy (kol-e-sis-to-du-o-den-os'to-mĭ). Surgical formation of a passage from gallbladder to duodenum.

cholecystogastrostomy (ko-le-sis-to-gas-tros'to-mĭ). Surgical formation of a passage from the gallbladder to the stomach.   [gallbladder.

cholecys'togram. An x-ray picture of the

cholecystography (ko-le-sis-tog'ră-fĭ). Examination of the gallbladder by x-ray.

cholecystoileostomy (ko-le-sis-to-ĭl-e-os'-to-mĭ). Forming a communication bet. the gallbladder and ileum.

cholecystojejunostomy (ko-le-sis-to-je-ju-nos'to-mĭ). Forming a communication bet. the gallbladder and jejunum.

cholecystokinin (ko″le-sĭs″tō-kī'nĭn). A hormone supposed to stimulate action of the gallbladder.

cholecystolithiasis (ko-le-sis-to-lith-i'ă-sis). Gallstones in the gallbladder.

cholecystolithotripsy (ko-le-sis-to-lith'o-trip-sĭ). Crushing of a gallstone in the unopened gallbladder.

cholecys'tomy. Cutting into the gallbladder. SYN: *cholecystotomy.*

cholecystopathy (ko-le-sis-top'ă-thĭ). Any gallbladder affection.

cholecystopexy (ko-le-sis'to-pek-sĭ). Suturing the gallbladder to the abdominal wall.

cholecystoptosis (ko-le-sis-top-to'sis). Displacement of the gallbladder downward.

cholecystorrhaphy (kō-lē-sis-tor'ă-fĭ). Suturing of the gallbladder.

cholecystostomy (ko-le-sis-tos'to-mĭ). Surgical formation of a permanent opening into gallbladder through abdominal wall.

cholecystotomy (ko-le-sis-tot'o-mĭ). Incision of gallbladder through the abdominal walls for removal of gallstones.

choledochectasia (ko-led-o-kek-ta'zĭ-ă). Distention of the common bile duct or *ductus choledochus.*

choledochitis (ko-led-o-ki'tis). Inflammation of common bile duct.

choledochoduodenostomy (ko-led″o-ko-du-o-den-os'to-mĭ). Surgical communication bet. the common bile duct and duodenum.

choledochoenterostomy (ko-led″o-ko-en-ter-os'to-mĭ). Surgical passage bet. common bile duct and intestine.

choledocholithiasis (ko-led″o-ko-lith-i'ă-sis). Calculi in the common bile duct.

choledocholithotomy (ko-le-do-ko-lith-ot'o-mĭ). Removal of a gallstone through an incision of the bile duct.

choledocholithotripsy (ko-le-do-ko-lith'o-trip-sĭ). Crushing of a gallstone in the common bile duct.

choledochoplasty (kol-e-do'ko-plas″tĭ). Operation for repair of common bile duct.

choledochorrhaphy (ko-led-o-kor'ră-fĭ). Suturing the severed ends of the common bile duct.

choledochostomy (kol-ed-o-kos'to-mĭ). Surgical formation of an opening into common bile duct through abdominal wall.

choledochotomy (kol-ed-o-kot'o-mĭ). Surgical incision of the common bile duct.

choledochus (ko-led'o-kus). The common bile duct. SYN: *ductus choledochus.*

cholehemia (ko-le-he'mĭ-ă). Bile in the blood. SYN: *cholemia.*

choleic (ko-le'ĭk). Cholic; pert. to the bile.

chol'elith. A bilestone.

cholelithiasis (ko-le-lith-i'as-is). Formation of, or presence of, calculi or bilestones in the gallbladder or gallduct.

cholelithic (ko-le-lith'ĭk). Pert. to or caused by biliary calculus.

cholelithotomy (kol-e-lith-ot'o-mĭ). Removal of gallstones through a surgical incision.

cholelithotrity (ko-le-lĭ-thot'rĭ-tĭ). Crushing of a biliary calculus.

cholemesis (kol-em'e-sis). Bile in the vomitus.

cholemia (ko-le'mĭ-ă). Bile salts in the blood.

cholepathia (ko-le-path'ĭ-ă). Faulty contractions of bile ducts.

   c. spas'tica. Spasmodic contraction of biliary ducts.

choleperitoneum (ko-le-per-ĭ-to-ne'um). Bile in the peritoneum.

cholepyrrhin (ko-le-pir'ĭn). Impure bilirubin. SYN: *biliphein.*

chol'era. An acute, specific, infectious disease characterized by diarrhea, painful cramps of muscles, and tendency to collapse.

   c. infantum. An acute disease of childhood, accompanied by vomiting, purging, and collapse.

   c. morbus. An acute, sporadic disease, resembling cholera, but not excited by the comma bacillus of Koch.

   c. sicca. A term sometimes applied to a fulminating variety of cholera which occurs without vomiting or purging.

choleraic (kol-ĕ-ra'ĭk). Pert. to cholera.

cholerase (kol'er-ās). The special bacteriolytic enzyme of cholera vibrio.

choleresis (kol-er-e'sis). The excretion of bile by the liver.

choleretic (kol-er-et'ĭk). Pert. to choleresis, or any agent that increases excretion of bile by the liver.

choleric (kol'er-ik). Irritable; quick-tempered without apparent cause.

choleriform (kol-er'ĭ-form). Appearing like cholera.

cholerigenous (kol-er-ij'en-us). Giving rise to cholera.

cholerine (kol'er-ēn). A mild form or initial stages of Asiatic cholera.

cholerization (kol-er-ĭ-za'shun). Inoculation against cholera.

cholerophobia (kol-er-o-fo'be-a). Morbid fear of acquiring cholera.

cholerrhagia (kol-er-ra'jĭ-ă). A flow of bile.

cholerythrin (kol-er'ĭ-thrin). 1. Cholerared. 2. Pigment in urine of tropical residents.

cholesta'sia. Arrest of the bile excretion.

chol''estat'ic. Caused by arrest of biliary excretion.

cholesteatoma (kol-es-te-ă-to'ma). 1. (Primary.) A pearl tumor or pearly nodules in brain. 2. (Secondary.) One of suppurative otitic origin in presence of marginal perforations.

choles'terase. A cholesterol ferment.

cholesteremia (ko-les-ter-e'mĭ-ă). Cholesterol in the blood.

cholesterin (ko-les'ter-in). S'erol; solid alcohol combined with fatty acids, forming a crystalline fat from bile and nerve tissue.

   DOSAGE: 3-5 gr. (0.2-0.3 Gm.).

cholesterinemia (ko-les-ter-in-e'mĭ-ă). Presence of cholesterol in the blood. SYN: *cholesterolemia.*

cholesterinuria (ko-les-ter-ĭn-u'rĭ-ă). Passing of cholesterin in the urine.

cholesterol (ko-les'ter-ol). A monatomic alcohol, $C_{27}H_{45}OH$, found in fats and oils, esp. in the bile, making up the greater part of gallstones.

   DOSAGE: 3-5 gr. (0.2-0.3 Gm.).

   holesterolemia (ko-les-ter-ol-e'mĭ-ă). Cholesterol in the blood.

cholesteroluria (ko-les-ter-ol-u'rĭ-ă). Cholesterol in voided urine.

cholesterosis (ko-les-ter-o'sis). Cholesterol deposition, esp. in excessive amounts, as in the gallbladder.

choletelin (ko-let'el-ĭn). Yellow coloring derived from bilirubin.

choletherapy (ko-le-ther'ă-pĭ). Use of oxgall as a medicine.

choleuria (ko-le-u'rĭ-ă). Bile in urine.

choleverdin (ko-le-ver'din). Green pigment appearing in gallstones and in urine in jaundice. SYN: *biliverdin.**

choline (kŏl'ēn). A ptomaine found in bile and suprarenal extract; a decomposition product of lecithin essential for functioning of the liver.

cholochrome (ko'lo-krōm). Any bile pigment.

cholohemothorax (ko-lo-hĕm-o-tho'raks). Bile and blood in the thorax.

chololith (kol'o-lith). A gallstone; biliary calculus.

chololithiasis (kol''o-lith-i'ăs-is). Presence of concretions in the gallbladder. SYN: *cholelithiasis.*

cholorrhea (kol-or-re'ă). Excessive secretion of bile.

choloscopy (ko-los'ko-pĭ). Testing the biliary function.

cholosis (ko-lo'sis). A perversion of bile secretion.

choluria (ko-lu'rĭ-a). Bile salts in the urine.

chondral (kon'dral). Pert. to cartilage.

chondralgia (kon-dral'jĭ-ă). Pain in or around a cartilage.

chondralloplasia (kon''dral-o-pla'zĭ-ă). Presence of cartilage in abnormal places.

chondrectomy (kon-drek'to-mĭ). Surgical excision of a cartilage.

chondric (kon'drik). Pert. to cartilage.

chondrification (kon-drĭ-n-ka'shun). Conversion into cartilage.

chon′drigen. Basal substance of cartilage, which turns into chondrin on boiling. SYN: *chondrogen.*

chondrin (kon′drĭn). Gelatinlike matter obtained by boiling cartilage.

chondriosome (kon′drĭ-o-sōm). A constituent of cytoplasm in the protoplasm of a cell. May be concerned in the production of germ cells.

chondritis (kon-dri′tis). Inflammation of cartilage.

chon″droadeno′ma. Cartilaginous tissue in an adenoma.

chon″droangio′ma. Cartilaginous elements in an angioma.

chondroblast (kon′dro-blast). Cell of primitive cartilage in the embryo.

chondroclast (kon′dro-klast). A cell concerned in the absorption of cartilage.

chondroconia (kon-dro-ko′nĭ-ă). Reddish granules in myelocytes.

chondrocostal (kon-dro-kos′tal). Pert. to costal cartilages.

chondrocranium (kon-dro-kra′nĭ-um). The cartilaginous embryonic cranium before ossification.

chondrocyte (kon′dro-sīt). A cartilage cell.

chondrodynia (kon-dro-dĭn′ĭ-ă). Pain in or about a cartilage.

chondrodysplasia (kon″dro-dis-pla′zĭ-ă). Abnormal cartilage growth.

chondrodystrophy (kon-dro-dis′tro-fĭ). Defect in cartilage formation at epiphyses of long bones.

chondrofibroma (kon-dro-fi-bro′mă). A mixed tumor with elements of chondroma and fibroma.

chondrogen (kon′dro-jen). The cement substance of cartilage.

chondrogenesis (kon-dro-jen′es-is). Formation of cartilage.

chondroid (kon′droid). Resembling cartilage; cartilaginous.

chondroituria (kon-dro-ĭ-tu′rĭ-ă). Chondroitic acid in urine.

chondrolipoma (kon-dro-lip-o′mă). Cartilaginous and fatty tissue tumor.

chondrology (kon-drol′o-jĭ). The science of cartilages.

chondrolysis (kon-drol′ĭ-sis). The breaking down and absorption of cartilage.

chondro′ma. A cartilaginous tumor of slow growth.
   It may occur any place where there is cartilage. It causes no pain.

chondromalacia (kon-drō-mal-a′sĭ-ă). Softness of any cartilage.

chondromalacosis (kon-drō-mal-ă-ko′sis). Cartilage softening. SYN: *chondromalacia.**

chondromatous (kon-dro′mă-tus). Pert. to chondroma, or tumor of a cartilage.

chondromucoid (kon-dro-mu′koid). Mucin in cartilage.

chondromyoma (kon-dro-mi-o′mă). Myoma and cartilaginous neoplasm combined.

chondromyxoma (kon-dro-mĭk-sō′mă). Chondroma with myxomatous elements.

chondromyxosarcoma (kon-dro-mĭk″sō-sar-kō′mă). A cartilaginous and sarcomatous tumor

chondropathology (kon-dro-path′ol-o-jĭ). Pathology of cartilages.

chondropathy (kon-drop′ath-ĭ). Any disease of cartilage.

chondrophyte (kon′dro-fīt). A growth from articular cartilage.

chondroplast (kon′dro-plast). Cell of primitive cartilage in the embryo. SYN: *chondroblast.*

chondroplas′tic. Pert. to plastic operations on cartilage.

chondroplasty (kon′dro-plas-tĭ). Plastic or reparative surgery on cartilage.

chondroporosis (kon-dro-po-ro′sis). The porous condition of cartilage, pathological or normal, during ossification.

chondroproteins (kon-dro-pro′te-ins). A group of glucoproteins found in cartilage, tendons, and connective tissue.

chondrosarcoma (kon-dro-sar-ko′mă). Cartilaginous sarcoma.

chondro′sis. The development of cartilage.

chon″droster′nal. Pert. to sternal cartilage.

chondrotome (kon′dro-tōm). Device for dissection of cartilage.

chondrotomy (kon-drot′o-mĭ). Dissection or surgical division of cartilage.

chondroxiphoid (kon-dro-zi′foid). Pert. to the ensiform cartilage or xiphoid.

chondrus (kon′drus). Cartilage.

Chopart′s amputation (sho-pars′). Disarticulation at the midtarsal joint.

chor′da. A string or tendon.
   c. dorsalis. Primitive spinal cord and backbone.
   c. tendinea. One of several tendinous cords bet. the ventricles.
   c. tympani. Tympanic nerve.
   c. umbilicalis. Umbilical cord connecting fetus and placenta.
   c. Willisii. One of several fibrous cords across the superior longitudinal sinus.

chordal (kor′dal). Pert. to a chorda, esp. the notochord.

chordée (kor-de′). Downward, painful curvature of the penis on erection in gonorrhea caused by inflammatory infiltration of the corpus spongiosum which interferes with its distensibility.

chorditis (kor-di′tis). Inflammation of a cord, esp. the spermatic, or a vocal cord.
   c. nodo′sa. Formation of small. whitish nodules on one or both vocal cords.

chordoskeleton (kor-do-skel′et-on). That part of the skeleton in the embryo formed about the primitive spinal cord.

chordot′omy. Division of any cord to relieve pain.

chorea (ko-re′ă). A nervous affection marked by muscular twitching. Known also as Sydenham's chorea (St. Vitus Dance).
   Occurs mostly in children.
   c., electric. Progressively fatal spasmodic disorder.
   ETIOL: Possibly of malarial origin. Occurs usually in Italy. SYN: *Dubini′s disease.*
   c., epidemic. Religious emotional neu-

rosis, manifest in the 14th century in Europe, exhibited in form of dancing mania. SYN: *dancing mania.*

c. gravidum. A form seen in some pregnant women, usually in those who have had chorea before, esp. in their first pregnancy.

c., Huntington's. A hereditary and chronic form manifested in adult life.

c., hyoscine. Movements simulating chorea, and sometimes accompanied by delirium, seen in acute hyoscine intoxication.

c. insaniens. Movements so violent patient is unable to walk, eat, or even lie down.

c., major. Chorea with violent hysterical muscular action.

c., mimetic. Chorea due to imitative movements.

c., minor. Ordinary form of chorea.

c., posthemiplegic; c., postparalytic. Involuntary movements of patients subsequent to a hemiplegic attack.

c., rhythmic. Chorea with movements at regulated times.

c., senile. Chorea developing in senility.

choreal (ko-re′al). Pert. to chorea.

choreic (ko-re′ik). Pert. to or of nature of chorea.

choreiform (ko-re′ĭ-form). Of the nature of chorea.

choreomania (ko-re-o-ma′nĭ-ă). Epidemic chorea, as the dancing mania of the middle ages.

chorioadenoma (ko-rĭ-o-ad-en-o′mă). Adenoma of the chorion.

chorioangioma (ko-rĭ-o-an-jĭ-o′mă). A vascular tumor of the chorion.

choriocapillaris (ko-rĭ′′o-kap-il-la′ris). Capillary layer of choroid.

choriocele (ko′rĭ-o-sēl). A protrusion of the chorioid coat of the eye through a defective sclera.

chorioepithelioma (ko-ri-o-ep-ĭ-the-lĭ-o′mă). Excessive proliferation of chorionic epithelium. SYN: *syncytioma malignum.*

chorioid (ko′rĭ-oid). Vascular coat of eye bet. sclera and retina. SYN: *choroid, q.v.*

chorioma (ko-rĭ-o′mă) (pl. *chorio′mata*). A tumor of the chorion.

choriomeningitis (ko-rĭ-o-men-in-ji′tis). Cerebral meningitis with cellular infiltration of the meninges.

c., acute lymphocytic. Disease resembling epidemic encephalitis, ant. poliomyelitis, and meningitis.

chorion (ko′rĭ-on). Membrane developed from the external epiblastic layer and an internal mesoblastic layer which together form the wall of the primitive blastocyte.

c. epithelioma. Very malignant cancer of uterus occurring most commonly after a vesicular mole and sometimes after abortion.

chorionic (ko-rĭ-on′ik). Pert. to the chorion.

c. villi. The vascular projections from the chorion.

chorionitis (ko-rĭ-on-i′tis). 1. Inflamma-

tion of the chorion. 2. Inflammation of the true skin, or corium.

chorioretinitis (ko-rĭ-o-ret′′in-i′tis). Inflammation of choroid and retina.

chorista (ko-ris′tă). An error of development showing separation from the rudiments in a developing embryo.

choristoma (ko-ris-to′mă). A neoplasm due to overdevelopment of embryonic rudiments.

choroid (ko′roid). Dark brown, vascular coat of eye bet. sclera and retina, extending from *ora serrata* to optic nerve.

choroideremia (ko-roy-der-e′mĭ-ă). Absence of the choroid coat of the eyeball.

choroiditis (ko-roid-i′tis). Inflammation of choroid.

c., anterior. When outlets of exudation are at the choroidal periphery.

c., areolar. In which inflammation spreads from around the macula lutea.

c., central. Exudation is limited to the macula.

c., diffuse or disseminated. When the fundus is covered with spots.

c., exudative. When covered with patches of inflammation.

c., metastatic. When due to embolism.

c. serosa. Increase of fluids in eyeball raising intraocular pressure, resulting in atrophy of optic nerve and blindness. SYN: *glaucoma.**

c., suppurative. When suppuration occurs.

choroidocycli′tis. Inflammation of the choroid coat and ciliary processes.

choroidoiritis (ko-royd-o-i-ri′tis). Inflammation of the choroid coat and iris.

choroidoretinitis (ko-royd-o-ret-in-i′tis). Inflammation of choroid and retina.

choromania (ko-ro-mă′nĭ-ă). Epidemic dancing mania; choreomania.

Christian Science. A religion and system of healing disease of mind and body which teaches that all cause and effect is mental, and that sin, sickness, and death will be destroyed by a full understanding of the Divine Principle of Jesus' teachings and healing. (Webster's *New Int. Dictionary,* 2nd ed.)

Chris′tison's formula. To estimate solids in urine per 1000 parts, multiply last 2 figures of specific gravity by 2.33.

Chrobak pelvis (kro′bak). A deformed pelvis caused by hip joint disease.

chromaffin (krō-măf′ĭn). 1. Staining readily with chromium salts. 2. Noting pigmented cells forming medulla of the suprarenal glands and the paraganglia.

c. system, c. tissue. The mass of tissue forming paraganglia and medulla of suprarenal glands, which secretes adrenalin and stains readily with chromium salts.

chromaffino′ma. A chromaffin cell tumor. SYN: *paraganglioma.*

chromaffinopathy (kro-maf-in-op′ă-thĭ). Any disease of chromaffin tissue.

chromaphil (kro′maf-ĭl). Pert. to a histological element or cell which stains readily with chromium salts. SYN: *chromaffin.*

chromate (kro'māt). A salt of chromic acid. SEE: *potassium chromate.*

chromatelopsia (kro"mat-ĕ-lop'sĭ-ă). Color blindness.

chromat'ic. Pert. to color.

chromatin (krō'mă-tĭn). Deeply staining substance of protoplasm in a cell nucleus which is considered as the physical basis of heredity.

chromatinolysis (kro"mă-tin-ol'ĭ-sis). 1. Destruction of chromatin. 2. The emptying of a cell, bacterial or other, by lysis.

chromatinorrhexis (kro"mă-tin-or-rek'sis). Splitting of chromatin.

chromatism (kro'mă-tĭzm). 1. Unnatural pigmentation. 2. Chromatic aberration.

chromatodysopia (kro-mă-to-dis-o'pĭ-ă). Color blindness.

chromatogenous (kro-mă-toj'en-us). Causing pigmentation or color.

chromatolysis (kro-mă-tol'ĭ-sis). 1. Lysis of a cell leaving nothing but an empty cell membrane. 2. Destruction of chromatin.

chromatometer (kro-mă-tom'et-er). A scale of colors for testing color perception.

chromatopathy (kro-ma-top'ă-thĭ). Any skin disease that is marked by pigmentation. [easily.

chromat'ophil, chromatophil'ic. Staining

chromatophore (kro-mat'o-fōr). A pigment bearing cell.

chromatopsia (kro-mă-top'sĭ-ă). Abnormally colored vision.

chromatoptometry (kro-mat-op-tom'e-trĭ). Measurement of color perception.

chromatosis (kro-mă-to'sis). Pigmentation.

chromaturia (kro-mă-tu'rĭ-ă). Abnormal color of the urine.

chro'micized. Mixed with a chromium salt.

chromidiosis (kro-mid-ĭ-o'sis). Overflow of chromatin and nuclear substance into cell protoplasm.

chromid'ium (pl. *chromidia*). Central chromatic body of a blood platelet.

chromidrosis (kro-mĭ-dro'sis). Excretion of colored sweat.

chromium (kro'mĭ-um). SYMB: Cr. At. wt. 52. A very hard, metallic element, steel gray in color.

    c. compounds. Largely used in industries.

    POISONING: SYM: A disagreeable taste in the mouth, pain, diarrhea, collapse, and cramping.

    TREATMENT: Chalk, magnesia, and other weak alkalies to neutralize its acid effects. Wash out stomach and give soothing drinks.

chro'moblast. An embryonic cell that becomes a pigment cell.

chromocholoscopy (kro-mo-ko-los'ko-pĭ). Examination of the biliary function by a pigment extraction test.

chromocrinia (kro-mo-krin'ĭ-ă). The secretion or excretion of pigmented matter.

chromocystoscopy (kro-mo-sis-tos'ko-pĭ). Determination of functional activity of kidneys by use of dyes.

chromocyte (kro'mo-sīt). Any colored cell.

chromocytometer (kro-mo-sī-tom'et-er). Instrument for determining the hemoglobin in red blood corpuscles.

chromodermatosis (kro-mo-der-mă-to'sis). Any pigmented skin disease.

chro"modiagno'sis. Diagnosis by change of color of the serum.

chromogen (kro'mo-jen). Any principle that may be changed into coloring matter.

chromogen'esis. Production of pigment.

chromogen'ic. Pigment producing.

chromolipoid (kro-mo-lip'oid). Any lipoid, such as carotin, that is pigmented. SYN: *lipochrome.*

chromolume (kro'mo-lŭm). Device for producing colored light rays.

chromolysis (kro-mol'i-sis). 1. Destruction of chromatin. 2. Lysis of a cell. SYN: *chromatolysis.*

chromo'ma. Neoplasm assumed to be derived from chromatophore cells.

chromomere (kro'mo-mēr). A minute granule of a chromatin.

chromometer (kro-mom'e-ter). Device for determining the pigment in a substance.

chromometry (kro-mom'et-rĭ). The estimation of coloring matter.

chromopar'ic. Producing color; chromogenic.

chromopex'ic. Fixing coloring matter, as the liver.

chromophage (kro'mo-fāj). A phagocyte that destroys pigment believed to be present in the blanching of hair. SYN: *pigmentophage.*

chromophane (kro'mo-fān). Retinal pigment.

chromophil(e (kro'mo-fil). 1. Any structure that stains easily. 2. Staining readily.

chromophilic (kro-mo-fil'ik). Staining readily; chromophilous.

chromophilous (kro-mof'il-us). Chromophilic.

chromophobe (krō'mō-fōb). Resistant to stain or a cell which does not stain.

chromophor'ic. Pert. to or bearing color.

chromophose (kro'mo-fōz). A subjective sensation of a spot of color in the eye. SEE: *centraphose, centrophose.*

chromophytosis (kro-mo-fi-to'sis). Pigmentation of skin due to a vegetable parasite. Tinea, or pityriasis versicolor.

chro'moplasm. The network of a cell nucleus.

chromoplas'tid. A pigment granule in protoplasm.

chromoprotein (kro-mo-pro'te-in). A pigmented conjugated protein made up of pigment and a simple protein, as hemoglobin. SEE: *proteins.*

chromop'sia. Chromatopsia; colored vision.

chromoptometer (kro-mop-tom'e-ter). Instrument for determining keenness of color vision.

chro"moradiom'eter. An instrument for measuring penetrative power of roentgen rays.

chromoscope (krō-mō-skōp). Instrument for determining color perception.

chromoscopy (krō-mos'kō-pǐ). 1. Examination for color vision 2. Administration of dyes to stain the urine and in this manner make a diagnosis of kidney function.

chromosome (kro'mō-sōm). 1. Microscopic rod-shaped body within the male and female germ cells which carries the parents' transmissible qualities. 2. The unit of chromatin in the nucleus of a cell.

   c., accessory. An unpaired monosome, which does not divide, but goes into only 1 of the daughter cells. SYN: *allosome, heterochromosome.*

   c., bivalent. Two chromosomes united temporarily.

   c., heterotropic. SEE: *accessory chromosome.*

   c., heterotypical. Chromosome different in appearance and behavior from an ordinary chromosome.

   c., sex. An accessory chromosome, so named because it is thought to transmit sexual characteristics.

   c., x-. SEE: *accessory chromosome.*

   c., y-. An accessory chromosome, sometimes seen in male cells, supposed to transmit the male sex factor in fecundation.

chro'mother'apy. The use of colored light in the treatment of disease.

chromotox'ic. Caused by toxic action on the hemoglobin.

chromoureteroscopy (kro-mo-ū-ret-er-os'-ko-pǐ). Inspecting orifices of ureters after giving a substance to dye the urine.

chronaxia (kron-ak'sǐ-ă). Time intensity relation of electrical stimuli.

chronaximeter (kron-aks-im'et-er). Device for measuring chronaxia.

chronaxy (kro'nak-sǐ). A number expressing the sensitiveness of a nerve to electrical stimulation.

chron'ic. Long drawn out; applied to a disease that is not acute.

chronicity (kro-nis'it-ǐ). State of being chronic.

chronobiol'ogy. Science of duration of life, and methods of prolonging it.

chronograph (kron'o-graf). Device for recording short intervals of time.

chronological (krŏn"ō-lŏj'ǐ-kăl). Occurring in natural sequence according to time.

   c. age. The number of years of one's life.

chron'oscope. Device for measuring extremely short intervals of time.

chronotrop'ic. Pert. to all that modifies periodically recurring action, such as the heartbeat.

   c. fibers. Those which control contraction of the heart.

chronot'ropism. Modification of periodical movements through external causes.

chrotoplast (kro'to-plast). An epithelial cell.

chrysarobin (kris-ar-o'bin) (goa powder). USP. A mixture of neutral principles obtained from a substance deposited in the wood of *Araroba,* a leguminous tree grown in South America.

chthonophagia (thon-o-fa'jǐ-ă). Eating clay or dirt; geophagy.

Chvostek's sign (shvos'teks). Local spasm following a tap on one side of face.

chylangioma (ki-lan-jǐ-o'mă). 1. Tumor of intestinal lymph vessels containing chyle. 2. Retention of chyle in lymphatic vessels with dilatation.

chyle (kīl). The milklike emulsion into which the fats of foods are transformed by the intestinal juices.

chylemia (ki-le'mǐ-ă). Chyle in the peripheral circulation.

chylidrosis (ki-li-dro'sis). A milklike sweat resembling chyle.

chylifacient (ki-li-fa'shent). Forming chyle.

chylifaction (ki-li-fak'shun). The formation of chyle.

chylifactive (ki-lif-ak'tiv). Forming chyle; chilifacient.

chyliferous (ki-lif'er-us). Carrying chyle.

chylification (ki-li-fǐ-ka'shun). Formation of chyle.

chylocele (ki'lo-sēl). Infused chyle in *tunica vaginalis testis.*

chylocyst (ki'lo-sist). The chyle bladder or reservoir of Pecquet.

chylocystic (ki-lo-sis'tik). Pert. to the *receptaculum chyli.*

chyloderma (ki-lo-der'mă). Lymph accumulated in the enlarged lymphatic vessels and thickened skin of the scrotum; lymph scrotum; scrotal elephantiasis.

chylology (ki-lol'o-jǐ). The study of chyle.

chylomediastinum (kī-lo"me-dǐ-as-tī'num). Chyle in the mediastinum.

chylomicron (ki-lo-mi'kron). Small particle of fat in the blood after digestion and absorption of fat in the food, and perceptible under a microscope.

chylopericardium (ki-lo-per-ǐ-kar'dǐ-um). Chyle in the pericardium.

chyloperitone'um. Effused chyle in peritoneal cavity.

chylophoric (ki-lo-for'ĭk). Conveying chyle; chyliferous.

chylopoiesis (ki-lo-poi-e'sis). Formation of chyle and absorption by lacteals in the intestines. SYN: *chylification.*

chylopoietic (ki-lo-poi-et'ĭk). Pert. to formation of chyle.

chylosis (ki-lo'sis). Formation of chyle. SYN: *chylifaction, q.v.*

chylotho'rax. Chyle in pleural cavities.

chylous (kī'lus). Pert. to or of the nature of chyle.

chyluria (ki-lu'rǐ-ă). Chyle or fat globules in the urine.

chymase (ki'mās). A gastric ferment that stimulates action of pancreatic juice.

chyme (kīm). The mixture of partly digested food and digestive secretions found in the stomach and small intestine during digestion of a meal; it is a varicolored, thick, but nearly liquid, mass. SEE: *"chym-" words, enchyma, oligochymia.*

chymifica'tion. 1. Formation of food into chyme. 2. Gastric digestion.

chymosin (ki'mo-sin). Milk curdling enzyme found chiefly in gastric juice. SYN: *rennet, rennin.*

chymosinogen (kī-mo-sin'o-jen). A substance from which chymosin is formed.

C. I. Abbr. for color index.

cibisitome (si-bis'it-ōm). Instrument for incision of capsule of the lens.

cicatricial (sik-ă-trish'al). Pert. to a cicatrix.

cicatricotomy (sik-ă-trik-ot'o-mĭ). Incision of a cicatrix or scar.

cicatrix (sik'a-triks, sik-a'triks). A scar left by a healed wound.

cicatrizant (sik-kat'riz-ant). Favoring or causing cicatrization.

cicatrization (sik-at-ri-za'shun). Healing by scar formation. SEE: *intention.*

cic'atrize. To heal by scar tissue.

cilia (sil'ĭ-ă). (sing. *cil'ium*). 1. Eyelashes. 2. Hairlike processes projecting from epithelial cells, as in the bronchi, which wave mucus, pus, and dust particles upward.

ciliariscope (sil-ĭ-a'ri-skōp). Instrument for examination of the ciliary region of the eye.

ciliarotomy (sil-ĭ-ar-ot'o-mĭ). Surgical section of the ciliary zone in glaucoma.

cil'iary. 1. Pert. to any hairlike processes. 2. An eyelid, and eyelash.

  c. arteries. Small arteries of eye.

  c. body. Extends from base of iris to ant. part of choroid; consists of ciliary processes and ciliary muscle.

  c. glands. Glands of Moll, a form of sweat glands of the eyelid.

  c. muscle. Accommodation muscle of eye.

  c. processes. Consist of about 70 folds arranged meridionally so as to form a circle, have same structure as rest of choroid and secrete nutrient fluids which nourish neighboring parts, as cornea, lens, vitreous body. SEE: *choroidocyclitis.*

  c. reflex. Normal movement of pupil in accommodation of eye.

cil'iate. Having hairlike projections resembling cilia.

ciliated (sil'ĭ-a-ted). Possessing cilia.

  c. epithelium. Epithelium with hairlike processes on surface. They waft only in one direction and line the respiratory tract and fallopian tubes.

ciliectomy (sil-ĭ-ek'to-mĭ). Excision of portion of ciliary muscle, body, or border of eyelid.

ciliospinal (sil-ĭ-o-spi'nal). Pert. to the ciliary body and spinal cord.

  c. center. Spinal cord center which controls dilatation of the pupil.

  c. reflex. Dilation of pupil following irritation of neck vein.

ciliotomy (sil-ĭ-ot'o-mĭ). Section of the ciliary nerves.

cilium (sil-ĭ-um). 1. An eyelash. 2. Hairlike process of certain cells.

cillosis (sil-o'sis). Twitching of an eyelid, spasmodically.

cimbia (sim'be-ă). Slender band of white fibers crossing the ventral surface of a cerebral peduncle.

Cimex lectularius (si'meks lek-tū-la'rĭ-us). The bedbug.

cinchona (sin-ko'nă). (Peruvian bark.) USP. The dried bark of the tree cinchona, the source of quinine. Its preparation, the tincture and compound tincture, useful as a bitter tonic.

  DOSAGE: 1 dram (4 cc.).

cinchonism (sin'kon-izm). Poisoning from cinchona or its alkaloids.

cinchonize (sin'ko-nīz). To bring under the influence of cinchona or its alkaloids, esp. quinine.

cinchophen (sin'ko-fen) (atophan). USP. Light yellow powder with slightly bitter taste; a dangerous drug to use.

  DOSAGE: 8 gr. (0.5 Gm.).

  c. poisoning. Out of 117 cases of poisoning reported there were 61 deaths.

cinclisis (sin'klis-is). Rapid winking, or quick, spasmodic movements of any part of the body.

cincture sensation (sink'tūr). Sensation of a tight girdle about the waist. SYN: *zonesthesia.*

cinemat'ics. Science of motion; kinematics.

cinematoradiography (sin-e-mat″o-rā-dĭ-og'ra-fĭ). Radiography of an organ in motion.

cineplas'tics. Formation after amputation of muscles of a stump, so that it is possible to impart motion and direction to an artificial limb.

cineraceous (sin-e-ra'shus). Like ashes.

cinerea (sin-e're-ă). The gray matter of the brain and nervous system.

cine'real. Pert. to gray matter of the nervous system.

cineritious (sin-er-ish'us). Ashen, as the gray matter.

cinesalgia (sin-es-al'jĭ-ă). Pain caused by movement of muscles.

cinesi-. Prefix: Motion. See also *kinesi-.*

cinesia (sin-e'sĭ-ă). Motion sickness, as car sickness, seasickness.

cinesthesia (sin-es-the'zĭ-ă). 1. The sense of motion. 2. The false sense of moving in space.

cinetocyte (si-net'o-sīt). A 4th element or wandering cell in the blood.

cinetocythemia (si-net″o-sī-the'mĭ-ă). Many cinetocytes in the blood.

cinetocytopenia (si-net″o-sī-to-pe'nĭ-ă). Having an abnormally small number of cinetocytes in the blood.

cinetocytosis (si-net″o-sī-to'sis). Many cinetocytes in the blood. SYN: *cinetocythemia.**

cingulum (pl. *cin'gula*) (sin'gu-lum). Association fibers in the brain.

cion (si'ŏn). The uvula.

cioni'tis. Inflammation of the uvula.

cionoptosia (si-on-op-to'sĭ-ă). A lengthened uvula.

cionotome (si-on'o-tōm). Instrument for excision of the uvula.

cionotomy (si-on-ot'o-mĭ). Excision of uvula.

circa (sir'kă). Prefix: About.

circinate (sur'si-nat). Circular.

cir'cle. Any ring-shaped structure.

  c. of diffusion. One or more on projection plane of an image not in focus of the lens.

c. of Willis. Union of the ant. and post. cerebral arteries (branches of the carotid) forming an anastomosis at base of the brain.

c., vascular. One around the mouth formed by inf. and sup. coronary arteries.

cir'cuit. Course or path of an electric current.

c. breaker. A safety device for opening an electrical circuit; a switch.

c., closed. A circuit through which electricity is passing or can pass.

c., electric. The path through conductors by which an electric current passes.

c., ground. Ground or earth as part of electric circuit.

c., high frequency. A spark gap, condenser, and the oscillatory transformer or resonator.

c., magnetic. The closed path of magnetic lines; e. g., the magnetic circuit of a transformer.

c., open. A circuit having some break in it so that current is not passing or cannot pass. This break may be intentional, as an open switch, or accidental, as a blown fuse, a loose connection, or a broken wire.

c., short. An accidental overflow of current due to the establishment of a low resistance bypass.

cir'cular. 1. Shaped like a circle. 2. Recurrent.

c. insanity. That in which manic and depressive attacks follow one another without intervals of lucidity.

circula'tion. Movement in a circular course.

c. of the aqueous humor of the eye. The aqueous humor is secreted by the ciliary process into the post. chamber of the eye.

c. of bile salts. The sodium glycocholate and taurocholate found in hepatic bile pass with it into the intestine, where they are absorbed along with the fats.

c. of the blood The blood leaving the left ventricle enters the aorta, from which it escapes into the various large arteries. It thus reaches the coronary arteries of the heart itself and the arteries of the head, body wall, abdominal viscera, and extremities. Passing through the various capillary systems, it is gathered into veins, of which there are 2 systems. (1) Most veins empty their blood into the *venae cavae superior* and *inferior*. (2) The veins from the stomach, pancreas, spleen, and intestine unite to form the *vena portae*, which runs to the liver. Here it breaks up into a new capillary system, which drains through the hepatic veins into the *vena cava inferior*. The combined blood of the *venae cavae* and the coronary veins enters the right atrium, passes through the right ventricle, and is forced out into the pulmonary artery. The pulmonary capillary system drains by way of the pulmonary veins into the left atrium and thence into the left ventricle.

c. of the cerebrospinal fluid. The cerebrospinal fluid, secreted by the choroid plexuses in the lateral ventricles of the cerebral hemispheres, passes through the interventricular foramina into the 3rd ventricle, thence through the cerebral aqueduct into the 4th ventricle.

c., collateral. Circulation through small vessels which enlarge to compensate for an obstruction in the large vessels.

c., enterohepatic. SEE: *circulation of bile salts.*

c., fetal. Blood of the fetus coursing through the placenta and umbilical cord.

c. of the lymph. The lymph is formed in vessels which are found in the viscera, the body wall, and the extremities. Many of these vessels empty into a passage in the abdomen (*cisterna chyli*).

c., portal. Veins from the pancreas, spleen, stomach, intestines unite behind the pancreas and form the portal tube or vein.

c., pulmonary. The venous blood which is received into the right auricle passes through the tricuspid valve into the right ventricle. From there into the pulmonary artery, which divides into 2 branches, 1 going to each lung. (This is the only instance when an artery contains venous or dark blood deficient in oxygen.) The artery breaks up in the lung into capillaries, and here, by means of the hemoglobin in the red corpuscles, takes up oxygen from the inspired air. Red arterial blood returns to the heart by the 4 pulmonary veins, 2 from each lung entering the left auricle. (This is the only instance where veins contain oxygenated blood.)

c., systemic. General circulation through the whole body except the lungs.

c., venous. Circulation of the blood via the veins.

circulation time. Determination of velocity of the blood.

cir'culatory. Pert. to circulation.

circum-. Prefix: Around, as *circumduction.*

circumarticular (sĭr″kŭm-ar-tĭk'ū-lar). Surrounding a joint. SYN: *periarthric.*

circumcision (ser-kum-sĭ'shun). Removal of the end of the prepuce by a circular incision.

circumclusion (ser-kum-klu'zhun). Acupressure by use of a pin under an artery and a wire loop over it, attached to each end of the pin.

circumcor'neal. Around the cornea.

circumcres'cent. Developing around or over a part.

circumduction (sir-kum-duk'shun). 1. The action or swing of a limb, such as the arm, in such a manner that it describes a cone-shaped figure, the apex of the cone being formed by the joint at the proximal end, while the complete circle is formed by the free distal end of the limb. 2. Circular movement of the eye.

circumflex (sir'kum-fleks). Winding around, as a vessel.

circumin'sular. Surrounding the island of Reil.

circumintes'tinal. Around the intestine.

circumlen'tal. Situated around the lens.

circumnu'clear. Surrounding the nucleus.

circumoc'ular. Surrounding the eye.

   c. core. A nucleus.

circumor'al. Encircling the mouth.

   c. pallor. White area around the mouth contrasting vividly with color of face, esp. seen in scarlet fever.

circumorbital (sĕr"kŭm-or'bĭt-ăl). Around an orbit.

circumpolariza'tion. The rotation of a ray of polarized light.

circumre'nal. Around or about the kidney.

cir'cumscribed. Limited in space.

cir"cumstantial'ity. The mention of irrelevant facts and details in conversation.

circumval'late. Surrounded by a wall or raised structure.

   c. papillae. V-shaped row of papillae at base of tongue.

circus movements (ser'kus). "Contraction or excitation wave traveling continuously in circular fashion around a ring of muscle or through the wall of the heart." (*Lewis.*)

cirrhonosus (sir-ron'o-sus). Disease of the fetus marked by a golden yellow color of the pleura and peritoneum.

cirrhosis (sir-ro'sis). An intestinal inflammation with hardening, granulation, and contraction of the tissues of an organ, more esp. the liver.

   c., alcoholic. That of the liver due to alcoholism.

   c., atrophic. One marked by atrophy of the liver.

   c., biliary. Affecting the liver and gallbladder.

   c., fatty. Cirrhosis with fatty infiltration of the liver cells.

   c., hypertrophic. In which the connective tissue hyperplasia starts from the periphery of the capillary bile ducts instead of from ramifications of portal vein as in atrophic form.

   c. of liver. A chronic disease characterized anatomically by a hyperplasia of the connective tissue and destruction of the secreting cells shown chiefly by symptoms of portal obstruction.

   c. of lung. A chronic disease of the lung characterized by an overgrowth of fibrous tissue.

   c., portal. Cirrhosis with inflammation and ensuing obstruction to portal circulation.

cirrhotic (sir-rot'ĭk). Pert to or affected with cirrhosis.

cirsectomy (sir-sek'to-mĭ). Excision of a portion of a varicose vein.

cirsenchysis (sir-sen'kĭ-sis). Injection of varicose veins.

cirsocele (sir'so-sēl). Dilation of veins of spermatic cord. SYN: *varicocele.*

cirsodesis (sir-sod'ĕ-sis). Ligation of varicose veins.

cirsoid (sir'soid). Resembling a varix. SYN: *varicose.*

cirsomphalos (sir-som'fă-los). Varicose veins around the navel.

cirsotome (sir'so-tōm). Instrument for cutting varicose veins.

cirsotomy (sir-sot'o-mĭ). Treatment of a varicosity by multiple incisions.

cister'na, cis'tern. Any reservoir cavity.

   c. chy'li. BNA. *Receptaculum chyli.* A dilated sac into which is emptied the intestinal 2 lumbar, and 2 descending lymphatic trunks; the origin of the thoracic duct.

cisternal (sĭs-ter'năl). Concerning a cavity filled with fluid.

   c. puncture. A spinal puncture with a hollow needle bet. the cervical vertebrae, through the dura mater into the cisterna at base of brain.

Citel'li's syndrome. Poor memory, mental backwardness, insomnia or drowsiness, and lack of concentration in those with adenoids or sphenoid sinusitis.

citochol reaction (sī'to-kol). The use of concentrated cholesterolized extract of heart muscle as the antigen for a rapid flocculation test.

citrate (sit'rāt). Compound of citric acid and a base.

   c. solution. Used to prevent clotting of blood that has been shed.

Cl. Symb. of chlorine.

cladosporiosis (klad"o-spo-rĭ-o'sis). Infection with *Cladospo'rium,* a fungus, marked by appearance of gummatous nodules.

cladothricosis (klad-o-thrĭ-ko'sis). Infection with *Cladothrix.*

Cladothrix (klad'o-thriks). A schizomycete having a clearly visible sheath and pseudobranching cell threads.

   C. foersteri. A species forming felted masses in the human tear ducts.

clamp (klamp). Device for compression of vessels.

clang. A loud, metallic sound.

   c. tint. A delicate tone.

clap. Popular term for gonorrhea.

   c. threads. Slimy threads of mucus and pus in urine during gonorrhea.

clapotage, clapotement (klă-po-tazh', klă-pot-mon'). Any splashing sound heard on succussion of a dilated stomach.

Clap'ton's lines. Green lines on dental margin of gums in copper poisoning.

clar'et stain or **cheek.** Capillary nevus of cheek. SYN: *nevus flammeus.*

clarificant (klar-if'ik-ant). Any agent that clears the turbidity of a liquid.

Clarke's bodies. Alveolar sarcomatous intranuclear bodies of breast.

   C.'s column. Gray matter, the trophic center for the direct cerebellar tract; the vesicular column.

clasmatoblast (klaz-mat'o-blast). A mast cell.

clasmatocyte (klaz-mat'o-sīt). A large, wandering, uninucleated cell, with many branches.

clasmatocytosis (klaz-mat-o-si-to′sis). Breaking up of clasmatocytes and islands of granules formed from their débris.

clasmatodendro′sis. A breaking up of astrocytic protoplasmic expansions.

clasmato′sis. Crumbling into small bits; fragmentation, as of cells.

clasp-knife rigidity. Spastic action in a joint in cerebral palsies.

clastic (klas′tik). Causing division into parts.

clastothrix (klas′to-thriks). Brittleness of the hair. Syn: *trichorrhexis*.

claudication (klaw-di-ka′shun). 1. Limping. 2. Loss of function, temporarily due to spasm (arterial) in brain or heart. 3. An obstruction.

  c., intermittent. Arterial spasm with subsequent painful cramping of the legs and lameness.

Claudius' cells (klaw′di-us). Large columnar cells external to the organ of Corti.

  C.'s fossa. Small depression in post. part of pelvis, on either side, in which lies the ovary.

claustrophilia (klaws-tro-fil′i-ă). Dread of being in an open space, as in neurasthenia, or of open spaces unprotected by the sun, as by those who have had a sunstroke or heatstroke.

claustrophobia (klaws-tro-fo′bi-ă). Fear of being confined in any space, as in a locked room. Opp. of *agoraphobia*.*

claustrum (klaws′trum). A barrier.

clausura (klaws-su′ră). Atresia of a passage, closure.

clava (kla′vă). (pl. *clavae*). Enlarged extremity of the *funiculus gracilis* in the post. portion of the medulla oblongata. *Tuberculum gracile*.

cla′vate. Clubshaped.

  c. nucleus. Collection of nerve cells within the clava.

clav′icle. The collarbone; a bone curved like the letter f, which articulates with the sternum and the scapula.

  c., fracture of. Sym: (1) Swelling, pain, protuberance with sharp depression over the injured bone. (2) Patient supports arm at the elbow, arm useless.

clavicular (kla-vik′u-lar). Pert. to the clavicle.

cla′vus. 1. A corn or callosity. 2. A sharp head pain like the driving of a nail into the head.

clawfoot (klaw′fut). Muscular wasting with distortion, giving foot appearance of a claw. Syn: *pescavus*.

clawhand. Muscular atrophy and clawlike flexion of fingers.

clear′ing agent. One that makes microscopical objects more transparent.

cleavage (kle′vej). 1. Splitting a complex molecule into 2 or more simpler ones. 2. Cell division following the fertilization of an egg. Syn: *segmentation*.

  c. cell. The blastomere.

  c., hydrolytic. Hydrolysis.

  c. lines. Those appearing in linear direction when a pin punctures a cadaver.

  c. nucleus. Segmentation of the vitellus.

cleft. A fissure.

  c. palate. A congenital palatine fissure forming 1 cavity for the nose and mouth.

  c. sternum. A congenital fissure of the breastbone.

  c. tongue. One with furrows.

cleido- (kli′do). Prefix: Pert. to the clavicle.

cleidorrhexis (kli-do-rek′sis). Fracture or bending the clavicles of the fetus for delivery.

cleidotomy (kli-dot′o-mi). Dividing a fetal clavicle to facilitate delivery.

cleptoma′nia. Impulsive stealing, the intrinsic value of the article not being the motive. Syn: *kleptomania, q.v.*

clergyman's sore throat. A form of granular pharyngitis.

Clev′enger's fissure. *Sulcus temporalis inferior* bet. 2nd and 3rd occipital convolutions.

climacteric (kli-mak′ter-ik, kli-mak-ter′-ik). That period that marks the cessation of a woman's reproductive period.

  c., grand. The 63rd year.

climatol′ogy. Branch of meteorology which is the study of climate and its relation to disease. See: *bioclimatology*.

climatotherapy (kli-mat-ō-ther′ap-i). Change of climate as a treatment of a disease.

cli′max. Period of greatest intensity.

cli′mograph. A graph of the effect of climate on health.

clinic (klin′ik). 1. Bedside examination. 2. A center for physical examination and treatment of those unable to pay for the same or for those able to pay a minimum fee.

clin′ical. 1. Pert. to the course of a disease, or the symptoms as opposed to anatomical changes. 2. Pert. to a clinic.

  c. thermometer. One which measures body temperature.

clinician (klin-ish′an). A practicing physician; clinicist.

clinoid (kli′noid). Resembling a bed in shape.

  c. processes. Three pairs of prominences on upper surface of sphenoid bone.

clinom′eter. Instrument for estimation of power of rotation of ocular muscles.

cli′noscope. Instrument for measuring the weakness of ocular muscles.

clinostat′ic. Caused by assuming a recumbent position.

clinostat′ism. The recumbent position.

cliseometer (klis-e-om′et-er). Device for measuring the female pelvic inclination.

clithrophobia (klith-ro-fo′bi-ă). Morbid fear of being locked in.

clition (klit′i-on). A craniometric point in center of highest part of the clivus on the sphenoid bone.

clitoridauxe (klit-or-id-awk′sĕ). Hypertrophy of the clitoris.

clitoridectomy (klit-or-i-dek′to-mi). Excision of clitoris.

clitoriditis (klit-or-id-i′tis). Inflammation of the clitoris.

clitoridotomy (kli-tor-ĭ-dot′ŏ-mĭ). Incision of the clitoris.

clitoris (kli′tor-is). The analogue of the penis in the female. An erectile organ practically covered by its prepuce and located bet. and behind the ant. parts of the labia minora.

   c. crises. Recurring crises of involuntary excess of sexual feeling culminating in a true orgasm with spasm of the clitoris followed by lancinating pains in the genital organs lasting for hours. Rare.

clitorism (klit′or-izm). The counterpart of priapism. A long continued, painful condition in the female with recurring erection of the clitoris with an occasional orgasm.

clitoritis (klit-o-ri′tis). Inflammation of the clitoris. SYN: *clitoriditis.*

cli′vus. A surface that slopes, as the sphenoid bone.

   c. blumenbach′ii. The slope at base of skull.

cloaca (klo-a′ka). 1. A fistulous area in bone. 2. A common outlet to the bladder and rectum.

clonic (klon′ik). Pert. to alternate contraction and relaxation of muscles.

   c. spasm. One marked by muscular contraction and relaxation. Occurs in 2nd stage of epilepsy.

clonicity (klon-isʹĭ-tĭ). Being clonic.

clonicotonic (klon-ĭ-ko-ton′ĭk). Both clonic and tonic, as some forms of muscular spasm.

clon′ism, clonis′mus. Condition of being affected with clonic spasms, or a succession of them.

clon′ograph. An instrument for registering spasmodic movements.

clon′ospasm. Rapid alternation of muscular contraction and relaxation.

clon′us. Spasmodic alternation of contraction and relaxation; opposite of *tonus.* SEE: *wrist clonus.*

Cloquet's canal (klo-kās′). An irregular passage (hyaloid) through center of the vitreous body in the fetus.

closed core transformer. A transformer having a continuous core of magnetic material (usually iron) without any air gap.

clot (klŏt). 1. To coagulate. 2. A thrombus; a coagulum, as of blood or lymph.

   c., agony. One formed in the heart when death ensues from prolonged heart failure.

   c., ante-mortem. One formed in the heart or its cavities before death.

   c., blood. A coagulum formed of blood.

   c., chicken fat. A yellow-colored blood clot.

   c., currant jelly. A clot of fibrin of reddish color and jellylike consistency.

   c., distal. One formed in a vessel on distal side of a ligature.

   c., external. One formed outside a blood vessel.

   c., heart. A thrombus within the heart.

   c., internal. One formed by solidification of blood.

   c., laminated. One formed in a succession of layers filling an aneurysm.

   c., muscle. One formed in coagulation of muscle plasma.

   c., passive. One formed in the sac of an aneurysm.

   c., plastic. One formed from the intima of an artery at the point of ligation.

   c., post-mortem. One formed in the heart or in a large blood vessel after death.

   c., proximal. One formed on the proximal side of a ligature.

   c., stratified. Thrombus consisting of layers of different colors.

clothes louse. *Pediculus corporis;* a body louse.

clouding of consciousness. PSY: A state of mental confusion characterized by insufficiency of perception and impaired attention, and resulting in loss of orientation of time and place, amnesia and ill-adjusted reactions. Occurs in toxic, febrile, and other deliria. SEE: *consciousness.*

clou′dy swelling. Degeneration in which the tissues swell and become turbid.

clove-hitch. A knot consisting of 2 contiguous loops which are placed around an object, the ends of the cord being toward each other; used for making traction on a part for the reduction of dislocations or for restraining mental or delirious patients.

clove, oil of (carophyllus). USP. A volatile oil distilled from the dried flower buds of the clove tree.

   ACTION AND USES: Antiseptic and aromatic. Useful also as an anodyne in dental practice.

clo′ven spine. Spina bifida. Congenital defect of spinal canal walls caused by lack of union bet. laminae of the vertebrae.

clown′ism. Grotesque actions and attitudes.

clubbed fingers. Rounding of ends and swelling of fingers in children with congenital heart disease and in older children and adults with long standing pulmonary disease.

clubfoot. Nontraumatic foot deviation. SEE: *kyllosis, talipes.*

clubhand. Deformity of the hand resembling clubfoot.

clumping. 1. Adhesion of wound surfaces. 2. Clumping of microörganisms in a culture when specific immune serum is added. SYN: *agglutination.*

clu′nes. The buttocks; nates.

clupeine (klŭ′pē-ēn). A protamine from the spermatozoa of the herring.

clysis (kli′sis). Injection of fluid for washing out the blood in a cavity.

clysma (klis′mă). An enema.*

cly′ster. Rectal injection or enema; a clysma.

C. M. Abbr. for *chirurgiae magister,* Master in Surgery.

cm. Abbr. for *centimeter.*

cnemial (ne'mĭ-al). Pert. to the leg, esp. the shin.

cnemis (ne'mis). Shin, lower leg, tibia.

cnemitis (ne-mi'tis). Inflammation of the tibia.

CO₂. Symb: Carbon dioxide.

CO₂ therapy. Therapeutic application of low temperatures with solid carbon dioxide. See: *refrigeration.*

co″activ′ity. Action that aids an enzyme to function, as the action of bile salts upon lipase, but not the same as that incited by an activator.

coadunation (ko-ad-u-na'shun). Union or junction of dissimilar substances in 1 mass.

coagglutina′tion. Clumping by an antigen and the homologous antibody of the corpuscles of another organism.

coagglu′tinin. An antibody that is effective on 2 or more organisms.

coag′ula. Plural of *coagulum.*

coagulable (ko-ag'u-lă-bl). Capable of clotting; apt to clot.

coagulant (ko-ag'u-lant). 1. That which causes a fluid to coagulate. 2. Causing coagulation.

coagulase (ko-ag'u-lāz). Any enzyme, such as thrombin, which causes coagulation. See: *coagulin, coagulum.*   [fluidity.

coag′ulate. To lessen the properties of

coag′ulated. Clotted or curdled.

  c. proteins. Derived proteins (insoluble), resulting from the action of alcohol on protein, or heat on protein solutions.

coagula′tion. The process of clotting.

  c. band. Weltmann's concentration at which flocculation occurs, designated as K.B. See: *K.B.*

coag′ulative. Causing coagulation.

coag′ulin. A specific substance, produced in the body of an animal by an injection of a substance, which will cause quickened coagulation in that of another. See: *coagulase.*

coagulinoid (ko-ag'u-lin-oid). A coagulin whose function has been destroyed by heating to 65°-70° C.

coagulometer (ko-ag-u-lom'et-er). Device for measuring the blood's coagulability.

coaguloviscom′eter. An instrument for determining the rapidity of the coagulation of the blood.

coag′ulum. 1. A blood clot. 2. A curd.

coalesce (ko-al-es'). To fuse; run or grow together.

coales′cence. Fusion or growing together of 2 or more parts of bodies.

coal tar. A tar that is produced in the destructive distillation of bituminous coal, as crude creosol.

coapta′tion. The adjustment of separate parts to each other, as the edges of fractures, or of a wound.

coarctate (ko-ark'tāt). To press or pressed together.

  c. retina. Funnel-shaped retina.

coarcta′tion. 1. Compression of the walls of a vessel. 2. Shriveling. 3. A stricture.

coarctotomy (ko-ark-tot'o-mĭ). Cutting or division of a stricture.

cobra venom solution (kō′brä vĕn′ŭm). Minute quantities of the secretion of the cobra in sterile physiological salt solution, and standardized so that 1 cc. is equivalent to 5 mouse units.

cocaine hydrochlor′ide (ko-kān'). USP. The hydrochloride of an alkaloid obtained from erythroxylin cocoa.

  Dosage: Topical application of ½ to 4%.

cocainism (ko-kān'izm). The habitual use of cocaine, which is more rare than morphinism.

cocainization (ko-kān-ĭ-za'shun). Inducing analgesia by use of cocaine.

cocainize (ko-kān'īz). To put under the influence of cocaine.

cocainomania (ko-kān-o-ma'ne-ă). Intense desire for cocaine and its results.

coccidiosis (kok-sid-ĭ-o'sis). Nodular formations scattered over the body due to infestation with Coccidium and resulting symptoms.

Coccidium (kok-sid′ĭ-um). A genus of protozoans.

  C. hominis. A species found in the human liver and intestines.

  C. oviforme. A species found in the bile ducts in man and causing cystic dilatation.

  C. sarkolytus. A supposed parasite of carcinoma.

  C. syphilidis. An organism assumed to be the cause of syphilis, *Spirochaeta pallida* being one stage of its life cycle.

coccinella (kok-sin-nel'ă). Coccus employed as a coloring agent. Syn: *cochineal.*

coccobacte′ria (sing. *coccobacterium*). Round, spheroid, or ovoid bacterium including the *gono-, meningi-, micro-, pneumo-, staphylo-,* and *streptococci.*

coccogenous (kok-oj′en-us). Produced by cocci.

coccoid (kok'oid). Resembling a micrococcus.

coccus (kok'us) (pl. *cocci*). 1. A capsule or cell. 2. A bacterial, spheroid, cell form, which includes *diplococcus,* * *gonococcus,* * *macrococcus,* * *meningococcus,* * *micrococcus,* * *pneumococcus,* * *staphylococcus,* * *streptococcus.* *

coccyalgia (kok-sĭ-al'jĭ-ă). Pain in the coccyx.

coccydynia (kok-sĭ-din'ĭ-ă). Pain in or around the coccyx; coccyalgia.

coccygeal (kok-sij'ē-al). Pert. to the coccyx.

coccygectomy (kok-sij-ek'to-mĭ). Excision of coccyx.

coccygodynia (kok-sĭ-go-din'ĭ-ă). Pain in the coccygeal region; coccyalgia.

coccyodynia (kok-sĭ-o-din'ĭ-ă). Pain in region of coccyx. Syn: *coccygodynia.*

coccyx (kok'siks). Last 4 bones of the spine. Usually ankylosed and articulating with the sacrum above.

cochineal (koch'in-ēl). Dried female insect, used as carmine coloring matter for pharmaceutical products, and as a dye in laboratory work.

cochlea (kok'lē-ă). A winding, cone-shaped tube, the inner part of the labyrinth of the ear. The auditory part of the inner ear.

cochlear (kok'le-ar). Pert. to the cochlea.

   c. nerve. One supplying the cochlea.

cochleare (kok-le-a're). Spoonful.

cochleariform (kok-le-ar'ĭ-form). Spoonshaped.

cochleitis (kok-le-i'tis). Inflammation of the cochlea. SYN: *cochlitis.*

cochleoörbicular reflex (kok-le-o-or-bik'u-lar). Contraction of orbicularis palpebrarum muscle resulting from sudden noise being produced near ear.

cochleopalpebral reflex (kok-lē-ō-pal'pĕ-bral). Contraction of orbicularis palpebrarum muscle resulting from sudden noise being produced near ear.

cochleovestibular (kok-le-o-ves-tib'u-lar). Pert. to the cochlea and vestibule of the ear.   [cochlea.

cochlitis (kok-li'tis). Inflammation of the

cock'roach. *Blatta orientalis.* Common beetlelike insect infesting houses.

COCL. Abbr. for cathodal opening clonus.

cocon'sciousness. A conscious objective state in which subconscious impressions rise to the surface.

cocontraction (kō-kon-trak'shun). Adjustment of 2 muscles during contraction, said of antagonist muscles in coördination.

coctolabile (kok-to-la'bĭl). Incapable of remaining unaltered when subject to boiling water.

coctoprecipitin (kok-to-pre-sip'it-in). A precipitin produced by injecting a serum that has been boiled.

coctostabile (kok-to-stab'ĭl). Incapable of being altered or destroyed by boiling water.

codeine (ko'de-ĭn). USP. An alkaloid obtained from opium.

   ACTION AND USES: Analgesic, hypnotic sedative with effects resembling morphine.

   DOSAGE: ¼ to 2 gr. (0.015-0.13 Gm.).

   c. phosphate. USP. Phosphate of the alkaloid codeine with a preference because of its free solubility in water. DOSAGE: Same as codeine.

   c. sulfate. USP. The sulfate of the alkaloid codeine. ACTION AND USES: Same as codeine. DOSAGE: Same as codeine.

Codivilla's extension (ko-di-vil'lă). One for fractures made by weight pulling on a nail passed through the lower end of the bone.

cod-liver oil (oleum morrhuae). USP. A fixed oil obtained from the fresh livers of the cod fish. The official oil is standardized for its vitamin A and D content.

   DOSAGE: 2½ drams (10 cc.).

coefficient (ko-ef-fish'ent). A figure put before a chemical formula to express amt. or degree of normal change in a substance under stated conditions.

   c. of absorption. Volume of gas absorbed by a unit volume of a liquid at 0° C. and a pressure of 760 mm.

   c., Baumann's. Ratio of ethereal sulfates to all sulfates in urine.

   c., biological. Amt. of potential energy used by body at rest.

   c., Bouchard's. Ratio bet. amt. of urine and total solids of the urine.

   c., Falta's. Percentage of ingested sugar eliminated from the system.

   c., isotonic. Number showing the amt. of salt to be added to distilled water to prevent the destruction of erythrocytes when it is added to blood.

   c., lethal. Concentration of disinfectant that will kill bacteria in the shortest length of time at 20-25° C.

   c., urotoxic. Number showing toxicity of the urine: *i. e.,* amt. of toxic matter produced by 1 Kg. of the poison in 24 hours.

coen'zyme. Enzyme activators. SEE: *co-activity.*

coetaneous (ko-e-ta'ne-us). Having the same age or date.

coexcitation (ko-ek-sī-ta'shun). Simultaneous excitation of 2 parts or bodies.

coferment (ko-fer'ment). A coenzyme.

coffee-ground vomit. Vomit similar to coffee in pigment and consistency, occurring in cancer of the stomach.

coffeurin (kof-e-u'rin). A principle said to exist in urine after excess use of coffee.

cogni'tion. Awareness, having perception and memory.

cog'wheel respira'tion. A sudden, brief halt in inspiration and expiration.

coherent (kō-hēr'ĕnt). 1. Sticking together, as parts of bodies or fluids. 2. Consistent; making a logical whole.

cohe'sion. The property of adhering.

cohe'sive. Adhesive; sticky.

Cohnheim's theory (kŏn'hīmz). Theory that tumors result from embryonal cells not utilized for fetal development.

coil. 1. A spiral formed by winding some substance. 2. A coil of wire for passage of electric impulses.

   c., Bris'tow. Small, portable faradic coil operated on 2 dry cells and the simple device of an iron core sliding in and out of the primary coil which allows a flexible regulation of the secondary current. It is used for muscle stimulation in weak but not paralyzed muscles.

   c., choke. Coil of wire which may or may not be provided with a movable laminated iron core, used to limit the flow of current in alternating current circuits. An electrical device using the inductive properties of the alternating current to limit or retard the current entering or leaving an apparatus.

   c., faradic. Device for the production of an induced current from a direct current source. Its essential parts are (1) a primary coil consisting of a few turns of insulated thick wire around a soft iron core, (2) a secondary coil consisting of many turns of insulated fine wire, (3) an interrupting device.

   c., gland. Sweat gland.

   c., induction. Large faradic coil.

c., Oudin (oo-dan'). A coil of fine wire with a large number of turns which increases voltage to such an extent that when the high frequency machine runs at full power there will be a corona discharge to the air from the Oudin (monoterminal) outlet.

c., primary. SEE: *faradic coil.*

c., Ruhmkorff (rŭm'korf). An apparatus consisting of 2 insulated coils, the primary made up of a few turns of coarse wire, the secondary consisting of many turns of fine wire, enclosing a core of soft iron wires. The primary coil is connected with current supply and an interrupter. Induction coil in which secondary coil is not movable but is fixed at point of maximum intensity.

c., secondary. SEE: *faradic coil or high frequency.*

a., spark. Specially designed faradic coil for graduated muscular contraction by electrical muscle stimulation.

c., Tesla. Coil in a modern diathermy apparatus magnetically coupled to the first coil, and the 2 together are known as the resonator.

coiled posture. A natural position with some, but esp. assumed in cerebral diseases, in hepatic, intestinal, or renal colic.

coilonychia (koy-lo-nik'ĭ-ă). Nails that have a concave outer surface.

coin counting. A sliding movement of tips of thumb and index finger over each other in paralysis agitans.

c. test. A metal-like sound heard in pneumothorax. SYN: *bell metal resonance, q.v.*

coital (ko'ĭ-tal). Pert. to coition.

coition (ko-ish'un). Cohabitation. Sexual intercourse* bet. man and woman. *Copulation, coitus, concubitus, q.v.*

coitophobia (ko-i-to-fo'bĭ-ă). Morbid fear of the sexual act.

coitus (ko'ĭ-tus). Coition, copulation, *q.v.* Sexual intercourse bet. man and woman.

c., à la vache. Coitus with woman in knee-chest position.

c. interrup'tus. Withdrawal of the penis from the vagina before the seminal emission occurs.

c. reservatus. 1. Same as *coitus interruptus.* 2. Onanism.*

colal'gia. Pain in the colon.

colation (ko-la'shun). Straining, filtering.

colauxe (kol-awks'e). Distention of the colon.

colchicum (kol'chik-um). Colchicum seed, USP. The seed of a plant of the same name.

DOSAGE: From 10 to 30 ℳ (0.6-1.8 cc.).

cold. 1. A catarrhal affection of the respiratory mucous membranes known as the common cold. 2. The opposite of heat, *q.v.*

c., asphyxia. Place body in cold room, rub with snow or ice water, use artificial respiration. SEE: *artificial respiration, asphyxia from cold, respiration.*

c., chest. Bronchitis.* Inflammation of the bronchial mucous membranes.

c. cream. USP. White flavored ointment used mainly as a cosmetic and for chapped skin, minor excoriations of the face, and herpes labialis.

c., head. Coryza,* rhinitis.* Acute catarrhal inflammation of the nasal mucous membranes.

c. pack. Used to reduce temperature.

c. sore. Fever blister. Eruption of vesicles on an inflammatory base. SEE: *herpes.*

colectomy (ko-lek'to-mĭ). Excision of part of the colon.

coleocele (ko'le-o-sēl). A vaginal hernia.

coleocystitis (ko-le-o-sĭs-ti'tĭs). Inflammation of the vagina and bladder.

coleot'omy. Incision into the pericardium or into the vagina.

colibacellemia (ko-lĭ-bas-ĭl-le'mĭ-ă). Colon bacillus in the blood.

colibacillo'sis. Infection with the colon bacillus.

colibacilluria (ko-lĭ-bas-ĭl-u'rĭ-ă). Colon bacillus in the urine.

colibacil'lus. The *Bacillus coli.*

colic (kol'ik). 1. Spasm in any hollow or tubular soft organ accompanied with pain. 2. Pert. to the colon.

SEE: *cholecystalgia, tormina.*

c., biliary. In bile ducts usually associated with a gallstone.

c., infantile. Occurring in infants, principally first few months. SYM: Extremities cold, abdomen distended and hard.

c., intestinal. Pain may occur throughout the abdomen and is frequently due to errors of diet.

c., lead. Associated with lead poisoning, occupational, painters, etc. Severe abdominal colic.

c., menstrual. Abdominal pain during menses due to some uterine disorder.

c., renal. In region of one of the kidneys and toward the thigh.

c., uterine. Painful menstruation. SYN: *dysmenorrhea.*

col'ica. 1. Abdominal colic. 2. Colic artery.

c. pictonum. Painter's colic.

c. scortorum. Abdominal pain in prostitutes.

colicoli'tis. Colon inflammation due to *Bacillus coli.*

colicople'gia. Lead poisoning with colic and lead paralysis.

colicystitis (ko"lĭ-sis-ti'tĭs). Inflammation of bladder. ETIOL: *Bacillus coli.*

colicystopyelitis (ko"lĭ-sis"to-pi-ē-li'tis). Inflammation of bladder and pelvis of kidney. ETIOL: *Bacillus coli.*

col'iform. 1. Sieve form; cribriform. 2. Pert. to microörganisms resembling the *Bacillus coli communis.*

co'li infection. Infection with *Bacillus coli communis.*

colilysin (ko-lil'ĭ-sin). A hemolysin formed by *Bacillus coli communis.*

colinephri'tis. Nephritis caused by the colon bacillus.

coliplication (ko-lĭ-pli-ka'shun). Operation for correcting a dilated colon.

colipuncture (ko-lĭ-punk'tŭr). Puncture

of the colon to relieve distention. SYN: *colocentesis.*

colipyuria (ko-lĭ-pī-u′rĭ-ă). Pus in urine due to *Bacillus coli.*

colisep′sis. Infection caused by the colon bacillus.

coli′tis. Inflammation of the colon.

    c., mucous. Colitis accompanied by large quantities of mucus. More common in women than in men and among nervous types. A secretory neurosis of the large intestine.

    c., ulcerative. Ulceration of inner lining of colon with dilatation.

colitoxemia (ko-lĭ-toks-e′mĭ-ă). Toxemia caused by the colon bacillus.

colitoxico′sis. Systemic poisoning caused by the colon bacillus.

colitox′in. A toxin generated by the colon bacillus.

coliuria (ko-lĭ-u′rĭ-ă). Presence of *Bacillus coli* in the urine. SYN: *colibacilluria.*

collagen (kol′aj-en). 1. A substance existing in the various tissues of the body, as in the white fibers of connective tissue. 2. A protein which can be prepared from connective tissue (tendons, etc.) and from which gelatin can be made.

collapse′. 1. An abnormal retraction of the walls of an organ. 2. A sudden failure of vital power due to reflex inhibition of the heart and respiratory system, or to loss of blood, low metabolism, or undue lowering of the blood pressure.

    c. of lung. Artificially induced by: (a) Artificial pneumothorax; (b) thoracoplasty, or (c) avulsion of phrenic nerve.

collap′sing. Falling into extreme and sudden prostration resembling shock.

    c. pulse. Pulse of aortic insufficiency or regurgitation; water-hammer pulse. SYN: *Corrigan's pulse.*

collapsother′apy. Treatment of pulmonary affections by unilateral pneumothorax and immobilization of affected lung.

collar (kol′ar). 1. A band worn round the neck. 2. Structure or marking formed like a neckband.

    c. of Venus, c., venereal. Mottled appearance of the skin of the neck occasionally seen in syphilis. SYN: *melanoleukoderma colli.*

col′larbone. The clavicle, *q.v.* SEE: *jugulum.*

collat′eral. 1. Accompanying, as side by side. 2. Subordinate or secondary. 3. Not related lineally. 4. An accessory nerve or blood vessel.

    c. circulation. That of small anastomosing vessels, esp. when a main artery is obstructed.

collat′erals. Minute side branches of processes of axone or axis cylinder processes.

collect′ing plates. The electronegative element of a galvanic battery.

    c. tubes. Ducts directly discharging into the calices or uriniferous tubules of the kidney.

collemia (kol-e′mĭ-ă). A colloidal form

of matter in the blood causing capillary obstruction.

Colles' fascia (kol′ez). Inner layer of superficial fascia of perineum.

    C.'s fracture. The transverse fracture of the distal end of radius (just above wrist) with displacement of hand backward and outward.

    C.'s law. A theory, long accepted (since the advent of the Wassermann test), that a syphilitic child may be born of a mother who is not affected by the nursing child who may affect others. Later in life it has been demonstrated that the mother may show signs of late tertiary syphilis, although her Wassermann was negative at the birth of child.

colliculectomy (kol-lik″u-lek′to-mĭ). Removal of the *colliculus seminalis.*

colliculi′tis. Inflammation of the *colliculus seminalis.*

collic′ulus. A little eminence.

    c. anteriores. The ant. corpora quadrigemina.

    c. bulbi, c. bulbi intermedius. Erectile tissue encircling the male urethra at the entrance to the bulb.

    c. cervicalis. Fold of mucous membrane extending posteriorly from the apex of the trigone of the bladder.

    c. facialis. Flat, thickened part of the eminentia medialis.

    c. glandis. Two protrusions on the lower portion of the corona of the glans penis, connected by the frenum.

    c. inferiores. The inferior corpora quadrigemina.

    c. posteriores. The post. corpora quadrigemina.

    c. rotundus anterior. Ant. division of the corpora quadrigemina.

    c. rotundus posterior. Post. division of the corpora quadrigemina.

    c. seminalis. The verumontanum. Eminence on male urethral floor, in front of the prostate.

    c. superiores. The ant. corpora quadrigemina.

    c. urethralis. Colliculus seminalis.

col′lier's lung. Pulmonary disease due to inhalation of coal dust. SYN: *anthracosis.*

Colling's elec′trotome. Apparatus for using cutting current to relieve fibrous obstruction of neck of bladder in prostatic hypertrophy by endovesical or transurethral operation.

Collip unit. Dosage unit of parathyroid extract. One-one hundredth of the quantity necessary to increase by 5 mg. the amount of calcium in 100 cc. of blood after 15 hours in a dog weighing 20 Kg.

colliquation (kol-ĭ-kwa′shun). 1. Abnormal discharge of a body fluid. 2. Softening of tissue due to liquefaction. 3. A wasting.

colliquative (ko-lik′wă-tiv). Pert. to a liquid and excessive discharge, as a *colliquative diarrhea.*

collo′dium, collo′dion. Preparation intended for external use (protective for surgical dressings), having for its base a solution of pyroxylin or gun cotton, in a mixture of ether and alcohol. Two are official.

c., flexible. USP. A more elastic preparation of collodium, containing camphor and castor oil.

colloid (kol'oid). 1. Gelatinous; like glue; opposite of crystalloid.* 2. A particle invisible to the naked eye, which, instead of dissolving, is held in a state of suspension. 3. Gelatinous substance developing in colloid degeneration and carcinoma. Colloids are insoluble, incapable of crystallization, and not diffusible through animal membranes.
SEE: *biocolloid, solutions, suspension.*

c. cancer. One in which the tumor cells have a gluelike appearance.

c. chemistry. This deals with such systems and substances, and with the problems of emulsions, mists, foams, and suspensions.

c. cyst. A sac containing a jellylike liquid.

c. degeneration. A mucoid degeneration seen in the protoplasm of epithelial cells.

c. milium. Colloid degeneration of the skin.

c., suspension. A mixture holding particles in suspension, the forms of which change with the forces acting upon them, such as milk, fat, etc.

colloidal (kol-loyd'ăl). Pert. to a colloid.

colloidin (kol-loi'din). A jellylike substance seen in colloid degeneration.

colloidoclasia (kol-oid-o-kla'sĭ-ă). A rupture of the colloid equilibrium of the body.

colloidopexy (kol-oid'o-pek-sĭ). Fixation of colloids during metabolism.

collo'ma. 1. A colloid degeneration of a cancer. 2. A cyst containing a gelatinous substance.

collonema (kol-o-ne'mă). Tumor of mucoid tissue. SYN: *myxoma, myxosarcoma.*

collopexia (kol-o-peks'ĭ-ă). Fixation of the *cervix uteri.*

col'lum. 1. The necklike part of an organ. 2. The neck.

collutory (kol'lu-to-rĭ). A gargle or mouthwash.

collyrium (kol-lir'ĭ-um). An eyewash.

colnocyte (kol'no-sīt). A multinucleated cell. Many nuclei in 1 mass of protoplasm with a cellular wall.

colobo'ma. A congenital fissure of the choroid iris, or eyelids.

colocentesis (ko-lo-sen-te'sis). Surgical puncture of the colon to relieve distention.

colocholecystostomy (ko-lo-kol-e-sis-tos'-to-mĭ). Surgical formation of a communication bet. colon and gallbladder. SYN: *cholecystocolostomy.*

colocleisis (ko-lo-kli'sis). Occlusion of the colon.

coloclysis (ko-lok'li-sis). A colonic enema.

coloclyster (ko-lo-klis'ter). A colonic enema.

colocolostomy (ko-lo-kol-os'to-mĭ). For-

mation of a connection bet. 2 portions of the colon.

colocynth (kol'o-sinth). USP. Dried pulp of unripe colocynth fruit.
ACTION AND USES: A drastic hydragogue cathartic.
DOSAGE: 1-5 gr. (0.065-0.32 Gm.).

coloenteritis (ko-lo-en-ter-i'tis). Inflammation of mucous membrane of small and large intestines.

colofixa'tion. Surgical suspension of the colon in ptosis.

co'lon. The large intestine from the cecum to the rectum, 4 to 6 feet long, and divided into the *ascending,* the *transverse,* and the *descending colon.*

c. bacteria. *Bacillus coli communis* is the most commonly found.

colonalgia (ko-lon-al'ji-a). Pain in the colon; colic.

colonic (ko-lon'ik). Pert. to the colon.

c. irrigation. Injection into the colon of a large amt. of fluid which is intended to fill colon and flush it.

colonitis (ko-lon-i'tis). Inflammation of the colon. SYN: *colitis.*

colonom'eter. Device for estimating colonies of bacteria on a culture plate.

colonopexy (ko'lon-o-pek-sĭ). Process of attaching part of colon to abdominal wall. SYN: *colopexy.*

colonorrhagia (ko"lon-or-ra'jĭ-ă). Hemorrhage from the colon.

colonorrhea (ko"lon-or-re'ă). Mucous colitis.

colonoscope (ko-lon'o-skōp). Instrument for examination of the colon.

colonos'copy. Examination of upper portion of rectum with an elongated speculum.

col'ony. A collection of microörganisms in a culture.

colopexos'tomy. Resection of the colon and fixation to abdominal wall to establish an artificial anus.

colopexotomy (ko-lo-peks-ot'o-mĭ). Incision and fixation of colon.

colopexy, colopexia (ko'lo-pek-sĭ, ko-lo-peks'ĭ-ă). Fixation of the sigmoid or cecum to the abdominal wall by suture.

coloplication (ko-lo-pli-ka'shun). Making a fold in the colon to reduce its lumen.

coloprocti'tis. Colonic and rectal inflammation.

coloproctostomy (ko-lo-prok-tos'to-mĭ). Making a communication bet. a segment of colon and the rectum.

coloptosia (ko-lop-to'sĭ-ă). Prolapsus of the colon, esp. of the transverse colon.

coloptosis (ko-lop-to'sis). A downward displacement of the colon.

colopuncture (ko'lo-punk-chur). Puncturing the colon.

col'or. A visible quality, distinct from form, and light and shade.

c. blindness. Inability to identify 1 or more of the primary colors. Daltonism.

c. hearing. A sense of color caused by a sound.

c. index. The hemoglobin content of red blood cells compared with the normal, found by dividing the percentage of hemoglobin by that of erythrocytes.*

colorectitis (ko-lo-rek-ti'tis). Inflammation of colon and rectum. SYN: *coloproctitis.*

colorectostomy (ko-lo-rek-tos'to-mĭ). Formation of passage bet. colon and rectum.

colorim'eter. Instrument for measuring amt. of pigments.

colostomy (ko-los'to-mĭ). Incision of the colon for purpose of making a more or less permanent fistula in treatment of carcinomatous stenosis of lower portion of colon, and in cases of inoperable carcinoma of rectum.
   c. diet. A low residue diet.*
   c., inguinal. Incision of colon to form artificial anus.

colostra'tion. Infant diarrhea assumed to be caused by colostrum.

colostrorrhea. (ko-los-tror-re'ă). Abnormal secretion of colostrum.

colos'trum. Secretion from the lactiferous glands before the onset of true lactation 2 or 3 days after delivery.

colotomy (ko-lot'o-mĭ). Incision of colon. SEE: *Callisen's operation.*

coloty'phoid. Typhoid fever with ulceration of colon.

colpalgia (kol-pal'jĭ-ă). Vaginal pain.

colpatresia (kol-pat-re'zĭ-ă). Occlusion or pathological closure of the vagina.

colpectasia (kol-pek-ta'sĭ-ă). Dilatation of the vagina. [gina.

colpec'tomy. Cutting out part of the va-

colpeurynter (kol-pu-rin'ter). A bag for dilatation of the vagina sometimes used instead of the intracervical hydrostatic bag for the induction of labor.

colpeurysis (kol-pu'ris-is). Enlarging of the vagina by surgery.

colpitis (kol-pi'tis). Vaginitis. Inflammation of the vagina.
   c. emphysematosa. Air bleb formation in the vagina as seen in *B. welchii* infection.
   c. mycotica. That due to the presence of yeasts and molds.
   c. senilis. That accompanied by atrophy of the mucous membrane with the formation of highly vascular papillae. Seen in elderly women who have passed the menopause.
   c., trichomonas. That due to the *Trichomonas vaginalis.* Characterized by punctate hemorrhagic spots in the vagina and a frothy yellowish leukorrhea.

colpocele (kol'po-sēl). Hernia into the vagina.

colpoceliotomy (kol'po-se-lĭ-ot'o-mĭ). Entering the abdomen surgically through the vagina.

colpocleisis (kol-po-kli'sis). Operation of occluding the vagina.

colpocystitis (kol-po-sis-ti'tis). Inflammation of vagina and bladder.

colpocystocele (kol-po-sis'to-sēl). Prolapse of the bladder into the vagina.

colpocys'toplasty. Treatment of vesico-vaginal fistula.

colpocystosyrinx (kol''po-sis-to-sir'inks). Fistula bet. bladder and vagina.

colpocystotomy (kol-po-sis-tot'o-mĭ). Cutting into the bladder through the vagina.

colpocystoureterocystotomy (kcl''po-sis''-to-u-re''ter-o-sis-tot'o-mĭ). Incision into the ureter through the walls of the bladder and vagina.

colpodesmorrhaphia (kol-po-des-mor-a'-fĭ-ă). Repair of the vaginal sphincter.

colpodynia (kol-po-din'ĭ-ă). Pain in the vagina. SYN: *colpalgia.*

colpohyperplasia (kol-po-hi-per-pla'zĭ-ă). Excessive growth of mucous membrane of the vagina.
   c. cystica. Infectious inflammation of the vaginal walls which is characterized by the production of small blebs.

colpo''hysterec'tomy. Removal of the uterus through the vagina.

colpohysteropexy (kol-po-his'ter-o-pek-sĭ). Fixation of uterus through the vagina.

colpohysterot'omy. Incision through the vagina into the uterus, as for excision of a fibroma.

colpomyomectomy (kol-po-mi-o-mek'to-mĭ). Removal of a fibroid tumor of the uterus through the vagina.

colpomyomotomy (-mot'o-mĭ). Incision of uterus through the vagina for removal of tumor.

colpopathy (kol-pop'ă-thĭ). Any pathology of the vagina.

colpoperineoplasty (kol-po-per-ĭn-ē'o-plas-tĭ). Plastic operation on vagina and perineum.

colpoperineorrhaphy (kol-po-per-in''e-or'-raf-ĭ). Operation for mending perineal tears in vagina. SYN: *colpoperineoplasty.*

col'popexy. Suture of a relaxed and prolapsed vagina to the abdominal wall.

colpoplasty (kol'po-plas-tĭ). Plastic operation upon vagina.

colpoptosis (kol-pop-to'sis). Prolapse of the vagina.

colporrhagia (kol-po-ra'jĭ-ă). Excessive vaginal discharge. Vaginal hemorrhage.

colporrhaphy (kol-por'ă-fĭ). Suture of vagina.

colporrhexis (kol-por-reks'is). Operative repair of defective vaginal floor.

colposcope (kol'po-skōp). An instrument for examining the fornices of the vagina and *cervix uteri.*

col'pospasm, colpospas'mus. Spasm of the vagina. SYN: *vaginismus.*

col'postat. Device for holding a radium applicator in the vagina.

colpostenosis (kol-po-sten-o'sis). Stenosis or narrowing of the vagina.

colpostenotomy (kol-po-sten-ot'o-mĭ). A cutting operation for dilating the lumen in stricture of the vagina.

colpotherm (kol'po-thurm). Electrical device introduced into the vagina to convey heat. [the vagina.

colpotomy (kol-pot'o-mĭ). An incision of

colpoureterocystotomy (kol-po-u-re''ter-o-sis-tot'o-mĭ). Exposure of the ureteral orifices by incision through the walls of the vagina and bladder.

colpoureterot'omy. Incision of the ureter through the vagina.

colpoxerosis (kol-po-ze-rō'sis). Abnormal dryness of the vulva and vagina.

columella (kol-ŭ-mel'lă). 1. A column. 2. BACT: Portion of the sporangiophore upon which are borne the spores.

    c. na'si. The ant. part of the septum of nose; *concha nasalis,* a turbinate bone.

column (kol'um). A supporting anatomical part resembling a cylinder.

    c., anterior. Ant. portion of gray columns on either side of the spinal column.

    c. of Clarke. A group of column cells in the cervix of the post. gray column of the spinal cord.

    c., direct cerebellar. A bandlike tract of ascending white fibers immediately in front of the line of entrance of the post. nerve roots on the posterolateral surface of the spinal cord.

    c. of Goll. Inner division of the white column of the spinal cord; contains sensory fibers.

    c. of Gowers. Tract of ascending fibers ant. to the direct cerebellar column, and on the lateral surface of the spinal cord.

    c., lateral. Lateral white column of the spinal cord bet. lines of entrance and exit of ant. and post. nerve roots.

    c. of Morgagni. One of several vertical ridges in mucous membrane at junction of anus and rectum.

    c., posterior. Post. portion of gray columns of spinal cord. [of Clarke.

    c., posterovesicular. Same as column

    c., respiratory. Longitudinal fibrous bundle starting at upper portion of medulla and running down to the 4th cervical nerve.

    c., Sertoli's. A columnar figure in testicle formed by collections of Sertoli's cells.

    c., spinal. The line of vertebrae from the head to the pelvis, making up the bony flexible case for the spinal cord.

    c. of Turck. A subdivision of the white column of the spinal cord.

    c., vesicular. Line of ganglion cells on inner side of post. column.

columna (ko-lum'na) (pl. *columnae*). A column or pillar.

    c. adiposa. Fat column.

    c. bertini. Interpyramidal extension or renal column supporting renal blood vessels.

    c. carnea. A muscular projection within the cardiac ventricles.

    c. nasi. Nasal septum.

    c. rugarum vaginae. Fold of mucous membrane of the vagina which is arranged in a columnar fashion.

colum'nar layer. Retinal rod-and-cone layer.

columning (kol'um-ing). Introduction of tampons in vagina to support the prolapsed uterus.

colyone (ko'lĭ-ōn). An autacoid which inhibits hormone or cellular activity. SYN: *chalone.*

colypeptic (ko-lĭ-pep'tĭk). Slowing up digestive processes.

colyphrenia (kol-ĭ-fre'nĭ-ă). Abnormal tendency to mental inhibition.

colyseptic (ko-lĭ-sep'tĭk). Antiseptic.

colytic (ko-lit'ĭk). Inhibitory.

co'ma. An abnormal deep stupor occurring in illness, or as a result of it, or it may be due to an injury. The patient cannot be aroused by external stimuli.

    c., alcoholic. Due to alcohol.

    c., apoplectic. Due to cerebral hemorrhage or apoplexy; one side of body, or the extremities, 1 or more, will be paralyzed.

    c., diabetic. Occurring in diabetes, due to presence of diacetic acid in system and to acidosis. Paralysis not present.

    c., uremic. The result of disturbed kidney metabolism, causing autointoxication through the retention of unknown substances in the blood and producing acidosis.

    c. vigil. Delirious lethargy with open eyes and partial consciousness.

co'matose. In a condition of coma.

comedo (kom'e-do) (pl. *comedon'es*). Blackhead; fleshworm. Discolored dried sebum plugging an excretory duct of the skin.

comes (ko'mēz) (pl. *com'ites*). A blood vessel which accompanies a nerve or another blood vessel.

com'ma bacillus. *Spirillum cholerae asiaticae.*

com'ma tract. A longitudinal bundle of descending fibers in the *fasciculus cuneatus* of the spinal cord. Schultze's bundle.

commen'sal. Pert. to a nonparasitic organism living on or within another.

comminute (kom'in-ūt). To break into pieces.

com'minuted fracture. A crushed bone.

comminution (kom-in-u'shun). Reducing a solid body to varying sizes by grating, pulverizing, slicing, granulating, and by other processes. SEE: *attenuation, dynamization.* [missure.

commissu'ra (pl. *commissurae*). A com-

    c. anterior alba. A narrow band of white substance near ant. median fissure of the spinal cord.

    c. anterior cerebri. White bundle crossing from side to side in the ant. wall of the 3rd ventricle.

    c. anterior grisea. Part of gray commissure in front of and bet. the *commissura anterior alba.*

    c. brevis. Post. portion of inferior cerebellar vermiform process.

    c. hippocampi. A little triangular space bet. the diverging crura of the fornix.

    c. magna. Corpus callosum.*

    c. simplex. Lobule on superior vermiform process of the cerebellum.

    c. superior. A large, transverse, fibrous tract in superior portion of the tuber cinereum.

commissu'ral. Pert. to a commissure.

commissure (kom'ĭ-shūr). Meeting point or fibrous band bet. two parts.

common bile duct. Duct carrying bile to the duodenum and receiving it from the cystic and hepatic ducts. SYN: *ductus choledochus.* SEE: *bile.*

commu'nicable disease. A disease which may be carried directly or indirectly from one individual to another.

commu'nicans. One of a number of communicating nerves.

  c. hypoglossi. Twelfth cranial nerve.

  c. peronei. Fibular connecting nerve.

  c. poplitei. Lateral sural cutaneous nerve.

  c. Willisii. Post. and ant. communicating cerebral arteries making up part of *circulus Willisii.*

com'mutator. A device for reversing the direction of an electric current; usually a segmental ring attached to a dynamo on which brushes slide. Also similar hand operated devices.

Comolli's sign (ko-mol'lĭs). A triangular swelling corresponding to the outline of the scapula when fractured.

comose (ko'mōs). Hairy. Having much hair.

compact'. Dense, packed, solid.

  c. tissue. The external, hard portion of bone.

compar'ative anat'omy. Human anatomy compared with that of animals.

compatibil'ity. State of suitability to be mixed or taken together without unfavorable results, as drugs.

compat'ible. Not opposed to; able to mix with another substance without destructive changes.

com'pensating. Making up for a deficiency.

  c. operation. Tenotomy of the associated antagonists in diplopia.

compensa'tion. Making up for a defect, as cardiac circulation competent to meet demands made upon it, regardless of valvular defect.

com'plement. A substance or body producing bacteriolysis or hemolysis which, by means of an amboceptor, is connected with a bacterial or animal cell.

  c. unit. Smallest quantity of complement required for hemolysis of a given amount of red blood corpuscles with 1 amboceptor unit present.

complement'al, complement'ary. Supplying something that is lacking.

  c. air. Amt. of air (1600 cc. or 3 pt.) that can be inspired over and above the tidal air by the deepest inspiration. SEE: *air.*

  c. colors. Any 2 primary colors which, when blended, produce white light.

complemen'toid. A complement, the lysis-causing power of which has been destroyed.

complementophil (kom-ple-ment'o-fil). Having the power to combine with a complement.

com'plex. 1. PSY: A subconscious idea (or group of ideas) which have become associated with a repressed wish or emotional experience and which may influence behavior although the person may not have any appreciation of the connection between the repressed desire and his thoughts or actions. 2. All the ideas, feelings, and sensations connected with a subject. 3. Intricate.

  c., castration. Morbid fear of being castrated.

  c., inferiority. A repressed state of mind in which one feels himself inferior to others.

  c., superiority. Exaggerated conviction of one's own superiority; also pretense of being superior to compensate for a supposed inferiority.

complex'us. The total indications or phenomena of a morbid state.

complica'tion. An added difficulty; a complex state.

com'pos men'tis. Of sound mind; sane.

com'pound. 1. Any substance composed of definite proportions of 2 or more elements so combined as to not exhibit only by chemical change. 2. Not simple, composed of 2 or more parts.

  c. astigmatism. Myopia of both vertical and horizontal meridians.

  c. cathartic pills. Ones composed of calomel, colocynth, gamboge, and jalap.

  c. fracture. One having an open wound into seat of fracture.

  c., inorganic. One of many compounds which, in general, contain no carbon.

  c. microscope. One consisting of 2 or more lenses.

  c., organic. One of many compounds containing carbon and usually found in carbohydrates, proteins, and fats.

compress (kom'pres). 1. Cloth, wet or dry, folded and applied firmly to a part to prevent hemorrhage or to relieve inflammation; made of cotton, oakum, marine lint, jute, etc. 2. (kŏm-prĕs'). To press together into smaller space. 3. To close by squeezing together, as a wound.

  c., abdominal. Three folds of linen reaching from sternum to pubis, overlapping sides of abdomen, wrung out of the water at 70° F., held in place by flannel binder little wider than linen, long enough to reach around the body.

  c., chest. Application of 2 pieces of old linen of sufficient size to fit the entire chest from the clavicles down to the umbilicus, wrung out of water at 60° F., and covered with flannel.

  c., cold. Linen cloth, several layers dipped in cold water, slightly wrung out, applied to given part. To secure constant temperature, compress is frequently renewed, ice bag or aluminum coil through which ice water is circulating is placed on it. Duration, 30-60 minutes.

  c., forehead. A soft towel wrung out of water below 60° F. renewed at least every 2 minutes.

  c., hot. Linen cloth folded into several layers, dipped in hot water (107-115° F.) slightly wrung out and placed on part to be treated, covered with a piece of flannel, large enough to overlap the linen slightly. Temperature is maintained at constant level by renewing compress or by coil through which hot water (107-115° F.) is circulating.

c., neck. Application of a soft towel wrung out of water bet. 42-60° F.

c., precordial. Pad of 4 layers of linen cloth, moistened in water 60-65° F., is applied over the heart region. On this is placed a coil through which water at 60-65° F. is circulating. This water temperature is reduced until ice water is used. Duration, 10-45 minutes. Twice daily.

c., Priessnitz. Cold wet compress.

c., spinal. Usually the application of a soft cloth wrung out of ice water, renewed every 2-3 minutes. Applied to cervical region for meningitis, cerebral congestion, and nervous asthenia; dorsal region for hysterical vomiting; and to lumbar region for renal and uterine hemorrhage.

c., throat. Application of 2 strips of linen 3 inches wide and long enough to reach from beneath 1 ear under the chin to the opposite ear, wrung out of water at 60° F., a piece of flannel ¼ inch wider covers it and overlaps at top of head.

c., trunk. Consists of 3 folds of linen from axilla to pubis and reaching around the trunk, wrung out of water 60-75° F., covering with flannel bandage secured by pins. Changed every hour.

c., wet. Application of 2 or more folds of old linen wrung out of water at prescribed temperatures and covered with flannel.

compres'sion. A squeezing together; state of being pressed together.

c. atrophy. That in a part due to steady compression.

c. of the brain. Same as cerebral compression, q.v.

c., cerebral. Pressure on the brain produced by increased intercranial fluids, embolism, thrombosis, tumors, and skull fractures. More serious than concussion.* [means of the fingers.

c., digital. Arterial compression by

c., myelitis. That due to pressure on the spinal cord, often due to a tumor.

compres'sor. 1. Instrument for making pressure on a part. 2. Contraction of a muscle, causing compression of another structure.

compul'sion. Act performed to relieve fear connected with obsession; dictation by the patient's subconscious, arising against the subject's wishes and, if denied, causing uneasiness. Impulsive actions, on the contrary, often seem to express the personality.

c. neurosis. Obsession or psychoneurosis urging one to perform an absurd act or to say something silly.

compul'sive. Exercising or applying compulsion.

c. ideas. PSY: An idea that continues to suggest against one's will the commitment of an overt act, such as murder or suicide.

compul'sory. Compelling action against one's will.

c. movements. Movements caused by injury to a nerve center.

con-. Prefix: Together with, as congenital.

conarium (ko-na'rĭ-um). The pineal gland. Corpus pineale (BNA).

conation (ko-na'shun). Any desire or impulse compelling action.

concassation (kon-kas-a'shun). 1. Shaking of a precipitate in a bottle or pulverizing by beating. 2. Mental distress.

Concato's disease (kon-kä'tōs). Progressive inflammation of serous membranes. ETIOL: Tuberculosis.

concave (kon'kāv). Having a spherically depressed or hollow surface.

concav'ity. A hollowed surface, with curved, bowl-like sides.

conca"vocon'cave. Concave on opposing sides.

concavocon'vex. Concave on 1 side and convex on opp. surface.

concentration (kon-sen-tra'shun). 1. Increase in strength of a fluid by evaporation. 2. Medicine strengthened by evaporation. 3. Fixation of mind on 1 subject to exclusion of all other thoughts.

con'cept. An idea.

concep'tion. The union of the male sperm and the ovum of the female.

concha (kong'kä). 1. The outer ear or the pinna. 2. The inferior turbinated bone.

c. auriculae. Floor of the auricle.

c. bullosa. Turbinated bone expansion, during chronic rhinitis.

c. nasalis inferior. Inferior turbinated bone.

c. nasalis media. Middle turbinated bone.

c. nasalis superior. Superior turbinated bone.

c. nasalis suprema. Supreme or highest turbinated bone.

c. Santorini. Concha nasalis suprema.

c. sphenoidalis. Roof of the nasal cavities.

conchitis (kong-ki'tis). Inflammation of any concha.

conchoidal (kong-koi'dal). Having the shape of a shell.

conchoscope (kong'ko-scōp). Instrument for examination of the nasal cavity.

conchotome (kong'ko-tōm). Device for excision of middle turbinated bone.

concoc'tion. The boiling of 2 or more substances together.

concom'itant. Accessory; taking place at the same time.

concrescence (kon-kres'ens). The union of separate parts; coalescence.

concrete (kon'krēt). Condensed, hardened, or solidified.

concre'tion. 1. A calculus. 2. Solidification of a fluid substance.

concub'itus. Copulation, coition, sexual intercourse.

concus'sion. "Shaking" from impaction against an object.

c. of the brain. Cerebral concussion. A common result of a blow to the head. or fall on the end of spine with transmitted force, usually causing uncon-sciousness, either temporary or pro-longed.

c. of labyrinth. Deafness resulting from a blow to the head or ear.

c., spinal. Lesion of spinal cord due to injury or jarring.

condensa´tion. 1. Making more solid. 2. Changing a liquid to a solid or a gas to a liquid. 3. PSY: The union of ideas to form a new mental pattern.

CHEM: A type of reaction in which 2 or more molecules of the same substance react with each other and form a new substance with higher molecular weight and different chemical properties.

conden´ser. Device for solidifying vapors and liquids. SEE: *capacitor.*

c., electrical. Device for storing of electricity by using 2 conducting sur-faces and a nonconductor.

con´diment. Appetizing ingredient added to food.

CLASSIFICATION: 1. *Aromatic:* Vanilla, cinnamon, cloves, chervil, parsley, bay leaf, etc. 2. *Acrid or Peppery:* Pepper, ginger, allspice, etc. 3. *Alliaceous or Al-lylic:* Onion, mustard, horseradish. 4. *Acid:* Vinegar, capers, gherkins, citron. 5. *Animal Origin:* Caviar, anchovies.

condi´tional reflex. An inherited reflex which is a physiological result of a non-specific stimulus that is automatic and instinctive, though commonly without the knowledge of the individual.

condi´tioned reflex. One acquired as result of training and repetition.

conduc´tance. The conducting ability of a body or a circuit for electricity.

conduc´tion. PHYS: The process whereby a state of excitation affects successive portions of a tissue or cell, so that the disturbance is transmitted to remote points.

c., bone. Sound conduction through cranial bones.

conductiv´ity. The specific electric con-ducting ability of a substance.

conductor (kon-duk´tor). 1. Medium trans-mitting a force. 2. A guide directing a surgical knife.

condylar (kon´dĭ-lăr). Pert. to a condyle.

condylarthrosis (kon-dĭl-ar-thro´sis). A form of diarthrosis;* an ovoid head in an elliptical cavity.

condyle, condylus (kon´dīl, -lus). A rounded protuberance at the end of a bone form-ing an articulation.

condylectomy (kon-dĭ-lek´to-mĭ). Excision of a condyle.

condylion (kon-dil´ĭ-on). Point on lateral (outer) surface of the mandibular con-dyle.

condyloid (kon´dĭ-loid). Pert. to or re-sembling a condyle.

c. process. *Capitulum mandibulae;* condyle.

condyloma (kŏn-dĭ-lō´mă). A wartlike growth of the skin, usually seen on the external genitalia or near the anus.

c. latum. A mucous patch on the vulva or anus, coated with gray exudate,

flattened in form, with delimited area, characteristic of syphilis.

condylomatous (kon-dĭ-lo´mat-us). Pert. to a condyloma.

condylotomy (kon-dĭ-lot´o-mĭ). Division without removal of a condyle.

cone (kōn). 1. A shape with circular base with sides sloping to a point above. 2. Retinal flask-shaped figure in layer of rods and cones.

c. of light. Triangular light areas on the membrana tympani extending down-ward from the umbo.

c. ocular. Cone of light in int. of eyeball.

confabula´tion. PSY: The relation of imag-inary experiences to fill in gaps in the memory.

confec´tio, confec´tion. Sugarlike soft solids in which 1 or more medicinal substances are incorporated with the object of affording an agreeable form for their administration and a con-venient method for their preservation.

confinement (kon-fīn´ment). The puer-peral state or period of childbirth.

con´flict. 1. Opposing action of incom-patibles. 2. PSY: The conscious or un-conscious struggle bet. two opposing de-sires or courses of action. A technical term applied to a state in which social goals dictate behavior contrary to more primitive (often subconscious) desires.

con´fluent. Running together, as when the pustules in smallpox merge.

conformator (kon´for-ma´´tor). Apparatus for establishing cranial outlines.

confrontation (kon-frun-ta´shun). The ex-amination of two patients together, one with a disease and the other from whom the disease was supposed to be contracted.

congelation (kon-je-la´shun). Freezing, or a frostbite.

congenerous (kon-jen´er-us). Possessing the same function, as synergistic mus-cles.

congen´ital. Occurring during fetal life; hereditary.

congested (kon-jes´ted). Hyperemic; con-taining an abnormal amt. of blood.

conges´tion. A localized inflammation which may or may not be accompanied by infection, such as a felon, a boil, a carbuncle. SEE: *affluxion, hyperemia.*

congestive (kon-jes´tiv). Pertaining to congestion.

c. fever. Malarial fever.

congius (kon´jĭ-us) (pl. *con´gii*). A gallon.

conglo´bate. In 1 mass, as lymph glands.

congloba´tion. Aggregation of particles in a mass.

conglom´erate. 1. An aggregation in one mass. 2. Clustered; heaped together.

c. gland. A gland with several lobes.

conglutin (kon-glu´tin). A protein resem-bling casein found in peas, beans, and almonds.

conglu´tinant. Promoting adhesion, as of the edges of a wound.

conglu´tinate. Having the quality of ad-hesiveness.

conglutination (kon-glu-tin-a'shun). 1. Coalescence, adhesion. 2. Reaction, such as agglutination.

coniasis (kon-i'ă-sis). Dustlike calculi in gallbladder and bile ducts.

conidia (ko-nid'ĭ-ă) (pl. of *conidium*). Asexual spores.

conidiophore (kon-id'ĭ-o-for). The stalk supporting conidia.

coniol'ogy. The study of dust and its effects.

conio'sis. Any condition caused by inhalation of dust.

coniza'tion. Coring and removal of the mucous lining of cervical canal and its glands by the cutting high frequency current for treatment of chronic endocervicitis.

conjuga'ta. Diameter of pelvis, measured from center of the promontory of the sacrum to the back of the symphysis pubis.

   c. vera. Sometimes written *c.v.* Same as conjugata, *q.v.*

conjugate (kon'jŭ-gāt). 1. Paired or joined. 2. An important diameter of the pelvis, measured from the center of the promontory of the sacrum to the back of the symphysis pubis.

   c. deviation. Deviation of both eyes to either side.

   c., diagonal. Measured from the lower edge of the symphysis to the sacrum, and can be determined during life, whereas the true conjugate cannot, except immediately after labor. It is about ½-¾ in. longer than the true conjugate, or about 5 in.

   c. diameter. Same as conjugate (2).

   c., external. Measured from the spine of the last lumbar vertebra to the front of the pubes (this can be done only with calipers), and is normally about 8 in.

   c., true. Same as conjugate (2). It should measure not less than 4¼ in. and is sometimes as large as 4½ or 4¾ in. If less than 4¼ in., the pelvis is a deformed one.

conjuga'tion. A sexual fusion of 2 cells having a partition of chromatin resulting in subsequent division into 2 cells.

   c., multiple. Conjugation of more than 2 similar cells.

   c. nucleus. Nucleus of a fertilized ovum.

conjuncti'va. Mucous membrane which lines eyelids and is reflected onto eyeball.

conjunctival reflex (kon-junk-ti'val). Closure of eyelids when conjunctiva is touched or threatened.

conjunctivitis (kon-junk-tĭ-vi'tis). Inflammation of conjunctiva.

   c., acute contagious. Pink eye. ETIOL: Koch-Weeks bacillus.

   c., catarrhal. One due to irritation or cold.

   c., follicular. Type characterized by pinkish round bodies in retrotarsal fold.

   c., gonorrheal. Acute conjunctivitis due to contact with the gonococcus.

   c., granular. Acute, contagious, inflammatory conjunctivitis with granular

elevations on the lids which ulcerate and cicatrize. SYN: *trachoma.*

   c., membranous. Acute conjunctivitis characterized by a false membrane; with or without infiltration.

   c., phlyctenular. Circumscribed type characterized by lymphoid tissue in small red nodules.

   c., purulent. That characterized by abundant purulent discharge. ETIOL: Gonorrhea. Ex: *Ophthalmia neonatorum.*

   c., vernal. One beginning in the spring and disappearing when cold weather begins.   [tiva.

conjunctivo'ma. A tumor of the conjunc-

conjunctivoplasty (kon-junk-tĭ'vo-plas-tĭ). Removal of part of cornea, but replacing with flaps from the conjunctiva.

connec'tive. That which connects or binds together.

   c. tissue. One of the 5 main tissues (framework) of the body, which can be further subdivided into 5 subgroups, viz.: (1) *Areolar* tissue; (2) *adipose* tissue; (3) *bone* and *dentine;* (4) *lymphoid* tissue; (5) *cartilage* tissue. These tissues are mainly concerned in supporting and connecting other bodily structures.

co'noid. Resembling a cone; conical.

   c. ligament. Lower and inner portion of coracoclavicular ligament.

   c. tubercle. Eminence on inf. surface of clavicle to which is attached the conoid ligament.

conomyoidin (ko-no-mi-oid'ĭn). Contractile protoplasm in cones of the retina.

consanguinity (kon-san-gwin'it-ĭ). Relationship by blood.

conscious (kon'shus). Being aware and having perception.

con'sciousness. PSY: A state of awareness.

   c., clouding of. A phase of delirium in which the patient's consciousness is cloudy or not clear.

consenescence (kon-sen-es'ens). The state of growing old.

consen'sual. Reflex stimulation from another part.

   c. light reflex. Contraction of unexposed pupil in sympathy with exposed pupil.

   c. reflex. Any reflex occurring on opposite side of body from point of stimulation.

consolidation (kon-sol-id-a'shun). The act of becoming solid. Esp. used in connection with the solidification of the lungs due to engorgement of the lung tissues, as occurs in acute pneumonia.

constella'tion. Ideas arising from unrepressed emotions.

constipation (kon-sti-pa'shun). A sluggish action of the bowels.

   c., atonic. Lack of muscle tone due to lack of exercise of abdominal muscles, and to abdominal ptosis.*

   c., obstructive. Due to an obstruction in the intestines. Surgical aid needed. Preoperative diet should contain low residue and no gas forming foods.

c., spastic. Constipation accompanied by intestinal spasms.

constitu'tion. The physical make-up and functional habits of the body.

constitu'tional. Pert. to the body as a whole.

c. disease. One which affects the entire body.

c. psychosis. Functional psychosis; not of organic origin.

constric'tion. 1. A binding or squeezing of a part. 2. The narrowing of the caliber of a vessel by pressure.

constric'tor. 1. That which binds or restricts a part. 2. A muscle, such as a sphincter, which can narrow or close a canal.

construc'tive metabolism. The building up or anabolic process.

consult'ant. A consulting physician or surgeon who acts only in an advisory capacity.

consulta'tion. Diagnosis and proposed treatment by 2 or more physicians at one time.

consumption (kon-sump'shun). 1. Tuberculosis.* 2. Wasting. 3. The using up of anything.

consump'tive. Pert. to or afflicted with tuberculosis.

con'tact. 1. Mutual touching or apposition of 2 bodies. 2. Closing of an electric current. 3. One who has been exposed to contagion.

c. complete. When entire surface of 1 tooth touches entire surface of an adjoining tooth, proximally.

c., direct. Communication of a contagious disease through a healthy person touching an infected body.

c., immediate. Same as direct contact.

c., indirect. The spread of a contagious disease by some medium other than direct touch of the sick person.

c., mediate. Same as indirect contact.

c., proximal or **proximate.** Touching of teeth on their adjacent surfaces.

c. surface. Proximal surface of a tooth.

con'tact breaker. Device for breaking a galvanic current.

conta'gion. The process of transferring a specific disease either by direct or indirect contact. SEE: *virulent, virus.*

contagios'ity. The state of being contagious.

conta'gious. That which is transmissible by contact, as "communicable diseases."

contagium (kon-ta'jĭ-um). The agent causing infection or contagion.

contiguity (kon-tĭ-gŭ'i-tĭ). Contact or proximity without continuity.

c., amputation in. Amputation through a joint.

c., law of. If 2 ideas occur in association they are apt to be repeated.

c., solution of. Dislocation or displacement of 2 normally contiguous parts.

con'tinence. Self-restraint, used esp. in connection with refraining from sexual indulgence.

continuity (kon-tĭ-nū'it-ĭ). The state of being continuous or intimately united.

c., amputation in. Amputation through a long bone.

c., solution of. Division of normally continuous parts by fracture, rupture, laceration, incision.

contin'uous. Without break, cessation, or interruption.

c. spec'trum. An unbroken series of wave lengths, either visible or invisible.

contour (kon'toor). Outline or surface configuration of a part.

contoured (kon'toord). Having an irregular, smooth, undulating surface resembling a relief map.

contra-. Prefix: Opposite; against, as *contraindication.*

contra-ap'erture. A 2nd opening made in an abscess.

contraception (kon-tra-sep'shun). The prevention of conception.

contracep'tive. Any agent or device used to prevent conception, such as condoms,* pessaries,* or medication. None can be guaranteed to prevent conception.

contract'. To draw together, reduce in size, or shorten.

contrac'tile. Able to contract, or shorten.

contractil'ity. Having the ability to contract or shorten.

contrac'tion. A shortening, as that of a muscle, or a reduction in size; a shrinking. SEE: *cholepathia spastica, chronotropism.*

contracture (kon-trak'chur). Permanent contraction of a muscle due to spasm or paralysis.

c., functional. Decrease of a contracture during anesthesia or sleep.

contrafissura (kon″tră-fĭ-shu'ră). A fracture at a point opp. from where the blow was received.

contraindication (kŏn″tră-ĭn-dĭ-kā'shŭn). Any symptom or circumstance indicating the inappropriateness of a form of treatment, otherwise advisable.

contralat'eral. Originating in, or affecting, the opposite side of the body. ANTO: *ipsilateral.*

c. reflexes. 1. Passive flexion of 1 part following flexion of another. 2. Passive flexion of 1 leg causing similar movement of opposite leg.

con'trast sprays. Those administered by sitting on side of bathtub, spraying feet and legs with warm water for 1 minute and cold water for 1 minute. Alternate for 10 minutes twice daily.

contravoli'tional. In opp. to or without the will; involuntary.

contrecoup (kon-trĕ-koo'). Injury of a part as a result of transmitted shock from a blow on the opposite side of the part or body. SEE: *contrafissura.*

contrectation (kon-trek-ta'shun). Impulse to embrace or sexually dally with one of the opposite sex; spooning.

control (kon-trōl'). 1. To regulate or maintain. 2. An experiment to test the correctness of an assumption.

c. animal. One not immune exposed to a virus, with an immune animal, at the same time.

c. experiment. Same as control (2).

contrude (kon-trūd'). 1. Abnormal lingual curve or line of dental arch. 2. To crowd together, as the teeth.

contru'sion. Having the teeth crowded.

contuse (kon-tuz'). To bruise.

contusion (kon-tu'zhun). An injury in which the skin is not broken.

F. A. TREATMENT: Apply cold applications. Follow with firm bandage to prevent swelling. Twenty-four to 48 hours later, heat is desirable followed by massage. SEE: *concussion*.

co'nus. 1. A cone. 2. Post. staphyloma of myopic eye.

c. arteriosus. Right cardiac ventricle's upper rounded ant. angle, where pulmonary artery arises.

c. medullaris. Conical portion of lower spinal cord.

convalescence (kon-val-es'ens). The period of recovery after the termination of a disease or an operation.

convales'cent. 1. Getting well. 2. One who is recovering from a disease or operation.

c. diet. A soft diet.

convection (kon-vek'shun). Movement of heat from the source of the heat to another part of a liquid or gas.

convec'tive discharge. Discharge from a high potential source in the form of visible or invisible stream of electrical energy passing through the air to the patient.

convergence (kon-ver'jens). 1. Visual lines directed to a nearby point. 2. The moving of 2 or more objects toward the same point.

convergent (kon-ver'jent). Tending toward a common point.

conver'sion. Change from one position or state to another.

c. symptom. PSY: A term for a repressed emotion that becomes manifested through a physical symptom; seen in hysteria.

converter, rotary. Apparatus used to convert a direct current into an alternating one or *vice versa*.

con'vex. Curved evenly; the segment of a sphere.

convex″ocon′cave. Concave on 1 side and convex on opp. surface. SYN: *concavo-convex*.

convexocon'vex. Convex on 2 opp. faces.

convolute (kon'vo-lūt). Rolled, as a scroll.

con'voluted. Convolute, rolled.

c. bone. Turbinated bone, *concha nasalis*.

c. tubule. The coiled or twisted part of a uriniferous tubule.

convolution (kŏn'vō-lū'shŭn). 1. A winding motion. 2. A turn or fold. 3. ANAT: A coil of tissue on the brain surface, separated by fissures.

c., angular. A gyrus forming post. portion of inf. parietal lobule.

c.'s, annectant. The 4 gyri connect-

ing the convolutions on upper surface of occipital lobe with parietal and temporosphenoidal lobes.

c., ant. central. SEE: *ascending frontal convolution*.

c., ant. choroid. Gyrus choroides.

c., anteroparietal. SEE: *ascending frontal convolution*.

c., ant. orbital. One which lies in front of the orbital sulcus.

c., Arnold's. Gyri posteriores inferiores.

c., ascending frontal. One forming ant. boundary of fissure of Rolando.

c., ascending parietal. One parallel with ascending frontal convolution, separated from it by fissure of Rolando except at extremities, where they are generally united.

c.'s, Broca's. The inf., or 3rd, frontal convolution.

c., callosal, callosomarginal. Gyrus fornicatus.

c.'s, cerebral. Those of the cerebrum.

c. of the corpus callosum. Gyrus fornicatus.

c., cuneate. Gyral isthmus.

c., dentate. A small, notched gyrus rudimentary in man, situated in dentate fissure, below tenia hippocampi.

c., ext. olfactory. Small projection forming outer boundary of the olfactory grooves.

c., hippocampal. Uncinate gyrus.

c., inf. frontal. The lower and outer part of frontal lobe.

c., inf. occipital. A small one lying bet. middle and inf. occipital fissures.

c., inframarginal. Superior temporosphenoidal convolution.

c., insular. One of a group of small convolutions forming the island of Reil, entirely concealed by the operculum.

c., int. orbital. The gyrus next out side of the gyrus rectus.

c.'s, intestinal. The coils of the intestines.

c., marginal. One beginning in front of locus perforatus anterior and bounding longitudinal fissure on mesial aspect of the hemisphere.

c., middle frontal. One continuous post. with ascending frontal convolution and extending forward over ant. end of hemisphere to its orbital surface.

c., middle occipital. One bet. 1st and 3rd occipital convolutions.

c., middle temporosphenoidal. A small gyrus continuous with the middle occipital or angular gyrus.

c., occipitotemporal. Two small convolutions on lower surface of temporosphenoidal lobe.

c., olfactory. Olfactory lobe.

c.'s, orbital. Small gyri on orbital surface of frontal lobe.

c.'s, parietal. Ascending parietal convolution and superior parietal convolution.

c., post. orbital. A small one on post. and outer side of orbital sulcus, and continuous with inf. frontal convolution.

c., second (or middle) frontal. One continuous post. with ascending frontal convolution.

c., sup. frontal. One which bounds great longitudinal fissure, arising post. from upper end of ascending frontal convolution.

c., sup. occipital. Upper of the 3 convolutions on sup. surface of occipital lobe.

c., sup. parietal. Portion of parietal lobe limited ant. by upper part of the fissure of Rolando, post. by ext. parieto-occipital fissure, and inf. by intra-parietal sulcus.

c., sup. temporosphenoidal. Upper of 3 convolutions forming temporosphenoidal lobe. It lies just below and is parallel with sylvian fissure.

c., supramarginal. The ant. portion of inf. parietal lobule behind inf. extremity of intraparietal fissure (sulcus), below which it joins the ascending parietal convolution.

c. of the sylvian fissure. The convolution that bounds the fissure of Sylvius.

c., transverse orbital. The gyrus occupying post. portion of inf. surface of frontal lobe, at ant. extremity of fissure of Sylvius.

c., uncinate. One extending from near post. extremity of occipital lobe to apex of temporosphenoidal.

convul'sant. 1. An agent which produces a convulsion. 2. Causing onset of a convulsion.

c. poisons. The common ones are strychnine and other drugs of the nux vomica groups, and various, special, infrequently used drugs, such as brucine, ignatia, picrotoxin.

convul'sion. Paroxysms of involuntary muscular contractions and relaxations generally in children.

c., clonic. One having intermittent contractions, muscles being alternately contracted and relaxed.

c., epileptiform. One accompanied by unconsciousness.

c., hysterical. Convulsion caused by hysteria.

c., puerperal. Eclamptic convulsion in pregnant or puerperal women.

c., salaam. Spasm of sternomastoid muscles causing bowing motions of the body.

c., tonic. One in which the contractions are maintained for a time, as in tetany.

c., toxic. Convulsion caused by action of a toxin on nervous system.

c., uremic. Convulsion caused by uremic condition.

convul'sive. Pert. to convulsions.

c. reflex. Incoördinate contraction of muscles in a convulsive manner.

c. tic. Spasm of face.

Coo'lidge tube. An x-ray tube whose cathode consists of a spiral tungsten wire surrounded by a molybdenum tube.

coördinated reflexes (ko-or'din-at-ed). The reverse of convulsive reflexes in that action occurs coördinately.

coördination (ko-or-din-a'shun). The working together of various muscles for the production of a certain movement.

copiopia (ko-pi-o'pi-ă). Eyestrain causing fatigue.

copodyskinesia (ko-po-dis-kin-e'sĭ-ă). Occupational neurosis.

cop'per (cuprum). SYMB: *Cu.* At. wt. 63.57. A metal, small quantities of which are utilized by the body. Its salts are an irritant poison.

copperas (kop'er-ăs). Green vitriol. Pale bluish-green crystals. SEE: *ferrous sulfate.*

cop'per sul'fate (blue vitriol). USP. Deep blue, shiny crystals or granular powder.

DOSAGE: As an astringent ¼ gr. (0.016 Gm.); as an emetic, 5 gr. (0.32 Gm.).

coprecip'itin. One which acts on 2 or more organisms.

copre'mia. Intestinal autointoxication, so called, caused by waste products in the blood.

coprohematol'ogy. Study of the blood in the feces.

coprolagnia (kop-ro-lag'nĭ-ă). An erotic satisfaction at the sight or odor of excreta.

coprolalia (kop-ro-la'lĭ-ă). PSY: A morbid desire to use sacrilegious or obscene words in ordinary conversation. Seen in obsessional neurosis or dementia precox.

coprolith (kop'ro-lĭth). Hard, inspissated feces.

coprology (kop-rol'o-jĭ). Examination of the feces. SYN: *scatology.*

coproma (ko-pro'mă). Accumulation of feces in the rectum. SYN: *fecaloma, scotoma, stercoroma.*

coprophagy (ko-prof'ă-jĭ). The eating of excrement.

coprophilia (kop-ro-fil'ĭ-ă). Abnormal interest in feces; a perversion in adults.

coprophobia (kop-ro-fo'bĭ-ă). A morbid disgust at the sight of filth of any kind.

coprostasis (kop-ros'tas-ĭs). The scybalous impaction of feces; constipation.

coprozo'a. Protozoa in fecal matter outside of the intestine.

coprozo'ic. Pert. to coprozoa; found in feces or fecal matter.

copula (kop'u-lă). 1. An immune body. 2. Sexual intercourse. 3. A narrow part bet. 2 structures.

copulation (kop-u-la'shun). Sexual intercourse bet. the sexes. SYN: *coition,* *coitus,* *cohabitation, concubitus.*

cor, cordis (kōr). The heart.

c. adiposum. Fatty degenerative tissue in the heart.

c. bovinum. Hypertrophied heart.

c. hirsutum. Shaggy heart surface appearance.

c. juvunum. Heart disorder combined with orthostatic albuminuria.

c. tomentosum, c. villosum. SEE: *cor hirsutum.*

coraco-acromial (kor″ă-ko-ă-kro′mĭ-ăl). Pert. to acromial and coracoid processes.

cor′acoid. Formed like the beak of a crow.

    c. ligament. Ligament in upper region of shoulder blade.

    c. notch. Notch in upper portion of scapula.

    c. process. Projection from the shoulder blade.

coramine (cō′ra-mēn). A 25% aqueous solution of pyridine - beta - carboxydiethylamide.

    USES: As a circulatory and respiratory stimulant.

    DOSAGE: Orally, hypodermically, intramuscularly, or intravenously, from 15 to 45 ㎖ (1-3 cc.), increased as condition demands.

Corbus' disease. Balanitis with gangrene.

corbus thermophore (kor′bus therm′ofōr). Small round instrument with tapering metal tip 2 inches long carrying a thermometer in center for insertion in cervix or urethra for application of medical diathermy.

cord. A stringlike structure.

    c., spermatic. One formed by the *vas deferens*.

    c., spinal (*medulla spinalis*). That portion of the central nervous system contained in the spinal canal.

    c., umbilical. One which connects the umbilicus of the fetus to the placenta.

cor′date. Shaped like a heart.

cor′diform. Shaped like a heart.

cordi′tis. Inflammation of a funiculus.

cor′dopexy. Operative fixation of an anatomical cord, esp. the vocal cords.

cordot′omy. Spinal cord section of lateral pathways to relieve pain. SYN: *chordotomy*.

corecleisis (kor-e-kli′sis). Occlusion of the pupil.

corectasia, corectasis (kor-ek-ta′zĭ-ă, -tasis). Dilatation of the pupil of the eye; corediastasis.

corectome (ko-rek′tōm). Instrument used for cutting or removing the iris. SYN: *iridectome*.

corectomedialysis (kor-ek″to-me-dĭ-al′ĭ-sis). Separating outer border of iris from its ciliary attachment.

corectomy (ko-rek′to-mĭ). Surgical removal of the iris. SYN: *iridectomy*.

corectopia (kor-ek-to′pĭ-ă). Having the pupil to one side of center of iris.

cored carbon. Electrode with carbon shell and core of metal or metal salt. SEE: *impregnated carbon*.

coredialysis (ko-re-di-al′is-ĭs). Separation of iris' outer border from its ciliary attachment. SYN: *corectomedialysis.**

corediastasis (kor-ed-ĭ-as′ta-sis). Dilatation of pupil. SYN: *corectasia.**

corelysis (kor-e-li′sis). Obliteration of pupil because of adhesions of iris to cornea.

coremorphosis (kor-e-mor-fo′sis). Establishment of an artificial pupil.

corencleisis (kor-en-kli′sis). Formation of an artificial pupil by ligating the iris through a corneal incision.

coreometer (ko-re-om′e-ter). Instrument for measurement of the pupil.

coreom′etry. Measurement of the pupil of the eye.

coreoncion (kor-e-on′sĭ-on). Double hooked iris forceps.

coreoplasty (ko′re-o-plas-tĭ). Any operation for forming an artificial pupil.

corestenoma (kor-e-sten-o′mă). Narrowing of pupil.

    c. congen′itum. Partial congenital obliteration of pupil by excrescences.

coretomedialysis (kor-et-o-mē-dĭ-al′is-is). Making of an artificial pupil through the iris.

coretomy (ko-ret′o-mĭ). Any cutting operation on the iris.

Corex-D glass. Window glass which transmits the solar ultraviolet rays more fully than any other glasses except quartz.

corium (ko′rĭ-um). The deep layer of the skin. The true skin.

corm. A short, solid, underground stem. EX: *Colchicum*. SEE: *heloma*.

corn. Horny induration and thickening of the skin, hard or soft, according to location. SYN: *clavus*.

cor′nea. Clear, transparent, ant., glasslike portion of coat of eyeball. It is pearly white in health. Curvature is greater than rest of eyeball.

cor′neal. Pert. to the cornea.

    c. reflex. Closure of eyelids resulting from direct corneal irritation.

corneitis (kor-ne-i′tis). Inflammation of the cornea. SYN: *keratitis*.

corneoiri′tis. Inflammation of iris and cornea.

corneomandibular reflex (kor-ne-o-mandĭb′u-lar). Deflexion of mandible toward opposite side when cornea is irritated while mouth is open and relaxed.

corneosclera (kor-ne-o-skle′ră). The cornea and sclera considered together.

corneous (kor′ne-us). Horny; hornlike.

    c. layer. Horny outer layer of the epidermis. SYN: *stratum corneum*.

    c. tissue. Substance of the nails.

cornic′ulum. A small, hornlike process.

    c. laryn′gis. Small, hornlike nodule on arytenoid cartilage.

cornifica′tion. The process of becoming hard.

Corning-glass. Window glass substitute for transmitting the antirachitic rays of sunlight.

cor′nu. Any excrescence like a horn.

    c. ammo′nis. Hippocampus major of brain.

    c. cuta′neum, c. huma′num. Hornlike excrescence on skin.

    c. of the uterus. 1. Prolongation of uterus into which the fallopian tubes open. 2. Oviducts.

cor′nual. Pert. to a cornu.

    c. myelitis. Myelitis of ant. cornua of spinal cord.   [crown.

coro′na. Any structure resembling a

    c. capitis. Crown of head.

    c. ciliaris. Circular figure on inner surface of ciliary body.

c. dentis. Crown of a tooth. [*penis.*
c. glandis. Post. border of *glans*
c. radiata. 1. Radiating fibers from optic thalamus. 2. Layer of cells placed radially about the ovum.
c. veneris. Blotches on forehead parallel to hairline. A lenticular syphilide.
co'ronal. Pert. to a corona.
c. suture. One which joins the parietal and frontal bones of the cranium.
coronary (kor'o-na-rǐ). 1. A term applied to blood vessels of the heart which supply blood to its walls. 2. Encircling; surrounding.
c. arteries. Those of the heart supplying the heart muscle. There are also a right and left coronary artery of the stomach. Narrowing and spasm of the coronary heart arteries produce angina pectoris.
cor'oner. County officer who investigates and holds inquests over those dead from unknown or violent causes.
cor'onoid. Shaped like a crow's beak or crown.
c. fossa. Seat of coronoid process of the ulna in humerus.
c. process. A process of the ulna projecting in front; also one of the lower jaw in front.
coroparelcysis (kor″o-par-el'si-sis). Bringing the pupil to one side in central corneal opacity.
coroscopy (ko-ros'ko-pǐ). Shadow test to determine refractive error of an eye. SYN: *skiascopy.*
corot'omy. Any cutting of the cornea.
cor'pora (sing: *corpus*). Bodies.
c. cavernosa penis. Two columns of erectile tissue on dorsum of the penis.
c. olivaria. Two oval masses behind pyramids of the oblongata.
c. quadrigemina. Four rounded bodies of gray matter in the midbrain making up the lamina quadrigemina. The ant. pair are called the *nates;* the post., the *testes.*
cor'porin. Hormone from the corpus luteum. SYN: *progesterone.*
corpulence (kor'pū-lĕns). Fatness of the body. SYN: *obesity.*
corpulent (kor'pū-lĕnt). Fat; obese.
cor'pus. The principal part of any organ; any mass or body.
c. albicans. Mass of scar tissue or white body that replaces the corpus hemorrhagicum following the rupture of the graafian follicle. It decreases in size and leaves a pitlike depression on the ovary's surface.
c. amylaceum. Mass having an irregular, laminated structure like a starch grain, found in the prostate, neuroglia, etc.
c. annulare. Pons Varolii.
c. Arantii. Tubercle found in center of semilunar valves.
c. bigeminum. Optic lobe.
c. callosum. The great commissure of the brain bet. the cerebral hemispheres.

c. cavernosum penis. One of 2 erectile tissues adjoining each other on the dorsum of the penis.
c. cavernosum urethrae. SEE: *corpus spongiosum, q.v.*
c. ciliare. Ciliary body.
c. dentale, c. dentatum. Gray layer in white substance of the cerebellum.
c. fimbriatum. White layer edging the lower cornu of the lateral ventricle.
c. flavum. A waxy body seen in the central nervous system.
c. geniculatum. Tubercle on lower portion of optic thalami.
c. hemorrhagicum. Blood clot formed in the cavity left by rupture of the graafian follicle.
c. highmorianum. Mediastinum testis.
c. interpedunculare. Gray matter bet. peduncles before the pons Varolii.
c. luteum. The yellow body which develops in the ruptured graafian follicular cavity after the ovum has been discharged, on or about the 13th or 14th day after menstrual flow begins.
c. mammillare. SEE: *corpus albicans.*
c. pampiniforme. Parovarium.
c. pyramidale. Pyramid of the oblongata.
c. restiforme. Column of the medulla extending to the cerebrum and cord.
c. rhomboidale. SEE: *corpus dentatum.*
c. spongiosum. Erectile tissue surrounding the urethra.
c. striatum. Gray body in lateral ventricle of brain.
c. subthalamicum. Lower portion of hypothalamus.
c. vitreum. Vitreous portion of eye
c. wolffianum. Wolffian body.
cor'puscle. 1. A cell. 2. A minute particle; corpusculum.
There are 2 varieties, red and white, found in the blood, *q.v.*
c., amniotic; c., amylaceous. Starch-like rounded body found in tissue, usually nervous, showing degeneration.
c., axile; c., axis. The center of a tactile corpuscle. [*cle.*
c., Bennett's. SEE: *Drysdale's corpus-*
c., Bizzozero's. Blood platelet.
c., blood. An erythrocyte or leukocyte.
c., bone. A bone cell.
c., Burckhardt's. Yellowish particles found in secretion of trachoma.
c., calcareous. A lime-containing cell found in dentine of a tooth.
c's., cancroid. Characteristic nodule in cutaneous epithelioma.
c., cartilage. A cell characteristic of cartilage.
c's., chorea. Hyaline bodies found in the corpora striata in chorea.
c., chromophil. Tiny body found in cytoplasm of a nerve cell. SYN: *Nissl's body.*
c's., chyle. Corpuscle seen in chyle.
c., colloid. SEE: *corpuscle, amniotic.*
c., colostrum. Large corpuscle found in colostrum.

c's., corneal. Connective tissue corpuscles found in fibrous tissue of cornea.

c. of Donne. SEE: *colostrum corpuscles.*

c's., Drysdale's. Elements found in the fluid of ovarian cysts.

c., educated. A cell derived from a mother cell which has overcome the toxic effects of bacteria of a disease.

c's., genital. Nerve terminals in the external genitalia.

c's., Gierke's. Particles seen in the nervous system.

c's., Gluge's. Particles seen in diseased nervous tissue.

c's., Golgi-Mazzoni. Tactile corpuscles with extensively branched nerve fibers and with few lamellae, found in subcutaneous tissue of the fingertips.

c's., Hassall's. Corpuscles found in the thymus gland.

c's., Krause's. Nerve endings in mucosa of genitalia, mouth, nose, and eyes.

c's., lymph. Leukocytes found in blood and lymph.

c's., malpighian. Corpuscles found in the spleen and kidney.

c's., Mazzoni's. Nerve endings resembling Krause's corpuscles.

c's., Meissner's. SEE: *tactile corpuscles.*

c's., Norris'. Invisible disks in blood serum.

c's., pacinian. Largest of the end organs of the skin, found in the subcutaneous tissues.

c., phantom. A red blood corpuscle which has lost its coloring matter.

c., tactile. A rounded nerve ending found in the papillae of the corium, esp. of the fingers and toes.

c., terminal. A nerve ending. SEE: *nerve.*

c., touch. SEE: *tactile corpuscle.*

c's., Wagner's. SEE: *tactile corpuscles.*

corpus'cular. Pert. to corpuscles.

corpus'culum. Corpuscle.

c. renis. Malpighian corpuscle and its capillaries in the kidneys, where secretion of the water in urine occurs.

correc'tant, correc'tive. 1. A drug that modifies action of another. 2. Pert. to such a drug.

Corrigan's disease. An abnormal condition caused by aortic regurgitation, and recognized by visible pulsation in the main arteries.

C.'s pulse. A full bounding pulse, which appears to be completely empty bet. beats; is associated with aortic insufficiency. SYN: *water-hammer pulse.*

corro'sion. Disintegration, esp. carious disintegration of a tooth.

corro'sive. Disintegrating, as eating away.

c. alkalies. These are corrosive hydroxides most commonly of sodium, ammonium, and potassium, as well as carbonates.

cor'tex. 1. The outer layers of an organ as distinguished from its inner substance. 2. Outer layer of a bone or of the skull.

c. cerebri. The cortex of the brain, composed mainly of gray or cineritious substance. SEE: *arm center.*

c. renis. The cortical substance of the kidney, made up of urinary tubes and blood vessels, supported by a stroma or matrix.

cortiadrenal (kor-tĭ-ad-re′nal). Pert. to cortex of adrenal gland.

cor′tical. Pert. to the cortex.

corticifugal (kor-tĭ-sif′u-gal). Passing from the cerebral cortex.

corticipetal (kor-tĭ-sĭp′e-tal). Passing toward the cerebral cortex.

corticoadre′nal. Pert. to cortex of adrenal gland.

corticoaf′ferent. Passing toward the cerebral cortex. SYN: *corticipetal.**

corticoef′ferent. Passing from the cerebral cortex. SYN: *corticifugal.**

corticopedun′cular. Pert. to cortex and cerebral peduncles.

corticopleuritis (kor-tĭ-ko-plū-ri′tis). Inflammation of outer parts of pleura.

corticospi′nal. Pert. to cerebral cortex and spinal cord.

corticotro′phin. The adrenotropic factor or principle in the ant. lobe of the pituitary gland. FUNCT: To maintain normal structure and functioning of adrenal cortex.

corticotro′pic. Pert. to corticotrophin.

cor′tin. An assumed hormone of cortex of suprarenal gland.

Corti's arches (kor′tēz). Arches formed by junction of Corti's rods.

C.'s canal. Spinal canal in organ of Corti.

C.'s cells. Hair cells of organ of Corti.

C.'s membrane. One that covers Corti's organ.

C.'s organ. Prominence on inner portion of basal membrane in cochlear duct and containing terminal auditory apparatus.

C.'s rods. Supporting pillars of organ of Corti.

C.'s teeth. Huschke's* teeth; tiny toothlike protuberances at edge of cochlear labium vestibulare.

C.'s tunnel. Corti's canal.

coryleur (kor-il-er′). Coryl sprayer.

Cory'nebacte'rium diphthe'riae. The diphtheria bacillus.

coryza (ko-ri′za). Cold in the head; an acute catarrhal inflammation of the nasal mucous membrane.

c. spasmod'ica. Hay fever.

cosen'sitize. To sensitize to more than 1 infection.

cosmetic (koz-met′ik). Powder or cream for improving complexion.

c. operation. One for correcting an unsightly skin formation or structural conformation of face.

cos'ta (pl. *costae*). Rib. SEE: *cartilage.*

cos'tal. Pert. to a rib.

c. cartilage. Cartilaginous part of a rib articulating with the sternum.

costal'gia. Pain in the region of a rib· pleuralgia.

costectomy (kos-tek′to-mǐ). Excision of a rib or part of one.

cos′tive. Constipated.

cos′tiveness. Constipation.

costochon′dral. Pert. to a rib and its cartilage.

costoclavic′ular. Pert. to ribs and clavicle.

costocor′acoid. Pert. to ribs and coracoid process of scapula.

costogenic (kos-to-jen′ĭk). Pert. to defect arising from bone marrow of ribs.

costopneumopexy (kos″to-nu′mo-pek-sĭ). Anchoring a lung to a rib.

costoster′nal. Pert. to a rib and the sternum.

costotome (kos′to-tōm). Knife or shears for cutting through a rib or cartilage.

costotomy (kos-tot′o-mǐ). Excision of a rib or part of one. SYN: *costectomy, q.v.*

costo″transverse′. Pert. to the ribs and transverse processes of articulating vertebrae.

costover′tebral. Pert. to a rib and a vertebra.

cot′ton. Fluffy covering of the plant *Gossypium.*

    c., absorbent. Cotton prepared to absorb liquids.

    c., styptic. Cotton impregnated with an astringent.

    c. wool sandwiches. These are used when a sharp pointed foreign body, such as a pin, has been swallowed.

cotyledon (kot-I-le′don). 1. Mass of villi on chorionic surface of the placenta. 2. Any of rounded portions into which the placenta's uterine surface is divided. 3. Seed leaf of a plant embryo.

cotyloid (kot′il-oid). Shaped like a cup.

    c. cavity. The acetabulum or socket receiving the head of the femur.

couching (kow′ching). Displacement of the lens downward in cataract.

cough. A violent expiratory effort preceded by a preliminary inspiration. The glottis is partially closed, the extraordinary muscles of expiration are brought into action, and the air is noisily expelled.

    c., aneurysmal. Brassy and clanging, heard in patients suffering from aneurysm.

    c., asthmatic. More like an attack of dyspnea than a cough.

    c., brassy. Met with in cases where there is pressure on the left recurrent laryngeal nerve, as in aortic aneurysm.

    c., bronchial. Heard in cases of bronchiectasis.*

    c., diphtherial. Heard in laryngeal diphtheria; noisy and brassy, with stridulous breathing.

    c., dry. One unaccompanied by moisture.

    c., effective. When sputum is brought up.

    c., hacking. A series of repeated efforts, as occurs in the early stages of pulmonary tuberculosis.

    c., harsh. A metallic cough occurring in laryngitis.

    c., hiccough. Singultus. Seen in forms of hysteria; unfavorable if seen toward end of acute disease.

    c., hysterical. Incessant and barking.

    c., ineffective. When there is no sputum.

    c., laryngeal. Seen in laryngitis.* shrill and husky. SPUTUM: Small plugs of mucus.

    c., loud. Hysterical cough, *q.v.*

    c., moist. A loose cough accompanied by moisture.

    c., painful. The suppressed cough of the early stages of pleurisy and pneumonia.

    c., paroxysmal. That occurring in whooping cough and bronchiectasis. Also described as spasmodic.

    c., pulmonary. Hard and painful in pneumonia.

    c., reflex. Due to irritation from the middle ear, pharynx, stomach, or intestine. It may occur singly or coupled, or it may be hacking in character.

    c., short. A dry cough seen in the early stages of a common cold or catarrhal influenza.

    c., whooping. Seen in pertussis.* Convulsive, short, followed by a whoop. SPUTUM: Tough mucus, followed by vomiting.

coulomb (koo-lom′). Unit of electrical quantity. It is the quantity of electricity transferred by 1 ampere in 1 second.

counterextension (kown-ter-eks-ten′shun). Back pull or resistance to extension on a limb.

counterir′ritant. An agent that is applied locally to produce inflammatory reaction with the object of affecting some other part, usually adjacent to or underlying the surface irritated. Ex: *Mustard, chloroform, cantharides.*

counterirrita′tion. Superficial irritation, or agent producing it, which relieves some other irritation of deeper structures.

countero′pening. A 2nd opening, as in an abscess, not draining satisfactorily from 1st incision.

coun′terpressure instrument. To provide counter-retraction to offset that exerted by exit of needle.

coun′terpuncture. Counteropening.* An additional opening made to help drainage, as an abscess.

coup de soleil (koo-da-sŏ-lay′). Sunstroke.

coup′ling. Slow pulse, heartbeats alternating strong or weak; seen in digitalis poisoning.

courses (kōr′siz). Menses; catamenia.

Coutard's method or **technic.** A method of x-ray irradiation consisting of 10 equal applications.

couveuse (koo-vuz′). Infant incubator.

cover cell (kŭv′ĕr). A cell which serves to protect another cell of specialized function. SEE: *cell.*

cov′erglass. Thin glass disc to cover a mounted object to be microscopically examined.   [glands.

cowperi′tis. Inflammation of Cowper's

Cowper's glands. A pair of compound tubular glands about the size of a pea beneath the bulb of the male urethra, and emptying a mucous secretion into it.

cowpox (kow'pox). Vaccinia; pustular eruption on teats and bag of a cow in form of bluish vesicles, containing a virus which may produce smallpox in a human being; also claimed to render a subject permanently immune from the disease.

cox'a. 1. The *os innominatum.* 2. The hip joint.

    c. valga. Opp. of *coxa vara.* Deformity produced when angle of head of femur with the shaft is increased above 120°.

    c. vara. A deformity produced by decrease in angle made by head of femur with the shaft. Normally it should be 120°; but in coxa vara it may be 80-90°. It occurs in rickets or may be due to bone injury.

coxal'gia. 1. Pain in the hip. SYN: *coxodynia.* 2. Hip joint disease. SYN: *coxitis.*

coxi'tis. Hip joint disease.

coxodyn'ia. Pain in the hip joint. SYN: *coxalgia.*

coxofem'oral. Pert. to the hip and femur.

coxo"tuberculo'sis. Tuberculous condition of the hip joint.

c. p. Abbr. Chemically pure.

Cr. SYMB: Chromium.

crab louse. *Phthirius inguinalis.* One that infests the pubic region.

crachotement (krȧ-shōt-mon(g)'). Inability to spit, even with a strong desire to do so; usually accompanied by syncope following uteroövarian operation.

cracked pot sound. Percussion sound resembling that heard when striking a cracked pot, indicative of a pulmonary cavity.

cra'dle. Frame for keeping bedclothes from pressing on a wound or fractured part.

craigi'asis. Infection with Craigia microorganism causing symptoms peculiar to dysentery.

cramp. A spasmodic, esp. a tonic, contraction of 1 or many muscles, usually painful.

    c., clonic. Wryneck caused by rheumatism. SYN: *rheumatic torticollis.**

cra'nial. Pert. to the cranium.

    c. bones. Those of the head. SEE: *skeleton.*

    c. nerves. These have their origin in the brain, 12 in number. Name, number and functions of cranial nerves are as follows:

    1st Pair—Olfactory. Special sense of smell.

    2nd Pair—Optic. Special sense of sight.

    3rd Pair—Oculomotor or *Motor Oculi.* Great motor of eye, supplies 5 of the 7 eye muscles.

    4th Pair—Patheticus or *Trochlear.* Motor of superior oblique muscle of eye.

    5th Pair—Trigeminus or *Trifacial.*

Great sensory nerve of head and face; divides into 3 portions, *viz.,* 1st Ophthalmic, Sensory; 2nd Sup. Max., Sensory; 3rd Inf. Max., Sensory, Motor and a lingual nerve of the sense of taste. Most difficult of all the cranial nerves to trace.

    6th Pair—Abducens. Motor of external rectus of eye.

    7th Pair—Facial or *Portio Dura.* Great motor nerve of face muscles; exclusively motor at its origin, but it subsequently receives fibers from the (5th) Trigeminus, which give it some sensory function.

    8th Pair—Acoustic or *Auditory,* or *Portio Mollis of 7th.* Special sense of hearing.

    9th Pair—Glossopharyngeal. In part a special nerve of taste, nerve of sensation, and also contains motor fibers.

    10th Pair—Pneumogastric Vagus or *Par Vagum* (a mixed nerve). At its origin it is exclusively sensory, but lower down it is also motor and capable of providing both for sensation and motion in organs to which distributed.

    11th Pair—Spinal Accessory. Considered to be exclusively motor, but some authorities claim for it sensory fibers. Accessory portion joins the vagus, to which it supplies its motor and some of its cardioinhibitory fibers. Spinal portion supplies the trapezius and sternomastoid muscles.

    12th Pair—Hypoglossal. Exclusively [motor.

craniectomy (kra-nĭ-ek'to-mĭ). Opening of skull for cerebral hemorrhage, tumor of brain, fracture of skull, or epilepsy.

craniocele (kra'nĭ-o-sēl). Protrusion of the brain from the skull.

craniocer'ebral. Rel. to skull and brain.

cranioclast (kra'nĭ-o-klast). Instrument for crushing fetal skull in delivery.

cra'nioclasty. Crushing of fetal head in dystocia.

craniocleidodysostosis (kra"nĭ-o-kli"do-dis-os-to'sis). Defective ossification of bones of head, face and clavicles; a congenital condition.

cra'niograph. Device for making graphs of the skull.

craniol'ogy. The study of the skull, its size, and shape, esp. in reference to different races.

craniomalacia (kra-nĭ-o-mal-a'sĭ-ȧ). Softening of the skull bones.

craniometer (kra-nĭ-om'et-er). Instrument for taking cranial measurements.

craniomet'ric points. Any prominences or marks on skull for defining the configuration of the cranium; for use in craniometry.

craniom'etry. Study of the skull and measurement of it without its soft parts.

craniopharyngeal (kra"nĭ-o-far-in'je-al). Pert. to cranium and pharynx.

craniopharyngioma (kra-nĭ-o-far-in"jĭ-o'mȧ). Tumor of portion of the *hypophysis cerebri.*

cranioplasty (kra'ne-o-plas-tĭ). Plastic operation on skull.

cra′niopuncture. Puncture of the skull.

craniorhachischisis (kra-nĭ-o-rak-is′kis-is). Congenital fissure of skull and spine.

craniostosis (kra-nĭ-os-to′sis). Congenital ossification of cranial sutures.

craniotabes (kra-nĭ-o-ta′bēz). Atrophy in infancy of cranial bones.

craniotome (kra′nĭ-o-tōm). Device for forcible reduction of fetal skull in labor.

craniotomy (kra-nĭ-ot′o-mĭ). Breaking up fetal skull to facilitate delivery in difficult parturition.

craniotonos′copy. Auscultatory percussion of cranium.   [ear.

craniotympan′ic. Pert. to skull and middle

cra′nium. The skull. The 8 bones of the head comprising the skull enclosing the brain. Generally applied to the 28 bones of the head and face.

crap′ulent, crap′ulous. Intoxicated.

crassamen′tum. Coagulum, blood clot.

crater′iform. BACT: Saucer-shaped, crater-like, or goblet-shaped.

cravat′ ban′dage. Triangular bandage folded to form a band around the injured part. SEE: *bandage*.

cream of tartar. Potassium bitartrate, $KHC_4H_4O_6$. An aperient and diuretic.
DOSAGE: 1-4 Gm. Usually given in hot water with lemon juice to flavor. SEE: *argol*.

crease (krēs). A line produced by a fold.
c., gluteofemoral, c., ileofemoral. The crease that bounds the buttocks below.

creatinase (kre-at′in-ās). An enzyme that decomposes creatinine.

creatine (kre′at-in). Methylglycocyamine, $NH:C(NH_2)N(CH_3).CH_2.COOH + H_2O$, a colorless, crystalline substance that can be isolated from various animal organs and body fluids.
DOSAGE: 1-2 gr. (0.06-0.12 Gm.).

creatinemia (kre-a-tin-e′me-ă). Excess of creatine in circulating blood.

creatinine (kre-at′in-in). Methylglycocyamidine, $C_4H_7ON_3$.
DOSAGE: 1-2 gr. (0.06-0.12 Gm.).

creatinuria (kre-ă-tin-u′rĭ-ă). Creatinine in urine.

creatorrhea (kre-ă-tor-re′ă). The presence of muscle fibers in the feces, seen in some cases of pancreatic disease.

creatotoxism (kre″ă-to-toks′ĭzm). Meat poisoning.

crèche (krāsh). A day nursery for children.

Crede′s method (kre′dĕs). 1. The means whereby the placenta is expelled by downward pressure on the uterus through the abdominal wall with the thumb on the post. surface of the fundus uteri and the flat of the hand on the ant. surface, the pressure being applied in the direction of the birth canal. 2. For treatment of the eyes of the newborn, the use of 1% silver nitrate solution instilled into the eyes immediately after birth for the prevention of *ophthalmia neonatorum* (gonorrheal ophthalmia).

cremas′ter. One of the fascialike muscles suspending and enveloping the testicles and spermatic cord.

cremaster′ic. Pert. to the cremaster muscle.
c. fascia. One of the coverings of the spermatic cord.
c. reflex. Retraction of testis when skin is stroked on front inner side of thigh.

cremation (kre-ma′shun). Reduction of bodies of the dead by heat as a substitute for burying.

cre′mor. Cream.
c. tar′tari. Cream of tartar.

crenate (kre′nat). Notched or scalloped, as crenated condition of blood corpuscles.

crena′tion. The conversion of normally round red corpuscles into shrunken, knobbed, starry forms, as when blood is mixed with salt solution of, say, 5% strength. SEE: *plasmolysis*.

creosote (kre′o-sōt). USP. A mixture of phenols obtained from wood tar.
DOSAGE: 4 ♏ (0.25 cc.).

crepitant (krĕp′ĭ-tănt). Crackling; having or making a crackling sound.

crepitation (krĕp-ĭ-tā′shŭn). 1. A crackling sound heard in certain diseases, as the râle heard in pneumonia. 2. A grating sound heard on movement of ends of a broken bone.

crep′itus. 1. The noise of gas discharged from the intestines. 2. Crepitation.*
c. redux. Râle indicating approaching recovery in pneumonia.

crepuscular (kre-pus′kŭ-lar). Pert. to twilight.   [moon.

cres′cent. Shaped like a sickle or the new
c. of Gianuzzi (jăn-noot′tse). Small granular cells or marginal corpuscles bet. secreting cells of a mucous gland and the basement membrane.
c., myopic. Grayish patch in fundus of eye due to atrophy of choroid.

crescentic (kres-en′tik). Sickleshaped.

cresol (kre′sol). USP. Yellowish brown liquid obtained from coal tar, having 4 times germicidal properties of phenol.
DOSAGE: 1 gr. (0.06 Gm.).

cresomania (kres-o-ma′nĭ-ă). Hallucination of possessing great wealth.

crest. The ridge or part surrounding a process or organ.

cre′tin. One afflicted with congenital myxedema; an idiotic dwarf.

cretinism (kre′tin-izm). Congenital affection, characterized by a lack of physical and mental development.
c., sporadic cases of. Present the same features but the thyroid instead of being larger is smaller. Found in various parts of world. SEE: *cretin*.

cretinoid (cre′ti-noid). Having the symptoms of cretinism, or resembling a cretin, due to a congenital condition.

cre′tinous. Pert. to a cretin or to cretinism.

crevice (krev′is). A small fissure, or crack.
c., gin′gival. The fissure produced by the marginal gingiva with the tooth surface.

crevicular (krev-ik′u-lar). Pert. to the gingival crevice.

crib'rate. Profusely pitted or perforated like a sieve.

cribra'tion. The state of being perforated.

crib'riform. Sievelike.

c. fascia. Inner superficial fascia of thigh.

c. plate. The thin, perforated, medial portion of the horizontal plate of the ethmoid bone.

cricoarytenoid (kri-ko-ă-rit'en-oid). Extending bet. the cricoid and arytenoid cartilages.

cricoderma (kri-ko-der'mă). Ring-shaped infiltrations in center of indurations on the skin.

cricoid (kri'koid). Ringlike.

c. cartilage. A ringlike cartilage forming the lower back part of the larynx.

cricoidectomy (kri-koid-ek'to-mĭ). Excision of cricoid cartilage.

cricoidynia (kri-koi-dĭn'ĭ-ă). Pain in cricoid cartilage.

cricopharyn'geal. Pert. to the cricoid cartilage and pharynx.

cricothyreotomy (kri-ko-thi-re-ot'o-mĭ). Division of the cricoid and thyroid cartilage.

cricothyroid (kri-ko-thi'roid). Pert. to the thyroid and cricoid cartilages.

cricot'omy. Division of the cricoid cartilage.

cricotracheot'omy. Division of the cricoid cartilage and upper trachea in closure of the glottis.

crinogenic (krin-o-jen'ĭk). Producing or stimulating secretion.

crisis (kri'sis). 1. The turning point of a disease; a very critical period often marked by a long sleep and profuse perspiration. 2. The term used for the sudden descent of a high temperature to normal or below; generally occurs within 24 hours. 3. Sharp paroxysms of pain occurring over the course of a few days in certain diseases, *e.g.*, gastric crisis, vesical crisis, Dietl's crisis, laryngeal crisis, etc. SEE: *lysis.*

c., blood. The appearance in the blood of large numbers of nucleated erythrocytes over the course of a few days.

c., Dietl's. In cases of floating kidney, the ureter becomes kinked and urine is obstructed, producing symptoms of renal colic.

c., false. When temperature falls and the pulse rate remains high, suggesting that later on the temperature may rise again.

c., true. One accompanied by a fall in the pulse rate.

crista. A crest or ridge.

c. ampullaris. A localized thickening of the membrane lining the ampullae of the semicircular canals; it is covered with neuroepithelium containing auditory cells.

c. galli. A ridge on the ethmoid bone to which the *falx cerebri* is attached.   [crest.

c. lacrimalis posterior. The lacrimal

c. spiralis. A ridge on the spiral lamina of the cochlea.*

critical (krit'ik-al). 1. Pert. to a crisis. 2. Dangerous.

c. reflex. Abnormal tension of an area resulting from direct stimulation of that area.

Crookes' dark space. Nonluminous region enveloping outline of the cathode in a discharge tube. SEE: *cathode, dark space.*

C. tube. An early form of vacuum discharge tube devised by Sir William Crookes and used by him for the study of cathode rays.

cross birth. Presentation of the fetus where the long axis of the fetus is at right angles to that of the mother and requiring version.

cross eye. Manifest deviation of one eye when looking at an object. SYN: *strabismus,* *squint.*

crossed reflexes (krŏst). 1. Passive flexion of 1 part following flexion of another. 2. Passive flexion of 1 leg causing similar movement of opposite leg.

cross knee. Knock knee. SYN: *genu valgum.*

crotaphion (kro-ta'fĭ-on). Tip of greater wing of sphenoid bone.

crotchet (krotch'et). Sharp hook for extracting fetus after craniotomy.

croton oil (kro'ton). USP. A fixed oil expressed from the seed of the croton plant.

DOSAGE: 1 ℳ (0.06 cc.) diluted with sugar or olive oil.

crounotherapy (kroo″no-ther'ă-pĭ). Use of mineral waters for therapeutic purposes.

croup (crōop). Disease characterized by suffocative and difficult breathing, laryngeal spasm, and sometimes by the formation of a membrane.

c., catarrhal. Acute catarrhal laryngitis.

c., membranous. Croupous laryngitis or true croup. Inflammation of larynx with exudation forming a false membrane.

c., spasmodic or **false.** Catarrhal laryngitis without formation of false membrane, but with spasm of the glottis. Occurs in children.

croupous (kroo'pus). Pert. to croup or having a fibrinous exudation.

c. membrane. False membranous formation found in croup.

c. pneumonia. Lobar pneumonia.

crown'ing. Stage in delivery when fetal head presents at the vulva.

crownwork. Artificial crown for a tooth.

crucial (krū'shal). 1. Cross shaped. 2. Decisive.

cru'cible. A vessel for melting substances with great heat.

cru'ciform. Shaped like a cross.

crude (krūd). Raw, unrefined, or in a natural state.

cru'ra (sing. *crus*). A pair of elongated masses or diverging bands, resembling legs.

c. cerebel'li. Cerebellar peduncles.

c. cer'ebri. Pair of bands joining cerebellum to medulla and pons.

c. of diaphragm. Two pillars connecting spinal column and diaphragm.

c. of the fornix. Arches made by division of the fornicate extremities.

crural (kru'ral). Pert. to the leg or thigh; femoral.

c. arch. Femoral arch.

c. hernia. Femoral hernia.

crus (pl. *cru'ra*). 1. The leg. 2. Any structure resembling the leg.

c. cerebri. Either of the 2 peduncles connecting the cerebrum with the pons.

crust, crust'a. 1. A scab. A secondary lesion; dry serous or seropurulent, brown, yellow, red or green exudations on a free surface. 2. An outer covering or coat.

c. lactea. Seborrhea of scalp in nursing infants. SEE: *galactophlysis.*

cryalgesia (kri-al-je'zĭ-ă). Pain from the cold. SYN: *crymodynia.*

cryanesthesia (kri-an-es-the'zĭ-ă). Loss of sense of cold.

cryesthesia (kri-es-the'zĭ-ă). Sensitiveness to the cold.

crymodynia (kri-mo-din'ĭ-ă). Pain from cold. SYN: *cryalgesia.*

crymophilic (kri-mo-fil'ĭk). Showing preference for cold, as certain microörganisms.

crymophylactic (kri-mo-fĭ-lak'tĭk). Resistant to cold.

crymother'apy. The use of cold in treating disease.

cryo-aerotherapy (kri-o-a-er-o-ther'ă-pĭ). Cold air bath in which, by degrees, the patient is accustomed to freezing temperature.

cryocautery (kri-o-kaw'ter-ĭ). Device for collection and application of solid carbon dioxide.

cry'ogen. Mixture of carbon dioxide snow at —176° F.

cryogenic (kri-o-jen'ĭk). Producing or pert. to low temperatures.

cryom'eter. A thermometer for measuring very low temperature.

cryophil'ic. Preferring low temperatures.

cryoscope (kri'o-skōp). Device for performing cryoscopy.

cryoscopy (kri-os'ko-pĕ). Comparison of freezing point of blood, urine, and other fluids with that of distilled water.

cryotherapy (kri-o-ther'ă-pĭ). The therapeutic use of cold.

cryotol'erant. Able to tolerate very low temperatures.

crypt (kript). A tubule; follicle or pit.

c. of Lieberkühn. Intestinal glands; tubular depressions in the intestinal mucous membrane. They are lined with columnar epithelium and have circular apertures opening upon the surface.

c's, Morgagni's. Recessions or pockets in rectal mucosa.

c., synovial. Pouch in a joint's synovial membrane.

cryptanamnesia (kript-an-am-ne'zĭ-ă). Subconscious memory.

cryptectomy (krip-tek'to-mĭ). Excision of a crypt.

cryptesthesia (krip-tes-the'zĭ-ă). Intuition.

cryptic (krip'tĭk). Having a hidden meaning; occult.

cryptitis (krip-ti'tis). Inflammation of a crypt or follicle.

cryptodidymus (krip-to-did'ĭ-mus). One fetus concealed within another.

cryptogenetic (krĭp-to-jen-et'ĭk). Of unknown or indeterminate origin.

c. infection. The invasion of bacteria without outward evidence of entry into the body. SEE: *infection.*

cryptoglio'ma. A glioma that has not yet revealed itself.

cryptolith (krip'to-lith). A concretion in a glandular follicle.

cryptomenorrhea (krip-to-men-o-re'ă). Monthly subjective symptoms of menses without flow of blood.

cryptomerorachischisis (krip''to-mer''o-rak-is'kis-is). *Spina bifida occulta* without a tumor but with bony deficiency.

cryptomnesia (krip-tom-ne'zĭ-ă). Subconscious memory.

cryptophthal'mus. Complete congenital adhesion of eyelids to globe of eye.

cryptoplas'mic. Having existence in a concealed form.

cryptopodia (krip-to-po'dĭ-ă). Fibromata of feet so diffuse as to resemble pads.

cryptopyic (krip-to-pi'ĭk). Having concealed suppuration, as a pyemia without apparent etiology.

cryptoradiom'eter. Device for estimating penetrative power of x-rays.

cryptorchid (kript-or'kĭd). One with testicles which have not descended into the scrotum.

cryptorchidectomy (kript-or-kĭ-dek'to-mĭ). Operation for an undescended testicle.

cryptorchidism (kript-or'kid-izm). Failure of testicles to descend into scrotum.

cryptorchis (kript-or'kis). One with undescended testicles. SYN: *cryptorchid.*

cryptorrhea (krip-to-re'ă). Excessive secretion of a ductless gland.

cryptorrheic (krip-to-re'ĭk). Pert. to internal secretions. SYN: *cryptorrhetic.*

cryptorrhet'ic. Pert. to the internal secretions.

cryptoscope (krip'to-skōp). Fluoroscope.

cryptotox'ic. Having unknown toxic properties.

cry reflex (krĭ). Sudden painful response cry during sleep.

crys'tal. A symmetrical shape produced by chemical compounds, certain salts, and by frost.

c., blood. One composed of hematoidin.

c., Böttcher's. SEE: *crystal, spermin.*

c., Charcot-Leyden. Found in asthmatic sputum, leukemic blood, etc. Octahedral and composed of a phosphate.

c., Charcot-Neumann. Spermin crystals found in semen and some animal tissues.

c., Charcot-Robin. A type formed in blood in leukemia.

c., spermin. Composed of spermine

phosphate and seen in prostatic fluid on addition of a drop of ammonium phosphate solution.

crystallin (kris'tăl-ĭn). Globulin of the crystalline lens.

crys'talline. Resembling crystal.

    c. deposits. ACID GROUP: Includes the urates, oxalates, carbonates, and sulfates. ALKALINE GROUP: Includes the phosphates, cholesterin, systine, ammonium urate.

    c. lens. The lens of the eye in the capsule behind the pupil. It separates the *aqueous* from the *vitreous* humor. It is transparent and refracts the rays of light, impinging them upon the surface to bring them to a focus on the retina.

crystalliza'tion. The formation of crystals.

crys'talloid. 1. Like a crystal. 2. Opposite of *colloid*; a substance capable of crystallization, which in solution can be diffused through animal membranes, and is readily soluble, *e. g.*, *salt*, *sugar*.

crystalloiditis (kris-tal-oid-i'tis). Inflammation of crystalline lens.

crystallopho'bia. Abnormal fear of glass or objects made of glass.

crys'tallose. A sweetening agent (saccharinate of sodium) said to be many times sweeter than sugar and to be used as a substitute for it.

crystalluridrosis (krist-al-ū-rĭd-ro'sis). Crystallization of urinary elements on the skin.

Cu. Symb. for *copper* (*cuprum*).

cubic measure. 1728 cubic inches (cu. in.) = 1 cubic foot (cu. ft.). 27 cubic feet = 1 cubic yard (cu. yd.).

cu'bital. Pert. to the ulna, or to the forearm.

cu'bitus. Elbow; forearm; ulna.

    c. valgus. An abnormal curvature of the humeral diaphysis; congenital or due to rickets.

    c. varus. Deformity due to fracture of either condyle of the humerus, the extended forearm deviating out from the axis of the arm; gunstock deformity; congenital.

cu'boid. Wedge-shaped.

    c. bone. *Os cuboideum.* Outer bone of tarsal or instep bones.

cucurbit (ku-ker'bit). Cupping glass.

cul-de-sac. A narrow cavity or vessel open only at 1 end, as of the eye.

    c., Douglas'. The peritoneal pouch bet. the ant. wall of the rectum and the post. wall of the uterus.

-cule, -cle. Suffix: Little, as *molecule*, *corpuscle*.

culicifuge (ku-lis'if-ūj). An agent to prevent mosquito attacks.

cul'men. Top or summit of a thing.

    c. cerebelli. Most prominent part of the vermis sup. near its ant. extremity.

cultiva'tion. Growing microörganisms in an artificial medium.

cultural (kul'tu-ral). Pert. to cultures of microörganisms.

cul'ture. BACT: A mass of microörganisms growing in laboratory culture media.

    c., blood. Used in the diagnosis of specific infectious diseases.

    c., gelatin. A culture of bacteria on gelatin.

    c., hanging block. A thin slice of agar seeded on its surface with bacteria, and then inverted on a cover slip and sealed in the concavity of a hollow glass slide. This method is used to study the mode of cell division.

    c., hanging drop. A culture accomplished by inoculating the bacterium into a drop on a cover glass, and mounting it in the depression on a concave slide.

    c. medium. A substance on which microörganisms may grow. Those most commonly used are broths, gelatin, and agar, which contain the same basic ingredients. Salt should be used in media if blood is added to them to prevent the blood from hemolyzing.

    c., negative. A culture made from suspected matter which fails to reveal the suspected organism.

    c., physical. The training of the body by means of gymnastics.

    c., positive. A culture which reveals the suspected organism.

    c., pure. The culture of a single form of microörganism uncontaminated by other organisms.

    c., stab. A bacterial culture made by thrusting into the culture medium a point inoculated with the matter under examination.

    c., stock. A permanent culture from which transfers may be made.

cu.mm. Abbr. for cubic millimeter.

cumulative (ku'mu-la-tiv). Increasing in effect.

    c. drugs. Those which, after being received into the body in small doses, often repeated, are not immediately eliminated, but tend to accumulate in the system and suddenly produce symptoms of poisoning. Carbolic acid and mercurial preparations are examples of drugs which act in this way.

cuneate (ku'ne-āt). Wedge-shaped.

    c. fasciculus, c. funiculus. Continuation of posteroexternal column of cord into the medulla.

    c. nucleus. Gray matter at end of cuneate fasciculus.

cuneiform (ku-ne'ĭ-form). Wedge-shaped bones of the tarsus, internal, middle, and external.

    c. cartilage. Cartilage along the arytenoid bone.

    c. hysterectomy. Excision of a wedge of uterine tissue.

cuneo-. Prefix: A wedge. [form bones.

cu"neocu'boid. Pert. to cuboid and cunei-

cuneohysterectomy (ku-ne-o-his-ter-ek'-to-mǐ). Excision of a wedge of tissue from the post. surface of the *cervix uteri* to correct abnormal anteflexion.

cu'neus. Wedge-shaped lobule of brain on mesial surface of occipital lobe.

cunic'ulus. Burrow in epidermis made by the itch mite.

cunnilingus (kun-nĭ-lin′gus). Application of tongue or mouth to the cunnus, *q.v.*, a practice not peculiar to either sex and also observed among various animals.

cun′nus. The vulva,* pudenda.*

cup. 1. Small drinking vessel. 2. A cupping glass.

   c. favus. Depression around a hair.

   c., glaucomatous. "Pressure excavation" of optic nerve in glaucoma.

cu′pola. The little dome at apex of cochlea and of spiral canal.

   c. space. Tympanic attic.

cupping. Application of glass vessel from which the air has been exhausted by heat or a special suction apparatus to the skin in order to draw blood to the surface.

   c., dry. Used to relieve kidney and in pneumonia to relieve congestion and pain, or to stimulate the kidneys; also to induce hyperemia in infected areas. DURATION: 10-20 minutes.

   c., wet. Application of cupping after incision of the skin. Seldom now used. The area for both forms of cupping should first be shaved and sterilized.

cu′prum. Abbr. Cu. Copper, *q.v.*

curare, curari (kū-rāh′rē). Toxic extract of *Strychnos* plant family used to paralyze motor nerve endings.

   DOSAGE: ½ gr. (0.005 Gm.).

curarization (kū″răh-rĭ-zā′shŭn). Condition following introduction of curare; eyelids heavy, nystagmus, husky voice, weak jaw and throat muscles, inability to raise head, arms, and legs.

cure. 1. Course of treatment of patients. 2. Restoration to health.

curet, curette (ku-ret′). Scraping instrument for removing foreign matter from a cavity.

curettage (ku-ret′aj). Scraping of a cavity.

   c., uterine. Scraping with a curette to remove impregnated ovum or its remnants clinging to uterine wall.

curettement (ku-ret′ment). The scraping of a part by means of a curette.

curie (ku-re′). The standard unit of quantity of radon, being the amt. in equi'ibrium with 1 Gm. of radium element.

cu′riegram. A radium photograph.

curietherapy (kū-rĭ-ther′ă-pĭ). Radium therapy.

curled. BACT: Said of parallel chains in wavy strands, such as in anthrax colonies.

cur′rant jelly clot. Post mortem, soft, red clot in heart and vessels.

cur′rent. A flow, as of water, or the transference of electrical impulses.

   c., alternating. A current which periodically flows in opposite directions.

   c., constant. SEE: *direct current*.

   c., continuous. SEE: *direct current*.

   c., cutting. Needle point or blade connected to 1 terminal of a high frequency machine producing current of undamped oscillations; large dispersive electrode is connected to other terminal.

   c., damped. An oscillating current of electricity in which the amplitude of successive alternations becomes less and less until it finally dies away.

   c., d′Arsonval direct. SEE: *diathermy*.

   c., de Watt′eville. Combined use of galvanic and faradic current made possible by use of special switch known as De Watteville switch.

   c., direct. A current that flows in 1 direction only.

   c., direct vacuum tube. A current obtained from a d.c. source by applying to the part to be treated a vacuum electrode connected to 1 terminal of the machine, the other terminal being grounded.   [*rent*.

   c., electric cutting. SEE: *cutting cur-*

   c., farad′ic. An intermittent, alternating current induced in the secondary winding of an induction coil.

   c., Frimandeau (frim-an′dō). Interrupted galvanic current obtained by use of Frimandeau coil. Is an unidirectional current.

   c., galvan′ic. A steady unidirectional current produced by chemical action in a single or multiple dry or wet cell, or obtained from a direct current lighting or power circuit ("main"), or from an alternating current circuit by the introduction of (a) motor generator, (b) rectifier, and (c) "B Battery" eliminator.

   c., grounded. Ground on earth, a part of an electric circuit.

   c., high frequency. A current having a frequency of interruption or change of direction sufficiently high so that tetanic contractions are not set up when it is passed through living contractile tissues.

   c., induced. An electric current generated in an adjacent coil by varying the magnetic field or by means of a moving magnetic field, or by motion of the coil in a fixed field.

   c., interrupted. A current which is frequently opened and closed. SEE: *interrupter*.

   c., inverse. A term used to describe current flowing through a tube in the wrong direction.

   c., Lapicque. Interrupted current of low frequency, unidirectional.

   c., leakage. SEE: *grounded current*.

   c., low frequency. An alternating current whose frequency in cycles per second is low in reference to a particular standard, such as the pitch frequency of "middle C" or, in some cases, the common frequency limit of audition.

   c., low tension. Same as low frequency currents.

   c., Morton wave. An interrupted current obtained from a static machine.

   c., os′cillating. A current alternating in direction, and of either constant or gradually decreasing amplitude.

   c., pulsating. A current pulsating regularly in magnitude. As ordinarily used, applies to a unidirectional current.

c., sinusoidal (si'nus-oid-al). SEE: *alternating current*. An alternating current following the sine law and of such frequency as to afford the opportunity of separate (clonic) muscular contractions.

c., static. Electricity produced by friction.

c., surging. Interrupted or alternating current in which the strength attained during each period of flow gradually increases to a maximum and then gradually decreases to zero.

c., undamped. An alternating current of electricity in which the amplitude of successive alternations is maintained.

c., unit of. Ampere, *q.v.*

c., Watteville. A faradic current reinforced by a constant current flowing through the secondary of the coil in the same direction as the current of break.

c., wave-o. Type of static current.

curriculum (kur-rik'u-lum). A course of study.

Curschmann's spirals (koorsh'mahnz). Coiled spirals of mucus seen in sputum of asthma, etc. SEE: *sputum*.

curtasal (kur-ta-säl'). An odorless, white, crystalline substance, composed of sodium and calcium formate, with a small amt. of magnesium citrate.

DOSAGE: To suit the taste, as a rule requiring twice the amt. of table salt.

curvature (kŭr'vă-chŭr). A bending or sloping away from a rectilinear surface, either normal or abnormal; a curve.

SEE: *kyphosis, lordosis, scoliosis.*

curve. A bend.

c. of Carus. An arc corresponding with the pelvic axis.

curvi-. Combining form, meaning curved.

Cus'co's spec'ulum. A duckbill vaginal speculum manipulated by a screw.

Cushing's disease. Degenerative state of the erythrocytes.

C.'s syndrome. A condition caused by hypopituitarism. SYN: *dystrophia adiposogenitalis.*

cusp (kusp). Point of the crown of a tooth. [crowns (canine).

cuspid (kus'pid). The 4 teeth with conic

cuspidate (kus'pĭ-dāt). Having cusps.

cuta'neous. Pert. to the skin.

c. respiration. The transpiration of gases through the skin.

c. pupillary reflex. Pupillary dilation when skin on any part of body is pinched.

c. reflex. Common gooseflesh.

cu'ticle. The outer portion of the skin; the epidermis or scarf skin; cuticula. SEE: *corium, cutis.*

cuticula (ku-tĭk'u-lă). Cuticle.

c. den'tis. A thin, transparent, dry membrane without nerves or vessels; epidermis, scarf skin.

cuticulariza'tion. Growth of epidermis over a sore or wound.

cutis (ku'tis). The derma, or true skin.

c. anserina. "Gooseflesh" caused by erection of skin papillae, as from cold or shock.

c. laxa. Dermatolysis, or hypertrophy of the skin and subcutaneous tissue.

c. pendula. Flabby skin.

c. vera. The corium*; deep layer of skin.

c. verticis gyrata. Looseness and hypertrophy of the skin which may hang in folds.

cutisector (ku-tis-ek'tor). Device for excision of skin.

cutitis (ku-ti'tis). Inflammation of skin. SYN: *dermatitis.*

cutization (kū-tĭ-za'shun). Skinlike condition of a mucous membrane as result of continued exposure.

cyanemia (si-an-e'mĭ-ă). Blue color of blood.

cyanephridrosis (si-ăn-ef-ĭ-dro'sis). Bluish sweat.

cyanide poisoning (si'an-īd). Cyanides are widely used in mining, electroplating, photography, for fumigation and in other industries. Cyanide is one of the most common and most deadly poisons known. [blue.

cyano-. Combining form, meaning *dark*

cyanochroia (si-an-o-kroi'ă). Cyanosis.

cyanoder'ma. Blue discoloration of skin. SYN: *cyanosis.*

cyanomycosis (si"an-o-mi-ko'sis). Development of blue pus due to *Micrococcus pyocyaneus.*

cyanopathy (si-an-op'ă-thĭ). Blue discoloration of skin. SYN: *cyanosis.*

cyanophil (si-an'o-fil). Blue staining substance of plants and animals.

cyanophilous (si-an-of'il-us). Having an affinity for blue dyes.

cyanopia, cyanopsia (si-an-op'ĭ-ă, -si-a). Vision in which all objects appear to be blue.

cy'anosed. Affected with cyanosis.

cyanosis (si-an-o'sis). Slightly bluish, grayish, slatelike, or dark purple discoloration of the skin.

c., congenital. Usually associated with stenosis of the pulmonary orifice, an imperfect ventricular septum, or a *patulous foramen ovale.*

c., entero'genous. Induced by intestinal absorption of toxins.

c., false. Due to abnormal pigment in the blood.

c. retinae. Bluish appearance of retina seen in congenital heart disease, polycythemia, and in certain poisonings, as dinitrobenzol.

cyanotic (si-an-ot'ik). Of the nature of, affected with, or pert. to, cyanosis.

cyasma (si-az'mă). Lenticular pigmentation of skin of pregnant women.

cyclarthrosis (si-klar-thro'sis). A lateral ginglymus or pivot joint which makes possible rotation.

cycle (sī'kl). A series of movements or events; a sequence.

c., cardiac. The series of consecutive movements through which the heart passes in performing 1 heartbeat.

cyclectomy (si-klek'to-mĭ). Excision of a portion of the ciliary body or muscle or ciliary border of eyelids.

cy′clic. Periodic.

    c. insanity. Manic depressive insanity; a form in which mania, melancholia, and sanity succeed each other at intervals; circular insanity.

cy′clical vomiting. Periodical and recurring attacks of vomiting met with in those of a nervous temperament. The condition is usually associated with acidosis.

cyclicot′omy. Cutting of the ciliary muscle.

cycli′tis. Inflammation of ciliary body.

    c., plastic. Ciliary body inflammation accompanied by that of entire uveal tract, giving rise to a fibrinous exudate in ant. chamber and vitreous.

    c., purulent. Suppurative inflammation of ciliary body and iris.

    c., serous. Simple inflammation without iritis.

cyclo-. Circle.

cycloceratitis (si-klo-ser-a-ti′tis). Inflammation of cornea and ciliary body.

cyclochoroiditis (si-klo-ko-roi-di′tis). Inflammation of ciliary body and choroid coat of eye.

cyclodial′ysis. Operation performed in certain types of glaucoma to produce communication bet. ant. chamber and suprachoroidal space for the escape of aqueous humor.

cycloduc′tion. Movement of a part, as the eyeball, produced by the oblique muscle.

cycloid (si′kloid). Extreme variations of mood from elation to melancholia.

cyclokerati′tis. Inflammation of cornea and ciliary body.

cyclomastopathy (si″klo-mas-top′ă-thĭ). Excessive tissue proliferation of the breast.

cyclophoria (si-klo-fo′rĭ-ă). Rotation of eyeball due to insufficiency of oblique muscles.

cyclople′gia. Paralysis of ciliary muscle.

cycloplegic (si-klo-ple′jik). Producing cycloplegia.

cyclople′gios. Agents which cause paralysis of ciliary muscle.

cyclopro′pane (C_3H_6). A gaseous anesthetic agent, colorless, slightly heavier than air, with a not unpleasant odor.

cyclo′sis. Movement of protoplasm and plastids within the protozoan cell.

cyclothymia (si-klo-thi′mĭ-ă). PSY: Cyclic insanity.

cyclothy′mic. Pert. to cyclothymia.

    c. personality. PSY: One in which periods of elation and sadness alternate. SYN: *syntonic.*

cyclotomy (si-klot′o-mĭ). Incision of ciliary muscle.

cyesedema (si-e-se-de′mă). Thickening of the cutis; bloating in pregnant women.

cyesiognosis (si-e-sĭ-og-no′sis). Diagnosis of pregnancy.

cyesiology (si-e-si-ol′o-gĭ). The study of pregnancy.

cyesis (si-e′sis). Pregnancy.

cyetic (si-et′ĭk). Pert. to pregnancy.

cylicotomy (sil-ik-ot′o-mĭ). To cut ciliary muscle. SYN: *cyclotomy.*

cylin″droadeno′ma. An adenoma containing cylindrical masses of hyaline material.

cylindroden′drite. Process from an axis cylinder or neuraxon. SYN: *paraxon.*

cylindroid (sil-in′droid). 1. Cylinder shaped. 2. A mucous, spurious cast in urine.

cylindro′ma. Malignant tumor containing a collection of cells forming cylinders.

cylindrosarco′ma. A tumor containing properties of cylindroma and sarcoma.

cylindruria (sil-in-dru′rĭ-ă). Cylindroids in the urine.

cyllosis (sil-o′sis). Clubfoot.

cymbocephalic (sim-bo-sef-al′ik). Having a boat-shaped head.

cynanche (sin-ang′ke). Severe sore throat.

    c. malig′na. Gangrenous sore throat.

    c. tonsilla′ris. Tonsillitis, quinsy.

cynan′thropy. Insanity in which the patient behaves like a dog.

cyn′ic spasm. Spasm of face muscles causing a grin or snarl like a dog.

cynobex (sin′o-beks). Dry, barking cough.

cynophobia (sin-o-fo′bĭ-ă). Unreasonable fear of dogs. SYN: *lyssophobia.*

cynorex′ia. Morbid appetite, bulimia.*

Cyon's experiment (si′onz). A stimulus to an intact ant. spinal nerve root resulting in a stronger muscle contraction than the same stimulus to the peripheral end of a divided nerve root.

    C.'s nerve. A filament of the vagus; depressor nerve of heart.

cyophoria (si-o-fo′rĭ-ă). Pregnancy.

cyopho′ric. Pert. to pregnancy.

cyotrophy (si-ot′ro-fĭ). Nourishment of the fetus.

cypridopathy (sĭ″pri-dop′ă-thĭ). Any venereal disease.

cypridophobia (si″pri-do-fo′bĭ-ă). 1. Morbid fear of venereal disease. 2. Abnormal fear of the sexual act. 3. False belief of having a venereal disease.

cypriphobia (sip-rĭ-fo′bĭ-ă). Morbid aversion to and fear of coitus.

cyrtometer (sir-tom′et-er). Instrument for measuring circumference of chest and comparison of chest curves.

cyrtosis (sir-to′sis). Having any abnormal curvature of the spine.

cyst (sist). 1. A bladder. 2. Any sac containing a liquid.

    c., adventitious. Cyst formation around a foreign body.   [*toma.*

    c., blood. Bloody tumor. SYN: *hema-*

    c., Boyer's. Subhyoid bursal cyst.

    c., chocolate. Ovarian cyst with darkly pigmented gelatinous content.

    c., colloid. Cyst with gelatinous contents.

    c., daughter. Cyst growing out of the walls of another cyst.

    c., dentigerous. One containing teeth. SYN: *follicular odontoma.*

    c., dermoid. One containing elements of hair, teeth, or skin.

    c., extravasation. Cyst arising from hemorrhage into tissues.

    c., follicular. Cyst arising from occlusion of small follicle or gland.

c., Gaertner's. Cyst of the remnants of the Wolffian duct.

c., intraligamentary. Cystic formation bet. the leaves of the broad ligament.

c., mucous. Retention cyst composed of mucus.

c., nabothian. Cystic formation caused by closure of the ducts of the nabothian glands in the cervix uteri by the healing of an erosion.

c., ovarian. Cystic formation in the ovary. SEE: *ovary.*

c., paraovarian. Cystic formation of the paraovarium.

c., piliferous. Same as dermoid cyst. Tumors made up of all 3 primary germ layers and containing hair, teeth, bone, sebaceous material, and skin.

c., retention. One retaining the secretion of a gland, as in a mucous or sebaceous cyst.

c., sebaceous. One of a sebaceous gland.

c., seminal. Cyst composed of semen.

c., unilocular. Cyst containing only 1 cavity.

c., vaginal. Cystic formation in the vagina.

cystadenoma (sist-ad-en-o′mă). An adenoma containing cysts. Cystoma blended with adenoma.

cystalgia (sis-tal′jĭ-ă). Paroxysms of pain in the bladder.

cystatro′phia. Atrophy of bladder.

cystauchenotomy (sis-taw-ken-ot′o-mĭ). Incision into the neck of bladder.

cystectasy (sis-tek′tă-sĭ). 1. An operation for extracting calculus from the bladder by dividing the membranous portion of the urethra, and then dilating neck of bladder. 2. Dilatation of bladder.

cystectomy (sis-tek′to-mĭ). Excision of cystic duct.

cysteine (sist′e-in). A sulfur-containing amino acid, beta-thio alpha-amino propionic acid, $C_3H_7NSO_2$, found among the decomposition products of proteins.

cyster′ethism. Irritability of the bladder; vesical irritation.

cysthitis (sis-thi′tis). Inflammation of the vulva.

cysthus (sis′thus). 1. Vulva. 2. Anus.

cysthypersarcosis (sist-hi-per-sar-ko′sis). Hypertrophy of muscular coat of the bladder. [bladder.

cys′tic. Pert. to a cyst, or to the urinary

c. duct. The duct of the gallbladder which unites with the hepatic duct from the liver to form the common bile duct.

c. tumor. Tumor composed of cysts.

cysticercosis (sis-tĭ-ser-ko′sis). Infestation by larva *Taenia solium.*

cysticercus (sis-tis-er′kus). Encysted larvae of tapeworms.

cysticolithectomy (sis″tĭ-ko-lĭ-thek′to-mĭ). Removal of an impacted stone from the cystic duct.

cysticorrhaphy (sis-tĭ-kor′ră-fĭ). Suture of the cystic duct.

cysticotomy (sis-tĭ-kot′o-mĭ). Incision of cystic bile duct. SYN: *choledochotomy.*

cystidolaparotomy (sis″ti-do-lap″ar-ot′o-mĭ). Incision into bladder through abdomen after abdominal section.

cystidotrachelotomy (sis″tĭ-do-tra″ke-lot′-o-mĭ). Incision into neck of bladder. SYN: *cystauchenotomy.**

cystifelleotomy (sis″tĭ-fel-e-ot′o-mĭ). Incision of gallbladder through abdominal walls. SYN: *cholecystotomy.*

cys′tiform. Having the form of a cyst; cystic; cystoid.

cystigerous (sis-tij′er-us). Containing cysts.

cystin(e ($C_9H_{12}N_2S_2O_4$). A sulfur-containing amino acid, which can be obtained by oxidation from cysteine and which is likewise obtained from proteins.

cystinemia (sis-tĭ-ne′mĭ-ă). Supposititious presence of cystine in the blood.

cystinuria (sis-tĭn-u′rĭ-ă). Cystine in the urine, seen in jaundice and hepatic disease.

cyst′is. 1. A cyst. 2. A bladder.

cystistax′ia. Blood oozing from the mucous membrane of the bladder.

cystitis (sis-ti′tis). Symptomatic inflammation of the bladder of 2 types: Nonbacterial (trauma, chemicals), and bacterial (acute or chronic, superficial, interstitial, or complicated by pericystitis).

c. cystica and **granulosa.** *Chronic:* Slight frequency of urination. Leukoplakia: Chronic pyuria and painful irritation, perhaps hematuria.

c., ulcerative. Aside from tuberculosis, carcinoma, syphilis, there are elusive ulcer (violent chronic irritation of bladder without gross evidence of cystitis), solitary ulcer, incrusted ulceration (bacterial, causing intense cystitis)

cystitome (sis′tĭ-tōm). Instrument for incision into sac of crystalline lens.

cystit′omy. 1. Incision of capsule of crystalline lens. 2. Incision into the gallbladder.

cysto-. Prefix: Pert. to the urinary bladder.

cystoadenoma (sis″to-ad-en-o′mă) A tumor containing cystic and aderomatous elements.

cystobubonocele (sis-to-bu-bo′no-sēl). Hernia involving the bladder.

cystocarcino′ma. Glandular tumor distended with fluid secretion of the gland.

cystocele (sis′to-sēl). A bladder hernia.

cystocolos′tomy. Formation of communication bet. the gallbladder and colon.

cystodiaphanoscopy (sis″to-di-ă-fan-os′ko-pĭ). Transillumination of abdomen by an electric light in bladder.

cystodyn′ia. Paroxysmal pains in the bladder. SYN: *cystalgia.*

cystoelytroplasty (sis″to-el′ĭ-tro-plas-tĭ). Repair of a vesicovaginal fistula.

cystoenterocele (sis″to-en′ter-o-sēl). Protrusion of a portion of the bladder and intestine.

cystoepiplocele (sis″to-ĕ-pĭp′lo-sēl). Protrusion of a portion of the bladder and the omentum.

cystoepithelio′ma. Epithelioma in stage of cystic degeneration.

cystofelleotomy (sis-to-fel-e-ot'o-mĭ). Incision of gallbladder through abdominal wall. SEE: *cholecystotomy.*

cystofibro'ma. Fibrous tumor containing cysts.

cystogram (sis'to-gram). A radiographic film of the bladder.

cystography (sis-tog'ră-fĭ). Making radiographs of the bladder.

cys'toid. Bladderlike.

cystolith (sis'to-lith). A vesical calculus.

cystolithectomy (sis-to-lith-ek'to-mĭ). Excision of a stone from the bladder.

cystolithiasis (sis-to-lĭ-thi'ă-sis). Calculi in the bladder.

cystolith'ic. Pert. to a vesical calculus.

cystolutein (sis-to-lu'te-in). Yellow coloring matter in cysts.

cysto'ma (pl. *cysto'mata, cysto'mas*). A cystic tumor; a growth containing cysts.

cystom'eter. Device for estimating the capacity of the bladder and its pressure reactions.

cystomor'phous. Cystlike; cystoid.

cystomyxoadenoma (sis"to-mik"so-ad-en-o'mă). Myxoma and adenoma with cystic degeneration.

cystomyxo'ma. Myxoma with cystic formation.

cystonephro'sis. Cystiform dilatation of kidney tubules.

cystoneural'gia. Neuralgia of the bladder or pain without apparent cause; cystalgia.

cystoparaly'sis. Paralysis of bladder.

cys'topexy. Surgical fixation of bladder to wall of abdomen.

cystophotog'raphy. Taking pictures of interior of bladder.

cystoplasty (sis'to-plas-tĭ). Plastic operation upon the bladder.

cystoplegia (sis-to-ple'jĭ-ă). Paralysis of the bladder.

cystopto'sia, cystopto'sis. Prolapse into the urethra of the vesical mucous membrane.

cystopyelitis (sis-to-pi-e-li'tis). Cystitis with pyelitis.

cystopyelonephritis (sis-to-pi-e-lo-nef-ri'tis). Inflammation of urinary bladder, kidney, and pelvis of kidney.

cystoradiog'raphy. Radiography of the gall- or urinary bladder.

cystorectostomy (sis-to-rek-tos'to-mĭ). Making a surgical communication bet. the bladder and rectum.

cystorrha'gia. Hemorrhage from the urinary bladder.   [bladder.

cystorrhaphy (sist-or'ă-fĭ). Suture of

cystorrhe'a. A discharge of mucus from the urinary bladder.

cystosarco'ma. Sarcoma containing cysts.

cystoscope (sist'o-skōp). Instrument for interior examination of bladder.

cystoscopy (sis-tos'ko-pĭ). Examination of the bladder with the cystoscope.

cys'tospasm. Spasmodic contractions of the urinary bladder.

cystospermitis (sis-to-sperm-i'tis). Inflammation of seminal vesicles.

cystos'tomy. Surgical incision into the bladder.

cystotome (sist'o-tōm). Knife for incision of bladder.

cystotomy (sist-ot'o-mĭ). Incision of bladder.

cystotrachelotomy (sis-to-trak-e-lot'o-mĭ). Incision into neck of bladder. SYN: *cystauchenotomy.*

cystoureteritis (sis-to-u-re-ter-i'tis). Inflammation of ureter and urinary bladder.

cystoureterogram (sĭst"o-ū-rē'tĕr-ō-grăm). A picture of the bladder and ureter.

cystoure'throscope. Device for examining the post. urethra and urinary bladder.

cytarrhagia (sit-ar-ra'jĭ-ă). Hemorrhage from socket of a tooth.

cytase (si'tās). A ferment in phagocytes.

cyto-. Indicating the cell.

cytoarchitectonic (si"to-ark-ĭ-tek-ton'ĭk). Pert. to structure and arrangement of cells.

cytobiology (si-to-bi-ol'o-jĭ). Biology of cells.

cytobiotax'is. Grouping and apparent coöperation bet. embryonic cells. SYN: *cytoclesis.*

cy'toblast. A cell nucleus. SEE: *cyton.*

cytoblaste'ma. Supposititious mother liquid of cells.

cytocan'nibalism. Absorption of 1 cell by another cell.

cytocentrum (si-to-sen'trum). Sphere of attraction.

cytoceras'tic. Pert. to cells changing to a higher form.

cytochemism (si-to-kem'izm). Reaction of body cells to chemical agents or the injections of antitoxin.

cytochem'istry. The chemistry of the living cell.

cytochrome (sĭ'to-krōm). 1. A pigment in the muscles and other tissues, receiving and giving off oxygen. 2. A nerve cell having only traces of a body with a nucleus.

cytochylema (si-to-ki-le'mă). The more fluid constituent of cell protoplasm.

cytoci'dal. Destructive of living cells.

cytocide (si'to-sīd). That which destroys cells.

cytoclas'tic. Destructive to cells.

cytoclesis (si-to-kle'sis). The apparent coöperation of cells with each other. SYN: *cytobiotaxis.*

cytocyst (si'to-sist). The remains of a cell enclosing a mature schizont.

cytode (si'tōd). A cell, esp. a nonnucleated cell, or a mass of protoplasm.

cytoden'drite. A dendrite given off from the body of a nerve cell.

cytodiagno'sis. Diagnosis by examination of the contents of an exudating cell.

cytodieresis (si-to-di-er'e-sis). Cell division, amitosis or mitosis.

cytodistal (si-to-dis'tal). Pert. to a neoplasm remote from the cell of origin.

cytofin (si'to-fin). An alloxur body allied to a purine formed by thymic acid.

cytogenesis (si-to-jen'es-is). Origin and development of the cell.

cytogenous (si-toj'en-us). Cell forming, esp. those of connective tissue.

cytoglobin (si-to-glo'bĭn). A globin from lymphocytes and leukocytes.

cytoglycopenia (si-to-gli-ko-pe'nĭ-ă). Deficient glucose of blood cells.

cytog'ony. The formation of the cell.

cytohistogen'esis. The structural development of cells.

cytohyaloplasm (si-to-hi'al-o-plazm). Reticular network of protoplasm.

cytoid (si'toid). Resembling a cell.

cytoinhibition (si"to-in-hi-bish'un). Phagocytic cell action in preventing the lysis of bacteria.

cytokeras'tic. Pert. to cellular development.

cytokine'sis. Changes in cellular protoplasm outside of the nucleus during mitosis.

cytology (si-tol'o-gĭ). The science of cell life and cell formation.

cytolymph (si'to-limf). Matrix of cytoplasm of cells.

cytolysin (si-tol'is-in). That which produces disintegration of cells.

cytol'ysis. Dissolution of cells by specific amboceptors and complements.

cytomachia (si-to-mak'ĭ-ă). Cellular activities and resistance during infection by microörganisms.

cytometaplasia (si"to-met-ă-pla'zĭ-ă). Change of form or function of cells.

cytometer (si-tom'et-er). Instrument for estimating cells.

cytom'etry. The counting and measuring of cells.

cytomicrosome (si-to-mik'ro-sōm). Minute granules in the protoplasm (cytoplasm) of the cell.

cytom'itome. Any part of the network of the cytoplasm.

cytomorphol'ogy. The study of the structure of cells.

cytomorphosis (si-to-mor-fo'sis). The cellular transformations resulting from senescence or senile changes.

cyton (si'ton). 1. A cell. 2. The body of a nerve cell; also called perikaryon.

cytopathology (si"to-păth-ŏl'ŏ-jĭ). Study of the cellular changes in disease.

cytope'nia. Diminution in cellular elements of blood.

cytophagocyto'sis. Destruction of other cells by phagocytes.

cytophagous (si-tof'ag-us). Devouring or destructive of cells.

cytophagy (si-tof'aj-ĭ). Cell destruction by phagocytes. Syn: *cytophagocytosis.*•

cytophil(e (si'to-fĭl). Having an affinity for or attracted by cells.

cytophylaxis (si-to-fĭ-lak'sis). The protection of cells against lysis.

cytophylet'ic. Pert. to genealogy of cells.

cytophys'ics. The physics of cellular activity.

cytophysiol'ogy. Physiology of the cell.

cytoplasm, cytoplasma (si'to-plazm, -plaz'-ma). 1. Protoplasm. 2. Cell plasm not including the nucleus.

cytoplas'tin. The plastin substance of the cytoplasm.

cytoproximal (si-to-proks'im-al). Pert. to a nerve fibril or axis cylinder nearest to the cell of origin.

cytoreticulum (si-to-ret-ik'u-lum). The fibrillar network supporting fluid of protoplasm.

cytoscopy (si-tos'kop-ĭ). Microscopic examination of cells.

cytosome (si'to-sōm). The cell body without its nucleus.

cytospongium (si-to-spun'jĭ-um). The network of a cell containing the fluid portion of protoplasm.

cytost (si'tost). A specific toxin from an injured cell.

cytostasis (si-tos'tă-sis). Stasis of white blood corpuscles, as in incipient stage of inflammation.

cytostromatic (si-to-stro-mat'ĭk). Pert. to the cellular stroma.   [taxia.

cytotactic (si-to-tak'tik). Pert. to cyto-

cytotax'ia, cytotax'is. Attraction or repulsion of cells for each other.

cytother'apy. Treatment by use of glandular extracts; organotherapy.

cytoth'esis. Restoration or repair of injured cells.

cytotoxin (si-to-toks'in). An exotoxin that attacks different organs and tissues, produced by injection of foreign cells.

cytotropic (si-to-trop'ik). Having an affinity for cells.

cytozo'ic. Living within or attached to a cell, as certain protozoa.

cytozyme (si'to-zīm). A supposed substance which produces thrombokinase.

cytrophoblast (sī-tro'fo-blast). A cuboidal cell composing an inner layer resulting from differentiation of trophoblasts; the outer layer being the plasmotrophoblasts. Syn: *Langhans' cells.*

cytula (si'tū-lă). The impregnated ovum.

cyturia (si-tu'rĭ-ă). Presence of any kind of cells in the urine.

Czermak's spaces (chăr'măks). The interglobular spaces in dentine because of failure of calcification.

Czerny-Lembert suture (chăr-nĭ-lam-bār'). An intestinal suture in 2 rows.

Czerny operation (chăr'nĭ). A radical hernia operation.

D

D. Abbr. for *da, detur*, let there be given; for *dexter*, right; in optics, for *diopter;* in dentistry, for *deciduous*. SYMB: For Vitamin D potency.

Da Costa's disease. Retrocedent gout.

dacrocystitis (dak″ro-sis-ti′tis). Inflammation of the lacrimal (tear) sac.

dacryadenal′gia. Pain in a lacrimal gland.

dacryadeni′tis. Inflammation of a lacrimal gland.

dacryadenoscirrhus (dak-rĭ-ad-en-o-skĭr′us). Induration of a lacrimal gland.

dacryagoatresia (dak′rĭ-a-gog-ă-tre′sĭ-ă). Occlusion of a tear duct.

dacryagogue (dak′rĭ-ă-gog). 1. A lacrimal duct. 2. That which stimulates the secretion of a lacrimal duct.

dacrycystal′gia. Pain in a lacrimal gland; dacryocystalgia.

dacryelcosis (dak-rĭ-el-ko′sis). Ulceration of the lacrimal apparatus.

dacryoadenal′gia. Dacryadenalgia; pain in a lacrimal gland.

dacryoadenitis (dak-rĭ-o-ad-en-i′tis). Inflammation of lacrimal gland.

dacryoblennorrhe′a. Discharge of mucus from a lacrimal sac, and chronic inflammation of the sac.

dacryocele (dak′rĭ-o-sēl). Protrusion of a lacrimal sac.

dacryocyst (dak′rĭ-o-sist). The lacrimal (tear) sac.

dacryocystalgia (dak-rĭ-o-sis-tal′jĭ-ă). Pain in the lacrimal sac.

dacryocystec′tomy. The excision of membranes of the lacrimal sac.

dacryocystitis (dak-rĭ-o-sis-ti′tis). Inflammation of the tear sac involving mucous membrane of the lacrimal sac, together with submucous membrane.

dacryocystoblennorrhea (dak-rĭ-o-sis″to-blen-or-re′ă). Chronic blennorrhea of the lacrimal sac.

dacryocystocele (dak-rĭ-o-sis′to-sēl). Protrusion of lacrimal sac.

dacryocystopto′sis. Prolapse of the lacrimal (tear) sac.

dacryocystorrhinostomy (dak-rĭ-o-sis-tor-rin-os′to-mĭ). Lumen of tear sac brought into direct communication with nasal cavity.

dacryocystosyringotomy (dak″rĭ-o-sis″to-sĭr-in-jot′ō-mĭ). Making an opening bet. the lacrimal sac and the nasal cavity.

dacryocystotome (dak-rĭ-o-sis′to-tōm). Device for incision of lacrimal sac.

dacryocystot′omy. Incision of the lacrimal sac.

dacryohemorrhea (dak″rĭ-o-hem-o-re′ă). Shedding of bloody tears.

dac′ryolin. An albuminous matter in tears.

dac′ryolite, dac′ryolith. Concretion in lacrimal passages.

dacryoma (dak-rĭ-o′mă). 1. A lacrimal tumor. 2. Obstruction of lacrimal puncta producing epiphora.

dacryon (dak′rĭ-on). The lacrimal point of juncture of the lacrimal, frontal, and upper maxillary bones.

dacryops (dak′rĭ-ops). Constant flow of tears; dacryorrhea.

dacryopyorrhea (dak″rĭ-o-pi-o-re′ă). Discharge of pus from lacrimal duct.

dacryopyo′sis. Suppuration in the lacrimal sac or duct.

dacryorrhe′a. Excessive flow of tears.

dacryosolenitis (dak″rĭ-o-so-len-i′tis). Inflammation of a lacrimal or nasal duct.

dacryosteno′sis. Stricture of a lacrimal or nasal duct.

dacryosyr′inx. A lacrimal fistula.

dactyl (dak′til). A finger or toe; a digit of the hand or foot.

dactyl′ion. Adhesions bet. or union of fingers or toes.

dactyli′tis. Chronic disease of bones of fingers and toes in very young children.

dactylocampsodynia (dak″tĭ-lo-kamp″so-din′ĭ-ă). Painful contraction of 1 or more fingers.

dactyl′ogram. A fingerprint.

dactylog′raphy. 1. The study of fingerprints. 2. The act of using a machine for blind deaf mutes to convey by touch the signs of speech.

dactylogryposis (dak-tĭ-lo-grĭ-po′sis). Permanent contraction of the fingers.

dactylology (dak-til-ol′o-jĭ). Representing words by signs made with the fingers.

dactylomeg′aly. Abnormal size of fingers and toes.

dactylos′copy. Examination of fingerprints for purpose of identification.

dactylospasm (dak′til-o-spazm). Cramp of a finger or toe.

dactylus (dak′ti-lus). A toe or finger.

Dakin's solution. A solution for cleansing wounds.

daltonism (dawl′ton-izm). Color blindness.

dam. A thin sheet of rubber to protect cavities or the field of dental operation from fluids.

damp (damp). 1. Moist, humid. 2. A noxious gas.

   d., after-. Air with large per cent of carbon dioxide.

   d., black, choke. A gas formed by oxygen and the giving off of carbon dioxide by the coal.

   d., cold. Vapor charged with carbon dioxide.

   d., fire. Methane, CH_4, found in coal mines.

   d., stink. Hydrogen sulfide.

   d., white. Carbon monoxide.

damped oscilla′tion. A current alternating in direction and of gradually decreasing amplitude. SEE: *current, oscillating*.

damping. The steady diminution of the

amplitude of successive vibrations, as of an electric wave or current.

dance, St. Vitus'. A disease characterized by involuntary and irregular jerkings and movements in diverse groups of muscles. SEE: *chorea.*

Dan'ce's sign. Slight retraction in the right iliac region in some cases of intussusception.

dan'cing disease. Epidemic dancing mania of Italy, supposed to have been caused by the bite of the tarantula. SEE: *tarantism.*

  d. mania. Epidemic chorea.

dan'druff (*dermatitis seborrheica*). Exfoliation of the epidermis of the scalp in the form of dry, white scales which fall. Scalp scurvy. Sometimes due to seborrhea.*

dandy fever (dan'dĭ). Dengue. An acute, epidemic, febrile disease occurring in southern U. S. and East and West Indies.

Danielssen's disease. Anesthetic leprosy.

d'Arsonvalism (ar-son-val'izm). Obsolete term indicating the employment of d'Arsonval current therapeutically.

d'Arsonvalization (ar-son-val-iz-a'shun). The employment of the d'Arsonval current in the form of autocondensation, autoconduction, or the direct biterminal method. SEE: *diathermy.*

dartoid (dar'toid). Resembling the *tunica dartos* in its slow, involuntary contractions.

dar'tos. The muscular, contractile tissue beneath the skin of the scrotum.*

  d. muscle reflex. Wormlike contraction of dartos muscle following sudden cold application to perineum.

dartre (dar'tr). Any chronic skin disease.

dar'trous. Of the nature of herpes; herpetic.

darwin'ian ear. Congenital deformity of the ear in which the helix is absent at upper angle.

  d. tubercle. A blunt point projecting from upper part of the helix.

dasetherapy (das-e-ther'ă-pĭ). Treatment of disease by residence in a region of pine and spruce trees.

dasym'eter. Device for estimating density of gases.

daturine (da-tu'rin). The active principle of stramonium. A poisonous alkaloid. USES: Manias, epilepsy, as a hypnotic in insanity, etc. Action resembles atropine, *q.v.*

daughter cell. One formed by the division of a mother cell.

  d. cyst. A small cyst growing out of the walls of a large cyst.

  d. nucleus. Formation of a new nucleus by a diaster.

  d. star. Double star found during mitosis. SYN: *amphiaster.*

  d. wreath. Daughter star seen from its surface view.

Davidson's reflex (dāv'ĭd-son). Light reflected through pupillary area when diagnostic light bulb is held in closed mouth.   [bright light.

day blind'ness. Inability to see well in a

de-. Prefix: Down or from.

deacidifica'tion. Neutralization of acidity.

deactiva'tion. The process of becoming inactive.

deaf mute. A deaf and dumb person.

deaf-mut'ism. The state of being both deaf and dumb.

deafness. Loss of ability to hear, complete or partial.

  d., bass. Inability to hear some of the low tones.

  d., cerebral. Due to brain lesion.

  d., cortical. Deafness due to disease of the cortical centers.

  d., mind. SEE: *psychic deafness.*

  d., occupational. That which is caused by working in places where noise is very deafening.

  d., psychic. Condition in which auditory sensations persist, but due to lesions in auditory centers the sounds are not comprehended.

  d., simulated. Malingering.

  d., tone. Inability to distinguish musical sounds.

  d., word. SEE: *psychic deafness.*

dealbation (de-al-ba'shun). Bleaching.

deamidiza'tion. The decomposition of amino acids.

deam'inase. An enzyme which causes deamidization.

de"amina'tion. Removing of amino group — NH₂ from an amino-body. SYN: *deaminization, q.v.*

deamination (de-am-in-i-za'shun). A chemical decomposition whereby substances like the amino acids and alkaloids lose their amino groups and form ammonia.

deanesthe'siant. That which will overcome anesthesia.

deaquation (de-ă-kwa'shun). Removal of water from anything; dehydration.

dearterializa'tion. Changing character of arterial into venous blood; deoxygenation.

death. Cessation of life.

  d., black. A term given to death from the plague.

  d., local. Gangrene or necrosis of a part.

  d., molar. SEE: *local death.*

  d., molecular. That of cell life.

  d. rate. This is the number of deaths occurring per 1000 of the population in a given area within a specified time.

  d. rattle. Sound heard in the throat of the dying.

  d., somatic. That of the entire organism.

debil'itant. 1. A remedy used to reduce excitement. 2. That which weakens.

debil'itate. To produce weakness or debility.

debil'ity. Weakness of tonicity in functions or organs of the body. SEE: *cataphrenia.*

debouchement (da-boosh-mon'). Opening or emptying into another part.

Debove's membrane (de-bōvz'). Layer of connective tissue cells bet. the epithelium and basement tissue of mucous membranes of air passages and intestinal mucosa.

débridement (da-bred-mon'). 1. Enlargement of a wound in operating. 2. Slitting of a constricting band of tissue.

deca-, dec-. Prefix: Ten.

decagram (dek'a-gram). A weight of 10 Gm. or 154.34 gr.

decalcifica'tion. Loss of lime salts in bone.

decal'cify. To soften bone by removal of calcium or its salts by acids.

decaliter (dek'a-le-ter). A measure of 10 liters; 610.28 cu. in.

decalvant (de-kal'vant). Destroying hair or making bald.

decameter (dek'am-e-ter). A measure of 10 meters; 393.71 in.

decanormal (dek-ă-nor'mal). Pert. to a solution 10 times as strong as a normal one.

decant'. To pour off liquid so the sediment remains in the bottom of the container.

de''canta'tion. The gentle pouring off of a liquid from its sediment.

decapita'tion. Separating the head of the fetus from the trunk to facilitate delivery.   [an organ.

decapsula'tion. Removal of a capsule of

decarboxylation, decarboxylization (de-kar-boks-il-a'shun, -i-za'shun). A chemical decomposition whereby substances like the amino acids lose their carboxyl (COOH) groups; the example of histidine is given under *aporrhegma.*

decay'. Decomposition of refuse organic matter by oxygen in the air; bacteria hastens the process. SEE: *cementoclasia, chemolysis.*

decerebra'tion. Removal of the brain.

dechlorina'tion. Removal of salt in a diet. SYN: *dechlorization.*

dechloriza'tion. Reduction or removal of salt in a diet.

dechlorura'tion. Decrease in chlorates excreted in the urine produced by diet. SYN: *dechlorization.*

decholesterolization (de-ko-les-ter-o-li-za'shun). Reducing cholesterol from the system.

decholin (dek'o-lin). An oxidation product of cholic acid, derived from ox bile. Recommended to be used in chronic cholecystitis and as a diuretic.

     DOSAGE: 3¾-7½ gr. (0.25-0.5 Gm.).

deci-. Prefix: *Decimus,* tenth.

decibel (des'ĭ-bel). The unit of intensity and volume of sound.

decidua (de-sid'u-ă). The name given to the endometrium or mucous membrane when conception occurs and which envelops the impregnated ovum.

     d. basalis (*serotina*). That part of the decidua which unites with the chorion to form the placenta.

     d. capsularis (*reflexa*). That part of the decidua which surrounds the ovum.

     d. graviditatis. The pregnancy decidua.

     d. menstrualis. The decidualike reaction in the endometrium that occurs during the premenstrual stage.

     d. reflexa. Same as capsularis.

     d. serotina. Part of the internal wall to which the ovum is attached.

     d. vera. The true decidua that is present throughout the entire endometrium during gestation. SEE: *caducous membrane.*

decidual (de-sid'u-al). Pert. to or resembling the decidua.

decidualitis (de-sid-u-al-i'tis). A bacterial infection of the decidua.

deciduation (de-sid-u-a'shun). The loss of the decidua during menstruation.

deciduitis (de-sid-u-i'tis). Inflammation of the decidua.

deciduoma (de-sid-u-o'ma). A tumor arising from fetal elements (chorion) and not derived from the decidua.

     d., benign. The more or less normal invasion of the uterine musculature by the syncytium which disappears after the gestation is completed.

     d., malignant. A tumor consisting of syncytial and Langhans cells which have a tendency to invade the general system by means of the blood stream, and having a high mortality.

deciduomatosis (de-sid-u-o-mă-to'sis). Excessive and irregular formation of decidual tissue in the nonpregnant state.

deciduosarco'ma. Chorioma malignum; a tumor of the chorion.

deciduous (de-sid'u-us). Falling off.

     d. teeth. The milk teeth or temporary teeth, 10 in each jaw; 4 incisors, 2 canines, and 4 molars. They usually appear at 6 months and fall out at the end of 6 years. Those of the lower jaw appear before the upper ones, as follows: *Lower central incisors,* at 6-9 months. *Upper incisors,* at 8-10 months. *Lower lateral incisors and first molars,* at 15-21 months. Canines, at 16-20 months. Second molars, at 20-24 months. SEE: *dentition.*

decigram (des'ig-ram). One-tenth of a gram, about 1.54 gr.

deciliter (des'ĭ-li-ter). One-tenth of a liter; 6.1 cu. in.

decimeter (des'im-e-ter). One-tenth of a meter; 3.93 in.   [ard strength.

decinor'mal. Having one-tenth the stand-

declinator (dek'lin-a-tor). Instrument used during trephining for holding apart the dura mater.

decline (de-klin'). 1. Progressive decrease. 2. Declining period of a disease.

decli'vis cerebel'li. Sloping post. portion of the monticulus of the sup. vermis of the cerebellum.

decoc'tion. A liquid preparation made by boiling vegetable substances with water.

decollation (de''kol-a'shun). Fetal decapitation. SYN: *detruncation.*

decollator (de'kol-ă-ter). Device for decapitation of the fetus.

décollement (de-kol-mon'). Separation of 2 normally adherent structures.

decompensa'tion. Failure of compensation, as in circulation of the heart.

decom'plementize. To take away the complement from.

decomposition (de-com-po-zish'un). 1. The putrefactive process; decay. 2. Reducing a compound body to its simpler constituents. See: *fermentation, resolution.*

d., double. A chemical change in which the molecules of 2 interacting compounds exchange a portion of their constituents.

d., hydrolytic. 1. Chemical change in substances due to addition of 1 molecule. 2. Complete dissolution of water, more or less.

d., simple. A chemical change by which a molecule of a single compound breaks into its simpler constituents or substitutes the entire molecule of another body for 1 of these constituents.

decompres'sion. The removal of pressure, as from gas in the intestinal tract. See: *Wangensteen's method.*

decortica'tion. Section of a rib or ribs for expansion or rest of a lung.

dec'rement. Declining period of a disease.

decrep'itate. To cause decrepitation or a crackling noise.

decrepita'tion. A crackling noise.

decrepitude (de-krep'ĭ-tud). Senile breaking down.

decubation (dé-ku-ba'shun). 1. The act of lying down. 2. The recovery stage of an infectious disease.

decu'bital. Pert. to a bedsore.

decubitus (de-ku'bi-tus). 1. A bedsore.* 2. A patient's position in bed. See: *Andral's decubitus.*

d., acute. Bedsore due to presence of cerebral lesions.

decussate (de-kus'at). To cross, or crossed, as in the form of the letter *x*. Interlacing or crossing of parts.

decussa'tion. 1. A crossing of structures in form of an x. 2. The place of crossing; chiasma.

d. of the pyramids. Crossing of fibers of pyramids of the medulla oblongata from 1 pyramid to the other.

decussorium (de-kus-o'rĭ-um). Instrument for depression of the dura following trephining.

deep reflexes (dēp). Opposite of superficial or skin reflexes; reflexes within, or fractional stretch reflexes.

deer fly. A biting fly which carries *Bacterium tularense* to man.

d. f. malady. Fever transmitted to man from rodents bitten by fly or other insects, or by direct contact. Syn: *tularemia.**

defatiga'tion. Extreme fatigue; exhaustion; weariness.

defat'ted. Deprived of fat.

defecalgesiophobia (def"e-kal-je-sĭ-o-fo'bĭ-ă). Fear of defecating because of pain.

defecation (def-e-ka'shun). Evacuation of the bowels.

defec'tive. 1. Not perfect. 2. A person deficient in 1 or more physical, mental, or moral powers.

defensive protein. An antibody, *q.v.*

d. reflex. Retraction or tension in defense against an action or threatened action.

def'erens. Ductus or *vas deferens.*

deferent (def'er-ent). Away from or downward. See: *afferent, efferent.*

d. duct. Vas deferens.

deferentectomy (def-ér-en-tek'to-mĭ). Cutting of the *vas deferens.*

deferential (def-er-en'shal). Pert. to or accompanying the ductus deferens.

deferentitis (def-er-en-ti'tis). Inflammation of the *vas deferens.*

deferred' shock. Delayed onset of symptoms of shock.

deferves'cence. The period that marks the subsidence of fever to normal temperature.

defibrina'tion, defibriniza'tion. Process of being deprived of fibrin. See: *coagulation.*

defi'ciency. A lack, something missing.

d. disease. One due to lack of essential constituents in the diet, such as vitamins, or one due to defective metabolism.

defi'ning power, defini'tion. The power of a lens to give a clear image.

defin'itive. Clear and final; without question.

deflagra'tion. Sudden, sharp combustion usually with a crackling sound.

defloration (def-lo-ra'shun). The destruction of the hymen.

defluvium (dē-flu'vĭ-um). Falling out of the hair.

defluxion (de-fluk'shun). A flowing down; copious discharge or loss of any kind.

deforma'tion. The act of deforming; a disfiguration.

deform'ities. If present after injury, usually imply presence of fracture or dislocation, or both.

deform'ity. An unnatural alteration in the form of a part or organ. Distortion of any part or general disfigurement of the body. It may be acquired or congenital.

d., anterior. Abnormal ant. convexity of the spine. Syn: *lordosis.**

d., gunstock. One in which the forearm when extended makes an angle with the arm, because of displacement of axis of the extended arm.

d., Madelung's. Distortion of the radius at its lower end, with ulnar displacement backward.

d., seal fin. Outward deflection of the fingers in rheumatoid arthritis.

d., silver-fork. The peculiar deformity seen in Colles' fracture.

d., Sprengel's. Congenital upward displacement of the scapula.

d., Velpeau's. Silver-fork deformity, *q.v.*

d., Volkmann's. Congenital tibiotarsal dislocation.

defunda'tion. Excision of the uterine fundus.

defurfura'tion. Shedding of epidermis in scales; branny desquamation.

Deg. Abbr. for *degeneration* or *degree.*

degan'glionate. To deprive of ganglia.

degen'erate. 1. A sexual prevert; loosely

applied to a low mental or moral type. 2. To deteriorate.

degen'erates. A term used to include all cellular masses whose staining reactions, form, size, etc., do not admit of classification.

degenera'tion. Deterioration or impairment of an organ or part in structure of cells and the substances of which they are a part.

   d., Abercrombie's. SEE: *amyloid degeneration.*

   d., adipose. SEE: *fatty degeneration.*

   d., albuminoid. SEE: *amyloid degeneration.*

   d., amyloid. Starch infiltration of tissue in various organs or parts, forcing the cells apart; a condition usually accompanied by pus and suppuration.

   d., ascending. Nerve fiber degeneration progressing to the center from the periphery.

   d., bacony. SEE: *amyloid degeneration.*

   d., calcareous. Deposits of lime salts in tissues and parts.

   d., caseous. Cheesy alteration in tissues seen in tuberculosis of same.

   d., cloudy swelling. A condition in which protein substances in cells become cloudy, the cells increasing in size, with minute droplets of protein substances.

   d., colloid. Jellylike disorganization of a part.

   d., cystic. Cyst formation accompanying degeneration.

   d., descending. Nerve fiber degeneration progressing toward the periphery from the original lesion.

   d., fatty. Disturbance of fat metabolism changing a part into an oily substance.

   d., fibroid. Change of membranous tissue into that of a fibrous nature.

   d., gray. Gray degeneration in nerve tissue due to chronic inflammation.

   d., hyaline. Caused by hyaline deposits, replacing musculoelastic elements of blood vessels with a firm, transparent substance which causes loss of elasticity.

   d., lardaceous. SEE: *amyloid degeneration.*

   d., mucoid. Disorganization of mucous cells.

   d., myxomatous. SEE: *mucoid degeneration.*

   d., parenchymatous. SEE: *cloudy swelling degeneration.*

   d., secondary. SEE: *wallerian degeneration.*

   d., senile. Bodily and mental changes of the aged.

   d., vitreous. SEE: *hyaline degeneration.*

   d., wallerian. Nerve fiber degeneration after separation from its nutritive center.

   d., waxy. Amyloid or lardaceous degeneration.

   d., Zenker's. Amyloid degeneration in muscular tissue.

degen'erative. Pert. to or accompanied by degeneration.

deglu'tible. Capable of being swallowed.

deglutition (deg-lu-tish'un). The act of swallowing.

deglu'titive. Pert. to deglutition.

degusta'tion. The sense of taste.

dehiscence (de-his'ens). A bursting open, as of a graafian follicle.

dehy'drate. Depriving, or to deprive, the body of chemical compounds of water or its elements.

dehydra'tion. Withdrawal of water from the tissues naturally or artificially.

Deiters's cells (di'terz). 1. Supporting cells in organ of Corti. 2. Spider cells of the neuroglia. 3. Neuro cells, the neuraxons of which become the axis cylinders of nerve fibers. SEE: *cell.*

   D.'s nucleus. Collection of cells back of the acoustic nucleus.

   D.'s process. Axis-cylinder process or neuraxon. [waste.

dejecta (de-jek'tă). Feces; intestinal

dejection, dejecture (de-jek'shun, -ŭr). 1. A cast down feeling, or mental depression. 2. Defecation or act of defecation.

Dejerine's disease (da-zhĕ-rēns'). Interstitial neuritis of infants.

   D.'s syndrome. Syndrome with deep sensitivity repressed but with normal tactile sense, caused by lesion of long root fibers of post. column.

dekanormal (dek-ă-nor'mal). Having 10 times the strength of normal, as a solution.

de Kraft blue pencil. Vulcanite fiber tube tightly packed with asbestos powder, metal cap at 1 end for attachment of ground chain, and blue metal tip covers end toward patient. Used for static brush discharge.

delacerate (de-las'er-āt). To tear or lacerate.

delacrima'tion. Epiphora; more or less constant overflow of tears.

delactation (de-lak-ta'shun). Weaning or cessation of lactation.

delamina'tion. The division into laminae, esp. that of a blastoderm into 2 layers, epiblast and hypoblast.

delayed reflex (dē-lād'). Any in which the response is abnormally delayed.

   d. symptoms. Delayed onset of symptoms, as of shock.

delectatio morosa. Dallying with voluptuous thoughts.

deligation (de-li-ga'shun). The application of ligatures.

delimita'tion. Determination of limits of an area or organ in diagnosis.

deliquesce'. To cause liquefaction.

deliquescence (del-ik-wes'ens). The process of becoming liquefied as result of absorption of water from the air.

deliquescent (del-ik-wes'ent). Pert. to a substance which absorbs water from the atmosphere.

delire de toucher (de-lĭr-dĕ too-shā'). An abnormal desire to touch things.

delir'iant. An agent that will produce delirium. Ex: *atropine, hyoscine.*

delirifacient (de-lir'i-fa'shi-ent). A drug causing delirium. SYN: *deliriant*.

delirium (de-lir'i-um). Disorientation for time and place, usually with illusions and hallucinations. A state of mental confusion and excitement.

d., acute. One developing suddenly and speedily, resulting in recovery or death.

d., alcoholic. SEE: *delirium tremens*.

d., chronic. Delirium of chronic psychoses, without febrile characteristics.

d. constantium. Delirium of patients with reiteration of same fixed idea.

d. cordis. Violent heartbeat.

d. epilepticum. Delirium either following an epileptic attack or appearing instead of an attack.

d. e potu. SEE: *delirium tremens*.

d. ex inanitione. Delirium in cases of anemia, occurring usually when fever subsides.

d., febrile. Delirium occurring with fever.

d. of grandeur. Condition in which patient exaggerates his own power and importance.

d. hystericum. Delirium of hysteria.

d., lingual. Form where meaningless sounds are muttered constantly.

d., maniacal. Often associated with high temperature and acute illness.

d. metabolicum. Form in which patient feels he is not using his own name and objects and people about him are not in their real characters and that they are spying upon him.

d. mussitans. Excitement causing lingual delirium.

d. of negation. Form in which patient thinks parts of his body are missing.

d., partial. Delirium reacting on only a portion of the mental faculties, causing only some of the patient's actions to be unreasonable.

d. of persecution. Delirium in which patient feels he is being persecuted by those about him.

d., toxic. Delirium produced by presence of toxins in the body.

d., traumatic. Delirium following injury or shock.

d. tremens. A psychic disorder involving hallucinations, both visual and auditory, found in habitual users of alcoholic beverages.

d., violent. Feverish delirium with exaltation and great strength.

delitescence (del-it-es'ens). An unusually complete and speedy resolution of an inflammation.

deliver. To aid in childbirth by removal of a fetus or placenta.

delivery. Expulsion of the child at birth with placenta and membranes from the mother. SEE: *labor*.

d., abdominal. Removal of the child by Cesarean section.

d., forceps. Delivery of the child by the use of tractor instruments.

d., post-mortem. Delivery of the child after death of the mother either by the abdominal or vaginal route.

d., precipitate. A precipitate delivery is one that occurs under nonaseptic conditions and when the physician is not present.

d., premature. Delivery of the child before the time of viability.

d., spontaneous. Delivery of the child without external aid.

delomorphous (del-o-mor'fus). Having definite form and shape.

d. cells. Granular cells which stain easily; found next to basement membrane in stomach; glands in cardiac region.

delousing (de-lows'ing). Ridding of lice by their destruction.

del'ta for'nicis. A triangular surface on lower side of fornix; *commissura hippocampi*.

del'toid. Shaped like the Greek letter △.

d. ligament. Internal lateral ligament of ankle joint.

d. muscle. The *musculus deltoideus*, which covers the shoulder prominence.

d. ridge. Ridge on humerus where deltoid muscle is attached.

de lunat'ico inquiren'do. Legal process to determine alleged incompetence of a person.

delusion (de-lu'shun). Hallucination. A false belief or sense.

d., depressive. One causing a saddened state.

d., expansive. Conviction of one's own fineness, power or importance.

d., fixed. Those that remain unaltered.

d., fleeting. These come and go.

d. of grandeur. A false sense of possessing wealth or power.

d. of negation. SEE: *nihilistic delusion*.

d., nihilistic (ni-hil-is'tik). One that causes the victim to believe that everything has ceased to exist.

d. of persecution. Delusion in which patient feels everyone about him is against him.

d., reference. One that causes the victim to read a meaning not intended in the acts or words of others, usually an interpretation of slight or ridicule.

d., systematized. Logical correlation with false reasoning and deduction.

d., unsystematized. Delusion without any correlation between ideas and surroundings.

delu'sional. Pert. to a delusion.

dement'. One who has lost his sanity.

demented (de-men'ted). Of unsound mind.

dementia (de-men'shi-ă). Irrecoverable deteriorative mental state, the common end result of many entities.

d., acute. A form affecting young persons; often curable.

d., alcoholic. Dementia in terminal portion of chronic alcoholic state.

d., apathetic. Dementia with diminished sensitivity, occurring in the last stages of disease, usually.

d., apoplectic. Form following cerebral hemorrhage or tumors.

d., catatonic. A form of dementia precox.

d., chronic. An incurable form occurring at any time of life.

d., epileptic. That accompanied by mental deterioration, and due to long continued epilepsy.

d. naturalis. Congenital form; idiocy.

d., organic. Dementia caused by lesions of nerve centers.

d., paralytic. Chronic brain disease with degeneration of the cortical neurons and progressive loss of physical and mental power.

d. paralytica (păr-ă-lit′ĭ-kă). A traumatic psychosis.

d. paranoides. Dementia precox with paranoid tendencies.

d., paretic. Paralytic dementia, q.v.

d., postfebrile. Dementia following severe cases of infectious diseases.

d. precox. It has been characterized as a "dream state," a psychosis represented by a dreaming mind in a sleeping body, the latter being easily aroused but not the former. SYN: schizophrenia.

d., presenile. One beginning in the 5th decade.

d., secondary. Dementia occurring after a primary mental disease, such as mania.

d., senile. That occurring in the aged.

d., syphilitic. Dementia caused by lesion of syphilis.

d., terminal. Dementia following another form of mental disease. SEE: secondary dementia.

d., toxic. That due to the excessive use of some drug.

demi-. Prefix: Half.

demilune cells (dem′ĭ-lūn). Collection of marginal cells in form of a half moon in submaxillary gland.

demineraliza′tion. Loss of salts by excessive secretion and excretion.

demise′. Death.

Dem′odex. Genus of mites and ticks of the class Arachnida and order Acarina.

D. folliculo′rum. The pimple mite, which often infests hair sacs and sebaceous follicles.

demog′raphy. Statistical study of births, marriages, and deaths, and physical, moral, and intellectual development.

demonoma′nia. Obsolete term for psychotic belief that one is possessed by demons.

demonop′athy. A mania in which one is convinced of being possessed of devils. SYN: demonomania.

Demours′ membrane (de-moorz′). A fine membrane bet. the endothelial layer of the cornea and the substantia propria.

demucosa′tion. Excision of mucosa of any part of body.

demul′cent. An agent that will soothe the part or soften the skin to which applied.

demutiza′tion. Overcoming mutism by teaching the patient to speak or to use the sign language.

dena′tured. Subject to having the nature of a substance changed, or to render unfit for consumption, as alcohol, q.v.

dendraxon (den-drak′son). Terminal filaments of the neuraxon of a nerve cell.

den′dric. Pert. to or possessing a dendron.

dendriform (den′drĭ-form). Branching or like a tree in shape.

den′drite. One of the branched, protoplasmic extensions of a neuron; usually several from each neuron.

dendrit′ic. Treelike in form.

d. calculus. A renal stone molded in the form of the pelvis and calyces.

dendroid (den′droid). 1. Dendriform, pert. to dendrites. 2. Arborescent, treelike.

dendron (den′dron). A dendrite. A protoplasmic branch from a nerve cell.

dendrophagocytosis (den′′dro-fag-o-sĭ-to′-sis). The absorption of portions of astrocytes by microglia cells.

Denecke's spirillum (den′ĕ-kes). Nonpathogenic organism similar. to V. comma, found usually in cheese. SYN: vibrio tyrogenus.

dener′vated. 1. Excision, incision, or blocking of a nerve supply. 2. A condition in which the nerve supply is blocked or cut off.

dengue (deng′ga). Acute, epidemic, febrile disease lasting 8 days, seldom fatal.

denidation (den-id-a′shun). Removal during menstruation of the nidus of a fertilized ovum.

dens (pl. dentes). A tooth.

d. bicuspidus. The bicuspid tooth, dens premolaris. BNA.

d. caninus. BNA. The canine tooth.

d. deciduus. BNA. Milk tooth, first tooth.

d. incisivus. BNA. Incisor tooth.

d. molaris. BNA. Molar tooth, grinder.

d. permanens. BNA. One of the 32 teeth making up the permanent denture.

d. sapientiae. Late tooth, wisdom tooth. dens serotinus. BNA.

densimeter (den-sim′e-ter). Instrument for measuring densities.

densitom′eter. A special densimeter for measuring bacterial growth and effect upon it of antiseptics and bacteriophages.

den′sity. 1. Relative weight of a substance compared with some other substance of equal bulk. 2. The quality of being dense.

dentag′ra. Toothache.

den′tal. Pert. to the teeth.

d. curve. The curve or bow of the line of the teeth in the jaw.

d. disk. A thin, circular piece of paper, or cloth, or other substance charged with abrasive powder for cutting or polishing teeth and fillings.

d. engine. A machine operated with foot power, or by an electric or a water motor, to give a swift rotary motion to drills, burs, and burnishers.

dentalgia (den-tal′jĭ-ă). Toothache.

dentaphone (den′tă-fōn). Device for conveying sound through the teeth.

dentate (den'tāt). Notched; having short triangular divisions of the margin; toothed.

den'tes. Teeth; plural of *dens, q.v.*

dentibuc'cal. Pert. to both the cheek and teeth.

dentic'ulate. Finely toothed.

    d., body. Corpus dentatum.

dentifica'tion. Conversion into dental structure.

dentifrice (den'tif-ris). A powder or other substance for cleaning teeth.

dentigerous (den-tij'er-us). Having or containing teeth.

dentila'bial. Pert. to both teeth and lips.

dentilin'gual. Pert. to both teeth and tongue.

dentim'eter. Device for measuring teeth.

den'tinal. Pert. to dentine.

dentine, dentin (den'tēn, den'tin). The osseous tissues of a tooth enclosing the pulp cavity.

dentinifica'tion. Formation of dentine.

dentini'tis. Inflammation of dentine.

den'tinoid. 1. Resembling dentine. 2. A tumor arising from dentine.

dentino'ma. A dentine tumor.

dentinos'teoid. Small tumor arising from dentine. SYN: *dentinoid.*

den'tist. A practitioner of dentistry.

den'tistry. The scientific care of teeth; dental surgery.

    d., operative. Phase dealing with dental operations on mouth as contrasted with dental laboratory work.

denti'tion. The process and time of teething.

dentoalve'olar. Pert. to alveolus of a tooth.

dentoalveoli'tis. A purulent inflammation of the tooth socket linings, characterized by looseness of the teeth and gum shrinkage. SYN: *pyorrhea alveolaris.*

den'toid. Dentiform; odontoid; tooth shaped.

dentoliva (dent-o-li'va). Olivary body.

dentor'din (den'chur). Organic substance of a tooth.

denture (den'chur). A set of 32 permanent or of 20 deciduous teeth, either natural or artificial.

    d., artificial. False teeth replacing natural teeth.

    d., full. Complete set of artificial teeth.

denucleated (de-nu'kle-āt-ed). Deprived of a nucleus.

denuda'tion. Removal of a protecting layer or covering.

denutrition (de-nu-trish'un). Malnutrition.

deob'struent. Having the property of removing obstructions.

deodorant (de-ō'dor-ant). An agent which destroys or neutralizes foul odors. Those in common use are: Chloride of lime, creolin, izal, iodoform, permanganate of potash, chlorine and hydrogen peroxide. SEE: *odor.*

deodorize (de-o'dor-īz). To remove foul odor.

deodorizer (de-o'dor-ī-zer). That which deodorizes.

deontology (de-on-tol'o-jī). Medical ethics.

deoppila'tion. The doing away with obstructions.

deor'sum. Downward or turning downward.

    d. ver'gens. Turning downward.

deorsumduction (de-or"sum-duk'shun). Bending downward.

deossifica'tion. Lacking in mineral constituents of bone.

deox'idate. To deprive a chemical of oxygen.   [oxygen.

deoxida'tion. Process of depriving of

deoxidizer (de-ok'sĭ-di-zer). A deoxidizing substance.

depersonaliza'tion. A sense of being someone else; a lessened sense of one's own identity.

depilate (dep'il-ate). To strip of hair.

depilation (dep-il-a'shun). The process of hair removal. SEE: *epilation.*

depil'atory. An agent used for the removal of hair.

deplete (de-plēt'). To empty, as in blood letting; to produce depletion.

depletion (de-ple'shun). Withdrawal of fluid, esp. the blood.

deplumation (de-plu-ma'shun). Falling of eyelashes as result of disease.

depolariza'tion. Preventing or destruction of polarity.

deposit (de-poz'it). 1. Sediment. 2. Matter collected in any part of an organism, normal or otherwise.

deprava'tion. 1. Deterioration, esp. of secretions. 2. Perversion.

depraved (de-prāvd'). 1. Perverted; abnormal. 2. Deteriorated.

depres'sant. An agent that will depress a body function or nerve activity. Ex: *Bromides, aconite, chloral hydrate.*

    d., cardiac. One which lessens heart action, so that it beats slower and weaker.

    d., cerebral. One lessening brain activity, making patient dull and less active. Large doses may produce sleep.

    d., motor. One which lessens contractions of involuntary muscles.

    d., respiratory. A drug lessening frequency and depth of breathing.

    d., secretory. One making gland secretions less.

depressed (de-prest'). 1. Hollowed. 2. Low in spirits.

depression (de-presh'un). 1. Lowered function, mental or physical. 2. A hollow.

    d., averse. Melancholia.

    d., cardiac. Notch in ant. margin of left lung for the cardiac apex.

depres'somotor. A drug which diminishes muscular movements by lessening the impulses for motion sent from the brain or spinal cord.

depressor (de-pres'or). Instrument for depressing a part.

    d. nerve. A nerve whose irritation causes a change in blood pressure.

    d. reflex. More or less transient stimulation of depressor fibers.

    d., tongue. Device used to flatten tongue for throat examinations.

dep'rimens oc'uli. *Musculus rectus inferior.*

depri'val. Deprived of or without organs, parts, or functions.

depriva'tion. Deprival.

deprive'ment. Being without function, parts, or organs. SYN: *deprival.*

depuliza'tion. Destruction of fleas which carry the plague bacillus.

dep'urant. A medicine that purifies through the removal of *excreta.*

depura'tion. Process of freeing from impurities.

dep'urative. Cleansing. [emunctory.

depura'tor. 1. That which purifies. 2. An

deradenitis (der-a-den-i'tis). Inflammation of a lymph gland of the neck.

deradenoncus (der-ad"e-non'kus). Swelling or tumor of a neck gland.

derangement (de-rānj'ment). Disorder of the mental functions.

deratization (de-rat"i-za'shun). Extermination of rats.

Derbyshire neck (dar'be-shēr). Goiter.

Dercum's disease (der'kŭm). Dystrophy of subcutaneous connective tissue; painful. SYN: *adiposis dolorosa, paratrophy.*

dereistic (de-re-is'tik). Pert. to overexercise of the imagination to the extent of ignoring reality, as seen in day dreaming.

deric (der'ik). Pert. to ectoderm as distinguished from enteric.

derivation (der-iv-a'shun). Diversion of fluids from 1 to another part.

deriv'ative. 1. Pert. to or producing a diversion of fluids. 2. Counterirritant.

derm, derma. The *cutis vera,* or true skin.

Dermacen'tor. A genus of ticks.

   D. anderso'ni. An oval, reddish brown tick, the conveyor of Rocky Mountain fever.

der'mad. Toward the skin; externally.

dermagra (der-mag'rä). A deficiency disease.

dermal. Relating to the skin or derma.

   d. muscle. A muscle controlling skin action.

dermalax'ia. Morbid relaxation or softness of the skin.

dermalgia (der-mal'jĭ-ă). Pain in the skin.

dermametropathism (der"mă-mĕ-trŏp'ă-thizm). Diagnosis of skin disease by observing the markings made by drawing a blunt pencil across the skin.

dermamyiasis (der-mă-mi-i'ă-sis). Skin disease caused by invasion of larva of dipterous insects.

dermanaplasty (derm-an'ă-plas-tĭ). Skin grafting.

dermapos'tasis. Abscess formation accompanying a disease of the skin.

dermat-, dermato-. Prefixes: Skin.

dermatagra (derm-ă-tag'rä). 1. Pellagra. 2. Dermatalgia. 3. Gouty affection of the skin.

dermatalgia (derm-ă-tal'jĭ-ă). Paresthesia with localized pain in the skin. SYN: *dermalgia.*

dermatatrophia (derm-at-ă-tro'fĭ-ă). Atrophy of the skin.

dermatauxe (der-mă-tawk'sē). Hypertrophy of the skin.

dermatitis (der-mat-i'tis). Irritation of skin evidenced by itching, redness, and various skin lesions.

   d. aestivalis. Hot weather dermatitis.

   d. calorica. That due to heat or cold, as sunburn, etc.

   d. congelationis. Frostbite, chilblain. SEE: *chilblain.*

   d. exfoliativa. Acute or subacute inflammation of the skin commonly involving whole surface and characterized by redness and abundant flaky desquamation.

   d. gangraenosa. Skin inflammation of gangrenous form.

   d. herpetiformis. Chronic, inflammatory disease characterized by erythematous, papular, vesicular, bullous, or pustular lesions with tendency to grouping and with itching and burning.

   d. hiemalis. Dermatitis occurring in cold weather.

   d. infectiosa eczematoides. Pustular eruption during or following a pyogenic disease. SYN: *Engman's disease.*

   d. medicamentosa. Drug eruption.

   d. multiformis. Form with lesions of a pustular nature.

   d. papillaris capillitii. Formation on scalp and neck of surface elevations interspersed with pustules and ending in scarlike elevations resembling keloids.

   d. repens. Inflammatory disease of the skin following injury.

   d. seborrheica. Acute or subacute inflammatory skin disease beginning on the scalp, characterized by rounded, irregular, or circinate lesions covered with yellowish or brownish-gray greasy scales.

   d. venenata. Any inflammation caused by local action of various animal, vegetable, or mineral susbtances on the surface of the skin. Commonly called ivy poisoning.

   d., x-ray. Skin inflammation due to overdose of x-ray.

dermatoautoplasty (der"mat-o-aw'to-plas-tĭ). Grafting of skin taken from some portion of the patient's own body.

dermatobiasis (der-mat-o-bi'as-is). The presence of *Dermatobia noxialis* in the tissues, and condition produced thereby.

dermatocele (der'mă-to-sēl). Tendency of hypertrophied skin and subcutaneous tissue to hang loosely in folds. SYN: *dermatolysis.*

   d. lipomato'sis. A pedunculated lipoma with cystic degeneration.

dermatocelidosis (der-mat-o-kel-i-do'sis). Freckles; a macular eruption.

dermatocellulitis (der-mat-o-sel-u-li'tis). Inflammation of subcutaneous connective tissue.

dermatoconiosis (der-mat-o-kon-i-o'sis). Occupational dermatitis caused by the irritation of dust.

dermatocyst (der'mat-o-sist). A skin cyst.

dermatodyn'ia. Pain in the skin; dermatalgia.*

dermatofibro'ma. A skin fibroma.

dermatogen (der-mat'o-jen). An antigen from any skin disease.*

dermatog'enous. Of the nature of or producing skin or disease of skin.

dermatoglyphics (der"mă-to-glif'ĭks). Surface markings of the skin.

dermat'ograph. 1. A device for marking the body for diagnosis. 2. A wheal made on the skin in dermatography.

dermatograph'ia, dermatog'raphy. 1. A treatise on the skin. 2. A form of urticaria in which wheals are made by pressure.

der"matohet'eroplasty. Grafting with grafts from another's skin.

dermatoid (der'mă-toid). Resembling skin.

dermatokelidosis (der-mat-o-kē-li-do'sis). A macular eruption; freckle.

dermatol'ogist. A skin specialist.

dermatol'ogy. The science of the skin and its diseases.

dermatolysis (der-mă-tol'is-is). Tendency of hypertrophied skin and subcutaneous tissue to hang in folds. Loose skin. SYN: cutis laxa, cutis pendula.

dermato'ma. Circumscribed thickening of skin. [incising the skin.

dermatome (der'ma-tōm). Instrument for

dermatomere (der'mă-to-mēr). A segment of embryonic integument.

dermatomucosomyositis (der"ma-to-mŭ-ko"so-mi-o-si'tis). Inflammation of the skin, involving mucosa and muscles.

dermatomycosis (der"mat-o-mi-ko'sis). A disease of the skin due to a vegetable parasite.

dermatomyo'ma. Myoma of the skin.

dermatomyositis (der"ma-to"mi-o-si'tis). Inflammation of the skin and muscles.

dermatoneuro'sis. Any skin disease of nervous origin.

dermatopath'ia. Any disease of the skin.

dermatopathol'ogy. Study of diseases of the skin.

dermatop'athy. Any skin disease. SYN: dermatopathia.

dermatopho'bia. Abnormal fear of having a skin disease.

dermatophyte (der'mat-o-fīt). A plant-growing parasite on the skin.

dermatophytide (der-mă-tof'ĭ-tēd). A toxic rash or eruption occurring in dermatomycosis.

dermatoplas'tic. Pert. to skin grafting.

dermatoplasty (der'mat-o-plas-tĭ). Transplanting living skin to cover cutaneous defects caused by injury, operation, or disease.

dermatorrhagia (der"mă-tor-ra'jĭ-ă). Hemorrhage into or from the skin.

dermatorrhea (der"mă-tor-re'ă). Excessive secretion of sebaceous glands.

dermatoscopy (der-mă-tos'ko-pĭ). Examination of the skin with a high powered lens.

dermatosiophobe (der-mă-to'sĭ-o-fōb). One having a morbid fear of acquiring a skin disease.

dermatosiophobia (der-mă-to"sĭ-o-fō'bĭ-ă). Dread of skin disease.

dermatosis (der-mat-o'sĭs). Any disease of the skin.

dermatosome (der'ma-to-sōm). Section of equatorial•plate in mitosis.

der"matother'apy. Treatment of skin diseases.

dermatothlasia (der"mă-to-thla'zĭ-ă). An uncontrollable tic or impetus to pinch the skin.

dermatotome (der'mă-to-tōm). 1. One of the fetal skin segments. 2. A knife for incising the skin or small lesions.

dermatotropic (der-mă-to-trop'ĭk). Acting esp. on the skin.

dermatoxerasia (der"mă-to-ze-ra'sĭ-ă). Roughening of skin. SYN: xeroderma.

dermatozo'on. Animal parasite of the skin.

dermatrophia (der-ma-tro'fĭ-ă). Atrophy of the skin.

dermic (der'mĭk). Pert. to the skin.

dermis (der'mis). The skin; cutis vera or true skin.

dermi'tis. Inflammation of skin.

der'moblast. Part of mesoblastic layer, developing into the corium.

dermography (der-mograf'ĭ-ă, -mog'raf-ĭ). The appearance of elevated red marks on the skin as the result of pressure or stroking its surface; seen in vasomotor ataxia.

der'moid. 1. A cyst containing elements of hair, teeth, and skin. 2. An ovarian tumor. SEE: cyst. 3. Resembling the skin.

dermoidec'tomy. Excision of a dermoid cyst.

dermol'ysin. A substance in the blood supposed to be capable of dissolving the skin.

dermol'ysis. A rare destructive disease of the skin.

dermomyco'sis. A skin disease produced by a vegetable parasite. SYN: dermatomycosis.

dermonosol'ogy. The pathology of skin affections.

dermopathy (der-mop'ath-ĭ). Any skin disease.

dermophlebitis (der-mo-fle-bi'tis). Inflammation of superficial veins and surrounding skin.

dermophylax'is. The protective function of the skin in warding off infections.

dermophyte (der'mo-fīt). A vegetable skin parasite. SYN: dermatophyte.

dermorrha'gia. Hemorrhage from or into the skin. SYN: dermatorrhagia.

dermoskel'eton. The skin, teeth, hair, and nails.

dermostenosis (der-mo-sten-o'sis). A tightening of the skin. SEE: scleroderma.

dermosynovi'tis. Malignant disease of the sole of the foot and synovial sheaths.

dermosyphilop'athy. Any syphilitic disease of the skin.

dermotrop'ic. Acting esp. on the skin.

dermovac'cine. A vaccine for skin inoculation.

desanimania (des-an-ĭ-ma'nĭ-ă). Amentia; dementia.

desatura'tion. A process whereby a saturated organic compound is converted into an unsaturated one.

Desault's appara'tus or ban'dage (de-sōz'). Bandage used for fracture of clavicle.

descemetitis (des-em-et-i'tis). Inflammation of Descemet's membrane on the corneal post. surface; serous cyclitis.

Descemet's membrane (des'māz). A fine membrane bet. the endothelial layer of the cornea and the substantia propia; *lamina elastica posterior.* SEE: *Demours' membrane.*

descemetocele (des-se-met'o-sēl). Protrusion of Descemet's membrane.

descendens (de-sen'dens). Descending; a descending structure.

    d. hypoglossi, d. noni. A branch of the hypoglossal nerve.

descensus (de-sen'sus). Falling, descent. SYN: *ptosis.*

    d. testis. BNA. Passage of the testicle down into the scrotum. SYN: *migration of testicle.*

    d. uteri. Defective pelvic floor allowing the uterus or part of the uterus to protrude out of the vagina.

desen'sitize. 1. To deprive of or lessen sensitivity by nerve section or blocking. 2. To abate anaphylactic sensitiveness.

desex'ualize. To castrate, or to perform ovariotomy or testectomy.

deshydre'mia. Lack of fluid elements of the blood.

desiccant (des'ĭk-ant). Causing desiccation or dryness.

des'iccate. To dry.

desicca'tion. The process of drying up. SEE: *electrodesiccation.*

    d., electric. Electric therapy to cure a lesion.

desiccative (des'ĭk-a″tĭv, des-sik'ă-tiv). Causing to dry up.

desmalgia (dez-mal'jĭ-ă). Pain in a ligament.

desmectasia, desmectasis (des-mek-ta'sĭ-ă, -tă-sis). The stretching of a tendon.

desmepithelium (des-mep-ith-e'lĭ-um). The epithelial lining of vessels and synovial cavities.

desmitis (des-mi'tis). Inflammation of a ligament.

desmo-. Prefix: A bond, a ligature.

desmobacte'ria. Group of bacteria of a filiform shape; similar to genus Bacilli.

desmocyte (dez'mo-sīt). A supporting tissue cell. SYN: *fibroblast, fibrocyte.*

desmocytoma (dez-mo-sī-to'ma). A tumor formed of desmocytes; a sarcoma.

desmodyn'ia. Pain in a ligament.

desmogenous (des-moj'en-us). Of connective tissue origin.

desmog'raphy. A description of or treatise on ligaments.

des'moid. 1. Tendonlike; fibroid. 2. A very tough and firm fibroma.

desmology (des-mol'o-jĭ). Science of tendons and ligaments.

desmo'ma. A tumor of the connective tissue.

desmoneoplasm (dez-mo-ne'o-plazm). A connective tissue tumor.

desmopathy (des-mop'ă-thĭ). Any ligament disease.

desmopexia (des-mo-peks'ĭ-ă). Fixation of round ligaments to the abdominal wall for the correction of uterine displacement.

desmoplas'tic. Causing or forming adhesions.

desmopyknosis (dez-mo-pik-no'sis). Dudley's operation. Shortening of round ligaments by attaching them by loops to the ant. uterine wall.

desmorrhexis (des-mor-reks'is). Rupture of a ligament.

desmosis (des-mo'sis). Any disease of the connective tissue, esp. of the skin.

desmosome (des'mo-sōm). A small thickening in an intercellular bridge.

desmotomy (des-mot'o-mĭ). Dissection of ligament.

despumation (de-spu-ma'shun). Separation of froth or scum from a liquid.

des'quamate. To shred or scale off the surface epithelium.

desquamation (des-kwa-ma'shun). Scaling of the skin or cuticle.

desquamative (des-kwam'ă-tiv). Of the nature of desquamation or pert. to, or causing it.

desquamous (des-kwam'us). Scaling or falling off, as the skin.

dessertspoon. One holding about 2 fluid drams. Spoons are not all uniform in capacity.

desudation (de-su-da'shun). Excessive sweating often followed by slight pustular eruption.

detelec'tasis. Lack of normal inflation; collapse of an organ.

deter'gent. A medicine that purges or cleanses; cleansing.

deteriora'tion. Retrogression; said of impairment of mental or physical functions.

determina'tion. 1. A tendency in a definite direction, as of blood, to a part. 2. A quantitative analysis.

deter'miners. Genes* or the element in chromosomes* supposed to be responsible for inherited traits.

determinism (de-term'in-izm). The theory that all human action is the result of innate urges although they may not be conscious ones.

deter'sive. Detergent; cleansing or purging.

dethy'roidism. Condition resulting from removal of the thyroid.

dethy'roidized. Without a thyroid gland.

de'tonating chamber. A muffler surrounding the discharging balls of a static machine or resonator to deaden the sound of a spark discharge.

detona'tion. A violent noise caused by an explosive combustion.

detox'icate. To remove the toxic principle of a substance. SYN: *detoxify.*

detoxify (de-toks'ĭ-fī). To remove the toxic quality of a substance. SYN: *detoxicate.*

detrition (de-trish'un). The wearing away of a part, esp. through friction, as that of the teeth.

detritus (de-tri'tus). Any broken down or degenerative tissue or carious matter.

detruncation (de-trun-ka'shun). Decapitation, esp. of a fetus. SYN: *decollation.*

detru'sor uri'nae. Ext. longitudinal layer of muscular coat of bladder.

detumes'cence. Subsidence of a tumor-like swelling.

deutencephalon (dūt-en-sef'ă-lon). The interbrain. SYN: *thalamencephalon.*

deuteranopia, deuteranopsia (du-ter-an-o'-pĭ-a, -op'sĭ-ă). Green blindness, so named because green is the 2nd of the primary colors. SEE: *protanopia, tritanopia.*

deuterium (dū-te'rĭ-um). Heavy hydrogen; the mass 2 isotope of hydrogen, symbol H² or D.

  d. oxide. Heavy water.

deuteroal'bumose. An albumose formed in peptic digestion of proteins.

deuteroelas'tose. A deuteroalbumose formed in the peptic digestion of elastin.

deuteromyosinose (du-ter-o-mĭ-o'sĭn-ōz). A product of myosin digestion.

deuteropathi'a, deuterop'athy. A disease caused by a preceding disease.

deu'teroplasm. The nonprotoplasmic material contained in the cytoplasm of cells.   [daughter cysts.

deutoscolex (du-to-sko'lex). Secondary

devasa'tion. Destruction of blood vessels.

devasculariza'tion. Loss or draining of blood from a part.

devel'opment. Growth to full size or maturity. Progress of an egg to the adult state. Evolution.

developmental (de-vel-op-men'tal). Pert. to development.

deviation (de-vī-a'shun). Going out of the way; departure from normal.

  d., conjugate. Deviation of face and eyes to the same side in paralytics.

  d., minimum. The smallest deviation that a prism can produce.

  d. of complement. Incapable of hemolysis.

deviom'eter. Device for estimating degree of strabismus.

devisceration (de-vis-er-a'shun). Removal of viscera. SYN: *evisceration.*

devitaliza'tion. 1. Destruction or loss of vitality. 2. Anesthetizing sensitive pulp of a tooth; known as "killing the nerve."

devolu'tion. Catabolism; degeneration.

dew cure. Walking with bare feet in grass wet with dew. SYN: *kneippism.*

  d. point. Temperature at which dew begins to form.

dexiocar'dia. Displacement of heart on right side of the body.

dexter (deks'ter). On the right side.

dextrad (dex'trad). Toward the right side.

dextral (dex'tral). Pert. to the right side.

dex'tran. C₆H₁₀O₅. A monodextrin.

dex'trase. An enzyme that splits dextrose and converts it into lactic acid.

dex'trin. A yellowish-white powder which forms mucilaginous solutions in water and can be prepared by the action of heat or acid on starch.

dextrinuria (deks-trin-u'rĭ-ă). Dextrin in the urine.

dextro-. Prefix: To the right.

dextrocardia (deks-tro-kar'dĭ-ă). Having the heart on the right side of body.

dextrocar'diogram. A cardiogram representing action of the right ventricle.

dextroc'ular. Having a stronger right eye than the left one.

dextrocularity (deks-trok-ŭ-lar'ĭ-tĭ). The condition of having the right eye stronger than the left.

dextroduc'tion. The movement of visual axis to the right.

dextrogas'tria. Having the stomach on right side of body.

dextrogyre (deks'tro-jīr). A substance turning to the right.

dextroman'ual. Righthanded.

dextrop'edal. Having greater dexterity in using the right leg than the left one.

dextropho'bia. Abnormal aversion to objects on right side of body.

dextrorotatory (deks-tro-ro'tă-tor-ĭ). Turning rays of light to the right.

dextrose (deks'troz). A simple sugar of the monosaccharose* group; also known as glucose, or grape sugar.

  DOSAGE: 6 oz. (180.0 Gm.) daily.

  NP: For rectal or subcutaneous injection 5% watery solutions are used: **1** oz. of glucose to 1 pt. of water, or added to normal saline.

dextrosinistral (deks-tro-sin-is'tral). From right to left.

dextrosuria (deks-trōs-ŭ'rĭ-ă). Dextrose **in** the urine.

dextrotrop'ic, dextrot'ropous. Turning **to** the right.

dextrover'sion. Turned toward the right.

dezymotize (de-zi'mo-tīz). To free of ferments or germs.

dho'bie itch. Tropical name for form of *Tinea cruris* that is more intense than that of temperate zone.

di-. Prefix: Twice.   [tion.

diabetes (di-a-be'tēz). A disease of nutri-

  d., acute. Form of diabetes mellitus, usually caused by nervous or morbid symptoms. A large amount of sugar shows suddenly in the urine.

  d., artificial. Type produced by piercing of floor of 4th ventricle or by dosing with phlorizin.

  d., biliary. Jaundice with hypertrophic cirrhosis of liver.

  d., bronzed. Diabetes with sclerosis of the liver and pancreas, and marked by pigmentation of the skin and viscera. SYN: *hemochromatosis.*

  d., conjugal. Form affecting husband and wife at the same time.

  d. descipiens. Diabetes mellitus minus polyuria.

  d., gouty. Diabetes in people leading a life of too much food and too little exercise.

  d. hepatogenes. Diabetes mellitus caused by liver disease.

  d., hysterical. Polyuria induced by a hysterical attack or state.

  d. insipidus. Polyuria.* SYM: Enormous amounts of urine, pale and watery. Sp. gr. 1.002-5. No sugar or albumen. More common in the young. Thirst, weakness, dry skin. PROG: Unfavorable.

  d. melli'tus. Persistent glucosuria.*

  d., pancreatic. Diabetes associated with disease of the pancreas.

d., phlorizin. Glycosuria caused by administration of phlorizin.

d., puncture. SEE: *artificial diabetes.*

d., true. SEE: *diabetes mellitus.*

diabetic (di-ab-et'ik). Pert. to diabetes.

d. center. An area in the median line of ant. half of 4th ventricle, a puncture of which causes glycosuria.

d. ear. Otitis media diabetica.

d. neuritis. Multiple neuritis of diabetes.

d. sugar. Glucose in the sugar of the urine of diabetics.

d. tabes. Diabetes with neuritic pains in leg and loss of knee jerk.

diabetide (di-ab-e'tĭd). A cutaneous form of diabetes.

diabetin (di-ă-be'tin). Pure crystallized levulose used as a substitute for cane sugar in diabetes.

diabetogenic (di-ab-et-o-jen'ik). Causing diabetes.

diabetogenous (di-ab-e-toj'en-us). Diabetogenic*; caused by diabetes.

diabetometer (di-ab-et-om'e-ter). A device for measuring sugar in diabetic urine.

diab"olep'tic. One professing to have supernatural communication, esp. with the devil.

diabro'sis. A corrosion causing perforation.

diabrot'ic. 1. Corrosive. 2. An escharotic or corrosive.

diacele (di'as-ēl). The 3rd ventricle of the brain.

diacetate (di-as'et-āt). A salt of diacetic acid.

diacetemia (di-as-et-e'mĭ-ă). Diacetic acid in the blood.

diace'tic acid. Acetoacetic acid, found in acidosis and in the urine of the diabetic. It is similar to acetone and is found in serious diabetes and in persistent vomiting after anesthesia.

diacetonu'ria. Diacetic acid in urine; diaceturia.

diaceturia (di-as-ĕ-tu'rĭ-ă). Diacetonuria; diacetic acid in urine.

diac'id. Having 2 atoms of hydrogen replaceable with a base.

diaclasia (di-ak-la'sĭ-ă). A fracture, esp. breaking a bone before surgery.

diaclast (di'ă-klăst). Device for perforating the fetal skull.

diacrinous (di-ăk'rin-us). Pert. to cells which secrete outwardly; exocrine.*

diacrisis (di-ăk'ri-sis). 1. A change in the character of a secretion. 2. Any disease having an altered secretion. 3. A critical discharge.

diacrit'ic, diacrit'ical. Diagnostic; said of symptoms.

diad (di'ad). An element or radical having an atomicity of 2; a bivalent.

di'aderm. Blastoderm composed of ectoderm and entoderm, and containing bet. them the segmentation cavity.

diadochokinesia (di-ă-dok"o-ki-ne'sĭ-a). Ability to make antagonistic movements, as pronation and supination, in quick succession.

di'agnose. To determine the cause and nature of a pathological condition; to recognize a disease.

diagnosis (di-ag-no'sis) (pl. *diagnoses*). Recognition of disease states from symptoms, auscultation, inspection, palpation, percussion, posture, reflexes, general appearances, abnormalities and abnormal attitudes and habits microscopic and chemical examinations, x-ray, mechanical, and other means.

d., clinical. One determined by symptoms alone.

d., differential. Comparison of symptoms of 2 similar diseases to determine from which the patient is suffering. SEE: *differential diagnosis.*

d. by exclusion. True diagnosis by elimination of all others.

d., pathological. Diagnosis of type of lesion, disregarding its location.

d., physical. Diagnosis by external examination only.

d., serum. Diagnosis by means of serum and its effects.

diagnos'tic. Pert. to a diagnosis.

diagnosti'cian, di'agnost. One skilled in diagnosis.

diagraph (di'ă-graf). Device for recording outlines, esp. of the cranium.

dial. A derivative of barbital,* but more active.

USES: Sedative and hypnotic.

DOSAGE: ½ gr. (0.03 Gm.) to 1½ gr. (0.1 Gm.). SEE: *barbital.*

dialectrol'ysis. Treatment by ionization.

Dialis'ter pneumosin'tes. A bacterium found in the nasal secretion at beginning of influenza.

dialy-. Prefix: To separate.

dialysate (di-al'is-āt). A liquid that has been dialyzed.

dialysis (di-al'is-is). 1. The passage of a solute through a membrane. 2. A process in which a liquid to be purified or studied is enclosed in a thin, membranous sack and exposed to water or any other solvent which continually circulates or changes outside the sack.

dialyt'ic. Belonging to or resembling the process of dialysis.

di'alyze. To make a dialysis or to have made one.

dialyzable (di-al-iz'ă-bl). Capable of dialysis.

dialyzer (di'al-īz-er). Membrane used in performing dialysis.

diamagnet'ic. Repulsion by the magnet.

diameter (di-am'et-er). The distance from any point on the periphery of a surface, body, or space to the opposite point.

d., anterior transverse, of the fetal head. SEE: *temporal diameter.*

d., anteroposterior, of the pelvic cavity. The distance bet. middle of symphysis pubis and upper border of 3rd sacral vertebra.

d., a., of the p. inlet. The distance from upper part of symphysis pubis to promontory of sacrum.

d., a., of skull. The distance in a straight line bet. the metopic point and the most remote point upon the external surface of the tabular portion of the occipital bone, or bet. most prominent point of the glabella and the most prominent point upon the external surface of the occipital bone.

d., basilobregmatic. Distance in a straight line bet. basilon and bregma.

d., Baudelocque's. SEE: *external conjugate diameter of pelvis.*

d., biauricular. 1. Distance in a straight line bet. 2 points on a line passing over the vertex and uniting the 2 auricular points, each immediately above the ridge which continues the zygomatic arch backward. 2. Transverse distance bet. the centers of external auditory meatuses, or bet. middle point of the upper margins of each external auditory meatus.

d., biglenoid. Distance bet. the center of 1 glenoid cavity of the temporal bone and that of the other.

d., bigoniac. Distance bet. the 2 gonions.

d., bijugal. Horizontal distance bet. 2 malar points.

d., bijugular. Transverse distance bet. 2 jugular points.

d., bimalar. The transverse distance bet. 2 malar points.

d., bimandibular. Transverse distance bet. tubercles on the inferior borders of the inferior maxilla.

d., bimastoid. Transverse distance bet. 2 mastoid processes of the temporal bone.

d., biparietal. Transverse distance bet. parietal eminences on each side.

d., bisacromial. Transverse distance bet. 2 acromial processes.

d., bisiliac. Transverse distance bet. most distant points of the crests of the 2 ilia. SYN: *intercristal diameter.*

d., bisischiadic. SEE: *transverse diameter of pelvis.*

d., bitemporal. Distance bet. 2 most distant points of the coronal suture.

d., bitrochanteric. Distance bet. the highest point of 1 trochanter major and that of the other. SYN: *intertrochanteric diameter.*

d., bizygomatic. Greatest transverse distance bet. most prominent points of the zygomatic arches.

d., cervicobregmatic. Distance bet. anterior fontanel and junction of the neck with floor of the mouth.

d., diagonal conjugate, of the pelvis. The distance from the upper part of the symphysis pubis to the most distant part of the brim of the pelvis.

d., external biorbital. Greatest transverse distance bet. outer borders of external orbital apophyses of the frontal bone.

d., external conjugate, of the pelvis. Anteroposterior diameter of the pelvic inlet measured externally; distance from the skin over the upper part of symphysis pubis to the skin over a point corresponding to the sacral promontory.

d. of fetal skull. Important diameters at full term are: Suboccipitobregmatic, 3¾ in.; cervicobregmatic, 3¾ in.; frontomental, 3½ in.; occipitomental, 5 in.; supraoccipitomental, 5½ in.; occipitofrontal, 4½ in.; suboccipitofrontal, 4 in.; biparietal, 3¾ in.; bitemporal, 3⅕ in.

d., frontomental. Distance from top of forehead to point of chin.

d., inial. Distance in a straight line in median line of skull, bet. most prominent points of the inion and the glabella.

d., internal biorbital. Greatest transverse distance bet. inner borders of the external orbital apophyses of the frontal bone.

d., interspinous. Distance bet. 2 anterior superior spines of the ilia.

d., maximum, anteroposterior, of the skull. Distance, in the median line, bet. the most prominent part of the glabella and the most prominent point in the middle line upon the tabular portion of the occipital bone.

d., m. frontal. Distance bet. 2 stephanions.

d., m. occipital. Distance in a straight line bet. 2 asterions.

d., m. transverse, of the skull. Longest horizontal transverse line that can be drawn within the cranium.

d., mentobregmatic. Distance from chin to middle of anterior fontanel.

d., minimum frontal. Distance bet. 2 extremities of supraorbital line.

d., occipitofrontal. That extending from root of the nose to most distant point of the occiput.

d., occipitomental. Greatest distance bet. occiput and chin.

d., sacrosubpubic. Distance bet. middle of promontory of sacrum and middle of lower border of the triangular ligament of pubic symphysis.

d., sagittal. SEE: *basilobregmatic diameter.*

d., sternovertebral. Distance from sternum to vertebral column, measured externally.

d., suboccipitobregmatic. That extending from middle of ant. fontanel to lowest accessible point of the occiput.

d., suboccipitofrontal. Greatest distance bet. forehead and junction of occiput with the neck.

d., subtemporal. Distance bet. point upon sphenotemporal suture which is crossed by the ridge upon the inferior surface on the greater wing of the sphenoid bone of 1 side and a similar point on the other side.

d., temporal. Greatest horizontal distance bet. 2 opposite points upon the line passing over the vertex and uniting the 2 auricular points, on surface of the temporal bones.

d., trachelobregmatic. Diameter bet. ant. fontanel and meeting point of neck with floor of mouth.

d., vertical, of fetal head. That extending from highest point of head to ant. margin of foramen magnum.

diamid(e (di-am′id). A double amide. SEE: *hydrazine.*

diamine (di-am′in). A chemical compound with 2 NH₂ radicals.

diaminu′ria. Diamines in the urine.

diapason (dī-ă-pa′sun). A diagnostic tuning fork used in diseases of the ear.

diapedesis (di-ă-ped-e′sis). Blood or leukocytes transuding through the intact blood vessel walls.

diaphane (di′ă-fān). The investing membrane of a cell.

diaphanometer (di″ă-fan-om′et-er). A device estimating amt. of solids in a fluid by its transparency.

diaphanom′etry. Determination of translucency of a fluid, as the urine.

diaphanoscope (di-ă-fan′o-skōp). Device for electric examination of body cavities.

diaphanos′copy. Examination of fluids by the diaphanoscope.

diaphemetric (dī″ă-fe-met′rĭk). Pert. to degree of tactile sensibility.

diaphoresis (di-ă-for-e′sis). Profuse sweating.

diaphoretic (di-ă-for-et′ic). A sudorific or an agent which increases perspiration.

   d., drugs. These produce their effects either by stimulation, or general applications, or both.

   d., nauseating. One, such as warm drinks or sweat baths, which dilates superficial capillaries and causes relaxation.

   d., refrigerant. One that acts on sweat centers in the spinal cord and medulla, and reduces circulation, *i. e.,* lobelia, tobacco.

   d., simple. One that stimulates sudoriferous glands, such as sulfur.

diaphragm (di′ă-fram). A musculomembranous wall separating the abdomen from the thoracic cavity with its convexity upward.

   d., hernia of. Protrusion of abdominal contents through the diaphragm. ETIOL: Congenital or through injury.

   d., pelvic. The musculofascial layer forming the lower boundary of the abdominopelvic cavity.

diaphragmal′gia. Pain in the diaphragm.

diaphragmat′ic. Pert. to the diaphragm.

diaphragmati′tis. Inflammation of the diaphragm.

diaphragmatocele (di″ă-frag-mat′o-sēl). Hernia of the diaphragm.

di″aphragmi′tis. Inflammation of the diaphragm. SYN: *diaphragmatitis.*

di″aphragmodyn′ia. Pain in the diaphragm.

diaph′ysary. Pert. to or affecting the shaft of a bone.

diaphysec′tomy. Removal of part of the shaft of a long bone.

diaphysis (di-af′is-is). The shaft or middle part of a long cylindrical bone. SEE: *apophysis, epiphysis.*

diaphysitis (di-ă-fi-si′tis). Inflammation of shaft of a long bone.

diaplasis (di-ap′la-sis). Reduction of a fracture or dislocation. SYN: *diorthosis.*

di′aplex. Choroid plexus of 3rd ventricle.

diaplex′al. Pert. to the diaplex.

diaplex′us. Choroid plexus of 3rd ventricle.

diapnoic (di-ap-no′ik). 1. Pert. to or causing perspiration, esp. insensible perspiration. 2. A mild sudorific.

diapoph′ysis. An upper articular surface of transverse process of a vertebra.

diapyesis (di-ap-i-e′sis). Suppuration.

diapyetic (di-ap-i-et′ik). Pert. to or causing suppuration.

diarrhea (di-ă-re′ă). Morbid frequency of bowel evacuation, due to diet, irritation, or inflammation of the mucous membrane of intestines.

   d., acid. Green, broken stools with sour odor.

   d., bilious. Bile in the stools.

   d., catarrhal. Diarrhea caused by degeneration in the intestines.

   d., choleraic. Diarrhea accompanying cholera in severe form with vomiting and collapse.

   d., colliquative. Variety causing collapse, due to frequency of evacuation.

   d., congestive. Form caused by congestion of alimentary tract.

   d., critical. Diarrhea causing a crisis, or occurring at the time of a crisis.

   d., dry. Variety in which stools are exceptionally small, but can cause death.

   d., dysenteric. Diarrhea with mucus and bloody discharge.

   d., emotional. Form caused by emotional stress.

   d., fatty. Diarrhea with stools containing undigested fat particles.

   d., infantile. In children under 2 years.

   TREATMENT: Water, woolen clothing, no food, warm baths, hot applications or mustard plaster, emetic enemas, cleanliness, fresh air.

   d., inflammatory. Type caused by increased vascularity of intestinal mucosa.

   d., intermittent. Diarrhea recurring, due possibly to malarial poisoning.

   d., lienteric. Watery stools with undigested food particles.

   d., membranous. Diarrhea with passage of pieces of intestinal mucosa.

   d., nervous. Nervous increase of peristalsis.

   TREATMENT: In general, heat externally, rest, enemas and cathartics if resulting from constipation; sedatives if of nervous origin.

   DIET: Starvation diet of broth, and hot water for a day or two.

   d., mucous. Diarrhea with mucus in stools.

   d., puerperal. Form occurring in puerperas, caused by septicemia or indigestion.

   d., purulent. Presence in stools of pus, due to intestinal ulceration.

   d., serous. Water stools.

   d., simple. Variety in which stools contain only normal excreta.

   d., summer. Diarrhea due to summer heat.

   d., ulcerative. Severe diarrhea with ulceration of mucosa of intestines.

diarthric (di-ar'thrik). Pert. to 2 or more joints.

diarthrosis (di-ar-thro'sis). An articulation in which opposing bones move freely; a hinge joint.

diartic'ular. Pert. to 2 joints.

diaschisis (dī-as'ki-sis). Disturbance or injury to 1 part of central nervous system may cause alteration in function of some distant part.

diascope (di'as-kōp). A glass held against the skin for ascertaining noncongestive changes.

diastal'sis. Ability to distinguish 1 thing from another.

diastal'tic. Denoting reflex action.

diastase (di'as-tas). A specific enzyme or ferment in plant cells, such as in sprouting grains and malt, and in the digestive juice which converts starch into sugar.

  d. index. Normal index in urine bet. 6.6 and 30. Lower if kidney is diseased. In acute disease of pancreas may be 200 or more, due to pancreatic obstruction.

diastasis (di-as'ta-sis). 1. In surgery, injury to a bone involving separation of an epiphysis. 2. In cardiac physiology, the last part of diastole.

  d. recti. A separation lateralward of the 2 halves of the m. rectus abdominis.

diaste'ma. 1. A fissure. 2. A space bet. 2 teeth.

diastematocrania (di-as″tem-at-o-kra'-nĭ-ă). Congenital sagittal fissure of the skull.

diastematomyelia (di-as″tem-at-o-mĭ-e'-lĭ-ă). Congenital splitting of the spinal cord.

diastematopye'lia. Median slit of the pelvis; congenital.

dias'ter. 1. Daughter star. 2. Figure formed by 2 aster-shaped masses of chromatin in a maturing ovum.

dias'tole. PHYS: The normal period in the heart cycle during which the muscle fibers lengthen, the heart dilates, and the cavities fill with blood, the atria before the ventricles; roughly, the period of relaxation alternating with systole or contraction, thus constituting the pulsation of the heart.

diastol'ic. Pert. to diastole.

  d. pressure. This is the point of the greatest cardiac relaxation.

diastrophia (di-as-tref'ĭ-ă). Psychosis exhibiting extreme cruelty.

diatax'ia. Ataxia of both sides of body.

  d. cerebra'lis infanti'lis. Birth palsy.

diatela, diatele (di-ă-te'lă, -lē). Membranous roof of 3rd ventricle.

diater'ma. Portion of the floor of 3rd ventricle.

diathermal (di-a-ther'mal). Permeable by radiant heat.

diather'manous. Diathermal*; permeable by heat.

diather'mia. An inferior term for diathermy. SEE: diathermy.

diather'mic. Of the nature of diathermy or of its results.

diathermy (di'ă-ther″mĭ). The therapeutic use of a high frequency current to generate heat within some part of the body.

  d., medical. The generation of heat within the body by the application of high frequency oscillatory current for medical purposes.

  d., short wave. Treatment by patient's being placed in the path of diathermic rays, but not in contact with either electrode.

  d., surgical. Diathermy of high degree for electrocoagulation, cauterization, etc.

diathesis (di-ath'e-sis). Constitutional predisposition to disease.

diathet'ic. Pert. to diathesis, or predisposition.

di'atom. One of a group of unicellular microscopical plants.

diatom'ic. 1. Containing 2 atoms; said of molecules. 2. Bivalent.

diato'ric. Artificial teeth attached with vulcanized rubber to their bases.

diax'on, diax'one. A neuron having 2 axons.

diazo-. A formative of names of compounds derived from 2 aromatic hydrocarbons, containing 2 atoms of nitrogen with phenyl.

  d. reaction. A deep red color in urine. SEE: Ehrlich's diazo reaction.

diba'sic. Containing in each molecule 2 atoms of hydrogen replaceable by a base; said of acids.

diblas'tula. A blastule containing the ectoderm and entoderm.

Dibothriocephalus (di-both″rĭ-o-sef'al-us). Flat worms with flat suckers; Pseudolphyllidea carus.

dical'cic. Containing 2 atoms of calcium in a molecule.

  d. orthophosphate. $CaHPO_4$. A salt, often found in the urine.

dichloramine-T (di-klor'a-mēn). USP. White powder containing about 28% chlorine.

  ACTION AND USES: Germicide and disinfectant.

dichloro-hexyl-resorcinol (dī-klō″rō-hek″-sĭl-rē-sor'sĭn-ōl). An antiseptic effective against streptococcus, staphylococcus and B. pyocyaneus.

dichot'omy, dichotomiza'tion. 1. Division into 2 parts, as bifurcation of the embryo. 2. Sharing of fees between practitioner and consultant.

dichroic (di-kro'ĭk). Pert. to dichroism.

dichroism (di'kro-izm). Property of a substance appearing to be 1 color by direct light and another by transmitted light.

dichro'masy. Able to see only 2 colors.

dichromat'ic. Being able to see only 2 colors.

dichromatopsia (di-kro-mat-op'sĭ-ă). Ability to distinguish only 2 primary colors.

dichro'mic. 1. Containing 2 atoms of chromium. 2. Seeing only 2 colors.

dichro'mophil. Double staining with both acid and basic dyes.

dichromophilism (di-kro-mof'il-izm). Having the capacity for double staining.

Dick method. A toxin-antitoxin injection for the prevention of scarlet fever.

D. test. *Negative Reaction*: Some slight inflammatory changes due to irritation by proteins in fluid administered. SEE: *Schick method; Schick test.*

dicliditis (dik-li-di'tis). Inflammation of a cardiac or other valve.

diclidostosis (di-klid-os-to'sis). Ossification of the venous valves.

diclidot'omy. Cutting a valve, esp. a rectal one.

dico'ria. Double pupil in each eye.

dicrotic (di-krot'ik). One heartbeat for 2 arterial pulsations; rel. to a double pulse. SEE: *pulse.*

dicrotism (di'krot-izm). The state of being dicrotic.

dictyoma (dik-ti-o'ma). A retinal tumor.

didac'tylism. The congenital condition of having only 2 digits on a hand or foot.

didial (di'di-ăl). Proprietary hypnotic.

didymalgia (did-im-al'ji-ă). Pain in a testicle.

didymitis (did-i-mi'tis). Inflammation of a testicle. SYN: *orchitis.*

didymodynia (did''i-mo-din'i-ă). Pain in a testicle.

didymus (did'i-mus). 1. A twin. 2. A double monstrosity. 3. A testicle.

diechoscope (di-ek'o-skōp). A stethoscope that gives 2 sounds in 2 different parts at the same time.

di''elec'tric. An insulating substance which offers great resistance to the passage of electricity by conduction but through which electric force may act by induction.

dielectrolysis (di''e-lek-trol'i-sis). The forcing of a drug or medicinal compound to a particular part of the body by osmosis brought about or accelerated with an electric current.

diencephalon (di-en-sef'ă-lon). The midbrain. SYN: *thalamencephalon.*

dieresis (di-er'es-is). 1. Breaking up or dispersion of things normally joined, as by an ulcer. 2. Mechanical separation of parts by surgical means.

dieret'ic. Dissolvable or separable.

diet. Selection of food materials necessary for the nourishment of the body, or suitable in disease states, or both.

d., balanced. One that will provide a favorable alkaline reaction or balance for the body, and maintain energy requirements.

dietary (di'ĕ-ta-rĭ). A regulated diet.

dietetic (di-ĕ-tet'ik). Pert. to diet.

dietet'ics. The science of the use of foods in health and disease. Some fundamental principles and facts of this science will be summarized here.

di-ethyl-stilboestrol (di''ĕth''ll-stĭl''bō-ĕs'trol). A synthetic estrogen.

dietitian (di-ĕ-tish'an). One scientifically trained in dietetics (which includes nutrition) and who is in charge of the diet of a hospital, or other institution.

Dietl's crisis (de'tlz). Renal colic; accompanied by scanty, bloodstained urine.

Dieulafoy's triad. Tenderness, muscular contraction, and skin hyperesthesia in acute appendicitis at McBurney's point.

differen'tial. Marked by differences.

d. blood count. Determination of the number of each variety of leukocytes in a cubic millimeter of blood.

d. diagnosis. Diagnosis based on comparison of symptoms of 2 or more similar diseases to determine which the patient is suffering from. SEE: *blood count, diagnosis.*

differentia'tion. Acquirement of functions different from those of the original type.

diffusate (dif'fu-săt). In the process of dialysis, that portion of a liquid which passes through a membrane and which contains crystalloid matter in solution. SYN: *dialysate.*

diffuse (dif-fūs'). Spreading, scattered, spread.

d. inflammation. One not localized.

diffusible (dif-fu'zib-l). Capable of being diffused.

diffu'sion. 1. Absorption of a liquid such as the absorption, by cells, of water from lymph when the percentage of salt is less in lymph than in the cells.

2. A process whereby different gases interpenetrate and become mixed, due to the incessant motion of their molecules.

digastric (di-gas'trĭk). Having 2 bellies; said of certain muscles.

digen'esis. Reproduction in which alternate generations are asexual.

digest'. 1. To undergo digestion. 2. To make a condensation of a subject.

diges'tant. 1. An agent that will digest food or aid in digestion.

diges'tible. Pert. to that which may be digested.

diges'tion. The process by which food is broken down, mechanically and chemically, in the gastrointestinal tract and is converted into absorbable forms.

d., artificial. Digestion outside the living organism by a ferment.

d., cecal. Digestive process in the cecum.

d., duodenal. The acid chyme is now made alkaline, and the fats it contains are emulsified by the action of bile.

d., extracellular. That occurring outside the body of the cell.

d., gastric. Portion of the digestive process taking place in the stomach.

d., intestinal. Hydrolytic processes continue here, and absorption of the products is active. SEE: *absorption.*

d., intracellular. Digestion within the cell body.

d., oral. Portion of the digestive process taking place in the mouth.

d., pancreatic. Portion of digestive process influenced by pancreatic juice.

d., peptic. SEE: *gastric digestion.*

d., primary. Digestion by gastrointestinal tract.

d., salivary. Digestive action by the saliva. SEE: *salivary digestion.*

d., secondary. Cellular assimilation of nutritive material.

d., tryptic. SEE: *pancreatic digestion.*

digestive (di-jes'tiv). Pert. to digestion.

    d. juice. One of several secretions which aid in processes of digestion.

dig'it (pl. *dig'iti*). A finger or toe.

digital (dij'it-al). Pert. to or resembling a finger or toe.

    d. reflex. Sudden flexion of terminal phalanx of a finger or thumb when nail is suddenly tapped.

digitalis (dij-it-a'lis). USP. Foxglove. The dried leaves of *Digitalis purpurea.*

    DOSAGE: 1½ gr. (0.1 Gm.). Infusion of digitalis: 1½ fluid dram (6 cc.). Tincture digitalis: 15 ♏ (1 cc.).

digitalism (dij'it-al-izm). The poisonous effects produced by digitalis.

digitalization (dij-it-al-iz-a'shun). Subjection of an organism to the action of digitalis.

dig'itate. Having fingerlike impressions or processes.

digitation (dij-it-a'shun). A fingerlike process, esp. of a muscle.

dig'itus. A finger or toe.

diglossia (dī-glos'sĭ-ă). State of having a double tongue.

dihydrotachysterol (dī″hī″drō-tăk-ĭ-ster′ōl). A hydrogenated tachysterol obtained by irradiation of ergosterol.

dihydrotheelin (dī″hĭ-drō-thē′ĕl-ĭn). Commercial hormone preparation obtained from hogs' ovaries and urine of pregnant mares or synthetically from estrone. SYN: *estradiol.*

dihysteria (di-his-ter'ĭ-ă). State of having a double uterus.

diktyo'ma. A ciliary epithelium tumor.

dilaceration (dī″las-er-a'shun). A tearing apart.

dilantin sodium (dī'lăn-tĭn). *Sodium diphenyl hydantoinate.* It is related to the barbiturates. A derivative of glyceryl urea. An anticonvulsant used in epilepsy.

dila'tant. Anything that causes dilation.

dilatation (di-la-ta'shun). 1. Expansion of an organ or vessel. 2. Expansion of an orifice with a dilator.

dila'tion. 1. Expansion of an orifice with a dilator. 2. Expansion of an organ or vessel. SYN: *dilatation.*

dilator (dī-lā'tor). Instrument for dilating muscles, stretching cavities or openings.

    d., Barnes. Rubber bag that is filled with fluid.

    d., Bossi. A multiple pronged instrument that dilates by separation of the prongs.

    d., Goodell. Similar to the Bossi except that it has but 3 prongs.

    d., gyn. An instrument for dilating the cervix uteri.

    d., Hegar's. Graduated metal sounds that are inserted into the cervical canal and cause a graded dilatation.

    d., Tent's. Small cones made of seaweed, sponge, or tree roots which are inserted into the uterine canal dry and, on absorbing moisture, expand to cause a slow dilatation.

dilaudid hydrochloride (dī-law'dĭd) (dihy-

dromorphinone hydrochloride). A white crystalline powder, odorless, and freely soluble in water.

    DOSAGE: As sedative or relief of pain, 1/24 gr. (0.0025 Gm.) orally; subcutaneously: 1/32 gr. (0.002 Gm.) being equivalent to 1/6 gr. (0.01 Gm.) morphine.

dil'uent. That which dilutes.

dilution (di-lu'shun). 1. Process of rendering a substance attenuated or diluted. 2. A diluted substance.

dimetria (di-me'trĭ-ă). A double uterus.

dimorphous (di-mor'fus). Occurring in 2 different forms.

dineuric (di-nu'rik). Having 2 axiscylinder processes.

dinical (din'ĭ-kal). Pert. to giddiness or vertigo.

dionin (dī'o-nin) (ethylmorphine hydrochloride). USP. A white, slightly bitter powder.

    USES: As a sedative, analgesic, and antispasmodic; externally, in iritis and other affections of the eye.

    DOSAGE: Internally: ¼ gr. (0.015 Gm.).

diopsimeter (dī-op-sim'et-er). Device for exploring the visual field.

diop'ter. Refractive power of lens with focal distance of 1 meter, used as unit of measurement in refraction.

dioptometer (di-op-tom'et-er). Device for measuring ocular refraction.

dioptom'etry. The determination of refraction and accommodation of the eye.

dioptral (di-op'tral). Pert. to a diopter.

dioptric (di-op'trik). 1. Dioptral; pert. to refraction of light. 2. A diopter.

diop'trics. The science of refraction of light.

diorthosis (di-or-tho'sis). Reduction of a fracture or dislocation. SYN: *diaplasis.*

diosmosis (di-oz-mo'sis). Passage of a fluid through a membrane. SEE: *dialysis, osmosis.*

dioxid(e (di-oks'ĭd). 1. A compound having 2 oxygen atoms to 1 of another element. 2. A gas given off by the lungs. Extraneous gases inhaled may be exhaled also.

dipeptid(e (di-pep'tid). A protein having 2 amino acids. SEE: *peptide, polypeptid.*

dipha'sic. Having 2 phases.

diphonia (di-fō'nĭ-ă). Simultaneous production of 2 different voice tones.

diphtheria (dif-the'ri-a). An acute infectious disease characterized by the formation of a false membrane on any mucous surface, and accompanied by great prostration.

    d. carrier. A person harboring in his body the Klebs-Loeffler bacillus without manifest symptoms, thus acting as a distributor of the infection.

    d., laryngeal. In this type, croupy cough, aphonia, stridulous respiration due to narrowing of glottic opening are early evidences of the disease.

    d., surgical or **wound.** Diphtheric membrane formation on wounds.

diphthe'rial. Pert. to diphtheria.

diphtheriaphor (dif-the'rĭ-ă-for). A diphtheria carrier or vector.

diphtheric (dif-the'rik). Pert. to diphtheria.

diphtherin (dif'the-rin). The toxin of diphtheria, from *Bacillus diphtheriae*.

diphtheritic (dif-ther-it'ĭk). Pert. to diphtheria.

diphtheritis (dif-ther-i'tis). Another name for diphtheria.

diphtheroid (dif'the-roid). Resembling or false diphtheria. SYN: *pseudodiphtheria*.

diphtherotox'in. The specific toxin of the diphtheria bacillus.

diphthongia (dif-thon'jĭ-ă). The simultaneous utterance of 2 vocal sounds of different pitch in pathological conditions of the larynx.

Diphyllobroth'rium. A genus of tapeworms, 3 species being found in the human.

    D. la'tum (*Taenia lata*). A large tapeworm with many segments infesting man.

diphyodont (dif'ĭ-o-dont). Having 2 sets of teeth; as man.

diplacusis (dip-lă-ku'sis). Variety of disturbed perception of pitch characterized by hearing 2 tones for every sound produced.

diplegia (di-ple'jĭ-ă). Paralysis of similar parts on both sides of the body. SYN: *double hemiplegia*.

diplegic (di-ple'jik). Pert. to diplegia.

diploalbuminu'ria. Coexistence of physiologic and pathologic albuminuria.

diplobacil'lus. A double bacillus, 2 being linked end to end.

diplobacte'rium. An organism made up of 2 adherent bacteria.

diploblastic (dip-lo-blas'tĭk). Having 2 germinal layers.

diplocar'dia. Having a double heart.

diplococcemia (dip″lo-kok-se'mĭ-ă). Diplococci in the blood.

diplococcus (dip-lo-kok'us). A coccus occurring in pairs.

diploe (dip'lo-e). Cancellated tissue bet. the tables of the skull.

diploet'ic, diplo'ic. Pert. to the diploe or cancellated tissue bet. cranial tables.

diplogen'esis. Having 2 parts or producing 2 substances.

diplomellituria (dip″lo-mel-ĭ-tu'rĭ-ă). Occurrence of diabetic and nondiabetic glycosuria in the body.

diplomyelia (dip-lo-mi-e'lĭ-ă). Lengthwise fissure of the spinal cord, with seeming duplication.

diploneu'ral. Having 2 nerves from different origins, as certain muscles.

diplophonia (dip-lo-fo'nĭ-ă). Having 2 different voice tones at the same time. SYN: *diphonia*.

diplopia (dip-lo'pĭ-ă). Double vision; monocular (astigmatism, subluxated lens, incipient cataract); binocular (due to derangement of extraocular muscles).

    d., binocular. Double vision occurs when both eyes are used.

    d., crossed. Binocular vision in which the images are reversed.

    d., direct. SEE: *homonymous diplopia*.   [lopia.

    d., heteronymous. SEE: *crossed dip-*

    d., homonymous. Double vision in which right-hand image appears on right side and left-hand image on left side. OPP: *crossed diplopia*.

    d., monocular. Double vision with 1 eye.

    d., unocular. SEE: *monocular diplopia*.

    d., vertical. Diplopia with 1 of 2 images higher than the other.

diplopiometer (dip-lo-pĭ-om'et-er). Device for estimating double vision.

dip'loscope. Device for study of binocular vision.

diplosoma'tia. Twins joined at 1 or more points. SYN: *diplosomia*.

diploso'mia. Twins joined together. SYN: *diplosomatia*.*

dipsomania (dip-so-ma'nĭ-ă). PSY: A morbid and uncontrollable craving for alcoholic beverages. SEE: *alcoholism*.

dipsopathy (dip-sop'ă-thǐ). 1. Dipsomania. 2. Limitation of intoxicants for purposes of cure.

dipsosis (dip-so'sis). Abnormal thirst.

dipsotherapy (dip-so-ther'ă-pǐ). Limitation of water to be drunk as a cure.

direct'. Immediate, uninterrupted.

    d. current. One flowing in 1 direction only. SEE: *current*.

    d. light reflex. One in which response occurs in area of stimulation.

    d. murmur. That due to stenosis of cardiac orifices.

    d. reflex. Prompt contraction of sphincter of iris when light entering through pupil strikes retina of eye.

director (dǐ-rek'tor). Grooved device for guiding a knife.

direc'toscope. Device for examination of the larynx.

dir″igomo'tor. Controlling or directing muscular activity.

dis-. Prefix: Free of, undo, as *disable*.

disaccharid(e (dis-ak'ĭ-rĭd). A member of the disaccharose* group of carbohydrates. SEE: *carbohydrates*.

disac'charose. A *complex* sugar that may be split into 2 molecules of monosaccharids.

disarticula'tion. Amputation through a joint.

disassimila'tion. Changing assimilated material into less complex compounds, freeing potential energy.

dis″asso'cia'tion. A mental condition in which ideas are split from the consciousness and which are no longer amenable to objective control such as amnesial somnambulism,* catalepsy,* dual personality,* fugues,* and trances.

disc. A round, flat, platelike structure. SEE: *disk*.

discharge (dis-charj'). 1. The escape (especially by violence) of pent up or accumulated energy or of explosive material. 2. The flowing away of a secretion or excretion of pus, feces, urine, etc. 3. The material ejected by discharge (2nd def.).

    d., brush. That from a static machine having a disruptoconvective character.

d., cerebral cortical. The violent action of a diseased portion of the cerebral cortex that gives rise to an epileptic paroxysm.

d., convective. One from a high potential source in the form of electrical energy passing through the air to the patient.

d., disruptive. A passage of current through an insulating medium due to the breakdown of the medium under electrostatic stress.

d., disruptoconductive. The static brush discharge simulating both the convective and the disruptive or spark discharge.

d., electric. A slow or instantaneous bringing back to a neutral electric condition, by which every highly electrified body loses its surplus electricity, giving it up to surrounding bodies less highly electrified.

d., lochial. Uterine excretion following childbirth. SEE: *lochia.*

d., silent. The gradual loss of electricity by even isolated bodies, owing to the conductibility of air and its contained vapors, together with that of the isolating bodies themselves.

discharge tube. A vessel of insulating material (usually glass) provided with metal electrodes, which is exhausted to a low gas pressure and permits the passage of electricity through the residual gas when a moderately high voltage is applied to the electrodes.

discharg'ing. Excreting.

d. lesion. A lesion of nerve center in brain suddenly discharging motor impulses.

dischrona'tion. Failure of relativity in the consciousness of time.

discission (dĭ-sĭsh'un). Rupture of the capsule of the crystalline lens in operation for cataract.

discitis (dis-kī'tis). Inflammation of any disk, esp. an interarticular cartilage. SYN: *meniscitis.*

discoblas'tic. Pert. to discoid segmentation of yolk in an impregnated ovum.

dis'coid. Like a disc.

discoplacen'ta. A disklike placenta.

discre'te. Separate; opposed to *confluent.** Said of certain eruptions on the skin.

dis'cus prolig'erus. Epithelial cells enveloping the ovum within the graafian follicle.

discuss'. To disperse, scatter, or cause to disappear.

discussion (dis-kush'un). Dispersal of a tumor or swelling.

discutient (dis-ku'shent). Agent which disperses a lesion or tumor.

disdiaclast (dis-dī'ă-klast). A doubly refracting element in the tissues of striated muscles.

disease'. Literally the lack of ease: a pathological condition of the body that presents a group of symptoms peculiar to it and which sets the condition apart as an abnormal entity differing from other normal or pathological body states.

disengage'ment. GYN: The displacement of the fetal head from within the maternal pelvis.

disequilib'rium. On unequal and unstable equilibrium.

disinfect (dis-in-fekt'). To free from infection by physical or chemical means.

disinfec'tant. A chemical which kills bacteria. Disinfectants include formaldehyde, sulfur dioxide, chlorine, phenol (carbolic acid), cresols, iodine, and mercurochrome.

CHEMICAL: *Liquid*: Chloride of lime, 2 parts to 100 of water. Corrosive Sublimate, 1 part to 1000 of water. Carbolic Acid, 1 part to 450 of water. Whitewash (milk of lime).

GASEOUS: Formaldehyde. Sulfurous acid must not be used in occupied room. SEE: *chlorite.*

HEAT: 150°-200° dry. Boiling water or steam may also be used.

disinfecting agents. SEE: *alcohol, borax, boric acid, chlorine preparations, cresols, formaldehyde, hydrogen dioxide, kreseptol, mercuric chloride, nitric acid, phenol, potassium permanganate, sulfur, urotropin.*

disinfec'tion. The application of disinfectants. It is not possible to insure a 100% disinfection of a room. Disinfestation, or the killing of vermin by chemicals and their vapors, however, is possible.

d. of blankets and woolens: May be steam disinfected, or soaked for 2 hours in 5% carbolic and then washed. Cotton goods may also be so treated, or boiled before washing.

d. of excreta. Should be soaked in 5% carbolic solution for 1 hour before disposal. All infected excreta should be burned, but sputum may be treated as excreta if impossible to burn.

disinfestation (dis-in-fes-ta'shun). The process of killing infesting insects or parasites.

disintegra'tion. The product of catabolism; the falling apart of the constituents of a substance.

disk. A round, flat, platelike structure.

d., blood. A red blood corpuscle.

d., Bowman's. Segment of a muscle fiber.

d., choked. Inflammation of the optic disk. SYN: *papillitis.*

d. diameter. Optic disk diameter.

d., epiphyseal. Disklike epiphysis at vertebral centrum's ends.

d., germinal. Area of central portion of blastoderm.

d. holder. Microscope joint to enable mobility in every direction.

d., intermediate. Fine membrane passing transversely across the stria of a striated muscle fiber.

d., interpubic. Disk of cartilage bet. the pubic bones at their symphysis.

d., optic. Area of the retina where optic nerve enters it.

d. proligerous. SEE: *germinal disk.*

d., Thorington's. Device used for retinoscopy.

dis'loca'tion. The displacement of any part, more esp. the removal temporarily of a bone out of its normal position in a joint.

d., closed. Simple dislocation, *q.v.*

d., complete. One which completely separates the surfaces of a joint.

d., complicated. One which is associated with other important injuries.

d., compound. One in which the joint communicates with the external air.

d., congenital. One which exists from or before birth.

d., consecutive. One in which the luxated bone has changed its position since its first displacement.

d., divergent. One in which the ulna and radius are dislocated separately.

d., habitual. One which often recurs after replacement.

d., incomplete. A subluxation; a slight displacement.

d., intrauterine. One which occurs to the fetus in the utero.

d., metacarpophalangeal joint. Disk of finger.
This is usually complicated by an interposition of tendons or other structures, and if reduced tends to slip out immediately.

d., Monteggia's. Dislocation of hip joint in which head of femur is near anterosuperior spine of the ilium.

d., Nelaton's. Dislocation of the ankle in which the astragalus is formed up bet. the end of the tibia and the fibula.

d., old. A dislocation in which no reduction has been accomplished, even after many days, weeks, or months.

d., partial. Same as incomplete.

d., pathologic. One which results from paralysis or disease of joint or supporting tissues.

d., primitive. One in which the bones remain as originally displaced.

d., recent. One in which there is no complicating inflammation.

d., simple. One in which the joint is not penetrated by a wound.

d., subastragalar. Separation of the calcaneum and the scaphoid from the astragalus.

d., thyroid. Displacement of the head of the femur into the thyroid foramen.

d., traumatic. One due to injury or violence. SEE: *Names of bones in alphabetical order.*

dislocation, words pert. to: ankle, anteresis, aparthrosis, cecoptosis, diarthrosis, elbow, neck, shoulder, wrist.

disocclude (dis-ŏ-klūd'). To grind a tooth so that it does not touch the opp. one in the other jaw.

disorganiza'tion. Alteration in an organic part, causing it to lose most or all of its distinctive characteristics.

disorientation (dis-o-ri-en-ta'shun). Inability to estimate direction or location, or to be cognizant of time or of persons.

disparate points (dis'par-at). Points on the 2 retinas which are not corresponding or identical, causing objects to appear double.

dispareunia (dis-par-ū'nĭ-ă). Pain in the female during coitus.

dispen'sary. Place or clinic for free dispensation of medicines and treatment.

dispen'satory. A commentary on medicines.

dispense (dis-pens'). To prepare or deliver medicines to those for whom they are prescribed.

disperse (dis-pers'). 1. To scatter. 2. The suspended particles in a colloid solution.

disper'sion. 1. Act of dispersing. 2. That which is dispersed.

d., coarse. Mechanical suspension.

d., colloidal. Colloid solution.

d. me'dium. Liquid in which a colloid is dispersed.

d. particles. Colloid particles in a colloid system.

d. system. A colloid solution.

disper'soid. A colloid or molecular disperse solution.

dispirem (di-spi'rem). Stage that succeeds the diaster and precedes division of cell body, when threads of daughter cell are convoluted.

displace'ment. 1. Removal from the normal or usual position or place. SEE: *cardianastrophe.* 2. Attachment of emotion from repressed conflict to some apparently indifferent idea.

distrac''tibil'ity. A disturbance of attention in which the direction of thought frequently changes because of external impressions.

dissect (dis-sekt'). To separate tissues and parts of a cadaver for anatomical study.

dissection (dis-sek'shun). The cutting of parts for purpose of separation and studying of the same.

dissem'inated. Scattered throughout an organ or the body.

d. sclerosis. A degenerative disease of the nervous system; insular sclerosis.

dissipation (dis-ĭ-pa'shun). Dispersion of matter.

dissociation (dis-so-sĭ-a'shun). Separation, as the separation by heat of a complex compound into simpler molecules.   [pure strains.

d., microbic. Substrains arising from

d. of personality. Split in consciousness resulting in 2 different phases of personality, neither being aware of the words, acts, and feelings of the other. SEE: *dual personality, multiple personality.*

d., psychological. Disunion of mind of which the person is not aware. Dual personalities, fugues, somnambulism, are so classified.

d. symptoms. Anesthesia to heat, cold, and pain, without loss of muscular sense or tactile sensibility.

dissolu'tion. Death; pathological resolution or breaking up of the integrity of an anatomical element.

dissolve (di-zolv'). To cause absorption of a solid in and by a liquid.

dissolvent (diz-ol'vent). 1. Having the power to dissolve. 2. That which is capable of disintegrating.

dissol'ving. To cause to enter into a solution.

distad (dis'tad). Away from the center.

distal (dis'tal). Farthest from the center, from a medial line, or from the trunk. Opposite of *proximal*.

distend'. 1. To stretch out. 2. To become inflated.

disten'tion. The state of being distended. SEE: *goblet cell, Wangensteen's method*.

distichiasis (dis-tǐ-ki'a-sis). Two rows of eyelashes, the post. of which is directed inward toward the eye.

distil'. To vaporize by heat, condensing and collecting the volatilized products.

dis'tillate. The portion of a substance subject to distillation which passes in the form of a vapor and condenses.

distilla'tion. Condensation of a liquid, heated to a volatization point, as the condensation of steam from boiling water.

   d., destructive. The process of decomposing complex organic compounds by heat in the absence of air, and condensing the vapor of the liquid products.

   d., dry. Distillation of solids without liquids.

   d., fractional. Separation of liquids based upon the difference in their boiling points.

distinctom'eter. Device for palpation of abdomen along its borders.

distobuccal (dis-to-buk'al). Pert. to the distal and buccal walls of bicuspid and molar teeth.

distoma, distomum (dis'to-ma, -mum). Trematode worm with a ventral and oral sucker. SEE: *distomiasis*.

distomiasis (dis-to-mi'as-is). Distoma in the body; may be hepatic, intestinal, pancreatic, or billiary. SEE: *distoma*.

distractibil'ity. PSY: A condition of mental wandering in which the thoughts are attracted by extraneous conditions or influenced by a disassociation of consciousness.

districhiasis (dis-trik-i'as-is). Two hairs growing from the same hair follicle.

distrix (dis'triks). The splitting of ends of the hairs.

dito'cia, dito'kia. Twin birth.

ditokous (dit'o-kus). Giving birth to twins.

Dittrich's plugs (dit'ricks). Small particles in fetid sputum composed of pus, detritus, bacteria, and fat crystals.

diuresis (di-u-re'sis). Abnormal secretion of urine.

diuretic (di-u-ret'ik). Increasing or an agent which increases the secretion of urine.

   d., alterative. One eliminated by the kidney which aids diseased urinary tract surfaces.   [flow.

   d., hydragogue. One increasing renal

   d., refrigerant. One which alleviates irritation from urine.

diuretin (dī-u-re'tin). A white, odorless powder, original soluble sodium salicylate salt of theobromine.

   DOSAGE: Average, 15 gr. (1 Gm.).

diur'nal. 1. Daily. 2. Happening in the daytime, or pert. to it; opposed to *nocturnal*.

divagation (div-a-ga'shun). Disconnected and incoherent speech.

divergence (di-ver'jens). Separation from a common center, esp. that of the eyes.

diver'gent. Radiating in different directions.

diver's paralysis. Occupational disease due to returning too suddenly under normal atmosphere after working under high air pressure. SYN: *bends, caisson disease, tunnel disease*.

divertic'ula. Plural of *diverticulum, q.v.*

   d. hernia. Hernia containing part of the intestine.

diverticulec'tomy. Surgical removal of a diverticulum.

diverticuli'tis. Inflammation of a diverticulum or of diverticula in the colon, causing stagnation of feces in little distended sacs of the colon (diverticula).

   d., acute. SYM: Similar to appendicitis.

   d., chronic. SYM: Constipation growing worse, mucus in stools, griping abdominal pains at intervals. Wall of bowels may thicken, which may produce chronic intestinal obstruction.

diverticulo'sis. Diverticula of the colon.

diverticulum (di-ver-tik'u-lum) (pl. *diverticula*). A sac or pouch in the walls of a canal or organ, esp. the colon.

   d., Meckel's. Vestiges of the vitelline duct sometimes appearing as an extended pouch at the lower portion of the ileum.

divulsor (di-vul'sor). Device for dilatation of a part.

   d., pterygium. Instrument for separating corneal portion of the pterygium.

   d., tendon. Device for separating tendon from surrounding tissue.

dizygotic twins (di-zi-got'ik). Twins who are the product of 2 ova and who are dissimilar in most ways.

diz'ziness. Giddiness, vertigo.

Dobell's solution (do'belz). Carbolic acid, borax, sodium bicarbonate, glycerine, and water in solution.

Dobie's globule (dŏ'bēs). A very tiny spherical body in a striated muscle fiber's light band.

dochmiasis, dochmiosis (dok-mi'as-is, -mi-o'sis). Hookworm disease. SYN: *ankylostomiasis, uncinariasis*.

Dochmius (dok'mĭ-us). A species of parasite. SYN: *ankylostoma*.

Dock's test meal. Shredded wheat biscuit and 9-12 oz. water. SEE: *Ewald's t. m.*

dodecadactylitis (do-dek-a-dak-til-i'tis). Inflammation of duodenum.

dodecadactylon (do-dek-a-dak'til-on). The duodenum.

dolichocephalic (dol'ĭk-o-se-fal'ĭk). Having a skull with a long ant. post. diameter.

dolichoceph′alism, dolichoceph′aly. The quality of having a low cephalic index.

dolichohieric (dol-ĭk-o-hi-er′ĭk). Having a slender sacrum.

dolichopellic, dolichopelvic (dol-ĭk-o-pel′-ĭk, -pel′vĭk). Having an abnormally long or narrow pelvis.

dolichosigmoid (dol-ĭk-o-sig′moid). Having an abnormally long sigmoid flexure.

doll′s head anesthesia. Anesthesia affecting the head, neck, and upper thorax.

dolor (do′lor). Physical or mental pain. SEE: *calor, rubor, tumor.*

   d. cap′itis. Headache.

dolorific (dol-o-rif′ik). Causing pain.

dolorogen′ic. Causing pain.

domatophobia (do-mat-o-fo′bĭ-ă). A form of claustrophobia; abnormal aversion to being in a house. [ment.

domicil′iary. Pert. to a house, as treatment.

dom′inant. That which is inherited from 1 parent developing to the exclusion of a contrasting character from the opp. parent.

donator (do′na-tor). One who or that which gives something.

   d., hydrogen. A substance which gives up hydrogen to another substance. SEE: *hydrogen acceptor.*

donee (dō-nē′). One who receives blood transfused from another, the donor.

Donné′s corpuscles (don-năz′). Bodies in colostrum having ameboid movements.

   D.′s test. To determine pus in urine, mix with 10% solution of potassium hydrate. Pus is present if a lumpy hyaline mass with air bubbles rising slowly is formed when mixture is shaken.

do′nor. One who furnishes blood for transfusion.

   d., universal. One whose blood is of Group O, and whose blood is not agglutinated by the blood of anyone.

Don′ovan body. Supposed causative agent of lymphogranuloma inguinale, *q.v.*

doraphobia (do-ra-fo′bĭ-ă). Abnormal aversion to touching the hair or fur of animals.

Dorel′lo′s canal. A bony canal in tip of temporal bone enclosing abducens nerve.

Dorendorf′s sign. A filling up or fullness of the supraclavicular groove in aneurysm of the aortic arch.

dorsabdom′inal. Pert. to the back and abdomen.

dorsad (dor′sad). Toward the back.

dor′sal. Pert. to the back.

   d. elevated position. Patient is on the back, head and shoulders elevated at an angle of 30° or more. Employed for digital examination of genitalia, and in bimanual examination.

   d. inertia posture. In which patient rests on the back showing tendency to turn to either side or to slip down in bed.

   d. nerves. Nerves emerging from the dorsal vertebrae.*

   d. recumbent position. Same as dorsal elevated, except extremities are moderately flexed and rotated outward, the soles of the feet resting upon bed or table, or legs may be extended.

   d. reflex. Irritation of the skin over the erector spinal muscles, causing contraction of muscles of the back.

   d. rigid posture. One in which both legs (or the right one) are drawn up.

   d. vertebrae. Twelve bones of the spinal column bet. the cervical and lumbar vertebrae. SEE: *position, posture.*

dorsalgia (dor-sal′jĭ-ă). Pain in the back. SYN: *notalgia, rachialgia.*

dorsi-, dorso-, dors-. Combining form for *dorsum,* back.

dorsiduct (dor′si-dukt). To draw toward the back or backward.

dorsiduc′tion. Drawing toward the back.

dorsiflect (dor′sĭ-flekt). Bending backward.

dorsiflex′ion. The act of bending backward.

dorsim′esad. In the direction of the dorsimeson. [back.

dorsim′eson. The median plane of the

dorsispinal (dor″sĭ-spi′nal). Pert. to the back and spine.

   d. veins. Veins around the vertebrae.

dorsoceph′alad. Situated toward the back of the head.

dorsodynia (dor-so-din′ĭ-ă). Rheumatism in the muscles of upper part of back.

dorsosa′cral. Pert. to lower back.

   d. position. Patient lies upon the back, same as in the dorsal recumbent position,* excepting that thighs are flexed upon abdomen and legs upon thighs which are abducted. Leg holders are used to support legs in position.

dor′sum. The back or post. surface of a part.

dos′age. The amt. of medicine to be administered to a patient at one time.

   d. meter. An instrument designed to estimate the quantity of radiation, so as to determine the duration of exposure when using roentgen rays.

dose (dōs). Amt. of a medicinal preparation to be taken at 1 time.

   d., divided. Fractional portions adm. at short intervals.

   d., lethal. A fatal dose.

   d., maximum. Largest dose it is safe to adm.

   d., minimum. Smallest dose that will be effective.

dosimeter (do-sim′e-ter). Device for measuring very small doses.

   d., Mecapion. Instrument registering 180 roentgens to determine x-ray dosage.

   d., Victoreen′. Apparatus which registers 256 roentgens to measure x-ray dosage.

dosimetric (do-sĭ-met′rik). Pert. to dosage.

   d. system. One of regular or determinate dosage.

dosimetry (do-sim′et-rĭ). Measurement of medicinal doses.

dossil (dos′il). A round lint pledget for cleansing wounds.

do′tage. Senility; feeblemindedness of very old age.

dothienenteritis (doth-i-en-en-ter-i′tis) Inflammation of Peyer′s patches. SYN: *typhoid fever.*

double (dŭb'l). Combining 2 things or qualities.

d. consciousness. Expression of 2 phases of personality.

d. personality. A split in consciousness, neither personality being aware of acts and words of other. SEE: *dual personality, multiple personality.*

d. touch. Exploration with a finger in 1 cavity and thumb in another.

d. uterus. State of having a double uterus. SYN: *dihysteria.*

d. vision. Seeing 2 images of an object at the same time. SYN: *diplopia.*

douche (doosh). A current of vapor or stream of water, hot or cold, directed against a part.

d., air. Air current directed on body for therapeutic purposes.

d., alternating. SEE: *Scotch douche.*

d., astringent. One containing substances for shrinking the mucous membrane, such as alum or zinc sulfate.

d., circular. Needle spray or application of water to body through horizontal jets size of a needle from number of small rose sprays so placed that the water is projected against the skin of bather from 4 directions simultaneously.

d., cleansing. One used for purposes of personal cleanliness; usually contains an alkaline substance. Temperature, 105° F.

d., deodorizing. One to deodorize the vagina and vaginal secretions when they have an offensive odor. Used most often in cancer cases. Potassium permanganate is the most commonly used agent.

d., fan. A fan-shaped spray obtained by placing index finger upon the stream of water as it emerges from distal end of douche hose.

d., high. One where the bag is at least 4 feet above the hips of the patient.

d., intrauterine. This is sometimes given immediately postpartum or postabortum when the cervix uteri is still patent. Hot water alone or water containing vinegar is used for the control of postpartum hemorrhage.

d., jet. A solid stream from the douche hose.

d., low. One where the bag is 1-1½ feet above the hips of the patient.

d., medicated. One containing a medicinal substance for the treatment of local conditions. Lysol, tincture of iodine, and bichloride of mercury are the most commonly used.

d., neutral. Douche given at average surface temperature of body—90°-97° F.

d., pail. General affusion with pails of water at 3 temperatures dashed over the patient in quick succession. Temperatures of 1st bath, 100°, 96° and 90° F., reduced 2 degrees each, given once or twice weekly.

d., perineal. One projected upward from a bidet* placed just above floor; patient sits in armchair, crescent-shaped seat, and receives douche upon perineum.

d., rain. Overhead shower.

d., Scotch. Alternating of hot and cold jets of water against local area of skin.

d. solutions. *Alum:* ½ to 1%. *Bichloride of Mercury:* 1:3000-1:10,000. *Boracic Acid:* 2%. *Carbolic Acid:* ⅛ to 1%. *Green Soap:* 1%. *Lysol:* ⅛ to ½%. *Potassium Permanganate:* 1/10 to 1%. *Silver Nitrate:* 1/10%. *Sodium Bicarbonate:* 2%.

d., stimulating. The use of copious amt. of hot or cold water in case of pelvic congestion.

d. temperatures. For a *cleansing douche,* 105° F. For a *hemorrhage douche,* 120° F. For an *inflammation douche,* 115° F. For a *neutral douche,* 92° to 97° F. For a *vaginal douche,* 98° to 115° F.

d., vaginal. Long, warm douche, 20 to 30 minutes, flowing slowly from height not greater than 15 in. above patient's pelvis, temperature from 98° to 115° F., from 3 qt. to 5 gal. daily.

d., vapor. Stream of vapor projected from the douche hose, given with or without intervening flannel clothes.

Douglas' cul-de-sac. Peritoneal sac which lies behind uterus and in front of rectum.

D.'s pouch. Same as Douglas' *cul-de-sac.*

douglasitis (dug-las-i'tis). Inflammation of the *cul-de-sac* of Douglas.

dow'el. Metal pin for fastening an artificial crown to a tooth root.

Dowell test. Injection of ant. pituitary in flexor surface of arm, which causes an erythema at point of injection in a pregnant woman.

Doyère's eminence (dwah-yair'). Elevation where a nerve filament enters a muscle.

D. P. Abbr. for Doctor of Pharmacy.

dr. Abbr. for dram or drachm.

D. R. Abbr. for reaction of degeneration.

drachm (dram). A unit of weight in apothecaries' system. SYMB: ℨ. SYN: *dram.*

dracontiasis (drak-on-ti'as-ĭs). Disease produced by infestation with *Filaria medinensis.*

drain (drain). 1. Exit or tube for discharge of morbid matter. 2. To draw off a fluid.

d., absorbable. One taken up by lymphatic and venous system.

d., capillary. Drawing off by capillary attraction. Never use in suppuration, etc.

d., nonabsorbable. One made from horsehair, gauze, rubber, glass, or metal. TYPES: *abdominal, antrum, perineal, suprapubic,* etc.

d., tubular. One prepared from bone. Absorbed 8-10 days.

drainage (dra'năj). The free flow or withdrawal of fluids, as pus from a cavity or wound. SEE: *autodrainage, drain.*

d., capillary. Drainage by method of capillary attraction.

d. funnel. Drainage with glass funnels.

d., postural. Drainage for draining nasal area and the sinuses.

The patient lies on his back on a bed with shoulders over the side and head hanging down.

d. tube. Device for allowing escape of pus, serum, blood, or other fluids from a wound, abscess, etc.

d. t. carrier. Device for placing drainage tube in position.

d. t. trocar. Device to introduce drainage tube without making a large incision.

dram. Sixty gr. or 1/8 oz. apothecary weight; 3.888 Gm., 27.34 gr. or 1/16 oz., avoirdupois.

d., fluid. A teaspoonful or 1/8 of a fluid ounce or 57.1 gr. of distilled water, the equivalent of 3.70 cc. In Great Britain 54.8 gr. of distilled water or 3.50 cc.

dram'atism. Dramatic behavior and lofty speech in insanity.

drapetomania (drap-et-o-ma'nĭ-ă). Insane impulse to wander from home.

dras'tic. 1. Acting strongly. 2. A very active purgative, usually producing many evacuations, and accompanied by pain and tenesmus. Ex: *croton oil, elaterin.*

draught (draft). 1. A drink. 2. Drawing liquid into the mouth.

draw sheet. One so arranged that it can be removed easily from under a patient.

drepanocyte (dre-pan'o-sīt). Sickle or crescent cell.

drepanocytemia (dre-pan-o-si-te'mĭ-ă). Sickle-cell anemia.

drepanocytic (dre-pan-o-sit'ĭk). Pert. to or resembling a sickle cell.

dressing. Covering, protective, or support for diseased or injured parts.

d., absorbent. Gauze, sterilized gauze, absorbent cotton, lint, lint cloth, paper lint, absorbent wool, wood wool, moose pappe, spongiopiline.

d., hot moist. Most common form is saturated hot boric solution, heated to as hot as can be borne by bare forearm of nurse.

Dreyer's tuberculin or **vaccine** (dri'erz). A tuberculosis vaccine prepared by removing the lipoid material from tubercle germs.

Drinker respirator. Apparatus in which alternating positive and negative air pressure upon the patient creates artificial respiration.   [drop by drop.

drip. 1. To fall in drops. 2. To instill

d., intravenous. Slow injection of glucose and saline solution, a drop at a time, intravenously.

d., Murphy. Slow rectal instillation of a fluid drop by drop.

drip sheet. Modified sheet bath. SEE: *bath drip sheet.*

drisdol (dris-dol'). Crystalline vitamin D, in solution of propylene glycol.

DOSAGE: Average adult, 3 drops daily.

dromomania (dro-mo-ma'nĭ-ă). Insane impulse to wander.

dromotrop'ic. Pert. to supposed fibers in cardiac nerves which influence conductivity of muscles.

drop. 1. A minute spherical mass of liquid. 2. Falling of a part from paralysis or injury.

d., ague. Fowler's solution.

d., black. Vinegar of opium.

d. culture. A bacterial culture in a drop of culture media.

d. finger. Baseball finger.

d. foot. Toes dragging in walking with falling of foot due to paralysis of dorsal flexor muscles.

d., knockout. A drug to cause unconsciousness; usually adm. for criminal purposes.

d. wrist. Paralysis of extensor muscles causing hand to hang down from forearm.

droplet. Very small drop.

d. infection. That conveyed by means of infective particles, as when carried in a spray from the nose or mouth. Usual mode of infection from common cold, etc.

drop'per. A pipet, bottle, or tube for dropping a liquid.

dropsical (drop'sik-al). Of the nature of or affected with dropsy.

dropsy (drop'sĭ). A condition rather than a disease. Morbid accumulation of water in the tissues and cavities; hydrops.

d. of amnion. OB: Abnormal increase in amt. of amniotic fluid. SYN: *polyhydramnios.*

d. of the belly. Ascites.

d. of brain. Hydrocephalus.

d., cardiac. That due to cardiac disease.

d. of chest. Hydrothorax.

d. of peritoneum. Hydroperitoneum.

d., ovarian. A collection of fluid in the ovary forming a crust.

d., tubal. A collection of fluid in the fallopian tube. SYN: *hydrosalpinx.*

d., uterine. A collection of fluid in the uterine cavity. SYN: *hydrometra.*

drowning. Result of prolonged submersion in water.

drug. A medicinal substance, used in the treatment of disease.

d. action, incompatible. Ill effects produced by 2 or more drugs antagonistic to each other.

drug addiction. Abnormal use of habit-forming drugs, such as absinthe, alcohol, cannabis, chloroform, cocaine, ether, nicotine, opium and its derivatives—morphine and heroin.

drug rashes. Drugs of which large doses are liable to produce a rash are: Arsenic, belladonna, bromides, chloral, iodides, opium, phenacetin, quinine, sera, sodium salicylate, turpentine (the nurse may notice the rash on the buttocks after a turpentine enema has been given), and the application of cyanide gauze to a wound (in this latter case the rash is confined to the area of the wound, which is surrounded by "sores").

Antipyrin: Papular, erythematous rash,

sometimes accompanied by edema and much irritation.

Arsenic: Papular or erythematous rash, sometimes urticarial. Prolonged use may produce pigmentation of skin.

Belladonna: Erythematous rash, usually accompanied by intense itching.

Bromides: Usually like acne vulgaris. Sometimes erythema.

Chloral: Papular erythema.

Enemata (soap) may cause erythema or urticaria if hard soap is used.

Iodides: Usually papular erythema, sometimes with acnelike pustules.

Phenolphthalein: Macular rash, sometimes purpuric.

Quinine: Very irritable erythema or urticaria.

Salicylate: Erythematous rash, possibly morbilliform.

Serum: Usually urticaria.

Sulfonal: Erythematous or urticarial rash.

drugs, handling of. Read the label or other printed instructions issued with medicine carefully; measure out accurately the doses (quantities) ordered, and never guess.

A measuring glass or spoon should be employed, marked either in drams and ounces only, or with the words teaspoon, dessertspoon, and tablespoon also.

One drop equals 1 minim. Symbol, ♏. One teaspoonful equals 1 dram. Symbol, ℨ. Two teaspoonfuls equal 2 drams or 1 dessertspoonful. Four teaspoonfuls equal ½ ounce or 1 tablespoonful. Two tablespoonfuls equal 1 ounce. Symbol, ℥.

Important Points: (1) The cork must never be left out of the bottle, as a necessary property may evaporate or the drug may become a dangerous concentration. (2) The drug compartment must be kept locked.

To Give a Dose of Medicine: Make quite sure: (a) To whom it has to be given; (b) what has to be given; (c) when it has to be given; (d) the amt. to be given.

Shake the bottle, measure the dose, again note label. Give to patient and see that it is swallowed. A small drink of water will take away unpleasant taste or medicine may be taken through a straw. As in feeding, the patient's head and shoulders should be well raised before the dose of mixture is given to him.

drum. The tympanic cavity of the ear.

    d. belly. Tympanites.

    d. head. Tympanic membrane.

drunkenness. Alcoholic intoxication.

druse (drūs). 1. Rupture of tissues with no lesion of surface. 2. Small, hyaline, globular pathological growths formed on optic papilla.

dry cells. A zinc container lined with thin blotting paper which serves as the negative electrode, carbon rod in center as positive electrode, a paste of ammonium chloride, zinc chloride, manganese dioxide, and granulated carbon fills space bet. electrodes, preventing polarization.

dry diet. A temporary high carbohydrate diet with measured liquid given bet. meals only.

dry ice. Solidified carbon dioxide used for commercial refrigeration.

dry measure. A measure of volume for dry commodities, as follows:

2 pints (pt.)	= 1 quart (qt.)
8 quarts	= 1 peck (pk.)
4 pecks	= 1 bushel (bu.)

Drys'dale's corpuscles. Nonnucleated, granular cells supposed to be in ovarian fluid.

du'alism. 1. The assumption that any chemical compound is made up of 1 electrified negative and an electrified positive. 2. The accepted belief that a hard and a soft chancre are the result of different diseases.

dual personality. A split in consciousness which results in the expression of 2 different phases of personality at various intervals, neither personality, as a rule, being aware of the words, acts, and feelings of the other. When this does rarely occur it has been called "co-consciousness."

Dubini's disease (doo-be′nĕz). Rhythmic, rapid contractions of a group or groups of muscles. SYN: *electric chorea, spasmus Dubini*.

duboisine (du-boi′sin). Alkaloid derivative of plant *Duboisea myoporoides*.

    DOSAGE: 0.0008-0.0015 Gm. (1/80-1/40 gr.).

    d., poisoning from. Resembles atropine, *q.v.*

Duchenne's disease (du-shen′). 1. Bulbar paralysis. 2. Tabes dorsalis.

Ducrey's bacillus (du-kray′). The cause of soft sore, or chancroid; small, rod-shaped organism found in pairs.

duct. Tubular vessel conveying blood or other secretions of the body.

    d., accessory pancreatic. Duct of the pancreas, leading into pancreatic duct or the duodenum near the mouth of the common bile duct.

    d., alimentary. SEE: *thoracic duct*.

    d's., alveolar. Expansions of the bronchioles.

    d., archinephric. SEE: *wolffian duct*.

    d., Bartholin's. The duct of Bartholin's gland, a vulvovaginal gland.

    d's., bile. Canals carrying bile in the body.

    d's., biliary. Ducts connecting lobules of the liver.

    d., Botallo's. Fetal blood vessel connecting the pulmonary artery and aorta.

    d., cochlear. Canal of the cochlea.

    d., common bile (*ductus choled'ochus*). Conveys bile to duodenum. SEE: *gallduct*.

    d., c. seminal. SEE: *ejaculatory duct*.

    d., Cuvier's. Fetal ducts in the auricle, 2 in number, right one becoming sup. vena cava.

    d., cystic (*ductus cys'ticus*). Excretory duct of gallbladder. SEE: *gallduct*.

    d's., definitive. Milk ducts in the nipple.

d., ejaculatory (*ductus ejaculatorius*). Conveys semen into urethra.

d., endolymphatic. A duct in the labyrinth of the ear.

d., excretory. Duct discharging secretions in the body.

d., galactophorous. Duct carrying milk in mammary glands' lobes.

d's., gall. SEE: *bile ducts.*

d., Gartner's. A remnant of the wolffian duct extending from the parovarium through the broad ligament into the vagina.

d., hepatic (*ductus hepat'icus*). Receives bile from liver. SEE: *gallduct.*

d's., intralobular bile. SEE: *biliary duct.*

d., lacrimal. Tear duct carrying tears from lacrimal sac to nose.

d's., lactiferous. SEE: *galactophorous duct.*

d., Leydig's. SEE: *wolffian duct.*

d., mammary. SEE: *galactophorous duct.*

d., mesonephric. SEE: *wolffian duct.*

d., metanephric. Ureter.

d., milk (*ductus lactiferus*). A mammary duct entering the nipple.

d., Müller's. Bilateral ducts in the embryo that go to form the uterus, vagina, and fallopian tubes.

d., nasal (*ductus lacrima'lis*). Carries tears from lacrimal sac.

d., omphalomesenteric. SEE: *umbilical duct.*

d., pancreat'ic (*ductus pancreaticus*). Conveys pancreatic juice to the duodenum.

d., parotid (*ductus parotide'us*). Discharges parotid secretions into mouth.

d., prostatic (*ductus prostat'ica*). One of 20 ducts which discharge prostatic secretion into the urethra.

d., right lymphatic. Duct carrying lymph near liver on right side of body.

d. of Rivini. A duct of the sublingual gland.

d., salivary (*ductus sublingua'lis minor and ductus submaxilla'ris*). Carrying from a salivary gland.

d., Santorini's. SEE: *accessory pancreatic duct.*

d., secretory. A gland's smaller canals.

d., segmental. A pair of embryonic tubes, located bet. visceral and parietal layers of mesoblast on each side of the body.

d., seminal. SEE: *ejaculatory duct.*

d., Skene's. Periurethral ducts, 2 straight tubular glands on the floor of the urethra.

d., spermatic. Vas deferens.

d., Stenson's, Steno's. Parotid gland duct.

d., sublingual. SEE: *Rivini's and Bartholin's ducts.*

d., submaxillary. SEE: *Wharton's duct.*

d., sudorif'erous. Sweat duct.

d., tear. SEE: *nasal duct.*

d., testicular. Vas deferens.

d., thoracic (*ductus thorac'ius*). Discharging into subclavian vein.

d., umbilical. Embryonic duct bet. cavity of intestines and umbilical vesicle.

d., vitelline. SEE: *umbilical duct.*

d., Wharton's. Submaxillary salivary gland duct.

d., Wirsung's (vēr'soong). Excretory duct of the pancreas.

d., wolffian. Ducts which, in the embryo, connect the wolffian body to the cloaca.

duct'less. Having no duct, secreting only internally.

d. glands. Ductless glands secrete internally one or more hormones which have a specific action upon the body. SEE: *endocrine, endocrinology, exocrine.*

ductule (duk'tŭl). A very small duct.

ductus. Latin for duct. Used in BNA.

d. arteriosus. A channel of communication bet. main pulmonary artery of the fetus and aorta.

d. choledochus. The common bile duct.

d. communis. One about 3 in. long formed by union of cystic and hepatic ducts; carries the bile to the intestine.

d. deferens. Excretory duct of the testicle. SYN: *vas deferens.*

d. hemithoracicus. Ascending branch of thoracic opening either into right lymphatic duct or close to angle of union of right subclavian and right internal jugular veins.

d. hepaticus dexter. One issuing from the right lobe of the liver, uniting with the ductus hepaticus sinister and forming the hepatic duct.

d. hepaticus medius. An occasional branch of the hepatic duct conveying bile from the quadrate lobe.

d. hepaticus sinister. One issuing with ductus hepaticus dexter to form hepatic duct.

d. prostatici. Ducts for secretion of prostate into the urethra.

d. sacculo-utricularis. Small tube connecting saccule of internal ear with utricle.

d. venosus. Smaller, shorter, and post. of 2 branches into which umbilical vein divides after entering the abdomen; joins left hepatic vein.

Duhrssen's incisions of the cervix uteri. Incisions made in the undilated cervix in order to allow for completion of the delivery of the fetus.

duipara (dū-ip'ăr-ă). A female pregnant for the 2nd time.

dulcin (dul'sin). A toxic substance (C_9H_{12}-N_2O_2), 200 times sweeter than sugar. SYN: *sucrol, dulcite.*

dull. 1. Not resonant on percussion. 2. Not mentally alert.

dullness, dulness (dul'nes). 1. Lack of normal resonance on percussion. 2. State of being dull.

dumb. Mute. Congenitally unable to speak.

d. ague. Latent malaria not expressed by ordinary signs.

dumb'bell crystals. Crystals shaped like a dumbbell.

dumb'ness. Muteness.

duode'nal. Pert. to the duodenum.

d. bulb. Area of duodenum just beyond the pylorus.

d. digestion. Process by which arrival of acid chyme in the duodenum results in the production of at least 2 substances whose composition is not exactly known but which get into the blood stream and act as chemical messengers.

d. ulcer. Broken mucous membrane, usually accompanied by suppuration and perhaps a sore is present which bleeds with more or less danger of perforation.

d. papilla. Raised surface near entrance of ductus choledochus communis into duodenum.

duodenectomy (du-o-den-ek'to-mǐ). Excision of part or all of the duodenum.

duodeni'tis. Inflammation of the duodenum.

duodenocholecystostomy (dū-od-en"o-kol-e-sis-tos'to-mǐ). Formation by surgical means of a fistula bet. duodenum and gallbladder.

duodenocholedochotomy (du-od-en"o-koled-o-kot'o-mǐ). Surgical incision of the duodenum to reach the gallbladder.

duodenocystostomy (du-od-en"o-sist-os'to-mǐ). Formation of a passage bet. the duodenum and the bladder.

duodenoenterostomy (du-od-en"o-en-teros'to-mǐ). Formation of passage bet. the duodenum and intestine.

duodenogram (du-o-de'no-gram). A roentgenogram of the duodenum.

duodenohepatic (du-o-den-o-he-pat'ik). Pert. to duodenum and liver.

duodenojejunostomy (du-o-den-o-jej-u-nos'to-mǐ). Making a passage bet. the duodenum and jejunum.

duodenos'copy. Inspection of the duodenum with an endoscope.

duodenostenostomy (du-o-den-o-sten-os'to-mǐ). The making of an opening through the abdomen into the duodenum.

duodenostomy (du-o-den-os'to-me). Operation of making a permanent opening into the duodenum through the wall of the abdomen.

duodenotomy (du-o-den-ot'o-me). An incision into the duodenum.

duodenum (du-o-de'num). The first part of the small intestines connecting with the pylorus of the stomach and extending to the jejunum.

duplica'tion, du'plicature. A doubling or folding, or state of being folded.

dupp (dŭp). Word denoting 2nd sound at cardiac apex heard in auscultation.

Dupuytren's contraction (du-pwē-tränz'). Contraction of palmar fascia causing ring and little fingers to bend into palm so that they cannot be extended.

du'ra. Dura mater.

d. mater. The outer membrane covering the spinal cord (*dura mater spina'lis*) and brain (*dura mater cer'ebri or enceph'ali*). SEE: *pia mater, tentorium.*

dural (du'ral). Pert. to the dura. [*dural.**]

durama'tral. Pert. to the dura. SYN:

du'raplasty. Plastic repair of the dura mater.

durematoma (dū-rem-at-o'mǎ). Accumulation of blood bet. arachnoid and dura.

duritis (du-ri'tis). Inflammation of the dura. SYN: *pachymeningitis.*

duroarachnitis (dū-ro-ar-ak-ni'tis). Inflammation of dura and arachnoid membrane.

durocaine (du'ro-kān). Spinal anesthetic. Procaine hydrochloride in pseudohypobaric solution.

Duroziez's murmur (du-ro-zǐ-ez'). Double murmur over femoral artery on pressure.

dust'ing powder. Any fine powder for dusting on skin.

Duverney's gland (doo-ver-nas'). The vulvovaginal gland.

dwarf. Congenital abnormally short person. A pigmy.

dwar'fishness. Condition of being a dwarf.

dyad (di'ad). A bivalent element.

dynamia (dī-nam'ǐ-ǎ). Vital energy or ability to combat disease.

dynamic (di-nam'ik). Pert. to vital force or inherent power, opp. of *static.*

d. psychology. A theory that energy is inherent in mind.

dynam'ics. The science of bodies in motion and their forces.

dynamization (di-nam-iz-a'shun). The attempt to add to the potency of medicine by agitation or comminution.* SEE: *attenuation.*

dy'namo. Apparatus for conversion of mechanical energy into electrical power.

dynamogen'esis. The capacity to call forth increased energy.

dynamogen'ic. Pert. to, or caused by, an increase of energy.

dynamograph (di-nam'o-graf). Device for recording muscular strength.

dynamometer (di-na-mom'e-ter). 1. A device for measuring muscular strength. Simple dynamometer is spring scales bet. segment to be examined and examiner's hand. 2. A device for giving the magnifying power of a lens.

dynamoneure (di-nam'o-nŭr). A motor, spinal nerve cell.

dynamoscope (di-nam'o-skōp). Instrument for auscultation of muscles.

dynamoscopy (di-nam-os'ko-pǐ). Auscultation of muscles.

dyne (dīn). A unit of force which would propel a mass of weight of 1 gram with a velocity of 1 cm. in a second. [ful.

dys-. Prefix meaning bad, difficult, pain-

dysacous'ia, dysacous'ma. Discomfort caused by loud noises.

dysacusia (dis-a-ku'si-a). Abnormal discomfort from noises; *dysacousma.*

dysadrenia (dis-ǎ-dre'nǐ-ǎ). Functional disorder of the kidneys.

dyse'mia. Blood deterioration.

dysalbumose (dis-al'bū-mōs). A variety of albumose insoluble in water or hydrochloric acid.

dysantigraphia (dis-an-tǐ-gra'fǐ-ǎ). Inability to copy writing or printed letters.

dysaphia (dis-af'ǐ-ǎ). Dullness of the sense of touch.

dysarteriotony (dis"ar-te-ri-ot'o-ni). Abnormal blood pressure, either too low or too high.

dysarthria (dis-ar'thri-ă). Difficulty in articulation of joints, as in amyostasia.

dysarthro'sis. Joint malformation.

dysbasia (dis-ba'zi-ă). A disease of the cord or brain resulting in ataxia, or difficulty in walking.

dys'bolism. Disordered metabolism.

dysbulia (dis-bu'li-ă). Inability to fix the attention; difficulty experienced in thinking; mind weariness. 2. Weak and uncertain will power.

dyschezia (dis-ke'zi-ă). Constipation due to habitual neglect to respond to stimulus to defecate.

dyschiria (dis-ki'ri-ă). Inability to tell which side of the body has been touched. If referred to the wrong side it is called *allochiria;** to both sides, *synchiria.** Syn: *achiria.*

dyscholia (dis-ko'li-ă). Morbid condition of the bile.

dyschromatopsia (dis-kro-mat-op'si-ă). Imperfect color vision.   [skin.

dyschro'mia. Discoloration, as of the

dyscinesia (dis-sin-e'zi-ă). Impairment of voluntary movements.

dyscoimesis (dis-koy-me'sis). Delay in falling asleep.

dysco'ria. Abnormal form of the pupil.

dyscrasia (dis-kra'si-ă). Morbid condition supposed to be caused by toxins in the blood.

dyscrasic (dis-kra'sik). Pert. to dyscrasia.

dyscri'nism. Any disorder of secretions, esp. of an endocrine gland.

dysdiadochokinesia (dis"di-ă-do"ko-kin-e'si-ă). Inability to quickly substitute antagonistic motor impulses.

dysdiemorrhysis (dis-di-em-or'i-sis). Sluggish circulation of capillaries.

dyse'mia. Any blood disease.

dysendocriniasis (dis-en-do-krin-i'a-sis). Faulty function of the endocrine glands.

dysendoc'rinism. Faulty function of the endocrine glands; dysendocriniasis.

dysendocrisi'asis. Faulty function of the endocrine glands; dysendocriniasis.

dysenteric (dis-en-ter'ik). Pert. to dysentery.

dysentery (dis'en-ter-e). Inflammation of intestinal mucous membrane accompanied by ulceration, fever, and bloody evacuations.

    d., amebic. Due to amebas. Sym: Similar to catarrhal dysentery with intermissions. Treatment: Also similar.

    d., catarrhal. Due to change of weather, diet, or water. Sym: Diarrhea, vomiting, abdominal pain, desire to stool, and fever. Increasing stool; bloody. Treatment: Liquid diet. Rest in bed. Irrigation of colon.

    d., diphtheric. Epidemic intestinal affection, caused by vegetable organism in drinking water. Sym: Intensified catarrhal dysentery symptoms. Treatment: Dietetic, same as other forms of the disease. Milk alone, 4 to 5 pt., lean meat, only.

dysergasia (dis-er-ga'si-ă). Inability to function properly. Syn: *neurasthenia.*

dysergastic (dis-er-gas'tik). Pert. to dysergasia.

    d. reaction. Hallucinations, fears, disorientation, dream states, and other mental disorders resulting from poor circulation and nutrition of the brain.

dysergia (dis-er'ji-ă). Lack of coördination in muscular voluntary movements.

dysesthesia (dis-es-the'zi-ă). 1. Sensations, as of the pricks of pins and needles, or of crawling. Syn: *formication.* 2. Failing sensitivity, esp. of touch.

    d., auditory. Abnormal discomfort from loud noises. Syn: *dysacusia.*

dysfunction (dis-funk'shun). Absence of complete normal function.

dysgalac'tia. Defective milk secretion.

dysgenesia, dysgenesis (dis-jen-e'si-ă, -sis). Impairment or loss of procreative powers. Syn: *sterility.*

dysgen'ic. Causing racial deterioration.

dysgen'italism. Condition caused by abnormal genital development.

dysgerminoma (dis-jer-min-o'mă). A neoplasm in sex cells in hermaphrodites and in undescended testicles or undeveloped ovaries.

dysgeusia (dis-gu'si-ă). Perversion or impairment of sense of taste.

dysglan'dular. Abnormal functioning of glands, esp. those of internal secretion.

dysglycemia (dis-gli-se'mi-ă). Faulty blood sugar metabolism.

dysgno'sia. Any anomaly of intellect. Syn: *dysthymia.*

dysgone'sis. 1. Functional disorder of the genital organs. 2. Poor growth of bacterial culture.   [growth.

dysgon'ic. Bacterial cultures of sparse

dysgraph'ia. Writer's cramp.

dyshematopoiesis (dis-hem"ă-to-poy-e'si-ă). Imperfect blood formation.

dyshidria (dis-hid'ri-ă). 1. Retention of contents of the sweat follicles. 2. Milk perspiration.

dyshor'monal. Caused by endocrine disturbance.

dyshor'monism. Deficiency of hormones or any internal secretions.

dysidrosis (dis-id-ro'sis). Disorder of the perspiratory apparatus. Never appears in the aged or children. Syn: *dyshidria.* See: *pompholyx.*

dysin'sulinism. Imperfect secretion of insulin.

dyskerato'sis. Epithelial alterations in which a certain number of isolated malpighian cells become differentiated.

dyskine'sia. Defect in voluntary movement.

    d. al'gera. Condition in which active movement is painful.

    d. intermit'tens. Limb disability occurring intermittently.

    d., uterine. Pain in the uterus on movement.

dyskinet'ic. Having disordered normal movement.

dyskoimesis (dis-koy-me'sis). Difficulty in going to sleep.

dyslalia (dis-lal'ĭ-ă). Impairment of speech due to defect of speech organs.

dyslexia (dis-leks'ĭ-ă). Difficulty in reading as result of brain lesion.

dyslochia (dis-lo'kĭ-ă). Disordered lochial discharge, or premature cessation.

dyslogia (dis-lo'jĭ-ă). Difficulty in expression of ideas.

dysmasesis (dis-mas-e'sis). Difficulty in masticating. Syn: *dysmastesis*.

dysmegalop'sia. Inability to visualize correctly the size and shape of things.

dysmenorrhea (dis-men-or-ē'ă). Painful or difficult menstruation, either primary or secondary.

  d., congestive. Condition caused by pelvic congestion.

  d., inflammatory. Condition caused by pelvic inflammation.

  d., mechanic. See: *obstructive dysmenorrhea*.

  d., membranous. A severe spasmodic dysmenorrhea which is accompanied by the passage of a cast of the uterine cavity.

  d., neurotic. Form caused by neurosis.

  d., obstructive. Dysmenorrhea caused by obstruction of menstrual flow.

  d., primary. Difficult menstruation starting from the first period and usually a result of maldevelopment of the uterus.

  d., secondary. When periods were, at the outset, normal, but, because of the development of some pathological state in the pelvis, there is a disturbance of menstruation.

  d., spasmodic. Dysmenorrhea caused by uterine contractions of spasmodic form.

dysmetria (dis-me'trĭ-ă). An inability to fix the range of a movement.

dysmetrop'sia. Inability to visualize correctly the size and shape of things. Syn: *dysmegalopsia*.

dysmimia (dis-mim'ĭ-ă). 1. Inability to express oneself by gestures or signs. 2. Inability to imitate.

dysmnesia (dis-ne'zĭ-ă). Any impairment of memory.

dysmorphophobia (dis-morf-o-fo'bĭ-ă). Morbid fear of deformity; a form of paranoia.

dysmorphosis (dis-mor-fo'sis). Not normal in form.

dysmyoto'nia. 1. Muscle atony. 2. Excessive muscle tonicity. Syn: *myotonia*.

dysneuria (dis-nu'rĭ-ă). Impairment of the nervous function.

dysodontiasis (dis-o-don-ti'as-is). Painful or difficult dentition.

dysontogenesis (dis-on-to-jen'es-is). Defective development of an organism.

dysontogenet'ic. Pert. to defective development.

dysopia (dis-o'pĭ-ă). Defective or painful vision.

dysop'sia. Defective vision. Syn: *dysopia*.

dysorexia (dis-o-rek'sĭ-ă). Perverted or lessened appetite.

dysosmia (dis-oz'mĭ-ă). Impairment of the sense of smell.

dysostosis (dis-os-to'sis). Defective bone formation.

  d., cleidocranial. A congenital ossification of the skull with partial atrophy of clavicles.

dysovarism (dis-o'var-izm). An abnormality due to disturbance in the ovarian internal secretion.

dysox'idizable. Not easy to oxidize.

dyspan'creatism. Impaired pancreatic function.   [tus.

dyspareunia (dis-pa-ru'nĭ-ă). Painful coi-

dyspepsia (dis-pep'sĭ-ă). Imperfect digestion. Not a disease in itself, but symptomatic of other diseases or disorders.

  d., acid. With excessive acid.

  d., acute. Due to dietary errors and of short duration.

  d., alcoholic. Caused by excessive use of alcoholic beverages.

  d., amylaceous. Form in which foods containing starch are not easily digested.

  d., atonic. Due to lack of gastric juice.

  d., biliary, bilious. Form in which there is insufficient quantity or quality of bile secretion.

  d., cardiac. Form occurring during heart disease.

  d., catarrhal. Due to inflammation of the stomach.

  d., fermentative. Dyspepsia caused by fermenting of food.

  d., gastric. Dyspepsia caused by faulty stomach function.

  d., gastrointestinal. Dyspepsia caused by faulty function of stomach and intestines.

  d., hepatic. Dyspepsia caused by liver disease.

  d., hysterical. Dyspepsia present during hysterical attacks.

  d., intestinal. Due to abnormal state of pancreatic, biliary, and intestinal secretions.

  d., nervous. Indicated by gastric pain and palpitation.

dyspeptic (dis-pep'tik). 1. Affected with or pert. to dyspepsia. 2. One afflicted with dyspepsia.

dyspeptone (dis-pep'tōn). An insoluble product of gastric digestion.

dysperma'sia. Difficult or painful orgasm during coitus.

dysper'matism. Difficult or painful orgasm during coitus. Syn: *dyspermasia*.

dysper'mia. Difficult or painful orgasm during coitus. Syn: *dyspermasia*.

dysphagia, dysphagy (dis-fa'jĭ-ă, -jĭ). Inability to swallow as a result of spasm of the esophagus, seen in hysteria.

dysphasia (dis-fa'zĭ-ă). Impairment of speech.

dysphemia (dis-fe'mĭ-ă). Stammering.

dysphonia (dis-fo'nĭ-ă). Difficulty in speaking; hoarseness.   [throat.

  d. clerico'rum. Clergyman's sore

  d. pu'berum. Change of voice in boys during puberty.

dysphoria (dis-fo'rĭ-ă). Exaggerated feeling of depression and unrest without apparent cause.

dysphrasia (dis-fra′zĭ-ă). Impairment of speech. SYN: *dysphasia.*

dysphrenia (dis-fre′nĭ-ă). Functional or constitutional psychosis; the opp. of the organic type.

dysphylaxia (dis-fi-laks′ĭ-ă). Waking too early from sleep.

dyspinealism (dis-pin′e-al-ism). Functional impairment of pineal gland.

dyspituitarism. Condition due to disorder of the pituitary body in which both hyperpituitarism and hypopituitarism are present at the same time.

dysplasia (dis-pla′sĭ-ă). Abnormal development of tissue. SYN: *alloplasia heteroplasia.*

dyspnea (disp-ne′a). Labored or difficult breathing usually accompanied by pain.

   d., expiratory. As in asthma and bronchitis; wheezing and painful expiration. Secretions in respiratory tract cause of sound.

dyspneic (disp-ne′ik). Affected with or due to dyspnea.

dyspragia. Difficulty in functioning.

dyspraxia. Painful functioning.

dysstasia. Difficulty in standing.

dysstatic. Showing difficulty in standing.

dyssynergia. Failure of muscular coördination. SYN: *ataxia.*

dyssystole (dis-sis′to-lĭ). Dilatation with cardiac insufficiency. Asystole; incomplete systole.

dystasia (dis-tax′ĭ-ă). Difficulty in standing.

dystaxia (dis-tax′ĭ-ă). Partial ataxia.

dysteleology (dis-te-le-ol′o-jĭ). The study of rudimentary organs.

dysthymia (dis-thim′ĭ-ă). 1. Mental perversion; melancholia. 2. Pain of psychic origin.

dysthyreosis (dis-thi-re-o′sis). Impaired functional activity of thyroid gland. SYN: *dysthyroidism.*

dysthyroidism (dis-thi′roi-dizm). Imperfect development and function of the thyroid gland.

dystith′ia. Difficulty or inability to nurse at breast.

dystocia (dis-to′sĭ-ă). Difficult labor. May be produced by either the passenger (the fetus) or the passage (the pelvis of the mother).

dystonia (dis-to′nĭ-ă). Impairment of tonicity.

dystonic. Pert. to distonia or hyper- or hypotonicity of tissues.

dystopia. Malposition; displacement of any organ.

dystopic (dis-top′ĭk). Not in place.

dystopy. Malposition of an organ. SYN: *dystopia.*

dystrophia. Progressive weakening of a muscle. SYN: *dystrophy.*

   d. adiposogenitalis. Disease of the anterior pituitary gland showing genital atrophy and obesity, Fröhlich's syndrome.

dystrophic (dis-trof′ik). Pert. to dystrophia.

dystrophodextrin. A starchy material in normal blood but slightly soluble.

dystrophoneurosis (dis-trof″o-nu-ro′sis). Defective nutrition accompanied by a nervous disease.

dystrophy (dis′tro-fĭ). Progressive atrophy or weakening of a part or organ.

   d., progressive muscular. Progressive atrophy of muscles beginning in terminals of motor nerves. ETIOL: Nutritional disorder.

   TREATMENT: Vitamin E.

dystrypsia (dis-trip′sĭ-ă). Impaired secretion of pancreas.

dsyuria (dis-u′rĭ-ă). Painful or difficult urination, symptomatic of numerous conditions. Vesical tenesmus.

dysuriac. One affected with dysuria.

dyszooamylia (dis-zo″o-am-il′ĭ-ă). Failure to transform dextrose into glycogen.

dyszoospermia. Imperfect formation of spermatozoa.

E

E. Abbr. for *electromotive force, emmetropia,* and *eye,* also symb. for *voltage* and *erbium.*

Eales' disease (ēlz). Repeated hemorrhages into the retina and vitreous.

ear. Organ of hearing. Consisting of external, middle, and internal ear.

   e., blood supply of. Ant. and post. auricular, stylomastoid, petrosal, and int. auricular arteries.

   e. bones. Bonelets of tympanic cavity. SYN: *ossicles.*

   e. drum. The tympanum, or cavity in middle ear.

   e. dust. Calcareous concretions in membranous labyrinth. SYN: *otoconia, otolith.*

   e., external. Comprises auricle and external auditory canal; is separated from middle ear by tympanic* membrane or drum.

   e., internal. Comprises organ of hearing or cochlea in which are endings of auditory nerve, and organ of equilibration or balance consisting of three semicircular canals.

   e., middle. An irregular cavity in temporal bone.

   e., nerve supply of. *External:* 5th, 7th, and 9th cranial nerves. *Middle:* 9th cranial. *Internal:* 9th cranial nerve.

   e., swelling in front or behind. ETIOL: Mumps, mastoid disease, scurvy, anthrax, or gangrenous stomatitis.

   e.-wax. Wax in the ear. SYN: *cerumen.*

earache. Aural pain. SYN: *otalgia.*

earth eating. Eating clay or dirt. Sometimes done by children who lack lime; also by the insane. SYN: *chthonophagia, geophagism, geotragia.*

ear trumpet. A tubular device to aid the deaf in hearing.

earwax. Secretion in external meatus of ear. SYN: *cerumen.*

eat. 1. To devour as food. 2. To take solid food. 3. To corrode.

Eberthel'la. A genus of *Bacteriaceae* causing intestinal inflammation.

   E. typhi. Eberth's bacillus, which is the specific cause of typhoid fever.

eberthe'mia. The presence of typhoid bacilli (*Bacillus typhi abdominalis,* or Eberth's bacilli) in the blood.

eber'thian. Pert. to or caused by Eberth's bacillus.

Eb'ner's glands. Mucous glands of the tongue which bathe the gustatory hairs.

   E.'s retic'ulum. Nucleated cells in seminiferous tubules.

ebona'tion. Removal of bony fragments from a wound.

Ebstein's diet. One used in the treatment of obesity. Very little carbohydrate is permitted.

   E.'s disease or lesion. Epithelial necrosis and hyaline degeneration of the renal tubules in diabetes mellitus.

   E.'s leukemia. A rapidly progressing form of leukemia.

ebullition (eb-u-lish'un). 1. Boiling. 2. Effervescence.

eburnation (e-bur-nā'shun). Changes in bone causing them to become dense like ivory and hardened.

eburneous (e-bur'ne-us). Resembling ivory; ivory-colored.

ecaudate (e-kaw'dāt). Without a tail.

ecbolic (ek-bol'ik). 1. Hastening labor by toning up uterine muscles. 2. Causing abortion. 3. Any agent producing or hastening labor or abortion.

eccentric (ek-sen'trik). 1. Peculiar, abnormal in action or ideas. 2. Proceeding away from a center. 3. Peripheral.

   e. atrophy. Atrophy with dilatation.

   e. convulsion. One caused by peripheral irritation.

   e. hypertrophy. Hypertrophy of a hollow organ with dilation.

   e. limitation. Having smaller visual field than normal.

eccentropiesis (ek-sen"tro-pi-e'sis). Pressure from within exerted outward for treatment of anal fistula.

ecchondroma, ecchondrosis (ek-on-dro'mǎ, -dro'sis). A chondroma or cartilaginous tumor.

ecchondrotome (ek-on'dro-tōm). Knife for excision of cartilage.

ecchymoma (ek-i-mo'mǎ). An extravasated blood tumor.

ecchymosis (ek-ĭ-mo'sis) (pl. *-ses*). A form of macula appearing in large irregularly-formed hemorrhagic areas of the skin. The color is red, changing to blue, greenish brown, or yellow.

   ETIOL: Extravasation of blood into areolar tissue.

ecchymotic (ek-i-mot'ĭk). Resembling or rel. to an ecchymosis.

eccrinology (ek-rin-ol'o-jĭ). The science of secretions.

eccrisis (ek'kris-is). The expulsion of morbid or waste products. SYN: *excretion.* [motes excretion.

eccrit'ic. Promoting or that which pro-

eccyclomastopathy (ek-si"clo-mas-top'ǎ-thĭ). A mass of lesions of the breast made up of connective tissue and/or epithelial cells. SYN: *cyclomastopathy.*

eccyesis (ek-si-e'sis). Extrauterine or ectopic pregnancy.

ecdem'ic. Not endemic nor epidemic, as a disease carried to a region from without.

ecdemomania (ek-de-mo-ma'nĭ-ǎ). Wanderlust; abnormal desire to wander. SYN: *drapetomania, dromomania, vagabondage.*

ecderon (ek'dĕ-ron). Epidermis, or outer portion of skin, as distinguished from *enderon,* or inner portion.

echinate (ek'ĭ-nāt). 1. Spiny. 2. In agar streak, a growth with pitted or toothed margins along the inoculation line; in stab cultures, coiled growth with pointed outgrowths.

echinococcosis (ĕ-kin-o-kok-ko'sis). Infestation with echinococcus.

echinococcotomy (ĕ-kin-o-kok-ot'o-mĭ). Operation for evacuation of an echinococcus cyst.

Echinococcus (e-kin-o-kok'us) (pl. *Echinococci*). A genus of tapeworm, *Taenia echinococcus.* In its larval form it occurs in man, causing hydatid tumors of the liver. SYN: *hydatid.*

  e. cyst. A cyst in organs and tissues formed by the larva of the *Taenia echinococcus* of the dog.

  e. cysticus. Echinococcus disease causing a lone hepatic cyst.

  e. disease. Presence of echinococci in the body, causing cystic growths, esp. in the liver.

  e. granulosus. Variety of Echinococcus causing hydatid cyst development in the body.

  e. hydatidosus. Variety of Echinococcus characterized by development of daughter cysts from the mother cyst.

Echinorhynchus (ĕ-kin-o-rin'kus). A genus of parasitic worms (*Echinorhynchus gigus*) sometimes found in human intestines.

echinosis (ĕ-kin-o'sis). Blood corpuscles appearing like a sea urchin, having lost their smooth outlines.

echinulate (ĕ-kin'u-lāt). A bacterial growth having lateral spines. Seen along line of inoculation.

echo (ĕk'ō). A reverberating sound.

  e. acou'sia. Subjective echoes of sounds just normally heard.

  e., amphor'ic. Amphoric sound sometimes heard in auscultation of chest. SEE: *chest, percussion of.*

  e. sign. Repetition of closing word of a sentence, a sign of epilepsy or other brain conditions.

  e. speech. Involuntary repetition of a sentence or word spoken by another. SYN: *echolalia.*

echokinesia (ek-o-kin-e'sĭ-ă). Involuntary repetition of another's gestures.

echolalia (ek-o-la'lĭ-ă). An involuntary, parrotlike repetition of words spoken by others, often accompanied by twitching of muscles, as seen in dementia precox.

echomatism (ĕ-ko'mă-tizm). Automatic repetition of another's actions.

echomimia (ĕ-ko-mim'ĭ-a). The imitation of the actions of others without meaning as seen in dementia precox.

echomotism (ĕ-ko-mo'tizm). Imitation of movements. SYN: *echomatism, echomimia, echopraxia.*

echopathy (ĕ-kop'ă-thĭ). Imitation of another's actions and repetitions of his words; a neurosis.

echophotony (ĕ-ko-fot'o-nĭ). Production of color sensations by stimulus of sounds heard.

echophra'sia. Patient's meaningless repeating of words spoken to him. May be accompanied by muscle twitching; seen in dementia precox.

echopraxia (ĕ-ko-praks'ĭ-ă). Imitation, without meaning, of motions made by others. SYN: *echomimia.*

echoprax'is. Senseless repetition by the patient of movements made by the physician in treatment.

eclabium (ek-la'bĭ-um). Eversion of a lip.

eclampsia (ĕ-klamp'sĭ-ă). A major toxemia of pregnancy accompanied by high blood pressure, albuminuria, oliguria, tonic and clonic convulsions, and coma. May occur pre-, intra-, or postpartum.

  e., albuminuric. Eclampsia caused by presence of albuminuria.

  e. gravidum. Eclampsia in women during pregnancy.

  e., puerperal. Eclampsia in women following childbirth.

  e., uremic. Eclampsia due to presence of uremic condition.

eclampsism (e-klamp'sizm). Puerperal eclampsia without convulsive seizures.

eclamp'tic. Rel. to, or of the nature of, eclampsia.

eclamptism (ĕ-klamp'tizm). Condition due to autointoxication incident to pregnancy.

eclamptogen'ic. Causing convulsions.

eclamptogenus (ek-lamp-toj'en-us). Producing convulsions. SYN: *eclamptogenic.*

eclectic (ek-lek'tik). Selecting from various sources what seems to be the best.

  e. school of medicine. One employing indigenous plants or "specifics" according to patient's symptoms.

eclecticism (ek-lek'ti-sizm). A system of medicine treating disease through specific remedies for individual pathological conditions, rather than by treating body as a whole. Remedies, principally botanical.

ecmnesia (ek-ne'zĭ-ă). Inability to remember recent events as seen in senility. The memory of before and after events not affected.

ecoid (e'koid). The framework of a red blood corpuscle.

ecology (e-kol'o-gĭ). The physiology of organisms as affected by their environment. SYN: *bionomics.*

ecomania (e-ko-ma'nĭ-ă). An extreme humbleness manifested before those in authority but a dominating, irritable attitude towards members of the family. Manifested in chronic alcoholism.

écouvillonage (a-koo-vĭ-yon-ahzh'). The cleansing and application of remedies to a cavity by means of a brush or swab.

ecphyadectomy (ek-fi-ă-dek'to-mĭ). Removal of vermiform appendix. SEE: *appendectomy.*

ecphyaditis (ek-fi-ad'i-tis). Inflammation of vermiform appendix. SYN: *appendicitis.* [phylaxis.]

ecphylactic (ek-fi-lak'tĭk). Pert. to ec-

ecphylax′is. Impotent antibodies or phylactic agents in the blood.

ecphyma (ek-fī′mă). An outgrowth or excrescence, as a wart.

écrasement (ā-krăz-mon′). Excision by means of an écraseur.

écraseur (ā-krā-zer′). A wire loop used for excisions.

ecstasy (ek′sta-sĭ). An exhilarated, trancelike, or exalted state.

ecstrophy (ek′stro-fĭ). Turning an organ inside out. SYN: *exstrophy.*

ec′tad. Toward the surface; outward; externally.

ec′tal. External, outer, on the surface.

ectasia, ectasis (ek-ta′sĭ-ă, -sis). Dilatation of any tubular vessel.

   e. ventriculi paradoxa. Hourglass stomach.

ectasin (ek′tas-in). A tuberculin-derived substance causing vasomotor dilation.

ectat′ic. Distensible or capable of being stretched.

ecten′tal. Pert. to entoderm and ectoderm.

   e. line. Point of entodermal and ectodermal junction.

ectethmoid (ekt-eth′moid). Lateral mass of the ethmoid bone.

ecthyma (ek-thī′mă). An acute, noncontagious, inflammatory, pustular, cutaneous eruption on a hardened base which may be followed by slight scarring or temporary pigmentation.

   e. scrofulosum. Form seen in scrofula.

   e. syphiliticum. Pustular eruption occurring in tertiary syphilis.

ecthyreosis (ek-thī-rē-ō′sis). Loss of thyroid gland function.

ectiris (ek-ti′ris). The external portion of the iris.

ecto-. Prefix: Outside.

ectoan′tigen. 1. Any toxin or stimulator of antibody formation. 2. An antigen assumed to have its origin in ectoplasm of bacterial cells.

ec′toblast. Outer wall of a cell. OPP: *mesoblast.* SEE: *ectoderm.*

ectocardia (ek-to-kar′dĭ-ă). Having the heart out of normal position.

ectochoroidea (ek″to-ko-roy′de-ă). Outer layer of choroid coat of the eye.

ectocinerea (ek-to-sin-e′re-ă). The outer gray matter of the brain.

ectocolos′tomy. Formation through the abdominal wall of an opening into the colon.

ectocon′dyle. The outer condyle of the bone.

ectocornea (ek-to-kor′ne-ă). External layer of the cornea.

ectocu′neiform. External cuneiform bone.

ectocytic (ek-to-si′tĭk). Outside of the cell.

ectodac′tylism. Lack of a digit or digits.

ectoderm (ek′to-derm). The outer layer of cells in the blastoderm.

ectoder′mal. Rel. to the ectoderm.

ectodermatosis (ek-to-der-mă-to′sis). Disorder due to faulty development of the ectoderm.   [*ectodermal.*

ectoder′mic. Pert. to the ectoderm. SYN:

ectodermoi′dal. Pert. to or resembling the ectoderm.

ectodermo′sis. Illness resulting from congenital maldevelopment of ectodermal structures. SYN: *ectodermatosis.*

ectoen′tad. From without inward.

ectoen′zyme. A cellular secreted enzyme.

ectogenous (ek-toj′en-us). Having its origin outside of a body or structure, as infection.

ectoglia (ek-tog′lĭ-ă): Superficial embryonic layer in beginning of stratification of the medullary tube.

ectoglob′ular. Not within blood cells or globular bodies.

ectog′ony. Influences on the mother's body and metabolism from the developing zygote.

ectokelostomy (ek-to-ke-los′to-mĭ). Making an external opening into a hernial sac to prepare for a radical operation.

ectolecithal (ek-to-les′ith-al). Pert. to ovum having food yolk placed near the surface.

ectol′ysis. Ectoplasmic lysis.

ectomere (ek′to-mēr). One of the blastomeres forming the ectoderm.

ectome′roblast. Cells from which will be developed the ectoblast and mesoblast.

ectomy (ek′to-mĭ). Excision of any organ or gland.   [cleus.

ectonu′clear. Occurring outside a cell nu-

ectoperitoni′tis. Inflammation beginning in the peritoneum next to the viscera.

ectopia (ek-to′pĭ-ă). A congenital displacement of an organ.

   e. testis. An abnormal position of the testicle. SYN: *parorchidium.*

ectopic (ek-top′ik). In an abnormal position; said of a fetus.

   e. beat. Cardiac beat beginning at a point other than sinoauricular node.

   e. gestation or **pregnancy.** Implantation of the fertilized ovum outside of the uterine cavity.

   e. rhythm. Any cardiac rhythm that is abnormal or irregular.

ec′toplasm. The outermost layer of cell protoplasm.

ec′toplas′mic. Pert. to ectoplasm.

ectoplas′tic. Formed at the periphery; ectoplasmic.

ectopotomy (ek-to-pot′o-mĭ). Removal of the fetus in ectopic pregnancy.

ectopterygoid (ek″to-ter′ĭ-goyd). *Musculus pterygoideus externus.*

ectopy (ek′to-pĭ). Displacement. SYN: *ectopia.*

ectoret′ina. Outer layer of retina.

ectos′copy. Diagnosis by study of thoracic movements when patient speaks, or by abdominal movements.

ectostosis (ekt-os-to′sis). Formation of bone beneath the periosteum.

ectotoxe′mia. Toxemia due to a cause outside the body.

ectozoon (ek-to-zo′on). Parasitic animal that infests the outer integument of the body.

ectrodactylism (ek-tro-dak′til-izm). Congenital absence of 1 or more fingers or toes.

ectropic (ek-tro'pĭk). Pert. to complete or partial eversion of a part, generally the eyelid.

ectropion (ek-tro'pĭ-on). OPHTH: Eversion, as the edge of an eyelid.

ETIOL: Old age; relaxation of skin; cicatrix following trauma; infection; palsy of facial nerve.

e. of the cervix uteri. GYN: A turning out of the edges of the cervix following laceration.

ectro'pionize. To evert, or cause an eversion.

eczema (ek'zĕ-mä). Cutaneous inflammatory condition, acute or chronic, with erythema, papules, vesicles, pustules, scales, crusts, or scabs alone or in combination, dry, or with watery discharge and with thickening or infiltration and more or less itching or burning. More a symptom than a disease. SYN: *dermatitis.*

e. capitis. That on the head. Oozing dermatitis seborrheica.*

e., erythematous. Dry, pinkish, ill-defined patches with itching and burning, slight swelling with tendency to spread and coalesce, branny scaling, roughness and dryness of skin. May become generalized.

e. fissum. Form of eczema with painful openings in the joint regions.

e., hypertrophied. Eczema with a permanent enlargement of papillae of the skin, or skin growths.

e., lichenoid. Eczema with a thickened condition of the skin.

e. madidans. Variety with raw, erythematous points exuding moisture.

e., marginal. Eczema caused by ringworm.

e., papular. Pinpoint to pinhead-sized reddish, pinkish, or violaceous papules with rounded or acuminate thin-walled vesicles which, when ruptured, become covered with thin yellowish crust of dried sebum or inspissated pus interspersed with raw areas of denuded epithelium. Skin as a result of irritation and chronic congestion becomes thick and infiltrated and dark red.

e., pustular. Includes many forms: Follicular, impetiginous or consecutive types, including *eczema rubrum* (red, glazed surface with little oozing); *eczema madidans* (raw, red, and covered with moisture); *eczema crustosum* (more or less crusting with exudate); *eczema fissum* (thick, dry, inelastic skin with cracks and fissures); *squamous eczema* (chronic on soles, legs, scalp; multiple, circumscribed infiltrated patches with thin, dry scales); *eczema sclerosum* (marked thickening, elephantiasislike papillary hypertrophy resulting in rough, horny, verrucose patches on legs, soles, and palms with fissuring); *furrowed eczema* (slightly erythematous skin, harsh and dry, with innumerable cracks on outer epidermal layer).

e. rubrum. SEE: *eczema madidans.*

e., seborrheic. Form marked by excessive secretion from the sebaceous glands. SYN: *seborrhea.*

e. squamosum. Eczema with scaly formation.

e., vesicular. Formation of vesicles on the scalp in eczema. [eczema.

eczem'atous. Marked by or resembling

Edebohl's position (ed'e-bōl). The dorsal recumbent position with the buttocks resting upon end of table, the lower limbs flexed backward toward the abdomen sufficiently to permit holding the position with legs supported from ankles in a support attached to 2 straight uprights extending 1 on each side at end of table.

ede'ma. Serous matter in areolar tissue causing swelling.

e., acute circumscribed. Form with separated swellings on the body, but usually on the face.

e., angioneurotic. Edema caused by vasomotor disorder.

e., blue. Hysteric paralysis inducing a swollen, bluish condition of a limb.

e. bullosum vesicae. Form affecting the bladder.

e. of glottis. An infiltration of the submucosa of the larynx, with cough, loss of voice, and feeling of suffocation.

e., inflammatory. Edema of inflamed tissues.

e., malignant. Edema characterized by a rapid course, and speedy destruction of tissue.

e., purulent. Edema caused by purulent infiltration.

e., salt. Form caused by increase of salt in the diet.

edematous (e-dem'at-us). Pert. to, or affected with, edema.

eden'tulous. Without or lacking teeth.

edeology (e-de-ol'o-jĭ). The study of the anatomy, physiology, and diseases of the genital organs.

edes'tin. A globulin from hemp and other seeds; used in estimating amt. of peptolytic ferment in gastric juice.

edible (ĕd'ĭ-bl). Suitable for food.

edul'corant. Sweetening.

edulcorate (e-dul'ko-rāt). 1. To sweeten. 2. To wash out salts or acids.

E. E. G. Abbr. for *electroencephalogram.*

effect'or. One of the nerve endings having the efferent process end in a gland or muscle cell. The terminal arborizations of efferent or motor nerves. OPP: *receptor.**

ef'ferent. Carrying impulses away from some nervous center. Generally synonymous with "motor."

e. nerves. Motor nerves. They can carry impulses having the following effects: (1) Motor, causing contraction of muscles; (2) secretory, causing glands to secrete, and (3) inhibitory, causing some organ to become quiescent.

effervesce (ef-er-ves'). To boil, or form bubbles on the surface of a liquid.

effervescence (ef-er-ves'ense). Formation of bubbles of gas coming up to surface of fluid.

efferves'cent. Bubbling. Rising in little bubbles of gas.

effleurage (ef-flūr-ahzh'). In massage, deep or superficial stroking.

efflorescence (ef-flor-es'ens). A rash; a redness of the skin. SYN: *exanthem.**

efflorescent (ef-flor-es'ent). Becoming powdery or drying from loss of water of crystallization.

effluve'. A conductive discharge of a high potential current through a dielectric.

effluvium (ef-lu'vĭ-um) (pl. *effluvia*). An invisible emanation or exhalation. SYN: *odor, vapor.*

effuse'. Thin, widely spreading; said of bacterial growth.

effu'sion. Escape of fluid into a part, as the pleural cavity, such as empyema, or pyothorax (pus), hydrothorax (serum), hemothorax (blood), chylothorax (lymph), pneumothorax (air), hydropneumothorax (serum and air), and pyopneumothorax (pus and air). RS: *cast, Charcot's arthropathy.*

egersim'eter. Device for testing excitability of nerves and muscles.

egertic (e-jer'tik). Producing wakefulness.

egesta (e-jes'tă). Waste matter eliminated from the body. SYN: *dejecta, excreta.*

egg albumen. The white of an egg. SEE: *vitellin, vitellus, yellow sac.*

egg and ether enema. One given to relieve distention, but usually only as a last resort. SEE: *enema.*

ego (e'go). PSY: That part of the unconscious that has been influenced by the senses and which has taken on consciousness in its contacts with reality. A sum total of the innate endowments, environmental impressions, and the reactive tendencies arising out of the conflict between them.

    e. ideal. The unconscious perfection of an individual's pattern or standard of character, usually identified with one greatly admired.

    e. instincts. All instincts not of a sexual nature.

    e. libido. One concentrated in and upon the ego and not manifested toward external objects. Manifested in narcissistic disorders.

    e., super. An inner censor (outside of the field of consciousness) of the ego.

egobronchophony (e″go-bron-kof'o-nĭ). A bleating sound with bronchophony. SEE: *egophony.*

egocen'tric. Pert. to a withdrawal from external world with concentration upon inner self.

egoma'nia. Abnormal self-esteem and self-interest.

egophony (eg-of'o-nĭ). A nasal sound somewhat like the bleat of a goat heard in auscultation when the subject speaks in a normal tone.

egotrop'ic. Interested chiefly in oneself; self-centered.

Eh'renritter's ganglion. The jugular ganglion.

Ehrlich's side-chain theory (air'lik). So named because the protoplasmic cell is said to possess the certain receptors or "side-chains" which are capable of becoming fixed to certain protein groups with which they have a chemical affinity.

    E.'s theory of immunity. A theory which attempts to explain the formation of antitoxin in the blood. Also known as Ehrlich's side-chain theory, *q.v.*

Ehrlich-Hata "606." A specific for syphilis SYN: *salvarsan.*

Eichhorst's corpuscles (ĭk'horst). Spherical, small blood corpuscles found in pernicious anemia.

    E.'s neuritis. Neuritis involving nerve sheath and interstitial muscular tissues.

eidoptometry (i-dop-tom'et-rĭ). Determination of visual acuteness.

eighth cranial nerve. Acoustic nerve, *q.v.*

eikonom'etry. Determination of distance of an object by measuring the image produced by a lens of known focus.

eiloid (i'loid). Having a coil-like structure.

Eimeria (i-me'rĭ-ă). A parasite of the order *Coccidea.*

    E. hominis. A species in the pleural exudate of man.

eisodic (i-sod'ik). Centripetal or afferent, as nerve fibers of a reflex arc.

eiweissmilch (i'vīs-milk). Milk with curd broken up and whey removed, mixed with malt sugar, and boiled buttermilk for infant feeding.

ejaculatio (e-jak-u-la'she-o). Sudden expelling, as of semen.

    e. precox (pre'kox). Premature ejaculation. Inability to prevent ejaculation of semen at the beginning of copulation, or prior to it.

ejaculation (e-jak-u-la'shun). Ejection of the seminal fluids from the male urethra, or of the secretions of the vaginal glands, esp. Bartholin's glands, in the female.

ejac'ulatory. Pert. to ejaculation.

    e. duct. The seminiferous canal conveying semen from the testicles; more esp. from the seminal vesicles into the urethra.

ejecta (e-jek'tă). Matter thrown off by the body. SYN: *dejecta, egesta.*

EK, EKG. Abbr. for *electrocardiogram.*

ekphorize (ek'fo-riz). PSY: A bringing back of the effect of a psychic experience in an attempt to reëxperience it in memory. SEE: *engram.*

elaiop'athy. Swelling of joints due to contusion, followed by fatty deposits. SYN: *eleopathy.*

elastic (e-las'tik). Capable of being stretched and returning to its original state; having elasticity.

    e. bandage. One which can be stretched.

    e. cartilage. Yellow cartilage such as is found in the epiglottis, pharynx, external ears, and auditory tube.

    e. lamina. Descemet's membrane.

    e. skin. Rare condition in which there is unusual elastic state of the skin.

    e. stocking. One worn to place pressure on surface of the foot, or portion of the leg.

e. tissue. Connective tissue supplied with elastic fibers as found in the middle coat of arteries.

elasticin (e-las'tis-in). An albuminoid substance present in yellow elastic tissues. SYN: *elastin*.

elasticity (e-las-tis'it-ĭ). The quality of returning to original size and shape after compression or stretching.

elastin (e-las'tin). 1. Albuminoid substance; principal part of protective tissue and of skeletal structures. 2. A protein which can be prepared from various connective tissues. SEE: *albuminoid*.

elas'tinase. A ferment that dissolves elastin.

elas'toid. Pert. to a substance formed by hyaline degeneration.

e. degeneration. Hyaline degeneration of elastic fibers of an artery.

elasto'ma. A chronic disease of the skin; pseudoxanthoma.

elastometer (e-las-tŏm'et-er). Device for measuring elasticity.

elastom'etry. The measurement of elasticity of tissues.

elas'tose. A peptone resulting from gastric digestion of elastin.

elaterin (e-lăt'er-in). The neutral principle obtained from *elaterium*, a plant grown in the Mediterranean region.

DOSAGE: From 1/20 to 1/10 gr. (0.003-0.006 Gm.).

ela'tion. PSY: Joyful emotion. It is pathologic when out of accord with patient's actual circumstances.

el'bow. Joint of arm and forearm.

e., dislocation, ant. TREATMENT: Reduction by direct pressure with moderate extension.

e., d., lateral. Frequently accompanied with fracture of condyle.

e., d., post. SYM: Olecranon projects. Arm flexed. Lower end of humerus felt at bend. Elastic fixation of elbow. Distance increased bet. olecranon and condyles.

e. jerk. Striking tendon of biceps or triceps muscle causes involuntary bending or jerk of elbow.

e. joint. Humerus, radius, and olecranon process of ulna.

e. reflex. Sharp extension of forearm resulting from tapping of triceps tendon while arm is held loosely in bent position.

elcosis (el-ko'sis). Fetid ulceration.

Electra complex. PSY: A group of symptoms due to suppressed sexual love of daughter for father.

OPP: *Oedipus complex, q.v.*

elec'tric. Pert. to, caused by, or resembling electricity.

e. baker. Device for placing intense heat on a part, as in arthritis. SEE: *baker*.

e. field. Field exerting force of one dyne on unit positive charge. SEE: *intensity of electric field*.

e. muscle stimulation. Two types of current, faradic used for stimulation of nerve to the muscle, and galvanic used for stimulation of nerve and muscle. Contraction of muscle with galvanic occurs only at *make* or if strong enough at *break*. Used for diagnosis and treatment in neuromuscular diseases.

e. shock. SYM: Burns, with loss of consciousness; contact or proximity to source of current are principal symptoms.

e. valve. A vacuum tube having for one electrode a hot filament. Often used in rectifying alternating to direct current, as in roentgen generators.

electri'city. "A form of energy which, when in motion, exhibits magnetic, chemical, mechanical, and thermal effects, and when at rest or in motion exerts a force on other electricity. Recent investigations indicate that it is discrete or granular in nature. Electricity may be of 2 kinds, namely, positive and negative."—Sheldon.

e., atmospheric. Electricity existing in the atmosphere.

e., faradic. SEE: *induced electricity*.

e., franklinic. SEE: *static electricity*.

e., frictional. Generation of static electricity by rubbing 2 articles together.

e., galvanic. Electricity generated by chemical action.

e., induced. Electricity generated in a body from another body close by, without contact.

e., magnetic. Electricity induced by means of a magnetic device.

e., medical. Generation of electricity by a device which can be adjusted for treating medical cases.

e., negative. Electric charge caused by an excess of electrons negatively charged.

e., positive. Electric charge caused by loss of negative electrons. [friction.

e., static. Electricity generated by

e., unit of. SEE: *ampere, coulomb, farad, ohm, volt, watt*.

elec'trify. To charge a body with electricity.

electriza'tion. The act of charging the body with electricity.

electroanesthesia. Local anesthesia induced by an anesthetizing substance injected into tissues by electricity.

electrobiol'ogy. Science of electric phenomena in the living body.

electrobios'copy. Electric test to determine if life is extinct.

electrocar'diogram. A graphic record of the variation in time and potential of the electric current associated with action of the heart muscles.

electrocar'diograph. Device for recording variations in action of heart muscles.

elec'trocardiog'raphy. The use of a galvanometer or electrometer to obtain a graphic record of the electric currents generated by the beating heart.

elec''trocar''diopho'nograph. Device for recording heart sounds.

elec″trocatal′ysis. Chemical decomposition produced by electricity.

electrocau′tery. An apparatus for cauterizing tissue, consisting of a holder containing a wire, which may be heated to a red or white heat by a current of electricity, either direct or alternating.

electrochem′istry. Science of chemical changes produced by electricity.

elec′trochemy. Therapy concerned with physical applications, such as electricity, which produce chemical effects in the tissues.

electrocis′ion. Excision by electric current.

elec″trocoagula′tion. Coagulation of tissue by means of a high frequency electric current. The heat producing the coagulation is generated within the tissue to be destroyed.

electrocontractility (e-lek″tro-kon-trak-til′ĭ-tĭ). Contraction of muscular tissue by electrical stimulation.

electrocryptectomy (e-lek″tro-krip-tek′to-mĭ). Destruction of tonsillar crypts by diathermy.

electrocu′tion. The destruction of life by means of electric current.

electrocystoscopy (e-lek″tro-sis-tos′ko-pĭ). The use of electric light to see the interior of the bladder.

elec′trode. A medium intervening bet. an electric conductor and the object to which the current is to be applied.

　e., active. SEE: *therapeutic electrode.*

　e., brush. A wire brush used to apply electricity to a part of the body.

　e., cataphoric. Electrode devised so that the current passes from the positive pole to the body through a medicated solution.

　e., Cherry's. Vaginal electrodes for medical diathermy treatments of pelvic infections.

　e., depolarizing. Electrode with greater resistance than the part of the body in the circuit.

　e., diffusion. SEE: *cataphoric electrode.*

　e., disper′sive. When electrodes may be applied in pairs dissimilar in size and shape, then the smaller electrode is called the active, and the larger, the dispersive, indifferent, or inactive electrode.

　e., exciting. SEE: *therapeutic electrode.*

　e., franklinic. Form used for the application of static discharge.

　e., Guttman. Electrode for intramural electrocoagulation of the inferior turbinate.

　e., Hyam's. Special cutting current instrument for "conization" by high frequency current in treatment of chronic endocervicitis.

　e., hydrogen. Form absorbing hydrogen gas.

　e., impregnated. SEE: *therapeutic electrode.*

　e., indifferent. SEE: *electrode, dispersive.*

　e., multiple point. Several sets of terminals providing for the use of several electrodes. SEE: *multiterminal.*

　e., negative. Cathode.

　e., nonpolarizable. Electrode constructed to prevent polarization.

　e., normal. Electrode with constant cross section of 10 square centimeters.

　e., point. An electrode with an insulating handle at one end and a metallic point at the other for use in applying static sparks.

　e., positive. Anode.

　e., prescription. Therapeutic electrode made according to a physician's prescription.

　e., Roblee. Pelvic diathermy electrode introduced by Roblee, consisting of hard rubber vaginal speculum.

　e., roller. Form of electrode made like a roller.

　e., silent. SEE: *dispersive electrode.*

　e., spark ball or point. An insulating handle having on one end a metallic ball or point. Used in giving static sparks.

　e., therapeutic. Electrode devised so the carbon is impregnated with medicinal preparations.

　e., vacuum. Hollow glass tubes or bulbs from which the air has been exhausted to varying degrees and to which the current is conveyed by a wire passing through one end or by a metal collar surrounding the stem without any internal connection. Used for high frequency and static currents.

　e., vaginal. SEE: *Cherry's electrode.*

　e., Ze′ner's. Cervicovaginal diathermy electrode with 4 blades closing about cervix concentrating heat in cervical canal and immediate parametrium.

　e., zinc. Used connected to positive pole of galvanic machine for ionic medication.

elec″trodesicca′tion. The destructive drying of cells and tissue by means of short high frequency electric sparks, in contradistinction to fulguration, which is the destruction of tissue by means of long high frequency electric sparks.

elec″trodiagno′sis. The determination of the functional states of various organs and tissues according to their response to electrical stimulation.

electrodynamometer (e-lek-tro-di-na-mom′et-er). An instrument to measure the strength of an electric current either alternating or direct, as by means of the interaction of 2 wire coils carrying the current.

electroencephalogram (ē-lĕk-trō-ĕn-sĕf′ă-lō-grăm). A tracing on an electroencephalograph.

electroencephalograph (ē-lĕk-trō-ĕn-sĕf′ă-lō-grăf). An instrument for recording electrical fluctuations of the brain after amplification of more than a billion times.

electrog′raphy. Making of an x-ray picture. SYN: *skiagraphy.*

electrol′ogy. The branch of science that deals with the phenomena and properties of electricity.

electrolysis (e-lek-trol′ĭ-sis). The electrical decomposition of a chemical compound.

electrolyte (e-lek′tro-līt). 1. A solution which is a conductor of electricity. 2. A substance which, in solution, conducts an electric current and is decomposed by the passage of an electric current.

    e., amphoteric. One which produces both hydrogen and hydroxol.

electrolytic (e-lek-tro-lit′ik). Caused by or rel. to electrolysis.

    e. conduction. In metals the electrical charges are carried by the electrons of inappreciable mass.

elec′trolyzer. Instrument for reducing stricture with electricity.

electromag′net. A magnet consisting of a length of insulated wire wound around soft iron core.   [net.

electromagnet′ic. Pert. to an electromagnet.

    e. induc′tion. Generation of an electromotive force in an insulated conductor moving in an electromagnetic field, or in a fixed conductor in a moving magnetic field.

electromag′netism. Science of mutual relations of electricity and magnetism.

electromassage′. Massage combined with application of electrization.

electrom′eter. An instrument for measuring pressure, quantity and intensity of electricity.

electromo′tive. Pert. to passage of electricity in a current, or motion produced by it.

    e. force (abbreviation, E. M. F.). That effect of difference of potential which, on the closing of a circuit, causes a flow of electricity from one place to another, giving rise to an electric current.

elec′tron. An extremely minute corpuscle or charge of negative electricity; the smallest that is known to exist.

electroneg′ative. The condition of being subject to repulsion by bodies negatively electrified, and to attraction by bodies positively electrified.

electron′ic. Pert. to electrons.

electroniza′tion. The use of radiation to restore electrical equilibrium.

elec′tropath. One skilled in practice of electrotherapy.

electropathol′ogy. Determining electrical reaction of muscles and nerves as means of diagnosis.

electrophoresis (e-lek-tro-for-e′sis). Diathermy or iontophoresis. SEE: *phoresis*.

electrophorus (e-lek-tro-for′us). An instrument for obtaining static electricity by means of induction.

electrophotother′apy. Treatment by means of electric light.

electropos′itive. The condition of being subject to repulsion by bodies positively electrified, and to attraction by bodies negatively electrified.

electrophysiol′ogy. Study of the effects of electricity upon living tissue.

electropneumatotherapy (e-lek″tro-nu″-mă-to-ther′ă-pĭ). Treatment of voice by faradic current into the larynx.

electroprogno′sis. Prognosis by means of electrical reactions.

elec′tropuncture. Piercing tissues with an electric needle.

electropyrexia (e-lek″tro-pi-reks′ĭ-ă). Elevation of temperature by electricity.

electroradiometer (e-lek″tro-ră-dĭ-om′e-ter). An electroscope for differentiation of radiant energy.

electroscission (e-lĕk″trō-sĭ′shŭn). Division of tissues by electrocautery.

electroscope (e-lek′tro-skōp). An instrument which detects positive or negative static electricity.

electrostat′ic. Pert. to static electricity.

    e. generator. A device that generates static electricity. SEE: *influence machine.*

    e. unit. Any unit of electrical measurement based on the attraction or repulsion of a static charge, as distinguished from an electromagnetic unit, which is defined in terms of the attraction or repulsion of magnetic poles.

electrosur′gery. Surgery accomplished by electricity.

electrotax′is. Reaction of cells to electricity.

electrotherapeutics (e-lek″tro-ther-ă-pu′-tĭks). The use of electricity in the treatment of disease.

electrotherapist (e-lek″tro-ther′a-pist). A medical graduate who has had special training and has acquired skill in the therapeutic use of electricity. The term is sometimes used incorrectly to designate anyone who administers electrical treatments.

elec″trother′apy. Use of electricity in treating disease. SYN: *electrotherapeutics.*

electrothermotherapy (e-lek″tro-ther″mo-ther′a-pĭ). The production of heat within the living tissues for therapeutic purposes by means of bodily resistance to the passing of an electric current.

electroton′ic. Of or pert. to electrotonus.

electroto′nus. The change in the irritability of a nerve or muscle during the passage of an electric current.

electrotropism (e-lek-trot′ro-pizm). Reaction of cells to an electrical current.

electuary (e-lek′tu-a-rĭ). Medicinal substance mixed with saccharine matter to form pasty mass.

eleidin (e-le′ĭ-dĭn). A substance forming granules of the stratum granulosum of the epidermis.

el′ement. In modern chemistry, a substance which cannot be separated into substances different from itself by ordinary chemical processes. They exist in a free and in a combined state. Over 90 have been identified.

eleoma (el-e-o′mă). A neoplasm sometimes following injection of oil into the tissues.

eleometer (el-e-om′et-er). Instrument for determining quality and spec. gravity of oils.

eleomyenchysis (el″e-o-mi-en′kis-is). 1. The intramuscular injection of oils for chronic local spasms. 2. Prosthesis* by paraffin injection.

eleop'athy. Swelling of joints due to fatty deposits. SYN: *elaiopathy.*

eleoptene (el-e-op'tēn). The fluid part of a volatile oil.

eleosaccharum (e"le-o-sak'ar-um). A mixture of powdered sugar with a volatile oil.

eleotherapy (el-e-o-ther'ă-pĭ). The use of oil for therapeutic purposes.

eleotho'rax. The injection of oil into the pleural cavity to compress a tuberculous lung.

elephantiasis (el-ĕ-fan-ti'as-is). Chronic affection of skin with hypertrophy of cellular tissue.

  e. arabum. SYN: *elephantiasis.*
  e. graecorum. Leprosy.
  e. telangiectodes. Elephantiasis with blood vessel enlargement.

el'evator. 1. Curved retractor for holding lid away from the globe of the eye. 2. One for raising depressed bones by levers or screws.

eleventh cranial nerve. Accessorius nerve, *q.v.*

eliminant (ē-lim'ĭ-nant). 1. Effecting evacuation. 2. Agent aiding in elimination.

eliminate (ē-lim'ĭ-nāt). To expel; to rid the body of waste material.

elimina'tion. Excretion of waste body products by the skin, kidneys, and intestines.

  e. diet. Based on patient's history of food sensitiveness and results of skin tests. The "elimination diet" found to relieve the patient's symptoms is increased by gradual addition of foods to which patient has been found to be nonsensitive, until in so far as possible all the essentials of an adequate diet are included.

elinguation (ē-lĭn-gwā'shun). The operation of removing the tongue from the oral cavity.

elixir. An aromatic, sweetened, spirituous solution containing small amounts of medicinal substances.

El'liott treat'ment. Treatment given by means of rubber bag that distends vagina when attached to machine delivering water at temperature of 115° to 128° F. maintained for 45 to 60 minutes; used in pelvic inflammatory disease.

elutriation (e-lū-trĭ-a'shun). The separation of insoluble particles from finer ones by decanting the fluid.

elytritis (el-ĭ-tri'tis). Inflammation of the vagina.

elytrocele (el'ĭ-tro-sēl). Hernia into the vagina. SYN: *colpocele.*

elytroclasia (el"ĭ-tro-kla'sĭ-a). Rupture of the vagina. [the vagina.

elytrocleisis (el"ĭ-tro-kli'sis). Closure of

elytronitis (el-ĭ-tro-ni'tis). Inflammation of the vagina.

elytroplasty (el'it-ro-plas"tĭ). Plastic operation upon the vagina.

elytroptosis (ĕl"ĭ-trŏp-tō'sĭs). Prolapse of the vagina.

elytrorrhaphy (el-ĭ-tror'rā-fĭ). Suture of vaginal wall.

elytrostenosis (el"ĭ-tro-sten-o'sis). Narrowing of the vagina.

elytrotomy (el-ĭ-trot'o-mĭ). Incision of vaginal wall.

emaciate (e-mā-sĭ-āt). To cause to become excessively lean.

ema'ciated. Excessively lean.

emacia'tion. Wasting of the flesh; state of being extremely lean.

emaculation (em-ak-u-la'shun). Removal of spots from the skin.

emailloid (em-a'loid). Tumor having its origin in tooth enamel.

emana'tion. 1. Something given off; radiation; emission. 2. A disintegration product.

  e., actinium. One given off by actinium. SYN: *actinon.*
  e., radium. A radioactive gas given off by radium. SYN: *niton.*
  e., thorium. One given off by thorium. SYN: *thoron.*

emansio mensium (em-an'sĭ-o men'sĭ-um). Amenorrhea in which menstruation has never occurred.

emasculation (e-mas-ku-la'shun). Castration;* excision of the testicles. RS: *spay.*

emballometer (ĕm-băl-ŏm'ĕt-ĕr). Device employed in connection with a stethoscope.

embalming (em-bahm'ing). Preservation of a dead body against putrefaction.

embed'ding. Fixation in a mass of solid material.

embola'lia. Meaningless language of the insane. SYN: *embolophrasia.*

embole (em'bo-lē). 1. Reduction of a dislocation. 2. Formation of the gastrula by invagination. 3. Enarthrosis. SYN: *emboly.*

embol'ic. Pert. to or caused by embolism.

embol'iform. 1. Resembling a nucleus. 2. Wedge-shaped, as the *nucleus emboliformis.*

embolism (em'bo-lizm). Obstruction of a blood vessel by a clot or a foreign substance. RS: *embolus, thrombosis, thrombus.*

  e., air. One caused by air bubble. SEE: *air embolism.*
  e., fat. Globules of fat obstructing blood vessels. [purulent matter.
  e., pyemic. Embolism caused by

embolophrasia (em"bol-o-fra'zĭ-ă). Meaningless speech. SYN: *embolalia.*

em'bolus (pl. *emboli*). Any material which enters the blood stream and obstructs a blood vessel.

  e., air. An air bubble in the veins, the right atrium, or ventricle, or in the capillaries. SEE: *air embolism.*
  e., coronary. May be complication of arteriosclerosis and cause angina pectoris. SYM: Similar to pulmonary embolus.
  e., pulmonary. The commonest embolus met with. SYM: Face gray, eyes staring and wild, look of distress, gasping for breath; sudden death.

em'boly. Formation of the gastrula from invagination. SYN: *embole*.

embrace reflex (em-brās'). A variety of defensive reflex. The throwing out of the arms in an attitude of embrace, in fearful response.

embrasure (em-bra'shur). An opening widening outwardly or inwardly.

   e., buccal. Opening spreading toward the buccal aspect.

   e., labial. Embrasure opening toward the labial aspect.

   e., lingual. One spreading to the lingual aspect.

   e., occlusal. Space mesially and distally bet. marginal ridges of approximating teeth.

embroca'tion. 1. Fomentation, such as the application of heat and moisture; a stupe. 2. A drug rubbed into the skin.

embryectomy (em-brĭ-ek'to-mĭ). Removal of an extrauterine embryo.

embryo (em'brĭ-o). The term given the product of conception during the first 3 months after fecundation, after which it is called a fetus.

embryocardia (em-brĭ-o-kar'dĭ-ă). Heart action in which first and second pause are equal, and resembling the fetal heart sounds. Another variety is an undue lengthening of the first sound followed by a long pause.

embryoctony (em-brĭ-ok'to-nĭ). Destroying the fetus *in utero*, as in cases where delivery is impossible, or for abortion. SEE: *craniotomy*.

embryogenet'ic, embryogen'ic. Pert. to or giving rise to an embryo.

embryog'eny. The growth and development of an embryo.

embryog'raphy. A treatise on the embryo.

embryol'ogy. The science of fetal life.

embryoma (em-brĭ-o'mă). A tumor developed from misplaced germinal cells.

embry'onal. Pert. to or resembling an embryo.

embryonic (em-brĭ-on'ĭk). Pert. to or in condition of an embryo.

embryoniza'tion. Reversion of a cell or tissue to an embryonic structure.

embryonoid (em'brĭ-on-oyd). Having the appearance of an embryo.

embryoplas'tic. Having a part in the formation of an embryo; said of cells.

embryotocia (em″brĭ-o-to'sĭ-ă). An abortion; delivery of an embryo.

embryotome (em'brĭ-o-tōm). Instrument used in dismemberment of the fetus *in utero*.

embryotroph (em'brĭ-o-trof). A fluid resulting from the enzyme action of the trophoblasts upon the neighboring maternal tissue and which nourishes the embryo from the time of implantation into the uterus.

embryotrophy (em-brĭ-ot'ro-fĭ). Nutrition of the fetus.

embryotomy (em-brĭ-ot'o-mĭ). The dissection of a fetus to aid its delivery.

embryotoxon (em-brĭ-o-tox'on). Congenital marginal opacity of the cornea.

embryulcia (em-bri-ul'sĭ-ă). Forcible removal of the fetus as by embryotomy or taking a dead fetus with instruments.

embryulcus (em-brĭ-ul'kus). Instrument for extracting a fetus.

emedullate (e-med'ul-āt). To remove the marrow from a bone.

emer'gency. An unexpected serious happening, demanding immediate action.

   e. light reflex. Marked pupillary contraction, frowning, and closure of eyelids, resulting from sudden powerful light stimulus of retina.

   e. theory. Formulated by Cannon: Adrenal secretion is stimulated by sympathetic nervous system activity to meet bodily emergencies, as emotional excitement, pain, etc.

emer'gent. 1. Growing from a cavity or other part. 2. Sudden, unforeseen.

emesis (em'es-is). Vomiting.

   e., irritation. Drugs, uremia, nephritis, some brain tumors, chloroform, ether.

   e., nervous. Tumor or abscess of brain, sea sickness, acute myelitis, meningitis, anemia and hyperemia of brain, concussion and contusion of brain, fracture of skull, Ménière's disease, migraine, paresis, sclerosis.

   e., reflex. Irritation of fauces and pharynx; coughing, removal of viscous secretion from nasopharynx, eyestrain, unpleasant odors and sights, shock, nervousness, anticipation, anxiety, hysteria, morning sickness, gastric crisis of tabes, various heart troubles, hiccough.

   e., systemic. Pulmonary tuberculosis, whooping cough, peritonitis, irritations of bowels, acute obstruction of bowels, renal or biliary colic, Addison's disease.

emetic (e-met'ik). Medicine that produces vomiting. Ex: *apomorphine, a. hydrochloride, ipecac, mustard, sodium chloride.*

   e., direct. Those acting directly on gastric nerves, *e. g., mustard.*

   e., indirect. Those acting on vomiting center of brain, as *apomorphine.*

   e., local. Those which act through nerve irritation, such as salt.

   e., systemic. Those acting through the circulation, irritating vomiting centers by stimulation, such as mustard, soapy water, syrup of ipecac.

em'etine. Powdered, white alkaloid obtained from ipecac, *q.v.*

emetine bismuth iodide (em'e-tin biz'muth i'o-dīd). A combination of emetine and bismuth containing about 25% emetine and 20% bismuth.

   DOSAGE: 3 gr. (0.2 Gm.).

   e. hydrochloride. USP. The hydrochloride of an alkaloid obtained from ipecac.

   AVERAGE DOSAGE: 1/3 gr. (0.02 Gm.).

em'etism. Poisoning from overdose of ipecac.

emetocathar'tic. Producing both emesis and catharsis.

emetol'ogy. Study of emetics and their action.

E. M. F. Abbr. for *electromotive force.*

emiction (e-mik'shun). The act of urination.

emigra'tion. Passage of white blood corpuscles through the walls of capillaries and veins during inflammation.

em'inence. A prominence or projection, esp. of a bone.

    e., arcuate. A rounded eminence on upper surface of petrous portion of temporal bone. SYN: *jugum petrosum.*

    e., articular, of the temporal bone. A rounded eminence forming ant. boundary of the glenoid fossa.

    e., auditory. A collection of gray matter on floor of 4th ventricle of brain at its lower part, forming the deep origin of the auditory nerve.

    e., bicipital. A tuberosity for insertion of biceps muscle on radius.

    e., blastodermic. An elevated mass of cells of a developing ovum forming the blastoderm.

    e., canine. A vertical ridge on the external surface of the superior maxilla.

    e., collateral. One bet. middle and post. horns in lat. ventricle of brain.

    e. of Doyère. Slight elevation of muscular fiber corresponding to entrance of a nerve fiber.

    e. of the aquaeductus Fallopii. A ridge which traverses the inner wall of the tympanum above the fenestra ovalis.

    e., frontal. A rounded prominence on either side of median line, a little below center of frontal bone (BNA, *tuber frontale*).

    e., germinal. The *discus proligerus.*

    e., hypothenar. One on ulnar side of palm, formed by muscles of little finger.

    e., iliopectineal, e., iliopubic. Eminence on upper aspect of pubic bone above the acetabulum, marking the junction of bone with the ilium (BNA, *eminentia iliopectinea*).

    e., mamillary. Projection of inner pillars of fornix.

    e., median. Ant. bodies of medulla oblongata separated by ant. median fissure.

    e., nasal. A prominence on vertical portion of frontal bone above the nasal notch and bet. the 2 superciliary ridges.

    e., occipital. Protuberance on occipital bone.

    e., olivary. Oval projection at upper part of medulla olivary, above extremity of lateral column.

    e., parietal. The marked convexity on outer surface of parietal bone (BNA, *tuber parietale*).

    e.'s, portal. The small median lobes on lower surface of liver.

    e., pyramidal. The pyramid of the tympanum.

    e., thenar. The ball of the thumb.

eminentia (em-in-en'shǐ-ă). An eminence.

    e. alveolaris. Bony prominence on mandible 1½ in. ant. and sup. to the tonsil; corresponds to the location of the last molar tooth.   [poral bone.

    e. articularis. Prominence on tem-

    e. collateralis. Prominence on inferior horn of the lateral ventricle.

em'issary. 1. Providing an outlet. 2. An outlet.

    e. veins. Small veins piercing the skull, carrying blood from the sinuses within to the veins without the skull.

emissio (e-mis'sǐ-o). A discharge; emission.*

    e. seminis. Discharge of semen.

emission (e-mish'un). The discharge, esp. involuntary, of semen by the male, particularly during sleep. SYN: *pollution.* SEE: *ejaculation.*

emmenagogue (em-en'ă-gog). An agent that stimulates the mentrual function. Ex: *ergot, preparations of iron, manganese dioxide, viburnum.*

    e., direct. Emmenagogue directly affecting the organs involved.

    e., indirect. Emmenagogue effective in alleviating the causative disorder, such as anemia.

emmenia (em-me'nǐ-ă). The menstrual flow.

emmen'ic. Pert. to the menses.

em'menin. A placental hormone causing precocious maturity.

emmenioapthy (em-me-nǐ-o'path-ǐ). Any disorder of the menstruation.

emmenol'ogy. Science of menstruation.

emmetrope (em'met-rōp). One endowed with normal vision.

emmetropia (em-me-tro'pǐ-ă). Normal condition of eye in refraction; with eye at rest parallel rays are focused on retina; ability to focus on the retina a luminous point from 3.9 to 4.7 in. from the eye.

emmetrop'ic. Normal in vision. SEE: *hypermetropic, myopic.*

Em'met's operation. 1. Uterine trachelorrhaphy. 2. Suturing of a lacerated perineum. 3. Converting a sessile submucous tumor of the uterus into a pedunculated one. 4. Operation for procidentia uteri.

emol'lient. An agent that will soften and soothe the part when applied locally. The term is usually confined to agents affecting the surface of the body. Ex: *ointment of rose water, olive oil, petrolatum.* SEE: *demulcent.*

    e. enema. One for the purpose of coating membranes and allaying local pain and irritation, in order to soften and protect tissues.

emotion or **affect** (e-mo'shun). These constitute the "drive" which brings about the motor adjustment necessary to satisfy instinctive needs.

emo'tional. Relating to any of the emotions.

    e. attitudes. Those which express any of the emotions, such as joy, sorrow, etc. Seen in hysteroepilepsy.

    e. instability. PSY: Pert. to a psychopathic personality given to easy rage, brooding, and vastly fluctuating moods.

emotivity (e-mo-tiv'ǐ-tǐ). One's capability for emotional response.

empathema (em-path-e'ma). (pl. *empath-*

emata). Ungovernable or dominant passion.

   e. atonicum. Hypochondriasis.

   e. entonicum. An active mania.

   e., inane. Passion and excitement without cause or purpose.

empath'ic. Pert. to, or characterized by, emotions.

empathy (em'pa-thǐ). Sympathetically trying to identify one's feelings with those of another.

emphlysis (em'flis-is) (pl. *emphlyses*). Any vesicular or exanthematous eruption.

emphractic (em-frak'tik). 1. Obstructive, as clogging of pores of skin. 2. Anything that obstructs a function.

emphysatherapy (em-fiz-ă-ther'ă-pǐ). Injection of gas into a cavity for therapeutic purposes.

emphysema (em-fi-se'mă). Distention of tissues by gas or air in the interstices. SEE: *boxnote.*

   e., atrophic. Principally in the aged.

   e., cutaneous. Air in subcutaneous tissues with consequent distention.

   e., gangrenous. Malignant variety of edema caused by a microbe.

   e., interstitial. Rupture of air cells from overdistention, and escape of air into interlobular tissue.

   e., pulmonary. Same as vesicular.

   e., surgical. Cutaneous emphysema due to operation, esp. after wounds of respiratory tract.

   e., vesicular. Overdistention of alveoli and smaller bronchial tubes with air.

emphysematous (em-fi-sem'at-us). Affected with or pert. to emphysema.

empir'ic. One who relies solely upon experience.

empirical (em-pir'ik-al). 1. Pert. to or based on experience. 2. Pert. to an empiric.

empiricism (em-pir'is-izm). 1. Experience, not theory, as basis of medical science. 2. Quackery.

emplastic (em-plas'tik). 1. A constipating medicine. 2. Fit to be used as a plaster or in one.

emplas'trum (pl. *emplastra*). Preparation for external application, and of such consistency that it requires heat to spread it, and adheres to the skin when applied.

emprosthotonos (em-pros-thot'o-nos). Lying with body incurved and resting upon forehead and feet with face downward.

emptysis (emp'tis-is). Hemorrhage from the lungs. SYN: *hemoptysis.*

empyema (em-pī-e'ma). Pus in a body cavity, esp. in the pleural cavity.

   e., interlobular. Form with pus bet. lobes of lung.

   e. necessitatis. Form in which pus can escape spontaneously.

   e., pulsating. Form with cardiac beats causing pulsation of chest wall.

emoyesis (em-pī-e'sis). A pustular eruption on the skin.

empyocele (em-pi'o-sēl). A purulent scrotal tumor.

emul'gent. Extracting or draining.

   e. vessel. Blood vessel of the kidney.

emulsifica'tion. 1. Process of making an emulsion. 2. The breaking down of fats in the intestines to fatty acids and glycerol.

emul'sifier. Anything used to make an emulsion.

emulsify (e-mul'sǐ-fī). To form into an emulsion.

emul'sion. A mixture of 2 liquids not mutually soluble.

emul'soid. A colloid dispersion in which the dispersed particles are more or less liquid, absorbing some of the fluid in which they are immersed.

emulsum (e-mul'sum). A fluid in which oil or resin is suspended by means of a mucilaginous substance.

emunctory (e-munk'to-rǐ). 1. Pert. to organ or duct having an excretory function. 2. An excretory duct, *i. e.,* pores of skin.

enamel (en-am'el). The hard, white, dense substance forming a covering for the crown of the teeth.

enanthem, enanthema (en-an'them, -the'-mă). Eruption of mucous membrane.

enanthematous (en-an-them'at-us). Of the nature of an enanthema.

enanthesis (en-an-the'sis). A skin eruption due to internal disease.

enanthrope (en'an-thrōp). The source of a disease originating internally.

enantiobiosis (en-an-ti-o-bi-o'sis). The condition in which associated organisms are antagonistic to each other. SEE: *symbiosis.*

enantiopathy (en-an-tǐ-op'ath-ǐ). Treatment of one disease by another disease antagonistic to it, as malaria in general paresis.

enarkyochrome (en-ar'kǐ-o-krōm). A nerve cell arranged like a network, taking a stain best in the cell body.

enarthri'tis. Inflammation of a ball-and-socket joint.

enarthrosis (en-ar-thro'sis) (pl. *enarthroses*). A ball-and-socket joint; a form of diarthrosis.

encan'this. An excrescence or new growth at the inner angle of the eye.

encapsula'tion. Inclosure in a sheath not normal to the part.

encatarrhaphy (en-kat-ar'raf-ǐ). Insertion of an organ or tissue into a part where it is not normally found.

enceinte (on-sant'). Pregnant.

encelial'gia. Abdominal pain.

encephalalgia (en-sef-al-al'jǐ-ă). Deep-seated head pain. SYN: *cephalalgia.*

encephalasthenia (en-sef''al-as-the'nǐ-ă). Deficiency in brain power.

encephalatrophy (en-sef-al-at'rof-ǐ). Cerebral atrophy.

encephalic (en-sef-al'ik). Pert. to the brain or its cavity.

encephalin (en-sef'al-in). A nitrogenous glucoside obtained from brain tissue by boiling.

encephalitis (en-sef-ă-li'tis). Inflammation of the brain.

e., cortical. Encephalitis of brain cortex only.

e., epidemic. SEE: *encephalitis lethargica.*

e., hemorrhagic. Hemorrhage in brain inflammation.

e. hyperplastica. Acute encephalitis without suppuration.

e., infantile. Brain inflammation in the young causing cerebral palsy.

e., influenzal. SEE: *encephalitis lethargica.*

e. lethargica (leth-ar'jĭ-ka). An infective disease accompanied by stupor, ocular paralyses, tremor, nocturnal wakefulness. Generally occurs in sporadic form.

e., meningo-. Encephalitis combined with meningitis.

e. neonato'rum. A form occurring in the newly born. ETIOL: Fatty cells in the brain.

e. periaxialis. Inflammation of the white matter of the cerebrum, occurring mainly in the young.

e., purulent. Encephalitis characterized by abscesses in the brain.

e., pyemic; e., pyogenic. SEE: *purulent encephalitis.*

encephalocele (en-sef'al-o-sēl). Protrusion of the brain through a cranial fissure.

encephalocystocele (en-sef-al-o-sis'to-sēl). Protrusion of brain distended by hernial sac containing fluid.

encephalodialysis (en-sef″al-o-di-al'is-is). Softening of the brain.

encephalogram (en-sef'al-o-gram). A roentgen ray picture of the brain.

encephalography (en-sef-al-og'ra-fĭ). 1. Examination of head following the introduction of air into the subarachnoid space as a means of diagnosis. 2. Roentgenography.

encephaloid (en-sef'ă-loid). 1. Resembling the cerebral substance. 2. A malignant neoplasm of brainlike texture.

e. cancer. Malignant brainlike tumor. SYN: *encephaloma.*

encephalolith (en-sef'al-o-lith). A calculus of the brain.

encephalology (en-sef-al-ol'o-jĭ). A description of the brain.

encephalo'ma. 1. Tumor of the brain. 2. Brain cancer.

encephalomalacia (en-sef-al-o-mal-a'sĭ-ă). Brain softening.

encephalomeningi'tis. Inflammation of the brain and its membranes.

encephalomeningocele (en-sef-al-o-men-in'go-sēl). Protrusion through the cranium of membranes and brain substance.

encephalomere (en-sef'al-o-mēr). Any one of the natural segments into which the brain is divisible.

encephalometer (en-sef-al-om'e-ter). An instrument for measuring the cranium and locating brain regions.

encephalomyelitis (en-sef-al-o″mĭ-el-i'tis). Encephalitis with myelitis.

encephalomyelopathy (en-sef-al-o-mĭ-el-op'a-thĭ). Any disease of brain and spinal cord.

encephalon (en-sef'ă-lon). The brain, including the cerebrum, cerebellum, medulla oblongata, and pons.

encephalop'athy. Any dysfunction of the brain.

enceph'alopuncture. Puncture into the brain substance.

encephalopyosis (en-sef-al-o-pi-o'sis). Abscess of the brain.

encephalorrhagia (en-sef-al-or-a'jĭ-a). Hemorrhage of the brain.

encephalosclerosis (en-sef″al-o-skle-ro'sis). Brain hardening.

encephalo'sis. A degenerative process of the brain.

encephalospi'nal. Pert. to brain and spinal cord.

e. axis. Cerebrospinal axis.

encephalotome (en-sef'al-o-tōm). Instrument for incising brain tissue.

encephalotomy (en-sef-al-ot'o-mĭ). Brain dissection.

enchondroma (en-kon-dro'mă). A cartilaginous tumor occurring generally where cartilage is absent or within a bone where it expands the diaphysis.

enchondrosarcoma (en-kon″dro-sar-ko'mă). Sarcoma made up of cartilaginous tissue.

enchylema (en-ki-le'mă). Fluid granular matter in interstices of cell body and nucleus. SYN: *cytochylema.*

enchyma (en'kĭ-mă). A fluid formed from chyme which elaborates and repairs tissues and cells.

enclave (en-klāv'). Free tissue in an enclosure surrounded by a different kind of tissue.

enclavement (en-klāv'ment). An impaction of the fetus in the pelvic strait.

enclitic (en-klit'ik). Having the planes of the fetal head inclined to those of the maternal pelvis.

encolpism (en-kol'pizm). Medication by vaginal suppositories and injections.

encolpitis (en-kol-pi'tis). Inflamed condition of the vaginal mucosa.

encra'nial. Intracranial or within the cranium.

encyesis (en-si-e'sis). Normal uterine pregnancy.

encyopyelitis (en-si-o-pi-e-li'tis). Inflammation of the renal pelvis occurring in normal pregnancy.

encysted (en-sist'ed). Surrounded by membrane; encapsulated.

end. A termination; extremity.

e. artery. An artery which does not anastomose directly or indirectly with other arteries, *e. g.*, in kidney and spleen, etc.

e. body. Substance that kills bacteria in immunity to typhoid. SYN: *complement.*

e. bud, e. bulb, e. capsule. The terminal of a sensory nerve.

e. result. The ultimate or final result.

Endamoeba (ĕn″dăm-ē'bă). A genus of parasitic amebae producing cysts. SYN: *Entamoeba, q.v.*

endangeitis, endangitis (end-an-je-i'tis, -ji'tis). Inflammation of the endangium.

endangium (en-dan'jĭ-um). Inmost coat or intima of blood vessels.

endaortitis (end"a-or-ti'tis). Inflammation of inner coat of the aorta.

endarterial (end-ar-ter'ĭ-al). Pert. to the inner portion of an artery.

endarteritis (end-ar-ter-i'tis). Inflammation of innermost coat or intima of an artery resulting from syphilis, trauma, pyogenic bacteria, or infective thrombi.

  e., acute. Of large arteries. Rare.

  e., chronic. Degeneration of arterial coats in the aged. SYN: *atheroma.*

  e. deformans. Thickening of intima or replacement with atheromatous or calcareous deposits.

  e. obliterans. Chronic progressive thickening of intima leading to stenosis or obstruction of lumen.

endeictic (en-dī'tĭk). Symptomatic.

endem'ic. Peculiar to a certain people, race, or community.

  e. neuritis. A form of polyneuritis. SYN: *beriberi.*

ende"moepidem'ic. Endemic, but becoming epidemic periodically.

endermat'ic, enderm'ic. Administering medicine through the skin.

endermo'sis. 1. Administration of medicines through the skin. 2. Herpetic affection of any mucous membrane.

en'deron. The true skin with nonepithelial portion of the mucous membrane.

endoaneurysmorrhaphy (en"do-an-ū-ris-mor'af-ĭ). Opening an aneurysmal sac and suturing its orifice.

endoangiitis (en"do-an-jĭ-i'tis). Inflammation of the coat of blood vessels. SYN: *endoarteritis, endophlebitis.*

en'doantitox'in. An antitoxin within a cell.

en'doappendici'tis. Inflammation of mucosa of the vermiform appendix.

endoarteritis (ĕn"dō-är-tĕr-ĭ'tis). Inflamed condition of innermost lining of an artery. SYN: *endarteritis.**

en'doausculta'tion. Auscultation by esophageal tube passed into the stomach.

endoblast (en'do-blast). 1. The nucleus cell. 2. Inner layer of the blastoderm. SYN: *endoderm, hypoblast.*

endobronchi'tis. Inflammation of bronchial mucosa.

endocar'diac, endocar'dial. Within or arising from the heart.

endocarditis (en-do-kar-di'tis). Inflammation of the lining membrane of the heart or *endocardium.*

  e., chronic. SEE: *ulcerative endocarditis.*

  e., exudative. Begins as an acute affection. Rheumatism chief cause. SYM: Auscultation may give only indication—a prolongation of heart sound. PROG: Guarded. TREATMENT: Absolute rest.

  e., malignant. Usually secondary to suppurative inflammation elsewhere. SEE: *ulcerative endocarditis.*

  e., ulcerative. A rapidly destructive form, characterized by necrosis or ulceration of the valves and the deposition of colonies of micrococci.

  e., vegetative. Fibrinous clots on ulcerated valvular surfaces. SEE: *exudative endocarditis.*

endocar'dium. Lining (serous) membrane of inner surface and cavities of the heart.

endocervical (en-do-ser'vĭ-kal). Pert. to the endocervix.

endocervicitis (en-dō-ser-vĭ-si'tis). Inflammation of mucous lining of the cervix uteri.

endocervix (en-do-ser'viks). The lining of the canal of the cervix uteri.

endochondral (en-do-kon'dral). Within a cartilage.

endochorion (en-do-ko'rĭ-on). The inner chorion; vascular layer of allantois.

endochrome (en'do-krōm). The coloring matter (not green) of a cell's endoplasm.

endocoli'tis. Inflammation of the mucosa of colon. SEE: *colitis.*

endocolpitis (en-do-kol-pi'tis). Inflammation of the vaginal mucosa. SYN: *encolpitis.*

endocom'plement. An intracellular complement or one contained within the erythrocyte.

endocorpus'cular. Within a corpuscle.

endocra'nial. 1. Intracranial or within the cranium. 2. Pert. to the endocranium.

endocrani'tis. Inflammation of endocranium. SYN: *pachymeningitis, external.*

endocra'nium. 1. Cerebral dura. 2. Inner surface of cranium.

endocrinasthenia (en"do-krin-as-the'nĭ-ă). Neurasthenia due to dysfunction of the endocrines.

endocrine (ĕn'dō-krĭn, -krĭn). 1. An internal secretion. 2. Endocrinous.

  e. gland. A ductless gland; one of internal secretion, although some endocrines have both an internal and external secretion.

endoc'rinism. Disease due to malfunction of one or more of the endocrine glands. SYN: *endocrinopathy.*

endocrinodontia (en"do-kri-no-don'shĭ-ă). The relation of internal secretions to development and preservation of teeth.

endocrinology (en-do-krin-ol'o-gĭ). The science of the endocrines, or ductless glands, and their functions.

endocrinopath (en"do-krin'o-path). One affected by a disorder of one or more glands of internal secretion.

endocrinopathic (en"do-krin-o-path'ĭk). Of the nature of endocrinopathy.

endocrinopathy (en"do-krin-op'ă-thĭ). A disease due to disorder of an endocrine gland or glands.

endocrinosis (en"do-krin-o'sis). Condition resulting from dysfunction of an endocrine gland.

endocrinotherapy (en"do-krin-o-ther'ă-pĭ). Treatment with endocrine preparations.

endocrinotropic (en"do-krin-o-trop'ik). Showing an endocrine tendency.

endocrinous (en-dok'rin-us). Pert. to internal secretions or endocrine glands.

endocrit'ic. Referring to internal secretions.   [hydatid cyst.

en'docyst. The innermost layer of any

endocystitis (en-do-sis-ti'tis). Inflammation of membrane of bladder.

endoderm (en'do-derm). Inner layer of cells of an embryo. Syn: *hypoblast*.

endodiascopy (en-do-di-as'kō-pī). X-ray examination of a cavity.

endodontitis (en"do-don-ti'tis). Inflammation of the dental pulp.

en"doenteri'tis. Inflammation of lining membrane of intestines.

endoen'zyme. An enzyme not excreted from the cell.

endogastrectomy (en-do-gas-trek'to-mĭ). Excision of the gastric mucosa.

endogastric (en-do-gas'trik). Pert. to the stomach's interior.

endogastritis (en-do-gas-tri'tis). Inflammation of the lining membrane of the stomach.

endogen'ic. Having origin within the organism. Syn: *endogenous*.

endogenous (en-doj'en-us). 1. Produced within a cell or organism. 2. Concerning spore formation within the bacterial cell. Syn: *endogenic*.

endoglob'ular. Within the blood corpuscles, as malarial germs.

endointoxica'tion. Poisoning due to an endogenous toxin.

endolabyrinthitis (en"do-lab-ĭ-rin-thi'tis). Inflamed condition of the membranous labyrinth.

endolaryn'geal. Within the larynx.

Endolimax na'na (en-do-li'maks). A parasitic ameba found in the intestines.

endolum'bar. In the lumbar portion of the spinal cord.

endolymph (en'do-limf). Pale, limpid fluid within the labyrinth of the ear.

endolymphat'ic. Rel. to the endolymph.

endolysin (en-dol'is-in). Bacterial substance within a leukocyte which destroys bacteria.   [plasm.

endol'ysis. Disintegration of cell cyto-

endomastoiditis (en"do-mas-toy-di'tis). Inflammation of mucosa lining the mastoid cavity and cells.

endometrectomy (en"do-me-trek'to-mĭ). Excision of uterine mucosa. See: *curettage*.

endometrial (en-do-me'trĭ-al). Pert. to the lining mucosa of the uterus.

    e. cyst. An ovarian cyst or tumor that bleeds, which may develop dense and extensive adhesions.

endometrioma (en-do-me-trĭ-o'mă). A tumor containing shreds of ectopic endometrium; found most frequently in the ovary, *cul-de-sac*, rectovaginal septum, and the peritoneal surface of the post. portion of the uterus.

endometriosis (en-do-me-trĭ-o'sis). Ectopic endometrium located in various sites throughout the pelvis or in the abdominal wall.

endometritis (en-do-me-tri'tis). Inflammation of the inner mucous lining of the endometrium, *q.v.*

    e., cervical. Inflammation of the inner portion of the cervix uteri.

    e., fungous. Endometrial enlargement with bleeding and granulations.

    e., septic. Form caused by septic poisoning.

    e., simple. Catarrhal inflammatory condition of the endometrium.

endometrium (en-do-me'trĭ-um). The mucous membrane lining the inner surface of the uterus.

endom'etry. Measurement of the interior of a cavity or organ.

endomix'is. Mixture of the cell nuclear and cytoplasmic substance.

endomyocarditis (en"do-mĭ-o-kar-di'tis). Inflammation of the endocardium and myocardium.

endomysium (en-do-mis'ĭ-um). Connective tissue binding muscle fibers together.

endoneuri'tis. Inflammation of the endoneurium.*

endoneurium (en-do-nu'rĭ-um). The connective tissue support surrounding nerves and capillaries in a nerve funiculus. See: *nerve*.

endoparasite (en-do-par'as-īt). Any parasite living within its host.

endopathy (en-dop'ath-ĭ). Any endogenous disease.

endopelvic (en-do-pel'vic). Within the pelvis.

    e. fasciae. The downward continuation of the parietal peritoneum of the abdomen to form the pelvic fasciae which have a very important part in the support of the pelvic viscera.

endopericarditis (en"do-per'ĭ-kar-di'tis). Endocarditis complicated by pericarditis.

endoperimyocarditis (en"do-per-ĭ-mī"o-kar-di'tis). Inflammation of the pericardium, myocardium, and endocardium.

endoperitonitis (en"do-per-ĭ-to-ni'tis). Superficial inflammation of the peritoneum.

endophlebitis (en"do-fle-bi'tis). Inflammation of inner coat of a vein.

    e. obliterans. Endophlebitis causing obliteration of a vein.

    e. portalis. Inflammation of the portal vein.

en'doplasm. The center of the cell protoplasm.

endoplast (en'do-plast). A cellular nucleus.

end organ. Peripheral apparatus related to a nerve, with sensory (receptor), and motor (effector) functions.

endorrhachis (en-do-rā'kis). Membrane lining the spinal canal and dura mater.

endorrhinitis (en-do-ri-ni'tis). Inflammation of the mucous membranes of the nose. Syn: *coryza*.

endosalpingitis (en"do-sal-pin-ji'tis). Inflammation of lining of fallopian tubes.

endoscope (en'do-skōp). Metal, rubber, or glass tube for examining cavities through natural openings.

endoscopy (en-dos'ko-pī). Inspection of cavities by use of the endoscope.

endosep'sis. Septicemia having its origin within the body.

endoskel'eton. Internal bony framework of the body. See: *exoskeleton*.

endosmometer (en-dos-mom'et-er). Device for estimating inward passage of liquid through a septum.

endosmose, endosmosis (en'dŏs-mōs", -mō'-sis). Osmosis in which flow of water is from the outside liquid to the solution within a membranous cell.

en'dospore. BIOL: Thick-walled spore within the bacterium.

endosteitis (en"dos-te-i'tis). Inflammation of the endosteum or of medullary cavity of a bone.

endosteo'ma. A tumor in the medullary cavity of a bone.

endos'teum. Membrane lining bone in the medullary cavity.

endostitis (en"dos-tī'tis). Inflammation of the medullary cavity of a bone.

endostoma (en-dos-to'mă). Osseous tumor within a bone.

endostosis (en-dos-to'sis). The development of an endostoma.

endothelial (en-do-the'lĭ-al). Pert. to or consisting of endothelium.

endotheliocyte (en"do-the'lĭ-ō-sīt). Large, phagocytic, wandering cell found in circulating blood and in tissue.

endotheliocytosis (en"do-the'lĭ-o-si-to'sis). Abnormal increase in endothelial cells.

en"dothe"lioino'ma. Tumorous growths arising from endothelium containing fibrous substance.

endotheliolysin (en"do-the-lĭ-ol'is-in). An antibody found in snake venom which dissolves endothelial cells.

endotheliolytic (en"do-the-lĭ-o-lit'ĭk). Capable of destroying endothelial tissue.

endothelioma (en"do-the-lĭ-o'mă). Malignant growth of lining cells of the blood vessels.

endotheliomyoma (en"do-the"lĭ-o-mi-o'ma). Muscular tumor with elements of endothelium.

endotheliomyxoma (en"do-the"lĭ-o-miks-o'mă). Myxoma with element from endothelium.

endotheliotoxin (en"do-the-lĭ-o-toks'in). A specific toxin which acts on endothelial capillary cells, causing hemorrhages.

endothe'lium. The flat cell layer, lining serous cavities, lymphatics, and blood vessels. SEE: mesothelium.

end'otherm knife. A knife devised for using the high frequency current.

endother'mal. 1. Pert. to production of heat within an organism. 2. Pert. to absorption of heat during formation of chemical compounds. SYN: endothermic.

endother'mic. 1. Storing up potential energy or heat. 2. Absorbing heat. 3. Accompanied by heat absorption.

endothermy (en'do-ther"mĭ). A term used as a synonym for surgical diathermy.

en'dothrix. The parasite causing tinea tonsurans.

endothyreopexy (en-do-thi're-o-peks"ĭ). Displacing the thyroid gland and fixing it to the side of the neck.

endothyroidopexy (en"do-thi"royd-o-peks'ĭ). Operative displacement of the thyroid gland and fixing it to the side of the neck. SYN: endothyreopexy.

endotoscope (end-o'to-skōp). An ear speculum. SYN: otoscope.

en"dotoxico'sis. Poisoning due to an endotoxin.

en'dotoxin. Bacterial toxin confined within the body of a bacterium, freed only when the bacterium is broken down. SEE: cytotoxin, erythrotoxin, exotoxin, leukotoxin, neurotoxin.

endotracheitis (en-do-tra-ke-i'tis). Inflammation of the tracheal mucosa.

endotrachelitis (en"do-tra-kel-i'tis). Inflammation of the endocervical tissues. SYN: endocervicitis.

en"dovasculi'tis. Inflammation of the endangium or inner coat of a blood vessel. SYN: endangeitis.

endove'nous. Within a vein. SYN: intravenous.

end plate. The terminal mass of a nerve fiber ending on a muscle cell.

end product. The final waste or excretory product of digestion that passes from the system.

endyma (en'dĭm-ă). Membranous lining of cerebral ventricles. SYN: ependyma.

en'ema (pl. enemas or enema'ta). Injection of water, either plain or containing various drugs, etc., into the rectum and colon to empty the lower intestine, or to introduce food or medicine for therapeutic purposes.

  e., analeptic. One with ½ teaspoonful of salt to a pint of tepid water; a "thirst" enema.

  e., anthelmintic. One given to expel worms. [rhea.

  e., antidiarrheic. One given for diar-

  e., antiseptic. One for the destruction of microörganisms.

  e., antispasmodic. One to counteract spasms.

  e., astringent. One given to contract intestinal tissue and to provoke subsequent evacuation of worms.

  e., blind. The insertion of a rubber tube to cause expulsion of gas or flatus. SEE: carminative enema.

  e., carminative. One given to relieve distention caused by flatus and to stimulate peristalsis.

  e., cleansing. One to empty the lower intestine or the colon.

  e., demulcent. SEE: emollient enema.

  e., Dobell's. One for nutritive purposes.

  e., egg and ether. Used as a last resort in the relief of distention.

  e., emollient. One given to soften and protect tissues by making a coating over membranes, allaying local pain and irritation, and to act as a vehicle for the rectal administration of drugs.

  e., evacuating. SEE: cleansing enema.

  e., Ewald's. A nutritive enema containing red wine, 20% grape sugar solution with wheat flour boiled in it, mixed with eggs.

  e., flatus. One to relieve gas pressure.

  e., lubricating. Administered after an operation for hemorrhoids, and in order to soften the feces and lubricate the passage or anal canal to the external orifice or anus.

e., m. and m. Eight ounces of milk, and 8 ounces of molasses. The mixture may also be in proportions of 6 to 6.

•e., Mayo. Granulated sugar, 2 ounces, 1 ounce of sodium bicarbonate, and 8 ounces of water.

e., medicinal. An enema to which some drug or medication has been added on order of attending physician.

e., Noble's. One dram of turpentine mixed well with glycerine, 2 ounces; mix 3 ounces of magnesium sulfate with 4 ounces of water, and pour the 2 mixtures together.

e., nutrient or nutritive. One to give sustenance to a patient unable to be fed otherwise.

e., olive oil. Mix 4 ounces of olive oil with 1 dram of turpentine, beating the mixture well so as to break the oil globules. This will cause sufficient peristalsis to move the bowels.

e., one-two-three. Magnesium sulfate, 1 ounce; glycerine, 2 ounces, and hot water, 3 ounces (115° F.).

e., pancreatic. One containing pancreatin.

e., physiological salt solution. One teaspoonful of salt to a pint of water is a normal salt solution.

e., purgative. This produces action when other enemas fail; it should be a *high enema.*

e., quantity of. For retention, 3-8 ounces. Cleansing: For a child: ½-1½ pints; infants: ½-2 ounces; adults: 2-4 pints.

e., retention. This is one to retain. It may be used to provide nourishment, to medicate a diseased mucous membrane, or for absorption purposes, or for general, local, or systemic action.

e., Rosenheim's. A nutrient one, containing cod-liver oil, sugar, and peptone in a 3% soda solution.

e., saline. One with solution of magnesium sulfate in warm water.

e., sedative. Retention enema given for its soothing action and to allay irritability.

e., shock. One to ward off shock.

e., simple mixed. A soapsuds enema to which is added 1 dram of salt and ½ ounce of molasses.

e., soapsuds. The soapsuds are either ready prepared, or may be made by placing soap particles in a shaker and agitating the water until the right consituency is obtained. The foam is not removed.

e., s. s. & p. A mixture of 1 dram of peppermint added to a soapsuds solution. The peppermint may be added to a plain water solution, 1 dram to 16 ounces; a good enema to relieve flatulence.

e., s. s. & t. A mixture of thick liquid soap; green soap is best. Add ¼ ounce or 1 dram of turpentine and beat the 2 ingredients thoroughly together. The emulsion of this mixture is stirred into 1 quart of water at 115° F.

e., stimulating. This may be grouped with the medicated and the retention enemas.

e., temperature of. Carminative, stimulating, and for inflammation, 115° F. For hemorrhage, 120° F. For others, 105° F.

e., thirst. Analeptic enema, *q.v.*

e., yeast. One quart of warm water and ½ cake of yeast, thoroughly mixed and given very warm.

enepidermic (en-ep-ĭ-der′mĭk). Pert. to drugs applied without friction. SEE: *inunction.*

energometer (en-er-gom′e-ter). An instrument for measuring blood pressure.

en′ergy. The capacity of a system for doing work or its equivalent in the strict physical sense.

e. changes. These may be physical or chemical, or both.

e., conservation of. The theory that no energy in the universe can be lost, but that it may be transformed into other forms.

e., latent. That which exists but which is not being used.

e., potential. SEE: *latent energy.*

e., radiant. That form of energy which is transmitted through space without the support of a sensible medium.

e., static. SEE: *latent energy.*

enerva′tion. Weakness; failure of nerve energy.

En′gelmann's disc. Thin disc or light transverse muscular fiber band.

englobe′. To absorb within a spherical body, as the ingestion of bacteria by the phagocytes.

Engman's disease. Pustular eruption resembling eczema, which often occurs simultaneously with a pyogenic process. SYN: *dermatitis infectiosa eczematoides.*

engorged (en-gorjd′). Distended, as with blood.

engorge′ment. Vascular congestion; distention.

engram (en′gram). 1. Suppositious traces on protoplasm made by irritants or stimuli which, when repeated, form a habit after the stimulus ceases; the mnemic hypothesis. 2. The result of a psychic experience supposed to have established a pattern in memory. SEE: *ekphorize, mnemic theory.*

engraphia (en-gra′fĭ-ă). The process of making engrams, *q.v.*

enhem′atospore. A spore of the malarial parasite. SYN: *enhemospore, merozoite.*

enhemospore (en-hem′o-spŏr). A spore of the malarial parasite. SYN: *enhematospore, merozoite.*

enkatarrhaphy (en-kat-ar′af-ĭ). Artificial implantation of a structure where it does not normally occur.

enomania (e″no-ma′nĭ-ă). Craving for alcohol; delirium tremens.

enophthalmus (en-of-thal′mus). Recession of eyeball into orbit.

enosto′sis. An osseous tumor within the cavity of a bone. [ture.

ensiform (en′sĭ-form). Swordlike struc-

e. cartilage. Lower part of sternum, below the gladiolus. SYN: *xiphoid cartilage or process.* SEE: *chondroxiphoid, xiphodynia.*

ensisternum (en-sĭ-ster'num). The tip of the sternum; ensiform or xiphoid appendix. SYN: *metasternum.*

enstrophe (en'stro-fe). Inversion; a turning inward, esp. of eyelids.

en'tad. Toward the inside; inwardly.

en'tal. Pert. to the interior; inside, central.

entamebiasis (ent-am-e-bi'as-is). Infestation with Entameba.

Entameba (ent-am-e'ba). Unicellular animal parasite, several distinct species of which are found in man.

    E. bucca'lis. Found in buccal secretions in case of dental caries.

    E. coli. Found normally in the upper intestinal tract.

    E. hystolit'ica. A parasitic form of ameba, the cause of amebic dysentery and tropical abscess.

    E. kartul'isi. Found in the pus of necrotic bone abscesses.

    E. tetrage'na. A species found in the stool of tropical dysentery in Africa and Asia.

    E. un'dulans. A species found in the intestine.

entasia (en-ta'sĭ-ă). Spasmodic muscular contraction.

entelechy (en-tel'e-kĭ). 1. Complete development. 2. The activating cause of everything.

enteradeni'tis. Inflammation of intestinal glands.

en'teral. Within the intestine as distinguished from *parenteral.*

enteralgia (en-ter-al'jĭ-ă). Neuralgia or pain in the intestines.

enterectasia (en-ter-ĕk-tā'sĭ-ă). Dilatation of the small intestines.

enterectomy (en-ter-ek'to-mĭ). Excision of a portion of the intestines.

enterelcosis (en-ter-el-ko'sis). Intestinal ulceration.

enterepiplocele (en-ter-ep-ip'lo-sēl). Hernia involving the bowel and omentum.

enteric (en-ter'ik). Pert. to the intestinal tract.

    e. fever. Typhoid fever.

    e. pills. Those which will not dissolve until they reach the intestines.

enter'icoid. Resembling typhoid fever.

enteritis (en-ter-i'tis). Inflammation of the intestines, more particularly of the mucous and submucous tissues, usually of the small intestines.

    e., acute catarrhal. Acute inflammation of ileum and colon with diarrhea and intestinal catarrh.

    e., chronic catarrhal. Chronic inflammation of intestines and colon with chronic diarrhea.

    e., croupous. Diphtheritic. A sequel of typhoid fever and other diseases. Often characterized by formation of false membrane.

entero-. Prefix: Noting some relation to the intestines.

enteroanastomosis (en″ter-o-an-as″to-mo'sĭs). Intestinal anastomosis.

enteroan'tigen. An antigen derived from the feces.

enteroapokleisis (en″ter-o-ap-o-kli'sis). Operation for exclusion of a part of the intestine.

enterobacteriotherapy (ĕn″tĕr-ō-băk-tē″-rĭ-o-ther'ă-pĭ). Use of vaccines containing intestinal bacteria.

enterobi'asis. Infection with pin worms (*Enterobius vermicularis*).

enterobil'iary. Pert. to the intestines and the bile passages. [tine.

enterobro'sia. Perforation of the intestine.

enterocele (en'ter-o-sēl). 1. A hernia of the intestine. 2. Post. vaginal hernia.

enterocentesis (en″ter-o-sen-te'sis). Puncture of intestine to withdraw gas or fluids.

enterochirurgia (en″ter-o-ki-rur'jĭ-ă). Intestinal surgery.

enterocholecystostomy (en″ter-o-ko″le-sistos'to-mĭ). Making an opening bet. the gallbladder and small intestine. SYN: *cholecystenterostomy.*

enterocholecystotomy (en″ter-o-ko″le-sistot'o-mĭ). Incision of both gallbladder and intestine.

enterocinesia (en″ter-o-sin-e'sĭ-ă). Intestinal movement. SYN: *peristalsis.*

enterocinetic (en″ter-o-sin-et'ik). Pert. to or promoting peristalsis.

enteroclysis (en-ter-ok'li-sis). 1. Injection of a nutrient or medicinal liquid into bowel. 2. Irrigation of colon with large amt. of fluid intended to fill the colon completely and flush it. SEE: *proctoclysis.*

en'teroclysm. A high enema. SYN: *enteroclysis.*

enterocoele (en″ter-o-se'le). The abdominal cavity.

enterocolitis (en″ter-o-ko-li'tis). Inflammation of intestines and colon, a disease of teething, principally during summer, bet. 6 and 18 months and often later.

enterocrinin (ĕn-tĕr-ok'rĭn-ĭn). Hormone in large intestine which aids digestion by stimulating gastric juice.

enterocyst (en'ter-o-sist). A cyst of the intestinal wall.

enterocystocele (en″ter-o-sis'to-sēl). Hernia of the bladder wall and intestine.

enterocysto'ma. Cystic tumor of the intestinal wall. SYN: *enterocyst.*

enterodyn'ia. Pain in the intestine. SYN: *enteralgia.*

en″teroenteros'tomy. Formation of a communication bet. 2 segments (not continuous) of the intestine.

enteroepiplocele (en″ter-o-e-pip'lo-sēl). Hernia of small intestine and omentum.

en″terogastri'tis. Inflammation of stomach (gastritis) and of the intestines (enteritis).

enterogastrone (en″tĕr-ō-gas'trōn). Hormone depressing gastric motility and secretion.

enterogenous (en-ter-oj'en-us). Originating in the intestines.

en'terogram. Tracing or graph of intestinal movements.

enterog'raphy. 1. A description of the intestines. 2. Making of an enterogram.

en"terohepat'ic. Pert. to intestines and the liver.

en"terohepati'tis. Inflamed condition of both intestine and liver.

enterohydrocele (en"ter-o-hi'dro-sēl). Hydrocele with loop of intestine in the sac.

enteroidea (en-ter-oyd'e-a). The intestinal fevers; those caused by intestinal bacilli including *enteric* and *parenteric* fevers.

enterokinase (en-ter-o-kin'āz). A substance or hormone occurring in the mucosa of the duodenum, necessary for the activation of the trypsinogen of the pancreatic juice which is converted into trypsin.
RS: *enzyme, prosecretin, trypsin, trypsinogen.*

en'terolite. Intestinal calculus.

enterolith (en'ter-o-lith). An intestinal concretion.

enterolithiasis (en"ter-o-lǐ-thi'ǎ-sis). The formation of existence of enterolites.

enterol'ogy. The study of the intestinal tract.

en"teromega'lia, en"teromeg'aly. Abnormal enlargement of the intestines. SYN: *megacolon, megaloenteron.*

enteromyco'sis. Disease of intestine due to bacteria.

enteron (en'ter-on). The intestine.

enteroneuri'tis. Neuritis of the intestine.

enteronitis (en-ter-on-i'tis). Inflammation of the small intestine. SYN: *enteritis.*

enteroparesis (en-ter-o-par'e-sis). Flaccidity of the intestinal walls with diminished peristalsis.

enteropathy (en-ter-op'ǎ-thǐ). Any intestinal disease.

enteropexy (en'ter-o-peks-ǐ). Fixation of the intestine to the abdominal wall.

enteroplasty (en'ter-o-plas-tǐ). Plastic operation on intestines.

enterople'gia. Paralysis of the bowels.

enteroplex (en'ter-o-pleks). Instrument for joining cut edges of intestines.

en'teroplexy. Union of divided parts of the intestine.

enteroptosis (en-ter-op-to'sis). Prolapse of the intestine or abdominal organs.

enterorrhagia (en"ter-or-ra'jǐ-ǎ). Hemorrhage from the intestines.

enterorrhaphy (en-ter-or'rǎ-fǐ). The stitching of the lips of an intestinal wound, or of the intestines to some other structure.

enterorrhexis (en-ter-or-reks'is). Rupture of the intestine.

enteroscope (en'ter-o-skōp). Device for examination of intestines.

enterosep'sis. Intestinal toxemia; sepsis developed from the intestinal contents.

enterospasm (en'ter-o-spazm). Painful peristalsis.

enterosta'sis. Intestinal stasis.

enterosteno'sis. Narrowing or stricture of the intestine.

enterostomy (en-ter-os'to-mǐ). Surgical formation of a permanent opening into the intestine through the abdominal wall.

enterotome (en'ter-o-tōm). Instrument for incision of intestines.

enterotomy (en-ter-ot'o-mǐ). Incision or dissection of the intestines.

enterotox'ism. Absorption of intestinal toxins. SYN: *enterosepsis.*

enterotrop'ic. Affecting or attracted by the intestines.

enterovac'cine. A vaccine composed of fecal bacteria.

enterozo'ic. Pert. to parasites inhabiting the intestines.

enterozo'on. Any intestinal animal parasite.

entheomania (en-the-o-ma'nǐ-ǎ). Religious insanity.

enther'mic. Promoting or pert. to warmth.

enthetic (en-thet'ik). Introduced from outside. SYN: *exogenous.*

ento-. Prefix, *entos,* within, inside.

en'toblast. The germinal spot. SYN: *entoderm, hypoblast.*

entocele (en'to-sēl). 1. Internal hernia. 2. Displacement of a part, inward.

entochondrostosis (en"to-kon-dro-sto'sis). The development of bone within cartilage.

entochoroidea (en"to-ko-roy'de-ǎ). The inner layer of the choroid; coat of the eye.

entocineria (en-to-sin-e'rǐ-ǎ). The internal gray matter of nerve centers, esp. of the brain.

entocone (en'to-kōn). The inner post. cusp of an upper molar tooth.

entocor'nea. Post. or inner lining membrane of cornea. SYN: *Descemet's membrane.*

entocyte (en'to-sīt). Int. part of a cell within the ectoplasm. SYN: *endoplasm.*

entoderm (en'to-derm). The inner layer of cells in the blastoderm.* SYN: *hypoblast.* SEE: *ectoderm.*

entoectad (en-to-ek'tad). From within outward.

entome (en'tōm). Knife for division of urethral stricture.

entomion (en-to'mǐ-on). The tip of mastoid angle of the parietal bone.

entomol'ogy. The study of insects.

entophyte (en'to-fīt). Any vegetable parasite within the body.

entophyton (en-tof'it-on). Vegetable parasite in the body. SYN: *entophyte.*

entopic (en-top'ik). Normally situated; in a normal place.

entoptic (en-top'tik). Situated in the eyeball.

entoptoscopy (en"top-tos'ko-pǐ). Inspection of intraocular shadows.

entoral (en-to'rǎl). An oral respiratory vaccine.
USES: For immunization against colds.

entoret'ina. Internal layer of the retina.

entorrhagia (en-tor-a'jǐ-ǎ). Internal hemorrhage. SEE: *enterorrhagia.*

entos'thoblast. Hypothetical nucleus of the nucleolus. SYN: *entoblast.*

entotic (en-to'tǐk). Pert. to int. of ear

or to perception of sound due to condition of the auditory apparatus.

entozoon (en-to-zo'on). Any animal parasite in any internal organ.

en'trails. The intestines.

entrophia (en-tro'fĭ-ă). Normal growth and nourishment.

entro'pion. Inward curling of eyelid, esp. lower lid, with lashes.

entro'pionize. To invert or correct by turning in.

entro'pium. Inward curling of eyelids. SYN: *entropion.*

enucleate (e-nu'kle-āt). To remove a tumor or an entire body without rupturing.

enucleation (e-nu-kle-a'shun). 1. Removal of a tumor from its capsule. 2. Act of unfolding.

enu'cleator. Instrument for separating a tumor mass, as a myoma.

enuresis (en-u-re'sis). Incontinence. Involuntary discharge of urine, complete or partial, diurnal or nocturnal, dependent upon pathologic or functional causes, although it may be voluntary as representative of a behavior pattern.

  e., diurnal. Urinary incontinence during the day and its etiology is of a pathological nature.

  e., nocturnal. Urinary incontinence during the night.

envi'ronment. External surroundings, circumstances, or influences.

enzygotic (en-zi-got'ĭk). Developed from the same ovum.

  e. twins. Identical twins; those developed from one ovum. SEE: *dizygotic.*

enzyme (en'zim). Complex chemical substance produced by animals and plants, found particularly in the digestive juices, acting upon other substances and causing them to split up into simpler substances, and capable of accelerating greatly the course of specific chemical reactions.

  e., amylolytic. Enzyme changing starch to sugar.

  e., autolytic. Enzyme producing autolysis, or cell digestion.

  e., bacterial. Enzyme developed by bacteria.

  e., coagulating. Enzyme converting insoluble proteins into soluble proteins.

  e., deamidizing. Enzyme dividing amino acids into ammonia compounds.

  e., extracellular. Enzyme beyond the confines of the cell secreting it.

  e., fermentation. SEE: *coagulating enzyme.*

  e., glycolytic. Enzyme oxidizing sugar.

  e., hydrolytic. A decomposing enzyme with the addition of elements of water.

  e., inorganic. A metallic colloidal solution, acting somewhat like an enzyme.

  e., intracellular. Enzyme within the cell protoplasm.

  e., inverting. Enzyme dividing sugar.

  e., lipolytic. Enzyme dividing fat.

  e., oxidation. SEE: *deamidizing enzyme.*

  e., polypeptolytic. Enzyme having a

hydrolytic action on the polypeptids.

  e., proteolytic. Enzyme changing proteins into peptones.

  e., reducing. Reductase. One that withdraws oxygen.

  e., steatolytic. SEE: *lipolytic enzyme.*

  e., sucrolastic. Enzyme dividing or decomposing sugar.

  e., uricolytic. Enzyme converting uric acid into urea.

enzymolysis (en-zim-ol'ĭ-sis). Chemical change caused by an enzyme. SYN: *enzymosis.*

enzymo'sis. Fermentation due to an enzyme. SYN: *enzymolysis.*

enzymu'ria. Enzymes in the urine.

eonism (e'on-izm). Desire to dress in the clothing of the opposite sex; a sexual perversion. SYN: *transvestitism.*

eosin(e (ē'ō-sĭn, -sēn). ($C_{20}H_5Br_4O_5$.) 1. A dye derived from action of bromine on fluorescein.

  2. Any of several similar dyes.

  3. Rosy-red; dawn colored.

eosin'oblast. A bone marrow cell which develops into a myelocyte. SYN: *myeloblast.*

eosinopenia (e''o-sin-o-pe'nĭ-ă). Abnormally small number of eosinophil cells in the peripheral blood.

eosinophil(e (e-o-sin-o-fĭl, or -fĭl). An element or cell, such as a leukocyte, that stains easily with the coal tar product *eosin;* acidophile.

eosinophilia (e''o-sin-o-fil'ĭ-ă). 1. Accumulation of unusual number of eosinophil cells in the blood. 2. Condition of being eosinophilic.

eosinophilic (e''o-sin-o-fĭl'ik). Readily stainable with eosin.

eosinoph'ilous. 1. Easily stainable with eosin. 2. Having eosinophilia.

eosinotactic (e-o-sin-o-tak'tĭk). Attraction or repulsion of eosinophil cells.

epacmastic (ep-ak-mas'tĭk). Denoting increase of symptoms.

epac'tal. Supernumerary.

  e. bone. Wormian bone.

eparsalgia (ep-ar-sal'jĭ-ă). Any disorder due to overstrain of a part. SYN: *epersalgia.*

epaxial (ep-ak'sĭ-al). Situated above or behind any axis.

epencephalon (ep-en-sef'al-on). Embryonic structure from which develop the pons and cerebellum.

ependyma (ep-en'dim-ă). Membrane lining the cerebral ventricles and central canal of spinal cord.

  e. medullae spinalis. The spinal portion of the ependyma.

  e. ventriculorum cerebri. The ventricular portion of the ependyma.

ependymitis (ep''en-dim-i'tis). Inflammation of the ependyma.

ependymoblast (ep-en'dĭ-mo-blast). An embryonic ependymal cell or ependymocyte.

ependymocyte (ep-en'dĭ-mo-sīt). A cell of the ependymal region.

ependymo'ma. A tumor arising from fetal inclusion of ependymal elements.

epersal'gia. Pain and soreness due to overuse or unaccustomed use of a part.

ephebic (ef-e'bik). Pert. to adolescence.

ephebology (e-fe-bol'o-jĭ). The study of puberty and its changes.

ephedrine (ef'ed-rin). An alkaloid obtained from *Ma huang*, a species of *Ephedra;* first isolated by Nagai in 1887.
  DOSAGE: From 1/4-5/6 gr. (0.015-0.05 Gm.). Some patients need carefully regulated doses. The least dose which will give the specific desired effect is desirable.
  e. hydrochloride. USP. A more soluble salt of the alkaloid, containing about 80% ephedrine.
  DOSAGE: From 1/4-1 gr. (0.015-0.06 Gm.); locally, in from 1/2 to 3%.
  e. sulfate. This contains about 75% ephedrine; dosage and uses same as *ephedrine hydrochloride*, but believed by some to be more irritant.

ephelis (ef-e'lis). Freckle, lentigo.*

ephemeral (e-fem'er-al). Of brief duration.

ephidrosis (ef-i-dro'sis). Abnormal amt. of sweating.
  e. cruenta. Sweat containing blood.
  e. saccharata. Diabetic condition in which sugar is present in sweat.
  e. tincta. Colored sweat. SYN: *chromidrosis.*

epi-, ep-. Prefix meaning upon, at, in addition to.

epiallopregnanolone (ĕp''ĭ-al''o-prĕg-nan'ō-lōn). Male sex hormone in urine of pregnant women, which helps to form male sex characteristics.

epiblast. Outer layer of cells of the blastoderm. SEE: *hypoblast.*

epiblastic (ep-ĭ-blas'tik). Pert. to the epiblast.

epibole, epiboly (ĕ-pib'o-lĭ). Inclusion of the hypoblast within the epiblast, due to swifter growth of the latter. SEE: *emboly.*

epican'thus. Fold of skin which sometimes covers the inner canthus; a congenital defect.

epicar'dia. That portion of the esophagus which passes through the diaphragm into the stomach.

epicar'dium. The inner or visceral layer of the pericardium.*

epicele, epicoelia (ep'is-ēl, -i-coy'lĭ-a). The fourth ventricle of the brain.

epicondylalgia (ep''ĭ-kon-dil-al'jĭ-ă). Pain in the region of the epicondyle attributed to tenositis.

epicon'dyle. The eminence at the articular end of a bone above a condyle.

epicra'nium. Soft parts covering the cranium. [tal muscle.

epicranius (ep-i-kra'nĭ-us). Occipitofron-

epicri'sis. A supplementary or secondary crisis following a return of morbid symptoms.

epicritic (ep-ĭ-krit'ik). Pert. to extreme sensibility, such as that of the skin when it discriminates between degrees of sensation caused by touch or temperature.

epicysti'tis. Inflammation of cellular tissue above the bladder.

epicystot'omy. Opening above the symphysis pubis into the bladder.

epicyte (ep'i-sīt). 1. An epithelial cell. 2. A cell membrane.

epidem'ic. Appearance of an infectious disease not of local origin which attacks many people at the same time in the same area. SEE: *Winckel's disease.*
  e. jaundice. Weil's disease.

epidemiog'raphy. Study of epidemic diseases.

epidemiologic (ep''ĭ-dem'ĭ-o-loj'ik). Pert. to the study of epidemics.

epidemiologist (ep''ĭ-dem-ĭ-ol'o-jist). One who specializes in epidemic diseases.

epidemiology (ep-i-dem-ĭ-ol'o-jĭ). The science of epidemic diseases.

epider'mal, epider'mic. Pert. to the epidermis.

epidermatoplasty (ep-ĭ-der-mat'o-plas-tĭ). Grafting with pieces of epidermis with the underlying layer of the corium.

epidermic (ep-ĭ-der'mĭk). Pert. to the external layer of the skin or epidermis.

epidermidaliza'tion. 1. Skin grafting. 2. Conversion of mucous or germinative cells into outer, horny layer of the epidermis. SYN: *epidermization.*

epidermidol'ysis. Loosening of the epidermis. SYN: *epidermolysis.*

epidermido'sis. Any disease of the skin. SYN: *epidermosis.*

epider'mis. Cuticle, or outer layer of skin; scarf-skin.

epidermi'tis. Inflammation of the superficial layers of the skin.

epidermization (ep-e-der-mĭ-za'shun). Skin grafting. Conversion of deeper germinative layer of cells into outer and horny layer of epidermis.

epidermoid (ep-ĭ-der'moyd). 1. Resembling or pert. to the epidermis. 2. A tumor arising from aberrant epidermal cells. SYN: *cholesteatoma.*

epidermolysis (ep-ĭ-der-mol'ĭs-is). Loosening of the epidermis.
  e. bullosa. A form characterized by formation of deep-seated bullae appearing after irritation or rubbing of a part.

epidermo'ma. An excrescence on the skin.

epidermomycosis (ep-ĭ-der''mo-mĭ-ko'sis). Skin disease caused by a vegetable micro-parasite. SYN: *dermatomycosis.*

Epidermophyton (ep-ĭ-der-mof'ĭ-ton). A genus of fungi causing tinea cruris or Dhobie itch, *q.v.*

epidermophytosis (ep-ĭ-der-mo-fĭ-to'sis). Infection by a species of Epidermophyton. SYN: *Dhobie itch, washerwoman's itch, tinea cruris, tinea inguinalis.*

epidermo'sis. Any disease affecting the skin.

epidi'ascope. Lantern used for projection of images on a screen. SYN: *episcope.*

epididymectomy (ep-i-did-ĭ-mek'to-mĭ). Removal of the epididymus.

epididymis (ep-ĭ-dĭd'ĭ-mis) (pl. *epididymidēs*). A small, oblong body resting upon and beside the post. surface of the testes, consisting of a convoluted tube

18-20 ft. long, enveloped in the tunica vaginalis, ending in the vas deferens.

epididymitis (ep-ĭ-dĭd-im-i′tĭs). Inflammation of the epididymis.

e., gonorrheal. In third to eighth week of gonorrhea, symptoms either acute (swelling increasing rapidly involving testes, scrotum, etc.) or subacute (moderate swelling developing slowly), with pain.

e., nongonorrheal. Resembles gonorrheal but often terminates in gross suppuration.

e., relapsing. Any acute form that becomes chronic.

epididymodeferentectomy (ep-ĭ-dĭd-ĭ-mo-def′er-en-tek′to-mĭ). Excision of epididymis and vas deferens.

epididymodeferen′tial. Concerning both the epididymis and vas deferens.

epididymoörchitis (ep-ĭ-dĭd-im-o-or-ki′tis). Epididymitis with orchitis.*

epididymot′omy. Incision into the epididymis.

epididymovasotomy (ep-ĭ-dĭd″im-o-vas-os′-to-mĭ). Making an anastomosis bet. the epididymis and the vas.

epidu′ral. Located over or upon the dura.

e. space. Space outside of dura mater of brain and spinal cord.

epifolliculitis (ep-i-fol-lik-u-li′tĭs). Inflammation of hair follicles of the scalp.

epigas′ter. Embryonic structure which develops into the large intestine. SYN: *hindgut.*

ep″igastral′gia. Pain in the epigastrium.

epigas′tric. Pert. to the epigastrium. SEE: *precordia.*

e. reflex. Critical reflex of that area.

epigastrium (ep-i-gas′trĭ-um). Region over the pit of the stomach. SEE: *Auenbrugger's sign.*

epigastrocele (ep-ĭ-gas′tro-sēl). Hernia in the epigastrium.

epigastrorrhaphy (ep-i-gas-tror′ă-fĭ). Suture of an abdominal wound in the epigastric area.

epigenesis (ep-ĭ-jen′es-is). Generation by successive changes.

epiglottid′ean. Pert. to the epiglottis.

epiglottidectomy (ep″i-glot-id-ek′to-mĭ). Excision of the epiglottis.

epiglottiditis (ep″ĭ-glot-tid-i′tis). Inflammation of the epiglottis. SYN: *epiglottitis.*

epiglot′tis (pl. *epiglottidēs*). Thin, leaf-shaped mucous membranous laryngeal cartilage at root of the tongue which covers the entrance to the larynx when swallowing. SEE: *aryepiglottic.*

epiglottitis (ep″ĭ-glot-ti′tis). Inflammation of the epiglottis. SYN: *epiglottiditis.*

epihy′al. Pert. to the arch of the hyoid.

e. bone. Ossified stylohyoid ligament.

epilate (ep′ĭ-lāt). To extract the hair by the roots.

ep′ilating. Depilating; extracting a hair.

e. dose. The quantity of roentgen rays of radium necessary to cause temporary loss of hair.

e. forceps. Tweezers for pulling out hairs.

epilation (ep-i-la′shun). Extraction of hair. SYN: *depilation.*

epilatory (e-pil′a-tor-ĭ). Pert. to removal of hairs, or that which removes them. SYN: *depilatory.*

epilemma (ep-ĭ-lem′ă). Neurilemma of small branches of nerve filaments.

ep″ilep′sy. An episodic disturbance of consciousness during which generalized convulsions may occur.

e., alcoholic. Epileptiform attacks take place but without apparent mental deterioration. These attacks clear up with the cessation of indulgence in alcoholic stimulants.

e., cardiac. Epilepsy causing severe interference with heart action.

e., central. Epilepsy caused by spinal cord or brain disease.

e., cortical. Epilepsy with spasm on only 1 side, patient retaining consciousness.

e., hemiplegic. SEE: *cortical epilepsy.*

e., idiopathic. Presence of epilepsy without known cause.

e., Jacksonian. SEE: *cortical epilepsy.*

e., maniacal. Irregular variety without convulsions, but marked by mental disturbance.

e., menstrual. Form in which attacks coincide with menstruation.

e., nocturnal. Occurs only during sleep. Symptoms similar to grand mal. PROG: Favorable.

e., partial. SEE: *cortical epilepsy.*

e., reflex. Epilepsy caused by reflex irritation.

e., sleep. Spasmodic uncontrollable desire to sleep. SYN: *narcolepsy.*

e., spinal. Epilepsy due to lateral sclerosis of the spinal cord. [ilis.

e., syphilitic. Epilepsy present in syph-

e., thalamic. Form with lesion of the thalamus, causing hallucinations.

e., toxemic. Epilepsy caused by toxic action.

e., traumatic. Epilepsy caused by trauma, particularly of the cranial vertex.

epilep′tic. 1. Concerning epilepsy. 2. Individual suffering from epileptic attacks.

epilep′tiform. Having the form of epilepsy.

epileptogen′ic, epileptog′enous. Giving rise to epileptoid convulsions.

e. zone. Certain motor tracts in cerebral cortex, irritation of which gives rise to an epileptic seizure.

epilep′toid. Resembling epilepsy. SYN: *epileptiform.*

epileptol′ogy. Study of epilepsy.

epileptosis (ep-ĭ-lep-to′sis). Any mental disease due to epilepsy.

epiloia (ep-il-oi′ă). A syndrome consisting of mental deficiency, adenoma sebaceum, epileptic fits, hypertrophic sclerosis of the brain, tumors in the kidneys, and nodules on floor of fourth ventricle.

epimandibular (ep″ĭ-man-dib′u-lar). Above or upon the lower jaw.

epimenorrhagia (ep-ĭ-men-o-ra′jĭ-ă). Profuse menstruation.

epimenorrhea (ep-ĭ-men-o-re'ă). Too frequent menstruation.

epimerite (ep-ĭ-mer'ĭt). An organ of certain protozoa by which they attach themselves to epithelial cells.

epimysium (ep-ĭ-mis'ĭ-um). Delicate, elastic, homogeneous sheath enclosing each striated muscular fiber exclusive of those of the heart. SYN: *sarcolemma*.

ep'inasty. More vigorous growth on the upper than on the under surface, leading to a downward curvature of an organ.

epinephrectomy (ep-ĭ-ne-frek'to-mĭ). Excision of the suprarenal gland. SYN: *adrenalectomy*.

epinephrine (adrenalin) (ep-i-nef'rĭn). USP. The active principle of suprarenal gland, occurring as a white or light brown powder, darkening on exposure to the air.
  DOSAGE: (1:1000 solut.): *Subcut.*, $\frac{1}{120}$ gr. (0.0005 Gm.).
  e. hydrochloride solution. USP. A 1:1000 solution of the drug.
  AVERAGE DOSAGE: Hypodermically, 8 ℳ (0.5 cc.).

epinephrinemia (ep″ĭ-nef″rĭ-ne'mĭ-ă). Epinephrine in the blood.

epinephritis (ep″ĭ-nef-ri'tis). Inflammation of a suprarenal capsule.

epinephro'ma. A lipomatoid tumor of the kidney. SYN: *Grawitz's tumor*, *hypernephroma*.

epineural (ep-ĭ-nū'ral). Located upon a neural arch.

epineurium (ep″ĭ-nu'rĭ-um). The general connective tissue sheath of a nerve. SEE: *nerve*.

epionychium (ep″ĭ-o-nik'ĭ-um). Horny condition of fetal epidermis. SYN: *eponychium*.

ep″iot'ic. Located above the ear.
  e. center. Ossification center of temporal bone forming upper and post. part of the auditory capsule.

epipas'tic. Resembling a dusting powder.

epipharynx (ep-i-far'inks). Nasal portion of pharynx. SYN: *rhinopharynx*.

epiphenom'enon. An exceptional and extraneous phenomenon in a disease.

epiphora (e-pif'o-ra). Abnormal overflow of tears down the cheek.

epiphylac'tic. Pert. to epiphylaxis.

epiphylax'is. Increase of defensive powers of the body.

epiphyseal (ep-ĭ-fiz'e-al). Pert. to or of the nature of an epiphysis.

epiphyseolysis (ep″ĭ-fiz-e-ol'is-is). Separation of an epiphysis.

epiphyseopathy (ep″i-fiz-e-op'ă-thĭ). Any disease of an epiphysis or of the pineal gland.

epiphysial (ep-ĭ-fiz'ĭ-al). Of the nature of or concerning an epiphysis.*

epiphysis (ep-if'is-is) (pl. *epiphysēs*). 1. A juvenile piece of bone separated from a parent bone in early life by cartilage, but later becoming a part of the larger (or parent) bone; a center for ossification at each extremity of long bones. SEE: *diaphysis*. 2. The pineal body.

epiphysitis (ep″ĭ-fiz-i'tis). Inflammation of an epiphysis, esp. that at the hip, knee, and shoulder in infants.

epipial (ep-i-pi'al). Situated above or upon the pia mater.

epiplocele (ep-ip'lo-sēl). Hernia containing omentum.

epiploenterocele (e-pip″lo-en'ter-o-sēl). Hernia consisting of omentum and intestine. [tum.

epiploic (ep-ĭ-plo'ĭk). Pert. to the omen-

epiploitis (e-pi-plo-i'tis). Inflammation of the omentum.

epiplomerocele (ep-ip-lo-mer'o-sēl). Femoral hernia containing omentum.

epiplomphalocele (ep-ip-lom'fal-o-sēl). Umbilical hernia with omentum protruding.

epiploon (ep-ip'lo-on). The omentum*; esp. the great omentum.

epiplopexy (ep-ip'lo-peks-ĭ). Suturing of omentum to the ant. abdominal wall.

epiplosarcomphalocele (ep-ip″lo-sar-kom'-fal-o-sēl). An umbilical hernia with protruding omentum. SYN: *epiplomphalocele*.

epiploscheocele (ep-ip-los'ke-o-sēl). Omental hernia into the scrotum.

episclera (ep-ĭ-skle'ră). Loose connective tissue between sclera and conjunctiva.

episcleral (ep-ĭ-skle'răl). Overlying the sclera of the eye.

episcleritis (ep-ĭ-skle-ri'tis). Inflammation of the subconjunctival layers of the sclera.

ep'iscope. Projection lantern for examination of an object on a screen. SYN: *epidiascope*.

episioclisia (ep-iz″ĭ-o-klis'ĭ-ă). Surgical closure of the vulva.

episioelytrorrhaphy (ĕ-pis″ĭ-o-el-ĭ-tror'ră-fĭ). Narrowing of vagina and vulva.

episioperineorrhaphy (e-pis″i-o-per-in-e-or'ă-fĭ). Suturing the vulva and perineum for the support of a prolapse of the uterus.

episioplasty (e-pĭ″si-o-plas'tĭ). Plastic surgery on the vulva.

episiorrhaphy (e-pis″ĭ-or'ră-fĭ). Sewing of a lacerated perineum.

episiostenosis (ĕ-pis″ĭ-o-stĕ-no'sis). Narrowing of the vulvar slit.

episiotomy (e-pis″ĭ-ot'o-mĭ). Incision of perineum at end of second stage of labor to avoid laceration of perineum.

episol (ep'is-ol). A preparation of sodium morrhuate.
  DOSAGE: From $\frac{1}{2}$ to 1 cc. by injection.

epispadias (ep-ĭ-spa'dĭ-as). Congenital opening of urethra on dorsum of penis, and in the female, opening by separation of the labia minora and a fissure of the clitoris.

epispas'tic. An agent that, applied locally, will produce a serous or puriform discharge by exciting inflammation.

episplenitis (ep″ĭ-sple-ni'tis). Inflammation of the splenic capsule.

epistasis (e-pis'ta-sis). 1. A substance rising to the surface instead of sinking; scum, as on the urine. 2. The checking of any discharge. SEE: *hypostasis*.

epistax'is. Hemorrhage from nose.

episternal (ep-ĭ-ster'nal). Situated above the sternum.

epister'num. Upper portion of the sternum. SYN: *manubrium*.

epistropheus (ep-ĭ-stro'fe-us) (pl. *epistropheī*). BNA. Second cervical vertebra. SYN: *axis*.

epitendineum (ep-ĭ-ten-din'e-um). The fibrous sheath enveloping a tendon.

epitenon (ĕp-ĭt'ē-non). The connective tissue holding a tendon within its sheaths. SYN: *epitendineum*.

epithalamus (ep-ĭ-thal'ă-mus). Post. part of thalamus.

epithalaxia (ep-ĭ-thal-aks'ĭ-ă). Desquamation of epithelial cells, esp. of lining of the intestine.

epithe'lia. Epithelial layer or cells.

epithelial (ep-ĭ-the'lĭ-al). Pert. to or composed of epithelium.

  e. cancer. Carcinoma composed of epithelial cells. SYN: *epithelioma*.

  e. casts. Aggregations of renal epithelium, with cells filled with granules or fat droplets. They often preserve their original form in the epithelial tubes.

  e. cells. Cells which are irregular in shape, having a single nucleus. Frequently 2 or 3 are joined together. May be hyaline or granular.

  e. tissue. Cells held together by collagen, arranged to form skin or membrane covering external surfaces and lining inner parts. It is devoid of blood vessels and is nourished by lymph.

epithe'lioblasto'ma. Epithelial cell tumor.

epithe'liocep'tor. A structure in a gland which receives a stimulus from nerve end organs.

epithe'liofib'ril. A tiny fiber in the protoplasm of epithelial cells.

epitheliogenic, epitheliogenetic (ep-ĭ-the'-lĭ-o-jen'ik, -jen-et'ik). Caused by epithelial proliferation.

epithelioid (ep-ĭ-the'lĭ-oyd). Resembling epithelium.

epitheliolysin (ep'ĭ-the-lĭ-ol'is-in). An antibody which dissolves epithelial cells.

epitheliolysis (ep-ĭ-the-lĭ-ol'ĭ-sĭs). Death of epithelial tissue.

epithelioma (ep-ĭ-the-lĭ-o'mă). A cancerous affection of the external layer of skin.

  TREATMENT: Caustics or excision in superficial form, x-ray, Finsen light, Roger's light. SEE: *chimney-sweep's cancer*.

  e., deep-seated. Involving lymphatic glands; irregular rounded ulcers, occurring after several months.

  e., papillary. Malignant, more often occurring in men and after middle life. Attacks genitals, nose, eyelids, or lower lip, etc.

  e., superficial. Papules, yellowish or brownish, degenerating and forming ulcers, secreting a yellowish fluid.

epitheliomatous (ep'ĭ-the-lĭ-ō'măt-ŭs). Pert. to epithelioma.

epitheliosis (ep-ĭ-the-lĭ-o'sĭs). Trachoma-like proliferation of the conjunctival epithelium.

epithelium (ep-ĭ-the'lĭ-um) (pl. *epithelia*). Cells contained in the skin, and covering mucous and serous membranes.
  This tissue may be squamous, columnar, or modified.

  e., ciliated. Epithelium with cilia at the free ends of the cells.

  e., columnar. Epithelium composed of cells shaped like pillars.

  e., cylindrical. SEE: *columnar epithelium*.

  e., glandular. Epithelium composed of cells which are part of a secretory process.

  e., maternal. Uterine epithelium contrasted with that of the embryo.

  e., neuro-. Epithelium terminating the nerves of special sense.

  e., pavement. Epithelium of flat, platelike cells.

  e., pigmented. Epithelium containing colored cells.

  e., rod. Epithelium with cells of rod-like appearance.

  e., squamous. SEE: *pavement epithelium*.

  e., stratified. Epithelium with the cells in layers.

  e., surface. Epithelium composing the surface of a part.

  e., transitional. A partially stratified epithelium.

epithem (ep'ĭthem). Any external application, as a poultice.

epitonic (ep-ĭ-ton'ik). Increased tonus.

epitox'oid. Any toxoid which has less affinity for an antitoxin than is possessed by the toxin. SYN: *toxon*.

epitrichium (ep-ĭ-trik'ĭ-um). Superficial layer of the epidermis of the fetus.

epitrochlea (ep-ĭ-trok'lē-ă). The inner condyle of the humerus.

epitrochlear (ep-i-trok'le-ar). Pert. to the inner condyle of the humerus.

epituberculo'sis. Resembling tuberculosis but without tubercle bacilli. SYN: *paratuberculosis*.

epitur'binate. The tissue upon or covering the turbinate bone.

epitympanum (ep-ĭ-tim'pan-um). The attic of middle ear; area above the drum membrane.

epityphilitis (ep'ĭ-tif-lĭ'tis). Appendicitis.

epizoic (ep-ĭ-zo'ik). Parasitic on the epidermis.

epizoicide (ep-e-zo'is-ĭd). That which destroys epizoa. SEE: *epizoon*.

epizoon (ep-ĭ-zo'on) (pl. *epizoa*). An animal organism externally parasitic.

épluchage (ā-plü-shazh'). Wound excision for removing contaminated tissues.

eponychium (ep-o-nik'ĭ-um). The horny embryonic structure from which the nail develops.

ep'onym. A name for anything (diseases, organs, functions, places) adapted from the name of a particular person.

eponym'ic. Pert. to eponym. SYN: *eponymous*.

epon'ymous. Named after a person.

epoöphorectomy (ep''o-o-fo-rek'to-mǐ). Removal of the parovarium.

epoöphoron (ep-o-of'o-ron). BNA. Cystic dilatation of the remnant of the wolffian duct. SYN: *parovarium*.

epsom salt (ep'sŭm). USP. SEE: *magnesium sulfate*.

epulis (ep-u'lis). A fibrous, sarcomatous tumor having its origin in the periosteum of the lower jaw.

    e., malignant. Jaw sarcoma made up of giant cells.

epuloid (ep'u-loid). 1. Like an epulis. 2. Tumor of the jaw or gum appearing like an epulis.

epulosis (e-pu-lo'sis). Cicatrization; a cicatrix.

epulot'ic. Promoting cicatrization.

equa'tion. A symbolic representation of a chemical reaction.

equa'tor. Line encircling a round body and equidistant from both poles.

    e. of a cell. The plane at which a cell is divided.

    e. oc'uli. The plane of the eyeball which bounds its central transverse vertical plane.

equato'rial. Pert. to an equator.

    e. plate. Mass of chromosomes at equator of the nuclear spindle during karyokinesis.

equi-. Prefix meaning *equal*.

equilibrating (e-kwil'i-brāt-ing). Maintaining equilibrium.

    e. operation. Section of the antagonist of a paralyzed ocular muscle. SEE: *tenotomy*.

equilib'rium. Equipoise. Condition in which contending forces are equal.

    e., nitrogenous. Having amt. of nitrogen in egesta equal to that of ingesta.

    e., physiological. Having egesta equal to the ingesta.

equilin(e (ek'wil-ĭn). Crystalline estrogenic hormone derived from pregnant mares' urine, which affects growth of female sex organs. SYN: *theelin*.

equina'tion. Inoculation with virus of horsepox.

equinia (e-kwin'ǐ-ă). Infectious disease of horses which can also affect man. SYN: *glanders*.

equinovarus (e-kwi''no-va'rus). A form of clubfoot with a combination pes equinus and pes varus.

equivalence (e-kwĭv'al-ens). 1. Quality of being equivalent. 2. Condition in which 2 radicals reacting are of the same valence and 1 displaces the other in a compound.

equivalent (e-kwĭv'a-lent). 1. Equal in power, force, or value. 2. Amount of weight of any element needed to replace a fixed weight of another body.

Er., E. R. 1. Abbr. for *external resistance*. 2. Symb. for *erbium*.

erasion (e-ra'zhun). 1. Laying open a diseased part and scraping away diseased tissue. 2. Scraping away morbid products.

Erben's reflex (erb'ens). Retardation of pulse when head and trunk are forcibly bent forward.

er'bium. A rare metallic element. SYMB: Er. Atomic weight, 166.

Erb's paralysis or palsy. Paralysis of group of muscles of shoulder and upper arm involving cervical roots of 5th and 6th spinal nerves.

    The arm hangs limp, the hand rotates inwards and normal movements are lost. SEE: *paralysis*.

erec'tile. Able to become erect.

    e. tissue. Vascular tissue which, when filled with blood, becomes erect or rigid, as the clitoris or penis; also in the nasal cavities.

erec'tion. The state of swelling, hardness, and stiffness observed in the penis and to a lesser extent in the clitoris of the female, generally during sexual excitement.

erec'tor. A muscle that raises a part.

    e. spinae reflex. Irritation of the skin over the erector spinae muscles causing contraction of muscles of the back.

erect posi'tion. One having the occiput and heels in line with nose, groin, and great toes in same relative plane.

eremacausis (er''em-ak-aw'sis). Slow oxidation of organic matter exposed to heat.

eremophobia (er-em-o-fo'bǐ-ă). Dread of being alone.

erep'sin. An enzyme found in the small intestine.

    A protease which converts proteoses and peptones into simpler products, such as amino acids and ammonia. SEE: *digestion, enzyme*.

erep'tic digestion. The breaking down of polypeptides to dipeptides and amino acids.

erethin (er'e-thin). The principle of tuberculin which causes fevers.

erethism (er'e-thizm). Abnormal excitement or irritation which may be combined with collapse.

erethis'mic. Pert. to or causing erethism. SYN: *erethitic*.

erethisophrenia (er-e-thī'-so-fre'nǐ-ă). Unusual mental excitability.

erethistic (er-e-this'tik). Erethismic, exciting.

erethitic (er-ě-thit'ĭk). Causing erethism; irritable, excited.

ereuthrophobia (er''u-thro-fo'bǐ-ă). Pathological fear of blushing. SYN: *erythrophobia*.

erg. In physics, the amount of work done when a force of 1 dyne acts through a distance of 1 centimeter.

ergasia (er-ga'sǐ-ă). Functions of the mind and behavior resulting therefrom in contrast to those depending upon physiological functions.

ergasiodermatosis (er-gas''ǐ-o-der-mă-to'-sis). Dermatosis due to occupational cause.

ergasiomania (er-gas'ǐ-o-ma'nǐ-ă). Active interest in a task without completing it; seen in certain phases of manic excitement.

ergasiophobia (er″gas-ĭ-o-fo′bĭ-ă). Abnormal dislike for assuming responsibility or for work of any kind.

ergasthenia (er-gas-the′nĭ-ă). Overwork and debility caused therefrom.

ergas′tic. Possessing potential energy.

ergastoplasm (er-gas′to-plazm). Cytoplasm with higher power than ordinary plasma. SYN: *kinoplasm.*

er′gin. A substance producing allergy or uniting with allergin.

ergograph (er′go-graf). An apparatus for recording the contractions of muscles and measuring the amount of work done.

ergom′eter. An apparatus for measuring the amount of work done by a human or animal subject.

ergopho′bia. Morbid dread of working.

ergophore (er′go-fōr). That part of an antigen on which the specific properties of the substance depend. SYN: *toxophore.*

er′goplasm. Protoplasm peculiar to the centrosome, and composing the attraction sphere. SYN: *kinoplasm.*

er′gostat. A machine for measuring work done by a contracting muscle.

ergos′terin, ergos′terol. A substance derived from yeast, ergot, and other fungi, and resembling cholesterol in composition.

   e., irradiated. Ergosterin subjected to ultraviolet radiation which develops vitamin D potency. A remedy for rickets.

ergot (er′got). A drug obtained from a parasitic growth on rye.

   DOSAGE: 30 gr. (2 Gm.). Fluid extract: 30 ℳ (2 cc.).

ergotamine tartrate (er-got′a-mēn). SEE: *gynergen.*

ergotherapy (er-go-ther′ă-pĭ). Work used as a treatment of disease.

   e., passive. Generalized muscular exercise excited by faradic current.

ergotism (er′go-tizm). Poisoning with ergot.

ergotrate (er′go-trāt). An active principle isolated from ergot.

   DOSAGE: ½₃₂₀ gr. (0.2 mg.) orally, intramuscularly, or intravenously.

ergotrop′ic. Pert. to ergotropy.*

ergotropy (er-got′ro-pĭ). Injection of nonspecific proteins to increase body resistance.

eriom′eter. Device for measuring minute particles.

erode (e-rōd′). 1. To wear away. 2. To eat away by ulceration.

erogenous (e-roj′en-us). Causing sexual excitement. SYN: *erotogenic.**

   e. zone. Any part of the body which by touching or stroking, causes sexual excitement.

erosion (e-ro′shun). An eating away of tissue; abrasion of mucous membrane which may result in an ulcer.

   e. of the cervix uteri. The alteration of the epithelium on a portion of the cervix as a result of irritation by infection.

erosive (e-ro′siv). 1. Able to produce erosion. 2. An agent that erodes anything.

erotic (e-rot′ik). Pert. to sexual passion. SYN: *lustful.*

erot′icism. Excessive or morbid libido; also intense but normal sex desire.

   e., oral. Sensation of pleasure experienced when nursing at the breast, modified and sublimated but continuing into adult life through normal contacts of the lips, mouth, and throat.

   e., auto-. 1. Self-gratification of the sexual instinct. 2. Self-admiration combined with sexual emotion, such as that obtained from viewing one's naked body, or one's genitals. SEE: *erotomania, zones, erotogenic.*

e′rotism. PSY: The emotional phases of the sexual impulse. Desire for stimulation of mucous surfaces.

   e., al′lo. Erotism directed to an external object rather than to self. SEE: *eroticism, erotomania.*

   e., anal. Sensations of pleasure experienced by the child through defecation, which later are inhibited.

   e., auto-. Erotism directed to oneself. OPP: *alloerotism.*

erotogenic (er″o-to-jen′ĭk). Producing sexual excitement. SEE: *erotic zones.*

erotology (er-o-tol′o-jĭ). The study of love and its manifestations.

erotomania (e-rot-o-ma′nĭ-ă). Unrestrained libido in the insane. SEE: *eroticism, zones, erotogenic.*

erotopathia (er-o-to-path′ĭ-ă). Any abnormal or perverted sex impulse.

erotophobia (er-o-to-fo′bĭ-ă). Aversion to sexual love or its manifestations.

erotopsychic (er-o-to-si′kik). Mental perversion of the sexual impulse.

errat′ic. Wandering, as from one part of the body to another part; roving, odd. SYN: *eccentric.*

errhine (er′ĭn). An agent that will increase the secretion of the mucous membrane lining the nose. SYN: *sternutatory.* Ex: *quillaja, salicylic acid.*

erubes′cence. Reddening of the skin; a blush.

eructa′tion. Raising of gas or acid fluid from the stomach; belching. SEE: *oxyrygmio.*

eruption (e-rup′shun). A skin lesion or rash caused by disease.

   e., primary. Blebs, macules, papules, pustules, tubercules, tumors, vesicles, wheals, or phomphi *q.v.*

   e., secondary. Crusts, excoriations, fissures, pigmentations, scales, scars, ulcers, *q.v.*

erup′tive. Breaking out, as with a rash.

erysipelas (er-is-ip′el-as). Acute, febrile disease with localized inflammation and swelling of skin and subcutaneous tissue accompanied by systemic disturbance of variable degree. SYN: *St. Anthony's fire.*

   e., ambulant. Erysipelas which disappears from one part of the body and reappears in another.

   e., erythematous. Erysipelas in a mild form. [face.

   e., facial. Form found mainly on the

e., idiopathic. Erysipelas which does not develop subsequent to trauma or injury.

e., migrans. Widely spread form of erysipelas.

e., phlegmonous. Purulent form of erysipelas.

e., surgical. Erysipelas developing in a wound.

e., traumatic. SEE: *surgical erysipelas.*

erysipelatous (er″ĭ-sĭ-pel′a-tus). Of the nature of or pert. to erysipelas.

erysipeloid (er-is-ip′e-loid). Infective dermatitis resembling erysipelas but without fever and due to absorption of putrescent animal matter by the skin.

Erysipelothrix. Member of Actinomycetaceae. Nonmotile, sporeless, microaerophilic organism shaped like a rod.

E. erysipelatus suis. Causative agent of swine erysipelas.

erythema (er-ith-e′mä). A form of macula showing diffused redness over the skin.

e. annulare. Erythema with rounded, raised marginal lesions.

e. circinatum. In red circles.

e. congestivum. Erythema with congestive state of skin.

e., diffuse. Widely spread over body.

e. dose. The amount of radiant energy sufficient to evoke perceptible redness of the skin.

e. hyperemicum. Caused by heat or cold (erythema caloricum, chilblain), sun (erythema solare), artificial heat, as from hot water bottle or electric pad.

TREATMENT: Removal of exciting cause, calamine lotion or oil containing phenol or menthol.

e. infectiosum. Contagious form with rose-colored eruption.

e. intertrigo. Chafing of opposing surfaces, with erythema and often with maceration and abrasion.

e. multiforme. A macular eruption with dark red papules or tubercles. Usually on extremities appearing in successive eruptions of short duration.

e. nodosum. Red and painful nodules on legs associated with rheumatism. Also caused by certain drugs and food poisoning.

e., punctate. In minute points, as scarlet fever rash.

e. symptomaticum. Hyperemia of the skin with level patches.

e. venenatum. Form caused by an irritation from minerals, poisons, etc.

erythematic, erythematous. Pert. to or marked by erythema.

erythemogenic. Pert. to erythema.

erythemomegalalgia. Painful redness of skin. SYN: *erythromelalgia.*

erythralgia (er-ĭ-thral′jĭ-ă). A condition of painful redness of the skin. SYN: *erythromelalgia.*

erythrasma (er-ĭ-thraz′mä). Reddish-brown eruption in patches in the axillae and groins due to a fungus.

erythredema (er″ĭ-thre-de′mä). Disordered digestion in infants accompanied by multiple arthritis, and swollen hands and feet. SYN: *acrodynia, Swift's disease.*

erythremia (er-ĭ-thre′mĭ-ă). Excessive increase of red blood corpuscles with cyanosis. SYN: *polycythemia rubra.*

erythrism. Redness of the hair and beard with ruddy complexion.

erythristic (er-ĭ-thris′tik). Ruddy complexion. Having reddish hair.

erythroblast (er-ith′ro-blast). A cell from which the red blood cells are derived; rudimentary red blood corpuscles; bone marrow nucleated, colorless cells.

erythroblastemia. An excessive number of erythroblasts in the blood.

erythroblastic. Pert. to erythroblasts.

erythroblastoma. A tumor (myeloma) with cells resembling megaloblasts.

erythroblastosis. A condition marked by many erythroblasts in the blood.

erythrochloropia (er″ĭ-thro-klo-ro′pĭ-ă) Partial color blindness with ability to see only red and green.

erythrochromia (er″ĭ-thro-kro′mĭ-ă) Hemorrhagic red pigmentation of the spinal fluid.

erythroclastic. Destructive to red blood cells.

erythroconte. An abnormal substance found in pernicious anemia in the erythrocytes.

erythrocyanosis. Red or bluish discoloration on the skin with swelling, itching and burning.

erythrocyte (e-rith′ro-sīt). Red blood corpuscle.

erythrocythemia (er″ĭth″ro-si-the′mĭ-ă) Enormous increase in red blood cells SYN: *erythremia, polycythemia.*

erythrocytolysis (er-ĭth″ro-si-tol′ĭ-sis) Dissolution of red blood corpuscles.

erythrocytometer. Instrument for counting red blood corpuscles.

erythrocytoöpsonin. A substance opsonin for red corpuscles.

erythrocytorrhexis (er-ĭ-thro-si-tor-reks′is). Rupture of a cell and escape of its plasma. SYN: *plasmorrhexis.*

erythrocytoschisis (er-ĭ-thro-si-tos′kis-is) Splitting discs like blood platelets. SYN: *plasmoschisis.*

erythrodermia (er-ĭ-thro-der′mĭ-ă). Abnormal redness in the skin. SYN: *erythema.*

erythrodextrin (er-ith-ro-dex′trin). Form of dextrin from splitting of a polysaccharide molecule. SEE: *achroödextrin.*

erythrogenesis. The development of red blood corpuscles.

erythrogranulose. A modified granulose stained red by iodine.

erythrokatalysis (er-ĭ-thro-ka-tal′ĭ-sis) Ingestion and digestion of red blood corpuscles.

erythrol tetranitrate (er′ith-rol tet-ra-nī′trāt). A white crystalline mass with explosive properties like nitroglycerin but used in medicine as a dilute powder or in tablets.

DOSAGE: ¼ to ½ gr. (0.015-0.03 Gm.).

erythroleukemia (er-ĭ-thro-lu-ke′mĭ-ă)

Many immature cells in the blood causing anemia.

erythroleukosis (er-ĭ-thro-lu-ko'sis). Abnormal increase of red cells and granulocytes.

erythrol'ysin. An agent causing erythrolysis. SYN: *hemolysin, erythrocytolysin.* SEE: *lysin.*

erythrol'ysis. Dissolution of red blood corpuscles. SYN: *erythrocytolysis.*

erythromelalgia (er-ĭ-thro-mel-al'jĭ-ă). A skin neurosis accompanied by burning and throbbing which come and go, affecting any one of the extremities, esp. the feet.

erythrome'lia. Erythema of extensor surfaces of extremities but without pain.

ery'thron. Circulating red blood cell tissue and cells from which it arises.

erythroneocytosis (er''ĭ-thro-ne''o-sĭ-to'sis). Regenerative forms of red blood cells in the blood.

erythronoclastic (er-ĭ-thron-o-klas'tĭk). Destructive to erythrons.

erythropar'asite. A red blood corpuscle parasite.

erythrop'athy. Disease of the red blood corpuscles.

erythropenia (er''ĭ-thro-pe'nĭ-ă). Deficiency of red blood corpuscles.

erythrophage (er-ith'ro-fāj). A phagocyte which destroys red corpuscles.

erythropha'gia. Destruction of red blood cells by phagocytes.

eryth'rophile, erythroph'ilous. Readily staining red.

erythrophobia (e-rith''ro-fo'bĭ-ă). Abnormal dread of blushing or fear of being diffident or of being embarrassed.

erythrophose (e-rith'ro-fōs). Any red subjective perception of a bright spot. SEE: *phose.*

erythrophthi'sis. Serious damage to the restorative power of the red corpuscles.

erythrophthor'ic. Rapid destruction of erythrocytes.

erythrop'ia, erythrop'sia. Condition in which objects appear to be red.

erythropoiesis (e-rith''ro-poy-e'sĭs). The formation of red blood corpuscles.

erythropoietic (er''ĭth''ro-poy-et'ĭk). Pert. to red blood cells.

erythroprosopalgia (er''ĭth''ro-pros-o-pal'-jĭ-ă). A neurosis marked by redness and pain in the face.

erythropsia (er-ĭ-throp'sĭ-ă). Perversion of color vision in which objects look red.

erythrop'sin. Pigment in the external portion of the rods of the retina. SYN: *rhodopsin, visual purple.*

erythropykno'sis. Alteration of red blood cells by malarial parasites; "brassy bodies." SYN: *pyknosis.*

erythrorrhex'is. Rupture of a cell and escape of its plasma. SYN: *erythrocytorrhexis, plasmorrhexis.*

erythro'sis. A reddish-purple discoloration of the skin and mucous membranes in polycythemia.

erythrotoxin (er-ith''ro-toks'in). An exotoxin that attacks red blood cells. SEE: *leukotoxin.*

erythruria (er-ĭ-thru'rĭ-ă). Red color of the urine.

Esbach's method (es'baks). A method of estimating quantity of albumin in urine.

eschar (es'kar). A slough, esp. one following a cauterization or burn. SEE: *escharotic.*

escharotic (es-kar-ot'ik). Agent used to destroy tissue and to cause sloughing which produces what is known as an *eschar.* The third degree of counter-irritation.

eschatin (es'kă-tin). An extract of suprarenal cortex.

DOSAGE: Average, 1-5 cc. subcutaneously.

Escherichia (esh-er-ik'ĭ-ă). A genus of bacteria, most of which are found in the intestine.

E. co'li. The *Bacillus coli communis,* a colon bacterium, usually nonpathogenic.

Escherich's reflex (esk'ĕr'ĭk). Pursing or muscular contraction of lips resulting from irritation of mucosa of lips.

eschrolalia (es-kro-lal'ĭ-ă). Utterance without meaning of obscene words. SYN: *coprolalia.*

Escudero's test. A test for gout.

es'culent. Suitable to be eaten.

escutcheon (es-kutch'un). The coarse pubic hair in the adult.

eserine (es'er-ĭn). USP. SEE: *physostigmine.*

Es'march's bandage. A rubber bandage for controlling bleeding.

esodic (es-od'ik). Centripetal or afferent; pert. to sensory nerves conducting impulses toward the brain and spinal cord.

esoenteritis (es''o-en-ter-i'tis). Inflammation of the mucous membrane of the intestine.

esoethmoiditis (es-o-eth-moy-di'tis). Inflammation of membrane of ethmoid cells.

esogastri'tis. Catarrhal inflammation of the gastric mucous membranes.

esophageal (e-sof-ă'je-al). Pert. to the esophagus.

esophagec'tomy. Excision of a part of the esophagus. [geal spasm.

esophagismus (e-sof-aj-is'mus). Esophageal spasm.

esophagitis (e-sof-a-ji'tis). Inflammation of the esophagus.

esophagocele (e-sof'a-go-sēl). Hernia of the esophagus.

esophagodyn'ia. Pain in the esophagus.

esophagoenterostomy (e-sof''a-go-en-ter-os'to-mĭ). Formation of communication bet. the esophagus and intestine with excision of stomach.

esophagogastros'copy. Inspection of esophagus and stomach through an illuminated instrument.

esophagogastrostomy (e-sof''ă-go-gas-tros'to-mĭ). Formation of a communication bet. the esophagus and stomach.

esophagomalacia (e-sof''ă-go-măl-a'sĭ-ă). Softening of the esophageal walls.

esophagomycosis (e-sof''a-go-mi-ko'sis). Bacterial or fungous disease of esophagus.

esophagoplasty (e-sof″ă-go-plas'tĭ). Repair of the esophagus by a plastic operation.

esophagoplication (e-sof″ă-go-plĭ-ka'shun). Reduction of dilation of the esophagus by taking tucks in its walls.

esophagopto'sia, esophagopto'sis. Relaxation and prolapse of the esophagus.

esophagoscope (e-sof'ag-o-skōp). Device for examination of esophagus.

esoph'agospasm. Spasm of walls of the esophagus.

esophagostenosis (e-sof″a-go-stĕ-no'sis). Stricture or narrowing of the esophagus.

esophagostomy (e-sof-ag-os'to-mĭ). Formation of esophageal fistula.

esophagotome (e-sof'a-go-tōm). Instrument for forming an esophageal fistula.

esophagotomy (e-sof-ag-ot'o-mĭ). Making of an incision in esophagus, so as to remove foreign substance.

esophagus (e-sof'a-gus) (pl. *esophagī*). A musculomembranous canal extending from the pharynx to the stomach. Length about 9 inches. RS: *epicardia, epicardium, gullet.*

esophoria (es-o-fo'rĭ-ă). OPHTH: Tendency of visual lines to converge. SEE: *exophoria.*

esophylac'tic. That which is phylactic or protective.

esophylaxis (es″o-fi-laks'is). The protective biological action against disease exercised by the fluids and cells of the body. SEE: *exophylaxis.*

esosphenoiditis (es″o-sfen-oy-di'tis). Osteomyelitis of the sphenoid bone.

esoteric (es-o-ter'ĭk). Coming from within the organism.

esotropia (es-o-tro'pĭ-ă). Marked turning inward of eye, crossed eyes.

-ess. Suffix noting female sex.

es'sence. 1. The spirit or principle of anything. 2. An alcoholic solution of volatile oil.

essen'tial. 1. Pert. to an essence. 2. Indispensable. 3. Specific; independent of a local morbid condition. SYN: *idiopathic.*

   e. oil. Any volatile oil of vegetable or animal origin.

es'ter. In organic chemistry, a compound formed by the combination of an organic acid with an alcohol.

esterase (es'ter-ās). Enzyme which hydrolyzes esters of the fatty acids.

es'terize. To convert into an ester.

esterol (es'ter-ol). Known also as benzyl succinate; a white, odorless powder.

   DOSAGE: 5 gr. (0.3 Gm.).

es″thematol'ogy. Science of the sense organs and their function.

esthesia (es-the'zĭ-ă). 1. Perception, feeling, sensation. 2. Any disease that affects the senses or perceptions. It forms the termination of many medical words.

esthe'sioblast. An embryonic ganglion cell. SYN: *ganglioblast.*

esthesiol'ogy. Science of sensory phenomena. SYN: *esthematology.*

esthesiomania (es-thez″ĭ-o-mā'nĭ-ă). Insanity with sensory hallucinations and perverted moral sensibilities.

esthesiometer (es-the-zĭ-om'et-er). Device for measuring tactile sensibility.

esthesioneurosis (es-the′zĭ-o-nu-ro'sis). A loss of feeling without any apparent organic lesion.

esthe″siophysiol'ogy. Physiology of the sense organs.

esthesioscopy (es-the′zĭ-os'ko-pĭ). Testing tactile and other forms of sensibility.

esthesod'ic. Carrying sense impressions.

estheticokinetic (es-thet″ĭ-ko-kin-et'ĭk). Being both sensory and motor.

esthiomene (es-thĭ-om'en-e). A chronic hypertrophic ulcerative vulvovaginitis of unknown origin.

esthiomenus (es-the-om'e-nus). Swelling and ulceration of perianal region and vulva.

es'tival. Relating to or occurring in summer.

estivo-autumnal. 1. Pert. to summer and autumn. 2. A term applied to a form of malarial fever.

Est'lander's operation. Resection of a part of 1 or more ribs and excision of diseased pleura in chronic empyema.

estradiol (ĕs-trā'dĭ-ŏl). Commercial hormone product from hogs' ovaries and pregnant mares' urine or synthetically from estrone. SYN: *dihydrotheelin.*

   e. dipropionate. An estrogen very effective in menopause.

es'trin. The estrus-producing hormone *theelin.* SYN: *female sex hormone, feminin, folliculin.*

es'triol. Hormone found in urine of pregnancy. SYN: *theelol.*

es'trogen. Commercial product containing estrin.

estrogenic (es-tro-jen'ĭk). Causing estrus.

es'trone. Hormone found in urine of pregnancy. SYN: *theelin.*

es'trual. Pert. to the rutting of animals.

estrua'tion. Rutting of animals during heat period

es'trum, es'trus. 1. Usually, a recurrent period of sexual activity in animals. 2. Less commonly, the orgasm or climax of sexual excitement during copulation.

estua'rium. Vapor bath.

état mamelonné (ā-tā' mă-mě-lon-nā'). Condition of gastric mucosa in chronic inflammation with nodular projections.

e'ther. 1. Hypothetical substance once regarded as permeating all space and capable of transmitting electromagnetic vibrations. 2. Any organic compound in which an oxygen atom links together 2 carbon chains.

   DOSAGE: 15 gr. (1.0 Gm.).

   e. anesthesia. The action of ether is slower than other general anesthetics and the margin of safety is greater.

   e. asphyxia. Suffocation during ether anesthetization. SEE: *ether anesthesia, gases, resuscitation.*

   e. bed. One prepared to prevent patient from injuring self, to keep patient warm, and to protect bedding.

   e. drunkenness. Intoxication produced by imbibing ether.

   e., ozonic. Ether, hydrogen, peroxide

and alcohol used in whooping cough and diabetes, and as local antiseptic in scarlatina.

DOSAGE: 30-60 gr. (2-4 Gm.) 3 times daily.

e. reflex. Rapidly increasing flow of duodenal secretion resulting from introduction by intubation of 3 or 4 cc. of ether.

ethereal (e-the're-al). Pert. to or made with ether.

e. oil. A volatile oil.

etherin (e'ther-in). A tuberculous toxin extracted by ether. SYN: *etherobacillin.*

etherion (e-the'rĭ-on). A gas of extreme tenuity in the atmosphere.

etherization (e''ther-ĭ-za'shun). Administering ether to induce anesthesia.

e'therize. To anesthetize by use of ether.

ə''therobacil'lin. Poison extracted from tuberculosis bacillus.

etheromania (e''ther-o-ma'nĭ-ă). Addiction to use of ether.

ethiopifica'tion. Pathological blackening of skin or production of argyria.*

ethmo-. Prefix denoting "connected with or pert. to the ethmoid bone."

ethmocardi''tis. Chronic inflammation and proliferation of cardiac connective tissue. SYN: *cardiosclerosis.*

eth'moid. Sievelike, cribriform.

e. bone. Sievelike spongy bone which forms a roof for the nasal fossae and part of floor of ant. fossa of skull, and containing air sinuses.

e. sinus. Air cells or space inside ethmoid bone.

ethmoi'dal. Pert. to the ethmoid bone or sinuses.

ethmoidectomy (eth-moy-dek'to-mĭ). Excision of ethmoid cells.

NP: Patient in sitting position, ice packs to nose often ordered.

ethmoidi'tis. Inflammation of ethmoidal cells. May be acute or chronic. SYM: Headache, acute pain bet. eyes, nasal discharge.

ethmyphitis (eth-mif-i'tis). Diffuse inflammation of cellular tissue. SYN: *cellulitis.*

ethnog'raphy. The description of the human race.

ethnol'ogy. The science of human races.

ethyl (eth'il). In organic chemistry, the radical C_2H_5 which enters into the constitution of many compounds such as ethyl ether, ethyl alcohol, and ethyl acetate.

e. alcohol. Transparent, colorless, volatile liquid of characteristic odor and a burning taste.

e. aminobenzoate. Same as benzocain.

e. chlor'ide. USP. A very volatile liquid with a pleasant odor.

e. nitrite, spirit of. Commonly known as sweet spirit of niter. USP. Oily liquid. DOSAGE: 30 ♏ (2 cc.).

e. salicylate. A volatile liquid, characteristic odor, same effects, but less irritant than methyl salicylate. DOSAGE: From 5-10 ♏ (0.3-0.6 cc.).

e'thylene. A colorless gas (CH_2CH_2) pre-

pared from alcohol by dehydration and found in illuminating gas to the extent of 4%.

e. anesthesia. A concentration of 90% ethylene and 10% oxygen is necessary to produce surgical anesthesia, but it later may be maintained by an 80% concentration.

etiolate (e'tĭ-o-lat). Pale or sickly from lack of light or long continued illness.

etiologic, etiological (e''tĭ-o-loj'ik, e-tĭ-o-loj'ik-ăl). Pert. to causes.

etiology (e-tĭ-ol'o-jĭ). The study of the causes of disease which result from an abnormal state producing pathological conditions.

etymology (et-ĭ-mol'o-jĭ). The science of the derivation of words.

Eubacteriales (ū-băk-tē-rĭ-a'lēs). An order of Schizomycetes, including spherical, spiral, and rod-shaped forms.

eubiotics (u-bi-ot'ĭks). Hygienic living.

eu'bolism. Normal metabolism.

eucaine hydrochloride (ū-kăn' hy-dro-chlō'-rĭd). USP. White, crystalline powder.

DOSAGE: Topically, in strengths from 2 to 5%.

eucalyptus, oil of (u-kal-ip'tŭs). USP. Oil distilled from fresh leaves of the plant.

DOSAGE: 8 ♏ (0.5 cc.).

eucalyptol. USP. A substance obtained from oil of eucalyptus.

DOSAGE: 5 gr. (0.3 Gm.).

euchylia (ū-ki'lĭ-ă). Normal condition of the chyle.

eudiaphoresis (ū-di''ă-fo-re'sis). Normal secretion of perspiration.

eudiemorrhysis (u''dĭ-em-or'ĭ-sis). The normal blood flow through the capillaries.

eudiom'eter. An instrument for testing purity of air and analysis of gases.

euesthesia (u-es-the'sĭ-ă). Having normal senses.

eugenics (u-jen'iks). The science which deals with the physical, moral, and intellectual improvement of the human race by careful and judicious mating. It is also concerned with (1) the sterilization of mental defectives; (2) intermarriages; (3) restriction of marriage bet. persons physically unfit; (4) birth control and allied problems. SEE: *aristogenics.*

eugenism (u'jen-ism). The circumstances of environment and heredity which tend to bring about happy and healthy existence.

euglobulin (ŭ-glŏb'ŭ-lin). One of the two constituents of paraglobulin, *q.v.*

eugon'ic. Pertaining to a luxuriant growth of bacteria.

eukinesia (u-kin-e'sĭ-ă). Normal power of movement.

eunoia (u-noy'ă). Soundness of mind.

eunuch (ŭ'nuk). Castrated male; one who has had his testicles removed.

eupancreatism (u-pan'kre-ă-tizm). Normal condition of the pancreas.

eupep'sia. Normal digestion, as distinguished from dyspepsia.

eupep'tic. Possessed of a good digestion.

euphoria (û-fo'rĭ-ă). 1. A condition of good health. 2. PSY: A feeling of well being; mild elation.*

euplas'tic. Healing quickly and well.

eupnea (up-ne'ă). Normal breathing, as distinguished from dyspnea and apnea.

eupraxia (û-prak'sĭ-ă). Normal capacity to execute a motor pattern. SEE: *paralysis.*

eupraxic (û-prak'sik). Contributing to proper functioning.

euquinine (û-kwĭ'nĭn) (quinine ethyl carbonate). USP. Nearly tasteless, light, fleecy crystals.

DOSAGE: Same as for quinine, but may be given in larger doses.

euresol (u're-sol). A trade name for resorcinol monacetate.

Euro'tium. A genus of molds.

E. malig'num. A species causing inflammation in ext. auditory meatus.

euryon (u're-on). Either end of bilateral diameter of head.

euryosomic, eurysomatic (û″rĭ-ō-sōm'ĭk, -rĭ-sōm-at'ĭk). Having a thick, squat body.

eu'rythrol. Extract of ox spleen; used in chlorosis and anemia.

DOSAGE: 60-120 ℔ (3.75-7.5 cc.).

eustachian (u-sta'kĭ-an). After Eustachio, an Italian anatomist. Pert. to the auditory tube.

RS: *salpingemphraxis, syringitis, syrinx.*

e. catheter. Instrument for introducing medicated vapor into the eustachian tube.

e. tube. The auditory tube (from the middle ear to the pharynx, 3-4 cm. long and lined with mucous membrane).

e. valve. Fold of membrane in the right auricle of the heart. SYN: *valvula venae cavae inferioris.*

eustachitis (u-sta-kī'tĭs). Inflammation of the eustachian tube.

eusystole (u-sis'to-lĭ). A state of the systole of the heart that is normal in time and force.

eutectic (u-tek'tĭk). Easily melted.

euthanasia (u-than-a'zĭ-ă). 1. An easy death. 2. The proposed practice of ending a life in case of incurable disease.

euthenics (û-then'ĭks). Study of all that might improve humanity.

eutocia (u-to'sĭ-ă). Normal or natural labor and childbirth.

eutonon (u'tō-non). Proprietary liver extract, possibly a hormone, suggested for use in treating vascular diseases.

evacuant (e-văk'û-ant). Drug which moves the bowels.

evac'uate. To discharge, esp. from the bowels.

evacuation (e-vak-u-a'shun). Emptying, esp. the bowels. RS: *absorption, feces, stool.*

evacuator (e-vak'u-a-tor). Device for emptying, as of the bowels or for irrigating the bladder and removing calculi.

evag'inate. Pert. to protrusion of some part or organ from its normal place.

evagination (e-vaj-in-a'shun). 1. Emergence from a sheath. 2. Protrusion of an organ or part. SEE: *invagination.*

evanes'cent. Not permanent; of brief duration; passing gradually.

Evans-Strang diet, modified. SEE: *reduction diet.*

evapora'tion. 1. Change from liquid form to vapor. 2. Loss in volume due to conversion of a liquid into a vapor.

evec'tics. Acquiring of bodily energy.

eventra'tion. 1. Partial protrusion of abdominal contents bet. the 2 recti muscles. 2. Removal of contents of the abdominal cavity.

e. of the diaphragm. Elevation of the diaphragmatic dome into the thoracic cavity.

eversion (e-ver'shun). Turning outward. SEE: *chilectropion.*

e. of the cervix. A turning out of the cervical edges subsequent to laceration. SYN: *ectropion of cervix.*

évidement (ă-vēd-mòn'). Scraping away morbid tissue.

evipal (e'vĭ-pal). A derivative of urea, occurring as a white powder.

DOSAGE: 4 gr. (0.259 Gm.) to be used cautiously in liver damage.

e., soluble. USES: In short surgical operations as an anesthetic, given intravenously.

eviration (e-vĭ-ra'shun). 1. Castration. 2. Effemination or defemination, or transformations of psychical personality due to the development of contrary sexual instincts.

evisceration (e-vis-er-a'shun). 1. Removal of the viscera. 2. Removal of the contents of a cavity. 3. Protrusion of the viscera. SEE: *embryoctomy.*

evis″ceroneurot'omy. Scleral evisceration of the eye with division of optic nerve.

evolu'tion. A process of orderly and gradual change or development.

e., doctrine of. Theory that slow and gradual change of lower forms of life, through external processes, is the origin of the human species, as differing from environment.

e., spontaneous. Spontaneous birth of a child in transverse presentation.

evul'sion. 1. Tearing away of a part or new growth. 2. Forcible extraction, as of teeth.

Ewald's test dinner. Chopped meat, 165 Gm.; stale bread, 35 Gm., with a small portion of butter. This content is withdrawn in 3 hours. In this test, further action is desired than just 1 hour's effect could produce.

E. t. meal. White bread or rolls (no crust), 40 Gm., and water or clear tea, 400 cc. No butter, sugar, milk, or cream taken with this portion. One hour after giving, the contents of the stomach are expressed. Time plays a very important part in the carrying out of the treatment.

ex-. Prefix: Out, away from.

exacerbation (eks″as-er-ba'shun). Aggravation of symptoms or increase in the severity of a disease.

exacrinous (eks-ak'rin-us). Concerning a gland's external secretion.

examina'tion, phys'ical. The act or process of examining the body and its products as to fitness or for symptoms of a disease.

exangia (eks-an'jĭ-ă). Any dilatation of a blood vessel. Ex: *aneurysm, varix.*

exanthem, exanthema (eks-an'them, -anthe'mă) (pl. *exanthema'ta*). Any eruption of the skin, accompanied by inflammation, *e. g.,* measles, scarlatina, erysipelas, *q.v.*

exanthematous (eks-an-them'ă-tus). Pert. to an exanthem, eruption, or rash.

exanthrope (eks'an-thrōp). Disease not originating in the body.

exarteritis (eks-ar-ter-i'tis). Inflammation of the outer coat of an artery.

exarticula'tion. Amputation of a limb through a joint.

excava'tion. 1. A hollow or depression. 2. Formation of a cavity.

    e. of optic nerve. A cupping of the optic disk.

excen'tric. Away from; efferent.

excerebration (eks-ser-e-bra'shun). Removal of brain.

excernant (eks-ser'nant). Bringing about an evacuation or excretion. SYN: *excretory.*

excip'ient. Any substance added to a medicine to give it form and consistency. SYN: *vehicle.*

exci'sion. An act of cutting away or taking out.

excitabil'ity. Sensitiveness to being stimulated.

    e., independent. Power of a muscle to respond to a stimulus without intervention of motor nerves.

    e., reflex. Sensitiveness to reflex irritation.

excit'ant. An agent that will excite a special function of the body; subdivided, according to action, as *motor, cerebral,* etc. Ex: *alcohol, cocaine, strychnine.*

excita'tion. 1. The act of exciting. 2. Condition of being stimulated or excited. The entire vasomotor system of nerves is involved.

    e., direct. Irritation of a muscle with an electrode.

    e., indirect. Irritation of a muscle *via* its nerve.

excit'ing. Causing excitement.

    e. cause. Acting immediately as a cause of disease.

excitoglan'dular. Increasing glandular function.

excitometabol'ic. Increasing metabolic changes.

excitomo'tor. Increasing rapidity of muscular activity.

excitomus'cular. Causing muscular activity.

excitonu'trient. Stimulating nutrition.

exci'tor. That which incites to greater activity. SYN: *stimulant.*

excitosecre'tory. Tending to bring about secretion.

excitovas'cular. Increasing circulation.

exclave (eks'klāv). Detached part of an organ.

excochleation (eks-kok-le-a'shun). Curettage of a cavity.

excoriation (eks-ko-rĭ-a'shun). Abrasion of the epidermis or of the coating of any organ of the body by trauma, chemicals, burns, or other causes.

excrement (eks'krĕ-ment). The feces, excreta, dejecta. SEE: *excretion.*

    e. menstruum. Menstrual discharge.

excrementitious (eks-kre-men-tish'us). Of the nature of excrement.

excrescence (eks-kres'ens). An outgrowth from the surface of a part. RS: *eruption, macula, nodule.*

excre'ta. Waste intestinal matter; dejecta; feces. Waste material cast off by the body.

excrete (eks-krēt'). To separate and expel useless matter not utilized by the body.

excre'tion. Waste matter, excreta, or the process of the body in elimination.

ex'cretory. Pert. to or bringing about excretion.

excur'sion. 1. Wandering from the usual course. 2. Extent of movement of the eyes from a central position.

excurva'tion. A curvature outward. SYN: *kyphosis.*

excystation (eks"sis-ta'shun). Removal from a cyst.

exemia (eks-e'mĭ-ă). Loss of blood from circulation, though accumulation in a part.

exencephalia (eks-en-sef-al'ĭ-ă). A term for *encephalocele, hydrencephalocele, meningocele,* and *synencephalocele.*

exenteration (eks-en-ter-a'shun). 1. Evisceration. 2. Removal of viscera of fetus in embryotomy.

exercise. Functional activity of the muscles, voluntary or otherwise.

    e., active. A form of bodily movement which the patient performs with or without the personal supervision of the operator.

    e., assistive. A form of bodily movement which the patient performs assisted by the operator or some mechanical means such as a pulley or weight.

    e., blowing. One in which water is blown from 1 bottle to another, thus increasing intrabronchial pressure which tends to aid in expansion of the lung. It is by this means that an empyema* cavity is obliterated.

    e., Buerger's postural (bur'gers). Used for circulatory disturbances of the extremities.

    e., Brandt's. Exercises for pelvic lesions. Fallen into disuse due to the attendant dangers.

    e., crawling. Devised for treatment of scoliosis,* essentially for children.

    e., free. Form of bodily movement which is carried through by patient against least possible resistance.

    e., Frenkel's. Used to teach tabetics to walk.

    e., Krida knee. In intertrochanteric fractures of femur, remove post. half of plaster cast from the knee to the toes; anterior portion of leg cast remains attached to spica, and maintains position of hip. When patient is face down, this permits knee to be flexed and extended and ankle exercised.

e., Lewin circulatory. Passive exercise for leg for circulatory disturbance of extremity.

e., Master's. Ascending and descending 2 steps a variable number of times. Used as a tolerance test for circulatory efficiency and as an exercise in heart disease.

e., Mosher's. For dysmenorrhea. Lie on back on floor with knees bent, feet on floor. Raise abdomen, relax it, contract it forcibly and relax. Repeat 10 times.

e., passive. Form of bodily movement which is carried through by the patient without the assistance or resistance of the patient. Same as relaxed movement.

e., resistive. Form of supervised bodily movement, with or without apparatus, which offers resistance to muscle action.

e., rhythm. Used in obstetrical paralysis. Exercise to song or music.

e., Schott's. Named after the Dr. Schott of Nauheim, who first scientifically administered Nauheim baths. It consists of slowly and evenly executed exercises with slight resistance, for cardiac diseases.

e., sling suspension. Method of supporting arm or leg to be exercised in a sling suspended from overhead, thus eliminating the weight of the extremity as a hindrance during movement.

e., static. Alternate contraction and relaxation of a muscle or group of muscles without movement of the joint. Also known as muscle setting.

e., Stokes-Oertel (er'tel). For arteriosclerosis. A system in which walking and hill climbing are combined with restrictions of fluids.

e., therapeutic. Scientific supervision of bodily movement, with or without apparatus, for purpose of restoring normal function to diseased or injured tissues.

e., water. Hydrogymnastics.

ex'ercise bone. Bony growth developing in a muscle due to overexercise.

exeresis (eks-er'es-is). Excision of any part.

exfetation (eks-fe-ta'shun). Ectopic gestation.

exflagella'tion. The formation of flagella from body of a male parasite, 1 of the motile threads entering the female and fertilizing its ovum, as in malaria.

exfolia'tion. The scaling off of dead tissue. RS: *apostasis.*

exhala'tion. The process of breathing outward; the opposite of inhalation; emanation of a gas or vapor.

exhaus'ter. A cataract evacuator for removal of loosened or fluid matter by vacuum pressure through a hollow needle.

exhaus'tion. Prostration of vital forces.

exhib'it. 1. To show. 2. To administer a drug. 3. Collection of objects for public inspection.

exhibi'tionism. 1. An abnormal impulse that causes one to expose the genitals to one of the opposite sex, seen in paretic and senile dementia, epilepsy, and other mental defects. 2. Tendency to attract attention in other ways.

exhibitionist (eks-i-bi'shun-ist). 1. One with an abnormal desire to attract attention. 2. One who yields to an impulse to expose the genitals to the view of one of the opposite sex.

exhilarant (eks-il'ă-rănt). That which is mentally stimulating.

exhuma'tion. Disinterment of a corpse.

Ex'ner's nerve. One from the pharyngeal plexus to the cricothyroid membranes.

E.'s plexus. One of axis cylinder terminals in superficial layer of the cerebral cortex.

exo-. Prefix: Without; outside of.

exocar'dia. Congenitally abnormal position of the heart.   [heart.

exocar'dial. Occurring outside of the

exocataphoria (eks-o-kat-ă-for'ĭ-ă). Ł. downward and outward turning of the visual axes.

exocoli'tis. Inflammation of the peritoneal coat of the colon.

exocrine (eks'o-krĕn). 1. The external secretion of a gland, opp. of endocrine. 2. Pert. to excretion of a fluid without other protoplasmic substances. OPP: *ptyocrine.**

exocystis (eks-o-sist'is). Prolapse of the urinary bladder.

exodic (eks-od'ik). Efferent, centrifugal. Transmitting impressions outward from the central nervous system.

exodontia (eks-o-don'shĭ-ă). 1. Extraction of a tooth. 2. Protrusion of teeth forward.

exodontol'ogy. Branch of dentistry concerned with extraction of teeth.

exoen'zyme. One that does not function within the cells from which it is secreted.

exogamy (eks-og'am-ĭ). 1. Marriage outside of same family; outbreeding. 2. BIOL: Conjugation bet. gametes of different ancestry, as in some protozoans. SEE: *heterosexuality.*

exogastri'tis. Inflammation of the peritoneal coat of stomach.

exogenous (eks-oj'en-us). Originating outside of an organ or part.

exohemophylaxis (eks"o-hem"o-fi-laks'is). Injection of one's own blood mingled with arsphenamine.

exohysteropexy (eks-o-his-ter-o-peks'ĭ). Fixation of the uterus by implanting the fundus into the abdominal wall.

exometritis (eks-o-me-tri'tis). Inflammation of the peritoneal coat of the uterus.

exomphalos (eks-om'fă-los). 1. Umbilical protrusion. 2. Umbilical hernia. SYN: *exumbilication.*

exopath'ic. Pert. to a disease originating outside of the body.

exophoria (eks-o-fo'rĭ-ă). OPHTH: Tendency of visual axes to diverge outward. SYN: *esophoria*.

exophthal'mia. Abnormal protrusion of the eyeball. SYN: *exophthalmos*.

   e. cachectica. Exophthalmic goiter.

   e. fungosa. Late stage of glioma retinae.

exophthalmic (eks-of-thal'mik). Pert. to protrusion of the eyeball.

   e. goiter. A goiter marked by protrusion of the eyeballs, increased heart action, and enlargement of the thyroid gland.

exophthal'mos, exophthal'mus. Abnormal protrusion of eyeball. SEE: *ophthalmocele*.

exophylac'tic. Pert. to exophylaxis.

ex"ophylax'is. Protection from disease originating outside the body, as by the skin.

ex'oplasm. Outer protoplasm of a cell. SYN: *ectoplasm*.

exorbitism (eks-or'bĭ-tizm). Protrusion of eyeball. SYN: *exophthalmos*.

exormia (eks-or'mĭ-ă). Any papular skin disease.

exosep'sis. Septic poison of external origin.

exoserosis (eks-o-ser-o'sis). An oozing of serum or discharging of an exudate.

exoskel'eton. The hard parts of the body developed from the ectoderm or mesoderm, such as teeth, nails, and hair. SYN: *dermoskeleton*.

exosmo'sis. Diffusion of a fluid from within outward, as from a blood vessel.

exosplenopexy (eks-o-sple'no-peks-ĭ). Suturing the spleen to opening in the abdominal wall.   [tumor.

exostosis (eks-os-tō'sis). Osteoma or bone

exoter'ic. Pert. to causes developing outside the body. SYN: *exopathic*.

exother'mal, exother'mic. Chemical reaction with production of heat.

exothy'mopexy. Suturing of an enlarged thymus gland to the sternum.

exothyreopexy (eks-o-thi're-o-peks-ĭ). Suture of the thyroid and external fixation to induce atrophy.

exothy'ropexy. Suture of the thyroid and external fixation to induce atrophy. SYN: *exothyreopexy*.

exotoxin (eks-o-toks'ĭn). A toxin secreted by and given off by the organism through the lymph, the blood, or by continuity of tissue producing effects remote from the seat of invasion by the bacteria.

exotro'pia. Divergent strabismus; abnormal turning of one or both eyes outward.

expansion (eks-pan'shun). Increase of volume; spreading out.

   e., coefficient of. Increase in length or in volume when temperature is raised 1° C. from zero.

   e. muscle. Degree a muscle may be stretched by an attached weight.

expansive delusion. Belief in one's power and wealth, accompanied by a feeling of well-being.

expec'tant. Waiting.

   e. treatment. Treatment of symptoms as they arise.

expecta'tion. Hoping, anticipation.

   e. of life. Probable duration of life after a given age.

expec'torant. An agent that facilitates the removal of the secretions of the bronchopulmonary mucous membrane.

expectoration (eks-pek'to-ra'shun). Expulsion of mucus or phlegm from the throat or lungs.

expel'. To drive out.

expira'tion. The expulsion of air from the lungs in breathing. Its sound is the shortest breath sound heard.

expiratory (eks-pi'ră-tor-ĭ). Pert. to expiration.

   e. center. The part of the respiratory center in the medulla controlling expiratory movements.

explant'. To transfer from the body to an artificial medium for growth.

explora'tion. Examination by various means of an organ or part.

explo'ratory. Pert. to an exploration.

explo'sive speech. Sudden and explosive utterance. SEE: *speech*.

express'. To squeeze out.

expres'sion. 1. Expelling anything by pressure. 2. Facial disclosure of feeling or emotion. SYN: *facies*. SEE: *face*.

expul'sive. Having a tendency to expel.

   e. pains. Labor pains which are effective, contracting the uterine muscle.

exsanguinate (eks-san'gwin-āt). 1. To deprive of blood. 2. Bloodless.

exsanguination (eks-san-gwin-a'shun). Expulsion of blood from a limb toward the trunk by bandaging.

exsanguine (ek-sang'win). Anemic; bloodless.

exsec'tion. Excision.

exsiccant (ek-sik'ant). Absorbing or drying up a discharge.

exsicca'tion. The act of drying by heat. SYN: *desiccation*.

exsic'cative. Causing to dry up or that which drys. SYN: *desiccative*.

exsicco'sis. Water impoverishment in tissues and its results.

exso'matize. To remove from the body.

exstrophy (eks'strof-ĭ). Eversion; turning inside out of a part.

ext. Abbr. of L. *extractum*, extract.

extempora'neous. Not prepared according to formula but devised for the occasion.

   e. mixture. A preparation to be taken at once because of tendency to deteriorate.

extension (eks-ten'shun). The movement by which the 2 ends of any part are pulled asunder. A movement which brings the members of a limb into or toward a straight condition.

   e., Buck's. A method of producing traction by applying adhesive tape or moleskin to the skin and keeping it in smooth close contact by means of circular bandaging of the part to which it is applied.

exten'sor. A muscle that extends a part.

exte'rior. Outside of; external.

extern(e (ek'sturn). A recently advanced medical student living outside of a hospital who assists in the medical and surgical care of patients. SEE: *intern.*

external. Exterior; lateral; opp. of medial or internal.

externa′lia. External genitalia.

exteroceptive (eks″ter-o-sep′tiv). Pert. to end organs receiving impressions from without.

exteroceptor (eks-ter-o-sep′tor). A sense organ adapted for the reception of stimuli from outside the body. Ex: The eye.

exterofec′tive. Reacting to external stimuli, as the cerebrospinal nerves.

ex′tima. The outer case of a blood vessel.

extirpation (eks-tir-pa′shun). Excision of a part—taking out by the roots.

extocardia (eks-to-kar′dĭ-ă). Displacement of the heart.   [outward.

extor′sion. Rotation of an organ or limb,

extra-. Prefix: Outside of, in addition to.

extraärtic′ular. Outside a joint.

ex′tract. 1. A solid or semisolid preparation made by extracting the solubles with water or alcohol and evaporating the solution. 2. Active principle of a drug obtained by distillation or chemical processes.

    e., alcoholic. One in which alcohol acts as the solvent.

    e., aqueous. One in which water is the solvent.

    e., aromatic fluid. Extract made from an aromatic powder.

    e., compound. Extract prepared from more than 1 drug.

    e., ethereal. Extract using ether as the menstruum.

    e., fluid. One made into a solution from a vegetable drug, which contains medicinal components.

    e., powdered. A crushed, dried extract.

    e., soft. Extract of the consistency of honey.

    e., solid. Extract made by evaporating the fluid part of a solution.

extrac′tion. 1. Pulling out, as a tooth. 2. The removing of the active portion of a drug.

extrac′tor. Instrument for removing foreign bodies.

    e., tissue. Needles, trocars, or pointed instruments with a form of barb for extracting soft tissue for examination.

    e., tube. Device for removing an intubation tube from trachea.

extrac′tum (ext.). Solid or semisolid preparations produced by evaporating solutions of vegetable principles.

extracys′tic. Outside of or unrelated to a bladder or cystic tumor.

extradu′ral. 1. On outer side of the dura mater. 2. Unconnected with the dura mater.

extragenital (eks-tră-jen′ĭ-tal). Outside of or unrelated to the genital organs.

extrahep′atic. Outside of or unrelated to the liver.

extraligamen′tous. Outside of or unrelated to a ligament.

extramalle′olus. The external or lateral malleolus.

extramar′ginal. Pert. to subliminal consciousness.

extramastoiditis (eks-tră-mas-toy-di′tis). Inflammation of outside tissues contiguous to the mastoid process.

extramedul′lary. Outside or unrelated to any medulla, esp. the medulla oblongata.

extraneous (eks-tra′ne-us). Outside and unrelated to an organism.

extranu′clear. Outside of a nucleus.

extrapo′lar. Outside instead of bet. poles, as the electrodes of a battery.

extrasys′tole. Contraction of the heart prematurely, although normal rhythm is maintained. SEE: *systole.*

extrau′terine. Outside the uterus.

extravag′inal. Outside the vagina.

extravasate (ek-strav′a-sāt). 1. To escape from a vessel into the tissues, said of serum, blood, or lymph. 2. Exudate so escaping.

extravasation (eks-tra-va-sa′shun). The escape of fluids into the surrounding tissue.

extravas′cular. Outside a vessel.

extraventric′ular. Outside of any ventricle, esp. one of the heart.

extrem′ital. Pert. to an extremity. SYN: *distal.*

extrem′ity. 1. The terminal part of anything. 2. An arm or leg.

extrin′sic. From or coming from without.

    e. muscles. Those partly attached to the trunk and partly to a limb.

extroversion (ek-stro-ver′shun). 1. Eversion; turning inside out. 2. PSY: The direction of energy to objects in the environment.

ex′trovert. A personality-reaction type; one who is interested mainly in ext. objects and actions.

extrude (eks-trūd′). To push out of a normal position or situation.

extru′sion. 1. Occupying an abnormal external position. 2. Position of a tooth pushed forward from line of occlusion.

extubation (eks-tu-ba′shun). Removal of a tube, as the laryngeal tube.

exudate (eks′u-dāt). 1. Accumulation of a fluid in a cavity, or matter that penetrates through vessel walls into adjoining tissue, or the passing out of pus or serum, or the matter so passed.

exuda′tion. Morbid oozing of fluids, usually the result of inflammatory conditions. SEE: *ant. choroiditis, central choroiditis, exudate, exudative choroiditis.*   [dation.

ex′udative. Having the property of exu-

exude′. To pass off slowly through the tissues; said of a semisolid or fluid.

exumbilica′tion. Protrusion of navel. SYN: *exomphalos.*

exuviae (eks-u′vĭ-e). Cast-off parts, as desquamated epidermis; a slough.

eye. Organ of vision; composed of 3 coats: (a) *Retina,* sensory for light; (b) *uvea* (choroid, ciliary body, and iris), nutritional; (c) *sclera* and *cornea,* serve to protect delicate retina.

    e. closure reflex. Contraction of orbicularis palpebrarum with closure of lids resulting from percussion above supraorbital nerve.

e., hare's. Condition affecting eye so that it can only be partially closed. SYN: *lagophthalmos.*

e., nerve supply of. *Retina,* 2nd, or optic nerve; *muscles,* 3rd, or motor oculi; 4th, or trochlear, and 6th, or abducens; 7th, or facial, to lid muscles; 5th, or trigeminus *sensory,* to lids, conjunctiva, and eyeball; sympathetic nerves to smooth muscles of ciliary body and Mueller's muscle in lid.

e., refracting surfaces of. (a) Cornea; (b) anterior and posterior surface of lens, *refracting media;* (c) vitreous.

eyeball. The body of the eye.

eye′brow. The arch over the eye; also its covering, esp. the hairs.

eye′glass. A glass lens used to aid the defective eye in seeing.

eye′ground. Fundus of eye, seen with ophthalmoscope.

eye′lash. Cilium.* A stiff hair on the margin of the eyelid. SEE: *capsulociliary,* "*cili-*" words, *phalangosis, trichiasis.*

eye′lid (*palpebra*). The loose, tegumentary fold which covers the front of the eyebrow when brought together.

eyestrain. Tiredness of the eye due to overuse or uncorrected defect. SYN: *asthenopia.*

eyetooth. A cuspid or upper canine tooth.

F

F. 1. Abbr. of *Fahrenheit, field of vision, formula, Fusiformis.* 2. Symbol for *fluorine.*

FA. Abbr. for *fatty acid.*

F. A. Abbr. for *field ambulance.*

F. and R. Abbr. for *force and rhythm.*

fabel'la. One of 2 sesamoid fibrocartilages of the gastrocnemius.

fabrication (fab-ri-ka'shun). Recital of that which is not true, seen in Korsakow's syndrome.

F. A. C. D. Abbr. *Fellow of the American College of Dentists.*

face. Anterior part of head which includes the features.

　　f. presentation. Fetal face presentation in childbirth.

　　f., spasms of. May be intermittent, continuous, bilateral or unilateral.

facet, facette (fas'et). A small, smooth area on a bone or other hard surface.

fa'cial. Pert. to the face.

　　f. center. Brain center causing facial movements.

　　f. nerve. Seventh cranial nerve, great motor nerve of facial muscles, exclusively motor at origin but subsequently receives fibers from the trigeminus, which gives it some sensory function.

　　f. paralysis. Affecting the muscles of the face. The 7th cranial nerve is involved.

　　f. reflex. Contraction of facial muscles following pressure on eyeball.

　　f. spasm. Tic. SEE: *cranial nerves, face, facies, paralysis, tic.*

facies (fash'i-ez). 1. Face. 2. Countenance. 3. Surface.

　　f. abdomina'lis. Pinched, anxious, shrunken and drawn expression seen in abdominal troubles.

　　f. adenoid. Stupid appearance with open mouth.

　　f. aor'tica. Expression seen in aortic valve insufficiency, bluish sclera, cheeks sunken, face sallow.

　　f. hepat'ica. Seen in liver affections: Skin sallow, conjunctivae yellow, and eyeballs sunken.

　　f. hippocrat'ica. Seen in those dying from long continued illness or from cholera; cheeks and temples hollow, eyes sunken, complexion leaden, and lips relaxed.

　　f. mitra'lis. Seen in mitral insufficiency. Capillaries more or less visible, cheeks pink, more or less cyanosis.

　　f., myopath'ic. Due to muscular weakness, esp. that of the face, lids drop and lips protrude.

　　f. ovari'na. Seen in women with ovarian tumor; face drawn and pinched.

　　f. tetanica. Senile appearance due to wrinkling in tetanus.

　　f., typhoid. Dusky complexion, in-

jected conjunctivae and dull expression.

facilitation (fas-il"it-a'shun). Making an action or process easier, the energy of an impulse being added to that of other impulses activated at the same time.

fa'cing. An inlay to form the outer surface of a tooth.

faciobrachial (fa-shī-o-bra'kī-al). Pert. to the face and arm, esp. to juvenile muscular dystrophy.

faciocer'vical. Pert. to the face and neck, esp. to progressive dystrophy of facial muscles.

faciolin'gual. Pert. to the face and the tongue, esp. a paralysis of them.

fa'cioplasty. Plastic surgery of the face.

facioplegia (fa"sī-o-ple'jī-a). Facial paralysis. SYN: *prosopoplegia.*

facioscapulohumeral (fa"shī-o-skap"u-lo-hu'mer-al). Pert. to the face, the scapula, and the upper arm.

F. A. C. P. Abbr. for *Fellow of the American College of Physicians.*

F. A. C. S. Abbr. for *Fellow of the American College of Surgeons.*

factitious (fak-tish'us). Not natural; esp. of certain skin lesions.

fac'ulta"tive. BIOL: 1. Able to live under conditions of temperature or oxygen supply which vary. 2. Able to do something not compulsory; voluntary.

fac'ulty. 1. A mental attribute or sense. 2. Ability to function.

　　f., affective. Capacity for expressing emotions.　　　　　　　　　　[develop.

　　f., germinative. Power of a germ to

fagopyrism (fag-ō-pīr'izm). Buckwheat poisoning.

Fahr. Abbr. for *Fahrenheit.*

Fahraeus' test. A measuring of the speed at which red blood corpuscles settle.

Fahrenheit scale. The one used in the U. S. A., and England. The freezing point of water is 32° and the boiling point 212°. Indicated by capital letter F. SEE: *thermometer.*

faint. 1. To feel weak, as though about to lose consciousness. 2. Weak. 3. Syncope. SEE: *fainting.*

fainting (fānt'ing). Loss of consciousness due to cerebral anemia or insufficient blood to the brain.

faint'ness. 1. A sensation of impending loss of consciousness. 2. A sensation due to lack of food. SEE: *lipòthymia.*

falcate (fal'kāt). Sickle-shaped.

falcial (fal'sī-al). Pert. to the falx.

fal'ciform. Sickle-shaped.

　　f. ligament. The triangular ligament attached to sides of the sacrum and coccyx by its base. SYN: *great sacro-ischiadic ligament.*

　　f. process. Process of the dura that divides the hemispheres of the cerebrum. SYN: *falx cerebri.*

fal'cula. The falx cerebelli.

fal'cular. 1. Sickle-shaped. 2. Pertaining to the *falx cerebelli.*

fallec'tomy. Cutting away part of the fallopian tube.

falling drop. 1. A metallic tinkle heard over the normal stomach and bowel when inflated. 2. The same sound heard over large cavities containing fluid and air, as observed in hydropneumothorax.

   f. sickness. Epileptic condition.

   f. of the womb. Dropping of the uterus, so that it protrudes into vagina. SYN: *descensus uteri.*

fallo'pian. Pert. to parts named for the Italian anatomist Fallopius.

   f. canal. Canal in petrous bone for *nervus facialis.*

   f. ligament. Round ligament of the uterus.

   f. tube. The tube or duct that passes from the cornu of the uterus to the ovary, 1 on each side of the uterus opening just below the fundus. It acts as a passage for the ovum to the uterus, and for the spermatozoa from the uterus to the ovary. SYN: *oviduct.*

fallostomy (fal-os'to-mĭ). Surgical opening of the fallopian tube.

fallot'omy. Division of the fallopian tubes. SYN: *salpingotomy.**

Fallot's tetrad (fal-lōz' tet'rad). Congenital defects of the heart continued during adult life.

false ribs. The lower 5 pairs of ribs. SEE: *ribs, vertebrae.*

falx. Any sickle-shaped structure.

   f. cerebel'li. The vertical partition bet. the hemispheres of the cerebellum.

   f. cer'ebri. The falciform process dividing the cerebellar hemispheres.

   f. inguina'lis. BNA. The conjoined or conjoint tendon.

   f. ligamento'sa. The broad ligament of the liver. SYN: *falciform ligament.*

F. A. M. A. Abbr. for *Fellow of the American Medical Association.*

famil'ial. Pert. to or common to the same family, as *familial symptoms.*

family (fam'il-e). 1. A group consisting of parents and their children. 2. In biological classification, the division bet. the *order* and *genus.*

   f., degenerate. One that produces offspring of low or subnormal mentality.

   f., Jukes. A family whose history covers 5 generations of degeneracy.

   f., Kallikak. An American family with 1 branch mentally unfit and another of average intelligence.

fam'ine fever. Relapsing fever.

fang. 1. A sharp-pointed tooth. 2. The root of a tooth.

   f.'s, poison. Two teeth in upper jaw of poisonous reptiles adjacent to their poison glands.

far'ad. A unit of electrical capacity. The capacity of a condenser which, charged with 1 coulomb, gives a difference of potential of 1 volt.

farad'ic. Pert. to induced electricity.

   f. contrac'tion, graduated. Produced by Smart or Bristow coils.

far'adism. The therapeutic use of an interrupted current to stimulate muscles and nerves. Such a current is derived from the secondary or induction coil.

faradiza'tion. The treatment of nerves or muscles with the faradic current; the condition of nerves or muscles so treated.

faradother'apy. Treatment of disease by the faradic current.

farastan (far'a-stan). A combination of iodine and cinchophen.

   DOSAGE: 3¾ gr. (0.25 Gm.) with same caution as with cinchophen.

far'cy. A form of glanders.

   f. bud. A glanderous tumor.

   f., button. Farcy marked by dermal tubercular nodules.

farina (far-i'nă). Meal or flour; also, cornstarch.

farina'ceous. 1. Starchy. 2. Pert. to flour.

far-point. The farthest point of vision at which objects can be distinctly seen with eyes in complete relaxation.

Farre's tubercles (fars). Carcinomatous masses on surface of the liver.

far-sight'ed. Pert. to far-sightedness. SYN: *hypermetropic, hyperopic.*

far-sight'edness. An error of refraction in which, with accommodation completely relaxed, parallel rays come to a focus behind the retina. SYN: *hypermetropia, hyperopia.*

fascia (fash'i-a) (pl. *fasciae*). 1. A fibrous membrane covering, supporting, and separating muscles. 2. A bandage. They also unite the skin to underlying tissue.

   f., anal. Fascia of connective tissue covering levator ani muscle from the perineal aspect.

   f., Buck's. A fascial covering of the penis, derived from Colles' fascia.

   f., cervical, deep. Fascia of the neck covering the muscles, vessels, and nerves.

   f., c., superficial. Fascia of the neck just inside the skin.

   f., Cloquet's. Femoral fascia.

   f., Colles'. Inner layer of the perineal fascia.

   f., cremasteric. Fascia covering the cremaster muscle of the spermatic cord.

   f., cribriform. The fascia of the thigh covering the saphenous opening.

   f., dentata. Gray matter in the cerebral dentate convolution.

   f., infundibuliform. Funnel-shaped fascia, derived from interior abdominal wall, encasing the spermatic cord and testis.

   f., intercolumnar. Fascia derived from external abdominal ring sheathing the spermatic cord and testis.

   f., ischiorectal. SEE: *anal fascia.*

   f. lata. Wide covering encasing thigh muscles.

   f., lumbodorsal. Deep investing membrane covering deep muscles of the trunk and back.

   f., pectineal. Pubic section of fascia lata.

   f., pelvis. Fascial tissues of extreme

importance in the maintenance of normal strength in the pelvic floor. SEE: *pelvic diaphragm under "diaphragm."*

f., thyrolaryngeal. Fascia covering thyroid gland.

f., transversalis. Fascia located between perineum and transversalis muscle.   [ture of fascia.

fascial (fash'e-al). Pert. to or of the na-

f. reflex. Muscular contraction resulting from percussing facial fascia.

fasciaplasty (fash'ĭ-ă-plas″tĭ). Plastic surgery of fascia.

fascicular (fas-sik'u-lar). 1. Arranged like a bundle of rods. 2. Pert. to a fasciculus.

fasciculus (fa-sik'u-lus) (pl. *fasciculi*). A bundle of nerve or muscle fibers. SYN: *fasciola.*

f., cuneate. Wedge-shaped continuation of spinal cord's dorsolateral column into medulla oblongata. SYN: *Burdach's tract.*

f., fundamental. Portion of ant. column of spinal cord continuing into medulla oblongata.

f. gracilis. Continuation of dorsomedian column of spinal cord into medulla oblongata.

f. macularis. Fasciculus in optic nerve.

f., olivary. Fasciculus extending toward back of olivary body.

f., posterior longitudinal. Nerve fiber bundle running bet. corpora quadrigemina and nuclei of 4th and 6th nerves.

f., pyramidal. Section of ant. spinal cord column continuing to the pyramid.

f. of Rolando. Head of post. horn of medulla oblongata's gray substance.

f., solitary. Nerve fiber bundle in post. part of the internal capsule.

f. teres. Column on both sides of median furrow on 4th ventricle's floor.

f. unciformis. Fibers within sylvian fissure connecting frontal and temporosphenoid lobes.

fasciectomy (fă-shĭ-ek'to-mĭ). Excision of strips of fascia.

fasciod'esis. Operation of attaching a fascia to a tendon or another fascia.

fasciola (fă-se'o-lă). A bundle of nerve or muscle fibers. SYN: *fasciculus, q.v.*

f. cinerea. Upper portion of fascia dentata.

Fasci'ola. A genus of flukes or Trematoda.

fasci'olar. Pert. to the fasciola cinerea.

fascioliasis (fas-she-o-li'as-is). Infection of the body with a genus of trematode worms. SYN: *distomiasis.*

fas'cioplasty. Plastic operation on a fascia.

fasciorrhaphy (fash-ĭ-or'af-ĭ). Suturing a fascia.

fasciotomy (fash-ĭ-ot'o-mĭ). Surgical incision and division of a fascia.

fascitis (fash-i'tis). Inflamed condition of a fascia.

fast. Resistant to toxic agents or staining; said of bacteria and certain immunizing agents.

fastidium (fas-tid'ĭ-um). Aversion to food or to eating.

Sometimes seen in hysteria but not as the result of delusions.

fastigatum (fas-tig-a'tum). The gray matter on both sides of the inf. vermiform process of the cerebellum. SYN: *nucleus fastigii.*

fastigium (fas-tij'ĭ-um). The highest point. The full period of development of acute, infectious diseases when the temperature reaches the maximum or *stadium* and all symptoms have developed.

fast'ing. Going without food for a stated period.   [tive agents.

fast'ness. Resistance to stains or destruc-

fat. 1. CHEM: A carbon compound consisting of a combination of the trihydric alcohol glycerol with fatty acids such as stearic. Glyceryl tristearate, stearin, is $C_3H_5(C_{17}H_{35}COO)_3$. 2. Adipose, obese, corpulent. 3. Greasy, oily.

f. column. Layer of adipose tissue between subcutaneous tissue and hair follicles and sweat glands.

f. low diet. Approximately 40 to 50 Gm. fat daily. SEE: *reduction diet.*

f. and protein-free diet. 1. Carbohydrates. 2. Honey. 3. Fruit juices. 4. Juicy fruits. 5. Melons. 6. Cucumbers. 7. Marmalades and jellies. 8. Rhubarb. 9. Fresh tomatoes.

fatigue (fa-tēg'). Lassitude, tiredness, weariness. The normal weariness of overexertion and also the pathological exhaustion of physical and psychic disease.

f. diseases. Those caused by the constant repetition of specific muscular movements.

f. fever. SEE: *fatigue disease.*

f. muscles. Those in which there is an accumulation of waste substances acting as poisons, and which suffer from the loss of nutritive material as the result of fatigue.

f. poisons. Toxins causing fatigue.

f. reaction. In tuberculosis, an elevation of temperature following exertion.

fatty acid. The combination of glycerine and an acid, such as stearic, palmitic, oleic, or butyric acid.

f. casts. Mass of fat droplets arranged frequently in groups and probably remains of a true epithelial cast.

f. degeneration. A change involving the deposition of fat in the cytoplasm. SEE: *fat, heart.*

fauces (faw'ses). The aperture leading from the mouth into the pharynx, or cavity of the throat.

fau'cial. Pert. to the fauces.

f. reflex. Gagging or vomiting resulting from irritation of fauces.

faucitis (faw-si'tis). Inflammation of the fauces.

faveolate (fav-e'o-lāt). Honeycombed. SYN: *alveolate.*

fave'olus. A depression or small pit, esp. on the skin.

favus (fa'vus). Contagious skin disease characterized by pinhead to pea-sized, saucer-shaped, yellowish crust usually over hair follicles and accompanied by musty odor and itching. It may spread all over the body.

F. C. S. Abbr. for *Fellow of the Chemical Society.*

Fe. Chem. symb. for iron (*ferrum*).

fear. PSY: Primitively, the emotional reaction to an environmental threat, it now also presents itself frequently as an indicator of inner problems.

febricide (feb'ri-sīd). Destructive to fever. SYN: *antipyretic.*

febric'ula. Mild fever of short duration without other pathology.

febrifacient (feb-ri-fa'si-ent). Producing fever.

febrific (fĕ-brif'ĭk). Producing or conveying fever.

febrifugal (feb-rif'u-gal). Reducing fever.

febrifuge (feb'ri-fūj). That which lessens fever. SYN: *antipyretic.*

feb'rile. Feverish; pert. to a fever. SEE: *fever.*

   f. state. A term used to describe constitutional symptoms which accompany a rise in temperature. Pulse and respiration usually rise with headache, pains, malaise, loss of appetite, concentrated and diminished urine, constipation, restlessness, hot dry skin, insomnia, irritability.

febripho'bia. Anxiety or fear induced by a rise in body temperature.

febris (fe'bris). Fever.

   f. acmastica. Continued fever.

   f. acuta. Ague.

   f. castrensis. Typhus and remittent fever.

   f. enterica. Typhoid fever.

   f. flava. Yellow fever.

   f. lactea. Milk fever.

   f. remittens. Remittent fever.

   f. undulans. Malta fever.

   f. variolosa. A form of smallpox.

fe'cal. Pert. to, or of the nature of, feces.

   f. vomit. Feces in vomitus.

   ETIOL: Strangulated hernia or intestinal obstruction preventing anal outlet.

fecalith (fe'kal-ith). A fecal concretion. SYN: *coprolith.*

fecaloid (fe'kal-oid). Resembling feces.

fecaloma (fe-kal-o'mă). A fecal tumor in the rectum. SYN: *coproma, scotoma, stercoroma.*

fecalu'ria. Fecal matter in the urine.

feces (fe'sez). Stools; excreta; dejecta; excrement. Body waste, such as food residue, bacteria, epithelium, and mucus, discharged from the bowels by way of the anus.

   f., sheep. Small masses broken off from stonelike feces remaining in colon too long.

Fe(C₃H₅O₃)₂. Ferrous lactate; lactate of iron.

Fe(C₆H₅O₇). Citrate of iron.

Fechner's law (fek'nerz). The magnitudes of sensation produced by given stimuli form an arithmetical progression, the stimuli forming a geometrical progression. SYN: *psychophysical law.*

FeCl₂. Ferrous chloride.

FeCl₃. Ferric chloride.

FeCO₃. Ferrous carbonate; carbonate of iron.

fec'ula. 1. Sediment. 2. Starch.

feculent (fek'u-lent). Having sediment.

fecundate (fe'kun-dāt). To fertilize or impregnate or render fertile.

fecundation (fe-kun-da'shun). Impregnation; fertilization.

   f., artificial. Impregnation by injecting the seminal fluid into the uterus by mechanical means.

fecundity (fe-kun'dit-ĭ). Ability to produce offspring; fertility.

feeblemind'edness. Arrested mental development as distinguished from temperamental abnormality.

feed'ing. Taking or giving nourishment, esp. extraorally.

   The latter is sometimes necessary because the patient either refuses or is unable to eat.

   f., artificial. This is accomplished through the *nostrils*, the *esophagus*, and the *rectum;* also through *gastrostomy* or *duodenostomy.*

   f., colonic. Less useful with psychotic than with physically sick patients but at times it can be utilized. It is now somewhat questionable owing to the limited ability for absorption in the colon.

   f., esophageal. Used after operations on tongue or jaw, diseases of mouth, in mental cases, and forcible feedings. Mouth gag needed in last 2 cases. Also used for test meals.

   f., forcible. This is by way of esophagus or rectum.

   f., nasal. Largely used for children, and when unable to take nourishment normally, such as in delirium, coma, and stupor, diseases of mouth and pharynx. Any strained liquid food that will pass through catheter can be used. Temperature of feeding, 100° F. Olive oil and swabs needed for cleaning nostrils.

   f., rectal. Commonest form used although it is admitted that little nourishment can be absorbed through colon.

   f., tube. Done through the mouth or nostril, the latter requiring a much smaller tube and a little more dexterity, but less likely to be successfully resisted.

feel'ing. The conscious phase of nervous activity. The (a) emotions or centrally stimulated feelings and (b) those sensations peripherally produced by excitation of peripheral nerves including those of the special senses.

feet (pl. of *foot*). The pedal extremities of the legs.

Fehl'ing's solution. A commercial solution for detecting the presence of sugar in the urine. It consists of pure copper sulfate, sulfuric acid, and distilled water; or Rochelle salts in sodium hydroxide solution.

   F.'s test. Add a few drops of urine to 5 cc. of the hot solution, and continue to add the drops until there is an equal amount of urine and solution. The presence of a red or yellow precipitate reveals sugar. If the solution stands the sugar will be precipitated to the bottom. SEE: *sugar, test for in urine*.

fel. Bile.

   f. bo'vis. Ox gall. USP. Dried fresh bile of the ox, used principally in form of an extract.
   DOSAGE: 6 gr. (0.4 Gm.).
   SYN: *bilis bovina*.

fellatio (fel-a'shi-o). A form of sex perversion in which gratification is accomplished by buccal intromission of the penis; buccal coitus.

fel'on. Suppuration of terminal joint of a finger. SYN: *paronychia,* runround, whitlow*.

felt'work. 1. Fibrous network. 2. A plexus of nerve fibrils. SYN: *neuropilem*.

fe'male. 1. A woman or girl-child. 2. Pert. to a woman. SEE: *genitalia, female*.
   f. sex hormone. Hormone secreted by the ova which develops the uterus, vagina, and breasts at puberty, aids in regeneration of mucosa following menstruation, stimulates uterine contraction. SYN: *estrin, q.v.*

fem'inin. The female sex hormone. SYN: *estrin*.

fem'inism. 1. The female character. 2. Possession of female characteristics by the male. 3. Social movement for female independence.

feminiza'tion. Adoption of female characteristics.

fem'inonu'cleus. Nucleus of the impregnated ovum. SYN: *thelyblast*.

fem'oral. Pert. to the thigh bone or femur.
   f. artery. One beginning at *ext. iliac artery*, terminating behind the knee as the popliteal artery, on inner side of femur.
   f. reflex. Extension of knee and flexion of foot resulting from irritation of skin over upper ant. third of thigh.
   f. vein. Continuation of the popliteal vein upward toward the *ext iliac vein*. SYN: *crural vein*.

fem'orocele. Femoral hernia.

femorotib'ial. Rel. to the femur and tibia.

fe'mur. The thigh bone.
   It extends from the hip to the knee and is the longest and strongest bone in the skeleton.

fenes'tra (pl. *fenestrae*). 1. An aperture frequently closed by a membrane. 2. An open area, as in the blade of a forceps.
   f. ovalis. Windowlike oval opening in inner wall of middle ear closed by the 3 ossicles.
   f. rotunda. Round opening in inner wall of middle ear.

fen'estrated. Having openings.
   f. membrane of Henle. Elastic tissue layer in intima of larger arteries.

fenestra'tion. Condition of having fenestra.

ferment'. 1. To decompose. 2. (fer'ment). A substance capable of producing fermentation in other substances. SYN: *enzyme, q.v.*

fermenta'tion. Decomposition of carbohydrates; the process of converting sugar into alcohol and carbon dioxide through

the action of a ferment, heat, air, and moisture.
   f., alcoholic. That in which certain sugars, esp. glucose, are converted into alcohol and carbon dioxide.
   f., acetic. A continuation of alcoholic fermentation.
   f., amylolyt'ic. The process of hydrolyzation of starch with the formation of sugar.
   f., autolyt'ic. One in the tissues which disintegrates them after death.
   f., diastat'ic. Same as amylolytic fermentation.
   f., invertin. One that converts cane sugar into dextrose and levulose by invertin.
   f., lactic. That which sours milk.
   f., proteolyt'ic. One that changes protein into a peptone or to simpler structures.
   f. test. A confirmation test for sugar in the urine. Gas forms in the fermentation tube if sugar is present.
   f., viscous. Production of gelatinous material by different forms of bacilli.

fermentemia (fer-men-te'mĭ-ă). The presence of a ferment in the blood.

fermentogen (fer-men'to-jen). Any substance which, by proper stimulus, such as pepsinogen, may be converted into a ferment.

fermen'toid. A ferment without fermentive power.

fermentum (fer-men'tum). Yeast; a ferment.

-ferous. Suffix meaning producing.

fer'ratin. Organic iron compound found in the body tissues.
   DOSAGE: 5-15 gr. (0.3-1.0 Gm.).

Ferrein's pyramids (fe'rīnz). Medullary rays of a cortical kidney lobule.
   F.'s tubule. Convoluted kidney tubules.

ferri-, ferro-. Prefix used to indicate *presence of iron*.

fer'ric. Pert. to or containing iron. SYN: *ferruginous*.

fer'ric ammo'nium cit'rate. USP. Thin, garnet-red crystals, containing about 17% of iron.
   DOSAGE: 10-30 gr. (0.6-2 Gm.).
   f. amm. cit. virides. USP. Thin green scales or granules, containing approximately 15% iron.
   DOSAGE: ¼-1½ gr. (0.015-0.1 Gm.).
   f. chlor'ide ($FeCl_3$). USP. Used principally in form of tincture.
   DOSAGE: 10 ℳ (0.6 cc.) freely diluted.

ferrom'eter. Device for estimating proportion of iron in the blood.

ferropectic (fer-o-pek'tik). Pert. to fixing iron.

ferropexia (fer-o-pek'sĭ-ă). Iron fixation.

ferrous (fer'ous). Pert. to iron. SYN: *ferruginous*.

fer'rous car'bonate ($FeCO_3$). Iron carbonate, used chiefly in form of Blaud's pills.
   DOSAGE: 5-10 gr.
   f. i'odide (FeI_2). USP. An unstable preparation of iron used in form of

syrup. Should be transparent, pale or yellowish-green liquid.

DOSAGE: 15 ℳ (1 cc.).

f. sulfate (FeSo₄). USP. Green vitriol. Pale, bluish-green crystals.

DOSAGE: 2-5 gr. (0.13-0.32 Gm.).

ferruginous (fer-ru′jin-us). Pert. to or containing iron. SYN: *chalybeate.*

fer′rule. A band or ring of metal applied to the end of root or crown of a tooth to strengthen it.

fer′rum. SYMB: Fe. Iron.

fer′tile. 1. Impregnated. 2. Capable of reproduction.

fertility (fûr-tĭl′ĭ-tĭ). Quality of being productive or fertile.

fertiliza′tion. 1. Fecundation; impregnation of an ovum with the spermatozoon of the male, the male sex cell being carried in the seminal discharge.

2. BOT: Union of pollen with the ovule in plants.

fervescence (fer-ves′ens). Increase of fever.

fes′ter. To become inflamed and suppurate.

festina′tion. Morbid acceleration of gait seen in some nervous afflictions such as paralysis agitans.

festoon (fes-tōōn′). The wreathlike curvature of the gums around the necks of the teeth.

fe′tal. Pert. to a fetus.

fetalism (fe′tal-izm). Retention of fetal structures after birth.

feta′tion. Pregnancy.

feticide (fe′tĭ-sīd). Intentional destruction of fetal life.

fet′id. Rank or foul in odor.

fetish, fetich (fe′tish). That which attracts one of the opposite sex to another, or which excites the libido.

fe′tishism. 1. Belief in some object as possessing power, or being capable of inspiring a stimulus. 2. Substitution for a normal love object (a person) of parts or possessions of such a one. Libido gratification from contact with articles of dress, braid of hair, etc.

fetom′etry. Estimation of size of the fetus or its head before delivery.

fetoplacen′tal. Pert. to the fetus and its placenta.

fe′tor. Stench; an offensive odor.

fe′tus. The child *in utero* after the 3rd month of development.

f. papyraceous. In twin pregnancy, the dead fetus pressed flat by the development of the living twin.

fe′ver. Pyrexia, or elevation of temperature above normal, 98.6° F.

CLASSIFICATION (Wunderlich): (a) Subfebrile, 99.5°-100.4°; (b) slightly febrile, 100.4°-101.3°; (c) moderately febrile, 101.3°-103.1°; (d) decidedly febrile, 103.1°-104°; (e) highly febrile, 103.1° A. M., 104.9° P. M.; (f) hyperpyretic, above 106°.

f., childbed. Puerperal sepsis. An infection of the genital tract following childbirth. SEE: *puerperium.*

f., continuous. As in scarlet fever, typhus, or pneumonia, in which there is a slight diurnal variation.

f. delirium. It corresponds to (a) the degree of temperature, (b) to the activity of the toxin giving rise to the fever, (c) to the rapidity of tissue change, (d) to the extent of circulatory disturbance, and (e) to the previous habits of the individual.

f., induced. That artificially produced to favorably modify the course of a disease, notably paresis. Sustained fever of 105° F., or even higher, maintained for 6 to 8 or 10 hours may be induced by the use of medical diathermy, etc. The production of malaria, and of rat-bite fever permit of a series of fever-reactions of fairly long duration, while protein injections are capable of arousing only acute and, at times, dangerous febrile reactions.

f., intermittent. As in malaria and Malta fever with minimum normal or subnormal temperature, and with marked diurnal variation.

f., remittent. As in typhoid fever, septic fever, or remittent fever, with minimum temperature above normal, and with marked diurnal variation.

f., septic. One due to septic matter in the body.

fi′at (pl. *fi′ant*). "Let there be made," a term used in writing prescriptions.

fi′ber. Threadlike or filmlike element, as a nerve fiber. A neurone or the axonal portion of a neurone.

f., accelerator. One causing increased heart pulsations.

f., afferent. One carrying incoming impulses to nerve cells.

f., efferent. One carrying outgoing impulses.

f., epicritic. One carrying sensations of heat and cold, making possible tactile discrimination and light pressure sensation, each according to its separate fibers.

f., inhibitory. One causing slower heart action.

f., medullated; f., myelinated. Nerve fiber in which axis cylinder is sheathed in myelin.

f., nonmedullated; f., unmyelinated. Nerve fiber in which there is no myelin sheath bet. axis cylinder and neurilemma.

f., nerve. The part of a nerve cell which carries impulses. SEE: *nerve.*

f., protopathic. One causing sensation of heat, cold, or pain.

fi′bra. A fiber.

fibralbu′min. Globulin.

fibremia (fī-bre′mĭ-ă). Fibrin formed in the blood, causing embolism or thrombosis. SYN: *inosemia.*

fi′bril. A small fiber.

f., nerve. Tiny filament found in cytoplasm of nerve cell.

fibril′la (pl. *fibrillae*). A fibril or small fiber.

fibril′lar, fib′rillary. Pert. to, or consisting of, fibrils.

fib′rillated. Composed of minute fibers. SYN: *fibrillar, fibrous.*

fibrillation (fi-bril-a′shun). 1. The formation of fibrils. 2. Quivering of muscular fibers. 3. Tremor or rapid action of the heart.

    f., auric′ular. Rapid contraction of the atrium without disturbance of rhythm. The opposite of ventricular fibrillation.

    f., ventric′ular. Irregularity in force and rhythm of the heart.

fibrillolysis (fi-bril-ol′is-is). Dissolution of fibrils.

fibrillolyt′ic. Dissolving fibrils.

fibril′oceptor. A receptor receiving stimuli at the terminals of neurofibrils.

fibrin. A nitrogenous, whitish, elastic substance formed by the action of thrombin on fibrinogen, causing the blood to clot.

    f. ferment. The substance in shed blood that converts fibrinogen to fibrin. SYN: *thrombin.*

fibrination (fib-rin-a′shun). Abnormal amt. of fibrin in the blood.

fibrinemia (fi-brin-e′mĭ-ă). Presence of fibrin in the blood. SYN: *fibremia.*

fibrinocel′lular. Consisting of fibrin and cells.

fibrinogen (fi-brin′o-jen). A protein which can be prepared from circulating blood and which, during clotting, is changed into fibrin.

fibrinogen′ic, fibrinog′enus. Producing fibrin.

fi′brinoid. Resembling fibrin.

fibrinolysin (fi-brin-ol′is-in). A substance formed in the blood which dissolves fibrin.

fibrinol′ysis. The redissolving of a blood clot due to a solution of fibrin.

fibrinolyt′ic. Pert. to the splitting up of fibrin.

fibrinope′nia. Fibrin and fibrinogen deficiency in the blood.

fibrinoplas′tic. Of the nature of fibrinoplastin.

fibrinoplas′tin. A globulin in blood serum and other body fluids. SYN: *paraglobulin.*

fibrinopu′rulent. Consisting of pus and fibrin.

fibrinos′copy. Physical and chemical examination of the fibrin of blood clots and exudates. SYN: *inoscopy.*

fibrino′sis. Excess of fibrin in the blood.

fibrinous (fi′brin-us). Pert. to, of the nature of, or containing, fibrin.

fibrinuria (fi-brin-u′rĭ-ă). Passage of fibrin in the urine.

fibro-. Prefix: Relation to fibers or fibrous tissues.

fibroadenia (fi-bro-a-de′nĭ-ă). Fibrous degeneration of glandular tissue.

fibroadenoma (fi-bro-ad-e-no′mă). Adenoma with fibrous tissue forming a dense stroma.

fibroad′ipose. Being fibrous and fatty.

fibroangio′ma. A fibrous tissue angioma.

fibroareolar (fi-bro-ar-e′o-lar). With fibrous tissue and areolar arrangement.

fi′broblast. Any cell or corpuscle from which connective tissue is developed. SYN: *desmocyte, fibrocyte.*

fibroblastoma (fi-bro-blas-to′mă). Tumor of connective tissue or fibroplastic cells.

fibrobronchi′tis. Croupous bronchitis.

fibrocarcino′ma. A carcinoma in which the trabeculae are resistant and thickened with granular degeneration of the cells.

    f. cysticum. A fibrocarcinoma with enclosed cysts.

fibrocar′tilage. A cartilage in which more or less elastic or white fibrous connective tissue is found in its matrix.

fibrocel′lular. Both fibrous and cellular. SYN: *fibroareolar.*

fibrochondritis (fi′bro-kon-dri′tis). Inflammation of fibrocartilage.

fibrochondro′ma. Tumor of fibrous tissue and cartilage.

fi′brocyst. A fibrous tumor that has undergone cystic degeneration or one which has accumulated fluid in the interspaces.

fibrocystic (fi-bro-sis′tik). 1. Consisting of fibrocysts. 2. Fibrous with cystic degeneration.

fibrocysto′ma. Fibroma combined with cystoma.

fibrocyte (fi′bro-sīt). A fibrous tissue cell. SYN: *desmocyte, fibroblast.*

fibrocytogenesis (fi-bro-si-to-jen′es-is). The growth of connective tissue fibrils.

fibroelas′tic. Partly composed of fibrous elastic tissue.

fibroenchondroma (fi-bro-en-kon-dro′mă). An enchondroma containing fibrous elements.

fibrofat′ty. Having fibrous tissue and fat corpuscles.

fi′brogen. A protein which can be prepared from circulating blood and which, during clotting, is changed into fibrin.

fibroglia (fi-bro′glĭ-ă). Basement substance of connective tissue.

fibroglio′ma. A fibroma partly glioma.

fi′broid. 1. Containing or resembling fibers. SEE: *degeneration.* 2. A tumor made up of fibrous and muscular tissue. SYN: *fibroma.*

    f., interstitial. Tumor in muscular wall of uterus which may grow inward and form a *polypoid fibroid,* or outward and become a *subperitoneal fibroid.*

    f., uterine. Caused by disturbed balance bet. follicular and luteal hormones.

fibroidectomy (fi-broi-dek′to-mĭ). Surgical removal of a fibroid tumor.

fibrolipo′ma. A lipoma having much fibrous tissue.

fibro′ma (pl. *fibromata*). A fibrous, encapsulated, connective tissue tumor.

    f. of breast. A benign tumor, nonulcerative and painless.

    f., intramural. Located in muscle tissue of uterus bet. peritoneal coat and endometrium.

    f. molluscum pedunculum of vulva. A pedunculated fibroid tumor of the vulva.

    f., submucous. Encroaching upon endometrial cavity; sessile or pedunculated.

    f., subserous. Lying beneath peritoneal coat of uterus, often pedunculated.

f., uterine. A fibroid tumor of the uterus.

fibromatosis (fi″bro-mă-to′sis). Abnormal formation of fibrous tissue. SYN: *fibrosis.*

fibromatous (fī-brō′mă-tŭs). Pert. to, or of the nature of, a fibroma.

fibromectomy (fi-bro-mek′to-mǐ). Removal of a fibroid tumor.

fibromem′branous. Having both fibrous and membranous tissue.

fibromus′cular. Consisting of muscle and connective tissue.

fibromyi′tis. Inflammation of the muscular system followed by fibrous degeneration of muscular fibers and atrophy.

fibromyoma (fi-bro-mi-o′mă). 1. Fibrous tissue myoma. 2. GYN: A fibroid tumor of the uterus that contains more fibrous than muscle tissue.

fibromyomectomy (fi-bro-mi-o-mek′to-mǐ). Removal of a fibromyoma from the uterus, leaving that organ in place.

fibromyosi′tis. Chronic muscular inflammation with hyperplasia of connective tissue. SYN: *inomyositis.*

fibromyotomy (fi-bro-mi-ot′o-mǐ). Opening of a fibroid tumor.

fibromyxoma (fi-bro-miks-o′mă). A fibroma that has partially undergone myxomatous degeneration.

fibromyxosarco′ma. 1. A sarcoma containing fibrous and myxoid tissue. 2. A mucoid degenerated sarcoma.

fibroneuroma (fi″bro-nu-ro′mă). A mixed neuroma and fibroma. SYN: *inoneuroma.*

fibroösteoma (fi″brō-ŏs-tē-ō′mă). Tumor containing bony and fibrous elements.

fibropapilloma (fi″bro-pă-pǐ-lo′mă). A mixed fibroma and papilloma sometimes occurring in the bladder.

fibropericardi′tis. Fibrinous pericarditis.

fibropla′sia. The development of fibrous tissue, as in wounds.

fibroplas′tic. Giving formation to fibrous tissue.   [coma.

f. tumor. Small spindle-celled sar-

fibroplastin (fi-bro-plas′tin). A globulin in blood serum and other body fluids. SYN: *fibrinoplastin, paraglobulin.*

fibropsammo′ma. A tumor containing fibromatous and psammomatous tissue.

fibropu′rulent. Pus containing flakes of fibrous tissue.

fibrosarco′ma. A spindle-celled sarcoma containing much connective tissue.

fibrosis (fi-bro′sis). Abnormal formation of fibrous tissue.

f., arteriocapillary. Arteriolar and capillary fibroid degeneration.

f. of lungs. Formation of scar tissue in connective tissue framework of lungs following inflammation, pneumonia, and in pulmonary tuberculosis.

f. uteri. A condition of the uterus manifested by excess of fibrous tissue, predominating symptom being menorrhagia.*

fibrositis (fi-bro-si′tis). Interstitial myositis.

fibrous (fi′brus). Composed of or containing fibers; as in contradistinction to (osseous) bony composition.

fibrot′ic. Marked by or pert. to fibrosis.

fib′ula. BNA. Calf bone (*peroneal bone*). One of the longest and thinnest bones of the body. The outer and smaller bone of the leg from the ankle to the knee, articulating above with the tibia, and below with the tibia and astragalus. SEE: *peroneal, peroneus, tibia.*

fib′ular. Rel. to the fibula.

fibulocalcaneal (fib″u-lo-kal-ka′ne-al). Pert. to the fibula and calcaneus, or *os calcis.*

field. A specific area in relation to an object.

f., au′ditory. The space or distance within the limit of hearing.

f. of vision. That portion of space which the fixed eye can see.

fifth cranial nerve. Trigeminus or trifacial nerve, *q.v.*

f. ventricle. Space separating layers of septum lucidum.

fila (fi′lă). Plural of *filum, q.v.*

filaceous (fil-a′she-us). Composed of filaments. SYN: *filamentous.*

fil′ament. A threadlike structure; a fine fiber.

f., spermatic. A spermatozoon, esp. its tail.

filamen′tous. BIOL: Made up of long, interwoven or irregularly placed filaments.

Filaria (fil-a′rǐ-ă). A genus of parasitic nematode worms.

F. Bancrof′ti. Long, whitish, filiform worms. SYN: *Filaria sanguinis hominis.*

F. san′guinis hom′inis. SEE: *Filaria Bancrofti.*

fila′rial. Pert. to or caused by Filariae.

filariasis (fil-ar-i′as-is). A chronic disease due to one of the Filariae.

filarici′dal. Pert. to that which is destructive to Filaria.

filaricide (fi-lar′ǐ-sīd). That which destroys Filaria.

Filatov's disease. An exanthematous affection resembling scarlatina analogous to German measles.

F.'s spots. Koplik's spots.

fil′iform. 1. BIOL: Pert. to a growth that is uniform along the inoculation line in stab or streak cultures. 2. Hairlike, filamentous.

f. papillae. Smallest tongue papillae.

fil′ipuncture. Insertion of a slender wire or thread in an aneurysm to induce coagulation.

fil′let. 1. A bandage shaped like a loop. 2. Two bundles of sensory fibers in the medulla, pons, and brain. SYN: *lemniscus.*

f. of corpus callosum. Fibers forming white substance of the gyrus fornicatus.

f., olivary. Nerve fasciculus surrounding olivary body.

filling (fǐl′ing). 1. The material for insertion in a tooth cavity; usually gold, amalgam, or cement. 2. The operation of filling tooth cavities.

filmogen (fil′mo-jen). A protective vehicle for applying drugs.

fil′opressure. Pressure on a blood vessel caused by a ligature.

filovaricosis (fi″lo-var-ik-o′sis). Dilatation or thickening of the axis-cylinder of a nerve fiber.

fil′ter. 1. To pass a liquid through any porous substance which holds solid particles suspended. 2. Device for filtering liquids; filtrum. SEE: *absorption, osmosis.**

f. bed. Large scale filter to purify the water supply.

f., Berkefeld. One of diatomaceous earth which will not pass bacteria.

f., infrared. Cell of water and red glass which confines radiation to spectral region from 600 to 1400 mu, red glass alone from 600 to 4000 mu.

f., Kitasato's. Suction variety of filter, using porcelain dilator.

f., Pasteur-Chamberland's. Variety using porcelain tube and pressure to force liquid through.

f. paper. Coarse form of paper used in filtering solutions.

fil′ters. In radiation therapy, screens or various substances which permit passage of some wave lengths while absorbing others.

fil′trable. Capable of passing through the pores of a porcelain filter, through which bacteria cannot pass.

fil′trate. The fluid which has been passed through a filter. The residue is the *precipitate.*

filtra′tion. The process of straining through a filter. SEE: *absorption, filter.*

f. of roentgen rays. The absorption of some of the relatively longer wave lengths of roentgen radiation by placing in the path of the rays some absorbing medium, such as aluminum, copper, or zinc.

filtratometer (fil-tra-tom′et-er). Device for measuring gastric filtrates.

fil′trum. A filter.

fi′lum. A threadlike structure.

f. terminale. A long, slender filament forming end of spinal cord.

fimbria (fim′bri-ă) (pl. *fimbriae*). Any structure resembling fringe.

f. ova′rica. The longest fringelike extremity of the fallopian tubes; extending from the infundibulum close to the ovary.

f. tubae. Fringelike portion at abdominal end of the fallopian tubes.

fimbriate (fim′brĭ-āt). 1. BIOL: Having fingerlike projections. 2. Fringed.

f. body. Corpus fimbriatum.

fim′briated. Fringed.

fimbria′tum. 1. Outer end of the oviduct. 2. White band on edge of the cornu inferius of lateral ventricle of the brain. SYN: *corpus fimbriatum.*

fimbriocele (fim′brĭ-o-sēl). Hernia including the fimbriated portion of the oviduct.

Finsen light. Blue and violet light with heat waves excluded. Used in treatment of lupus and other skin affections.

first aid. The administration of emergency assistance to individuals who have been injured or otherwise disabled, prior to the arrival of a doctor, or transportation to a hospital or doctor's office. In no sense assume to be the substitution for medical care.

first cranial nerve. Olfactory nerve, *q.v.*

fish skin. A condom made of a fish bladder.

f. s. disease. A disease of the skin characterized by increase of the horny layer and deficiency of the skin secretions. SYN: *ichthyosis, q.v.*

fission (fish′un). 1. Splitting into 2 or more parts. 2. Division of a cell; method of cellular reproduction.

fissip′arous. Reproducing by fission.

fissura (fis-u′ră) (pl. *fissurae*). Fissure. SYN: *cleft, sulcus.*

fis′sural. Pertaining to a fissure.

fissure• (fish′ur). 1. A groove or natural division, cleft or slit, deep furrow in the brain. 2. Ulcer or cracklike sore. 3. A break in the enamel of a tooth.

f., anal. A linear cleft on the margin of the anus.

f., auricular. Fissure of petrous portion of the temporal bone.

f. of Bichat. A fissure below the corpus callosum in the cerebellum.

f., Broca's. Fissure encircling the 3rd left frontal convolution.

f., Burdach's. Fissure connecting lateral surface of insula and inner surface of operculum.

f., calcarine. Fissure extending from the cerebrum's occipital end to the occipital fissure.

f., callosomarginal. Fissure dividing the cerebrum into the callosum and margin.

f., central. SEE: *Rolando's fissure.*

f., Clevenger's. Fissure of inferior occipital region.

f.'s, Henle's. Connective tissue areas bet. the muscular fibers of heart.

f., hippocampal. Fissure of brain extending from post. part of corpus callosum to the tip of temporal lobe.

f., interparietal. Fissure separating parietal convolutions of the brain.

f., longitudinal. The deep cleft bet. the 2 hemispheres of the cerebrum.

f., occipitoparietal. The fissure bet. the occipital and parietal lobes of the brain.

f., palpebral. Opening separating the upper and lower eyelids.

f., portal. The opening into the liver on its undersurface; continues into the liver as the portal canal.

f., Rolando's. Fissure separating frontal and parietal lobes.

f., sphenoidal. Fissure separating the wings and body of the sphenoid.

f. of Sylvius. Fissure dividing middle and ant. cerebral lobes.

f., transverse. The fissure bet. the cerebellum and cerebrum of the brain.

f., umbilical. Ant. portion of liver's longitudinal fissure.

f., Wernicke's. Fissure dividing the temporal and parietal lobes from the occipital lobe.

fistula (fis′tu-la). Abnormal tubelike passage from a normal cavity or an abscess to a free surface or to another cavity or abscess.

f., anal. Fistula near the anus.

f., biliary. One through which bile is discharged after a biliary operation.

f., blind. One open at only 1 end.

f., complete. Fistula with both external and internal opening.

f., cervical. An abnormal opening into the cervix uteri.

f., cervicovaginalis laqueatica. Fistula in the vaginal portion of the cervix uteri bet. the uterine canal and the vagina.

f., enterovaginal. One bet. the bowel and vagina.

f., fecal. One in which there is a discharge of feces through the opening.

f., metroperitoneal. Fistula bet. uterine cavity and the peritoneum.

f., parotid. One through which there is an abnormal leakage of saliva onto ext. surface of cheek.

f., perineovaginal. Opening from vagina through the perineum.

f., rectovaginal. Opening bet. rectum and vagina.

f., ureterovaginal. Opening bet. ureter and vagina.

f., vesicouterine. Opening bet. uterus and bladder.

f., vesicovaginal. Opening from bladder into the vagina.

fistulatome (fis′tu-la-tōm). Instrument for incising a fistula.

fistulectomy (fis′tu-lek′to-mĭ). Excision of a fistula. [fistulous.

fistulization (fis″tu-li-za′shun). Becoming

fistuloenterostomy (fis″tu-lo-en-ter-os′to-mĭ). Operative closure of a biliary fistule and formation of new passage of bile into the intestine.

fistulous (fis′tu-lus). Pert. to, or containing, a fistula.

fit (fit). A sudden attack, convulsion, or paroxysm.

fixa′tion. 1. The act of holding or fastening in a fixed position. The condition of being fixed. Immobilizing, making rigid.

2. PSYCH: A phase of psychosexual development in which the libido is arrested at an inferior or presexual level.

f. of complement. The action of a complement, a constituent of fresh blood serum, on an antigen, which, in turn, has been acted on by its antibody. During the uniting of antigen, antibody, and complement, the complement is rendered inactive or destroyed, and this process is known as fixation of complement.

f. forceps. Forceps for holding a part.

f. point. Point of clearest vision, for which eye accommodation is focused.

fix′ative. 1. A substance that serves to make firm or fixed. 2. One used to harden and preserve pathological specimens.

fix′ing. Rapid killing of tissue elements so that their normal living form is preserved.

fix′ity. OB: The stage when the head of the fetus enters the mother's pelvis.

Fl. Symb. of *fluorine.*

flabel′lum. White fibers in form of a fan-shaped bundle in corpus striatum.

flaccid (flak′sid). Relaxed, flabby, having defective or absent muscular tone.

fla′gellant. 1. Pert. to flagella. 2. Pert. to stroking in massage. 3. One who practices flagellation.

flagellate (flaj′el-āt). 1. With 1 or more flagella. 2. A protozoon with 1 or more flagella. [pulsion.

f. cell. One with long cilia for pro-

flagella′tion. 1. Flogging. 2. Massage by strokes. 3. Applying electricity by tapping the body. 4. A form of sexual perversion through which the libido is stimulated by striking the gluteal region with a whip or lashes.

flagellospore (flaj-el′o-spor). A spore with 1 or more flagella. SYN: *flagellula.*

flagel′lula. Flagellated spore. SYN: *flagellospore.*

flagellum (fla-jel′um) (pl. *flagella*). A hairlike, motile process on the extremity of a bacterium or protozoon.

flail joint. One with no ant. post. lateral stability after resection.

flames, inhalation of. SYM: Intense irritation of nose, throat, pharynx, windpipe, and lungs; with choking, coughing, interference with respiration; intense swelling of throat; breathing is markedly limited. **Shock.**

flank. The part bet. ribs and upper border of ilium. SEE: *latus.*

f. bone. The ilium.

flap. A mass of partly detached tissue attached at the base after resection.

f. amputation. A flap covering the end of a part left after an amputation.

f. extraction. Removal of cataract so as to make a flap in the cornea.

flarim′eter. A modified spirometer for estimating vital capacity, blood pressure, heart rate, etc.

flash method. Means of pasteurizing milk by rapidly raising temperature of milk to 178° F., maintaining it there for a few minutes and letting it fall to 40° F.

f. point. The temperature at which a substance will burst into flame.

flatfoot. Abnormal flatness of sole and arch of foot.

f., spasmodic. The foot is held everted by spasmodic contraction of the peroneal muscle.

flat′ness. Resonance heard on percussing over solid organs, or fluid in the thoracic cavity.

flatulence (flat′u-lens). Gas in the digestive tract due to fermentation or decomposition.

flatulent (flat′u-lent). Affected with or caused by gas in the alimentary tract.

fla′tus. 1. Gas in digestive tract. 2. Expiration of air; eructation. SEE: *borborygmus.*

f. tube. A rectal tube to procure expulsion of flatus in distention and before a saline enema.

f. vaginalis. GYN: Expulsion of air from a voluminous vagina.

flave'do. Yellowness, as of the skin; sallowness; jaundice.

flavescent (fla-ves'ent). Yellowish.

fla'vism. Having a yellow tinge to the hair.

flavo-. Prefix: Yellow.

flax'seed. Seed of *Linum usitatis simum.* SYN: *linseed.*

fl. dr. Abbr. of *fluidram.*

flea (flē). Insect of order *Siphonaptera.* It carries the bacillus of plague to humans.

    f. bites. Hemorrhagic puncta* surrounded by erythematous* and urticarial patches, as the result of the injection of their saliva.

    PREVENTION: Dust the skin with powdered camphor or naphthalene.

    f., chigger. The *Dermatophilus penetrans.*

    f., man. *Pulex irritans.*

    f., rat. *Pulex cheopis.*

fleam (flēm). Lancet used in venesection.

Flechsig's areas (flekh'zig). Ant., lateral, and post. areas of each lateral half of the medulla.

fleece of Stilling. Meshwork of white fibers that surrounds the dentate nucleus of the cerebellum.

flesh. The soft tissues of the animal body, esp. the muscles. SEE: *carnivorous, carnophobia, meat, meat poisoning.*

    f., proud. 1. Fungous growth. 2. Excessive granular tissue in a wound or ulcer.

fletch'erism. Taking small amounts of food a time with excessive mastication.   [flexion, bending.

flex. To bend upon itself, as a muscle;

flexibilitas cerea (fleks-ĭ-bil'it-as se're-a). Having the limbs act as if made of plastic material; a muscular reaction to psychic causes.

flexibil'ity. Quality of being bent without breaking; adaptability. SYN: *pliability.*

flex'ible. Capable of being bent without breaking.

flexile (fleks'il). Pliant; flexible.

flexion (flek'shun). The act of bending or condition of being bent, in contrast to extending. SEE: *antecurvature, clawfoot, clawhand.*

flex'oglass. Window glass substitute for transmitting antirachitic rays of sunlight.

flex'or. A muscle that bends a part, in a generally proximal direction; as opposed to an extensor.

flex'ure, flex'ura. A bend.

    f., duodenojejunal. Curve at meeting point of jejunum and duodenum.

    f., hemal. Inclination of vesicles of the cerebrum toward the hemal aspect.

    f., hepatic. The bend on right side forming junction of the ascending with the transverse colon.

    f., lumbar. Ventral curve of back in lumbar area.

    f., sigmoid. The s-like loop (in *left iliac fossa*) of the descending colon as it meets the rectum. SEE: *colon.*

f., splenic. Bend at junction of transverse with descending colon.

flight of ideas. PSY: Continuous but fragmentary stream of talk.

    Connection can be followed but direction is frequently changed, often by chance stimuli from the environment.

flint disease. Deposit of fine particles in the lungs. SYN: *chalicosis.*

floating. Moving about. Out of normal location.

    f. kidney. One movable from its normal bed of fat.

    f. ribs. The 11th and 12th ribs which do not articulate with the sternum.

floats. Glass capsules containing labels to float in an exposed liquid to designate its nature.

floccillation, floccitation (flok-sĭ-la'shun, -ta'shun). Semiconscious pricking at bedclothes in fevers and stupors. SYN: *carphologia, carphology.*

floccose (flok'os). BIOL: Pert. to a growth made up of short and densely but irregularly interwoven filaments.

floc'cular. Pert. to the flocculus of the cerebellum.

floc'culence. State of being flocculent or resembling shreds or tufts of cotton.

flocculent (flok'u-lent). Resembling the white portion of "floating island" or a fluid or culture containing whitish shreds of mucus.

flocculoreac'tion. Flocculation of a serum reaction.

floc'culus (pl. *flocculi*). 1. A lobe below and behind the middle peduncle of the cerebrum on each side of the median fissure. 2. A small tuft of wool-like fibers.

    f. retinae. Ciliary process of retina.

flooding (flŭd'ing). Profuse uterine bleeding.

Flood's ligament. A band of ligaments attached to lower part of lesser tuberosity of the humerus.

floor cell. One of the auditory cells in the floor of the arch of Corti.

flora (flō'ra). 1. Plant life as distinguished from animal life.

    2. Plant life occurring or adapted for living in a specific environment.

flour. Finely ground meal obtained from wheat. SEE: *bread, cereal.*

Flourens' theory (floo-ronz'). That thought is a process dependent upon the entire cerebrum.

flow. 1. Action of flowing; said of liquids. 2. The menstrual discharge. Bleeding from the uterus, but not as profusely as in flooding. SEE: *cholerrhagia, cholorrhea, osmosis.*

flower. That part of a plant which comprises the organs of reproduction. Ex: *anthemis, arnica, matricaria.*

flucticuli (fluk-tik'u-lī) (sing. *flucticulus*). Wavelike markings on lateral wall of 3rd ventricle.

fluctua'tion. A wavy impulse felt in palpation and produced by vibration of body fluid.   [stance.

flu'id. A nonsolid, liquid, or gaseous sub-

    f., amniotic. GYN: The fluid that fills

the fetal membranes in pregnancy. A clear, yellowish fluid. Spec. grav., 1.006. It is composed of albumin, salts (chiefly urea), and water, and suspended in it are lanugo, epidermal cells, *vernix caseosa*, and meconium.*

f. balance. Regulation of amount of water in the body by its controlling mechanism.

f., cerebrospinal.* That found in central canal of spinal cord and in the ventricles of the brain.

f. diet. One for postoperative cases for the first 2 days following an operation, carbonated water, ginger ale, tea, albumin, water, beef tea, broth, coffee. Raw fruit juices and milk should not be given unless ordered. SEE: *liquid diet.*

f. retention. Failure to expel fluids of the body normally. OPP: *fluid balance.*

fluidextract, fluidextractum (flext.). Solution of the soluble constituents of organic drugs of such strength that each cc. represents 1 Gm. of the drug.

flu'idounce. Eight fluidrams. SYMB: f ℥.

flu'idram. Measure of capacity equal to 57.1 gr. of distilled water; equal to 3.70 cc. SYMB: f ℨ.

fluke (flook). One of many kinds of trematode worms parasitic in man.

flu'mina pilo'rum. The curved lines along which the hairs of the body are arranged esp. in the fetus.

flu'or al'bus. White discharge from the uterus or vagina. SYN: *leukorrhea.*

fluorescein (flū-or-es'ein). A red crystalline powder.

fluorescence (flu-or-es'ens). Luminescence of a substance when acted on by short wave radiation.

fluorescent (flu-or-es'ent). 1. BIOL: Having 1 color by transmitted light and another by reflected light. 2. Luminous when exposed to other rays.

f. screen. 1. A sheet of cardboard, paper, or glass coated with a material which fluoresces visibly, such as calcium tungstate, used as the chief part of a fluoroscope when roentgen rays, radium rays, or electrons impinge upon it; a substitute for a fluoroscope in a darkened room. 2. A sheet of cardboard, paper, or glass, coated with anthracene or other fluorescing materials, to observe ultraviolet radiations.

fluoride (flu'or-īd). A compound of fluorine with a radicle; a salt of hydrofluoric acid.

fluorine (flu'or-en). Gaseous, chemical element. SYMB: F. Atomic weight, 19.

fluorometer (flu-o-rom'et-er). Device for adjusting the shadow in skiagraphy.

fluoroscope (flu'or-ō-skōp or flu-or'o-skōp). A device consisting of a fluorescent screen suitably mounted, either separately or in conjunction with a roentgen tube, by means of which the shadows of objects interposed between the tube and the screen are made visible.

fluoros'copy. The use of a fluoroscope for medical diagnosis or for testing various materials by roentgen rays.

fluorosis (flu-or-o'sis). Chronic fluorine poisoning, sometimes marked by mottling of tooth enamel. Often results from too much fluoride in drinking water.

flush. Sudden redness of the skin.

f., hec'tic. Redness of the cheeks seen in some chronic affections, such as pulmonary tuberculosis, and due to rise of temperature.

f., hot. One accompanied with sensation of heat; common in neuroses and psychoneuroses.

flut'ter. A tremulous movement, esp. of the heart, as auricular and ventricular flutter.

flux. 1. Flow of any fluid from a body cavity; diarrhea. 2. Discharge from the bowels.

f., bloody. Dysentery.

f., monthly. The menses.

f., radiant. Radiant power.

fly. Flying insect of the order *Diptera.* It is a carrier of disease.

f., blow. *Calliphora erythrocephala,* one which lays its eggs in wounds, openings of the body, or decaying matter.

f., horse. *Tabanus atratus.* May transmit Filariae and trypanosomes.

f., house. *Musca domestica.* May transmit typhoid, cholera, plague, dysentery, etc.

f., tsetse. *Glossina palpalis.* One which transmits African sleeping sickness or trypanosomiasis.

SEE: *blister.*

F. M. (*fi'at mistu'ra*). Abbr. for "let a mixture be made."

fo'cal. Pert. to a focus.

f. infection. One occurring near a focus, such as the cavity of a tooth.

f. lesion. A limited central lesion.

fo'cus (pl. *foci*). The point of convergence of light rays or waves of sound.

f., real. Point at which convergent rays intersect.

f., virtual. The point at which divergent rays would intersect if prolonged backward.

fog'ging, fog'ging sys'tem. A method of testing vision, used particularly in testing astigmatism, and in postcycloplegic examination. [*plica.*

fold. A ridge; a doubling back. SYN:

f., amniotic. Folded edge of the amniotic membrane where it rises over and finally encloses the embryo.

f., genital. Fold of skin in the embryo on each side of the genital tubercle which develops into the labia minora in the female.

f., mesouterine. Fold of peritoneum supporting the uterus.

fo'lia (pl. of *folium*). Leaves.

foliaceous (fo-li-a'she-us). Resembling or pert. to a leaf.

fo'lian proc'ess. The processus gracilis of the malleus.

folie (fol-e'). Mania; psychosis.

f. circulaire. Frequent repetition of excited and depressed phases of insanity. SYN: *circular insanity.*

f. du doute (fol-e′ du doot). Abnormal doubts about ordinary acts and beliefs; inability to decide upon definite standards of conduct.

folium (pl. *folia*). Thin, broad, leaflike structure.

foll′icle. A small excretory duct or sac or tubular gland.

f., graafian. GYN: Small excretory organ in the cortex of the ovary. The complete development of the primary oocyte to the stage where the ovum is fully developed. SEE: *ovary*.

f., intestinal. Lieberkühn's follicle, *q.v.*

f's., Lieberkühn's. Small tubelike depressions on mucosa of small intestine. SYN: *crypts of Lieberkühn*.

f., lymph. Accumulation of adenoid tissue found mainly on mucous membranes.

f., nabothian. Dilated cyst of the glands of the cervix uteri.

f., sebaceous. Oil gland of the skin.

f., solitary. Secreting lymph follicle of the intestinal mucosa.

folliclis (fol′ik-lis). Indolent papulonecrotic lesion, esp. on the extremities and possibly the face.

follic′ular. Pert. to a follicle or follicles.

f. tonsillitis. Inflammation of follicles on surface of the tonsil which become filled with pus.

f. tumor. A sebaceous cyst.

follic′ulin. An internal secretion of the ovary which, with lutein and ovulin, forms the oophorin hormone. SEE: *estrin*.

folliculitis (fol-ik-u-li′tis). Inflammation of a follicle or follicles.

f. barbae. Inflammation of the follicles of the bearded parts. SEE: *sycosis vulgaris*.

f. decalvans. Purulent follicular inflammation of the scalp resulting in irregular alopecia and scarring. SYN: *acne decalvans, Quinquad's disease*.

f. sebacea. Inflammation of the sebaceous glands, with accumulation of secretion. SYN: *acne*.

folliculoma (fol-ik-u-lo′mă). A tumor of the ovary originating in a graafian follicle, in which the cells resemble the cells of the zona granulosa layer.

folliculose (fol-ik′u-lōs). Composed of follicles.

folliculo′sis. Presence of an abnormal quantity of lymph follicles.

folliculus (fŏ-lik′u-lus) (pl. *fol′liculi*). A follicle.

f. oophorus vesiculosus. A graafian follicle, *q.v.*

fomentation (fo-men-tā′shun). A hot, wet application for the relief of pain or inflammation. SEE: *stupe*.

f., boracic. This may be prepared with boracic lint, which is already impregnated with boracic acid, and is colored pink as a distinguishing mark; or boracic acid may be added to lint, either in form of powder or crystals, and then wrung out of boiling water as before.

f., medical. Instead of lint, 2 or 3 thicknesses of flannel are used, and the fomentation is applied to unbroken skin, otherwise procedure is same as for a surgical fomentation; it is unnecessary to boil it; flannel is used because it retains the heat better than lint. This fomentation is also called a *stupe, q.v.*

f., surgical. SEE: *hot moist dressing*.

fom′es (pl. *fomites*). A porous substance that absorbs and transmits infectious material.

fom′ites (sing. *fomes*). Porous substances capable of absorbing and transmitting infectious material.

Fontan′a's spaces. Spaces bet. the processes of ligamentum pectinatum of the iris.

fontanel, fontanelle (fon-tan-el′). A space, or "soft spots" of unossified bone between sutures of the skull in the fetus and in infants.

Delayed closing is said to be evidence of disease. SYN: *fonticulus*.

f., anterior. At the junction of the coronal, frontal, and sagittal sutures.

f., posterior. At the junction of the sagittal and lambdoid sutures.

fonticulus (fon-tik′u-lus). Unossified bone or space bet. cranial sutures in the fetus and in infants. SYN: *fontanel*.

food. Sing. of *foods, q.v.*

food ball. Gastric stone made up of fruit and vegetable skins, seeds and fibers. SYN: *phytobezoar*.

food fever. Sudden rise in temperature accompanying digestive disturbances in children, supposed to be result of intestinal autointoxication. Lasts from 3 or 4 days to several weeks.

food poisoning. An attack of illness due to some injurious food, drink, or property.

f. p., bacterial. Food poisoning may be caused by: (a) The presence of bacteria; (b) by the poisonous products of bacteria, which is the case in *botulism, q.v.*; (c) paratyphoid germs may be found in the body of some animals, and if the meat from them is not thoroughly cooked it may produce an illness known as paratyphoid.

f. rashes. In those with an idiosyncrasy to some protein, certain rashes may be the only symptom of toxemia.

foods. Nutritive substances necessary to nourish, protect, and maintain the body.

f., analysis of.

f., composition of. 1. Organic foods: Such as (a) proteins, (b) carbohydrates, (c) fats, *q.v.* 2. Inorganic foods: (a) Water, (b) minerals, phosphates, carbonates, chlorides, fluorides, silicates. 3. Refuse: Undigested material such as waste, fiber, cellulose, etc. *Protective Foods:* These are foods containing vitamins A, C, and G, and calcium, such as milk, fruits, and vegetables and, to a lesser degree eggs.

foot. Termination of the leg. SEE: *skeleton*.

f. arches. Four arches: (a) Int. longitudinal; (b) outer longitudinal and (c) 2 transverse ones.

f. bath, mustard. AIM: To aid action

of hot water in relieving congestion in some distant part of the body.

f., fracture of. Should be splinted for about 4 wk., then gradually use foot, but weight should not be borne under 2 months. Arches must be restored.

f., Madura. Bone hypertrophy and degeneration, frequently followed by suppuration or gangrene.

foot candle. Amt. of light radiated 1 ft. from a standard candle. SYN: *light unit.*

footdrop. A falling or dragging of the foot from paralysis of the flexors of the ankle.

foot'ling presentation. Presentation of feet foremost in labor.

foot plate. Base of the stapes; an ossicle of the tympanum.

foot pound. Amt. of energy required to raise 1 pound 1 foot from a level.

forage (for-azh'). Cutting a channel by diathermy through an enlarged prostate.

foramen (for-a'men) (pl. *foram'ina*). A passage or opening; an orifice, a communication between 2 cavities of an organ, or a hole in a bone for passage of vessels or nerves.

f., intervertebral. Opening bet. every 2 articulated vertebrae for passage of nerves to and from spinal cord.

f. magnum. It pierces the occipital bone through which passes the spinal cord from the brain.

f. of Monro. Opening bet. 3rd and lateral ventricles.

f. obturator. Large oval foramen below acetabulum bounded by the pubis and ischium. SEE: *Magendie's foramen.*

f. ova'le. 1. Opening at lower post. of septum in fetus, bet. 2 cardiac auricles. 2. Oval opening in post. margin of great sphenoidal wing, for inf. maxillary nerve and small meningeal artery.

force, unit of Amount of force necessary to move a weight of 1 Gm. 1 cm. in 1 second. SYN: *dyne.*

forceps (for'seps). Pincers for holding, seizing or extracting. There are at least 100 distinct varieties of forceps, varying according to the operation for which they are intended.

forcipate (for'sip-āt). Forceps shaped.

for'cipressure. Arresting hemorrhage by pressure on an artery with forceps.

fore-. Prefix meaning *before* or *in front of.*

forearm (fōr'arm). The part of arm between elbow and wrist.

forebrain (fōr'brān). Ant. portion of the brain of the embryo. SYN: *prosencephalon.*

fore'finger. The first or index finger.

fore'gut. First part of the digestive tube whence pharynx, esophagus, stomach, and duodenum are formed. SYN: *protogaster.*

forehead (for'ed). The brow. SYN: *frons, metopon.*

for'eign bod'ies. Slivers, cinders, dirt, or small objects in the skin, ears, eyes, nose, and internally frequently lead to infection, and if not removed lead to unsightly marks or tattooing of the skin and inflammation of the organ involved.

forensic (for-en'sik). Pert. to the law. legal.

f. medicine. Legal medicine or medicine in relation to the law.

fore'pleasure. A psychoanalysis term indicating substituted sexual gratification or phantasy anticipation of the orgasm

fore'skin. Prepuce* or loose skin at and covering the end of the penis.

-form. Suffix meaning *having the form of*

formaldehyde (for-mal'de-hīd). USP. A colorless, pungent, irritant gas commonly made by oxidation of methyl alcohol; the simplest member of the group of aldehydes.* It is used in medicinal form of a solution of 40% formaldehyde or formalin.

f., casein. Antiseptic product.

f., gelatin. Antiseptic wound dressing

for'malin. Wood alcohol with a 40% content of formaldehyde. SYN: *aldehyde.*

formate (for'māt). A salt of formic acid.

formatio (for-ma'shĭ-ō). A structure with definite arrangement and shape.

f. reticula'ris. Dorsal part of the medulla oblongata.

forme fruste (form früst). An aborted form of disease arrested before running its course.

for'mic. Pert. to ants.

f. acid. Irritant fluid without color which is present in the red ant and some other insects, in some animal secretions, and in the "stings" of the nettle.

DOSAGE: 20-40 ɱ (1.3-2.5) of the spirit.

f. aldehyde. Formaldehyde.

f. ether. Volatile anesthetic liquid.

formica'tion. A sensation as of ants creeping upon the body; a form of paresthesia.

formiciasis (for-mis-i'as-is). Symptoms caused by ant bites.

formilase (for'mil-ās). A ferment which converts acetic acid into formic acid.

formin (for'mĭn). SEE: *methenamine.*

for'mula. 1. A rule prescribing ingredients with proportions for the preparation of a compound. 2. CHEM: An expression by symbols of the constitution of a molecule consisting of letters, each denoting 1 atom of 1 elementary substance, with figures denoting the number of atoms present.

f., Arneth's. Method of estimating number of immature leukocytes by means of an elaborate differential blood count.

f., official. One in a pharmacopeia.

form'ulary. A book of formulas.

f., national. One issued by the *American Pharmaceutical Association.*

for'nicate. 1. Arched or vaultlike. 2. To indulge in unlawful cohabitation.

fornica'tion. The act of illicit sexual intercourse.

for'nicolumn. The ant. pillar of the fornix.

fornicommissure (for-nĭ-kom'is-ŭr). The commissure or body of the fornix uteri.

for'nix (pl. *fornices*). 1. A fibrous, vaulted band connecting the cerebral lobes. 2. Any body with vaultlike or arched shape.

f. conjunctivae. OPHTH: Loose fold

connecting palpebral and bulbar conjunctivae.

f. uteri. Ant. and post. spaces into which the upper vagina is divided. These recesses are formed by protrusion of the cervix uteri into the vagina.

fortifica'tion spectrum. Appearance of dark patch with zigzag outline in visual field. SYN: *scintillating scotoma, teichopsia.*

Foshay's serum. One used in the treatment of tularemia.

fossa (fos'a) (pl. *fossae*). A furrow or shallow depression.

f., axillary. The armpit.

f., Claudius'. Triangular area harboring the ovary.

f., iliac. One of the concavities of the iliac bones of pelvis. The right one contains the appendix.

f. lacrimalis. Hollow of frontal bone holding the lacrimal gland.

f. navicularis. One bet. the hymen and fourchette.

f. ovalis. 1. BNA. Opening in thigh for large saphenous vein. 2. Remnant of embryonic foramen ovale in right cardiac auricle.

f., Rosenmuller's. Depression in pharynx posterior to opening of eustachian tube.

f. supratonsillaris. Space bet. anterior and posterior pillars of the fauces above the tonsil.

fossette (fos-et'). 1. A small depression or fossa. 2. A small but deep corneal ulcer.

foulage (foo-lazh'). Kneading with pressure of the muscles.

fourchet, fourchette (foor-shet'). A tense band or transverse fold of mucous membrane at the post. commissure of the vagina, connecting the post. ends of the labia minora.

fourth cranial nerve. Trochlear nerve, *q.v.*

fovea (fo've-ă). A pit or cuplike depression. SEE: *fossa.*

f. centralis. Pit in the middle of macula lutea.

foveate (fo'vē-āt). Pitted; having depressions.

foveation (fo-ve-a'shun). Pitting, as in smallpox.

foveola (fo-ve'o-la). A minute pit or depression.

Fowler-Murphy method. Elevation of head of bed with tube through an incision in right iliac fossa for drainage in diffuse suppurative peritonitis. Continuous rectal irrigation with a physiological salt solution accompanies the treatment.

Fow'ler's position. This places the patient in a semi-sitting position.

The head of bed may be raised on blocks, pins, or other support, or the backrest may be elevated, or patient may rest upon 4 or 5 pillows. It is more easily maintained if the patient sits in a swing or hammock, made by folding a bedsheet lengthwise, placing center of sheet tightly across the buttocks, with 1 end on each side. The ends are fastened securely at head of the bed, or as high as ends will reach.

F.'s solution. One containing 1% arsenic trioxide.

fractional test meal. A method of examining the gastric contents by withdrawing them at intervals, after a standard meal and subsequently submitting them to chemical analysis.

fracture (frak'tŭr). 1. A sudden breaking of a bone. 2. A broken bone.

fragilitas (fra-jil'i-tas). Fragility.

f. crin'ium. Brittleness, as of the hair, showing splitting and breaking of the shaft. Cause unknown.

f. os'sium. Brittleness of bones. SYN: *osteopsathyrosis.*

f. sanguinis. Blood fragility.

fragil'ity. State of brittleness.

f. of the blood. Tendency of blood corpuscles to divide up or dissolve.

fragmenta'tion. Breaking up into fragments.

frambe'sia. Infectious tropical disease. SYN: *yaws.*

frambesioma (fram-be-zĭ-o'mă). Primary lesion of yaws.

Frankenhäuser's ganglion (frang'ken-hoy-zerz). A nerve ganglion sometimes found in lateral walls of the cervix uteri.

Frank'lin glasses. Bifocal spectacles.

franklin'ic electric'ity. Electricity produced by friction. SEE: *electricity, static.*

Fraunhofer's lines (frown'ho-fer). Dark lines of the solar spectrum.

freckle (frek'l). Small local pigmentation, brownish or yellowish, of the skin.

free associa'tion. 1. Uncontrolled ideas when not under mental restraint or direction. 2. PSY: The procedure which requires the patient to speak aloud his thought flow, word for word, without censorship.

freez'ing. Frigidity of a limb due to cold.

f. microtome. One for cutting frozen objects.

f. mixtures (for ice bags). 5 oz. sal ammoniac, 5 oz. niter and 1 part of water.

Equal parts of sal ammoniac, salt, and niter.

f. point. Temperature at which liquids freeze.

Frei's disease. Venereal disease affecting the inguinal area, chiefly, with formation of buboes. SYN: *lymphogranuloma inguinale or venerea, Nicolas - Favre disease.*

F.'s test. Test given to confirm diagnosis of lymphogranuloma inguinale.

fremitus (frem'it-us). Vibratory tremors felt by palpation through the chest wall.

f., vocal or tactile. The transmission of the vibrations of the voice to the hand.

fre'nal. Pert. to the frenum.

frenose'cretory. Exercising an inhibitory power over the secretions.

frenotomy (fre-not'o-mĭ). Division of any frenum, esp. for tongue-tie.

fren'ulum (pl. *frenula*). A membranous fold acting as a check, as the one (*frenulum linguae*) from the lower gum to the root of tongue. SYN: *vinculum.*

f. clitoridis. The union of inner parts of the labia minora on undersurface of the clitoris, q.v.

f. labiorum pudendi. Fold of membrane connecting post. ends of labia minora.

f. praepu'tii. One that unites the foreskin (prepuce) to the glans penis.

f. of tongue. One attaching lower side of tongue to the gum.

frenum (fre'num) (pl. *frena*). A fold connecting parts and restricting their separation.

f. clitoridis. A stringlike structure at lower border of the 2 layers of the 2 labia minora forming the *praeputium clitoridis.*

f. glandis. Median folds connecting lower surface of glans penis with skin of the body of penis.

f. linguae. Fold on lower side of tongue attached to the gum.

f. puden'di. Membranous fold connecting post. ends of labia minora. SYN: *fourchet.*

fre'quency. The rate of oscillation or alternation in an alternating current circuit, in contradistinction to periodicity in the interruptions or regular variations of current in a direct current circuit.

fret'um of Haller. Constricted space between auricles and ventricles in the fetal heart.

freudian (froy'di-an). Pert. to Sigmund Freud or his theories of unconscious or repressed libido or past sex experiences or desires as the cause of various neuroses, the cure for which is the restoration of such conditions to consciousness through psychoanalysis.

Freund's operation (froyndz). Total abdominal hysterectomy for cancer of uterus. SYN: *laparohysterectomy.*

fri'able. Easily broken or pulverized.

fric'tion (in massage). Strong, circular manipulations always followed by centripetal stroking.

f., dry. Friction using no liquid.

f., moist. Friction using a liquid or oil.

f. murmur, f. sound. A frictional sound heard in pleurisy.

fric'tional electric'ity. Electricity produced by friction. SEE: *electricity, static.*

Friedländer's bacillus (frēd'len-derz). *Bacterium pneumoniae.*

F.'s disease. Extreme degree of fibrous tissue in the intima closing the lumen. SYN: *endarteritis obliterans.*

Fried'man's test. The injection, in 4 cc. doses twice a day for 2 days, of the urine of a woman suspected of pregnancy into an unmated female rabbit will cause the formation of corpora lutea and corpora hemorrhagica in the rabbit at the end of 2 days if the woman is pregnant. [spastic spinal paralysis.

Fried'mann's disease. Relapsing infantile

Fried'reich's ataxia (freed'rix). Rare disease resembling locomotor ataxia occurring in the children of a family, esp. girls. SYN: *family ataxia, hereditary ataxia.*

F.'s disease. SEE: *Friedreich's ataxia.*

F.'s sign. Sudden collapse of the cervical veins previously distended, at each diastole, caused by an adherent pericardium.

fright. Extreme, sudden fear.

f. neuroses. Traumatic hysteria.

f. precordial. Anxiety felt before melancholic frenzy.

frigid (frij'id). 1. Cold. 2. Irresponsive to emotion, applied esp. to the inability to feel sex desire on the part of a woman.

frigid'ity. Sexual coldness; inhibited libido.

frigolabile (frī-go-la'bĭl). Capable of being destroyed by low temperature.

frigorific (frig-o-rif'ik). Generating cold.

f. nerve. The vasoconstrictor.

frig'orism. A condition due to long exposure to cold.

frigostabile (fri-go-sta'bĭl). Incapable of being destroyed by high temperature.

frigotherapy (frig-o-ther'ă-pĭ). The use of cold in treatment of disease.

Frisch's bacillus. A microörganism said to be the cause of rhinoscleroma.

frit. 1. The material from which glass or the glazed portion of pottery is made. 2. A similar material for making the glaze of artificial teeth.

frog'belly. Flaccid abdomen in children afflicted by rickets, and atony of abdominal cells resulting from dyspepsia, accompanied by flatulence.

f. face. Flatness of face ~esulting from intranasal disease.

Fröhde's reagent (freh'dez). A test for alkaloids; 1 part of sodium molybdate in 1000 parts of strong sulfuric acid.

Fröhlich's syndrome (fra'liks). Result of pituitary disturbance creating feminine appearance in the male, accompanied by atrophy of genital organs.

Froin's syndrome (fro-wahn'). Yellow cerebrospinal fluid which rapidly coagulates. It contains an excess of lymphocytes, and also globulin.

frolement (frol-mon'). 1. Very light friction with the hand in massage.* 2. A sound resembling rustling heard in auscultation.

Frommann's lines (from'mahnz). Transverse lines in the axis-cylinder of medullated nerve fibers after being stained by silver nitrate.

frons (fronz). The forehead.

fron'tad. Toward the frontal aspect.

frontal (fron'tal). 1. Anterior. 2. The forehead bone.

f. bone. Forehead bone.

f. lobe (of the cerebrum). Four main convolutions in front of the central *sulcus.*

f. plane. That determined by an imaginary line when standing erect with feet apart, the line running from tip of nose, tip of right great toe, and tip of left great toe.

f. sinuses. Hollow spaces above the supraorbital margin (over the eyes). They are filled with air, and open into the nasal cavity.

fronto-. Prefix: Ant. position, or relationship with the forehead.

frontoma'lar. Rel. to the frontal and malar bones.

frontomax'illary. Rel. to the frontal bone and maxillary bones.

frontoparietal (fron"to-pă-ri'ĕ-tăl). Pert. to the frontal and parietal bones.

frontotem'poral. Pert. to frontal and temporal bones.

front-tap reflex. Contraction of gastrocnemius muscles resulting from percussing stretched muscles of extended leg.

frost'bite. Freezing or effect of freezing of a part of the body.

f.-itch. Itching skin disease in cold climates. SYN: *pruritus hiemalis.*

frottage (fro-tazh'). 1. A condition of *hyperesthesia sexualis* often associated with lowered virility inducing an irresistible impulse of pressing up behind women in crowds, thus producing an orgasm. 2. Massage technic using rubbing.

frotteur (fro-ter'). One who practices frottage.

frozen sleep. Hypothermia, *q.v.*

fruc'tose. Levulose. Fruit sugar.

fructosuria (fruk"to-su'ri-ă). Fructose in the urine.

fruit. The product of a plant for propagation of its kind. It is the seed usually with the part containing it.

fruit sugar. Fructose, levulose, *q.v.*

frumentaceous (fru-men-ta'she-us). Resembling or belonging to grain.

frumenti, spiritus. Whisky.

frumentum (fru-men'tum). Wheat or other grain.

frustra'tion. The failure of libido to find adequate outlet.

Ft. Abbr. of L. *fiat,* or *fiant,* let there be made. Also for *florentium.*

fuel value. Energy to be produced by oxidation of edible foods after eating. SEE: *calory, energy, food requirements.*

-fuge. Suffix meaning to *expel.*

fugitive (fu'jit-iv). 1. Temporary, transient. 2. Wandering; pert. to inconstant symptoms.

fugue (fūj). 1. Flight automatism. Leaving home or surroundings on a hysterical impulse generally with loss of memory as to identity and the past. 2. PSY: A form of consciousness similar to that produced by dual or multiple personality, purpose and direction of conduct and action being retained.

Fuld's test. A test for the antipyretic power of the blood serum.

fulgurant (ful'gu-rant). Severe and sudden, as a *fulgurant pain.*

ful'gurating. Pert. to fulguration. SYN: *fulgurant.*

fulgura'tion (ful-gu-ra'shun). Destruction of tissue by means of long high frequency electric sparks. SEE: *electrodesiccation.*

fuliginous (fu-lij'in-us). Resembling soot, esp. in color. [ing.

full'ing. A movement in massage; kneading-Palms hold a limb bet. them, the fingers extended, the limb being rolled backward and forward.

full term. Normal end of pregnancy, when the fetus is 20-21 in. long, has finger- and toenails reaching to end of digits, and, if a boy, with both testicles descended. It should weigh from 7 lb. upward and have been nourished in the womb for not less than 40 weeks.

ful'minant. Fulgurant. Coming in lightninglike flashes of pain, as in tabes dorsalis.

ful'minating. Fulgurant; occurring with very great rapidity, said of certain pains.

fumes. Vapors, esp. those having irritating qualities.

f., nitric acid. Used in various chemical processes.

fumiga'tion. The disinfecting of rooms by gases.

fu'ming. Having a visible vapor.

function (fung'shun). The normal action of any organ or set of organs.

func'tional. A word applied to disturbances of function in a variety of ways.

f. disease. One not organic, or in which changes of an organ are not in evidence; a disturbance of any organ's functions.

f. psychosis. One exhibited in manicdepressive psychosis, in which no pathology of the central nervous system is apparent.

funda (fun'dă). A four-tailed bandage.

fundal (fun'dal). Pert. to a fundus.

fund'ament. 1. A foundation. 2. The anús.

fun'diform. Sling-shaped or looped.

fun'dus (pl. *fundi*). 1. The larger part, base, or body of a hollow organ. 2. Cardiac end of the stomach.

f. glands. Minute tubelike glands of the gastric mucosa in the cardiac section.

f. uteri. The body of the uterus from the internal os of the cervix upward above the fallopian tubes.

f. oculi. Post. inner part of eye as seen with ophthalmoscope.

fundusectomy (fun-dus-ek'to-mĭ). Excision of the fundus of the stomach. SYN: *cardiectomy.*

fun'gate. To grow like a fungus.

fungating (fun'găt-ing). Of a fungous appearance, as some ulcers.

fungi (fun'ji). Plural of fungus.

fungicide (fun'ji-sĭd). Bactericide; that which destroys bacteria or fungi.

fungiform (fun'jif-orm). Fungus-shaped.

f. papillae. Small, rounded eminences on middle and ant. parts of dorsum and esp. along sides of tongue.

fungista'sis. A condition in which the growth of fungi is inhibited. SEE: *fungicide.*

fun'gistat. That which inhibits the growth of fungi.

fungistat'ic. Inhibiting the growth of fungi.

fungoid (fun'goid). Having the appearance of a fungus.

f., chignon. Bacterial growth of the hair. SEE: *chignon fungoid.*

fungosity (fun-gos'it-ĭ). A soft excrescence

fungous (fun'gus). 1. Fungoid, *q.v.* 2. Swiftly growing, as a soft excrescence.

fungus (fun'gus). 1. A vegetable cellular organism that subsists on organic matter, such as bacteria and molds. 2. A succulent morbid excrescence on the body resembling fungus. SEE: *actinomycosis, cladosporiosis.*

   f. haematodes. Malignant bleeding growth.

fu'nic. Pert. to the umbilical cord.

   f. souffle. SYM: The purring sound heard over the pregnant uterus, and having the same rate as the fetal heart beat.

fu'nicle. A small, threadlike structure. SYN: *funiculus.*

funicular (fū-nik'ū-lar). Pert. to the spermatic, or umbilical cord.

   f. process. That part of the tunica vaginalis that covers the spermatic cord.

funiculitis (fu-nik-u-lī'tis). Inflammation of the spermatic cord.

funiculopexy (fū-nik'ū-lo-peks-ĭ). Suturing the spermatic cord to the tissues in cases of undescended testicle.

funiculus (fu-nik'ū-lus) (pl. *funiculī*). 1. The umbilical cord. 2. The spermatic cord. 3. Any small structure resembling a cord. 4. Bundle of nerve fibers. SEE: *fasciculus.*

fu'niform. Ropelike.

fu'nis. 1. A cordlike structure. 2. The umbilical cord.

fun'nel. Conical, wide, open-mouthed device for pouring through its open tube at end into another vessel.

   f. drainage. Drainage by funnels.

   f. breast. Sternal depression of chest walls resembling a funnel.

funny bone. The internal condyle of the humerus.

fur. A deposit forming on the tongue, *q.v.*

fur'cal. Forked.

furfur (fur'fur). Scurf; dandruff.

furfuraceous (fur-fu-ra'shus). Scaly, or resembling scales.

furibund (fū'rĭ-bund). Maniacal; raging, as in certain types of insanity.

fu'ror. PSY: Extremely violent outbursts or anger, often without provocation.

   f. amatorius. Insatiable sexual desire.

   f. epilepticus. Epileptic insanity, or sudden anger as expressed by epileptics.

   f. femininus. Nymphomania.*

   f. genitalis. Erotomania.*

   f. uterinus. SEE: *furor femininus.*

furuncle (fu'rung-kl). A boil. SYN: *furunculus.*

furunc'ular. Pert. to a boil.

furunculoid (fū-rung'kū-loid). Resembling a furuncle or boil. SYN: *furunculous.*

furunculosis (fū-rung-kū-lo'sis). A condition resulting from boils.

furunc'ulous. Pert. to or of the nature of a boil or boils.

furunculus (fu-rung'ku-lus). Boil, furuncle. Acute, deep-seated phlegmonous inflammation formed in the skin usually ending in suppuration and necrosis.

Fusarium (fū-za'rĭ-um). A genus of fungus.

fuse. A safety device comprising a strip of wire of easily fusible metal, the conductance of which is predetermined. The metal fuses and breaks circuit when excess of current passes through. Convenient forms mounted in plugs, bet hard metal ends under screwheads.

fu'sible. Capable of being melted.

fu'siform. 1. Tapering at both ends. 2. BIOL: Pert. to gelatin which liquefies in parsnip form

Fusifor'mis. A genus of *Mycobacteriaceae* containing spindle-shaped organisms.

   F. ac'nes. *Corynebacterium acnes.*

   F. den'tium. Long, spindle-shaped organisms associated with *Borrelia vincenti* in ulcerative stomatitis.

fusion (fu'shun). Meeting and joining together through liquefaction by heat.

   f. faculty. Blending of the images of binocular vision into a single perception having the quality of depth.

fusocel'lular. Spindle celled.

fusospirillosis (fū"so-spir-il-o'sis). Vincent's angina.

fusospirochetal (fū"zo-spi-ro-ke'tăl). Pert. to fusiform bacilli and spirochetes such as found in Vincent's angina.

fusospirocheto'sis. Infection with fusiform bacilli and spirochetes.

fusostreptococcosis (fū"so-strep"to-kok-ko'sis). Infection with fusiform bacteria and streptococcus.

fustiga'tion. In massage, beating with light rods.

fututio (fū-tū'shĭ-o). Sexual intercourse.

fututrix (fū-tū'triks). A girl or woman who practices tribadism, *q.v.*

G

G. Abbr. for *gingival;* chemical symb. for *glucinum.*

Ga. Chemical symb. for *gallium.*

gad'fly. An insect which lays eggs under the skin of its victim, which cause swellings simulating a boil. Multiple furuncles appear with hatching of larva.

gadolinium (gad-o-lin'ĭ-um). SYMB: Gd. A very rare element; at. wt., 157.3.

Gaertner's canal or **duct** (gärt'nerz). Incorrect spelling for *Gartner's.*

Gaffkya (gaf'kĭ-ä). A genus of bacteria of the family *Coccaceae.*

  G. tetrag'ena. Found associated with the tubercle bacillus and pseudomembranous angina. SEE: *lactation.*

gag. 1. Device for keeping the jaws open or forcibly opening the mouth. 2. To retch or cause to retch.

  g. reflex. Gagging and vomiting resulting from irritation of fauces.

gait (gāt). Manner of walking.

  g., ataxic. Raising foot high, striking ground suddenly with entire sole.

  g., brachybasic. Shuffling gait of partial paraplegia.

  g., cerebellar. A staggering movement.

  g., cow. Swaying due to knock-knees.

  g., equine. Raising foot by flexing thigh on abdomen. Characteristic of peroneal paralysis. Slow, awkward.

  g., festinating. Body bent forward and rigid. Walks on toes as though pushed. Starts slowly, increases and does not stop until patient meets an obstruction. Seen in paralysis agitans.

  g., flat-footed. Toes everted, legs often bowed.

  g., frog. That of infantile paralysis; hopping.

  g., hemiplegic. Patient abducts paralyzed limb, swings it around and brings it forward so foot comes to ground in front of him.

  g., Huntington's chorea. A few normal paces, a long slow one, and then one or two hops.

  g., multiple neuritis. That of a high-stepping horse. Steppage gait, *q.v.*

  g., paralysis agitans. Tendency to begin slowly, then rapidly, falling forward.

  g., paralytic. Feet dragged with slow movements. Stumbles easily. Seen in chronic myelitis.

  g., scissor. One in which legs cross in walking.

  g., spastic. A stiff movement, toes seeming to catch and drag, legs held together, hips and knee joints slightly flexed. Seen in spastic paraplegia, sclerosis of lateral pyramidal columns of cord. Also in tumor of spinal cord and arachnoiditis.

  g., steppage. Foot and toes lifted high, heel brought down first. Seen in

peripheral neuritis, late stages of diabetes, alcoholism, chronic arsenical poisoning.

  g., waddling. Feet wide apart and walk resembling that of a duck. Seen in coxa vera and double congenital displacement of hip when lordosis is present.

gala-, galact-, galacto-. Combining forms, pert. to *milk.*

galactacrasia (gal-ak-tak-ra'zĭ-ă). An abnormal composition of milk.

galactag'ogin. The hormone of the placenta acting as a galactagogue.

galactagogue (gal-ak'tag-og). Agent that promotes the flow of milk. Ex: Mild malted milk. SEE: *lactation.*

galactan (gal-ak'tan). A complex carbohydrate forming galactose upon hydrolysis.

galac'tase. An enzyme or proteolytic ferment of milk.

galacte'mia, **galacthemia** (gal-ak-the'mĭ-ă). Milky condition of the blood.

galactic (gal-ăk'tĭk). Pert. to flow of milk.

galactidrosis (gal-ak-tid-ro'sis). A milk-like sweat.

galactin (ga-lak'tin). A basic amorphous substance in milk. SYN: *prolactin.*

galactoblast (gal-ak'to-blast). Body found in mammary acini; contains fat globules.

galactocele (gal-ak'to-sēl). 1. A tumor caused by the retention of fluid in a milk duct. 2. Hydrocele containing a milk-like liquid.

galactogogue (gal-ak'to-gog). Agent that promotes the flow of milk.

galactoma (gal-ak-to'ma). Cystic tumor of female breast. SYN: *galactocele,* 1.

galactom'eter. Device for measuring amt. of cream in milk by its specific gravity and degree of opacity. SYN: *lactometer.*

galactop'athy. 1. Treatment of nursing infants by drugs administered to the mother. 2. Use of a milk poultice.

galactopex'ic. Making galactose permanent.

galac'topexy. The fixation of galactose.

galactophagous (gal-ak-tof'ag-us). Feeding upon milk.

galactophlysis (gal-ak-tof'lis-is). 1. Eruption of vesicles containing milklike contents. 2. Infantile seborrhea of scalp. SYN: *crusta lactea.*

galac'tophore. A milk duct.

galactophoritis (gal-ak-tof-or-i'tis). Inflammation of a milk duct.

galactophorous (gal-ak-tof'or-us). Giving milk. [mammae.

  g. ducts. Excretory ducts of the

galactophthisis (gal-ak-tof'this-is). Debility and emaciation as result of excessive milk secretion.

galactophygous (gal-ak-tof'ig-us). Arresting flow of milk.

galactoplania (gal-ak-top-la'nĭ-ă). Secretion of milk in some abnormal part due to suppression of normal lactation.

galactopoietic (gal-ak"to-poy-et'ĭk). Having to do with the production of milk.

galactopyra (gal-ak-to-pi'ră). Milk fever.

galactorrhea (gal-ak-tor-e'ă). 1. Continuation of lactation, or flow of milk, at intervals after cessation of nursing. 2. Excessive flow of milk.

galactoschesia, galactoschesis (gal-ak-tos-ke'sĭ-ă, -tos'ke-sis). A stopping of the milk secretion.

galactoscope (gal-ak'to-skōp). Device for measuring quality of milk. SYN: *galactometer, lactoscope*.

galactose (ga-lak'tōs). A monosaccharide or simple sugar.

    g. test. Forty Gm. orally. Three Gm. in urine indicates liver impairment.

galactosis (gal-ak-to'sis). The secretion of milk.

galactostasis (gal-ak-tos'ta-sis). Cessation or checking of milk secretion. SYN: *galactoschesia*

galactosuria. Galactose in the urine.

galactotherapy (gal-ak-to-ther'ă-pĭ). Treatment of a nursing infant by drugs administered to the mother. SYN: *galactopathy*.

galactotoxin (gal-ak"to-toks'in). A poison in milk produced by bacteria.

galactotox'ism. Milk poisoning.

galactotrophy (gal-ak-tot'ro-fĭ). Feeding with nothing but milk.

galactoxism (gal-ak-toks'izm). Poisoning by milk. SYN: *galactotoxism*.

galactozymase (gal-ak-to-zi'mās). A starch hydrolyzing ferment in milk.

galactu'ria. The passing of milky urine. SYN: *chyluria.**

ga'lea. The epicranial aponeurosis which connects the bellies of the occipitofrontal muscle.

galeanthropy (ga-le-an'thro-pĭ). A delusion that one has become transformed into a cat.

galenicals, galenics (gă-lĕn'ĭ-kăls, -ĭks). Herb and vegetable medicines.

Ga'len's veins. The veins running through the tela chorioidea formed by the joining of the terminal and choroid veins, and forming the v. cerebri magna. SYN: *venae cerebri internae*.

galeophilia (gal-e-o-fil'ĭ-ă). Fondness for cats.

galeophobia (gal-e-o-fo'bĭ-ă). Abnormal aversion to cats.

galeropia, galeropsia (gal-er-o'pĭ-ă, -rop'-sĭ-ă). Unusual clearness of vision.

gall. 1. An excoriation. 2. The bitter secretion of the liver stored in the gallbladder.

gallate (gal'āt). A salt of gallic acid.

gall'bladder. Pear-shaped sac on undersurface of right lobe of liver holding bile from the liver until discharged through cystic duct; ¾ in. long, 1 in. greatest diameter; capacity, 50-75 cc. concentrated bile or 1½ pt. liver bile.

gall'duct. Tube carrying bile from the liver and gallbladder.

gal'lon. Four quarts; 231 cubic inches.

gal'loping. Pursuing a rapid course.

    g. consumption. Miliary tuberculosis.

gall'stone. Concretion formed in the gallbladder or bile ducts generally after 35th year.

Gal'ton's whistle. A whistle with which a note may be changed; used to test the hearing.

galvan'ic. Pert. to galvanism.

    g. battery. A series of cells, giving a combined effect of all the units, and generating electricity by chemical reaction.

    g. cell. One of a series of cells generating electricity through chemical reaction.

gal'vanism. Therapeutic use of direct current of electricity.

galvanization (gal-van-i-za'shun). Employment of a galvanic current.

galvanocau'tery. Cauterization of tissue by means of an electric current. SEE: *electrocautery*.

galvanocontractil'ity. Capability of a muscle of contracting under a galvanic stimulation.

galvanofaradiza'tion. Combined use of galvanic and faradic current made possible by use of a De Watteville switch.

galvanom'eter. An instrument that measures current by electromagnetic action.

galvanoner'vous. Pert. to the effect of a galvanic current upon a nerve.

galvanopalpa'tion. A method of measuring tactile sensibility of the nerves of the skin by the electric current.

galvanopunc'ture. Introduction of needles to complete a galvanic current.

galvanoscope (gal-van'o-skop). Instrument which shows the presence and direction of a galvanic current.

galvanosur'gery. Use of galvanism in surgery.

galvanotax'is. The tendency of a living organism to arrange itself in a medium so that its axis bears a certain relation to the direction of the current in the medium.

galvanotherapeu'tics, galvanother'apy. Treatment by means of electricity. SYN: *electrotherapy*.

gal'vanotherm''y. Treatment by the heat from a galvanic battery.

galvanot'onus. Tonic contractions caused by a galvanic current.

galvanotro'pism. The tendency of an organism to grow, turn, or move into a certain relation with an electric current.

gamete (gam'ēt). Any reproductive body; a germ cell.

gamet'ic. Pert. to gametes.

gametocide (gam'et-o-sĭd). An agent destructive to malarial gametocytes.

gametocyte (gam'et-o-sīt). The sexual cell which forms the gamete.

Gam'gee tissue. A dressing made of a thick layer of absorbent cotton between 2 layers of absorbent gauze; used for surgical dressing.

gam'ma. A term adopted to indicate a minimum quantity less than grains. One grain is estimated as equal to 6400 gammas.

g. rays. Light waves of extremely short wave length. They have 100 times greater penetrating power than beta particles. Almost completely absorbed by 6 in. of lead. SEE: *rays.*

gam′macism. Inability to pronounce correctly *g* and *k* sounds.

Gamna's disease. Splenomegaly with slow, progressive enlargement of the spleen.

G.'s nodules. Nodules stained yellow or brown in certain varieties of splenic enlargement. SEE: *Gamna's disease.*

gamo-. Combining form from *gamos*, marriage.

gamogenesis (gam-o-jen′ĕ-sis). Sexual reproduction.

gamogenet′ic. Pert. to sexual reproduction.

gam′ont. A sexual form of certain protozoans.

gamophobia (gam-o-fo′bĭ-ă). Psychoneurotic aversion to the marriage relationship.

gampsodactylia (gamp″so-dak-til′ĭ-ă). Deformity of the toes resembling claws. SYN: *clawfoot.*

ganglial (gang′glĭ-ăl). Pert. to a ganglion. SYN: *ganglionic.*

gangliasthenia (gang-lĭ-as-the′nĭ-ă). Neurasthenia due to disease of a ganglion. SYN: *ganglionic asthenia.*

gangliated (gang′lĭ-at-ed). 1. Having ganglia. 2. Intermixed.

g. cord. Main trunk of sympathetic nervous system.

gangliec′tomy. Excision of a ganglion.

gangliform (gang′lĭ-form). Formed like a ganglion.

ganglioglioma (gang-lĭ-glĭ-o′mă). Lymphatic glandular tumor.

ganglii′tis. Inflammation of a nervous or lymphatic gland. SYN: *ganglionitis.*

gang′lioblast. An embryonic cell of the ganglionic nervous system.

gangliocyte (gang′lĭ-o-sīt). A nerve cell.

gangliocyto′ma. A ganglion cell tumor.

ganglioform (gang′lĭ-o-form). Shaped like a ganglion. SYN: *gangliform.*

ganglioglio′ma. A ganglion cell glioma.

ganglioglioneuroma (gang″glĭ-o-glĭ″o-nŭ-ro′mă). Ganglion cells, glia cells, and nerve fibers in a nerve tumor.

ganglioma (gang-lĭ-o′mă). 1. Tumor of a lymphatic gland. 2. A swelling of lymphoid tissue.

ganglion (gang′lĭ-on) (pl. *ganglia*). 1. A mass of nerve tissue which receives and sends out nerve impulses, *e. g.*, the ganglionic masses forming the sympathetic nervous system. 2. Cystic tumors developing on a tendon or aponeurosis; sometimes occur on the back of the wrist due to strain, such as excessive practice on the piano. 3. An enlargement on the course of a nerve, such as is found on the receptor nerves before they enter the spinal cord. 4. An enlarged lymphatic gland.

g., abdominal. Any one of the abdominal ganglia.

g., ant. cerebral. Corpus striatum.

Corpus striatum and corpus lenticulare together.

g., Arnold's auricular. Tiny ganglion located beneath foramen ovale. SYN: *otic ganglion, otoganglion.*

g., auricular. SEE: *Arnold's auricular ganglion.*

g., azygous. 1. A single or unpaired ganglion. 2. Ganglion in which union of 2 parts of the sympathetic nerve takes place.

g., basal optic. Mass of gray matter beneath 3rd ventricle.

g., cardiac. Tiny ganglion toward which converge the fibers of superficial cardiac plexus.

g., carotid. Ganglion formed by filamentous threads from the carotid plexus beneath the carotid artery.

g., cephalic. Tiny ganglion situated upon the cranial ant. communicating artery.

g., cerebral. Main cerebral nerve centers.

g., cervical. One of 3 ganglia in cervical region.

g., cervicouterine. Ganglion of uterine cervix.

g., ciliary. Tiny ganglion located in the rear portion of the orbit.

g., diaphragmatic. Tiny ganglion joining the semilunar ganglion.

g., gasserian. Large ganglion located on ant. surface near apex of the petrous portion of the temporal bone.

g., geniculate. Ganglion in the fallopian aqueduct.

g., inf. cardiac. One of 2 small ganglia which occasionally take place of cardiac ganglia.

g., intercrural. Gray matter mass lodged in the crura cerebri.

g., interoptic. Interoptic lobe gray matter.

g., interpeduncular. SEE: *intercrural ganglion.*

g., intervertebral. Enlarged area on post. root of spinal nerve, close to the intervertebral foramen.

g., jugular. Ganglion located in upper portion of jugular foramen.

g., lenticular. SEE: *ciliary ganglion.*

g., lumbar. Ganglia in lumbar area, in sympathetic system.

g., marginal. Ganglion in cranial trunk, of sympathetic system.

g., Meckel's. SEE: *sphenopalatine ganglion.*

g., mesenteric. Ganglion composed of filamentous threads from sup. mesenteric plexus, close to the foot of the sup. mesenteric artery.

g., Müller's. SEE: *jugular ganglion.*

g., ophthalmic; g., optic. SEE: *ciliary ganglion.*

g., otic. SEE: *Arnold's auricular ganglion.*

g., petrous. Ganglion located on lower margin of temporal bone's petrous portion.

g., pharyngeal. Ganglion in contact with the glossopharyngeal nerve.

g., phrenic. One of a group of ganglia joining the phrenic plexus.

g., plexiform. SEE: *gasserian ganglion.*

g., renal. One of a group of ganglia joining the renal plexus.

g., respiratory. Ganglion of the respiratory centers.

g., reticular. Disseminated mass of gray matter in the oblongata.

g., sacral. One of a group of sympathetic ganglia on the sacral ventral surface.

g., semilunar. SEE: *gasserian ganglion.*

g., sensory. Ganglion joining the sensory nerves.

g., spermatic. One of the tiny ganglia joining the inner spermatic plexuses.

g., sphenopalatine. Ganglion in sphenomaxillary fossa connected with sympathetic and facial nerves.

g., spinal. Ganglionic enlargement of spinal nerves' dorsal roots.

g., sublingual; g., submaxillary. Ganglion in the submaxillary gland.

g., superior cardiac. SEE: *inferior cardiac ganglion.*

g., suprarenal. Ganglion situated in the suprarenal plexus.

g., temporal. Tiny ganglion joining the ant. branches of sup. cervical ganglion.

g., thoracic. One of 12 ganglia of thoracic area of sympathetic nerve.

g., tympanic. On tympanic portion of the glossopharyngeal nerve.

g., vestibular. Ganglion in fallopian aqueduct.

gang'lionated. Furnished with ganglia. SYN: *gangliated.*

ganglionectomy (gang-lĭ-o-nek'to-mĭ). Excision of a ganglion.

ganglionervous (gang-glĭ-o-ner'vus). Pert. to the sympathetic nervous system.

    g. system. Sympathetic nervous system.

ganglioneure (gang'lĭ-o-nŭr). A nerve cell within the cerebral or spinal ganglia.

ganglioneuroma (gang"glĭ-o-nŭ-ro'mă). A neuroma containing ganglion cells.

ganglionic (gang-lĭ-on'ĭk). Pert. to or of the nature of a ganglion.

g. asthenia. Neurasthenia caused by a diseased ganglion.

g. canal. One around the cochlear modiolus for the spinal ganglion.

g. centers. Gray matter bet. floor of lateral ventricles and ant. pyramids of the cord.

ganglionitis (gang-lĭ-on-i'tis). Inflamed condition of a ganglion.

gangrene (gan'grēn). The putrefaction of soft tissue; a form of necrosis. SYN: *mortification.*

g., anemic. Gangrene resulting from an obstructed circulation in the part.

g., angioneurotic. State resulting from thrombotic arteries and veins.

g., diabetic. Moist gangrenous condition arising in some diabetics.

g., dry. This results when the part that dies has little blood and when it remains aseptic. The arteries but not

the veins are obstructed. The tissues dry and drop off, the process continuing for weeks or months.

g., embolic. Gangrenous condition arising subsequent to an embolic obstruction.

g., gas. This is gangrene in a wound infected by the gas bacillus (*bacillus Welchii*), a microörganism.

g., hospital. Variety developing in crowded hospital, usually fatal.

g., humid. SEE: *moist gangrene.*

g., idiopathic. When the cause is unknown.

g., infective. Due to infection, as in carbuncle necrosis, cancrum oris, and cancrum noma.

g., moist. This occurs after a crushing injury, usually at distal part of an extremity, or when dry gangrene is infected with putrefactive bacteria, and when the part is full of blood.

g., primary. Gangrene developing in a part without previous inflammation.

g., secondary. Gangrene developing subsequent to local inflammation.

g., senile. Gangrene developing in the limbs of the senile.

g., symmetric. Gangrene on opposite sides of the body in corresponding parts.

g., traumatic. Result of extensive injuries.

g., white. Moist gangrene developing in patients with anemia and lymphatic obstruction.

gangrenosis (gang-gren-o'sis). Condition of mortification or gangrene.

gan'grenous. Of the nature of gangrene.

gan'oblast. An enamel cell. SYN: *ameloblast.*

Ganser's syndrome (gan'zerz sin'drōm). "Nonsense syndrome." Absurd acts and speech seen in prison psychosis, hysteria, and other states.

gargarism (gar'gar-izm). A gargle or throat wash.

gargle (gar'gl). 1. A wash for the throat. 2. To wash out the throat with a throat wash.

garlic. An edible, strongly flavored bulb, used mainly for seasoning. COMP: The active principle of garlic is sulfide of allyl.

    INDICATIONS: Its sulfurated essence is anticatarrhal.

gar'rot. A form of tourniquet.

Gart'ner's duct. A straight duct running from the parovarium to the vagina; ductus epoophori longitudinalis.

gas. An airlike fluid subject to expansion and convertible into a liquid by cold or compression.

g. bacillus. *Bacillus Welchii.* SEE: *gangrene.*

g., digestive tract. Among the gases in the digestive tract are: Oxygen, nitrogen, hydrogen, carbon dioxide, methane, and in decomposition of proteins, hydrogen sulfide, indol, skatol, ammonia, etc.

g., distention. Abdominal distention is result of abnormal gaseous, fluid, or solid accumulation in abdominal cavity.

It may be: (a) Acute; (b) chronic; (c) local, or (d) general. The abdominal wall, the cavity, or the intraäbdominal viscera may be involved. *Postoperative*: Result of complication following an operation. Limited to lower part of small, and all of large intestines.

g. excretions. Oxidation produces carbon dioxide or carbonic acid gas, from one-half to two-thirds of a cubic ft. per hr. being produced by an adult male of average weight.

g. gangrene. That caused by the gas bacillus. SEE: *gangrene.*

g., illuminating. This is a mixture of various combustible gases including hydrogen and carbon monoxide. Its poisonous effects are largely due to carbon monoxide, *q.v.*

g. in the blood. Dissolved gases are found in the blood in the form of oxygen, nitrogen, and a small portion of carbon dioxide, with carbonic acid from the tissues.

g., laughing. Nitrous oxide.

g., marsh. Methane.

g., mustard. Poisonous gas used in warfare (dichlorethyl sulfide).

g., refrigerant. A number of these gases are used in ordinary household mechanical refrigerators. Poisoning due to leaks, faulty connections or breakage, and gas dissipated into the atmosphere. Among these gases are methyl chloride, ammonia, sulfur dioxide, and more than 20 other gases. Most of these are toxic.

g., tear. A gas that irritates the conjunctiva and which produces a flow of tears.

gas′ator. Device for adm. chlorine gas for respiratory infections.

gaseous (gas′e-us). Of the nature or form of gas.

gases, war. Any chemical substances whether solid, liquid, or vapor, used to produce poisonous or irritant effects.

g., lewisite. Contains arsenic and smells of geraniums.

g., lung irritant. Chlorine and phosgene.

g., mustard. Dichlorethyl sulfide. SEE: *gas, vesicant.*

g., nose irritant. Diphenylchloroarsine. An irritant smoke.

g., suffocating. Made from chlorine compounds.

g., tear. Substance which, when dispersed into the air, causes the eyes to be blinded by tears. EX: *Bromoacetone.*

g., toxic. Hydrocyanic acid type.

g., vesicant. Attack every part of body; clothing and boots are infected and a source of danger.

gas′oline″. A product of the destructive distillation of petroleum.

gasomet′ric. Pert. to measurement of gases.

gasometry (gas-om′et-rĭ). Estimation of amount of gas present in a mixture.

gasserectomy (gas-er-ek′to-mĭ). Excision of the gasserian ganglion.

gasse′rian arteries. A branch from the int. carotid artery and one of the middle meningeal arteries to the gasserian ganglion. SEE: *ganglion.*

gas′sing. The use of war gases, *q.v.*

gasteral′gia. Pain in the stomach.

gasterangiemphraxis (gas″ter-an″jĭ-emfraks′is). 1. Congestion of blood vessels of stomach. 2. Pyloric obstruction.

gasterasthenia (gas-ter-as-the′nĭ-ă). Debility of stomach. SYN: *gastrasthenia.*

gasterhysterotomy (gas″ter-his-ter-ot′o-mĭ). Incision of uterus through abdomen. SEE: *cesarean operation.*

gastorrhagia (gas-tor-a′jĭ-ă). Hemorrhage from the stomach.

gastradenitis (gas-trad-en-i′tis). Inflammation of the stomach glands.

gastralgia (gas-tral′jĭ-ă). Paroxysmal epigastric pain without gastric lesion.

gastralgokenosis (gas-tral-go-ken-o′sis). A sensory neurosis of the stomach.

gastraneuria (gas-tra-nŭ′rĭ-ă). Defective action of nerves of the stomach.

gastrasthe′nia. Debility of the stomach. SYN: *gasterasthenia.*

gastratrophia (gas-tra-tro′fĭ-ă). Atrophy of the stomach.

gastrecta′sia, gastrec′tasis. Dilatation of the stomach. May be acute or chronic.

gastrectomy (gas-trek′to-mĭ). Surgical removal of a part of the stomach.

gas′tric. Pert. to the stomach.

g. analysis. Determines quality of secretion, amount of free and combined hydrochloric acid, absence or presence of blood, bile, bacteria, fatty acids. Esp. necessary if gastric ulcer or carcinoma is suspected.

g. digestion. As food passes through the cardiac orifice into the stomach, it tends to accumulate in the lowest part of the major curvature.

g. fever. Fever accompanied by gastric disturbances.

g. glands. Cardiac, fundic or oxyntic, and pyloric glands of the stomach.

g. juice. The digestive secretion of the stomach, containing gastrin which stimulates the gastric glands. Its reaction is acid.   [ach.

g. lavage. Washing out of the stom-

g. motor meals. These meals are used to test the motor activity of the stomach and intestines. SEE: *Boas motor meal, test meal, Von Leube meal.*

g. mucin (mu′sin). A fine, straw-colored powder, prepared from hog stomach.

USES: As a protective in peptic ulcer.

DOSAGE: Varies according to the severity, from 1 teaspoonful to 1 tablespoonful in warm water or milk ½ hour before meals.

g. reflex. Critical reflex in this area.

g. ulcer. An ulcer of the stomach. SYN: *peptic ulcer, q.v.*

gastricism (gas′tris-izm). Any gastric disorder.

gas′trin. A hormone that stimulates secretion of the glands in the cardiac end of the stomach. It is formed at the pyloric end of the stomach.

gastritis (gas-tri'tis). Inflammation of the stomach.

g., acid deficiency. May be due to improper mastication or mouth infection, and it is less frequent in the young and younger adult.

g., acute. SYM: Moderate fever; anorexia, coated tongue, intense pain in epigastrium, persistent vomiting, thirst; prostration.

g., atrophic. Chronic gastritis with atrophied mucosa and glands.

g., chronic. SYM: Weight and distress after eating; often tenderness on palpation. Eructations of gas and some liquid, nausea and vomiting frequently, constipation.

g., hypertrophic. Gastritis combined with glandular hypertrophy and infiltration.

g., phlegmonous. Acute gastritis with suppuration of the abdominal wall.

g., polypous. Gastritis characterized by knoblike projections on the surface.

g., pseudomembranous. Gastritis marked by membranous patch formation.

gastro-. Used in compounds to denote the *stomach*.

gastroanastomosis (gas″tro-an-as″to-mo'sis). Formation of passage bet. 2 pouches of stomach for relief of hourglass contraction.

gastroblennorrhea (gas-tro-blen-or-e'ă). Excessive secretion of gastric mucus.

gastrobrosis (gas-tro-bro'sis). Perforating ulcer of the stomach.

gastrocele (gas'tro-sēl). Hernia of the stomach.

gastrochronorrhea (gas-tro-kron-or-re'ă). Chronic gastric disease marked by permanent hypersecretion with dilatation and thickening of stomach walls and hypertrophy of glands. SYN: *Reichmann's disease.*

gastrocnemius (gas-trok-ne'mĭ-us). The large muscle of the leg. Extends foot and helps to flex knee upon thigh.

gastrocol'ic. Pert. to stomach and omentum.

g. omentum. The great omentum. SYN: *epiploon.*

g. reflex. Peristaltic wave in colon induced by entrance of food into fasting stomach.

gastrocoli'tis. Inflammation of stomach and colon.

gastrocoloptosis (gas-tro-kol-op-to'sis). Downward prolapse of stomach and colon.

gastrocolostomy (gas-tro-kol-os'to-mĭ). Establishment of permanent passage bet. stomach and colon.

gastrocolotomy (gas-tro-ko-lot'o-mĭ). Incision into stomach and colon.

gastrocolpotomy (gas-tro-kol-pot'o-mĭ). An incision of abdomen into upper part of vagina.

gastrodiaphane (gas-tro-di'af-ān). Device for electrically illuminating stomach interior, making visible its outlines through the abdomen.

gastrodiaphanos'copy, gastrodiaph'any. Examination of interior of the stomach by rendering its walls translucent by an electric light introduced into the organ.

gastroduodenitis (gas″tro-dŭ-od-en-i'tis). Inflammation of stomach and duodenum.

gastroduodenostomy (gas″tro-du-o-den-os′to-mĭ). Formation of an artificial opening between the stomach and duodenum.

gastrodynia (gas-tro-din'ĭ-ă). Pain in the stomach. SYN: *gastralgia.**

gastroelytrotomy (gas-tro-el-it-rot'o-mĭ). Cesarean section through linea alba into upper portion of vagina. SYN: *gastrocolpotomy.*

gastroenteralgia (gas″tro-en-ter-al'jĭ-ă). Pain in stomach and intestines.

gastroenter'ic. Pert. to stomach and intestines or to a condition involving them both.

gastroenteritis (gas-tro-en-ter-i'tis). Inflammation of the stomach and bowels.

gastroenterocolitis (gas″tro-en″ter-o-kol-i'tis). Inflammation of stomach, small intestine, and colon.

gastroenterocolostomy (gas-tro-en-ter-o-ko-los'to-mĭ). Creation of a passage bet. the stomach, small intestine, and colon.

gastroenterol'ogy. The pathology of the stomach and intestine.

gastroenteroptosis (gas″tro-en-ter-op-to'sis). Prolapse of stomach and intestines.

gastroenterostomy (gas-tro-en-ter-os'to-mĭ). Surgical anastomosis between the stomach and small bowel.

gas″troenterot'omy. Incision of stomach and intestine through abdominal wall.

gas″troepiplo'ic. Pert. to stomach and epiploon.

gastroesophagitis (gas-tro-e-sof-aj-i'tis). Inflammation of stomach and esophagus.

gastroesophagostomy (gas″tro-es-o-fa-gos'to-mĭ). Formation of passage from the esophagus into the stomach.

gastrogastrostomy (gas-tro-gas-tros'to-mĭ). Formation of passage in hourglass contraction bet. the 2 gastric pouches. SYN: *gastroanastomosis.*

gastrogavage (gas-tro-ga-vazh'). Artificial feeding through an opening into the stomach.

gastrogen'ic. Having its origin in the stomach.

gastrograph (gas'tro-graf). Device for determining the stomach's mechanical action.

gastrohelcosis (gas″tro-hel-ko'sis). Ulcer of the stomach.   [liver.

gas″trohepat'ic. Pert. to stomach and

gastrohepatitis (gas-tro-hep-ă-ti'tis). Combination of gastritis and hepatitis at same time.

gastrohydrorrhea (gas-tro-hi-dro-re'ă). Excretion of much watery fluid, other than gastric juice, into the stomach.

gastrohyperneuria, gastrohypernervia (gas-tro-hi-per-nū'rĭ-ă, -ner'vĭ-ă). Abnormal activity of gastric nerves.

gastrohyponeuria, gastrohyponervia (gas-tro-hi-po-nū'rĭ-ă, -ner'vĭ-ă). Defective activity of the gastric nerves.

gastrohysterectomy (gas-tro-his-ter-ek'-to-mĭ). Removal of the uterus through an abdominal incision.

gastrohysteropexy (gas"tro-his"ter-o-peks'ĭ). Ventrofixation of the uterus.

gastrohysterorrhaphy (gas-tro-his-ter-or'-af-ĭ). Fixation of uterus to the abdominal wall. SYN: *gastrohysteropexy.*

gastrohysterotomy (gas-tro-his-ter-ot'o-mĭ). Incision of uterus through abdomen. SYN: *gasterhysterotomy.*

gastroiliac (gas-trō-ĭl'ĭ-ak). Pert. to stomach and ilium.

   g. reflex. Physiologic relaxation of ileocecal valve resulting from food in stomach.   [intestine.

gastrointes'tinal. Pert. to stomach and

   g. decompression. Drainage of gases from the body cavities and tissues by use of suction through a tube inserted through the nostrils and into the digestive tract. SEE: *Wangensteen method.*

   g. system. The organs and parts concerned with digestion and nutrition.

gastrojejunostomy (gas-tro-je-ju-nos'to-mĭ). Surgical anastomosis between the stomach and jejunum.

gastrolith (gas'tro-lith). A concretion in the stomach.

gastrolithiasis (gas"tro-lith-i'ă-sis). Formation of calculi in the stomach.

gastrology (gas-trol'o-jĭ). Study of diseases of the stomach.

gastrol'ysis. Breaking adhesions bet. stomach and adjoining structures.

gastromalacia (gas-tro-mal-a'sĭ-ă). Softening of the stomach walls.

gastromegaly (gas-tro-meg'ă-lĭ). Enlargement of abdomen or of stomach.

gastromenia (gas-tro-me'nĭ-ă). A form of vicarious menstruation through the stomach.

gastromycosis (gas-tro-mi-ko'sis). Disease of the stomach due to fungi.

gastromyotomy (gas-tro-mi-ot'o-mĭ). Incision of circular muscular fibers of stomach below a gastric ulcer.

gastromyxorrhea (gas-tro-miks-or-e'ă). Excessive secretion of gastric mucus.

gastronephritis (gas-tro-nef-ri'tis). Inflammation of the stomach and kidney at same time.

gastronesteostomy (gas-tro-nes-te-os'to-mĭ). Formation of communication bet. jejunum and stomach. SYN: *gastrojejunostomy.*

gastropancreatitis (gas"tro-pan"kre-ă-ti'tis). Inflammation of the stomach and pancreas at same time.

gastroparalysis (gas"tro-pa-ral'is-is). Paralysis of the stomach.

gastroparesis (gas"tro-par'e-sis). Mild form of gastroparalysis.

gastropathy (gas-trop'ă-thĭ). Any disorder of the stomach.

gastroperiodynia (gas"tro-per"ĭ-o-din'ĭ-ă). Periodic pain in the stomach. SYN: *gastralgia.*

gastropexy, gastropexis (gas-tro-peks'e, -is). Suture of the stomach to the abdominal walls for correction of displacement.

gastrophrenic (gas-tro-fren'ĭk). Rel. to the stomach and diaphragm.

gastroplasty (gas'tro-plas"tĭ). Plastic operation on the stomach.

gastroplegia (gas-tro-ple'jĭ-ă). Paralysis of the stomach.

gastroplication (gas-tro-pli-ka'shun). Stitching the walls of the stomach to reduce dilatation.

gastroptosia, gastroptosis (gas-tro-to'-sĭ-ă, -sis). Abnormal falling of the stomach, Glenard's disease.

   Usually accompanied by the displacement of other organs, the abdomen being pendulous. SEE: *bathygastry.*

gastroptyxis, gastroptyxy (gas-trop-tiks'-is, -ĭ). Reduction of a dilated stomach. SYN: *gastroplication.*

gastropylorectomy (gas-tro-pi-lor-ek'to-mĭ). Excision of stomach at pyloric end.

gastropylor'ic. Rel. to stomach and pylorus.

gastroradiculitis (gas-tro-rad-ik-ŭ-li'tis). Inflammation of the post. spinal nerve roots, the sensory fibers of which supply the stomach.

gastrorrhagia (gas-tror-ra'jĭ-ă). Hemorrhage from stomach.

gastrorrhaphy (gas-tror'ă-fĭ). Suture of a stomach wall.

gastrorrhea (gas-tror-re'ă). An excessive secretion of gastric juice.

gastrosalpingotomy (gas-tro-sal-pin-got'-o-mĭ). Incision of the oviduct by abdominal section.

gastroschisis (gas-tros'kis-is). A congenital fissure in wall of abdomen which remains open.

gastroscope (gas'tro-skōp). Device for inspecting stomach's interior.

gastros'copy. Examination of the stomach and abdominal cavity.

gastro'sia. Excessive hydrochloric acid in the stomach. SYN: *gastroxia.*

   g. fungo'sa. Gastrosia in which fungi in the stomach give rise to organic acids.

gastro'sis. Any disease of the stomach or abdomen.

gas'trospasm. A gastric spasm.

gastrosplen'ic. Of or pert. to stomach and spleen.

gastrostaxis (gas-tro-staks'is). Hemorrhage of blood from membrane of the stomach.

gastrostenosis (gas-tro-sten-o'sis). Contracted state of the stomach.

   g. cardiaca. Stenosis of cardiac orifice.

   g. pylorica. Stenosis of pylorus.

gastrostogavage (gas-tros"to-gă-vazh'). Injection through a gastric fistula of food.

gastros'toma. A fistula of the stomach.

gastros'tomize. To perform a gastrostomy

gastrostomy (gas-tros'to-mĭ). Surgical creation of a gastric fistula through the abdominal wall.

   NP: Teach patient to care for self after hospitalization. Help patient to make mental adjustment. Care of mouth.

gastrosuccorrhea (gas-tro-suk-or-e'ă). An

excessive secretion of gastric juice with increased acidity; hypersecretion.

gastrother'apy. 1. Treatment of gastric diseases. 2. Treatment with extract of gastric mucosa; used esp. in pernicious anemia.

gastrotome (gas'tro-tōm). Instrument for incising stomach or abdomen.

gastrotomy (gas-trot'o-mĭ). Gastric or abdominal incision.

gastrotonometer (gas-tro-to-nom'e-ter). Instrument for measuring intragastric pressure by insufflation of air or carbonic acid gas.

gastrotrachelotomy (gas-tro-tra-kel-ot'o-mĭ). Cesarean section in which the uterus is opened by a transverse incision across the cervix.

gastrotrop'ic. Attracted to or affecting the stomach.

gastrotubotomy (gas-tro-tu-bot'o-mĭ). Incision into fallopian tube through abdomen. SYN: *gastrosalpingotomy*.

gastrotympanites (gas″tro-tim-pan-i'tes). Gaseous distention of the stomach.

gastrox'ia. Abnormal acidity of contents of stomach.

gastroxynsis (găs-trŏks-ĭn'sĭs). Excessive hydrochloric acid secretion by stomach. SYN: *hyperchlorhydria*.

gastrula (gas'tru-lă). Blastoderm when its cavity becomes the primitive alimentary canal.

gastrula'tion. The development of the gastrula.

gas tube. A discharge tube which depends on the presence of residual gas in the tube for the supply of electrons.

Gatch bed. A bed in which the patient can be raised and held into a half-sitting position.

gath'ering. An abscess or swelling.

ga'tism. Vesical or rectal incontinence.

gatophilia (gat-o-fil'ĭ-ă). Abnormal love for cats.

gatophobia (gat-o-fo'bĭ-ă). Aversion to cats. SYN: *ailurophobia, galeophobia*.

Gaucher's disease (go-shāz'). Primary epithelioma of the spleen or splenic anemia.

gauge (găj). Device for measuring size, capacity, amount or power of an object or substance; a standard of measurement.

Gault's reflex (galt). Contraction of orbicularis palpebrarum muscle resulting from sudden noise being produced near ear.

gauntlet (gawnt'let). A glovelike bandage which fits the hand and fingers.

gauss (gaws). The unit of intensity of a magnetic flux.

Gauss' sign (gaws). Unusual mobility of the uterus in the early weeks of pregnancy.

gauze (gawz). Thin, transparent fabric used in surgery.

    g., absorbent. Gauze from which oily matter and sizing has been removed.

    g., antiseptic. Gauze containing antiseptic material.

gavage (ga-vazh'). Feeding with a stomach tube, or with a tube passed through the nares, pharynx, and esophagus into the stomach; the food is in liquid or semiliquid form at a temperature of about 100° F. SEE: *gastrostogavage*.

Gavard's muscle (ga-varz'). The oblique muscular fibers of the stomach's coat.

Gawalowski's test (gav-al-ov'skĭ). Test for sugar made by use of ammonium molybdate and indicated by a blue color.

Gayet's disease (gă-yas'). A lethargic sleep resembling sleeping sickness. It is rare and fatal.

Gay-Lussac's' law. All gases on heating expand equally and on cooling contract equally, according to temperature relation. SEE: *Charles' law*.

Geigel's reflex (gī'gel). Reflex in females resembling cremasteric reflex* in males.

Geisböck's disease or **syndrome** (gĭs'beck). Abnormal number of red corpuscles in blood with cardiac hypertrophy and elevated blood pressure, without splenic enlargement. SYN: *polycythemia hypertonica*.

Geissler tube (gĭs'ler). The original discharge tube for showing the luminous effects of discharges through rarefied gases. The density of the gas in the tube is roughly one-thousandth that of atmospheric pressure.

gel (jel). 1. A semisolid condition of a precipitated or coagulated colloid. Jelly. A jellylike colloid. 2. Coagulum of a sol.

gelatin(e (jĕl'ă-tĭn). A derived protein prepared from bone and connective tissue.

    g. culture. Gelatinous base for bacterial growth.

    g. disk. Gelatin circlet for eye therapy.   [gelatin.

    g. peptone. Digestive product of

    g., nutrient. SEE: *gelatin culture*.

gelat'inase. An enzyme that liquefies gelatin.

gelatiniferous (jel-at-in-if'er-us). Producing gelatin.

gelatiniza'tion. Transformation into a gelatinous mass.

gelatinize (jel-at'in-īz). To convert into gelatin.

gelatinoid (jel-at'in-oyd). Resembling a gelatin; colloid.

gelatinolytic (jel-at″in-o-lit'ĭk). Dissolution or splitting up of gelatin.

gelatinosa (jel-at-in-o'să). A gelatinous, translucent substance capping the post. cornu of spinal cord on both sides. SYN: *Rolando's substance, substantia gelatinosa*.

gelat″inotho'rax. Injection of gelatin solution intrapleurally.

gelatinous (jel-at'in-us). Containing or of the consistency of gelatin.

gelation (jel-a'shun). The transformation of a sol into a gel.

Gellé's test (zhel-ās'). A tuning fork is connected with a rubber tube inserted in the ear. Pressure is produced by an attached bulb and, if ear is normal, vibrations are felt. SEE: *test*.

gelodiagno'sis. Identification of bacteria by means of a gelose culture medium.

gelose (jĕ'lōs). 1. Gelatinous element of agar, $C_6H_{10}O_5$. 2. Bacterial culture medium.

gelosis (jel-o'sis). A hard lump appearing to be frozen.

gelotherapy (jel-o-ther'ă-pĭ). Inducing hilarity in treatment of certain morbid states of the mind.

gelotripsy (jel'o-trip-sĭ). The massaging away of indurated swellings.

-gels. A termination to indicate colloids in a solid state.

Gély's suture (zhā-lē'). One for closing intestinal wounds employing cross stitches. SYN: *cobbler's suture.*

gemellus (jem-el'us). Either of 2 muscles inserted in the obturator internus tendon.

geminate (jem'ĭ-nāt). In pairs.

gemmation (jem-ma'shun). Fission by budding.

gemmule (jem'ul). 1. A fundamental structural cell unit. 2. The bud, or daughter cell, projecting from the parent cell. 3. A determinant.

gen (jen). The determining factor in transmission of characteristics. SYN: *gene.*

gena (je'na). The side of the face or cheek.

genal (je'nal). Pert. to the cheek. SYN: *buccal.*

gene (jēn). The agent in gametes determining a certain character in the zygote resulting. SYN: *gen, q.v.*

genea (je'ne-ă). 1. Generation. 2. Birth. 3. Descent.

general or house diet. A diet supplying the normal nutritive requirements of an ambulatory patient with no restriction of food articles.

gen'eralize. 1. To become or render general. 2. To become systemic, as a local disease.

gen'erating plate. That plate which is chemically acted upon in an electric cell.

generation (jen-er-a'shun). An act of forming a new organism.

  g., alternate. One of several sexless generations bet. the sexual ones. SYN: *digenesis.*

  g., asexual. Production of offspring without union of parents of distinct sex. SYN: *agamogenesis.*

  g., sexual. Reproduction by the union of male and female cells.

  g., spontaneous. Formation of a living organism from inanimate matter. SYN: *abiogenesis.*

  g., viviparous. Normal method of generation among higher animals, of bringing forth live offspring.

generative (jen'er-a-tiv). Concerned in reproduction of or affecting the species.

gen'erator, mo'tor. Combination of motor and dynamo.

generic (jen-er'ik). 1. General. 2. Pert. to a genus. 3. Distinctive or characteristic of a genus.

generin (jen'er-in). Supposed oxidizing agent causing the induction of menstruation and gestation.

genes (jēns) (sing. *gene*). Determiners which make up the chromosomes, and which are supposed to impart inherited traits.

gene'sial, genes'ic. Pert. to generation.

genesiology (jen-e-sĭ-ol'o-jĭ). The science of reproduction.

genesis (jen'es-is). Act of reproducing; generation.

genetic (jen-et'ik). Pert. to generation.

geneticist (jen-et'i-sist). One who specializes in genetics.

genet'ics. The science that accounts for natural differences and resemblances among organisms related by descent, as distinguished from those resulting from artificial selection. SEE: *eugenics.*

genetopathy (je-ne-top'ath-ĭ). Disease affecting the generative function.

genetous (jen'et-us). From birth. SYN: *congenital, q.v.*

Geneva Convention. An international agreement made in Geneva, Switzerland, in 1864 and 1906 safeguarding the wounded and those engaged in aiding them in warfare. Resulting in establishing of the Red Cross Society.

genial (je'nĭ-al). Rel. to the chin.

  g. tubercle. A nodule on the lower jawbone on either side of the symphysis.

geniculate (jen-ik'u-lāt). 1. Kneed. 2. Bent as a knee. 3. Pert. to the ganglion or geniculum of the facial nerve.

  g. neural'gia. Spasmodic form of facial neuralgia. SYN: *tic douloureux.*

  g. otalgia. Pain transmitted from the facial nerve to the ear.

geniculum (jen-ik'u-lum). A structure resembling a knot, or a knee.

genion (je'nĭ-on). Apex of the spina mentalis.

genioplasty (je'nĭ-o-plas"tĭ). Plastic surgery of the chin or cheek.

genital (jen'ĭ-tal). Pert. to the genitals.

  g. reflex. Functional nervous manifestations, masturbation, and convulsions, resulting from any form of genital irritation.

genitalia, gen'itals (jen-it-al'ĭ-ă). Organs of generation; reproductive organs.

  g., female. With the hymen acting as line of boundary, the female generative organs are divided into external and internal.

    g., male. Two bulbourethral (Cowper's) glands, 2 ejaculatory ducts, 2 glandular organs producing spermatozoa (the testes or gonads), 1 penis with urethra, 2 seminal ducts (vasa deferentes or ductus deferentes), 2 seminal vesicles, 2 spermatic cords, 1 scrotum, 1 prostate gland, *q.v.*

  g. reflex. Erection and ejaculation resulting from genital stimulation or indirectly from emotion whether asleep or awake.

gen'itoplas"ty. Reparative surgery on the genital organs.

gen"ito'rinary. Pert. to the genitals and the urinary organs.

  g. system. Organs and parts concerned with the kidneys, urinary bladder, and organs of generation and their accessories.

gen'oblast. 1. The nucleus of an impregnated ovum. 2. An ovum or spermatozoon.

gen'oceptor. The ceptor in a cell responsible for reproductivity.

genodermatosis (jen″o-der-mă-to'sis). Any congenital disease of the skin.

genoneme (jen'o-nēm). That part of a chromosome in which the genes are found.

genoplasty (jen'o-plas-tĭ). Any plastic surgery of the cheek.

genotype (jen'o-tĭp). 1. Basic hereditary combination of genes of an organism. 2. A type species. 3. Group marked by same hereditary characteristics.

genotypic (jen-o-tip'ik). Rel. to heredity.

Gensoul's disease (zhahn'soolz). A phlegmonous inflammation of the mouth floor and the subcutaneous and intermuscular tissue of the submaxillary region. SYN: *Ludwig's angina.*

gentian (jen'shĭ-an). USP. Dried rhyzome roots of the plant.
    DOSAGE: 1 dram (4 cc.).
    g. violet. A dye derived from coal tar. Used in indelible pencils and in 5% solution in treatment of burns and indolent ulcers.

gen'tianophil(e, gen″tianoph'ilous. Easily and readily staining with gentian violet.

genu (je'nu). 1. The knee. 2. Any structure of angular form resembling a bent knee.
    g. extrorsum. SEE: *genu varum.*
    g. introrsum. SEE: *genu valgum.*
    g. recurvatum. Hyperextension at the knee joint.
    g. val'gum. Knock-knee.
    g. va'rum. Bowleg.

genuclast (jen'u-klăst). Instrument for breaking knee joint adhesions.

genucu'bital. Pert. to the elbows and knees, esp. the knee-elbow position.
    g. position (knee-elbow). One with the patient on the knees, thighs upright, body resting on elbows, head down on hands; employed when not possible to use the knee-chest position.

genupectoral (jen″u-pek'to-ral). Pert. to the chest and knees.
    g. position. Knee-chest position.
    A position assumed by the female patient in which the patient is supported upon her knees and chest, and when the vaginal lips are open the vagina fills with air. This position is used for purposes of examination, treatment, and as an orthopedic aid in retroversion of uterus.

ge'nus. BIOL: The division between the species and the family.

genyantralgia (jen″ĭ-an-tral'jĭ-ă). Pain in the antrum of Highmore.

genyantritis (jen″ĭ-an-tri'tis). Inflammation of the antrum of Highmore.

genyoplasty (jen'ĭ-o-plas-tĭ). Any plastic operation on the chin.

geode (je'ōd). A lymph space connected with the lymphatic system.

geograph'ical tongue. Numerous scaly patches on dorsal surface of tongue coalescing into gyrate figures. SEE: *tongue.*

geophagia, geophagism, geophagy (je-o-fa'jĭ-ă, -of'a-jĭzm, -of'a-jĭ). A condition in which the patient eats unedible substances, as chalk or earth. SYN: *chthonophagia.*

geotragia (je-o-tra'jĭ-ă). Earth eating. SYN: *chthonophagia, geophagism.*

gephyrophobia (jef-ĭ-rō-fo'bĭ-ă). Aversion to bodies of water, or to crossing over bridges over water, or to traveling on boats.

geratic (je-rat'ik). Rel. to old age.

geratology (jer-ă-tol'o-jĭ). The study of old age. SYN: *gereology.*

Gerdy's fibers (zher'dēz). The superficial transverse ligament of the fingers.

gereology (je-re-ol'o-jĭ). The science of old age.

geriatrics (jer-ĭ-at'riks). Study and treatment of the diseases of old age.

Gerlach's network (ger'laks). Nerve fibers in gray substance of the spinal cord. SEE: *fiber.*

Gerlier's disease (zher-le-āz'). Paralyzing vertigo.

germ. 1. The first rudiment of an organism. 2. An ovum. 3. A microbe.
    g. cell. An ovum or spermatozoon.
    g., disease. Microörganism or its products said to be the cause of various infectious diseases.
    g. disease. Disease caused by a microörganism.
    g. epithelium, g. ridge. Ridge of epithelium in the embryo from which develops the sexual portions of the body.
    g. plasm. That part of a germ cell which contains the hereditary principle. SYN: *id.*
    g. theory. The hypothesis that certain bacteria or microbes may infect the body and cause disease states, each one exuding its own toxins.

German measles. Acute contagious disease with rash of short duration, resembling measles and scarlet fever. SYN: *rötheln, rubella.*

germicidal (germ-ĭ-si'dal). 1. Destructive to germs. 2. Pert. to an agent destructive to germs.

germicide (jer'mis-īd). A substance that destroys germs.

germ'inal. Pert. to a germ or ovum, or to germination. [*q.v.*
    g. spot. The nucleolus of an ovum.
    g. vesicle. Nucleus of an ovum, *q.v.*

germina'tion. Development of an impregnated ovum into an embryo.

ger'minative. Pert. to germination. SYN: *germinal.*

gerocomia (jer-o-ko'mĭ-ă). The hygiene of old age, or old men.

geroder'ma, gerodermia (je-ro-der'mĭ-ă). An appearance of senility brought about by premature loss of hair, wrinkling of the skin, and general atrophy.

geromorphism (je-ro-mor'fĭzm). Appearance of age in youth.

gerontal (jĕ-ron'tal). Pert. to an old man or to the aged. SYN: *senile*.

gerontology (je-ron-tol'o-jĭ). The study of the phenomena of old age. SYN: *geriatrics*.

gerontopia (je-ron-to'pĭ-ă). Second sight due to change in the refractive power of the lens. SYN: *senopia*.

gerontoxon (jĕ-ron-toks'on). Degenerative circle about corneal ext. surface seen in the aged. SYN: *arcus senilis*.

Gerota's capsule. The perirenal fascia.

gestaltism. The theory that the objects of mind come as wholes which cannot be split up into parts and which are unanalyzable.

gestation (jes-ta'shun). Period of intra-uterine fetal development. SYN: *fetation, gravidity, pregnancy*.

  g., abdominal. Ectopic gestation in which the product of conception is lodged in the peritoneal cavity.

  g., cervical. The temporary retention of the ovum within canal of cervix uteri after its expulsion from the uterus in abortion.

  g., cornual. Gestation in an ill-developed cornu of a bicornuate uterus.

  g., ectopic. Conception outside the uterus.

  g., interstitial. Tubal gestation in which the ovum is developed in that portion of oviduct that traverses wall of uterus.

  g., ovarian. A form of ectopic gestation in the ovary.

  g., plural. Gestation with more than 1 embryo.

  g., prolonged; g., protracted. Gestation prolonged beyond the usual period.

  g. sac. The amnion and its contents.

  g., secondary abdominal. Extrauterine gestation in which the fetus, originally situated in oviduct or elsewhere, has become lodged in abdominal cavity because of the rupture of the fetal sac.

  g., secondary. The ovum becomes dislodged from original seat of implantation, and continues to develop in a new situation.

  g., tubal; g., tubarian. Ectopic gestation in which the product of conception is lodged in the oviduct.

  g., tuboabdominal. Extrauterine gestation in which fetal sac is formed partly of the abdominal extremity of the oviduct and partly of plastic exudation in the neighborhood.

  g., tuboövarian. Extrauterine gestation in which the fetal sac is made up of the ovary and the abdominal end of the oviduct.

  g., uterotubal. Gestation in which the ovum is developed partly in uterine portion of oviduct and partly within cavity of uterus.

gestosis (jes-to'sis). Any disorder of pregnancy.

gherkin. A form of pickle. COMP: It is more of a condiment than a vegetable or a food.

Ghon's primary lesion. A bean-shaped shadow in the x-ray of the lung seen in certain cases of pulmonary tuberculosis in children.

ghost corpuscle. Depigmented red blood corpuscle. SYN: *phantom corpuscle*.

giant cell. One of large size with several nuclei, appearing to be made up of many cells, but not clearly outlined, found in both kinds of marrow, esp. in red marrow. SEE: *osteoblast*.

  g. c. tumor. Rare, benign, encapsulated tumor in lower jaw or on alveolar process of upper jaw in the young.

giantism (ji'an-tizm). Abnormal development of the body or its parts. SYN: *gigantism*.

Gianuzzi's cells or crescents (jan-oot'sez). Crescentic granular cells in mucous glands concerned with functional activity of the gland. SYN: *demilune cells*.

Giardia (gĭ-ar'dĭ-ă). Genus of protozoa with flagella, occasionally causing intestinal infection, although not known as pathogenic, usually seen in the intestinal passages.

  G. enterica, G. intestinalis, G. lamblia. Form with 4 pairs of flagella and a sucking disk, with a shape like a pear. SYN: *Cercomonas intestinalis, Lamblia intestinalis*.

giardiasis (gĭ-ar-di'as-is). Infection with *Giardia intestinalis*. SYN: *lambliasis*.

Gibbon's hydrocele (gĭb'ŏn). A hydrocele and large hernia combined.

gibbosity (gĭ-bos'ĭ-ty). 1. Condition of having a humpback. 2. A hump or gibbus, as the deformity of Pott's disease.

gibbous (gĭb'bus). Humped; protuberant or humpbacked. [*tigo*.

giddiness. State of dizziness. SYN: *ver-*

Giemsa stain (gēm'zah). One for demonstrating spirochetes, malarial organisms, and Negri bodies.

Gifford's reflex (gĭf'ford). Pupillary contraction resulting from endeavoring forcibly to close eyelids which are held apart.

gigantism (ji'an-tizm). Abnormal development of the body or of a part. SYN: *giantism*.

gigantoblast. A very large nucleated red corpuscle.

gigantocyte (ji-gan'to-sīt). 1. A giant cell. 2. A very large red blood corpuscle.

gigantosoma (ji-gan-to-so'mă). Abnormal size of the body. SYN: *giantism, gigantism*.

Gimbernat's ligament (zham-bār-nahz'). Ligamentum lacunare.

gin-drinkers' liver. Atrophic cirrhosis of the liver resulting from alcoholism. SYN: *hobnailed liver*.

ginger. USP. Dried root of the plant. DOSAGE: 30 ℔ (2 cc.).

gingiva (jin-ji'vă). The gum surrounding the alveolar processes of the jaws and teeth.

gingival (jin'jiv-al). Rel. to the gums.

gingivalgia. Pain in the gums.

gingivally. Toward the gums.

gingivectomy (jin"jĭ-vek'to-mĭ). Excision of gum tissue in pyorrhea. SYN: *ulectomy*.

gingivitis (jin-jĭ-vi'tis). Inflammation of the gums. SYN: *ulitis*.

gingivoglossitis (jin'ji-vo-glos-si'tis). Inflammation of the gums and tongue. SYN: *stomatitis*.

ginglyform (jin'glĭ-form). In the form of a hinge. SYN: *ginglymoid*.

gin'glymo-arthro'dial. Pert. to a joint that is both hinged and arthrodial. SEE: *arthrodia*.

ginglymoid (jing'lĭ-moyd). Pert. to or shaped like a hinged joint.

ginglymus (jing'lĭ-mus). A hinge joint; diarthrosis.* SEE: *joint*.

Giraldès' organ (zhir-al-dās'). A vestige of the wolffian body at post. side of the testicle. SYN: *paradidymis*.

girdle (gir'del). 1. A zone or belt; cingulum, the waist. 2. Shingles or herpes zoster.

    g. anesthesia. A portion around the body without sensation.

    g., Neptune. Stimulating or heating compress of linen covered by flannel encircling trunk from lower end of sternum to pubes.

    g. pain. Painful sensation around the body.

    g. sensation. Same as girdle pain.

    g. symptom. A symptom in tabes as of a tight girdle, such as a feeling of constriction about the chest; also found in compression of the cord due to collapse of the vertebrae as in Pott's disease.

glabel'la. Smooth space bet. the eyebrows above the nose.

gla'brate. 1. Bald. 2. Smooth.

glabrificin (glab-rif-is'in). A variety of antibody which exposes a capsulated bacterium to the action of lysin.

gla'brous. 1. Bald. 2. Smooth. SYN: *glabrate*.

glacial (gla'shal). Glassy; resembling ice.

glad'iate. Sword-shaped. SYN: *ensiform, xiphoid*.

gladi'oline. An alkaloid from tissue of the brain.

gladiolus (glad-i'o-lus). The intermediate and principal segment of the sternum, *q.v.*

glairin (glār'in). Gelatinous substance in water of some sulfur springs.

glair'y. Viscous, mucoid.

gland. 1. A secretory and excretory structure of *external* and *internal* secretion. 2. A lymphatic node.

    g., absorbent. Any one of the lymphatic glands.

    g., accessory. Gland functioning as an accessory to another gland.

    g., acinotubular. A gland structurally midway bet. an acinous and a tubular gland.

    g., acinous. Compound gland made up of many acini.

    g's., aggregate. Lymphatic glands in patch formation found mainly in ileum. SYN: *Peyer's patches*.

    g's., agminated. SEE: *aggregate glands*.

    g's., albuminous. Digestive tract glands secreting a fluid containing albumin.

    g's., anal. Glands in anal mucosa producing sweat and odor.

    g's., auricular. External otic lymph nodes.

    g's., axillary. Axillary lymph nodes.

    g's., Bartholin's. Tiny glands on both sides of the vagina. SYN: *vulvovaginal gland*.

    g's., Blandin's; g's., Blandin - Nuhn's. Tiny racemose glands secreting mucus and saliva, near the tip of the tongue on the undersurface.

    g's., Bowman's. Nasal glands in olfactory area.

    g's., brachial. Glands in the arm and forearm.

    g's., bronchial. Bronchial root lymph glands.

    g's., Bruch's. Conjunctival lymph nodes in lower lids.

    g's., Brunner's. Glands in the duodenal submucosa secreting intestinal juice.

    g's., buccal. Acinous glands in the cheek tissue.

    g., carotid. Tiny gland at fork of carotid artery.

    g's., cecal. Cecal lymph nodes.

    g's., ceruminous. Glands in auditory canal excreting cerumen.

    g's., cervical. Lymph glands situated in the neck.

    g., ciliary. SEE: *Moll's glands*.

    g's., Cobelli's. Glands in the esophageal mucosa.

    g., coccygeal. SEE: *Luschka's gland*.

    g., compound. Gland composed of numerous acini or pouches.

    g., c., tubular. Gland composed of numerous minute tubules leading to a lone duct.

    g., conglobate. Lymphatic gland.

    g., conglomerate. SEE: *acinous gland*.

    g's., Cowper's. Two small glands above the bulb of corpus spongiosum, whose secretion forms part of seminal fluid.

    g's., cutaneous. Dermal glands.

    g's., decidual. Glands contained in decidua in the uterus.

    g., ductless. Gland possessing no secretory duct.

    g's., duodenal. SEE: *Brunner's glands*.

    g's., Duverney's. SEE: *Bartholin's glands*.

    g's., Frankel's. Tiny glands located below the margin of the vocal cords.

    g's., fundus. Stomach glands secreting gastric juice.

    g's., Gay's. Multiple sweat glands developed to a great extent.

    g., genal. Gland in buccal submucosa.

    g's., genital. SEE: *sexual glands*.

    g's., gingival. Glands at gum margins.

    g's., hair. Sebaceous glands opening into each hair follicle.

    g's., haversian. Glands secreting synovial fluid.

    g's., hematopoietic. Glands participating in blood production.

    g's., hemolymph. Modified glands containing blood and lymph sinuses, which probably participate in the formation of the leukocytes and the destruction of red blood corpuscles.

g's., hepatic. Lymph nodes located in front of the portal vein.

g's., inguinal. Lymph nodes in the inguinal region.

g., interscapular. Embryonic lymphatic tissue.

g., interstitial. Gland in connective tissue of seminiferous tubules of testes and those ovarian tissues which produce internal secretions. SYN: *interstitial* or *Leydig's cells.*

g's., intestinal. Single glands scattered through the intestinal mucosa.

g's., jugular. SEE: *cervical gland.*

g's., Krause's. Conjunctival mucous glands.

g's., labial. Multiple acinous glands bet. the mucosa of the lips and the opening on the inner lip.

g., lacrimal. Gland secreting tears.

g's., lactiferous. SEE: *mammary glands.*

g's., Lieberkühn's. Tiny tubular glands on the intestinal mucosa.

g's., Littré's. Tiny mucous glands in the urethral mucosa in the cavernous area.

g's., lumbar. Lymphatics located behind the peritoneal region and the lower section of the diaphragmatic post. part.

g., Luschka's. Gland located near the coccygeal tip.

g., lymph; g., lymphatic. Nodule of lymphatic tissue, found along the path of a lymphatic vessel.

g's., mammary. Glands secreting milk.

g's., meibomian. Glands situated in the eyelid secreting sebaceous substance which keeps the lids from adhering.

g's., Mery's. SEE: *Cowper's glands.*

g's., Moll's. Modified sweat glands in the eyelid.

g's., Montgomery's. Mammary sebaceous glands in the areola.

g's., Morgagni's. SEE: *Littré's glands.*

g's., muciparous; g's., mucous. Glands secreting mucus.

g's., nabothian. Dilated mucous glands in the uterine cervix.

g's., odoriferous. Gland exuding odoriferous materials, as those around the prepuce or anus.

g's., oxyntic. Gastric glands usually found in the abdominal cardiac region.

g's., pacchionian. Small masses along the surface of the dura mater in the cranium.

g's., palatine. Mucous glands in the tissue of the palate.

g., parotid. Largest salivary gland located in front of the ear.

g's., Peyer's. SEE: *aggregate glands.*

g., pineal. Tiny glandular body of conical shape located bet. 2 sup. quadrigeminal bodies, connected with the thalamus, but not a part of the brain.

g., pituitary. Two-lobed body situated in a depression of the sphenoid bone.

g's., preputial. SEE: *Tyson's glands.*

g., prostate. Gland surrounding male bladder neck and urethra.

g's., pulmonary. Glands in lung tissue.

g's., pyloric. Gastric glands near the pylorus secreting pepsin.

g., racemose. SEE: *acinous gland.*

g's., Rivini's. SEE: *sublingual glands.*

g., salivary. Any gland secreting saliva, as parotid, sublingual, and submaxillary. SEE: *salivary glands.*

g., sebaceous. Racemose gland secreting sebum, located in the skin.

g's., seminal. Testicles.

g's., serous. SEE: *albuminous glands.*

g's., Skene's. Two glands in female urethra.

g's., solitary. SEE: *intestinal glands.*

g's., sublingual. Tiny salivary glands situated on either side of the tongue.

g's., submaxillary. Tiny salivary glands on either side of the tongue in the submaxillary triangles.

g's., sudoriferous; g's., sudoriparous. Glands secreting perspiration situated in the skin.

g., suprarenal. Tiny ductless gland above kidney secreting adrenalin.*

g's., sweat. SEE: *sudoriferous glands.*

g., thymus. Two-lobed gland in the neck of young children.

g., thyroid. Ductless gland situated in the neck in front of the trachea.

g's., tracheal. Acinous glands of the tracheal mucosa.

g., tubular. Gland of tubular formation.

g's., Tyson's. Tiny sebaceous glands found on penis and on corona of glans penis.

g's., urethral. SEE: *Littré's glands.*

g's., vaginal. Acinous glands in the vaginal mucosa.

g's., vulvovaginal. SEE: *Bartholin's glands.*

g's., Waldeyer's. Glands in the eyelid.

g's., Weber's. Glands in the tongue mucosa.

g's., Zeiss'. Small sebaceous glands lubricating the eyelids.

g., Zuckerkandl's. Tiny, tawny lobe occasionally seen bet. geniohyoid muscles.

glanders (glan'derz). Contagious infection of *Bacillus mallei* in horses and mules, communicable to man.

glandula (glan'du-la) (pl. *glandulae*). A small gland. SYN: *glandule.*

glan'dular. Pert. to or of nature of a gland.

g. therapy. Treatment of disease with endocrine glands or their extracts. SYN: *organotherapy.* SEE: *endocrinology, gland.*

glandule (glan'dŭl). A small gland. SYN: *glandula.*

glans. 1. A gland. 2. Goiter. 3. A nut.

g. clitoridis. The head of the clitoris.

g. penis, g. phalli. Bulbous end of the penis. SEE: *clitoris, penis.*

glare. Temporary blurring of vision, with possible permanent injury to retina from intense light (visible radiation) emanating from highly reflecting objects, such as sunlight reflected from water or snow, or projected by automobile headlight, or by a therapeutic lamp.

glase′rian artery. A section of internal maxillary artery; goes to tympanum. SYN: *tympanic artery*.

g. fissure. A fissure in the temporal bone.

glass, polarized. A medium that permits the exiting light waves to vibrate in only one direction.

g., swallowing. F. A. TREATMENT: SEE: *cotton-wool sandwiches*.

g., ultraviolet transmitting. Glass designed to admit ultraviolet radiation through it.

glass′es. 1. Transparent refractive device worn to correct eye defects. 2. Device worn to protect eye from glare. Federal specifications are "shade No. 3 filter lens." SEE: *glare, lens*.

glas′sy. Hyaline; vitreous; like glass, smooth and shiny.

Glau′ber's salt. Crystalline salt used as a hydragogue purgative. SEE: *sodium sulfate*, USP.

glauco′ma. Disease of eye characterized by increase in intraocular pressure which results in atrophy of optic nerve and blindness of 2 general types, *primary*, which sets in without cause, and *secondary*, in which there is an increase in intraocular pressure due to other eye disease.

SEE: *ciliarotomy*.

g. absolutum. Eye completely blind, cornea insensitive, ant. chamber shallow, excavated optic disc, eye as hard as stone, extremely painful.

g., chronic. Pressure up to 45-50, enlargement of ant. ciliary veins, cornea clear, dilated pupil, pain, poor vision during attacks, field may be normal, no cupping early.

g., infantile. Buphthalmos resulting in uniform enlargement of eye with increased pressure.

g. simplex. Pressure not high, contracted field, glaucomatous cupping, blindness, no acute attacks.

glaucomatous (glaw-ko′ma-tus). Pert. to glaucoma.

gleet. A mucous discharge from the urethra in chronic gonorrhea.

Glénard's disease (gla-narz′). Prolapse of 1 or more of the internal organs. SYN: *enteroptosis, splanchnoptosis*.

glenohumeral (gle-no-hu′mer-al). Pert. to the humerus and the glenoid cavity.

g. ligaments. Three ligaments in shoulder.

gle′noid. Having the appearance of a socket.

g. cavity. The socket which receives the head of the humerus, below the acromion process at the head of the shoulder.

gli′a. Supporting structure of nerves and cells of spinal cord and brain.

g. cell. Branched cell occurring in 3 forms, *macroglia, oligodendroglia*, and *microglia*, found in neuroglia, the sup-

porting tissue of the nervous structure. SEE: *cell, glia, neuroglia*.

gliacyte (gli′as-īt). A neuroglia cell.

gli′adin. A protein separable from the gluten of wheat.

It is deficient in lysine. It contains 94.11% amino acid.

glial (gli′al). Concerning glia or neuroglia.

gliarase (gli′ar-ās). Astrocytic mass with fission of cytoplasm.

gliobacte′ria. A zooglear mass containing bacilli.

glioblasto′ma. A neuroglia cell tumor. SYN: *glioma*.

gliococ′cus. A micrococcus in a mass of zooglea.

gliocyte (gli′o-sīt). A neuroglia cell. SYN: *gliacyte*.

gliocyto′ma. A neuroglia cell tumor.

gliogenous (gli-oj′en-us). Of the nature of neuroglia.

glio′ma (pl. *glio′mata*). 1. A sarcoma of neurogliar origin. 2. Neoplasm or a tumor composed of neuroglia cells.

g. retinae. Malignant tumor of retina; occurs in children under 5 years of age; metastasizes late. SYN: *pseudoglioma*.

gliomatosis (gli-o-mat-o′sis). Formation of a glioma.

gliomatous (gli-o′mă-tus). Affected with or of the nature of a glioma.

gliomyoma (gli-o-mī-o′mă). A mixed glioma and myoma.

glioneuroma (gli-o-nū-ro′mă). A tumor having the characteristics of glioma and neuroma.

gliosarco′ma. Glioma combined with fusiform cells of sarcoma.

gliosis (gli-o′sis). Excessive overgrowth or tumors of neurogliar tissue.

gliosome (gli′o-sōm). One of the rounded bodies seen in neuroglia cells.

glischrin (glis′krin). Mucin substance formed by *Bacillus glischrogenes*.

glischruria (glis-kru′rī-ă). Glischrin in the urine.

glisso′nian cirrhosis. Inflammation of peritoneal coat of the liver. SYN: *perihepatitis*.

glissoni′tis. Inflammation of Glisson's capsule.

Glisson's capsule (glis′uns). The outer capsule of fibrous tissue investing the liver. SYN: *capsula fibrosa hepatis*.

glo′bin. A protein constituent of oxyhemoglobin. It yields a large amt. of histidine by hydrolytic cleavage.

globinom′eter. Device for estimating the number of blood corpuscles in a given amount of blood. SYN: *cytometer*.

glo′boid. Spheroid; resembling a globe.

g. bodies. Minute ultramicroscopical microörganisms such as pathogens of poliomyelitis.

globular (glob′u-lar). Resembling a globe or globule; spherical.

globule (glob′ūl). Any small rounded body.

globulicidal (glob′u-lis-i′dal). Destructive to red blood corpuscles.

globulim′eter. Device for determining relative proportions of hemoglobin.

globulin (glob'u-lin). A simple protein soluble only in neutral salt solution.

g., serum. That found in blood serum.

glob″uline′mia. Globulin in the blood.

glob″ulinu′ria. Excretion of globulin in the urine.

glob′ulism. 1. Abnormal amt. of red corpuscles in the blood. 2. Administration of medicine in globules.

globulolysis (glob-u-lol′is-is). Red blood corpuscle destruction. SYN: *hematolysis.*

gobulolytic (glob-u-lol-it′ik). Capable of destroying red blood corpuscles.

globulose (glob′u-lōs). Albumose or proteid produced by the digestion of globulins.

globu′lysis. Destruction of red blood corpuscles. SYN: *globulolysis, hemolysis.*

globus. A globe or sphere.

g. hystericus. A lump in the throat in hysteria and other neuroses.

g. major. Head of epididymus.

g. minor. Lower end of epididymus.

g. pallidus. Pale section within the lenticular nucleus. SEE: *paleostriatum.*

glome. A small, round swelling made up of tiny blood vessels in a fibroid stroma containing many nerve fibers. SYN: *glomus.*

glom′erate. Conglomerate, clustered, grouped.

glomer′ular. Clustered. Pert. to a glomerulus.

glomerule (glom′er-ul). Mass of vascular tufts forming renal malpighian bodies with Bowman's capsule. SYN: *glomerulus.*

glomer′uli (sing. *glomerulus*). 1. Small structures in the malpighian body of the kidney made up of capillary blood vessels in a cluster and enveloped in a thin wall, giving off uriniferous tubules. 2. Plexuses of capillaries. Twisted secretory parts of sweat glands.

glomerulitis (glom-er-ū-li′tis). Inflammation of glomerulus, esp. of the renal glomeruli. SYN: *glomerulonephritis.*

glomerulonephri′tis. Lesions in the glomeruli with parenchymatous nephritis. SYN: *glomerulitis.*

glomer′ulus (pl. *glomeruli*). A cluster of vascular tufts which, with Bowman's capsule, form the malpighian bodies of the kidney.

glomus (glo′mus). A small, round swelling made up of tiny blood vessels and found in a stroma containing many nerve fibers.

g. caroticum. The carotid gland.

glos′sa. The tongue.

glos′sal. Rel. to the tongue.

glossalgia (glos-sal′ji-ă). Pain in the tongue. SYN: *glossodynia.*

glossectomy (glos″ek′to-mĭ). Partial or complete excision of tongue. SYN: *elinguation, Kocher's operation.*

glossi′tis. Inflammation of the tongue.

g., acute. Associated with stomatitis, *q.v.* The tongue is covered with ulcers and is tender and painful. Another form affects the parenchyma of tongue

and is characterized by edema, which may spread to surrounding structures, producing asphyxia and necessitating tracheotomy operation.

g. areata exfoliativa. Geographical tongue.

g., chronic. Sometimes while suffering from chronic ill health, chronic dyspepsia, and septic teeth, this condition arises.

g. desic′cans. A painful, raw, and fissured tongue.

g. parasit′ica. Black tongue. SYN: *glossophytia.* [tongue.

glosso-. Prefix: Signifies *pert. to the*

glossocele (glos′so-sēl). Swelling and protrusion of the tongue due to disease or malformation.

glossodynamometer (glos″so-din-a-mom′e-ter). Device for measuring contractile power of the tongue muscles.

glossodynia (glos-so-din′ĭ-ă). Pain in the tongue. SYN: *glossalgia.*

glos″soepiglot′tic. Pert. to the ligament bet. base of tongue and epiglottis.

glossoepiglottidean (glos″o-ep-ĭ-glŏ-tid′e-an). Rel. to the tongue and epiglottis.

g. folds. Three mucous membrane folds from base of tongue to the epiglottis. SYN: *plicae epiglotticae.*

g. ligament. Elastic band from base of tongue to the epiglottis in middle glossoepiglottidean fold.

glossograph (glos′o-graf). A graph for showing the tongue's movements in speaking.

glossohyal (glos-o-hi′al). Rel. to tongue and hyoid bone. SYN: *hyoglossal.*

glossolalia (glos-so-lal′ĭ-ă). Repetition of senseless remarks not related to the subject or situation involved.

glossology (glos-sol′o-jĭ). 1. Study of the tongue and its diseases. SYN: *glottology.* 2. Science of nomenclature. SYN: *onomatology.*

glossolysis (glos-sol′is-is). Paralysis of tongue. SYN: *glossoplegia.*

glossopathy (glos-sop′ă-thĭ). Disease of the tongue.

glossopharyngeal (glos″o-far-in′je-ăl). Rel. to tongue and pharynx.

g. nerve. Ninth cranial nerve. FUNCT: Taste, sensation, motor, vasomotor.

glossophytia (glos-so-fĭ′tĭ-ă). Black tongue caused by microphytes and dead epithelium.

glossoplasty (glos-so-plas′tĭ). Reparative surgery of the tongue.

glossople′gia. Paralysis of tongue, usually unilateral.

glossopto′sis. A dropping of the tongue downward out of normal position.

glossorrhaphy (glos-sor′ă-fĭ). Suture of wound of the tongue.

glossos′copy. Inspection of the tongue.

glossospasm (glos′so-spazm). Spasmodic contraction of muscles of the tongue.

glossotomy (glos-ot′o-mĭ). Incision of tongue.

gloss′y. Smooth and shining.

g. skin. An atrophy of skin due to nerve lesion or injury.

glot'tic. Of or pert. to the tongue, or the glottis.

glottis (glot'is). The vocal aperture of the larynx; the fissure bet. the vocal cords, the narrowest segment of the air passages.

g., edema of. An infiltration of serous fluid into the submucous membrane of the larynx.   [false vocal cords.

g. spuria. Space situated bet. the

glotti'tis. Inflammation of the tongue. SYN: *glossitis*.

glottol'ogy. The study of the tongue and its diseases. SYN: *glossology*.

Glover's stitch or suture (gluv'erz). The continuous suture used in intestinal wounds.

glucase (glu'kās). A ferment converting starch into glucose.

glucatonia (glu-ka-to'nĭ-ă). Reduction of blood sugar brought about by insulin therapy.

glucide (glŭ'sĭd). 1. One of a large class of organic compounds including the carbohydrates and glucosides.* 2. USP. White crystalline powder 500 times sweeter than sugar having no food value. One-quarter gr. (0.015 Gm.) in the place of an ordinary lump of sugar.

gluciphore (glu'sĭ-fōr). An atomic group which, when combined with other tasteless atoms called auxoglucs, forms sweet compounds. SEE: *auxogluc*.

glucohe'mia. Sugar in the blood. SYN: *glycosemia*.

gluco'neogenesis. The formation of glucose in the body from available fat or protein.

glu'cose. Dextrose or grape sugar.

glucose (glu'cōs). USP. A colorless or yellow, thick, syrupy liquid, obtained by the incomplete hydrolysis of starch.

g., dextrose. USP. Colorless crystals or powder.

DOSAGE: Orally, 6 oz. (180 Gm.); rectally, a solution, 5 to 10% strength, is sometimes employed intravenously (which should be exceedingly slow, and prepared under very careful technic, preferably from ampoules), varies; a 5 to 10% solution of 300 cc. frequently used.

glucose tolerance test. "Used to determine percentage of blood sugar at which the kidney begins to excrete sugar in the urine. It is of value in determining diet necessary, and amount of insulin required to balance this, in a patient suffering from diabetes, *q.v.*

glucoside (glu'ko-sĭd). Active principle from plant drug (usually ending in "in"), capable of being split into 2 or more simpler bodies.

glucosin (glu'ko-sĭn). Any one of a series of bases derived by action of ammonia on glucose.

glucosu'ria. Abnormal amt. of sugar in the urine. SYN: *glycosuria*.

gluelike tumor. Glioma. Also a colloid degenerative cancer or colloma.

Glu'ge's corpuscles. Granular cells containing fat droplets.

glu'side. Saccharin, said to be 300 times as sweet as cane sugar. SYN: *glusidum*.

DOSAGE: ½ gr. (0.03 Gm.).

glusidum (glŭ-sĭ'dŭm). Saccharin. Substance employed as a sugar substitute. SYN: *gluside.**

glutathione (glŭ-ta-thi'on). A tripeptide of glutamic acid, cystein, and glycine.

gluteal (glŭ'tē-ăl). Pertaining to the buttocks.

g. fold. Crease between the thigh and the buttocks. SEE: *rump*.

g. reflex. Contraction of gluteal muscles from stimulation of their skin.

glutelin (glŭ'tĕ-lĭn). A simple protein found in grain seeds, soluble in alkalies and dilute acids, but not in neutral solutions. SEE: *protein*.

glu'ten. Vegetable albumin, a protein which can be prepared from wheat, corn, and other grain.

glu'tin. The viscid portion of wheat gluten. SYN: *gliadin*.

glutinous (glŭ'tin-us). Adhesive; sticky.

gluti'tis. Inflammation of muscles of buttocks.

glu'tolin. An albumoid substance found in small amts. in paraglobulin.

glycase (gli'kās). The enzyme that converts maltose into dextrose. SEE: *enzyme, ferment*.

glycemia (gli-se'mĭ-ă). Sugar or glucose in the blood. SYN: *glycosemia.**

glycemin (gli'sem-ĭn). A substance, secreted by the liver of diabetics, which counteracts insulin.

glyceride (glis'er-id). An ester of glycerin compounded with an acid.

glycerin (glis'er-ĭn). USP. A clear, colorless liquid formed during the manufacture of soap, or by direct hydrolysis of fat. SYN: *glycerol*.

DOSAGE: 60 ₥ (4.0 cc.).

glycerite (glis'er-īt). Drug dissolved in glycerin. Four official.

glyceri'tum (pl. *glycerita*). Medicinal substance mixed or dissolved in glycerin.

glycerol (glis'er-ol). Clear, colorless, syrupy liquid formed by hydrolysis of fat. SYN: *glycerin, q.v.*

g. trinitrate. Nitroglycerin, USP.

DOSAGE: 1 ₥ (0.6 cc.) Tablets, 1/100 gr. (0.6 mg.).

glycine (gli'sēn). Aminoacetic acid* derived from gelatin and from many proteins. SYN: *glycocin, glycocoll.*

glyco-. Prefix from G. *glykus*, sweet. Used in chemical compounds to indicate the presence of glycerol or similar substance.

gly'cocin. Any fatty amino acid.

glycoclas'tic. Pert. to the hydrolysis and digestion of sugars.

glycocoll (gli'ko-kŏl). Aminoacetic acid derived from gelatin and from many proteins.

DOSAGE: Daily, 300-450 gr. (20.0-30.0 Gm.).

glycogen (gli'ko-jen). Animal starch, a whitish powder which can be prepared from mammalian liver and muscle, and other animal tissues.

glycogenase (gli'ko-jen-ās). An enzyme in the liver.
Its end product is dextrose.

glycogenesis (gli-ko-jen'es-is). The formation of glycogen, as occurs in man after the eating of a carbohydrate meal.

glycogenet'ic. Pert. to the formation of glycogen.

glycogen'ic. Rel. to glycogen.

glycogenolysis (gli''ko-jen-ol'is-is). Conversion of glycogen into dextrose in the liver.

glycogenolytic (gli-ko-jen-o-lit'ik). Pert. to the hydrolysis of glycogen.

glycogenosis (gli-ko-jen-o'sis). Abnormal amt. of glycogen in children resulting in an enlarged liver.

glycogenous (gli-koj'en-us). Pert. to glucose formation. SYN: *glycogenetic, glycogenic.*

glycogeusia (gli-ko-ju'sĭ-ă). A sweet taste.

glycohemia (gli-ko-he'mĭ-ă). Abnormal amt. of sugar in the blood. SYN: *glycosemia.*

glycol (gli'kol). Any one of the dihydric alcohols related to ethylene glycol, $C_2H_4\cdot(OH)_2$. The general formula is $C_2H_2n\cdot(OH)_2$.

glycolipid(e (gli''ko-lip'id). Compound of fatty acids with a carbohydrate, containing nitrogen, but no phosphoric acid.

glycolysis (gli-kol'i-sis). Hydrolysis of sugar by a ferment, esp. in the blood after death.

glycolyt'ic. Pert. to hydrolyzing sugar.
    g. enzyme or **ferment.** The enzyme having the property of destroying sugar in the blood.

glycometabol'ic. Rel. to the metabolism of sugar.

glycometabolism (gli''kō-mĕt-ăb'ō-lĭzm). Utilization of sugar* by the body. SYN: *saccharometabolism.* SEE: *metabolism.*

glyconeogenesis (gli''ko-ne-o-jen'e-sis). The formation of carbohydrates from noncarbohydrates, such as fat or protein.

glyconucleopro'tein. A carbohydrate group unduly developed in a nucleoprotein.

glycopenia (gli-ko-pe'nĭ-ă). Having a tendency to hypoglycemia.

glycopex'ic. Pert. to the fixing or storing of sugar.

glycopex'is. The storing of glycogen in the liver.

glycophe'nol. Saccharin, a very sweet crystalline substance. SYN: *gluside.*

glycophilia (gli-ko-fil'ĭ-ă). A condition in which there is a marked tendency to hyperglycemia.

glycopolyuria (gli''ko-pol-ĭ-ū'rĭ-ă). Diabetes mellitus with *polyuria* greater than *glycosuria.*

glycopri'val, glycopri'vous. Lacking in or without carbohydrates.

glycoprotein (gli-ko-pro'te-in). A compound or conjugated protein such as mucin. SEE: *protein.*

glycoptyalism (gli-ko-ti'al-ĭzm). Excretion of glucose in the saliva.

glycoregula'tion. The dietary and insulin control of sugar metabolism.

glycoreg'ulatory. Rel. to glycoregulation.

glycorrhachia (gli-ko-rak'ĭ-ă). Sugar in the cerebrospinal fluid.

glycorrhea (gli-kor-re'ă). Discharge of sugar from the body. SEE: *glycosuria.*

glycosecretory (gli''ko-se-kre'to-rĭ). Pert. to or determining the secretion of glycogen.   [in the blood.

glycose'mia. Abnormal amount of sugar

glycosialia (gli-ko-si-al'ĭ-ă). Sugar in the saliva.

glycosialorrhea (gli''ko-si-al-or-re'ă). Excessive secretion of saliva containing sugar.

glycosin (gli'kos-in). 1. A pancreatic principle said to be a substitute for insulin. 2. Compound sometimes forming uric acid in kidneys by combining with urea. SEE: *acid*

glycosom'eter. Device for determining proportion of sugar in urine in glycosuria.

glycosuria (gli-ko-su'rĭ-ă). The presence of sugar (glucose) in the urine.
    g., alimentary. Following ingestion of large amounts of starches or sugars.
    g., renal. When glucose is persistent and not accompanied by hyperglycemia.
    g., temporal. Appears during convalescence from acute fevers.
    g., transient. Found in the obese and in those under mental strain.

glycuresis (gli-ku-re'sis). Presence of sugar (glucose) in the urine. SYN: *glycosuria.**

glycuronuria (gli-kŭ-ro-nu'rĭ-ă). Glycuronic acid in the urine.

glycylglycine (glis-il-glis'in). The simplest form of a polypeptide

glycyltryptophan (glis''il-trip'tof-ăn). A dipeptide of glycine and tryptophan.

Gm. Abbr. for *gram*

gnathalgia (nath-al'jĭ-ă). Pain in the jaw. SYN: *gnathodynia*

gnathic (nath'ĭk). Pert. to an alveolar process or to the jaw.

gnathion (nath'ĭ-on). Lowest part of middle line of lower jaw; a craniometric point.

gnathitis (na-thi'tis). Inflammation of the jaw or adjacent soft parts.

gnatho- (nath'o). Prefix: Pert. to jaw or cheek.

gnathodynia (nath-o-din'ĭ-ă). Pain in the jaw. SYN: *gnathalgia.*

gnathoplasty (nath'o-plas-tĭ). Reparative surgery of jaws or cheek.

gnathoschisis (nath-os'kis-is). Congenital jaw cleft.

gnosia (no'sĭ-ă). The perceptive faculty of recognizing persons, things, and forms.

goat-leap pulse. Term applied to an irregular and bounding pulse. SEE: *pulse.*

gob'let cell. The simplest form of cell, beaker-shaped, and resulting from mucoid secretions forming a modification of an epithelial cell; glandular cell. SYN: *mucous cell.* SEE: *cell.*

gog'gle eyed. Having an abnormally protruding eye. SYN: *exophthalmic, strabismic.*

goiter (goi'ter). An enlargement of the thyroid gland.   [enlargement.

g., aberrant. Supernumerary thyroid

g., acute. Goiter growing rapidly.

g., adenomatous. Thyroid enlargement due to growth of encapsulated adenomata.

g., basedowified. SEE: *toxic goiter*.

g., colloid. One in which there is a great increase of follicular contents.

g., cystic. Bronchocele. It may be enlargement of a single vessel or liquification of an adenoma.

g., diver; g., diving. Movable goiter.

g., endemic. Goiter development in certain localities.

g., exophthalmic. A disease of the vegetative nervous system, causing excessive thyroid secretion.

g., fibrous. Goiter with hyperplastic capsule and stroma of the thyroid gland.

g., follicular. SEE: *parenchymatous goiter*.

g., lingual. Hypertrophied mass forming a tumor at post. portion of dorsum of tongue.

g., parenchymatous. Uniform enlargement of thyroid, common in the young.

g., perivascular. Goiter surrounding a large blood vessel.

g., retrovascular. Goiter development behind a large blood vessel.

g., simple. Thyroid gland hyperplasia.

g., substernal. Enlargement of lower part of thyroid isthmus.

g., suffocative. Goiter causing shortness of breath due to pressure.

g., toxic. One that produces an excessive toxic secretion.

g., vascular. Goiter due to distention of blood vessels.

gold-beaters' skin. A membrane from the cecum of the ox for surgical use.

Gold'berger's diet. One for pellagra. Eggs, lean meat, and brewer's yeast.

Gold'flam's disease. Excessive tiring of voluntary muscles and rapid decrease of contractility. SYN: *myasthenia gravis pseudoparalytica*.

gold seed. Thin capillary glass tube covered with gold containing some form of radium.

Golgi's cells. Nerve cells in the cerebral cortex and post. horns of spinal cord.

G.'s corpuscles. Special tactile corpuscles at insertion of tendons.

Goll's tract (golz). One in post. white column of spinal cord. SYN: *fasciculus gracilis*.

gomphi'asis. Loosening of the teeth.

gomphosis (gom-fo'sis). A conical process fitting into a socket in immovable (synarthrosis*) joint. SEE: *joint*.

gon'ad. A generic term referring to both the female sex glands, or ovaries, and the male sex glands, or testicles.

gonadal (gon-ă-dal). Pert. to a gonad. SYN: *gonadial*.

gonadectomy (gon-ă-dek'to-mĭ). Excision of a testicle or ovary.

gonad'ial. Pert. to a reproductive gland. SYN: *gonadal*.

gonadoad'vent. The advent at puberty of gonadal activity.

gonadogen (gon-ad'ō-jĕn). Commercial gonadotropic substance from pregnant mare's serum.

gonadokinetic (gon-ad-o-kin-et'ĭk). Stimulating the activity of the sexual glands.

gonadop'athy. Any disease of the sexual glands.

gonad'opause. Cessation of sexual activity with advent of senility.

gonadother'apy. Treatment by injection of extract of testicular or ovarian hormones.

gonadotrope (gon-ad'o-trōp). One dominated by the sex instinct.

gonadotropic (go-nad-o-trop'ik). Rel. to abnormal sex impulses.

gonadotro'pin, gonadotroph'in. Substance stimulating the gonads.

gonadotropism (go-nad-ot'ro-pizm). Domination by the sex impulse.

gon'aduct. The seminal duct or the oviduct.

gonagra (gon-a'grä). Gout in the knee.

gonal'gia. Pain in the knee.

gonangiectomy (gon-an-ji-ek'to-mĭ). Excision of the vas deferens or a part of it. SYN: *vasectomy*.

gonarthritis (gon-ar-thri'tis). Inflammation of the knee joint.

gonarthrocace (gon-ar-throk'ă-se). White swelling of knee joint.

gonarthromeningitis (gon-ar"thro-men-in-ji'tis). Synovitis of the knee joint.

gonarthrotomy (gon-ar-throt'o-mĭ). Incision of knee joint.

gonatag'ra. Gout in the knee.

gonatocele (gon-at'o-sēl). White swelling; tumor of the knee.

gonecyst, gonecystis (gon'e-sist, gon-e-sis'tis). A seminal vesicle.

gonecystitis (gon-e-sis-ti'tis). Inflammation of seminal vesicles.

gonecystolith (gon-e-sis'to-lith). A concretion or calculus in a seminal vesicle.

gonecystopyosis (gon-e-sist"o-pi-o'sis). Suppuration in a seminal vesicle or gonecyst.

goneitis (go-ne-i'tis). Inflammation of the knee.

gonepoiesis (gon-e-poi-e'sis). The secretion of the semen.

goniometer (gon-ĭ-om'et-er). Apparatus to measure joint movements and angles.

gonion (go'nĭ-on). Point of angle of the mandible or lower jaw.

gonioscope (go'nĭ-o-skōp). An instrument for inspecting angle of ant. chamber of eye and for determining ocular motility and rotation.

gono-, gon-. Prefix meaning *generation, offspring, semen*.

gonocide (gon'o-sĭd). Destructive to the gonococcus.

gonococ'cal. Rel. to or caused by gonococci.

gonococcemia (gon-o-kok-se'mĭ-ă). Gonococci in the blood.

gonococcic (gŏn-ō-kŏk'sĭk). Pert. to the gonococcus.

g. smears. Gonococci are in pairs

and tetrads, never in chains. They are biscuit-shaped with concave adjacent surfaces, Gram negative and intracellular. *Stains*: Gram's method, methylene blue.

gonococcide (gon-o-kok'sĭd). Destructive to or that which kills gonococci.

gonococcin (gon-o-kok'sin). A glycerin extract of gonococci used in the cutireaction test for gonorrhea.

gonococ'cocide. Destructive to or an agent which kills gonococci.

gonococcus (gon-o-kok'us). The organism causing gonorrhea.

gon'ocyte. 1. The primitive reproductive cell. 2. Lymphoidocyte, myeloblast.

gonohemia (go-no-he'mĭ-ă). General gonorrhea infection. SYN: *gonococcemia*.

gonophage (gon'o-fāj). The bacteriophage produced by the gonococcus.

gon'ophore. Any body that stores up or activates sex cells, as the spermatic duct, seminal vesicle, oviduct, or uterus.

gonorrhea (gon-o-re'ă). A specific, contagious, catarrhal inflammation of the genital mucous membrane of either sex.

gonorrhe'al. Of the nature of or pert. to gonorrhea.

   g. arthritis, g. rheumatism. Arthritis, or rheumatism resulting from gonorrheal infection.

gonotoxe'mia. Toxin generated by the gonococcus in the blood.

gonotox'in. Toxin produced by the gonococcus.

gonycamp'sis. Abnormal curvature of the knee or ankylosis.

gonycrote'sis. Knock-knee.

gonyectyposis (gon″ĭ-ek-tĭ-po'sis). Bowlegs. SYN: *genu varum*.

gonyocele (gon'e-o-sēl). Tuberculous synovitis of the knee. SYN: *white swelling*.

gonyoncus (gon″ĭ-on'kus). Tumor of the knee. SYN: *white swelling*.

goose flesh. A skin reaction caused by erection of skin papillae from cold or shock. SYN: *cutis anserina*.

Gordon's reflex (gord'ŏn). Extension of great toe when sudden pressure is made on deep flexor muscles of calf of leg.

gorget (gor'jet). A grooved instrument to protect soft tissues from injury from point of knife.

gouge (gowj). Instrument for cutting away hard tissue of bone.

Goulard's extract (goo'lars). USP. An aqueous solution of lead subacetate, containing 18% lead.

gout (gowt). Paroxysmal metabolic disease marked by acute arthritis and inflammation of the great toe and of the joints.

   g., chronic. Persistent form of gout.

   g., latent; g., masked. Lithemia without regular symptoms of gout.

   g., misplaced; g., retrocedent. Subsidence of joint symptoms followed by severe constitutional upsets.

   g., poor man's. Gout due to exposure and privation.

gout'y. Of the nature of, or rel. to gout.

   g. diathesis. Predisposition to gout.

Gowers' tract (gow'erz). One formed of fibers from post. roots of lateral tract of the spinal cord reaching the cerebellum by way of the sup. peduncle.

gr. Abbr. for *grain*.

graaf'ian fol'licle. BNA. One of the vesicles of the ovaries which contain and discharge an ovum.

gracile (gras'il). Slender; slight.

   g. fasciculus, g. funiculus. Inner division of post. white column of spinal cord containing sensory ascending fibers.

   g. nucleus. Mass of medullary gray matter terminating the funiculus gracilis.

grada'tim. Gradually or by degrees.

Gradenigo's syndrome (grah-den-e'goz). Suppurative otitis media with abducens paralysis and pain in temporal region.

graduate (grad'u-āt). 1. A vessel marked by lines for measuring liquids. 2. One who has been awarded an academic or professional degree from a college or university. [lines on a vessel.

grad'uated. Consisting of a succession of

   g. tenotomy. Partial surgical division of tendon of an eye muscle.

Graefe's, von, sign (graf'fes). Failure of the upper lid to follow a downward movement of the eyeball when the patient changes his vision from upward, downward. Seen in Graves' disease.

graft. Skin or other living substance inserted into a similar substance to supply an absence or defect by attachment and growth into an integral part of the original substances.

   g., autoplastic. One taken from another part of the patient.

   g. bone. A piece of bone generally taken from the tibia and inserted elsewhere in the body to replace another osseous structure.

   Bones for grafting can be kept in icebox until needed.

   g., heteroplas'tic. One taken from another person.

   g., ovarian. Implantation of a section of an ovary into the muscles of the abdominal wall.

   g., skin. Removal of small sections of skin to a raw, clean surface such as a large superficial burn.

   g., sponge. Small piece of sponge placed over an ulcerating part to stimulate epidermal growth.

   g., Thiersch's. One in which only epidermis and small amt. of dermis are used.

   g., Wolfe's. One in which the whole thickness of the skin is used.

   g., zooplas'tic. One taken from an animal.

grain. 1. Seed of a plant. 2. A weight; 0.065 of a gram. 3. Direction of fibers or layers.

   g. poisoning. Poisoning due to a fungus which develops on grain, as ergot. *Gangrenous*: Tingling, pain, spasmodic muscular contractions, blood stasis and gangrene, fingers, toes, nose or ears.

gram. The unit of weight (mass) employed by science.

It is equal to 15.4 gr. apothecary weight; 28.4 Gm. equal 1 oz. avoirdupois.

gramicidin (grăm-ĭ-sĭd'ĭn). A substance produced by soil-borne bacteria effective in treating wounds, sinus, and bladder infections and ulcers. As it breaks down red blood cells it must be heated if it is to come in contact with the blood.

gram mol'ecule. The gram quantity equal to the molecular weight of a substance.

gram neg'ative. Not Gram staining.

gram pos'itive. Staining by Gram's method.*

Gram's method. A method of staining bacteria.

Gran'cher's disease. Massive pneumonia.

G.'s sign. Raised pitch of expiratory murmur in pulmonary consolidation.

grand mal (grahn mal). The typical epileptic attack with or without coma.

gran'ular. Of the nature of granules. Roughened by prominences like those of seeds.

g. cast. Coarse or fine granule, short and plump, sometimes yellowish, similar to hyaline cast.

granula'tion. 1. Formation of granules, or state or condition of being granular. 2. Fleshy projections formed on the surface of a gaping wound that is not healing by first intention* or indirect union.

gran'ule. 1. A small, grainlike body. 2. In histology: (a) A minute mass in a cell, which has an outline, but no apparent structure; (b) any minute mass; (c) the crossing points of an intracellular reticulum endwise. 3. In pharmacy, a small globule of sugar and gum tragacanth, combined with a medicinal substance. SEE: *chondroconia, chromomere.*

g., agminated. Small round or angular particle of disintegrated red blood corpuscle in the blood.

g., albuminous. Cytoplasmic granule in many normal cells, not affected by ether or chloroform, but disappears from view when acetic acid is added.

g., aleuronoid. Pigment cell granule; colorless, myeloid, and colloidal.

g., alpha. Albuminous granule in leukocytes. Coarse, eosinophil, and highly refractive. SYN: *eosinophil granule, oxyphil granule.*

g., Altmann's. Found in glandular cells; may be concerned with secretory activity. Round in shape and stain with acid fuchsin. SYN: *fuchsinophil granule, plasmosome.*

g., azurophil. One which takes a stain with azure dyes easily. Found in lymphocytes; coarse and reddish in appearance.

g., basal. Small chromatin mass formed in certain protozoal nuclei. SYN: *blepharoplast.*

g., beta. A cell granule staining with both acid and basic dyes.

g., carbohydrate. Particle of carbohydrate in cells or fluids of the body in course of assimilation.

g., central. One in the cytoplasm of the cell. SYN: *centrosome.*

g., chromatic. Chromatin granule within a cell or nucleus.

g., cone. Retinal cell nucleus which is connected with a cone.

g., delta. Uninuclear plasma cell granule; basophilic.

g., elastin. One of elastic substance, sometimes fused to form fibers or membranes.

g., elementary. Blood dust. SYN: *hemokonia.*

g., eosinophil. SEE: *alpha granule.*

g., epsilon. Neutrophilic one found in protoplasm of polynuclear leukocytes.

g., fatty. Fat particles in a cell in course of assimilation or in a cell undergoing fatty degeneration, or produced by a cell in process of forming a fat cell.

g., Fauvel's. Peribronchitic abscess, *q.v.*

g., fuchsinophil. SEE: *Altmann's granule.*

g., gamma. Found in basophil connective tissue cells; occur in leukemic blood.

g., Grawitz's. Found in lead poisoning basophilia, in the red blood corpuscles.

g., gustatory. Minute nuclear mass in the gustatory papillae.

g., infective. One carrying trypanosomiasis infection.

g., iodophil. Found in polymorphonuclear leukocytes and staining easily with iodine. Seen in various acute infectious diseases.

g., osseous. Minute granule of inorganic matter in animal matrix of bones.

g., Kölliker's interstitial. Appears in various sizes in muscle fiber sarcoplasm.

g., lymph. Nucleated ameboid cells in lymph and chyle.

g., metachromatic. Found in protoplasm of numerous bacteria. Stains deeply; irregular in size. SYN: *Babes-Ernst body, metachromatic body.*

g., Much's. Rod found in sputum of tuberculosis which stains with Gram stain; considered to be a modified tubercle bacillus.

g., osseous. Minute granule of inorganic matter in animal matrix of bones.

g., oxyphil. SEE: *alpha granule.*

g., pigment. Particle of coloring matter seen esp. in pigment cells.

g., Plehn's. Basophilic and seen in conjugating form of *Plasmodium vivax.*

g., protein. Anabolic and catabolic particles of minute size in various proteins.

g., rod. Nucleus of the rod visual cell found in the external nuclear layer of the retina; connected with the rods.

g., Schridde's. Reddish granule occurring in myelocytes.

g., Schüffner's. Polychrome methylene blue-staining granule found in parasitized erythrocytes of tertian malaria; coarse and red.

g., seminal. Minute particles in semen, supposed to derive from disintegrated nuclei in nutritive cells from seminiferous tubules.

g., starch. One of the many granules which make up starch.

g., vitelline. SEE: *yolk granule.*

g., yolk. Albuminous granule in the vitellus forming the nutritive yolk. SYN: *vitelline corpuscle.*

g., zymogen. One in cells of pancreas supposed to give rise to pancreatic ferments.

granulitis (gran-u-li'tis). Acute miliary tuberculosis.

granuload'ipose. Pert. to granules of fat.

gran'uloblast. Mother cell of a granulocyte.

granulocyte (gran'u-lo-sīt). A granular leukocyte.

granulocytopenia (gran″-lo-si″to-pe'nĭ-ă). Abnormal reduction of granulocytes in the blood. SYN: *granulopenia.*

granulocytopoiesis (gran″u-lo-si″to-poi-e'sis). The formation of granulocytes.

gran'ulofatty. Composed of or containing fat granules as in fatty degeneration. SYN: *granuloadipose.*

granulo'ma. A granular tumor or growth, usually of lymphoid and epitheloid cells.

g. malignum. Multiple granuloma development.

granulomato'sis. The development of multiple granulomas.

g. sidero'ica. Brownish (Gamna) nodules in the enlarged spleen.

granulope'nia. Abnormal decrease of granulocytes in the blood. SYN: *granulocytopenia.*

gran'uloplasm. The inner substance of a unicellular organism surrounding the nucleus.

granuloplastic (gran″u-lo-plas'tik). Developing granules.

granulopoiesis (gran″u-lo-poi-e'sis). The formation of granulocytes.

granulopo'tent. Potentially capable of forming granules.

gran'ulose. The soluble portion of starch. It is converted into sugar by hydrolysis.

granulo'sis. A mass of minute granules.

g. ru'bia na'si. Disease of the skin of the nose.

gra'num. Grain. A seed or berry.

grape cure. Treatment by a diet of grapes. SYN: *ampelotherapy.*

grape sugar. Dextrose.

-graph. Suffix: Pert. to *a writing or treatise.*

graphite (graf'īt). A soft form of carbon. SYN: *plumbago.*

grapho-. Prefix: To write.

graphology (graf-ol'o-jĭ). Examination of handwriting in diseases of the nerves as a means of diagnosis.

graphorrhea (graf-o-re'ă). Writing of many meaningless words and phrases; manifested in dementia precox.

graphospasm (graf'o-spazm). Writer's cramp.

grattage (grat-ahzh'). Removal of morbid growths by rubbing with a brush or harsh sponge.

gravative (grav'a-tiv). Having a sense of weight, as in pressure pains of growths.

grave. Serious; dangerous; severe.

g. wax. Waxlike matter on flesh caused by exposure to moisture with exclusion of air, as a body in the water or underground. SYN: *adipocere.*

gravedo (grav-e'do). 1. Coryza. 2. Muscular rheumatism of the head.

gra'vel. Crystalline dust, or concretions of crystal from the kidneys, distinguished from true calculi by the absence of definite structural arrangement.

Generally made up of phosphates, calcium, oxalate, and uric acid.

graveolent (grav'e-o-lent). Fetid; having an unpleasant, strong odor.

Graves' disease. Exophthalmic goiter. SEE: *Moebius' sign.* [child.

gravid (grav'id). Pregnant; heavy with

gravida (grav'id-ă). A pregnant woman.

grav'idin. A substance on surface of standing urine, once considered a sign of pregnancy in women. SYN: *kyestein.*

grav'idism. State of being pregnant.

gravid'ity. Pregnancy.

gravidocardiac (grav″id-o-kar'dĭ-ak).Pert. to cardiac disorders resulting from pregnancy.

gravimet'ric. Determined by weight.

g. method. Examination of blood by weighing.

gravistatic (grav-is-tat'ik). Resulting from gravitation, as in a form of congestion.

gravita'tion. Force and movement tending to draw every particle of matter together.

grav'ity. Property of possessing weight.

g., specific. Weight of a substance compared with that of water, air, or hydrogen.

gravocaine (grav'o-kān). Spinal anesthetic mixture used in obstetrics.

gray. Black or brown mixed with white.

g. hair. Hair which is becoming white. SEE: *canities.*

g. matter. Nerve tissue containing neuron cell bodies with a grayish tint.

It is arranged on outer surface of the convolutions and in the basal ganglia and nuclei of the brain; in the spinal cord in the interior in a form like the letter H on cross section.

gray powder. USP. Mercury with chalk, containing about 38% mercury.

USES: Most frequently as a cathartic for children, sometimes as an alterative.

DOSAGE: As a laxative, 4-10 gr. (0.25-0.65 Gm.). As an alterative, ½-1 gr. (0.03-0.06 Gm.).

great toe reflexes. Comprehensive term referring to the many reflexes involving the great toe.

green. A color intermediate bet. blue and yellow, afforded by rays of wave length bet. 0.000491 and 0.000535 mm. SEE: *"chloro-"* words.

g. sickness. A form of anemia in adolescent girls, perhaps due to faulty diet during puberty. SYN: *chlorosis.*

g. soap. A solution of soft soap in alcohol, molded and dried.

soft'ening. Cranial abscess with f a greenish hue.

vit'riol. Ferrous sulfate. SYN: *eras.*

tick fracture. One involving only of the thickness of a bone. SEE: *nplete fracture.*

ome (gref'o-tōm). Instrument for ing tissue grafts.

rays. Roentgen rays with an aver-wave length of 2 angströms. SEE:

des orteils (grēf daz or-ta'). Muscu-atrophy of foot with contraction. *: clawfoot.*

r (grin'der). A molar tooth. SYN: *s molaris.*

ers' disease. An asthma due to dust alation. SYN: *siderosis.*

grippe (grĭp). Acute, infectious dis-e marked by fever, prostration, pains head and back, and by catarrh of piratory tract. SYN: *influenza, q.v.*

., devil's. Epidemic disease charac-ized by sudden epigastric or thoracic n, brief febrile stage, and recurrence symptoms after a short period of atement.

s (grĭps). Intermittent severe pains bowels. SYN: *colic; tormina, q.v.*

ootoxin (grip-po-toks'in). The toxin of the influenza bacillus.

gris'tle. Cartilage.

gro'cers' itch. Eczema or psoriasis of the hands due to irritation from handling flour, sugar, etc.

Groff electrosurgical knife. Device for use of cutting current.

groin. The depression between the thigh and trunk. The inguinal region. SEE: *bubonalgia, venereal bubo.*

groove. A furrow or elongated channel. SYN: *sulcus.*

  g., bicipital. Depression for long ten-don of the triceps located on ant. sur-face of humerus.

  g., Blessig's. A trace in the embryonic eye corresponding in position with the future *ora serrata.*

gross. Not minute; in mass.

  g. anatomy. That of organs and parts seen without the aid of a microscope.

  g. lesion. One visible to the eye with-out the aid of a microscope.

Grotthuss, law of. Light is absorbed when its wave length is in resonance with the atoms on which it falls.

ground bundle. The principal bundle of nerve fibers in a mass, as those of the ventral and lateral columns of the spi-nal cord. SYN: *fasciculus.*

ground itch. Invasion of skin by larvae of *Uncinaria duodenale*, causing a derma-titis.

group'ing. Classification.

  g., blood. Classifying blood of differ-ent individuals according to agglutinat-ing and hemolyzing qualities before making a blood transfusion.

group test. Any mental or aptitude test given to a group, the answers being written by those tested

grow'ing pains. Pains in the limbs of young persons, probably rheumatic.

growth. The development or increase in size of a living thing, as cyst, excres-cence, tumor, benign or malignant.

  g. quotient. Constant fractional part of total energy utilized for growth.

gru'el. Any cereal boiled in water.

gru'mose, gru'mous. 1. BACT: Made up of coarse granular bodies in the center. 2. Lumpy, clotted

Grunfelder's reflex (grün'feld-ĕr). Fan-like spreading of toes with upward flexion of great toe resulting from pres-sure over post. fontanel.

grutum (gru'tum). 1. Small pink and white patches most frequently on skin of face and scrotum caused by inspissated sebum beneath the horny epidermis. SYN: *milium.* 2. Oaten grits.

gry'ochrome. A nerve cell with fine granu-lar staining matter in the cell body.

gtt. Abbr. of *guttae*, drops.

guaiacol (gwi'ak-ol). USP. A phenol ob-tained from wood creosote.

  DOSAGE: 8 ℳ (0.5 cc.).

  g. carbonate. USP. A white crystal-line powder used internally as a taste-less, nonpoisonous substitute for guaia-col.

  DOSAGE: 15 gr. (1 Gm.).

guanase (gwan'ās). An enzyme in a num-ber of glands; it converts guanine into xanthine.

guanidine (gwan'id-in). A crystalline or-ganic compound, $NH:C(NH_2)_2$, found among the decomposition products of proteins.

guanidinemia (gwan'id-ĕn-e'mĭ-ă). Guani-dine in the blood.

guanine (gwah'nin). An organic com-pound, $C_5H_5N_5O$, which can be extracted from guano and is related to guanidine and xanthine.

guanophore (gwan'o-fōr). A cell in part consisting of guanine crystals.

guard cells. Lining of stomata of serous membranes made up of endothelial cells.

gubernaculum (gu-ber-nak'u-lum). Saclike membrane around generative buds or uniting 2 structures.

  g. testis. The structures supposed to guide the testicles into the scrotum from the abdomen.

Gubler's line (goob'lerz). The level of su-perficial origin of the trigeminus or 5th nerve.

  G.'s paralysis. Hemiplegia affecting parts on opposite sides of the body. SYN: *alternate* or *crossed hemiplegia.*

  G.'s tumor. A fusiform swelling on wrist in lead palsy.

Gudden's inferior commissure (good'enz in-fe'ri-or com'mis-sure). Fibers of op-tic tract. SYN: *arcuate commissure.*

  G.'s law. Lesions of the cerebral cor-tex are not responsible for lesions of peripheral nerves.

guillotine (gil'o-tēn) Instrument for ex-cising tonsils and laryngeal growths.

gul'let. The esophagus, *q.v*

gum. The fleshy substance or tissue covering the alveolar processes of the jaws.

gumboil (gum′boyl). Gum abscess.

gumma (gum′mä). Infectious soft tumor of the tissues seen in tertiary stage of syphilis.

gummatous (gum′at-us). Pert. to gumma.

gummose (gum′ōs). A sugar from animal gum. $C_6H_{12}O_6$.

gum′my. Sticky, swollen, puffy.

gun′shot wound. Penetrating or perforating wound which may contain a foreign body, as a bullet. SEE: *wound*.

gun′stock deform′ity. Deformity in which the long axis of the extended forearm turns outwardly from the arm, caused by fracture at the elbow.

gustation (gus-ta′shun). Sense of taste.

gustatory (gus′tat-o-rĭ). Pert. to sense of taste.

gustom′etry. Measurement of the degree of the sense of taste.

gut. The bowel or intestine.

    g., blind. Cecum.

gut′ta. A drop. The amount in a drop varies with the nature of the liquid, being about a minim of water.

    g. rosacea. Chronic inflammation of skin of face and nose. SYN: *acne rosacea*.

    g. serena. Blindness. SEE: *amaurosis*.

guttadiaphot (gut-ä-dĭ′ä-fŏt). Examination of blood by transmitted light as test for its pathological condition.

gutt′ate. Resembling a drop, said of certain cutaneous lesions.

gutta′tim. Drop by drop.

gut′tur. The throat.

guttural (gut′u-ral). Pert. to the throat.

gutturotet′any. Laryngeal spasm of throat with temporary stutter.

Guyon's sign (gwy-onz′). Ballottement of kidney.

Gwath′mey's meth′od or technic. Adm. of rectal anesthetic of ether and olive oil solution in labor. SEE: *anesthesia*.

gymnas′tics. Systematic bodily exercise, esp. in a gymnasium.

    g., circulatory. Exercises to increase circulation.

gymnocyte (jim′no-sīt). A cell with no limiting wall.

gymnophobia (jim-no-fo′bĭ-ä). Abnormal aversion to viewing a naked body.

gymnospore (jim′no-spŏr). Spore without a protective coat.

gynander (jin-an′der). An effeminate type of man.

gynandrism (jin-an′drizm). Hermaphroditism.

gynandroid (ji-nan′droyd). A female having sufficient hermaphroditic sexual characteristics to be mistaken for a man.

gynandromorphous (jin-an-dro-morf′us). Having the characteristics of both the male and female.

gynandry (jin-an′dry). Condition of hermaphroditism, *q.v.*

gynatresia (jin-a-tre′zĭ-ä). Atresia* of the vagina.

gynecic (jin-e′sik). Pert. to women.

gyneco-, gyno-. Prefix meaning *woman, female*.

gynecologic, gynecological (jin-e-ko-lo′jik, -ji-kal; gin-e-). Pert. to gynecology, or study of women's diseases.

gynecologist (jin-e-kol′o-jist; gin-e-kol′o-jist). Physician who specializes in the diseases of women.

gynecology (jin-e-kol′o-jĭ; gin-e-kol′o-jĭ). The study of the diseases of the female, particularly of the genital, urinary, or rectal organs.

gynecomania (jin-e-ko-ma′nĭ-ä; gin-e). Abnormal sex desire in the male. SYN: *satyriasis, q.v.*

gynecomastia, gynecomasty, gynecomazia (ji-ne-ko-mas′tĭ-ä, -tĭ, -ma′zĭ-ä). Abnormally large mammary glands in the male; sometimes may secrete milk.

gynecopathy (ji-ne-kop′ä-thĭ). Diseases peculiar to women.

gynecophonus (jin-e-kof′on-us). Having an effeminate voice.

gynephobia (jin-e-fo′bĭ-ä). Abnormal aversion to the company of women, or fear of them.

gynergen (ji′ner-jĕn). Known as *ergotamine tartrate*, is a salt of one of the alkaloids of ergot.

    DOSAGE: For oral use, 1/60 gr. (0.001 Gm.). Hypodermically, 1/240 gr. (0.00025 Gm.) with the same caution as with ergot.

gynesic (ji-ne′sik). Pert. to the diseases of women.

gyniatrics (jin-ĭ-at′riks). Treatment of diseases of women.

gynopath′ic. Pert. to disease of women.

gynoplastics (jin-o-plas′tiks). Reparative surgery of female genitalia.

gynoplasty (jin″o-plas′tĭ). Plastic surgery of the female reproductive organs.

gyrate (jī′rāt). 1. Ring-shaped, convoluted. 2. To revolve.

gyration (ji-ra′shun). A rotary movement.

gyre (jīr). Convolution. SYN: *gyrus*.

gyrencephalic (ji-ren-sef-al′ik). Having a brain marked by numerous convolutions.

gyri (ji′ri) (sing. *gyrus*). 1. Convolutions of the brain. 2. Spiral internal ear cavities.

gyro-. Combining form meaning a *circle, spiral, ring*.

gyrochrome (ji′ro-krōm). A nerve cell in which the stainable substance occurs in rings.

gyroma (ji-ro′mä). Ovarian tumor consisting of a convoluted mass.

gyromele (ji′ro-mēl). Revolving sound for massage and cleansing of stomach, determining its location, size, and condition.

gyrometer (ji-rom′et-er). A device for measuring the cerebral gyri.

gyrosa (ji-ro′sä). Gastric vertigo causing one to close one's eyes to prevent falling, as everything turns round when standing.

gyrose (ji′rōs). BACT: Marked by wavy lines or circles.

gyrospasm (ji′ro-spasm). Spasmodic rotary head movement.

gyrotrope (ji′ro-trōp). Cord connecting

an electrode with source of an electric current. Syn: *rheotrope.*

gyrous (ji′rus). Marked by circular lines. Syn: *gyrose.*

gyrus (ji′rus). A convolution of the brain.

g., angular. Gyrus in proximity with dorsal terminus of supertemporal fissure.

g., annectent. Any 1 of 4 gyri connecting the occipital and parietotemporal lobes.

g., basirrhinal. Gyrus close to temporal lobe tip situated bet. hippocampal and amygdaline fissures.

gyri breves insulae. (BNA.) Preinsular gyrus.

g., Broca's. Ant. frontal gyrus.

g., callosal. Gyrus on the margin of the corpus callosum.

g. centralis. Middle convolution.

g. cerebelli. Layer of the cerebellum.

g. cerebri. Convolution of the cerebrum.

g. chorioides. Portion of lateral recess of 4th ventricle in the embryo.

g. cochleae. Cochleal gyrus of internal ear.

g., dentate. Convolution situated in the dentate fissure.

g., descendens; g., Ecker's. Convolution at the margin of the occipital lobe.

g. fornicatus. See: *callosal gyrus.*

g., frontal, ascending. Ascending frontal lobe of cerebrum.

g., frontal, inferior. Convolution on external surface of frontal lobe of cerebrum located bet. the sylvian fissure and the inferior frontal sulcus.

g., frontal, middle. Gyrus bet. the superior and inferior frontal sulci.

g., frontal, superior. Convolution of cerebral frontal lobe situated above the superfrontal fissure.

g., fusiform. Gyrus beneath the collateral fissure joining the occipital and temporal lobes.

g., geniculi. Rudimentary gyrus at inferior end of corpus callosum.

g., Heschl's. Transverse temporal gyrus.*

g., hippocampal. Gyrus situated bet. the hippocampal and collateral fissures.

g., infracalcarine. Gyrus on the undersurface of the temporal lobe.

g., lingual. Gyrus bet. the calcarine and collateral fissures.

g. longus insulae. Lengthy gyrus composing the postinsula.

g., marginal. See: *frontal superior gyrus.*

g., mediofrontal. Gyrus located bet. the superfrontal and the subfrontal fissures.

g., mediotemporal. Gyrus located bet. the mediotemporal and supertemporal fissures.

g., occipital. Any 1 of the 3 gyri in the occipital lobe (inferior, middle, superior).

g., occipitotemporal. See: *fusiform gyrus.*

g., orbital. Section of orbital surface of frontal lobe.

g., paracentral. Area on mesial aspect of the cerebrum.

g., parietal. Gyrus of the parietal lobe (ascending and inferior).

g., paroccipital. Superior occipital cerebral gyrus.

g., postcentral. Gyrus situated bet. the central and postcentral fissures.

g., preinsular. One of the gyri composing the preinsula.

g., primary. Fetal cerebral regions marked by the primary fissures.

g. profundi cerebri. Very deep gyri of the cerebrum.

g., quadrate. Gyrus extending upward on the parietal lobe surface.

g. rectus. Gyrus on the orbital aspect of the frontal lobe, located bet. the mesial margin and the olfactory fissure.

g., Retzius'; g., sagittal. Gyrus paralleling the cranial sagittal suture.

g. subcallosus. Convolution of the corpus callosum.

g., subcollateral. See: *fusiform gyrus.*

g. supracallosus. Gray matter layer covering the corpus callosum.

g., supramarginal. Gyrus in the inferior parietal convolution twisting about the upper terminus of the sylvian fissure.   [lobe.

g., temporal. Gyrus in the temporal

g. transitivus. See: *annectent gyrus.*

g., uncinate. Ant. hooked portion of the hippocampal gyrus.

H

H. Symb. of *hydrogen;* abbr. for *haustus* (a draft), *hypermetropia, horizontal, Holzknecht unit,* and L *hora,* hour.

H+. The symb. for hydrogen ion concentration.

Haab's reflex. Contraction of pupils without alteration of accommodation or convergence when gazing at a bright object. A sign of a cortical lesion.

habena (ha-be′nă). 1. A frenum. 2. Bandage for a wound. 3. Pineal gland peduncle. SYN: *habenula, 2.*

habe′nal, habe′nar. Pert. to the habena or habenula.

habenula (hab-en′u-lă). 1. A frenum. 2. A peduncle of the pineal gland. BNA.

    h. urethra′lis. One of 2 whitish bands between the clitoris and *meatus urethra.*

hab′it. The result of an impulse passing through a certain set of neurons, then synapses many times.

    h. chorea. SEE: *habit spasm.*

    h., full. Full bloodedness, as in a disease.

    h. spasm. A spasmodic voluntary movement that has become involuntary. Often due to something irritating; sometimes from mimicry. SYN: *tic.**

    h. training. Schedule for 24 hr., adapted and rigidly enforced to train mental cases in habits of cleanliness and to stimulate mental activity.

habitua′tion. Act of becoming accustomed to anything from frequent use.

hab′itus. Indications in appearance of tendency to disease or abnormal conditions.

    h. apoplecticus. Full bloodedness, as in a disease.

    h. enteropticus. Physical state marking enteroptosis.

    h. phthisicus. Predisposition to pulmonary tuberculosis characterized by poor bone development, pallor, etc.

habromania (hab-ro-ma′nĭ-ă). A psychosis accompanied by pleasant delusions.

hachement (hash-mon′). Strokes with edge of hand in massage. SYN: *hacking.*

hack′ing. Strokes with edge of hand in massage. SYN: *hachement.*

    h. cough. A frequent, short cough.

had′dock. An edible fish.

Haemophilus (hem-of′il-us). A genus of Bacteriaceae growing best in hemoglobin.

    H. conjunctivit′idis. The cause of "pink eye." SYN: *haemophilus of Koch-Weeks.*

    H. ducrey′ii. The probable pathogenic agent of chancroid. SYN: *Ducrey's bacillus* and *Bacillus ulceris mollis.*

    H. haemolyt′icus. A nonpathogenic agent in the respiratory tract.

    H. influen′zae. Influenza bacillus or Pfeiffer's bacillus found in respiratory tract during influenza and other diseases.

    h. of Koch-Weeks. Same as *Haemophilus conjunctivitidis.*

    H. lacuna′tus. The cause of mild conjunctivitis.

    H. melaninogen′icus. A Gram-negative organism found on the genitalia and in oral cavities.

    H. pertus′sis. The possible cause of whooping cough. SYN: *Bordet-Gengou bacillus.*

haf′nium. A rare chemical element of at. wt. 178.6. SYMB: Hf.

Hagedorn needle (hă′ge-dorn). A curved surgical needle with flattened sides.

Haines formula. The number of grains of solid in a fluidounce of urine determined by multiplying the last 2 figures of the sp. gr. of a specimen by 1.1.

hair. A hirsute outgrowth from the skin.

    h. bulb (*bulbus pili*). Lower expanded portion of a hair root.

    h. cell. Epithelial cell possessing cilia.

    h. dye. May contain silver nitrate or aniline dyes which are often irritating to skin or eyes, causing severe dermatitis or conjunctivitis. Occasionally results in blindness.

    h. follicle (*folliculus pili*). An inversion of the skin forming a cylindrical depression, penetrating the corium* into the connective tissue which holds the hair root.

    h. papilla. Corium point extending into hair bulb.

    h., pubic. That over the pubes. It assumes the form of a triangle in the female. SYN: *escutcheon.* SEE: *pubic.*

hair′y heart. A heart covered with a rough exudation.

    h. tongue. One covered with hairlike papillae.

hala′tion. Blurring of vision due to light from a wrong direction.

halazone (hăl′ă-zon). A white powder, with properties like chlorine, but, being stable, in solid form.

    DOSAGE: 0.004 Gm. recommended to be added to 1 liter of water.

half-value layer. SEE: *half-value thickness.*

    h.-v. thickness. The thickness of a substance which, when placed in the path of a given beam of rays, will lower its intensity to ½ of the initial value.

halisteresis (hal-ĭ-ste-re′sis). Lime deficiency in the bones. SEE: *malacosteon, osteomalacia.*

    h. ce′rea. Waxy softening of the bones.

halistere′tic. Rel. to or affected with halisteresis, *q.v.*

halitosis (hal-i-tos′is). Offensive breath.

halituous (hal-it′u-us). Covered with moisture. SYN: *vaporous.*

hal'itus. 1. The breath. 2. Warm vapor.

haliver (hal'ĭ-ver). Oil from the halibut's liver. Rich in vitamins A and D.

   h. oil. The expressed oil from fresh halibut livers, standardized to contain approximately 100 times the amount of vitamin A, and 10 to 30 times the amount of vitamin D as standard cod liver oil.

   DOSAGE: Adults, 10 to 20℞ daily; children, 10 drops.

   h. o. with viosterol. Haliver oil to which has been added sufficient viosterol to assure a potency of not less than 10,-000 vitamin D units per Gm.

   DOSAGE: For infants, 8 to 10 drops daily; older children and adults, proportionately increased.

Hal'ler's cir'cles. Circles of veins and arteries in the eye.

hal'lex (pl. *hal'lices*). The great toe. SYN: *hallus, hallux.*

hallu'cination. PSY: False perception having no relation to reality and not accounted for by any ext. stimuli. May be *visual, auditory, olfactory,* etc.

   h., extracampine. Hallucination of hearing words spoken at a great distance.

   h., haptic. One pert. to touching the skin, or to sensations of temperature or pain.

   h., hypnogogic. Pre-sleep phenomena having the same practical significance as a dream but experienced while consciousness persists. Includes sense of falling, sinking, or of the ceiling moving.

   h., kinetic. Sensation of flying or moving the body or a part of it.

   h., microptic. One in which things seem reduced in size. [movement.

   h., motor. Imaginary perceptions of

   h., somatic. Sensation of pain attributed to visceral injury.

   h., teleologic. One which advises or guides the subject, such as those of Jeanne d'Arc.

hallucinosis (hăl-lū″sĭn-ō'sĭs). The state of having hallucinations more or less persistently. SEE: *hallucination.*

   h., acute. PSY: Alcoholic psychosis.

hal'lus, hal'lux (pl. *hal'luces*). The great toe.

   h. doloro'sus. Pain in the metatarsophalangeal joint of the great toe due to flat foot.

   h. flexus. Hammer toe.

   h. valgus. Displacement of great toe toward other toes.

   h. varus. Displacement of great toe away from other toes.

halmatogenesis (hal″mă-to-jen'e-sis). A sudden deviation of type from one generation to the other one.

ha'lo. 1. The areola, esp. of the nipple. 2. A ring surrounding the macula lutea in ophthalmoscopic images.

   h. glaumato'sus. A whitish ring surrounding the optic disk; seen in glaucoma.

   h. symptom. Colored circle around lights in glaucoma.

hal'ogen. A salt former; one of a group of elements (chlorine, Cl.; bromine, Br.; iodine, I., and fluorine, F.), having very similar properties.

haloid (hal'oid). Resembling salt.

   h. salt. A salt made up of a base and a halogen, resembling common salt.

halometer (ha-lom'ē-ter). 1. Device for measuring diffraction halo of a red blood cell. 2. Device for measuring the halo around optic disk.

halosteresis (ha-lo-ster-e'sis). Deficiency of lime salts in the bones. SYN: *halisteresis.*

Hal'sted's opera'tion. Operation for inguinal hernia and one for amputation of breast with carcinoma.

   H.'s suture. An interrupted one for intestinal wounds.

Hal'stern's disease. Endemic syphilis.

hamarthri'tis. Arthritis of the joints. SYN: *polyarthritis.*

hamartia (ham-ar'shĭ-ă). Error in development due to imperfect tissue combination.

hamartoma (ham-ar-to'mă). 1. A tumor due to new growth of blood vessels; opp. to dilatation of preëxisting vessels. 2. A tumor due to failure of development.

hamartomatosis (ham-ar-to-mă-to'sis). Existence of multiple hamartomas.

hama'tum. The unciform bone, *os hamatum.*

ham'mer toe. A toe with dorsal flexion of 1st phalanx and plantar flexion of 2nd and 3rd phalanges.

Hamp'son unit. X-ray unit of measurement.

   It is one-fourth of the erythema dose.

ham'string. A tendon which binds the popliteal space laterally.

   h., inner. Tendons of gracilis, sartorius, and 2 other muscles. [femoris.

   h., outer. Tendon of biceps flexor

ham'ular. Unciform; hook-shaped.

ham'ulus. 1. Any hook-shaped structure. 2. Hooklike process on the unciform bone.

hand. That part of the body which is distal to but attached to the forearm at the wrist.

hang'ing drop culture. Inoculating a drop of bouillon under a coverglass for a bacterial culture.

hang'nail. 1. Partly detached piece of skin at root of a fingernail. 2. A corn. 3. Whitlow. SYN: *agnail.*

Hanot's disease (han'os). Hypertrophic cirrhosis of liver with jaundice.

Han'son unit. One one-hundredth of the quantity of parathyroid extract solution necessary to elevate by 1 mg. the amt. of calcium in blood serum of a parathyroidectomized dog whose weight is 15 Kg.

hapalonychia (hap-al-o-nik'ĭ-ă). Lack of rigidity of the nails. SYN: *onychomalacia.*

haphalgesia (haf-al-ge'zĭ-ă). A sensation of pain upon touching the skin with an object which is not an irritant.

haphephobia (haf-e-fo'bĭ-ă). Aversion to being touched by another person.

haplodermatitis (hap"lo-der-mă-ti'tis). Simple inflammation of the skin. SYN: *haplodermitis.*

hap'lodermi'tis. Uncomplicated inflammation of the skin.

haplopathy (hap-lop'a-thĭ). Any uncomplicated disease.

hap'ten(e. The portion of an antigen containing the grouping on which the specificity depends.

haptic (hap'tik). Pert. to touch. SYN: *tactile.*

hap'tics. The science of the touch sense.

haptin (hap'tin). A cast off receptor.

haptophil(e (hap'to-fil, -fĭl). That portion of a receptor that unites with the haptophore group of a toxin.

haptophore (hap'to-fōr). The atom group of an antigen causing a combination with its corresponding antibody. SEE: *Ehrlich's side-chain theory.*

haptophor'ic, haptoph'orous. Pert. to the action of a haptophore.

har'dening. 1. Rendering a pathological or histological specimen firm or compact for making thin sections for microscopic study.
2. Increased resistance to changes in temperature of the atmosphere.
    Hardening is induced by bathing to cause a prompt skin vascular reaction.

hard'ness. 1. Strange quality shown by water containing certain dissolved salts.
2. That quality of x-rays determining their penetrating power. Hardness lessens as wave lengths become longer.

    h. of a gas tube. A term used to qualify the condition of a tube according to the degree of rarefaction of the residual gas.

hare'lip. Congenital vertical fissure of the upper lip, often found with cleft palate.

    h. suture. A twisted suture.

harlequin fetus (har'lĕ-kwin). A newly-born infant with *ichthyosis congenita.* SYN: *hyperkeratosis congenitalis.*

harmo'nia. A firm apposition of 2 smooth bony surfaces. SYN: *harmonic suture.*

Har'rison's groove. Depression on lower edge of the thorax caused by tug of the diaphragm; seen in adenoids and rickets.

Has'ner's valve or fold. Fold of mucosa at inf. meatus of nasal duct. SYN: *plica lacrimalis.*

Has'sall's corpuscles or bodies. Small, concentric, flattened cells of epithelium in follicles of the thymus.

Hath'cock's sign. Tenderness just beyond the angle of the jaws when the finger follows on the undersurface of the mandible towards the angle. Found in mumps before any swelling can be detected.

haunch (hawnsh). The hips and buttocks.

    h. bone. The ilium. SYN: *os coxae.*

Haus'man's stagna'tion test meal. Four tablespoonfuls of boiled rice and a glass of water are given at 9 o'clock at night (a little sugar and milk can be taken on the rice).

haustra (haws'tra) (sing. *haustrum*). The sacculated elevations of the colon.

    h. coli. Sacculations of the colon resembling tucks caused by the fact that the gut is longer than the longitudinal bands or taeniae.

haustral (haw'stral). Pert. to the colonic haustra.

    h. churning. Agitation of the intestinal contents.

haustrum (haw'strum) (pl. *haus'tra*). One of the sacculations of the colon caused by longitudinal bands shorter than the gut which causes formation of pouches in the colon. SYN: *haustra coli.*

haus'tus. A draught of medicine.

haut-mal (o'mahl). Grand mal when at its height.

haver'sian canal. Minute vascular canal found in osseous tissue.

    h. canaliculi. Chain of tiny canals joining the haversian canal.

    h. gland. Synovial membrane within joint.

    h. system. Architectural unit of bone, consisting of a central tube (*haversian canal*) with alternate layers of intercellular material (*matrix*) surrounding it in concentric cylinders. Alternating layers of matrix and cells are called *haversian lamellae.* SEE: *bone.*

hay fever. An allergic disease of mucous passages of nose and upper air passages induced by external irritation.

Hay'garth's deformities, nodes or nodosities. Exostoses or bony tumors on joints in arthritis deformans.

H. D. Abbr. for *hearing distance.*

head. 1. Caput. That part of the animal body containing the brain and organs of the sight, hearing, smell, and taste. It includes the facial bones. 2. The proximal end of a bone. 3. The larger extremity of any structure or body.

    h., abnormal fixity of. May be caused by postpharyngeal abscess, occipitocervical myelalgia, arthritis deformans, swollen cervical glands, rheumatism, traumatism of neck, sprains of cervical muscles, congenital spasmodic torticollis, caries of a molar tooth, cicatrices of burns.

    h., abnormal movement of. Habit spasms, such as noddings.

    h., black. A comedo, *q.v.*

    h. fold. Blastodermic fold in embryonic cranium.

    h. gut. Part of embryo which develops into stomach, duodenum, and esophagus.

    h., inability to move the. May be due to caries of cervical vertebrae and diseases of articulation bet. occiput and atlas.

    h. kidney. Embryonic kidney.

    h. lock. Interlocking of chins in twin birth.

    h., retracted. Seen in acute meningitis, cerebral abscess, tumor, thrombosis of sup. longitudinal sinus, acute encephalitis, laryngeal obstruction, tetanus, hydrophobia, epilepsy, spasmodic torticollis, strychnine poisoning, hysteria, and rachitic conditions. Also in painful neck lesions at the back.

h., rhythmical nodding of. Seen in aortic regurgitation, chorea, torticollis, q.v.

h. scald. Affection of scalp accompanied by crusts or scales.

head'ache. A diffuse pain in different portions of the head and not confined to any nerve distribution area.

h., sick. A nervous headache occurring periodically, usually on 1 side of the head, accompanied by nausea and vomiting.

SEE: *megrim, migraine.*

heal (hēl). To cure; to make whole or healthy.

heal'ing. The restoration to a normal condition, esp. of an inflammation or a wound.

health (helth). A condition in which all functions of body and mind are normally active.

h., bill of. Public health certificate certifying that passengers on a public conveyance or ship are free of infectious disease.

H., Board of. A public body in charge of the health of a community.

H., Department of. Branch of a government (city, county, or nation) for regulation and protection of the people's health.

h. nurse, public. One employed by a Board or Dept. of Health to serve the public.   [U. S. Treasury Dept.

H. Service, Public. A Bureau of the

health'y. Being in a state of health or enjoying it.

h. pus. Pus of a form without odor, which is less dangerous than the other types.

h. ulcer. Ulcer which heals easily.

hear'ing. The act or power of perceiving sound.

h. distance. That at which a given sound can be heard. On the prairies a voice may be heard for 2 miles or more.

h., functional tests for. 1. Hearing test, spoken voice, whisper voice (use only residual air). 2. Caloric test, cold water, 68° F. (nystagmus to opposite side); hot water, 110° F. (nystagmus to same side). 3. Turning test, produces nystagmus to the side opposite that toward which the turning took place. 4. Fistula symptom, nystagmus on compression or aspiration of air in external canal.

h., sense of. SYM: Subjective symptoms concerned with the sense of hearing, like those of sight, are of mental origin, such as "hearing voices" when none exist.

heart (hart). Hollow, muscular, contractile organ, the center of the circulatory system, enclosed within the *pericardium,* * made up of muscular substance called the *myocardium* * and lined with the *endocardium.* *

h., auscultation of. Shows intensity, quality, and rhythm of heart sounds and detects the presence of any adventitious sounds, as murmurs.

h. block. Loss of every other, or of every 3rd beat, the auricular systole not always being followed by the ventricular systole, the bundle of His failing to transmit the regular systolic impulse. The ventricle contracts regularly at a much slower rate than the auricle.

h. block, complete. Wrist pulse consists of ventricular contractions only, averaging from 30-40 beats a minute.

h. block, partial. One of 2 or 3 impulses passes to ventricle; pulse is thus 40-50.

h., dilatation of. Enlargement of heart due to stretching of its walls.

h. disease. Any pathological disorder of the heart.

Intravenous injections of epsom salt are being tried to detect the early stages.

h. failure. Sudden stoppage of heart's circulation due to interruption in normal balance.   [anginal pains.

h. f., anginal. Form beginning with

h. f., congestive. Cessation of heart's action due to presence of congestion.

h., fatty degeneration of. In which cardiac muscle has been metamorphosed into fat.

h., fatty, infiltration of. Abnormal amount of fat deposited in and upon heart.

h., fibroid. SYM: Same as fatty degeneration, condition dependent upon atheroma or sclerosis of coronary arteries.

h., hypertrophy of. Enlargement due to overgrowth of its muscle. VARIETIES: 1. *Simple Hypertrophy*: Thickened muscle and cavities normal size. 2. *Excentric Hypertrophy*: Thickened muscle and cavities dilated. 3. *Concentric Hypertrophy*: Thickened muscle and cavities diminished in size. Always congenital.

h., palpation of. Not only determines position, force, extent, and rhythm of apex beat, but also detects existence of any fremitus or thrill.

h., palpitation of. May result from dyspepsia; excitement, mental or physical; organic heart disease; exophthalmic goiter; overwork, as the "irritable heart" of untrained recruits; anemia; hysteria; or an independent neurosis. Also: *Endocarditis, myocarditis, pericarditis* due to infection, to trauma, circulatory disturbances, disorders of metabolism, nutrition, and growth.

h., percussion of. Determines shape and extent of cardiac dullness.

h. reflex. Reduced heart rate following pressure on post. fontanel.

h. test. Master has determined the efficiency of the heart by the number of steps a normal individual can ascend in a given time without increasing the heart rate more than 10 beats per minute and without increasing the blood pressure.

heart'burn. Acid liquid raised from the stomach, causing sensation of burning in the esophagus. SYN: *pyrosis.* SEE: *ardor ventriculi.*

heat. 1. Condition of being hot; warmth. 2. High temperature. 3. A form of energy manifested to the senses, as in the effects of fire, sun's rays, etc. 4. Sexual excitement in lower mammals; period of such excitement. SYN: *estrus*. 5. To make hot. 6. To become warm.

h., atomic. That amount which will raise an atom from 0° to 1° C.

h., body, loss of. The skin is supposed to lose 87.5 cal., the lungs 10.7 cal., and through excreta, 1.8 cal.

h., conductive. A term applied to heat transferred by conduction from poultices, bags, etc.

h., convective. That supplied from heated particles of gases or liquids, such as superheated air, melted paraffin, incandescent light apparatus, or the whirlpool bath.

h., conversive. A term used to designate heat generated in the tissues by a current of electricity or by some form of radiant energy.

h. cramps. Severe, intermittent, spasmodic cramping of muscles in abdomen and extremities.

h., diathermy. Electrical energy is converted into heat by the use of diathermy and short wave.

h., dry. May be adm. in form of hot, dry pack; hot water bottle; electric light bath; heliotherapy; hot bricks; resistance coil; electric pad or blanket; hot air bath, or therapeutic lamp.

h. exhaustion. Must not be mistaken for heatstroke, *q.v.* Usually affects adults, esp. the debilitated and fatigued.

h., initial. Muscular heat produced during tension development.

h., latent. The heat which is required to convert a solid into a liquid or a liquid into a gas at the same temperature.

h., latent, of fusion. That which is required to convert 1 Gm. of a solid into liquid at the same temperature, *e. g.,* when 1 Gm. of ice at 0° C. is converted into water at 0° C.; this process requires 80 calories, and until it is completed there will be no rise of temperature.

h., latent, of vaporization. That required to change 1 Gm. of a liquid at its boiling point to vapor at the same temperature. The latent heat of steam is 540 calories; therefore, when steam cools to liquid, each Gm. gives out 540 calories. This explains why it is that a scald from steam is much more severe than one caused by boiling water.

h., luminous. That derived from light. This may be borne better than other forms of radiation.

h., moist. May be applied as hot bath pack, hot wet pack, hot foot bath, fomentations, poultices or vapor bath.

h., molecular. Result of multiplying a substance's molecular weight by its specific heat.

h., prickly. Vesicles due to obstruction or acute inflammation of sweat glands. SYN: *miliaria.*

h., radiant. Heat given off from a heated body and which passes through the air in form of waves.

h. rays. Visible rays from 4000-7000 A. U. and infrared rays from 6000-14,000 A. U.

h., recovery. Portion of heat evolved after shortening muscular contraction has begun.

h., sensible. Heat producing a temperature rise when absorbed by a body.

h., specific. That amt. needed to raise 1° C. a substance's unit volume.

h. therapy. Use of heat in treatment of the body.

h. therapy, wet. Application of heat by hot water, steam and mud baths, and the hot pack, etc.

h. unit. A calorie, *q.v.*

heat'er. Any apparatus which gives off heat.

h., radiant. Infrared radiator. Consists of concave reflector at focus of which is incandescent filament lamp or a heater consisting of an electrically heated solid rod or resistance wire embedded in or wound on an electrically nonconducting refractory material.

heat'stroke. Result of direct exposure to high temperatures or to sun, usually in adults; esp. those who have been taking alcoholic beverages or who are debilitated or fatigued.

hebeosteotomy (he″be-os-te-ot′o-mĭ). Section of the pubic bone in order to enlarge the pelvic opening for facilitation of delivery. SYN: *pubiotomy.*

hebephrenia (he-be-fre′nĭ-ă). 1. Distortions of the countenance, smiling and laughing without cause, unnatural actions and speech; a syndrome of dementia precox. 2. Insanity about the time of puberty. [phrenia.

hebephrenic (he-be-fren′ĭk). Pert. to hebe-

Heb′erden's asthma. Paroxysms of severe pain about heart and down left arm, with sense of oppression. SYN: *angina pectoris, q.v.*

H.'s disease. Arthritis deformans.

H.'s nodes. Hard nodules or enlargements of tubercles of last phalanges of fingers; seen in osteoarthritis.

hebetic (he-bet′ik). Pert. to or occurring at the time of puberty.

hebet'omy. Section through pelvis to aid obstructed delivery. SYN: *pubiotomy.*

hebetude (heb′e-tŭd). Mental dullness, as seen in exhaustive conditions.

heb′in. Gonadotropic hormone.

heboid-paranoid. A name for that class of mental diseases which consists of the juvenile insanities, dementia precox, and paranoia.

heboidophre′nia. A simple form of dementia precox.

hebosteotomy (he-bos-te-ot′o-mĭ). Enlargement of pelvic diameter by section of the pelvis to aid delivery. SYN: *hebotomy, pubiotomy.*

hebot′omy. Section through the pubis to facilitate labor. SYN: *hebeosteotomy, pubiotomy.*

hecateromeric (hek-a″ter-om-er′ĭk). Having processes on a spinal neuron, one supplying each side of the spinal cord.

hecatomeric (hek-at-o-mer′ik). Having processes on a spinal neuron, one supplying each side of the spinal cord.

hectic (hek′tik). Habitual or constitutional.

   h. fever. A form of fever that occurs in connection with some organic disease, that is attended by some continuous and exhausting drain upon the system, as in pulmonary consumption or abscess of liver or kidney.

   h. flush. The bright pink-red spot that appears on the cheek during a paroxysm of hectic fever.

hec′togram. One hundred grams, or 1543.7 grains.

hec′toliter. One hundred liters.

hec′tometer. One hundred meters.

hedge′hog crys′tals. Globular crystals of ammonium urate with spines found in urine.

hedonism (he′don-izm). A theory or standard of conduct in which the principal object of life is pleasure.

hedrocele (hed′ro-sēl). Hernia; prolapse through the anus. SYN: *proctocele.*

heel. Post. extremity of foot. SYN: *calx.*

   h. bone. Bone at back of tarsus. SYN: *os calcis; calcaneum, calcaneus.*

Hegar's sign (hay′garz). Sign present during 2nd and 3rd month of pregnancy, due to: (1) Softening of uterus and esp. of cervix; (2) at this stage, the ovum does not fill the uterine cavity, so there is an empty space in its lower part. On bimanual examination the lower part of uterus is easily compressed bet. fingers in the vagina and those of the other hand.

Heidenhain's crescents and demilunes (hi′-den-hīnz). Marginal corpuscles, small, flattened and granular, bet. the secreting cells of a mucous gland and the basement membrane. SYN: *Giannuzzi's cells.*   [*uriniferous tubules.*

   H.'s rods. Columnar cells in the

height (hīt). Distance to which anything rises above that surface on which it rests.

Heine-Medin disease (hi′ne-ma′dĭn). Acute infectious disease accompanied by motor paralysis and muscular atrophy, frequently with permanent deformity. SYN: *acute anterior poliomyelitis.**

Heister's valves (hīs′terz). Crescentic mucous membrane folds of the gallbladder.

helcoid (hel′koid). Resembling an ulcer.

helcology (hel-kol′o-jĭ). The study of ulcers.

helcoplasty (hel-ko-plas′tĭ). Grafting healthy skin on ulcers. SEE: *dermatoplasty.*

helco′sis. The development of an ulcer. SYN: *ulceration.*

helicine (hel′is-in). Pert. to a helix or coil; spiral.

   h. arteries. Spiral arteries to the erectile tissue of the penis.

helicoid (hel′ĭ-koyd). Resembling a helix or spiral.

helicopodia (hel″ĭ-ko-po′dĭ-ă). The peculiar dragging gait in which the foot describes a partial gait; seen in certain paralyses.

helicotrema (hel-ĭ-ko-tre′mă). A semilunar foramen bet. the edges of the modiolus and hamulus of the lamina spiralis ossea, making a communication bet. the scala tympani and scala vestibuli.

heliencephalitis (he″li-en-sef-al-i′tis). Inflammation of the brain as the result of sunstroke.

heliopho′bia. Abnormal morbid fear of the sun's rays esp. by one who has suffered a sunstroke.

helio′sis. Sunstroke.

heliotherapy (he-lĭ-o-ther′ă-pĭ). The therapeutic application of radiation from the sun which includes infrared, ultraviolet, and visible radiation. SEE: *solarium.*

heliotropism (he-lĭ-ot′rō-pĭzm). Chemotropism induced by the action of sunlight; the tendency of an organism to turn toward or grow toward sunlight.

he′lium. A gaseous element (He).

   Radium and its emanations give it off in the form of alpha rays.

he′lix. 1. Margin of the external ear. 2. Margin of the auricle.

Hel′ler's test. A test for the presence of albumin in urine.

   Pour ½ in. of pure nitric acid into a clean test tube, and carefully overlay it with an equal quantity of urine. The presence of albumin is indicated by the appearance of an opaque ring at the junction of the fluids; also known as the "cold" test.

Hel′lin's law. Occurrence of twins once in 80 pregnancies, triplets once in 6400 pregnancies, quadruplets once in 512,000 pregnancies.

Helm′holtz's axis ligament. One about which the malleus rotates.

   H.'s line. The one perpendicular to the plane of the axis of rotation.

hel′minth. An intestinal vermiform parasite.

helminthagogue (hel-minth′ag-og). A remedy that expels worms. SYN: *vermifuge.*

helminthemesis (hel-min-them′e-sis). The vomiting of intestinal worms.

helminthiasis (hel-min-thi′a-sis). Having intestinal parasites or worms.

helmin′thic. Pert. to that which expels worms. SYN: *anthelmintic; vermifugal.*

helminthicide (hĕl-mĭn′thĭ-sīd). A worm-expelling drug. SYN: *vermicide.*

helminthol′ogy. The study of intestinal vermiform parasites.

helmintho′ma. A parasitic worm tumor.

helminthophobia (hel-min-tho-fo′bĭ-ă). Morbid dread of worms or delusion of being infested by them.

helmitol (hel′mi-tol). A methenamine compound, claimed to be well tolerated, and suitable for prolonged use.

   DOSAGE: From 5-10 gr. (0.3-0.6 Gm.) dissolved in water.

heloma (he-lo'mă). A callosity or corn. SYN: *clavus.*

helosis (he-lo'sis). The state of having corns.

helotomeia (he-lo-to-mi'ă). Corn surgery.

helot'omon. Surgical knife for cutting corns.

helotomy (he-lot'o-mĭ). Surgical treatment of corns.

hemabarometer (hem″ab-ar-om'et-er). Device for determining sp. gr. of blood.

hemachrome (hem'a-krōm). The red coloring substance of blood. SEE: *hemoglobin.*

hemachro'sis. Abnormal redness of blood.

hemacytom'eter. Apparatus for counting blood corpuscles.

hemacytozoon (hem-a-sī-to-zo'on). A protozoan parasite infesting red blood corpuscles.

hemad (he'mad). Toward the ventral or hemal aspect of the body. Opp. to neural or dorsal.

hem'aden. A ductless gland.

hemadenology (hem″ă-de-nol'o-jĭ). The study of internal secretions. SYN: *endocrinology.*

hemadostenosis (hem″a-do-sten-o'sis). Contraction of blood vessels.

hemadromom'eter. Device for recording rapidity of flow of blood. SYN: *hemodromometer.*

hemadynamometer (hem″a-di″na-mom'e-ter). Device for determining blood pressure.

hemadynamometry (hem″a-di-nă-mom'e-trĭ). Measurement of blood pressure.

hemafa'cient. A blood producing agent. SYN: *hemopoietic, sanguifacient.*

hemafecia (hem-ă-fe'sĭ-ă). Feces containing blood.

hemagglutination (hem″ag-glu-tin-a'shun). The clumping of red blood corpuscles.

hem″agglu'tinin. An antibody that induces clumping of red blood corpuscles.

hemagogue (hem'ag-og). An agent that favors the flow of blood or of the menses. SYN: *emmenagogue.*

he'mal. 1. Pert. to the blood or blood vessels. 2. Pert. to side of the body in which the heart is located.

  h. **arch.** The ribs, breastbone, and that part of the vertebrae, which together enclose the heart and viscera.

  h. **spine.** Linea alba and sternum.

hemalex'in. A blood alexin.

hemalex'is. The fabrication or development of alexin of the blood.

hemanal'ysis. A blood analysis. SEE: *blood.*

hemangiectasis (hem″an-jĭ-ek'ta-sis). Dilatation of blood vessels.

hemangioblastoma (hem-an″ji-o-blas-to'mă). Hemangioma of the brain of a capillary nature.

hemangioendothelioma (hem″an-jĭ-o-en″do-the-lĭ-o'ma). An overgrowth of the endothelium of the minute capillary vessels frequently on the cerebral meninges.

hemangioma (hem-an-jĭ-o'ma) (pl. *hemangiomata*). An angioma consisting of blood vessels.

hemangiomatosis (hem″an-jĭ-o-ma-to'sis). Multiple angiomata of blood vessels.

hemangiosarcoma (hem″an-jĭ-o-sar-ko'mă). A mixed sarcoma and hemangioma. SYN: *angiosarcoma.*

hemaphein (hem-af-e'in). Brown coloring matter in the blood; a decomposition product of hematin.

hemapoiesis (hem-ap-oi-e'sis). Blood formation. SYN: *hematopoiesis.*

hemapoietic (hem-ap-oi-et'ĭk). Pert. to hemapoiesis. SYN: *hematogenic, hematoplastic.*

hemapophysis (hem-ă-pof'is-is). A costal cartilage.

hemarthros (hem-ar'thros). Bloody effusion into cavity of a joint. SYN: *hemarthrosis.*

hemarthrosis (hem-ar-thro'sis). Effusion of blood in a joint cavity.

hem'ase. An enzyme in the blood.

hemasthenosis (hem-as-then-o'sis). Deterioration of the blood.

hematachometer (hem-at-ak-om'et-er). Device for determining rapidity of the circulation.

hemataerom'eter. Device for measuring gases in the blood.

hematalloscopy (hem-at-al-os'ko-pĭ). Examination to distinguish one kind of blood from another.

hematapostasis (hem-at-ap-os'tas-is). Unequal pressure of blood with effusion or congestion in some part of body.

hematapostema (hem″at-ap-os-te'mă) (pl. *hematapostemata*). Abscess containing extravasated blood.

hemateikon (hem-ăt-ī'kon). A microscopic picture of the blood.

hematemesis (hem-at-em'e-sis). Vomiting of blood.

hematencephalon (hem-at-en-sef'a-lŏn). Cerebral hemorrhage.

hematherapy (hem-a-ther'ă-pī). Adm. of fresh blood in treatment of disease.

hemather'mal. Warm blooded.

hemather'mous. Warm blooded. SYN: *hemathermal, hematothermal.*

hemathidrosis (he-mat-hi-dro'sis). Condition of sweating blood.

hematic (he-mat'ik). 1. Rel. to the blood. 2. A remedy for anemia.

hematim'eter. Apparatus for counting blood corpuscles in a cu.mm. of blood. SYN: *hematometer, hemocytometer.*

hem'atin. An acid radicle or brown amorphous substance that unites with globin in the formation of hemoglobin.

  h. **hydrochloride.** The hydrochloric acid ester of hematin, crystalline in form.

hematinemia (hem-ă-tin-e'mĭ-ă). Hematin in the circulating blood.

hematinic (hem-a-tin'ĭk). Pert. to blood. SYN: *hematic.*

hematinometer (hem-at-in-om'et-er). Device for determining quantity of hemoglobin in blood.

hematinu'ria. Hematin in the urine. SYN: *hemoglobinuria.*

hematischesis (hem-ă-tis'ke-sis). Arrest of bleeding or hemorrhage.

hemato'bium. A parasite that lives in the blood. SYN: *hematozoon.*

hem´atoblast. A blood platelet.

hematocele (hem´at-o-sēl). 1. A blood cyst. 2. Effusion of blood into a cavity. 3. Swelling due to effusion of blood into the *tunica vaginalis testis.*

h., parametric, pelvic, retrouterine. Tumor formed by blood effusion in the *cul-de-sac* of Douglas walled off by adhesions.

h., pudendal. A bloody tumor of the labium.

hematocelia (hem´´ă-to-se´li-ă). Hemorrhage into the peritoneal cavity.

hematoceph´alus. Fetus born with infusion of blood in the head.

hematochezia (hem´´ă-to-ke´zĭ-ă). Passage of stools containing blood.

hematochromato´sis. A condition showing staining of tissues with blood pigment. SYN: *hemochromatosis.*

hematochyluria (hem´´ă-to-ki-lū´rĭ-ă). Blood and chyle in the urine in *Filaria* infections.

hematocolpometra (hem´´at-o-kol´´po-me´tra). Retention of menstrual blood in the vagina and uterus.

hematocolpos (hem-at-o-kol´pos). Retained menstrual blood in the vagina from an imperforate hymen.

hematocrit(e (hem´ă-to-krĭt). Centrifuge for separating solids from plasma in the blood.

hematocryal (hem-at-o-kri´al). Possessing cold blood.

hematocrystallin (hem-at-o-kris´tal-in). The coloring matter of the blood. SYN: *hemoglobin.*

hematocyst (hem´at-o-sist). A blood cyst.

hematocyte (hem´at-o-sīt). A blood corpuscle.

hematocytoblast (hem´ă-to-si´to-blast). A cell in bone marrow.

hematocytolysis (hem´´ă-to-si-tol´is-is). Dissolution of blood corpuscles freeing hemoglobin. SYN: *hemolysis.*

hematocytometer (hem-at-o-si-tom´et-er). Device for determining number of corpuscles in given quantity of blood.

hematocytozoon (hem´´ă-to-si-to-zo´on). A parasite which lives in red blood corpuscles.

hematocyturia (hem´´ă-to-si-tū´rĭ-ă). Red blood corpuscles in urine; hematuria* as differentiated from hemoglobinuria.*

hematodystrophy (hem´´ă-to-dis´tro-fĭ). Any disorder of blood, such as anemia.*

hematogenesis (hem´´ă-to-jen´es-is). The development of blood corpuscles. SYN: *hematopoiesis.*

hematogenic, hematogenous (hem-a-to-jen´ik, -ă-toj´en-us). Pert. to formation of blood. SYN: *hematopoietic.*

hematoglob´ulin. Coloring matter of blood. SYN: *hemoglobin, oxyhemoglobin.*

hematogonia (hem´´ă-to-go´nĭ-ă). A bone marrow cell. SYN: *hematocytoblast, q.v.; leukoblast; lymphoidocyte; myeloblast.*

hematohidrosis (hem´´ă-to-hī-dro´sis). Excretion of bloody sweat. SYN: *hemathidrosis.*

hematohistioblast (hem´´a-to-his´ti-o-

blast). A polymorphous white blood cell of large size forming connective tissue.

hematoid (he´mă-toid). Looking like blood.

hematoidin (hem-ă-toy´dĭn). An iron-free principle in remains of old blood clots.

hematokolpos (hem-at-o-kol´pos). Collection of blood in the vagina. SYN: *hematocolpos.*

hematokrit (hem´at-o-krĭt). Device for determining number of corpuscles in the blood. SYN: *hematocrit.*

hem´atolith. Concretion in a blood vessel wall. SYN: *hemolith.*

hematology (hem-at-ol´o-gĭ). The science of the blood.

hematolymphangioma (hem´´ă-to-limf-an´´jĭ-o´mă). A tumor consisting of dilated blood vessels and lymphatics.

hematolysis (hem-at-ol´is-is). A term applied to (a) diminished coagulability, or (b) to the destruction or disorganization of the blood and its corpuscles. SEE: *hemolysis.*

hematolytic (hem-ă-to-lit´ik). Pert. to hematolysis. SYN: *hemolytic.*

hematoma (hem-ă-to´mă). A blood tumor.

h. auris. One beneath perichondrium of ear cartilage.

h., pelvic. One affecting cellular tissue of pelvis.

h., vulvar. Hematoma occurring on the vulva.

hematomediastinum (hem´´ă-to-me´´dĭ-ă-sti´num). Blood effusion into the mediastinum.

hematometer (he-mă-tom´et-er). Device for determining the properties of blood.

hematometra (he´´mă-to-me´tră). 1. Hemorrhage in the uterus. 2. Accumulation of menstrual blood in the womb. SEE: *hematocolpos, hydrometra, pyometra.*

hematom´etry. Determination of varieties and number of blood cells and percentage of hemoglobin in the blood.

hematomphalocele (hem´´at-om-fal´o-sēl). Effusion of blood into an umbilical hernia.

hematomyelia (he-mă-to-mī-e´lĭ-ă). Hemorrhage of blood into the spinal cord.

hematomyelitis (hem´´ă-to-mi-el-i´tis). Inflammation of spinal cord with bloody effusion.

hematomyelopore (hem-at-o-mi´el-o-pōr). Porous condition of the spinal cord resulting from hemorrhages.

hematonephrosis (hem-ă-to-nē-fro´sis). Blood distending the pelvis of the kidney.

hematon´ic. A blood tonic given to raise the percentage of hemoglobin.

hematopathol´ogy. The study of morbid conditions of the blood.

hematopericar´dium. Bloody effusion into the pericardial sac.

hematoperitone´um. Bloody effusion into the peritoneal cavity. SYN: *hemoperitoneum.*

hematopex´in. That which coagulates blood. SYN: *hemopexin.*

hematopex´is. Coagulation of the blood. SYN: *hemopexia.*

hem´atophage. A phagocytic cell which destroys red blood corpuscles.

hematophagia (hem-at-o-fa'jĭ-ă). 1. Subsistence on blood. 2. Adm. of blood as a treatment.

hematophagous (hem-ă-tof'ag-us). Living on blood.

hematophilia (hem-at-o-fil'ĭ-ă). Congenital condition characterized by defective blood coagulation causing copious hemorrhages. SYN: *hemophilia*.

hematophobia (hem″ăt-o-fō'bĭ-ă). Abnormal aversion to the sight of blood.

hematophthalmia (he-ma-tof-thal'mĭ-ă). Blood in the vitreous humor.

hematophyte (hem'ă-to-fīt). Plant organism or bacteria in the blood.

hematopla'nia. Condition of vicarious menstruation.

hematoplas'tic. Pert. to formation of blood. SYN: *hematopoietic*.

hematopneic (hem-ă-to-pne'ĭk). Rel. to oxygenation of the blood.

hematopoiesis (he″mă-to-poi-e'sis). The formation of red blood corpuscles.

hematopoietic (hem″ă-to-poy-et'ĭk). Rel. to blood-making processes. SYN: *hematogenic· hematoplastic*.

hematoporphyrin (hem″at-o-por'fĭr-ĭn). Iron-free hematin; a decomposition product of hemoglobin in the urine in certain conditions.

hematoporphyrinuria (hem″ă-to-por″fi-rin-u'rĭ-ă). Hematoporphyrin in urine.

hematoposia (hem″ă-to-po'sĭ-ă). Drinking of blood. SEE: *hematophagia*.

hematorrhachis (he-mă-tor'ă-kis). Hemorrhage into the spinal cord.

hematorrhea (he-mă-tor-re'ă). Profuse hemorrhage.

hematosalpinx (he-mă-to-sal'pinks). Retained menstrual fluid in the fallopian tube.

hematoscheocele (he-ă-tos'ke-o-sēl). Blood accumulated in the scrotum.

hematoscope (he'mat-o-skōp). Device for examining the blood.

hematoscopy (hem-at-os'ko-pĭ). Examination of the blood.

hematose (hem'at-ōs). Full of blood.

hematosepsis (hem-at-o-sep'sis). Blood toxemia. SYN: *septicemia*.

hematosin (hem-at-o'sin). Decomposition product of hemoglobin. SYN: *hematin*.

hematosis (he-ma-to'sis). 1. The formation of blood and the development of the red blood corpuscles. 2. Arterialization of blood.

hematospec'troscope. Spectroscope for inspecting the blood.

hematospectros'copy. Examination of the blood with the hematospectroscope.

hematospermatocele (hem″ă-to-sper-mat'-o-sēl). A blood-filled spermatocele.

hematospermia (he-mă-to-sper'mĭ-ă). Bloody semen.

　　h. spuria. When coming from the prostatic urethra.

　　h. vera. When coming from the seminal vessels.

hematostatic (he-mat-o-stat'ĭk). Retaining blood in a part.

hematosteon (hem-ă-tos'te-on). Bleeding into the medullary cavity of a bone.

hematother'mal. Warm blooded. SYN: *hemathermal; hemathermous*.

hematothorax (hem-at-o-tho'raks). Blood in the chest. SYN: *hemothorax*.

hematotox'ic. Pert. to toxemia.

hematotrachelos (he″mat-o-trak'e-los). Retained menstrual blood in cervix uteri causing distention.

hematotympanum (hem-at-o-tĭm'pan-um). Blood in the middle ear.

hematozoon (he-mat-o-zo'on). Any living organism in the blood.

hematozymosis (hem-at-o-zi-mo'sis). Blood fermentation.

hematuria (he-ma-tu'ri-ă). Blood in the urine.

　　h., renal. Urine smoky, sometimes bright red.

　　h., urethral. Always bright red. Precedes urination.

　　h., vesical. Urine bright red, not uniform.

hemaurochrome (hem″ă-u'ro-krōm). A hematin derivative found in the urine in sarcoma and carcinoma, malaria, anemias, and other disorders. Supposed to result from dissolution of red blood corpuscles.

hemeralopia (hem-er-al-o'pĭ-ă). Day blindness or night blindness, found particularly in macular lesions.

hemi-. Prefix meaning *half*.

hemiachromatopsia (he-mĭ-ak-ro-mat-op'-sĭ-ă). Color blindness in one-half, or in corresponding halves, of the visual field.

hemialbumin (hem-ĭ-al-bu'min). A product resulting from the digestion of albumin. SYN: *antialbumin*.

hemialbumose (hem-ĭ-al'bū-mōs). An albumoid product from the digestion of certain proteins. It occurs in bone marrow.

hemialbumosu'ria. Hemialbumose in the urine.

hemialgia (hem-ĭ-al'jĭ-ă). Pain in one-half of the body.

hemiamaurosis (hem″ĭ-am-aw-ro'sis). Blindness in one-half the visual field. SYN: *hemianopia*.

hemiamblyopia (hem″ĭ-am-blĭ-o'pĭ-ă). Blindness in half the visual field. SYN: *hemianopsia*.

hemiamyosthenia (hem″ĭ-am″i-os-the'nĭ-ă). Absence of normal muscular power on 1 side of the body. SYN: *hemiparesis*.

hemianacusia (hem″ĭ-an-a-kū'sĭ-ă). Deafness in 1 ear.

hemianalgesia (hem″ĭ-an-al-ge'sĭ-ă). Lack of sensibility to pain (analgesia) on 1 side of the body.

hemianesthesia (hem″ĭ-an-es-the'zĭ-ă). Anesthesia of one-half of the body.

hemianopia, hemianopsia (hem-ĭ-an-op'ĭ-ă, sĭ-ă). Blindness for one-half field of vision in 1 or both eyes.

　　h., altitudinal. Blindness in upper or lower half in each eye.

　　h., binasal. Affection of nasal half of visual field in each eye.

　　h., bitemporal. Affection of temporal half of visual field in each eye.

h., complete. Hemianopia of half of each eye.

h., crossed. Bitemporal or binasal hemianopsia.

h., heteronymous. SEE: crossed hemianopia.

h., homonymous. Blindness of nasal half of 1 eye and temporal half of the other or right-sided or left-sided hemianopia of corresponding sides in both eyes.

h., incomplete. Hemianopia of less than half of each eye.

h., quadrant. Affection of symmetrical quadrant of the field in each eye.

h., unilateral, uniocular. Hemianopsia affecting only 1 eye.

hemianosmia (hem″ĭ-an-os′mĭ-ă). Loss of smell in 1 nostril.

hemiapraxia (hem″ĭ-ă-prak′sĭ-ă). Incapacity to exercise purposeful movements on 1 side of the body.

hemiarthrosis (hem-ĭ-ar-thro′sis). A false articulation bet. 2 bones. SYN: synchondrosis.

hemiasynergia (hem″ĭ-as-in-er′jĭ-ă). Lack of coördination of parts affecting 1 side of the body.

hemiataxia (hem-ĭ-ă-taks′ĭ-ă). Impaired muscular coördination causing awkward movements of the affected side of the body.

hemiathetosis (hem″ĭ-ath-et-o′sis). Slow change of position; athetosis of 1 side of the body.

hemiatrophy (hem-i-at′ro-fĭ). Impaired nutrition resulting in atrophy of 1 side of the face or other part; marked by white or yellow macules on affected side.

hemiballism (hem-ĭ-bal′izm). Jerking and twitching movements of 1 side of the body. SYN: hemichorea.

he′mic. Pert. to blood. SYN: hemal.

hemicanities (hem″ĭ-kan-ish′ĭ-ēz). Grayness (canities) of hair on 1 side only.

hemicardia (hem-ĭ-kar′dĭ-ă). Half of a 4-chambered heart.

hemicellulose (hem-ĭ-sel′lu-lōs). A name for all the carbohydrates in the cell wall soluble in a dilute mineral acid.

hemicentrum (hem-ĭ-sen′trum). Either lateral half of the centrum of a vertebra.

hemichorea (hem-ĭ-ko-re′ă). Convulsive movements (chorea) of but 1 side of the body.

hemichromatopsia (hem″ĭ-kro-mat-op′-sĭ-ă). Blindness to color in one-half of the visual field. SYN: hemiachromatopsia.

hemicrania (hem-ĭ-kra′nĭ-ă). 1. Unilateral head pain, usually migraine. 2. Monstrosity having only one-half of the skull developed.

hemicraniectomy (hem″ĭ-kra-nĭ-ek′to-mĭ). Surgical division of cranial vault from before, backward, exposing half of the brain.

hemicraniosis (hem″ĭ-kra-nĭ-o′sis). Enlargement of half of cranium or face.

hemidiaphoresis (hem″ĭ-dĭ-ăf-or-e′sis). Sweating on 1 side of the body.

hemidi′aphragm. Paralysis affecting only one-half of the diaphragm.

hemidro′sis. Bloody sweating. SYN: hemathidrosis.

hemidyser′gia. Lack of coördination of muscles (dysergia) on 1 side of the body.

hemidysesthesia (hem″ĭ-dis-es-the′sĭ-ă). Impaired sensation (dysesthesia) of one-half of the body.

hemidystrophy (hem″ĭ-dis′tro-fĭ). Inequality in development of the 2 sides of the body.

hemiep′ilepsy. Epilepsy with convulsions confined to 1 lateral half of the body.

hemifa′cial. Pert. to 1 side of the face.

hemigastrectomy (hem″ĭ-gas-trek′to-mĭ). Excision of pyloric end of the stomach for hourglass contraction.

hemigeusia (hem-ĭ-gu′sĭ-ă). Loss of sense of taste on 1 side of the tongue.

hemiglossi′tis. Vesicular eruption on one-half of the tongue and inner surface of cheek. Herpetic in character.

hemihidro′sis. Sweating on only 1 side of the body. SYN: hemidiaphoresis.

hemihyperesthesia (hem″ĭ-hī-per-es-the′-sĭ-ă). Abnormal tactile and painful sensitiveness of 1 side of the body.

hemihyperidrosis (hem″ĭ-hī-per-i-dro′sis). Excessive perspiration confined to 1 side of the body.

hemihyperto′nia. Exaggerated tonicity of muscles on 1 lateral half of the body.

hemihyper′trophy. Muscular overgrowth (hypertrophy) of one-half of the body or face.

hemihypesthesia (hem″ĭ-hī-pes-the′sĭ-ă). Diminished sensibility on 1 side of the body.

hemihypotonia (hem″ĭ-hī-po-to′nĭ-ă). Partial loss of tonicity of muscles on 1 side of the body.

hemilat′eral. Rel. to 1 side only.

hemin (he′min). A brownish-red crystalline salt of hematin. SYN: hematin hydrochloride.

hemineurasthenia (hem″ĭ-nū-răs-the′nĭ-ă). Neurasthenia affecting 1 side of the body only.

hemiopia (hem-ĭ-o′pĭ-ă). Blindness in half of the visual field. SYN: hemianopia.

hemiopic (hem-ĭ-op′ik). Pert. to hemiopia.

hemiparal′ysis. Paralysis of 1 side of the body only.

hemiparanesthesia (hem″ĭ-par-an-es-the′-sĭ-ă). Anesthesia of 1 lower extremity or lower half of 1 side.

hemiparaplegia (hem″ĭ-par-ă-ple′jĭ-ă). Paralysis of the lower half of 1 side or of 1 leg.

hemipar′esis. Slight paralysis of 1 side of the body.

hem″iparesthe′sia. Numbness of 1 side of body.

hemipeptone (hem-ĭ-pep′tōn). One of the 2 compounds of peptone in pepsin digestion which later forms leucin, tyrosin, and amino acids.

hemiplegia (hem-i-ple′jĭ-ă). Paralysis of only one-half of the body.

h., alternate. Affecting 1 side of face and trunk and opposite of extremities

h., cerebral. Due to brain lesion.

h. cruciata. Medulla lesion involving the crossed arm and uncrossed leg fibers of the pyramids paralyzing 1 arm and the opposite leg.

h., facial. Paralysis of motor nerves of 1 side of face.

h., hephestic. Spasmodic form affecting blacksmiths.

h., spastic. Of infants, accompanied by spasms.

h., spinal. Brown-Sequard's paralysis.

hemiplegic (hem-i-ple'jik). Pert. to hemiplegia.

hemiprotein (hem-ĭ-pro'te-in). One containing only the group digested by trypsin.

hemisec'tion. Section of one-half of a part or organ. SYN: *bisection*.

hemispasm (hem'ĭ-spazm). Spasm of only 1 side of the body or face.

hemisphere (hem'is-fēr). Either half of the cerebrum or cerebellum.

Hemis'pora stella'ta. A variety of fungus causing mycosis.

hemispore (hem'ĭ-spōr). A spore which reproduces by division of terminal part of a hyphus.*

hemisporosis (hem-ĭ-spo-ro'sis). Infection with a fungus (*Hemispora stellata*) resulting in swellings of bone and other tissue of a gummatous nature. They may later ulcerate.

hemistrumectomy (hem"ĭ-strŭ-mek'to-mĭ). Excision of about one-half of a goiter.

hemisyndrome (hem-ĭ-sin'drōm). One indicating a unilateral lesion of the spinal cord.

hemisystole (hem-i-sis'to-le). One pulse beat to every 2 heartbeats.

hemiteric, hemiteratic (hem-ĭ-ter'ĭk, -ter-at'ik). Congenitally deformed, but not marked as monstrous.

hem'lock. 1. A species of fir tree. 2. Volatile oil extracted from hemlock tree.

hemo-. Prefix: Blood.

hem"oagglutina'tion. The clumping of red blood corpuscles.

hem"oagglu'tinin. An agglutinin which clumps the red blood corpuscles.

hemoalkalim'eter. A device for estimating degree of alkalinity of blood.

hemobilinuria (hem"o-bĭl-ĭn-ū'rĭ-ă). Urobilin in the blood and urine.

hem'oblast. Immature red blood corpuscles; a blood platelet. SYN: *hematoblast*.

hemoblastosis (hem-o-blas-to'sis). Changes occurring in or increase in amount of the blood forming tissues.

hemocatatonistic (hem"o-kat-at-on-is'tĭk). Diminishing the cohesion bet. the hemoglobin and red blood corpuscles and erythrocytes.

hemocatheresis (hem"o-kath-er-e'sis). Dissolution of red blood corpuscles.

hemocatheretic (hem"o-kath-er-et'ik). Destructive to blood corpuscles.

hemochromatosis (hem"o-krō-mat-ō'sis). A disease of pigmentation of the skin and viscera, sometimes associated with diabetes and has been called *bronzed diabetes*.

hem'ochrome. The red pigment of the blood.

hemochro'mogen. Decomposition product of hemoglobin.

hemochromomometer (hem-o-kro-mom'et-er). Device for making color test in estimation of quality of the blood.

hemoci'dal. Destructive to blood cells.

hemocla'sia, hemoc'lasis. Disintegration of red blood corpuscles. SYN: *hemolysis*.

hemoclas'tic. Destructive of erythrocytes. SYN: *hemolytic*.

hemoco'nia. Minute, colorless bodies in blood. SYN: *hemokonia*.

hemoconio'sis. Having an abnormal amt. of hemokonia in the blood. SYN: *hemokoniosis*.

hemocrinia (hem-o-krĭn'ĭ-a). Hormones in the blood.

hemocrinotherapy (hem"o-krĭn-o-ther'ă-pĭ). Injection of an endocrine extract combined with the patient's own blood.

hemocrystallin (hem-o-kris'tal-in). The coloring substance of the blood. SYN: *hemoglobin*.

hem'oculture. A bacteriological blood culture.

hemocyte (hem'o-sīt). Blood corpuscle.

hemocy'toblast. An embryonic blood cell from which all others are derived.

hemocytoblastoma (hem"o-si"to-blas-to'mă). A tumor containing embryonic blood cells.

hemocytocatheresis (hem"o-si"to-kath-er-e'sis). The dissolution of blood corpuscles.

hemocytogenesis (hem"o-si"to-jen'e-sis). The formation of erythrocytes.

hemocytology (hem-o-si-tol'o-jĭ). The science of blood cells.

hemocytolysis (hem-o-si-tol'is-is). Dissolution of the blood corpuscles. SYN: *hematocytolysis, hemolysis*.

hemocytometer (hem-o-si-tom'et-er). Device for determining relative number of corpuscles in the blood.

hemocytopoiesis (hem"o-si"to-poy-e'sis). The development of blood cells.

hemocytotripsis (hem"o-si"to-trip'sis). Fragmentation of the red blood corpuscles.

hemocytozoon (hem"o-si"to-zo'on). An animal microparasite of the blood cells. SYN: *hematobium*.

hemodiagno'sis. Examination of the blood for diagnostic purpose.

hemodi'astase. An amylolytic ferment in the blood.

hemodromometer (hem"o-dro-mom'et-er). Device for determining the blood's velocity.

hemodynam'ics. The study of circulation of the blood.

hemodynamometer (hem"o-di-na-mom'et-er). Device for measuring blood pressure.

hemodystrophy (hem-o-dis'tro-fĭ). Imperfect nutrition of the blood. SYN: *hematodystrophy*.

hemoferrum (hem-o-fer'um). The iron element of hemoglobin. SYN: *oxyhemoglobin*.

hemofuscin (hem-o-fus'in). Brown coloring matter derived from hemoglobin.

hemogenesis (hem-o-jen'es-is). Blood formation. SYN: *hematogenesis*.

hemoge'nia. A hemorrhagic condition of the blood forming apparatus.

hemogen'ic. Rel. to the production of blood.

hemoglobin (hem-o-glo'bin). A chromoprotein of red color; the coloring substance of the red blood corpuscles.

　　h. casts. Brown granules of hemoglobin found in paroxysmal hemoglobinuria. Determination may be made with the Sahli's method.

　　SEE: *achroiocythemia, blood, cell color, ratio.*

　　h. test. A patient with a low percentage of hemoglobin is a poor operative risk, and for this reason a test is made preoperatively if the condition is suspected.

hemoglobinemia (hem″o-glob-in-e'mi-ă). Presence of hemoglobin in the blood plasma.

hemoglobinocholia (hem″o-glo″bin-o-ko'lĭ-ă). Hemoglobin in the bile.

hemoglobinolysis (hem″o-glo-bin-ol'ĭ-sis). Dissolution of hemoglobin.

hemoglobinometer (hem″o-glo-bin-om'et-er). Device for determining the hemoglobin in the blood.

hemoglobinopepsia (hem″o-glo″bin-o-pep'-sĭ-ă). Destruction of hemoglobin. SYN: *hemoglobinolysis.*

hemoglobinophilic (hem-o-glo-bin-o-fil'ik). Pert. to substances which grow better in presence of hemoglobin.

hemoglobinorrhea (hem″o-glo″bin-or-re'ă). Flow of hemoglobin from the red blood corpuscles.

　　h. cutis. Effusion of hemoglobin into the skin.

hemoglo'binous. Pert. to or containing hemoglobin.

hemoglobinuria (hem″o-glo-bin-u'rĭ-ă). The presence of hemoglobin in the urine, but free from red blood corpuscles.

　　SEE: *Buhl's disease, Winckel's disease.*

hem″oglobinu'ric. Rel. to or marked by hemoglobinuria.

　　h. fever. Malarial hemoglobinuria.

hem'ogram. A graph of the differential blood count. SEE: *Schilling's hemogram.*

hemohistioblast (hem″o-his'tĭ-o-blast). A polymorphous white blood cell of large size which forms connective tissue. SYN: *hematohistioblast.*

he'moid. Having the appearance of blood.

hemoko'nia (pl. *hemokoniae*). Minute, highly refractive body in the blood, said to be disintegrated particle of blood corpuscle. SYN: *blood dust, blood mote.*

hemokoniosis (hem″o-ko-nĭ-o'sis). Abnormal amount of hemokoniae in the blood.

hemoleukocyte (hem-o-lŭ'ko-sĭt). A white blood corpuscle.

hem'olith. A calculus in the wall of a blood vessel.

hem'olymph. Blood and lymph.

　　h. glands. Glands bet. the hemogenic (spleen) and lymphatic glands.

hemol'ysin. An agent in a serum destructive of erythrocytes.*

hemolysis (hem-ol'ĭ-sis). Dissolution, generally in spleen, of the red blood corpuscles which renders the blood "laked," as, for example, when dilute hydrochloric acid or a serum containing hemolysin is added to the blood, the red corpuscles are destroyed.

hemolytic (hem-o-lit'ik). Pert. to the breaking down of red blood corpuscles.

　　h. unit. The amount of inactivated immune serum which causes complete hemolysis of 1 cc. of a 5% emulsion of washed red blood corpuscles, in the presence of complement.

hemolytopoietic (hem-ol-it″o-poi-et'ik). Rel. to processes of production and destruction of blood cells.

hemomediastinum (hem″o-me-dĭ-as-ti'-num). Effusion of blood into mediastinal spaces. SYN: *hematomediastinum.*

hemom'eter. Instrument for measuring blood pressure within the arteries. SYN: *hema-* or *hemodynamometer.*

hemometra (he-mo-me'trā). Retention of blood within the uterus. SYN: *hematometra.*

hemonephro'sis. Blood in pelvis of the kidney. SYN: *hematonephrosis.*

hemopath'ic. Rel. or due to disease of the blood.

hemopathol'ogy. The science of blood disorders.

hemop'athy. A disease of the blood.

hemoperitone'um. Effusion of blood into the peritoneal cavity.

hemopex'in. Enzyme which coagulates the blood.

hemopex'is. Blood coagulation.

hem'ophage. Cell destroying red blood corpuscles.

hemophagocyte (hem-o-fag'o-sĭt). A white blood corpuscle which ingests other blood corpuscles, esp. red.

hemophilia (hem-o-fil'ĭ-ă). A hereditary blood condition transmitted by females, who are not generally affected by it, but act as sex-linking carriers, and, in severe form, occurring exclusively in males SYN: *bleeder's disease.*

hemophiliac (hem-o-fil'ĭ-ak). One afflicted with hemophilia.

Hemophilus (he-mof'ĭ-lus). A genus of bacterial organisms which grow best on blood media.

　　H. influen'zae. The influenza bacillus.

hemophobia (he-mo-fo'bĭ-ă). Aversion to seeing blood or to bleeding.

hemophor'ic. Conveying blood.

hemophthal'mia, hemophthal'mus. Effusion of blood into eyeball.

hemoplas'tic. Blood-forming. SYN: *hematoplastic, hematopoietic.*

hemopneumothorax (hem″o-nu-mo-tho'raks). Blood and air in the pleural cavity.

hemopoie'sis. Formation of red blood corpuscles. SYN: *hematopoiesis.*

hemoptysis (hem-op'tis-is). Expectoration of pure blood; hemorrhage from the lungs.

hemorrhage (hem'o-raj). Abnormal discharge of blood, either external or internal; venous, arterial, or capillary from blood vessels into tissues, into or from the body.

h., accidental. OB. AND GYN: Hemorrhage caused by premature rupture of the placenta. SEE: *ablatio placentae.*

h., antepartum. Hemorrhage appearing before the onset of labor.

h., armpit. Place sterile gauze sponge into wound; apply pressure over pad and bandage over shoulder and under armpit. Also bandage under opposite armpit over shoulder already bandaged.

h., armpit and elbow (between). Insert sterile gauze sponge into wound and apply pressure over pad; or tourniquet.

h., arterial. In arterial bleeding (red) the blood ordinarily comes through in waves or spurts, unless the torn artery is deep or buried, when the flow may be steady.

h., capillary. Bleeding from minute blood vessels, present in all bleeding; when large vessels are not injured they may be controlled by simple elevation and pressure as with sterile compress.

h., carotid artery. Usually accompanied by bleeding from the jugular veins and may be fatal in a short time.

h., cerebral. Escape of blood into tissues of brain.

h., consecutive. Some time after an injury, 20 to 24 hours after an operation.

h., contact. Hemorrhage from the cervix uteri coming on as a result of exertion, or contact during coitus, douching, or instrumentation.

h., elbow and hand (bet.). Put pad in elbow, apply bandage over it as a tourniquet.

h. of foot. Apply pad and pressure and bandage.

h. of hand. Fill hand with sterile gauze sponge, clasp fingers around it and bandage; apply bandage just above elbow.

h. of knee. At the knee, or below, apply pad as stated with pressure, or put a pad under knee and bandage leg at that place.

h., lung. Blood bright red and frothy, frequently coughed up.

h., pancreas. Hemorrhage of dark blood in vomitus with slimy mucus, coming from pancreas, usually occurring in inflammation of pancreas. SEE: *hemorrhagic pancreatitis.*

h., postmenopausal. Bleeding from the vagina after the menopause has been established.

h., postpartum. SEE: *uterine hemorrhage.*

h., primary. Immediately following any trauma.

h., secondary. After 24 hours or at time of separation of ligature, usually bet. 7th and 10th day. Due to sepsis.

h., stomach. Blood dark, perhaps clotted or mixed with stomach contents, usually vomited

h., thigh. Upper part near groin. Insert pad of iodoform gauze into wound and apply pressure or press thumb in center of fold of groin against bone until bleeding stops below groin. Pad as above or tourniquet with pad under.

h., typhoid. It occurs in about 7% of cases. Loss may be 1 quart. It may occur singly or in succession, the latter being more serious than large hemorrhages. They take place at the end of the 2nd week and during the 3rd week of the disease.

h., unavoidable. Ceaseless, painless bleeding. SEE: *placenta previa.*

h., uterine. One into cavity of uterus.

h., venous. Characterized by steady, profuse bleeding of rather dark blood.

h., vicarious. Hemorrhage from a part due to suppression in another part. SEE: *vicarious menstruation.*

hemorrhagenic (hem-o-ră-jen'ĭk). Producing hemorrhage.

hemorrhagic (hem-or-aj'ĭk). Pert. to or marked by hemorrhage.

h. disease of the newly born. Tendency to spontaneous hemorrhages from umbilicus or mucous membranes. Vitamin K relieves condition.

hemorrha'gin. An element in venom of snakes and other toxins responsible for hemorrhages and effusion of blood by effecting solvent action upon capillary endothelium.

h. unit. Quantity of venom needed to produce vascular hemorrhage in 3-day-old chick embryos.

hemorrhagiparous (hem-o-ră-jip'ă-rus). Producing hemorrhage. SYN: *hemorrhagenic.*

hemorrhea (hem-or-e'ă). Hemorrhage.

hemorrhoid (hem'o-roid). A tumor in form of dilated blood vessels in the anal region. SEE: *hemorrhoidectomy, piles.*

h., external. Cutaneous and thrombotic, outside the sphincter.

h., internal. Venous, arterial, and capillary, within the sphincter but beneath the mucous membrane.

hemorrhoidal (hem-o-roy'dal). 1. Rel. to hemorrhoids. 2. Pert. to certain anal arteries, *arteria hemorrhoidalis.*

hemorrhoidectomy (hem-o-roi-dek'to-mĭ). Surgical excision of hemorrhoids.*

hemosal'pinx. Blood accumulated in an oviduct. SYN: *hematosalpinx.*

hemosozic (hem-o-so'zĭk). 1. Protective of blood corpuscles. 2. Rel. to an antiserum (*antihemolysin*) that prevents hemolysis.

hemospasia (hem-os-pa'zĭ-ă). Withdrawal of blood by cupping or leeching.

hemosper'mia. Bloody semen. SYN: *hematospermia.*

hemosta'sia, hemos'tasis. 1. Arrest of bleeding or of circulation. 2. Stagnation of blood.

hem'ostat. 1. Device or medicine which arrests the flow of blood. 2. Compressor for controlling hemorrhage of the tonsils.

hemostatic (hem-o-stat'ĭk). 1. Checking

hemorrhage. 2. Any substance which checks bleeding without being directly applied to the bleeding areas. Ex: *calcium lactate, ergot, whole blood.*

hemostyp'tic. An astringent that stops bleeding; chemically hemostatic.

hemotachometer (hem-o-tak-om'et-er). Device for measuring velocity of the blood.

hemotherapeu'tics. The use of blood, by transfusion or otherwise, in treatment of disease.

hemother'apy. Blood transfusion or drinking as a therapeutic measure. SYN: *hemotherapeutics.*

hemothorax (hem-o-tho'raks). Bloody fluid in the pleural cavity caused by rupture of small blood vessels, due to inflammation of the lungs in pneumonia, or to pulmonary tuberculosis, or to a malignant growth.   [murder.

hemothy'mia. An irresistible impulse to

hemoto'nia. The tension of the solid elements of the blood.

hemotox'in. A toxin destructive of red blood cells. SYN: *hemolysin.*

hemotrip'sia. Hemorrhage in 1 part that induces hemorrhage in another part.

hemotym'panum. Blood in the middle ear.

henbane (hen'bān). SYN: *Hyoscyamus, q.v.*

Henle's ampul'la. A vas deferens dilatation just above the ejaculatory duct.

    H.'s cells. Large granular ones with small nuclei in the tubuli seminiferi.

    H.'s glands. Tubular ones in the palpebral conjunctiva.

    H.'s layer. Outer layer of cells of inner root sheath of hair follicle.

    H.'s loop. U-shaped loop of the uriniferous tubule near apex of a medullary pyramid of the kidney.

    H.'s membrane. Bruch's layer forming inner boundary of the choroid.

    H.'s sheath. Connective tissue support of individual nerve fibers in a funiculus.

    H.'s sphincter. Muscular fibers encircling the prostatic and membranous parts of the urethra.

He'noch's angina. Form of angina with gangrenous patches found in mucosa of air passages in scarlet fever and diphtheria. SYN: *necrotic angina.*

    H.'s purpura. Purpura with intestinal disturbances. Infectious disease of children.

henry (hĕn'rē). Unit designating electrical inductance.

Hen'sen's disk, H.'s line. Light line in middle of dark band of sarcous elements.

    H.'s prop cells. Columnar epithelial cells in organ of Corti.

he'par. The liver, *q.v.*

heparin (hep'ar-ĭn). A substance (*phosphatide*) formed in the liver which inhibits the coagulation of the blood.

hep'arinize. To inhibit coagulation of blood with heparin.

hepatalgia (hep-at-al'jĭ-ă). Pain in the liver. SYN: *hepatodynia.*

hepatal'gic. Pert. to hepatalgia.

hepatatrophia (he-pat-ă-tro'fĭ-ă). Atrophied condition of the liver.

hepatauxe (hep"at-awk'se). Enlargement or hypertrophy of the liver.

hepatectomy (hep-ă-tek'to-mĭ). Excision of part or all of liver.

hepat'ic. Pert. to the liver.

    h. duct. The canal that receives bile from the liver.

    h. flexure. The right bend of colon under the liver. The junction of the ascending and transverse colon.

    h. lobes. Divisions of the liver.

    h. veins. The 3 vessels returning blood from the liver and discharging into the inferior vena cava.

    h. zones. Venous, arterial, and portal hepatic regions.

hepaticoduodenostomy (he-pat"ĭ-ko-du"-o-de-nos'to-mĭ). Making an artificial opening bet. hepatic duct and duodenum.

hepaticoenterostomy (he-pat"ĭ-ko-en-ter-os'to-mĭ). Operation for artificial opening bet. hepatic duct and intestine.

hepaticogastrostomy (he-pat-ĭ-ko-gas-tros'to-mĭ). The operation for a passage bet. the hepatic duct and the stomach.

hepaticolithotripsy (he-pat-ĭ-ko-lith'o-trip-sĭ). The crushing of a biliary calculus in the hepatic duct.

hepaticos'tomy. Establishment of permanent fistula into hepatic duct.

hepaticot'omy. Incision into the hepatic duct.

hepatin (hep'at-in). 1. Carbohydrate formed in the liver, which is changed to dextrose to meet body requirements. SYN: *glycogen.* 2. A hepatic hormone supposed to be useful in reducing high blood pressure. SYN: *hephormone.*

hepatitis (hep-ă-ti'tis). Inflammation of the liver.

    h., acute parenchymatous. Acute yellow atrophy of liver.   [liver.

    h., chronic interstitial. Cirrhosis of

    h. externa. Perihepatitis.

hepatiza'tion. The 2nd and 3rd stages in consolidation in lobar pneumonia, the tissue changing into a liverlike substance.

hepato-. Prefix: The liver.

hepatocele (he-pat'o-sēl). Hernia of the liver.

hepatocholangiocystoduodenostomy (hep"-at-o-ko-lan"jĭ-o-sis"to-du-o-de-nos'to-mĭ). Establishment of drainage of bile ducts into the duodenum through the gallbladder.

hepatocholangioduodenostomy (hep"at-o-ko-lan"jĭ-o-du-o-de-nos'to-mĭ). Establishment of drainage of bile ducts into the duodenum.

hepatocholangioenterostomy (hep"at-o-ko-lan"jĭ-o-en-ter-os'to-mĭ). Establishment of a passage bet. the liver and intestine.

hepatocholangiogastrostomy (hep"at-o-ko-lan"jĭ-o-gas-tros'to-mĭ). Establishment of drainage of bile ducts into the stomach.

hepatocholangiostomy (hep"at-o-ko-lan-jĭ-os'to-mĭ). Establishment of free drainage by opening into the gall duct.

hepatocirrhosis (hep-ă-to-sĭ-ro′sis). Cirrhosis of liver.

hepatocol′ic. Rel. to both liver and colon.

hepatocys′tic. Rel. to the liver and gallbladder, or the gallbladder.

hepatoduodenos′tomy. Establishment of an opening from the liver into the duodenum. SYN: *hepaticoduodenostomy.*

hepatodynia (hep-at-o-din′ĭ-ă). Pain in the liver.

hepatodys′entery. Inflammation of the liver causing dysentery.

hepatoenter′ic. Rel. to the liver and intestines.

hepatogas′tric. Rel. to the liver and stomach.

hepatogenic (hep-ă-to-jen′ik). Having its origin in the liver.

hepatogenous (hep-a-toj′en-us). Originating in the liver.

hepatog′raphy. Treatise on human liver.

hepatohemia (hep″ă-to-he′mĭ-ă). Liver congestion.

hep′atoid. Having the structural form of the liver.

hepatolentic′ular. Rel. to lenticular nucleus and the liver.
   h. degeneration. Progressive lenticular degeneration in cirrhosis of the liver. SYN: *Wilson's disease.*

hepatolith (hep′at-o-lith). A biliary concretion in the liver.

hepatolithiasis (hep-a-to-lĭth-i′a-sis). Calculi or concretions in the liver.

hepatol′ogist. A specialist in diseases of the liver.

hepatolysin (hep-ă-tol′ĭ-sin). A cytolysin destructive to hepatic cells.

hepatol′ysis. Liver cell destruction.

hepatolyt′ic. Destructive to tissues of the liver.

hepatoma (hep-ă-to′mă). A tumor of the liver.

hepatomalacia (hep″a-to-mal-a′sĭ-ă). Softening of the liver.

hepatomegaly (hĕ-pă-to-meg′ă-lĭ). Enlargement of the liver.

hepatomelanosis (hep″ă-to-mel-an-o′sis). Pigmented deposits or melanosis in the liver.

hepatonephri′tis. Inflammation of both liver and kidneys.

hepatonephromegaly (hep″ă-to-nef″romeg′ă-lĭ). Hypertrophy of both liver and kidney or kidneys.

hepatopathy (hep-a-top′ă-thĭ). Disease of the liver.

hepatoperitonitis (hep″ă-to-per″ĭ-to-ni′tis). Inflammation of the peritoneal covering of the liver. SYN: *perihepatitis.*

hep′atopexy. Fixation of a movable liver to abdominal wall.

hepatophag(e (hep′ă-to-fāj). A phagocyte that attacks liver cells.

hep″atopto′sia, hepatopto′sis. Downward displacement of the liver.

hep″atopul′monary. Rel. to both liver and lungs.

hepatore′nal. Pert. to both liver and kidneys.

hepatorrhaphy (hep-a-tor′ă-fĭ). The suturing of a wound of the liver.

hepatorrhea (hep-at-o-re′ă). 1. Bilious diarrhea. 2. Morbid flow from the liver.

hepatorrhex′is. Rupture of the liver.

hepatos′copy. Inspection of the liver.

hepatosplen′itis. Inflamed condition of both liver and spleen.

hepatosplenomegaly (hep″ă-to-sple″no-meg′ă-lĭ). Enlargement of both liver and spleen.

hepatostomy (hep-a-tos′to-mĭ). The making of an artificial fissure into the liver.

hep″atother′apy. 1. Treatment of liver disease. 2. The use of liver or liver extract.

hepatotomy (hep-ă-tot′o-mĭ). Incision into the liver.

hepatotoxemia (hep″ă-to-toks-e′mĭ-ă). Autointoxication due to malfunctioning of the liver.

hepatotox′in. A cytotoxin specific for liver cells.   [smith.

hephestic (he-fes′tik). Pert. to a black-
   h. hemiplegia, h. spasm. A hemiplegia and spasm of blacksmiths and of others, marked by paresis of arm muscles.

hephormone (hep′hor-mōn). A hepatic hormone supposed to reduce high blood pressure. SYN: *hepatin.*

heptachromic (hep″tă-kro′mĭk). Possessing normal color vision.

hep′tad. Any element with a valency of seven.

hep′toses. Sugars of the glucoses. $C_7H_{14}O_7$.

heptosu′ria. Heptose in the urine.

herb. A plant of tender, juicy nature, living only 1 season. Ex: *lobelia, pennyroyal, peppermint.*

herbiv′orous. Vegetarian; living on grasses and herbs.

herd. Any large aggregation of people or animals.
   h. instinct. The urge to remain one of the social group and to conform to social patterns and general opinions. An aversion to excessive individualism.

hered′itary. Transmitted from one's ancestry, or by inheritance.
   h. ataxia. Hereditary spinal ataxia.* SYN: *Friedreich's ataxia.*

heredity (he-red′i-tĭ). Inborn qualities or capacities, either ascribed to parents, or to racial impulses *in toto.*

heredo-. Prefix: *heredity.*

heredoataxi′a. Hereditary spinal ataxia. SYN: *Friedreich's ataxia.*

heredoluetic (her″e-do-lŭ-et′ik). Rel. to hereditary syphilis.

her″edosyph′ilis. Syphilis acquired before birth.

her″edotuberculo′sis. Tuberculosis assumed to be inherited.

Her′ing's the′ory. Doctrine that the visual substance in retina represents disassimilation for white, red, and yellow, and restitution for black, green, and blue.

heritage (her′it-aj). All the characteristics transmitted by parents to their children.

Her′mann's fluid. A fluid used to harden tissues for microscopic study.

hermaphrodism (her-maf'ro-dizm). Existence in an individual of elements of both ovaries and testicles.

h., complex. Having internal and external organs of both sexes.

h., dimidiate; h., lateral. Having the organs of 1 side male and of the other female.

h., spurious. Of 1 sex but with the outward signs of the other sex.

h., transverse. Having the outward organs indicating 1 sex, and the internal ones the other.

h., true. Double sex.

h., unilateral. Having an ovary or a testicle on 1 side, and a doubling of sex characteristics on the other.

hermaphrodite (her-maf'ro-dīt). One possessing genital and sexual characteristics of both sexes. SYN: *androgyne.*

h., complex. One with both internal and external organs of both sexes.

h., dimidiate. One who is male on 1 side, female on the other.

h., spurious. One sex with appearance of the other.

h., transverse. One who is externally 1 sex, internally the other.

h., unilateral. One who has an ovary and testicle on 1 side and either on the other side.

hermaph'roditism. Double sex. SYN: *hermaphrodism.*

hermet'ic. Airtight.

hermetical (her-met'ik-al). Airtight.

hernia (her'ni-a). External projection of a part from its natural cavity.

h., abdominal. Hernia through the abdominal wall.

h., bladder. Protrusion of the bladder or a part of bladder through normal or abnormal orifice.

h., cerebral. Of the brain through a cranial wound. [nia.

h., Cloquet's. A type of femoral hernia.

h., complete. Hernia in which sac and its contents have passed through the aperture.

h., concealed. Hernia that is imperceptible when palpated.

h., congenital. Hernia existing from birth.

h., crural. SEE: *femoral hernia.*

h., cystic. Bladder hernia. SYN: *cystocele.*

h., diaphragmatic. Hernia protruding through the diaphragm.

h., diverticular. Protrusion of intestinal congenital diverticulum.

h., encysted. Scrotal protrusion, which, enveloped in its own sac, passes into the tunica vaginalis.

h., femoral. Descending of intestines besides femoral vessels and through femoral ring.

h., funicular. Hernia into the umbilical or spermatic cord.

h., Holthouse's. SEE: *inguinocrural hernia.*

h., inguinal. Passing of intestines through inguinal canal. Occurs in 80% of cases of hernia.

h., inguinocrural. Hernia which is femoral and inguinal.

h., incarcerated. Hernia completely obstructing the bowels.

h., incomplete. Hernia which has not gone completely through the aperture.

h., irreducible. Hernia which cannot be returned to its original position out of its sac by manual methods.

h., labial. Protrusion of a loop of bowel into the labium majus.

h., lumbar. In lumbar regions or loins.

h., mesocolic. Hernia bet. the layers of the mesocolon.

h., nuckian. Hernia into canal of Nuck.

h., obturator. Hernia through the obturator foramen.

h., omental. Hernia enveloping the omentum.

h., ovarian. Presence of an ovary in a hernial sac.

h., phrenic. Projecting through the diaphragm into 1 of the pleural cavities.

h., posterior vaginal. Hernia of Douglas' sac downward bet. rectum and post. vaginal wall. SYN: *enterocele.*

h., properitoneal. Protrusion through the peritoneum and into the abdominal wall.

h., reducible. Hernia which can be replaced by manipulation.

h., retroperitoneal. Hernia into peritoneal sac extending behind the peritoneum into the iliac fossa.

h., Richter's. Hernia with a portion of the lumen remaining open.

h., scrotal. One that descends into the scrotum.

h., strangulated. One so tightly constricted that gangrene results if operation does not relieve. Not reducible by ordinary means.

h., umbilical. Occurring at the navel. More frequent in women.

h., uterine. Presence of the uterus in the hernial sac. [vagina.

h., vaginal. Hernial protrusion of the

h., vaginolabial. Hernia of a viscus into the posterior end of the labium majus.

h., ventral. If stretching and thinning of an abdominal scar occur, pressure from the abdomen may cause protrusion of part of the gut. It is then protected only by a layer of thin scar tissue.

her'nial. Pert. to a hernia.

h. sac. The pouch of peritoneum pushed before a hernia and into which it descends.

her'niated. Having a hernia.

herniation (her-nĭ-a'shun). Development of a hernia.

her"nioenterot'omy. Herniotomy at same time as enterotomy.

her'nioid. Resembling a hernia.

herniolaparotomy (her"nĭ-o-lap-ă-rot'o-mĭ). Abdominal section for the cure of hernia.

herniol'ogy. The science of hernia.

her'nioplasty. Surgical operation for hernia.

her″niopunc′ture. Puncture of a hernia with hollow needle for withdrawal of fluid or gas.

herniorrhaphy (her-nǐ-or′ră-fǐ). Surgical operation for hernia.

herniotomy (her-nǐ-ot′o-mǐ). Cutting for hernia. Operation for strangulation (intestinal) and radical cure.

hero′ic. Pert. to treatment which, if not successful, increases danger.

heroin (her′o-in). A narcotic derived from morphine, commonly used by addicts.

he′roinism. Addiction to habitual use of heroin.

herpangina (her-pan′jǐ-nä). A disease of children marked by fever and small ulcers in the throat.

herpes (her′pez). 1. A form of vesicles appearing in clusters on inflammatory base but with no tendency to rupture; in *herpes zoster* they are distributed along the nerve trunks. 2. Inflammatory skin disease characterized by formation of groups of vesicles. SEE: *tetter, zona.*

  h. facialis. SEE: *herpes simplex.*

  h. febrilis. Fever sores on lips.

  h. genitalis. Herpetic lesions on the female genitalia.

  h. gestationis. Herpes of pregnancy.

  h. labialis. Fever blister, cold sore, herpes of the face.

  h. menstrualis. Herpetic lesions seen on the lips at the time of the menstrual period.

  h. praeputialis. Herpes of the male genitals.

  h. simplex. So-called fever blisters.

  h. zoster. Acute inflammatory disease of the skin.

herpet′ic. Pert. to herpes.

  h. neuralgia. Painful neurosis with herpes zoster.

  h. sore throat. Herpetic tonsillitis.

herpet′iform. Resembling herpes.

her′petism. Predisposition to herpetic eruption.

hersage (ār-sazh′). Splitting of a nerve trunk into separate fibers.

hertz′ian waves. Electromagnetic vibrations that have wave lengths of a centimeter or longer.

Hesselbach's hernia (hes′el-bakhs). A lobated hernia which passes through the cribriform fascia.

  H.'s triangle. The triangular space bounded by Poupart's ligament below, ext. border of rectus muscle internally, and epigastric artery ext.

heteradenia (het-er-ad-e′nǐ-ä). 1. Glandular substance in a part not provided with glands. 2. Abnormal glandular tissue.

heteradenic (het-er-ad-e′nǐk). Pert. to or consisting of heteradenia.

heteradenoma (het″er-ad-en-o′mä). A heteradenic tissue tumor; any hyaline cylindroma.

heterecious (het-er-e′shus). Living upon different hosts at different stages of development.

heterecism (hět″er-ē′sǐzm). Development

of different cycles of existence on different hosts, said of certain parasites.

heteresthesia (het-er-es-the′zǐ-ä). Variation in degree (plus or minus) of sensory response to cutaneous stimuli.

heteral′bumose. Albumose insoluble in water but soluble in saline solutions, in acid or alkaline solutions. SYN: *hemialbumose.*

heteroautoplasty (het″er-o-aw′to-plas-tǐ). Grafting skin from 1 person to another.

heteroblas′tic. Having origin in tissue of another kind. Opp. of homoblastic.

heterochromatosis (het″er-o-kro-ma-to′sis). 1. Pigmentation of skin from foreign substances. 2. Difference in color. SYN: *heterochromia.*

heterochromia (het-er-o-kro′mǐ-ä). A difference in color.

  h. iridis. Different color of iris in the 2 eyes; the lighter colored iris is atrophic due to previous iridocyclitis, congenital or otherwise.

het″erochrom′osome. Chromosome differing from the ordinary one.

heterochromous (het-er-ō-krō′mŭs). With abnormal difference in coloration.

heterochro′nia. Denoting an abnormal time for the occurrence of a phenomenon or production of a structure.

heterochron′ic. Occurring at different or at abnormal times.

heterochylia (het-er-o-ki′lǐ-ä). A change in character of the gastric juice without apparent cause.

heterocinesia (het-er-o-si-ne′sǐ-ä). Movements the reverse of those the patient is instructed to make.

heterocri′sis. Irregular crisis with abnormal symptoms.

heterocyclic (het-er-o-si′klǐk). Pert. to ring compounds which contain other atoms in addition to carbon atoms as part of the ring.

heteroder′mic. Pert. to a method of skin grafting when grafts are taken from another person. SEE: *dermatoheteroplasty.*

het′erodont. Having teeth of various shapes.

heteroecious (hět″er-ē′shŭs). Existing upon different hosts during different phases of development.

heteroecism (hět″er-ē′sǐzm). Existence during different phases of development upon different hosts, said of certain parasites.

heteroer′otism. Sexual desire for another person.

heterogeneous (het-er-o-je′ne-us). Of unlike natures.

heterogen′esis. 1. Production of children unlike the parents. 2. Spontaneous generation.

heterogenet′ic. Rel. to heterogenesis.

heterogenous (het-er-oj′e-nŭs). Differing in nature or kind.

  h. vaccine. That made from some source other than patient's own organism. Opp. of *autogenous.*

het′erograft. A graft taken from another individual or an animal of a different

species than the one for whom it is intended. SEE: *autograft, isograft.*

heterog′raphy. Writing different words from those the writer intended.

heteroinfec′tion. Infection by virus not within the organism.

het″eroinocula′tion. Inoculation from other organisms.

heterola′lia. The use of meaningless words instead of those intended.

heterol′ogous. Made up of cell tissue not normal to the part, as certain new growths.

heterol′ogy. Difference from the normal in structure or method of growth.

heterolysin (het-er-ol′is-in). Lysins formed from an antigen from an animal of a different species. SEE: *autolysin, hemolysin.*

heterolysis (het-er-ol′is-is). Hemolytic action of blood serum of an animal upon corpuscles of another species. SEE: *isolysis.*

heteromeric (het-er-o-mer′ik). 1. Pert. to spinal neurons with processes to opposite side of cord. 2. Possessing a different chemical composition.

heterometaplasia (het″er-o-met-ă-pla′zĭ-ă). Transformation of tissue to a tissue foreign to the part where produced.

heteromorphous (het-er-o-mor′fus). Deviating from the normal type.

heteronomous (het-er-on′o-mus). Abnormal; differing from type.

heteronymous (het-er-on′ĭ-mus). 1. Expressed in or having different names. 2. On opposite sides.

    h. diplopia. Having a false image on same side as the sound eye.

heteroös′teoplasty. Grafting of bone, esp. with a graft from an animal.

heteropathy (het-er-op′ă-thĭ). 1. Abnormal reaction to irritation or to stimuli. 2. Creation of a morbid condition to neutralize another disorder.

heterophany (het-er-of′ă-nĭ). Having different expressions of the same disorder.

heterophasia (het-er-o-fa′zĭ-ă). Expression of meaningless words instead of those intended. SYN: *heterolalia, heterophemy.*

heterophe′mia, heteroph′emy. Expressing 1 thing when another is intended. SYN: *heterolalia, heterophasia.*

heterophil(e (het′er-o-fĭl). 1. Pert. to an antibody reacting with other than the specific antigen. 2. Pert. to a tissue or microörganism that takes a stain other than the ordinary one.

heterophonia (het-e-ro-fo′nĭ-ă). Change of voice.

heterophoralgia (het-er-o-for-al′jĭ-ă). Deviation of 1 eye accompanied by pain.

heteropho′ria. Extraocular muscle insufficiency. Muscle imbalance.

heterophthalmos (het-er-of-thal′mus). Difference in appearance of the eyes due to the irides differing in color. SEE: *heterochromia.*

heteroplasia (het-er-o-pla′sĭ-ă). Production of a part where it does not belong.

heteroplastic (het-er-o-plas′tĭk). Rel. to heteroplasia.

het′eroplasty. Grafting with tissue from another person or an animal.

heteropsia (het-er-op′sĭ-ă). Incquality of vision in the 2 eyes.

heteros′copy. Finding range of vision in strabismus.

heteroserotherapy (het-er-o-se-ro-ther′ă-pĭ). Treatment by serum from another person.

heterosex′ual. Having normal attraction for the opposite sex. SEE: *homosexual.*

het″erosexual′ity. The normal state of love for one of the opposite sex.

heterotax′ia. Abnormal position of organs or parts.

heteroto′pia. Displacement of an organ or part.

heterotop′ic. Misplaced; pert to heterotopia.

heterotopous (het-er-ot′o-pus). Pert. esp. to teratomata consisting of tissues out of normal placement.

heterotopy (het-er-ot′o-pĭ). Displacement of an organ or a portion of the body.

heterotox′in. A toxin introduced from without the patient's body.

heterotrans′plant. A transplant of tissue from another individual of different species.

heterotrichosis (het″er-o-tri-ko′sis). Growth of different kinds or color of hairs on the scalp, or body.

heterotro′pia. Manifest deviation of the eyes due to absence of binocular equilibrium. SEE: *strabismus.*

heterovac′cine. A vaccine from a source other than that of the disease for which it is intended.

heteroxanthine (het″er-o-zan′thin). Methyl xanthine found in the urine.

hettocyrtosis (het-o-sir-to′sis). A slight curvature of the spine.

Heubleim method (hoyb′lĭn). Low voltage doses of x-ray given over the entire body for cancer.

Heubner's disease (hoib′ners). Syphilitic endarteritis of the brain.

heurteloup (hert-loo′). An artificial leech; a cupping apparatus.

hexa-. Prefix: *Six.*

hexaba′sic. Having 6 replaceable hydrogen atoms.

hexachro′mic. Not being able to distinguish more than 6 of the 7 colors of the spectrum or to distinguish violet from indigo.

hexad (heks′ad). The atom of an element having a quantivalence of 6.

hexatomic (heks-ă-tom′ĭk). Consisting of 6 replaceable atoms.

hexavac′cine. A vaccine made from 6 different microörganisms.

hexavalent (heks″ă-vā′lĕnt). Capable of combining with 6 atoms of hydroxyl or its equivalent. SYN: *sexivalent.*

hex′one, or **hex′one base.** One of the amino acids, as histidine, arginine and lysine, so called because they contain chains of 6 carbon atoms.

hexon′ic. Rel. to hexone bases.

hex'oses. Monosaccharoses* of the general formula $C_6H_{12}O_6$; the group includes particularly *dextrose* and *levulose*, *q.v.*

hexosephosphate (hex-ŏs-fos'fāt). A substance that is converted into lactic and phosphoric acid during contraction of muscle.

hexyl-chloro-m-cresol (hĕks″ĭl-klō″rō-m-krĕs'ŏl). New antiseptic effective against staphylococcus and *Streptococcus pyocyaneus*.

Hex'ylresor'cinol solu'tion. S.T. 37. SEE: *caprokol*.

Hey's lig'ament. Femoral ligament; a falciform expansion of the fascia lata.

Hg. SYMB: *mercury* (*hydrargyrum*).

HgCl₂. Mercuric chloride; corrosive sublimate.

Hg₂Cl₂. Mercurous chloride; calomel.

HgI₂. Mercuric iodide.

HgO. Mercuric oxide.

HgS. Mercuric sulfide.

HgSO₄. Mercuric sulfate.

hia'tus. 1. An opening, a foramen. 2. The vulva.

> **h. Fallopii.** Groove on petrous portion of temporal bone into which fallopian canal opens.

> **h. semilunaris.** The groove in the external wall of middle meatus of nasal fossa into which the antrum of Highmore, frontal series, and ant. ethmoid cells open.

hiccough, hiccup (hik'up). Spasmodic periodic closure of the glottis following spasmodic lowering of the diaphragm, causing a short, sharp, inspiratory cough. SYN: *singultus*.

> **h., chemical.** Occurring after a drink, due to irritation of the stomach walls.

> **h., epidemic.** Hiccough occurring in connection with mild febrile attack of nasopharyngeal catarrh simulating influenza, and also in association with epidemic encephalitis.

> **h., hysterical.** Due to minor causes or of a secondary nature.

> **h., irritative.** Other forms due to irritation in lungs or pleura near the diaphragm, the liver peritoneum, stomach, and parts below. May be due to a tumor or disease of brain in the section controlling the diaphragm and stomach, or to the prostate gland.

Hicks' (Braxton) sign. Uterine intermittent contractions at end of 3rd mo. of pregnancy, or in presence of tumor.

hide'bound disease'. Hardening and thickening of the skin with loss of elasticity. SYN: *scleroderma*.

hidradenitis (hi-drad-en-i'tis). Inflammation of sweat glands by staphylococcus, usually in the axillae.

hidradenoma (hi-drad-e-no'mă). Adenoma of the sweat glands.

hidroa (hi-dro'ă). 1. Vesicles due to retention of sweat. SYN: *sudamina*. 2. Any bullous eruption. SYN: *hydroa*.

hidrocystoma (hi-dro-sis-to'mă). A cystic tumor of a sweat gland.

hidropoiesis (hi-dro-poy-e'sis). The development of sweat.

hidropoiet'ic. Pert. to hydropoiesis. SYN: *sudorific*.

hidrorrhea (hi-dro-re'ă). Abnormal sweating.

hidrosadenitis (hi-dros-ad-en-i'tis). Inflammation of sweat glands. SYN: *hidradenitis*.

hidroschesis (hi-dros'kes-is). Retention of perspiration.

hidrosis (hi-dro'sis). 1. Formation and excretion of sweat. 2. Excessive sweating.

hieralgia (hi-er-al'ji-ă). Pain in the region of the sacrum.

high blood pressure. Abnormal pressure in arteries at height of pulse wave.

high Calory diet. One that provides maintenance and extra heat and energy. *Indicated*: 1. To prevent loss of weight. 2. In wasting diseases. 3. In high basal metabolism. 4. After long illness. 5. In deficiency caused by anorexia, poverty, poor dietary habits. 6. During lactation when 1000 to 1200 extra Cal. are indicated.

high cellulose diet. The general diet plus the following: *Breakfast*: Bran muffin or a tablespoon of bran added to a cereal, and extra large serving of fruit. *10 A.M.*: Fruit juice. *Dinner*: Salad, extra serving of vegetables, fruit. *Supper*: Salad, extra serving of vegetables and fruits.

high frequency treatment. High frequency current passed through the body to produce heat in the tissues.

High'more, antrum of. The air sinus in the maxillary bone. SEE: *antracele, antrum*.

> **H.'s body.** Fibrous tissue mass, a prolongation of albuginea testis, projecting forward along posterior border of testis. SYN: *mediastinum testis*.

highmori'tis. Inflammation of the maxillary sinus or antrum of Highmore. SYN: *antritis, sinusitis maxillaris*.

Hil'ton's law. The nerve trunk supplying a joint also activates the muscles moving the joint and the skin over the insertion of the muscles.

> **H.'s line.** A white one at junction of skin of perineum and anal mucosa.

> **H.'s muscle.** The compressor sacculi laryngis muscle.

> **H.'s sac.** Pit along external portion of false vocal cords. SYN: *sacculus laryngis*.

hi'lum, hi'lus. 1. Depression or recess at exit or entrance of duct into a gland, or of nerves and vessels into an organ. 2. The root of the lungs at level of 4th and 5th dorsal vertebrae.

himantosis (hi-man-to'sis). Abnormal lengthening of the uvula.

hind'brain. Those parts of embryonic brain which develops into the pons and cerebellum. SYN: *epencephalon, metencephalon*.

> **h. gut.** Embryonic endgut from which a large part of the ileum and colon is formed.

> **h. kidney.** The metanephros or primordial kidney.

hinge joint. An articulation that moves freely as that bet. the innominate bone and the femur. SYN: *diarthrosis,** *ginglymus.**   [syphilis.

Hin'ton's test. Agglutination test for

hip. 1. Upper part of thigh, formed by the femur and innominate bones. 2. The region on each side of the pelvis.

h. bone. *Os coxa* or *os innominatum.* Its 3 portions are: (a) The ilium (pl. *ilia*); (b) ischium (pl. *ischia*), and (c) pubis (pl. *pubes*).

h., dislocation of. Dislocations of the hip are very often accompanied by a fracture and it is extremely difficult even for a well-trained surgeon to distinguish a pure dislocation from a fracture dislocation without an x-ray.

hip joint. Articulation bet. femur and innominate bone.

h. j., arthritis of. Usually occurring before age of 14 years. VARIETIES: Arthritic acetabulum, femoral. SYM: Divided into 3 stages, cardinal symptoms, wasting, spasm, lameness, pain, swelling, deformity. PROG: Influenced by circumstances. Tendency toward recovery. TREATMENT: Tonics, hygiene, mechanical and surgical treatment.

h. j. disease. May be: 1. Tubercular. 2. Pustular (pyogenic). 3. Fracture. 4. Congenital deformities. 5. Dislocation of. 6. Dystrophies of (internal glandular). 7. Perthe-Legge's of. SYM: *General:* 1. Early—pain, limp, muscle spasm. 2. Later—muscle wasting, swelling, deformity. TREATMENT: *General:* Build up patient's general health by: 1. Diets. 2. Fresh air and sunshine. 3. Tonics. *Specific:* Varies with disease. *General to all:* Put on spica plaster cast, surgery or mechanical manipulation.

hippocam'pal. Pert. to the hippocampus.

h. fissure. Fissure above the temporal lobe on mesial surface of cerebrum.

hippocam'pus, ma'jor. Elevation of floor of inf. horn of lat. ventricle of the brain, occupying nearly all of it.

h. minor. A white projection on mesial side of post. cornu of lateral ventricle.

Hippocrates (hĭ-pŏk'ră-tēz). Greek physician who is referred to as the "father of medicine."

hippocrat'ic fa'cies. The appearance of the face before impending death.

h. oath. Oath exacted of his students by Hippocrates in which they swore to revere him as they would a parent, prescribe for the good of the patient, give no deadly drug, perform no abortions, cut no stones, leaving that work to the stone cutter, act only for the welfare of the patient and keep his secrets, and also to keep themselves from intentional illdoing and seduction.

hip'pulin(e. An estrogenic substance, obtained from urine of pregnant mares.

hippu'ria. Large quantities of hippuric acid in the urine.

hippu'ric acid. An acid formed and excreated by the kidneys.

DOSAGE: 4-15 gr. (0.25-1.0 Gm.).

hippus (hip'us). Rhythmical and rapid dilatation and contraction of the pupils. Tremor of iris, spasmodic in character.

h., respiratory. Dilatation during inspiration, and contraction of pupil during expiration.

Hirschberg's reflex (hĭrsh'bĕrg). Adduction of foot when sole at base of great toe is irritated.

Hirschsprung's disease (hirsh'sprungs). Congenital hypertrophic dilatation of the colon.

hirsute (hĭr-sût'). Hairy.

hirsuties (hur-su'shĭ-ēz). Excessive growth of hair.   [that destroys leeches.

hirudicide (hi-ru'dis-īd). Any substance

hirudo (hi-ru'do). A blood-sucking aquatic worm; a leech.

His, bundle of. A bundle of muscles (*auriculoventricular*) helping to form the muscular tissue of the myocardium.*

histaffine (his'tă-fēn). 1. Having affinity for tissues. 2. A hypothetical substance in the blood serum assumed to fix certain constituents of normal and esp. pathological tissues.

histaminase (his-tam'ĭn-as). Substance inhibiting action of histamine.

histamine (his'ta-mēn). 1. A substance in the body found wherever tissues are damaged. Red flush of a burn is due to the local production of histamine; product of histidine catabolism.

2. An amine found in almost all animal tissues, and produced by the action of putrefactive bacteria; originally an ingredient found in ergot.

h. cataphoresis. Method of treating rheumatic afflictions in which histamine solution is applied to the skin by the positive pole of the galvanic current.

h. phosphate. USP. A chemically made product, which may be produced from citric acid by a lengthy process.

DOSAGE: From 1/120-1/30 gr. (0.0005-0.002 Gm.). 0.1% sol. *parent.*, 5 gr. (0.3 Gm.).

histamine'mia. Histamine in the blood.

histamin'ia. Shock induced by histamine in the body.

his'tase. An enzyme which digests tissue.

histen'zyme. An enzyme in renal tissues which splits up hippuric acid into benzoic acid and glycocol. SYN: *histozyme.*

histidine (his'tid-ēn). An amino acid. $C_6H_9N_3O_2$, obtained by hydrolysis from tissue proteins and necessary for tissue repair and growth.

his'tiocyte. A tissue cell. SYN: *histocyte.*

histiogenic (his-tĭ-o-jen'ĭk). Formed by the tissues. SYN: *histogenous.*

his'tioid. Resembling or composed of 1 of the body tissues. SYN: *histoid.*

his"tioir'sitative. Irritative to connective tissue.

histio'ma. A tissue tumor.

histo-. Prefix: *Relation to tissue.*

his'toblast. A tissue cell.

histochromatosis (his"to-kro-mă-to'sis). Name of disorders of reticuloendothelial system.

histoclas'tic. Decomposing tissue.

histocyte (his'to-sīt). A tissue cell. SYN: *histoblast.*

histocyto'sis. Histocytes in the blood in unusual numbers.

his"todiagno'sis. Diagnosis made from examination of the tissues.

histodial'ysis. Disintegration of tissue. SYN: *histolysis.*

histogenesis (his-to-jen'e-sis). Development into differentiated tissues of the germ layer; origin and development of tissue.

histogenetic (his-to-jen-et'ik). Pert. to histogenesis.

histogenous (his-toj'en-us). Made by the tissues.

histogram (his'to-gram). A graph showing frequency distributions.

histog'raphy. A written description of the tissues.

histohem'atin. A hemoglobin pigment in various tissues.

histohematogenous (his"to-hem-ă-toj'en-us). Arising from both the tissues and the blood.

histoid (his'toid). 1. Resembling one of the tissues. 2. Developed from a single tissue, as *fibroma.*

histokinesis (his-to-kin-e'sis). Movement through the tissues of the body.

histolog'ical. Pert. to microscopic tissue anatomy.

histol'ogy. Study of the microscopic structure of tissue.

   h., normal. Study of healthy tissue.

   h., pathologic. Study of diseased tissue. [tissues.]

histolysis (his-tol'is-is). Disintegration of

histolyt'ic. Pert. to histolysis.

histo'ma. A tumor composed of tissue. SYN: *histioma.*

his'ton(e. A class of simple proteins derived from cell nuclei which interferes with coagulation, yielding certain amino acids (the histone or hexone bases) as a result of hydrolysis.

histonec'tomy. Periarterial excision of parts of the sympathetic nerve.

histon'omy. The law governing development and structure of tissues.

histonu'ria. Excretion of histon in the urine seen in leukemia and certain fevers.

histopathol'ogy. Histology of diseased tissues.

histophysiol'ogy. Study of functions of cells and tissues.

histoplasmo'sis. A disease due to infection by *Histoplasma capsulatum.*

historeten'tion. Retention of substances in the tissues.

historrhexis (his-tor-rek'sis). Disintegration of tissue by a noninfectious agent.

histother'apy. Administration of animal tissues. SYN: *cytotherapy, organotherapy.*

histothrom'bin. A thrombin derived from connective tissue.

histotome (his'to-tōm). Instrument for cutting tissue for study of its minute structure. SYN: *microtome.*

histotomy (his-tot'o-mĭ). Dissection of organic tissue.

his'totribe. Instrument for crushing the tissues to stop bleeding.

histotrophic (his-to-trof'ik). Pert. to or favoring the formation of tissue.

histotrop'ic. Having attraction for tissue cells, as certain parasites, stains, or chemicals.

histozyme (his'to-zīm). A renal enzyme which converts hippuric acid into benzoic acid and glycocol, causing fermentation.

histrion'ic. Theatrical, dramatic.

   h. mania. Dramatic gestures, expressions, and speech in certain psychiatric states.

   h. spasm. Facial spasm, tics.

hives. Eruption of very itchy wheals, caused by an allergic substance or food. SYN: *nettle rash, urticaria, q.v.*

Hl. Abbr. for *latent hyperopia.*

Hm. Abbr. for *manifest hyperopia.*

HNO₂. Symb. for *nitrous acid.*

HNO₃. Symb. for *nitric acid.*

H₂O. Symb. for *water.*

H₂O₂. Symb. for *hydrogen peroxide.*

hoarse'ness. A rough quality of the voice.

hob'nail liv'er. One with irregular surface.

Hochsinger's sign (hŏk'zing-ers). 1. Indicanuria as a sign of tuberculosis in children. 2. Closure of fist in tetany caused by pressure on inner side of biceps muscle.

hodegetics (hod"e-jet'iks). Medical ethics and etiquete.

Hodgkin's disease (hoj'kins). A chronic, infectious disease producing enlargement of lymphoid tissue, spleen, and liver, and sometimes kidneys.

hodoneuromere (hod-o-nu'ro-mēr). Portion of the primitive trunk including neurons and processes.

Hoffman's anodyne (Hoff'man). A solution of ethereal oil and ether in alcohol.

   DOSAGE: Average, 60 ℳ (4 cc.).

hol'agogue. 1. A medicine hypothetically capable of expelling all diseases from the body. 2. Any radical remedy.

holarthritis (hol-ar-thri'tis). Inflammation of all or many joints. SYN: *polyarthritis.*

Hol'den's line. A wrinkle or indistinct furrow in the groin.

holergastic (hol'er-gas'tik). Pert. to major psychoses affecting the personality by great excitement, fits of depression, stupor, and confusional states.

hol'low-back. Ant. post. spinal curvature. SYN: *lordosis.*

Holm'gren's test. Matching colored skeins of yarn for testing color blindness.

holoblas'tic ova. Ova with segmentation of the entire yolk.

holocaine (hō'lo-kān). Brand of phenacaine.

   DOSAGE: Frequently used in 1% solutions.

holocrine (hol'o-krin). Pert. to a secretory gland or its secretions consisting of altered cells of the same gland. Opp. of *merocrine, q.v.*

holodiastol'ic. Rel. to the entire diastole.

holomastigote (ho-lo-mas'tĭ-gŏt). Having flagella all over the surface.

holorrhachischisis (hol-o-ră-kis'ki-sis). Complete spina bifida.

holoschisis (hol-os'kis-is). Simple cellular cleavage. SYN: *amitosis.*

holosystol'ic. Rel. to the entire systole.

holotetanus (hol-o-tet'an-us). General tetanus. SYN: *holotonia, q.v.*

holoto'nia. Muscular spasm of the entire body. SYN: *holotetanus.*

holoton'ic. Pert. to or affected by holotonia.

Holt'house's hernia. Inguinal hernia protruding along folds of the groin.

Holtz static machine. Machine for producing static electricity by induction.

Holzknecht unit (holts'knekt). Abbr. *H.* An x-ray unit of measurement; 1/5 the erythema dose.

homatropine hydrobromide (ho-ma'tropen). USP. The hydrobromide of a synthetic alkaloid.
    DOSAGE: As a mydriatic 1-2% aqueous solution.
    h. hydrochloride. USES: Same as homatropine hydrobromide. DOSAGE: 1% solution.

homax'ial. Having all axes alike, as a sphere.

homaxon'ic. Having all axes alike, as a sphere. SYN: *homaxial.*

homeo-. Prefix: Likeness or resemblance.

homeomorphous (ho-me-o-mor'fus). Of like shape but not of same composition.

hom"eoös'teoplasty. Grafting of a piece of bone like the one upon which it is grafted.

homeopathic (ho-me-o-path'ĭk). Pert. to homeopathy.

homeopathist (ho-me-op'ă-thist). One who practices homeopathy.

homeopathy (ho-me-op'ă-thĭ). School of medicine founded by Dr. S. C. F. Hahnemann which assumes that such agents cure disease, as in health produce similar symptoms, expressed by the phrase: *Similia similibus curatur,* or "Like cures like."

homeoplasia (ho-me-o-pla'zĭ-ă). Formation of new tissue similar to that already existing in a part.

homeoplas'tic. Rel. to or resembling the structure of adjacent parts.

homeostasis (ho-me-os'tă-sis). Equilibrium of fluid content, chemical reaction, and temperature.

homeostat'ic. Pert. to homeostasis.

homeotherapy (ho"me-o-ther'ă-pĭ). Treatment or prevention of disease with a substance similar but not identical with the active causative agent. Ex: *jennerian vaccination.*

homeothermal (ho-me-o-ther'mal). Pert. to maintaining even temperature, said of warm-blooded animals. SYN: *homothermal.*

homeotransplant (ho"me-o-trans'plant). Tissue from one individual transplanted into another.

homeotransplantation (ho"me-o-trans-

plan-ta'shun). Tissue transplantation from one to another of the same species.

homeotypical (ho"me-o-tip'ik-al). Of the usual or normal type.

homergy (hom'er-jĭ). Normal metabolism and its results.

homesickness. Abnormal desire to return home. SYN: *nostalgia.*

Home's lobe (hŏm). Median lobe of prostate gland which frequently hypertrophies in older men.

homicide (hom'i-sĭd). 1. Murder. 2. A murderer.

homiculture (hom'ĭ-kult-chur). Application of the laws of breeding to the human species. SYN: *eugenics, stirpiculture.*

homo-. Prefix: Likeness.

homoblastic (hō-mō-blăst'ĭk). Arising from the same type of tissue. SEE: *heteroblastic.*

homocen'tric. Having the same center.
    h. rays. Light rays from the same center.

homocerebrin (ho-mo-ser'e-brĭn). A substance from brain tissue resembling cerebrin.

homogeneous (ho-mo-je'ne-us). Uniform in structure, composition or nature.

homogenesis (ho-mo-jen'e-sis). Reproduction of offspring similar to the parents. Opp. of *heterogenesis.*

homogentis'ic acid. Alkaptone; an acid in the urine due to incomplete oxidation of tyrosine.

homogeny (ho-moj'en-ĭ). Reproduction of offspring similar to parents.

homoglandular (ho-mo-glan'du-lar). Rel. to the same gland.

homoiopodal (ho-moi-op'o-dal). With only 1 kind of process, as nerve cells.

homolat'eral. Pert. to or on the same side. SYN: *ipsilateral.**

homolog, homologue (ho'mo-log). 1. An organ or part common to a number of species. 2. One that corresponds to a part or organ in another animal.

homologous (ho-mol'o-gus). Pert. to a fundamental type; or series.
    h. series. Compounds with a similar chemical structure and properties, arranged in order of their molecular complexity, such as *methane* and *ethane.*
    h. tissues. Those identical in structure.
    h. vaccine. One from the microorganism infesting the patient. SYN: *autogenous vaccine.*

homology (ho-mol'o-jĭ). Similarity in function and origin.

homolysin (ho-mol'is-in). Lysin from injection of an antigen from an animal of same species. SYN: *hemolysin.* SEE: *heterolysin.*

homonomous (ho-mon'om-us). Having similar structure and form, as the fingers or toes.

homonymous (ho-mon'im-us). Having the same name.
    h. diplopia. Diplopia in which the image seen by the right eye is on the right side and *vice versa.*

homophil (ho′mo-fĭl). Pert. to an antibody reacting only with a specific antigen.

homoplas′tic. Having similar form and structure.

ho′moplasty. Repair by tissue similar to the one replaced.

homorgan′ic. Produced by the same organs.

homosex′ual. 1. An invert, one sexually attracted to another of the same sex. 2. Pert. to attraction to another of same sex.

    h. neurosis. Pert. to the paranoid form of psychosis.

ho‴mosexual′ity. A condition in which the libido is directed toward one of the same sex.

homostim′ulant. Stimulating the organ that an extract is derived from.

homother′mal. Continuously maintaining same heat, said of warm-blooded animals.   [tension.

homotonic (ho-mo-ton′ĭk). Of uniform

homotype (ho′mo-tĭp). One organ or part similar in form and function to another, as 1 of 2 paired parts or organs.

homotypic (ho-mo-tip′ĭk). Of the same form and type.

honorarium (hon-or-a′rĭ-um). A professional fee, esp. one that is a gift, or for which no charge has been made.

hook. A curved instrument.

    h., blunt. One used in extraction of fetus or in embryotomy.

hook-up. Term used in speaking of the method of arranging circuits, appliances, and electrodes in the giving of any particular treatment; as, for instance, the hook-up for direct sparks.

hook′worm disease. A condition brought about by the presence of the hookworm in the intestinal tract. SYN: *ankylostoma, uncinariasis.*

hoop′ing cough. An acute, infectious disease characterized by a catarrhal stage, followed by a peculiar paroxysmal cough, ending in a prolonged crowing or whooping inspiration. SEE: *pertussis, whooping cough.*

hordeolum (hor-de′o-lum). Inflammation of a sebaceous gland of the eyelid. SYN: *sty, q.v.*

    h. internum. Suppuration of Zeiss or meibomian glands.

horismascope (hor-iz′mă-skōp). A U-shaped tube for an acid test for albumin in the urine.

horizocardia (ho-ri″zo-kar′dĭ-ă). Horizontal position of the heart on the diaphragm.

horizon′tal posi′tion. Lying supine with feet extended. Employed in palpation and auscultation of fetal heartbeat and in operative procedures.

    h. p., abdominal. The patient lies flat on the abdomen with feet extended. Employed in examination of back and spinal column.

hor′mion. Junction of post. border of the vomer with the sphenoid bone.

hormo′nagogue. That which increases the production of hormones.

hor′monal. 1. Rel. to or acting as a hormone. 2. Intestinal peristaltic stimulant

hor′mone. 1. A chemical substance originating in an organ, gland, or part, which is conveyed through the blood to another part of the body, stimulating it to increased functional activity, and increased secretion.

    2. The secretion of the ductless glands, such as insulin, by the pancreas.

    h., adrenotropic. Hormone regulating function of the adrenals.   [*mone.*

    h., Allen-Doisy. SEE: *estrogenic hor-*

    h., A. P. L. Ant. pituitary hormone seen in urine and placenta of pregnant women.

    h., Aschheim-Zondek. Ant. pituitary hormone found in urine, which ripens ovarian follicles and forms corpora lutea.

    h., bleeding. Ant. pituitary hormone which supposedly causes uterine bleeding.

    h., capillary. Pressor constituent of post. pituitary which is regulator bet. blood and tissues.

    h., cardiac. Hormone found in the heart muscle which causes dilation of the arteries.

    h., chromaffin. Constituent of medulla of adrenals which slows up heart rate, increases blood pressure and increases urinary sugar output. SEE: *epinephrine.*

    h., chromatophorotropic. Intermedin, *q.v.*

    h′s., circulatory. Term for muscle and tissue constituents which function as vasodepressors and vasodilators.

    h., diabetogenic. Hormone antagonistic to insulin.

    h., estrogenic. Estrin, *q.v.*

    h., follicle; h., follicular. Estrin.

    h., gametokinetic. Hormone stimulating follicles.

    h., gonadotropic. Ant. pituitary hormone affecting the gonads.

    h., growth. Ant. pituitary hormone promoting normal growth.

    h. hunger. A condition resulting from failure of an organ or part to receive enough of a special hormone necessary for its functioning.

    h., inhibitory. Hormonal substance which inhibits the functioning of a hormone. SYN: *antihormone.*

    h., ketogenic. Hormone regulating fat storage.

    h., lactation. Ant. pituitary hormone supposed to be the regulator of lactation.

    h., langerhansian. Pancreatic internal secretion supposed to aid sugar metabolism.

    h., luteal. Progestin, *q.v.*

    h., luteinizing. Prolan B.

    h., mammary. Mammin.

    h., metabolism. Prephyson.

    h., mucifying. Corpus luteum hormone affecting the vaginal mucosa.

    h., orchidic. Androsterone.

    h., ovarian. Estrin.

    h., parathyroid. Hormone obtained from cattle which is used to treat tetany.

h., placental. Any placental hormone.

h., progestional. Progestin.

h., sex, female. Estrin, q.v.

h., s., male. Hormone controlling changes at puberty. SYN: *androsterone.**

h., sinus. Hormone from a frog's heart which is used in regulating the heart.

h., Swingle and Pfiffner's. Cortin.

h., sympathetic. Epinephrine.

h., thyrotropic. Ant. pituitary hormone stimulating the thyroid gland.

h., wound. Traumatin.

hormon′ic. Rel. to or acting as a hormone. SYN: *hormonal.*

hormonogenesis (hor″mon-o-jen′e-sis). Production of an internal secretion. SYN: *hormonopoiesis.*

hormonogenic (hor″mon-o-jen′ik). Producing hormones. SYN: *hormonopoietic.*

hormonol′ogy. The study of hormones.

hormonopoiesis (hor″mo-no-poy-e′sis). The production of hormones or internal secretions.

hormonopoietic (hor-mo-no-poy-et′ik). Pert. to the internal secretions and their production.

hormopoiesis (hor-mo-poi-e′sis). The production of hormones. SYN: *hormonopoiesis.*

hormopoietic (hor-mo-poi-et′ik). Rel. to hormones and their formation. SYN: *hormonopoietic.*

hormothyrin (hor-mo-thi′rin). An ant. pituitary hormone.

hor′motone. Thyroid, pituitary, pancreas, spleen, ovary, and testes extracts in combination given for neurasthenia.

hor′mozone. A hypothetical substance in the body supposed to regulate its chemical processes.

Hor′ner's syndrome. Anidrosis, enophthalmos, miosis, and ptosis from paralysis of cervical sympathetic nerves.

hor′net sting. Sting by a hornet.

   A general urticaria may result from the sting of this insect.

hor′ny. Resembling or consisting of horn.

h. epithelium. The horny granulations in trachoma of the skin.

h. layer. Horny layer of the skin. SYN: *stratum corneum.*

horopter (hor-op′ter). Sum of all points in the binocular vision.

horripilation (hor-ĭ-pi-la′shun). Goose flesh. SYN: *cutis anserina.*

horse′shoe fis′tula. A fistulous tract in a semicircle in front or behind the anus.

h. kidney. A congenital abnormality. The 2 kidneys are united at their lower poles, forming a horseshoe mass generally at a lower level than normal.

hos′pital. Institution for treatment of the sick and wounded.

h., base. A hospital unit within the lines of an army for reception of wounded and patients from the front, as well as for cases within the line itself.

h., camp. An immobile military unit for care of sick and wounded in camp.

h., cottage. A collection of detached cottages for care of the sick.

h., evacuation. A mobile advance hospital unit to take the place of field hospitals and to supplement base hospitals.

h., field. A portable military hospital beyond the zone of conflict and beyond the dressing stations.

hos′pitalism. Morbid conditions due to lack of ventilation in a hospital.

host. The organism or part which sustains the life of a parasite. SEE: *cenosite.*

hot eye. Temporary eye congestion in gout.

Hot′tentot ap′ron. Excessive elongation of the labia minora seen in Hottentot women. SYN: *velamen vulvae.*

H. deformity. Abnormal fatness of the buttocks. SYN: *steatopygia.*

hot′tentotism. Abnormal form of stuttering.

hot water bag. Rubber bag of various shapes and sizes for applying dry heat to circumscribed areas and for keeping moist applications warm.

hot wire meter. A type of meter used to measure the amperage in high frequency circuits.

hourglass contrac′tion. Excessive, irregular contraction of an organ at its center, as the pregnant uterus during 3rd stage of labor.

h. stomach. Division of stomach (in form of an hourglass) by a muscular constriction; often associated with gastric ulcer.

house fly. An insect transmitting disease; *Anthomyia canicularis; Musca domestica.*

house′maid's knee. A traumatism resulting from kneeling which produces a swelling of the bursa, ant. to the patella.

house physician. The senior interne in a hospital responsible for the orders of the attending physician.

house staff. The internes and externes of a hospital acting under direction of the general staff.

house surgeon. The senior surgical member of the hospital staff who acts for the attending surgeon in his absence.

Houston's muscle (hūs′tonz). The ant. part of the *musculus bulbo-cavernosus.*

H.'s valves. The folds of mucous membrane or valves formed by them in rectum; supposed to keep feces from entering the anus too rapidly. SYN: *plica transversalis recti.*

How′ship's fove′olae or lacunae. Small pits on surface of bone beneath periosteum in process of resorption. SEE: *osteoclast.*

H.'s symptom. Paresthesia, or pain in obturator hernia, on inner side of thigh.

HPO₃. Metaphosphoric acid.

H₃PO₂. Hypophosphorous acid.

H₃PO₃. Orthophosphorous acid.

H₃PO₄. Orthophosphoric acid.

H₄P₂O₆. Hypophosphoric acid.

H. S. Abbr. for *house surgeon.*

H₂S. Hydrogen sulfide, sulfureted hydrogen.

H₂SO₃. Sulfurous acid.

H₂SO₄. Sulfuric acid.

Ht. Symb. for *total hyperopia.*

Hub'bard tank. One used for underwater exercises.

Hughes reflex (ūs). Sudden downward movement of penis when the prepuce or gland of a completely relaxed penis is pulled upward.

Húguier's canal (ü-ghe-a'). A canal through which the chorda tympani nerve exits from the cranium.

    H.'s circle. Anastomosis around the isthmus of the uterus.

    H.'s diseases. Lupus of vulva, and uterine fibroma.

    H.'s glands. Two tiny vaginal glands.

Huhner test. One for sterility in the male. SEE: *test.*

hum. A soft continuous sound.

    h., venous. Sound from large veins in certain anemias. SYN: *bruit de diable.*

hu'man. Pert. to or characterizing man or mankind.

    h. bite. Wound caused by human teeth.

hu'manol. Liquid human fat used to prevent adhesions in operations on tendons and nerves.

humeral (hu'mer-al). Pert. to the humerus.

humeroradial (hū″mer-o-ra'dĭ-ăl). Pert. to humerus and radius, esp. in comparison of their length.

humeroulnar (hu″mer-o-ul'năr). Pert. to the humerus and ulna, esp. in comparison of their length.

hu'merus. Upper bone of arm from the elbow (articulating with the ulna and radius) to the shoulder joint, where it articulates with the scapula.

hu'mid. Moist, damp.

    h. gangrene. Gangrene with serous exudation and rapid decomposition. SEE: *gangrene.*

humidifier (hu-mid′i-fi-er). Apparatus to increase moisture content of the air in a room.

humid'ity. Moisture in the atmosphere.

hu'mor. A body fluid. The 4 humors of medieval pathology were blood, phlegm, yellow bile, and black bile.

    h., a'queous. The fluid in the chamber of the eye.

    h., crystalline. The fluidlike substance of the crystalline lens of the eye.

    h., vit'reous. The fluid in the vitreous body of the eye.

hu'moral. Pert. to or depending upon the body fluids.

    h. reflex. Any physiologic response to action of a hormone.

humpback. Curvature of the spine. SYN: *kyphosis.*

hung'er. Want of food, as distinguished from *appetite,* the ability to enjoy food. During hunger there are periods of increased activity of the stomach.

    h., air. Dyspnea, breathlessness.

    h. contractions. Those observed, and often felt, in the normal empty stomach. They may be painful. A series of such contractions is followed by a period of rest, after which they may return with greater intensity unless food is taken. Digestion may be activated under such conditions.

    h. cure. Restricted diet or fasting for cure of disease. SYN: *nestiatria, nestitherapy.*

    h. day. One on which a diabetic is restricted to broth only.

    h., hormone. Deficiency of special hormone in an organ.

hunte'rian chancre. Indurated, syphilitic chancre. SEE: *chancre.*

Hun'ter's canal. *Canalis adductorius.*

    H.'s chancre. Hunterian chancre.

Huschke's canal (hoosh'kēz). One formed by juncture of the *annulus tympanicus* tubercules.

    H.'s foramen. Perforation found in arrested development near inner extremity of tympanic plate.

    H.'s teeth. Tiny, toothlike protuberances at edge of cochlear labium vestibulare.

    H.'s valve. Plica lacrimalis.

Hutchinson's patch (hŭtsh'ĭn-sŏn). Salmon-colored area in the cornea seen in syphilitic keratitis. SYN: *salmon patch.*

    H.'s teeth. A congenital condition; pegged, lateral incisors and notched central incisors along the cutting edge. A sign of congenital syphilis.

Hux'ley's layer. Inner layer of nucleated cells forming the inner root sheath of a hair follicle.

hyalin (hi'al-in). 1. A substance obtainable from the products of amyloid, colloid, or hyaloid degeneration. 2. Basement substance of hyaline cartilage.

hyaline (hi'al-en, hi'al-ĭn). Crystalline, glassy, translucent. SEE: *casts, degeneration.*

    h. bodies. Homogeneous substance; the result of colloid degeneration and found in degenerated cells.

    h. cartilage. The true cartilage. Smooth and pearly. It covers the articular surfaces of bones.

    h. casts. The commonest form of cast. They are transparent, pale, and homogeneous with rounded ends, and they indicate nephropathy.

hyalino'sis. Waxy or hyaline degeneration.

hyalinu'ria. Hyalin present in the urine.

hyalitis (hi-al-i'tis). Inflammation of the vitreous humor.

    h., asteroid. Spherical bodies in the vitreous.

    h. puncta'ta. A form marked by minute opacities in the vitreous humor.

    h. suppurati'va. A purulent inflammation of the vitreous humor.

hyalo-. Prefix: Transparent.

hyaloenchondroma (hī″a-lo-en-kon-dro'mă). A chondroma composed of hyaline cartilage.

hyalogen (hi-al'o-jen). A protein substance in cartilage and the vitreous humor.

hyaloid (hi'al-oid). Hyaline, glassy.

h. artery. Present in the fetus. Supplies nutrition to lens. Disappears in later months of gestation.

h. canal. Lymph channel in vitreous extending from optic disc to post. capsule of lens; contains hyaloid artery in fetus.   [the vitreous humor.

h. membrane. That which envelops

hyaloiditis (hi″al-oid-i′tis). Inflammation of the hyaloid membrane of the vitreous humor. SYN: *hyalitis.*

hyaloma (hi-al-o′mă). 1. Conversion of the eye into hyalin. 2. Colloid degeneration of the skin. SYN: *colloid milium.*

hyalomere (hi′al-o-mēr). Homogeneous part of a blood platelet, pale in color, as contrasted with the chromomere.

hyalomitome (hi″al-om′ĭ-tōm). Fluid portion of the protoplasm. SYN: *hyaloplasm, hyalotome.*

hyalomu′coid. Mucoid in the vitreous body.

hyalonuria (hi″al-o-nu′rĭ-ă). Hyaline bodies in the urine.

hyalonyxis (hi″al-o-niks′is). Puncture of the vitreous body.

hyalophagia (hi″al-o-fa′jĭ-ă). The eating of glass by the demented.

hyalophagy (hi-al-of′aj-ĭ). Eating of glass by the demented. SYN: *hyalophagia.*

hyalopho′bia. Fear of touching glass.

hyaloplasm (hi′al-o-plazm). The fluid portion of protoplasm. SYN: *hyalin, hyalonitome.*

   h., nuclear. Clear substance filling the meshes of the nuclear reticulum. SYN: *karyolymph, nuclear sap.*

hyaloserositis (hi″al-o-se-ro-si′tis). Inflammation of a serous membrane with fibrinous exudate undergoing hyaline transformation.

   h., progressive multiple. "Phthisis of serous membranes." SYN: *polyorrhomenitis.*

hyalosome (hi-al′o-sōm). A body resembling a nucleolus, but staining slightly with nuclear or plasmatic dyes.

hyalotome (hi-al′o-tōm). Fluid portion of protoplasm. SYN: *hyaloplasm, paramitome, paraplasm.*

hyclorite (hĭ-clō′rĭt). A concentrated solution containing not less than 3.85% available chlorine.

   DOSAGE: For irrigation of body cavities, from 1:2000 to 1:200 dilution; for irrigation of infected wounds, usually 1 part to 7 parts water.

hydan′toin. A colorless base, glycolyl urea, $C_3H_4N_2O_2$, from urea or allantoin.

hydatid (hi′da-tid). 1. A vesicle similar to an echinococcus cyst. 2. An echinococcus cyst. SEE: *liver.*

   h. fremi′tus. A tremulous sensation felt on palpating a hydatid tumor.

   h. mole. Degenerative process in chorionic villi, which gives rise to multiple cysts and rapid growth of uterus with hemorrhage.

   h. of Morgagni. Cystlike remnant of the mullerian duct which is attached to the fallopian tube.

   h., sessile. Morgagnian hydatid connected with a testicle.

   h., stalked. Morgagnian hydatid connected with a fallopian tube.

hydatidiform (hi-dat-id′if-orm). Having the form of a hydatid.

hydatidocele (hi-dat-id′o-sēl). Hydatid cyst of scrotum or testicle.

hydatido′ma. A tumor consisting of hydatids.

hydatidosis (hi-dat-ĭ-do′sis). Condition caused by infestation with hydatids.

hydatidostomy (hi-dat-id-os′to-mĭ). Evacuation of a hydatid cyst.

hydat′iform. Having the form of a hydatid.

hy′datism. The sound produced by fluid in a cavity.

hydradenitis (hi-drad-en-i′tis). Inflammation of a sweat gland.

hydradeno′ma. Tumor of a sweat gland.

hydraeroperitoneum (hi-dra-er-o-per-it-o-ne′um). Collection of fluid and gas in the peritoneal cavity.

hydragogue (hy′dra-gog). Drug promoting watery evacuation of the bowels.

hydramnion, hydramnios (hi-dram′nĭ-on, -os). An excess of liquor amnii which leads to overdistention of the uterus and the possibility of malpresentations.

hydrargyrum (hi-drar′jir-um). Mercury or quicksilver. SEE: *mercury.*

hydrarthrosis (hi-drar-thro′sis). Serous effusion in a joint cavity; white swelling.

hydrate (hi′drat). 1. The result of water passing into a cell, thereby causing it to swell or burst. 2. A crystalline substance formed by water combining with various compounds.

hydrated (hi′dra-ted). Combined chemically with water.

hydrazine (hi′draz-in). 1. A colorless gas, H_4N_2, with peculiar odor; soluble in water. 2. One of a class derived from hydrazine.

hydre′mia. Excess of watery fluid in the blood.

hydrencephalocele (hi-dren-sef′al-o-sēl). Watery tumor protruding from the brain.

hydrencephalus (hi-dren-sef′al-us). Accumulation of fluid in the cerebral ventricles or outside of the brain. SYN: *hydrocephalus.*

hydrepigastrium (hi-drep-ĭ-gas′trĭ-um). Accumulation of fluid bet. the peritoneum and the abdominal muscles.

hydriatics (hi-drĭ-at′ĭks). Application of water in treatment of disease. SYN: *hydrotherapeutics.*

hydriatric (hi-dri-at′rik). Pert. to treatment of disease with water, as hydriatric procedures or hydriatric institutions.

hydriat′rist. One who practices hydrotherapy.

hy′drid. Chemical compound containing hydrogen and an element or radical.

hydro-. Prefix: Water; also hydrogen.

hydro′a. Chronic inflammatory skin disease.

   SYN: *dermatitis herpetiformis, pemphigus pruriginosus.*

hydroappen′dix. Watery fluid distending the vermiform appendix.

hydrobilirubin (hi″dro-bil-Ĭ-ru′bĭn). A brownish red bile pigment perhaps identical with stercobilin and urobilin.

hydrobromate (hi-dro-bro′māt). A salt of hydrobromic acid.

hydrocar′bon. A compound made up of hydrogen and carbon. The hydrocarbons may be classified as: 1. The methane series. 2. Ethylene series. 3. Alcohols. 4. Oxidation products of an alcohol.

    h. sat′urated. One with no free valences because of the great number of hydrogen atoms contained.

hydrocele (hi′dro-sēl). Serous fluid in the tunica vaginalis testis, or serous tumors of the testes or their parts.

    h., congenital. SYM: Increased size of head, emaciation of body. Prominent eyes with downward glance, wrinkled face, weakness, inability to walk, feeble voice. [the canal of Nuck.

    h. muliebris. A watery distention of

hydrocenosis (hi-dro-sen-o′sis). Evacuation of a dropsical fluid by tapping or by a hydragogue. SYN: *paracentesis.*

hydrocephal′ic. Pert. to hydrocephalus.

hydrocephalocele (hi-dro-sef′al-o-sēl). Watery hernia of the brain. SYN: *hydrencephalocele.*

hydroceph′aloid. Resembling or pert. to hydrocephalus.

    h. disease. One of infants similar to hydrocephalus.

hydrocephalus (hi-dro-sef′a-lus). Collection of serous fluid in the head. Dropsy of the brain.

hydrochlorate (hi-dro-klo′rāt). Any salt of hydrochloric acid.

hy″drochlo′ric acid (HCl). A normal acid in the gastric juice, amounting to 0.4 to 0.5%.

hydrocholecystis (hi-dro-ko-le-sis′tis). Dropsy of gallbladder.

hydrocirsocele (hi-dro-sir′so-sēl). Hydrocele with varicose veins of spermatic cord.

hydrocollidine (hi-dro-kol′id-ēn). A poisonous ptomaine from putrefying fish or animal flesh.

hydrocolpos (hi-dro-kol′pos). Retention cyst of the vagina containing watery, nonsanguineous fluid, or mucus.

hydroconion (hi-dro-ko′nĬ-on). An atomizer.

hydrocra′nia. Water on the brain. SYN: *hydrocephalus.*

hy′drocyst. A cyst containing watery fluid.

hydrocysto′ma. Disease marked by small hydrocysts. Sudamina on the face, esp. in women after middle age. SYN: *hidrocystoma.*

hydrodiascope (hi-dro-di′ā-skōp). Device to correct astigmatism.

hydrodictiotomy (hi″dro-dik-ti-ot′o-mĬ). Incision of retina for edema.

hydroelec′tric bath. Administration of an electrically charged bath.

hydroencephalocele (hi″dro-en-sef′al-o-sēl). Brain substance expanded into a watery sac protruding through a cleft in the cranium. SYN: *hydrencephalocele.*

hy′drogel. A colloid containing water that solidifies in gelatinous form.

hy′drogen (H). An element found chiefly in water.

hy′drogenate. To bring about a combination with hydrogen.

hydrogenation (hi-dro-jen-a′shun). A process of changing an unsaturated fat to a solid, saturated fat by the addition of hydrogen in the presence of a catalyst, as olein and stearin.

hydrogen dioxide (di-oks′ĭd). H_2O_2. USP. Used in form of 3% aqueous solution.

hydrogen ion or pH scale. A means of indicating accurately any degree of acidity or alkalinity.

    h. i. concentration. The pH value is the negative logarithm of the hydrogen ion concentration of the solution, expressed in gram ions for each liter.

hydrogen peroxide. An antiseptic and cleansing agent. SYN: *hydrogen dioxide, q.v.*

    h. p., solution of. The action kills bacteria because of its oxidizing power.

hydroglossa (hi-dro-glos′ă). Cystic tumor beneath the tongue. SYN: *ranula.*

hydrogymna′sium. Pool for underwater exercises.

hydrogymnas′tics. Underwater exercises.

hydrohematonephrosis (hi″dro-hem″at-o-nef-ro′sis). Blood and urine in pelvis of the kidney.

hydrohepatosis (hi″dro-hep-at-o′sis). Accumulation of fluid in the liver.

hydrohymenitis (hi″dro-hi-men-i′tis). Any inflammation of a serous membrane.

hydrokinet′ics. Science of fluids in motion.

hydrolase (hi′dro-lās). An enzyme that causes hydrolysis. SYN: *hydrolyst.*

hydrology (hi-drol′o-jĬ). The science of treatment of disease by water.

hydrolysis (hi-drol′Ĭ-sis). Combination of water with a salt to produce an acid and a base, one of which is more dissociated than the other. The reverse of neutralization.

hydrolyst (hi′drol-ist). A ferment that produces hydrolysis.

hydrolyt′ic. Rel. to hydrolysis.

hydroma (hi-dro′mă). A collection of serous fluid in a cyst.

hydromel (hi′dro-mel). Mixture of honey and water.

hydromeningitis (hi-dro-men-in-ji′tis). 1. Inflammation of membranes of brain with serous effusion. 2. Inflammation of Descemet's membrane.

hydromeningocele (hi″dro-men-in′go-sēl). Protrusion of meninges or spinal cord in a sac of fluid.

hydrom′eter. An instrument which measures the density of a liquid by the depth to which a graduated scale sinks into the liquid.

hydrometra (hi-dro-me′tră). Collection of watery fluid or mucus in the uterus.

hydromphalus (hi-drom′fal-us). Watery tumor at the umbilicus.

hydromyelia (hi″dro-mi-e′lĬ-ă). Increased fluid in central canal of spinal cord. SYN: *hydrorrhachis.*

hydromyelocele (hi-dro-mi'el-o-sēl). Protrusion of sac with cerebrospinal fluid through a spina bifida.

hydromyoma (hi-dro-mi-o'mǎ). Cystic fibroid, usually uterine, filled with fluid.

hydronephrosis (hi''dro-nef-ro'sis). Collection of urine in the kidney pelvis owing to obstructed outflow, forming a cyst by production of distention and atrophy of organ.

hydroparasalpinx (hi''dro-par-ǎ-sal'pinks). Accumulation of serous fluid in the accessory tubes of the fallopian tube.

hydroparoti'tis. Accumulation of fluid in the parotid gland.

hydropath'ic. Rel. to hydropathy.

hydropathy (hi-drop'a-thǐ). A term now used to denote the empirical application of water in the treatment of disease. SEE: *hydrotherapy.*

hydropericardi'tis. Serous effusion accompanying pericarditis.

hydropericardium (hi''dro-per-ǐ-kar'dǐum). Pericardial dropsy. Accumulation of water in pericardial sac without inflammation.

hydroperinephrosis (hi''dro-per-ǐ-ne-fro'-sis). Accumulation of serum of connective tissue surrounding the kidney.

hydroperion (hi-dro-per'ǐ-on). Fluid supposedly present bet. decidua reflexa and decidua vera.

hydroperitone'um. Accumulation of fluid in peritoneal cavity. SYN: *ascites.*

hydrophilous (hi-drof'ǐl-ŭs). Taking up moisture. SYN: *bibulous.*

hydrophobia (hi-dro-fo'bǐ-ǎ). Disease due to bite of a rabid dog. SYN: *lyssa.* SEE: *rabies.*

hydrophthalmos (hi-drof-thal'mos). Congenital glaucoma, enlarged eyeball. SYN: *buphthalmos.*

hydrophysometra (hi''dro-fi-so-me'trǎ). Presence of water and gas in the uterus.

hydrop'ic. Dropsical or pert. to dropsy.

hydropigenous (hi-dro-pij'en-us). Producing dropsy.   [plasm.

hydroplas'ma. The fluid part of protoplasm.

hydropneumatosis (hi''dro-nu-mǎ-to'sis). Liquid and gas in the tissues producing combined edema and emphysema.

hydropneumogony (hǐ-dro-nu-mog'ŏ-nǐ). Diagnosis of joint effusion by injecting air in joint.

hydropneumopericardium (hǐ-dro-nu''mo-per-ǐ-kar'dǐ-um). Serous effusion with gas in the pericardium.

hydropneumoperitoneum (hi''dro-nu''mo-per-ǐ-to-ne'um). Gas and serous fluid in the peritoneal cavity.

hydropneumothorax (hi''dro-nu''mo-tho'raks). Gas and serous effusion in pleural cavity. SYN: *pneumohydrothorax.*

hy'drops, hydrop'sy. Dropsy.
    h. tubae. Collection of fluid in an oviduct.
    h. t. profluens. A hydrops of the tube in which the distention becomes so great that the tube is forced to empty itself by the pressure, the emptying taking place *via* the uterine cavity. SYN: *intermittent hydrosalpinx.*

    h. vesi'cae fel'leae. Fluid in the gallbladder causing distention.

hydropyonephrosis (hi''dro-pi''o-nef-ro'sis). Dilatation of kidney pelvis with pus and urine.

hydrorheostat (hi-dro-re'o-stat). A rheostat with water resistance.

hydrorrhachis (hi-dro'rǎ-kis). Condition of increased cerebrospinal fluid bet. membranes and spinal cord or its central canal or cavities.

hydrorrhachitis (hi-dro-ra-ki'tis). Serous effusion from the spinal cord or its membranes with inflammation of the cord.

hydrorrhea (hi-dror-re'ǎ). 1. Copious watery discharge from any part. 2. Nasal, watery discharge from the nose.
    h. gravidarum. A condition during early months of pregnancy in which there is an excessive amount of fluid produced by the fetus.

hydrosalpinx (hi-dro-sal'pinks). Distention of fallopian tube by clear fluid. Watery discharge in gushes from the uterus and vagina.
    h., intermittent. A discharge of watery fluid from the oviduct. SYN: *hydrops tubae profluens.*

hydrosarcocele (hi-dro-sar'ko-sēl). Hydrocele with chronic swelling of testis.

hydroscheocele (hi-dros'ke-o-sēl). Dropsy of the scrotum.

hy'droscope. Device for inspection of water.

hydrosphygmograph (hi-dro-sfig'mo-grǎf). A sphygmograph with indicator consisting of a column of water.

hydro'sis. A wrong spelling of hidrosis.

hydrostat'ic. 1. Stagnated fluid. 2. Pert. to the pressure of liquids in equilibrium and that exerted on liquids.
    h. test. Putting lungs of a dead infant in water. If they float, the infant was born alive.

hydrostat'ics. Science of properties of fluids in equilibrium.

hydrosudotherapy (hi''dro-sū''do-ther'a-pǐ). Treatment of disease by sweating and hydrotherapy.

hydrosul'fosol. Substance for treating burns. Stimulates growth of new cells by laying down a thin, pliable coating over the burned areas. Reduces pain by excluding oxygen from the burned areas and speeding up healing.

hydrosyringomyelia (hǐ''dro-sir-in''go-mi-e'lǐ-ǎ). Distention of central canal of spinal cord with effusion of fluid and formation of cavities.

hydrotherapeu'tics. Treatment of disease with water. SYN: *hydrotherapy.*

hydrotherapist (hi-dro-ther'ǎ-pist). One who practices hydrotherapy.

hydrotherapy (hi-dro-ther'ǎ-pǐ). Scientific application of water in treatment of disease.

hydrothermostat (hi-dro-ther'mo-stat). Device for providing a continuous degree of heat.

hydrothioammonemia (hi''dro-thǐ''on-am-o-ne'mǐ-ǎ). Ammonium sulfide in the blood.

hydrothionemia (hi″dro-thi-on-e′mĭ-ă). Condition caused by hydrogen sulfide in the blood.

hydrothionuria (hi-dro-thi-on-u′rĭ-ă). Condition caused by hydrogen sulfide in the urine.

hydrothorax (hi-dro-tho′raks). Dropsy of the chest, or effused fluid in pleural cavity.

hydro′tis. Serous effusion in the internal ear or tympanum.

hydrotomy (hi-drot′o-mĭ). Dissection of tissue by forcible injection of water into the vessels.   [ear.

hydrotym′panum. Dropsy of the middle

hydroure′ter. Dropsy of the ureter.

hydrovarium (hi-dro-va′rĭ-um). Dropsy or cyst of the ovary.

hydroxide (hi-droks′ĭd). A basic radical combined with 1 or more hydroxyl groups.

hydroxy acids (hi-droks′ĭ). Acids containing 1 or more hydroxyl groups in addition to the carboxyl group, as *lactic acid*.

hydroxyethylapocupreine (hĭ-drok″sĭ-ĕth″-ĭl-a″pō-ku′pre-ĭn). Derivative of quinine effective in stopping growth of all types of pneumonia germs.

hydrozone (hi′dro-zōn). A bactericide of an aqueous solution of pure hydrogen dioxide.

hydruria (hi-dru′rĭ-ă). Increase of watery constituents of the urine with diminished solids in proportion. SYN: *polyuria*.

hygiene (hī′jēn). The study of health and observance of health rules.
  h., mental. Science of developing and maintaining mental health, preventing neurosis and mental unsoundness.
  h., oral. Scientific care of teeth and mouth.
  h., social. The prevention and treatment of venereal disease.

hygienic (hi-jĭ-en′ik). 1. Pert. to health or its preservation. 2. In a healthy condition.

hygien′ics. A system for promoting health.

hygienist (hi′ji-en-ĭst). A specialist in hygiene.
  h., dental. One trained in dental prophylaxis to assist a dentist.

hygienization (hī″jĕn-i-za′shun). The establishment of sanitary conditions and rules of hygiene.

hy′gric. Pert. to moisture.

hygro-. Prefix: Rel. to moisture.

hygrogogue (hi′gro-gog). A substance which has the property of absorbing moisture, *e. g.,* glycerine, when injected into the bowel, draws water from the tissues, thereby increasing the bulk in the rectum and so causes an action of the bowel. It is also applied to septic areas to draw fluid from tissues and so wash out toxins.

hygroma (hi-gro′mă) (pl. *hygromata*). A sac or bursa containing fluid.

hygroscopic (hi-gro-skop′ik). 1. Pert. to hygroscopy. 2. Absorbing moisture readily. SYN: *bibulous, hydrophilous.*

hygros′copy. Estimation of the quantity of moisture in the atmosphere.

hygrostomia (hi-gro-sto′mĭ-ă). Excess flow of saliva. SYN: *ptyalism, salivation.*

hyla (hi′lă). A lateral extension of the *aquaeductus cerebri.* SYN: *paraqueduct.*

hy′le. The primitive undifferentiated mass constituting all matter.

hy′lic. Pert. to matter or embryonic pulp tissues.

hylo′ma. A tumor composed of or in the hylic tissues, such as *hypohyloma,* and *mesohyloma.*

hymen (hi′men). A membranous fold wholly or partially occluding the vaginal orifice.
  h. annularis. Hymen with a ring-shaped opening in the center.
  h. biforis. One with 2 parallel openings with a thick septum between.
  h. cribriformis. One with many small perforations.
  h. denticulatis. One with an opening with serrated edges.
  h., fenestrated. Same as cribriform.
  h. imperforatus. A hymen with no opening in it.
  h., lunar. Hymen shaped like the moon.
  h., ruptured. Hymen that has been torn by coitus, injury, or operation.
  h. septus or **h., septate.** Hymen in which the opening is separated by a thin septum.
  h., unruptured. The normal hymen.

hymenal (hi′me-nal). Pert. to the hymen.

hymenectomy (hi-men-ek′to-mĭ). 1. Removal of a membrane. 2. Removal of the hymen.

hymenitis (hi-men-i′tis). Inflammation of the hymen or a membrane.

Hymenolepis (hi-men-ol′ep-is). A genus of tapeworm.
  H. nana. Tapeworm about an inch long found in human intestines.

hymenology (hi-men-ol′o-jĭ). Science of the membranes and their diseases.

hymenorrhaphy (hi-men-or′af-ĭ). Plastic operation on the hymen, occluding the vagina.

hymenotome (hi-men′ō-tōm). Knife used to divide membranes.

hymenotomy (hi-men-ot′o-mĭ). 1. Incision of the hymen. 2. Dissection of a membrane.

hyo-. Prefix: Connection with hyoid bone.

hyobasioglossus (hi″o-ba″sĭ-o-glos′us). The part of hyoglossal muscle attached to the hyoid bone. SYN: *basioglossus.*

hyoepiglottic (hi″o-ep-ĭ-glot′ik). Rel. to hyoid bone and epiglottis.

hyoepiglottidean (hi″o-ep-i-glot-id′ē-an). Rel. to hyoid bone and epiglottis. SYN: *hyoepiglottic.*

hyoglos′sal. 1. Pert. to the hyoglossus. 2. Extending to the tongue from the hyoid bone.

hy′oid. Bone at ant. surface of neck at root of the tongue, suspended from styloid processes by the stylohyoid ligament. SYN: *os hyoideum.* SEE: *basihyal.*
  h. arch. Second branchial arch.

hyopharyngeus (hi-o-far-in'je-us). Middle pharyngeal constrictor.

Hyoscyamus (hi-o-si'am-us). USP. Dried leaves of the plant *Hyoscyamus niger*.
DOSAGE: Tincture, 30 ♏ (2 cc.), and of the extract, from ½-2 gr. (0.03-0.13 Gm.).
POISONING: Related to atropine, *q.v.*
SYN: *henbane*.

hypacousia, hypacusia, hypacusis (hip-ă-koo'si-ă, -kŭ'si-ă, -sis). Impaired hearing.

hypalbuminosis (hip''al-bū-min-o'sis). Deficiency in proportion of albumin in blood.

hypalgesia (hi-pal-je'zĭ-ă). Lessened sensitivity to pain. SEE: *hyperalgesia*.

hypalgia (hi-pal'jĭ-ă). Lessened sensitivity to pain. SYN: *hypalgesia*.

hypamnios (hi-pam'nĭ-os). Deficiency in amt. of amniotic fluid.

hypanakinesis (hi-pan-a-kin-e'sis). Lowered rate of movement of stomach or intestines.

hypaxial (hi-paks'ĭ-al). Situated beneath the body axis.

hyper-. Prefix: Above, excessive, or beyond.

hyperacidaminuria (hi''per-as''id-am-in-ū'rĭ-ă). Presence of an excess of amino acids in the urine. SYN: *acidaminuria*.

hyperacid'ity. 1. An excess of acid. 2. An excess of acid in the stomach. SEE: *hyperchlorhydria*.

hyperacuity (hi-per-a-ku'ĭ-tĭ). Abnormal acuteness, as of vision.

hyperacusis (hi-per-a-ku'sis). Abnormal sensitivity to sound. Sometimes found in hysteria.

hyperadenosis (hi''per-ad-en-o'sis). Lymph gland enlargement. SEE: *Hodgkin's disease*.

hyperadiposis, hyperadiposity (hi-per-ad-i-po'sis, -pos'ĭ-tĭ). Excessive fatness.

hyperadrenalemia (hi''per-ad-re''nal-e'-mĭ-ă). Excess of adrenal secretion in the blood. [cretion.

hyperadre'nalism. Excess of adrenal se-

hyperadre'nia. Condition caused by abnormal activity of adrenal glands.

hyperalbuminosis (hi''per-al-bu-min-o'sis). Increased albumin in the blood.

hyperalgesia (hi-per-al-je'zĭ-ă). Excessive sensibility to pain; opp. of hypalgesia.

hyperalgia (hi-per-al'jĭ-ă). Excessive sensitivity to pain.

hyperanacinesia, hyperanacinesis (hi''per-an''ă-sin-e'si-ă, -sis). Unusual movement, as of the intestines or stomach.

hyperanakine'sis. Unusual mechanical activity, as of the stomach or intestines.

hyperaphia (hi-per-a'fĭ-ă). Excessive sensitiveness to touch.

hyperaphic (hi-per-af'ĭk). Marked by extreme sensitiveness to touch.

hyperazoturia (hi-per-az-ot-u'rĭ-ă). Excessive amt. of nitrogenous matter in the urine.

hyperbilirubinemia (hi''per-bil-ĭ-rū-bĭn-e'-mĭ-ă). Excessive amt. of bilirubin in the blood.

hyperblastosis (hi-per-blas-to'sis). Abnormal growth of a specific tissue.

hyperbrachycephaly (hi''per-brak-ĭ-sef'a-lĭ). Excessive degree of brachycephaly, having a cephalic index over 85.

hyperbu'lia. Morbid wilfulness.

hypercalcemia (hi-per-kal-se'mĭ-ă). An excessive amt. of calcium in the blood.

hypercalciuria (hĭ''pĕr-kăl-sĭ-ū'rĭ-ă). An excessive quantity of calcium in the urine.

hypercap'nia. Undue amt. of carbon dioxide in the blood.

hypercatharsis (hi-per-ka-thar'sis). Excessive bowel movement.

hypercementosis (hi''per-se-men-to'sis). Overgrowth of tooth cement (*cementum*).

hypercenesthesia (hi-per-sen-es-the'sĭ-ă). Exaggerated feeling of well-being.

hyperchloremia (hi-per-klor-e'mĭ-ă). Increase in chloride content of the blood.

hyperchlorhydria (hi-per-klor-hid'rĭ-ă). An excess of hydrochloric acid in the gastric secretion.

hyperchlorida'tion. A dosing with large amounts of sodium chloride.

hypercholestere'mia. Excess of cholesterol in the blood. SYN: *hypercholesterinemia*.

hypercholesterine'mia. Excess of cholesterol in the blood.

hypercholesterolemia (hi''per-ko-les''ter-ol-e'mĭ-ă). Excessive amt. of cholesterol in the blood.

hypercholesterolia (hi''per-ko-les''ter-o'-lĭ-ă). Excessive cholesterol in the bile.

hypercholia (hi-per-ko'lĭ-ă). Abnormal secretion of bile.

hyperchromasia (hi''per-kro-ma'sĭ-ă). Excessive pigmentation. SYN: *hyperchromatism*.

hyperchromatic (hi''per-kro-mat'ĭk). Overpigmented.
h. cell. One containing too many chromosomes.

hyperchro'matin. The azurophil part of the chromatin.

hyperchro'matism. 1. Excessive pigmentation. 2. Increased staining capacity of any structure. SYN: *hyperchromatosis*.

hyperchromatopsia (hi''per-kro-ma-top'-sĭ-ă). Defect of vision in which all objects appear colored.

hyperchromato'sis. Increased staining capacity.

hyperchromemia (hi''per-kro-me'mĭ-ă). Condition of a high color index of the blood.

hyperchromia (hi-per-kro'mĭ-ă). Excessive pigmentation. SYN: *hyperchromatism*.

hyperchromic (hĭ-pĕr-krōm'ĭk). Pert. to excessive pigmentation.

hyperchylia (hi-per-ki'lĭ-ă). Abnormal secretion of gastric juice.

hypercinesia (hi-per-sin-e'si-ă). Abnormal mobility.
h., professional. Occupational neurosis.

hypercrine (hi'per-krīn). Hyperfunction of an endocrine gland.

hypercrinia (hi-per-krin'ĭ-ă). Excessive activity of any endocrine gland. SYN: *hypercrinism*.

hypercri'nism. Condition due to excessive activity of any endocrine gland.

hypercryalgesia (hi-per-kri-al-je'sĭ-ă). Excessive allergy to cold. SYN: *hypercryesthesia.*

hypercryesthe'sia. Excessive allergy to cold. SYN: *hypercryalgesia.*

hypercyanosis (hi″per-si″an-o'sĭs). Extreme cyanosis.

hypercyanotic (hi-per-si-an-ot'ĭk). Denoting extreme cyanosis.

hypercyesis (hi-per-si-e'sĭs). Presence of more than 1 fetus in a uterus because of fertilization of a second ovum within a short time, at different menstrual periods. SYN: *superfetation.*

hypercythemia (hi-per-si-the'mĭ-ă). Condition of having an excessive number of red blood corpuscles.

hypercytosis (hi-per-si-to'sĭs). Abnormal increase in leukocytes in the blood. SYN: *hyperleukocytosis.*

hyperdactyl'ia. State of having supernumerary fingers or toes.

hyperdiastole (hi″per-di-as'to-le). Extreme cardiac diastole.

hyperdicrot'ic. Abnormally dicrotic.

hyperdistention (hi″per-dis-ten'shun). Excessive inflation.

hyperdiure'sis. Excessive urination. SYN: *polyuria.*

hyperdyna'mia. Muscular restlessness or extreme violence.

    h. uteri. Abnormal uterine contractions in labor.

hypereccrisia, hypereccrisis (hi-per-ek-kris'ĭ-ă, -ek'kris-is). Abnormal amt. of excretion.

hypereccritic, hyperecritic (hi-per-ek-rit'-ĭk). Pert. to an abnormal amt. of excretion or hypereccrisis.

hyperemesis (hi-per-em'e-sis). Excessive vomiting.

    h. gravidarum. One of the toxemias of early pregnancy characterized by excessive vomiting.

    h. lactentium. Vomiting in nursing infants.

hyperemia (hi-per-e'mĭ-ă). 1. Congestion. An unusual amount of blood in a part. 2. A form of macula; red areas on skin which disappear on pressure. 3. PT: Increase in the quantity of blood flowing through any part of the body; as undue redness of the skin, caused by the application of heat.

    h., active; h., arterial. Hyperemia caused by increased blood inflow.

    h., Bier's; h., constriction. Passive hyperemia* produced by application of an elastic bandage and by suction.

    h., leptomeningeal. Pia-arachnoid congestion.

    h., passive; h., venous. Hyperemia caused by decreased blood outflow.

hyperemization (hi″per-e-mi-za'shun). Hyperemia produced artificially for therapeutic purposes.

hypermotiv'ity. Excessive emotivity or response to stimuli.

hyperendocrin'ia. Pert. to hyperendocrinism.

hyperendocrinism (hi″per-en-dok'rĭ-nizm). Abnormal increase of internal secretion.

hyperendocrisia (hi″per-en-do-kris'ĭ-ă). Excessive increase of internal secretions. SYN: *hyperendocrinism.*

hypereosinophilia (hi″per-e″o-sin-o-fil'ĭ-ă). Excessive leukocytosis with increase of eosinophils.

hyperephidrosis (hi″per-ef-ĭ-dro'sis). Abnormal sweating.

hyperepinephrinia (hi″per-ep″ĭ-nef'rĭ-ă). Excessive adrenal secretion with arterial tension.

hyperepinephrine'mia. Undue proportion of adrenalin in the blood. SYN: *hyperadrenalemia.*

hy″perequilib'rium. A tendency to vertigo when turning.

hypererethism (hi-per-er'eth-izm). Excessive irritability.

hyperergasia (hi-per-er-ga'sĭ-ă). Unusual functional activity.

hyperergia (hi-per-er'jĭ-ă). Excessive or increased functional activity. SYN: *hyperergasia.*

hyperergy (hi'per-er-jĭ). Allergy to bacteria to a toxic degree.

hypererythrocythemia (hi″per-er-ith″ro-si-the'mĭ-ă). Excess of red corpuscles in the blood.

hyperesophoria (hi″per-es-o-fo'rĭ-ă). A tending of visual lines upward and inward. SYN: *heterophoria.*

hyperesthesia (hi″per-es-the'zĭ-ă). Unusual sensibility to sensory stimuli, such as pain or touch. SYN: *algesia.*

    h., acoustic; h., auditory. Abnormal sensitivity to sound.

    h., cerebral. Hyperesthesia caused by a cerebral lesion.

    h., gustatory. Oversensitivity of taste.

    h., muscular. Muscular sensitivity to pain and tiredness.

    h., optic. Abnormal sensitivity to light.

    h. sexualis. Abnormal increase in the sexual impulse.   [touch.

    h., tactile. Abnormal sensitivity of

hyperesthet'ic. Pert. to hyperesthesia.

hyperexophoria (hi″per-eks-o-fo'rĭ-ă). A tendency of visual lines upward and outward.

hyperextension (hi″per-eks-ten'shun). Extreme or abnormal extension.

hypergalactia (hi-per-gal-ak'shĭ-ă). Excessive milk secretion.

hypergenesis (hi-per-jen'es-is). Redundancy of organs or parts; overproduction. SYN: *hyperplasia.*

hypergenitalism (hi-per-jen'it-al-izm). Abnormal activity of the internal secretion of the genital glands, usually seen in precocious puberty and genital overdevelopment.

hypergeusesthesia, hypergeusia (hi″per-gu-ses-the'sĭ-ă, -gu'sĭ-ă). Excessive acuteness of sense of taste.

hyperglan'dular. Having excessive glandular secretions.

hyperglobu'lia. Having an excessive number of red blood corpuscles. SYN: *hypercythemia, polycythemia.*

yperglobulinemia (hi-per-glob-u-lĭn-e'-mĭ-ă). Excessive globulin in the blood.

yperglycemia (hi-per-gli-se'mĭ-ă). Increase of blood sugar from 0.15 to 0.2 or 0.3% or more, as in diabetes.
SEE: *hypoglycemia.*

yperglycistia (hi-per-glis-isʹtĭ-ă). Excess of glucose in the tissues.

yperglycogenolysis (hi-per-gli-ko-jen-ol'-is-is). Excessive conversion of glycogen into glucose by hydrolysis.

yperglycoplasmia (hi"per-gli"ko-plas'-mĭ-ă). Excessive sugar in the plasma of the blood.

yperglycorrhachia (hi"per-gli"ko-ra'kĭ-ă). Excess of sugar in the cerebrospinal fluid.

yperglycosemia (hi-per-gli-ko-se'mĭ-ă). Excessive sugar in the blood. SYN: *hyperglycemia.*

yperglycosuria (hi-per-gli-ko-su'rĭ-ă). Excessive sugar in the urine. SEE: *glycosuria.*

ypergnosis (hi'per-no-sis). All that is involved in projection of conflicts with the environment, evidenced in paranoia, *q.v.*

ypergonadism (hi-per-gon'ad-izm). Excessive internal secretion of the sexual glands.

yperguanidinemia (hi"per-gwan-ĭ-dēn-e'-mĭ-ă). Abnormal amt. of guanidine in blood.

yperhedonia, hyperhedonism (hi-per-he-do'nĭ-ă, -he'don-izm). 1. Abnormal pleasure in anything. 2. Abnormal sexual excitement.

yperhepatia (hi"per-he-pa'shĭ-ă). Overfunctioning of the liver.

y"perhidro'sis. Excessive sweating.

yperhor'monism. Excessive activity of the endocrine glands.

yperhydro'sis. Excessive sweating. SYN: *hyperidrosis.*

   h. oleosa. Increased and altered sebaceous secretion. SYN: *seborrhea.*

yperhypercytosis (hi"per-hi"per-sī-to'sis). Excessive increase of white blood corpuscles, esp. with increase of neutrophils.

yperhypocytosis (hi"per-hi"po-si-to'sis). Decrease of white corpuscles (leukopenia), esp. with relative increase of neutrophils.

yperidrosis (hi"per-id-ro'sis). Excessive sweating, symptomatic or idiopathic, acute or chronic, generalized or circumscribed.

yperinose'mia. Abnormal coagulability of the blood; excess of fibrinogen in the blood. SYN: *hyperinosis.*

yperino'sis. Excessive fibrinogen in the blood. SYN: *hyperinosemia.*

yperinsulinism (hi-per-in'su-lin-izm). Deficient amount of sugar in the blood.

yperinterrenopathy (hi"per-in-ter-ren-op'ă-thĭ). Any condition resulting from cortical overactivity of the suprarenal gland.

yperinvolution (hi-per-in-vo-lu'shun). 1. Reduction in size of uterus below normal after childbirth. 2. Reduction in

size below normal of any organ following hypertrophy. SYN: *superinvolution.*

   h. uteri. Extreme atrophy of the uterus seen following prolonged lactation or severe puerperal sepsis.

hyperisotonia (hi"per-i-so-to'nĭ-ă). Condition of greater degree of tension of muscles and arteries.

hyperisoton'ic. Noting 1 of 2 solutions having greater osmotic pressure. SYN: *hypertonic.*

hyperkeratomycosis (hi"per-ker"at-o-mi-ko'sis). Hypertrophy of horny layer of the epidermis due to a parasitic fungus.

hyperkerato'sis. 1. Overgrowth of cornea. 2. Overgrowth of the horny layer of the epidermis. SYN: *keratodermia, keratosis.*

   h. congenitalis. Hyperkeratosis in the harlequin fetus.

hyperkine'sia, hyperkine'sis. Excessive amt. of mobility. SYN: *hypercinesia.*

hyperlacta'tion. Excessive milk secretion. SYN: *superlactation.*

hyperleukocyto'sis. Excessive quantity of leukocytes. SYN: *leukocytosis.*

hyperlipemia (hi-per-lip-e'mĭ-ă). Fat droplets in the blood.

hyperlipo'sis. 1. Abnormal fat; adiposity. 2. Excessive fatty degeneration.

hyperlithuria (hi-per-lith-u'rĭ-ă). Excessive excretion of lithic (uric) acid in the urine.

hypermas'tia. 1. Excessively large mammary gland. 2. Presence of abnormal number of mammary glands. SYN: *polymastia, polymazia.*

hypermature (hi-per-mat-ūr'). Overmature; past maturity.

hypermegasoma (hi"per-meg-ă-sō'mă). Excessive bodily development. SYN: *gigantism.*

hypermenorrhea (hi-per-men-o-re'ă). 1. Too frequent menstrual periods. 2. Abnormal menstrual flow.

hypermetaplasia (hi-per-met-ă-pla'sĭ-ă). Overactivity in tissue replacement or transformation from one type of tissue to another, as cartilage to bone.

hyperme'tria. Unusual range of movement.

hypermetrope (hi-per'met'rŏp). One who is farsighted. SYN: *hyperope.*

hypermetro'pia. Farsightedness. Opp. of *myopia.* SYN: *hyperopia.*

hy"permetrop'ic. Pert. to farsightedness.

hypermnesia (hi-perm-ne'zĭ-ă). 1. Great ability to remember names, dates, and details. 2. An exaggeration of memory involving minute details of a past experience. It may occur in mentally unstable individuals after a shock.

hypermorph (hi'per-morf). One whose length of limb and consequent standing height is high in proportion to the sitting height. SEE: *hypomorph, mesomorph.*

hypermotil'ity. Unusual motility. SYN: *hyperkinesia.*

hypermyatrophy (hi"per-mi-at'ro-fĭ). Unusual wasting of muscle.

hypermyesthesia (hi"per-mi-es-the'sĭ-ă). Muscular sensitivity.

hypermyotonia (hi-per-mi-o-to'nĭ-ă). Excessive muscular tonus.

hypermyotrophy (hi-per-mi-ot'rō-fĭ). Abnormal muscular development.

hyperneocytosis (hi''per-ne''o-sī-to'sis). Abnormal increase of leukocytes in the blood (leukocytosis) including immature forms. SYN: hyperleukocytosis.

hypernephro'ma. Secondary or malignant tumor made up of adrenal tissue.

hyperneurotization (hi-per-nŭ-rot-i-za'-shun). Grafting of a motor nerve into a muscle to increase its energy.

hypernitremia (hi-per-nĭ-tre'mĭ-ă). Excess of nitrogen in the blood.

hypernoia (hi-per-noy'ă). Excessive mental activity or imagination. SYN: hyperpsychosis.

hypernor'mal. Abnormal.

hypernormocytosis (hi''per-nor''mo-sī-to'sis). An increased proportion of neutrophils in the blood.

hypernutri'tion. Supernutrition; overfeeding.

hyperontomorph (hi-per-on'to-morf). One with a tendency to hyperthyroidism.

hyperonychia (hi-per-o-nik'ĭ-ă). Overgrowth (hypertrophy) of the nails.

hyperope (hi'per-ōp). One who is far-sighted. SYN: hypermetrope.

hypero'pia. Farsightedness.
Parallel rays come to a focus behind the retina due to flattening of the globe of the eye, or to error in refraction. SYN: hypermetropia.

h., absolute. Hyperopia in which the eye cannot accommodate.

h., axial. Hyperopia caused by shortness of the eye's anteroposterior axis.

h., facultative. Hyperopia which can be corrected by accommodation.

h., latent. Hyperopia in which the error of refraction is overcome and disguised by ciliary muscle action.

h., manifest. Total amount of hyperopia which can be measured by a convex lens.

h., relative. Hyperopia in which vision is clear only when excessive convergence is made.

h., total. Complete hyperopia combining both latent and manifest types.

hyperorchidism (hi-per-or'kid-izm). Abnormal activity of testicular secretion.

hyperorexia (hi-per-o-reks'ĭ-ă). Abnormal hunger.

hyperorthocytosis (hi''per-or''tho-si-to'sis). Increased white blood cells with normal proportion of various forms and without immature forms.

hyperos'mia. Abnormal sensitiveness to odors.

hyperosto'sis. Abnormal growth of osseous tissue. SYN: exostosis.

hyperova'ria. Precocity of libido in young girls due to excessive ovarian secretion as the result of unusual and premature development of the ovaries.

hyperpancreatism (hi''per-pan'kre-ă-tizm). Abnormal activity of the pancreas with trypsin in excess of other ferments.

hyperparathyroidism (hi''per-par-a-thi'-roy-dizm). Condition due to increase of the parathyroid secretions.

hyperpep'sia. 1. Unusually rapid digestion. 2. Indigestion with hyperchlorhydria.

hyperpepsinia (hi''per-pep-sin'ĭ-ă). Excess of pepsin in the gastric secretion.

hyperperistalsis (hi''per-per-ĭ-stal'sis). Overactive peristalsis.

hyperphalangism (hi-per-fal'an-jizm). Having an extra phalanx on a finger or toe. SYN: polyphalangism.

hyperphasia (hi-per-fa'zĭ-ă). Loss of control of the organs of speech.

hyperphonesis (hi-per-fō-ne'sis). Increase in voice or percussion sound in auscultation.

hyperphonia (hi-per-fo'nĭ-ă). Stuttering or stammering due to excessive innervation of vocal muscles.

hyperphoria (hi-per-fo'rĭ-ă). Tendency of 1 eye to turn upward. SEE: anophoria.

hyperphosphatemia (hi-per-fos-fă-te'mĭ-ă). Abnormal amt. of phosphorus in the blood. SYN: hyperphospheremia.

hyperphosphaturia (hi''per-fos-fă-tū'rĭ-ă). Increased amt. of phosphates in the urine.

hyperphospheremia (hī''per-fos-fer-e'-mĭ-ă). Abnormal amt. of phosphorous compounds in the blood. SYN: hyperphosphatemia.

hyperphrenia (hi-per-fre'nĭ-ă). 1. Unusual intellectual activity. 2. Genius.

hyperpiesia, hyperpiesis (hi''per-pi-e'zĭ-ă, -sis). Abnormally high blood pressure.

hyperpietic (hi''per-pi-et'ik). Rel. to extremely high blood pressure.

hyperpinealism (hi-per-pin'e-al-izm). Excessive secretory activity of pineal gland.

hyperpituitarism (hi''per-pit-u'ĭ-tar-ism). Overactivity of the hypophysis cerebri or its ant. lobe.

hyperplasia (hi-per-pla'zĭ-ă). Rapid growth, abnormal increase of cells without formation of tumor, but with increase in size of an organ or part. SEE: hypertrophy.

h., fibrous. Connective tissue cell increase following any inflammation or in chronic visceral fibrosis.

h., lipoid. Increase in cells containing lipoid.

hyperplas'mia. 1. Abnormal increase within certain organs of leukocytes which do not appear in the blood. SYN: aleukemia. 2. Increase in size of red blood cells through absorption of fluids.

hyperplastic (hi-per-plas'tik). Rel. to hyperplasia.

hyperpnea (hi-perp-ne'a). An increased respiratory rate or breathing which is deeper than that seen in resting subjects. A certain degree of hyperpnea is normal after exercise.

hyperporo'sis. Excessive callous formation after a bone fracture.

hyperpragic (hi-per-pra'jĭk). Denoting excessive activity.

hyperprax'ia. Excessive activity.

hyperprochoresis (hi''per-pro-ko-re'sis). Unusually rapid passage of food through the alimentary tract due to increased peristalsis. SYN: *hyperperistalsis, hyperanacinesia, tormina nervosa.*

hyperprosexia (hi-per-pro-seks'ĭ-ă). PSY: Fixation of an idea to the exclusion of other ideas, as in compulsion states.

hyperproteinemia (hi″per-pro″te-in-e′mĭ-ă). Excess of protein in the blood plasma.

hy″perpro″teinu′ria. Excess of protein in the urine.

hyperproteosis (hi″per-pro-te-o′sis). A condition resulting from an excess of protein in the diet.

hyperpselaphesia (hi″perp-sel-af-e′zĭ-ă). Morbid sensitivity to touch.

hyperpsycho′sis. Overfunctioning of the mind.

hyperpyre′mia. Excess of heat and energy producing substances in the blood.

hyperpyretic (hi″per-pi-ret′ik). Pert. to high body temperature (hyperpyrexia).

hyperpyrexia (hi″per-pi-reks′ĭ-ă). Elevation of systemic temperature, above 106° F.

Produced by following physical agents: Baths, diathermy, radiofrequency current, hot air, radiant heat, electric blankets.

hyperpyrex′ial. Denoting high body temperature.

hyperreflex′ia. Increased action of the reflexes.

hyperres′onance. Increased resonance caused by percussion.

hypersecretion (hi-per-se-kre′shun). Abnormal amt. of secretion.

hy″persensibil′ity. Hypersensitivity of the body to a foreign protein or drug. SYN: *anaphylaxis, q.v.*

hypersensitiveness (hĭ″per-sĕn′sĭ-tĭv-nĕs). Excessive and abnormal susceptibility to the action of a given agent, as pollen or foreign protein. SEE: *allergy, anaphylaxis, hay fever.*

hypersensitiza′tion. An abnormally increased susceptibility to infection.

hypersialosis (hi-per-si-ă-lo′sis). Increased salivary secretion.

hyperskeocytosis (hi″per-ske″o-si-to′sis). Leukocytosis with many immature forms. SYN: *hyperneocytosis.*

hypersom′nia. A toxic condition conducive to sleeping an excessively long time.

hypersphyxia (hi-per-sfiks′ĭ-ă). High blood pressure with increased activity of the circulation.

hypersthe′nia. Abnormal strength or excessive tension, as in the insane.

hypersthen′ic. Denoting excessive strength, or tension.

hypersthenuria (hi″per-sthen-u′rĭ-ă). Dilute condition of the urine with elevation of the freezing point.

hy″persuscep″tibil′ity. Unusual susceptibility to a disease or to physical, esp. pathological, conditions. SEE: *allergic, allergy, anaphylactin, anaphylactogenic, anaphylaxis, anatoxic.*

hypersystole (hi-per-sis′to-lē). Unusual force or duration of the systole.*

hypersystol′ic. 1. Pert. to hypersystole. 2. Person with undue heart contractions.

hypertarachia (hi-per-tă-rak′ĭ-ă). Excessive irritability of the nervous system.

hypertelorism (hi-per-tel′or-izm). Abnormal width between 2 paired organs.

h., ocular. Abnormal width bet. the eyes.

hyperten′sion. 1. Tension or tonus above normal. 2. A condition in which patient has a higher blood pressure than normal for his age.

hyperten′sive. Marked by a rise in blood pressure.

h. diseases. Noninfectious ones with increased blood pressure.

hyperthe′lia. The presence of more than 2 nipples.

hyperthermalgesia (hi″per-therm-al-je′zhĭ-ă). Unusual sensitiveness to heat.

hyperthermia (hi-per-ther′mĭ-ă). Unusually high fever. SYN: *hyperpyrexia.*

hyperthermoesthesia (hi-per-therm-o-es-the′sĭ-ă). Unusual sensitiveness to heat. SYN: *hyperthermalgesia.*

hyperthrombinemia (hi″per-throm-bin-e′mĭ-ă). Excess of thrombin in the blood causing coagulation.

hyperthymergastic reaction (hi″per-thi-mer-gas′tik). A syndrome of a psychic disorder in which circumscribed attacks exhibit elated excitement, delusions of self-exaltation, euphoria, and other symptoms, including inability to conform to environment, and rebellion against inhibitions.

hyperthymia (hi-per-thi′mĭ-ă). 1. Morbid sensitiveness. 2. Cruelty or foolhardiness. 3. Moral insanity.

hyperthy′mism, hyperthymiza′tion. Excess secretion of the thymus gland.

hyperthyrea (hĭ-per-thi′re-ă). Excessive activity of the thyroid.

hyperthyreosis (hi″per-thi-re-o′sis). Overactivity of the thyroid. SYN: *hyperthyrea, hyperthyroidation.*

hyperthyroidation (hi″per-thi-roy-da′-shun). Excessive action of thyroid gland. SYN: *hyperthyrea.*

hyperthyroidism (hi-per-thi′roid-izm). A condition caused by excessive secretion of the thyroid glands which overstimulates the basal metabolism, causing an increased demand for food to prevent oxidization of body tissues.

hyperthyro′sis. Excess of thyroid secretion in the blood. SYN: *hyperthyroidation.*

hyperto′nia. Abnormal tension of arteries or muscles.

hyperton′ic. 1. Having a higher osmotic pressure than blood. Pert. to a solution of higher osmotic pressure than another.

2. Being in a state of greater than normal tension or of incomplete relaxation. Said of muscles. Opp. of *hypotonic.**

hypertonic′ity. Excess muscular tonus or intraocular pressure. SYN: *hypertonia.*

hypertonus (hi-per-to′nus). Increased tension, as muscular tension in spasm.

hypertoxic′ity. The state of being excessively poisonous.

hypertrichiasis (hi″per-tri-ki′a-sis). Abnormal growth of hair.

hypertrichophobia (hi″per-trik-o-fo′bĭ-ă). Fear of hair on the body.

hypertrichophrydia (hi″per-trik-of-rid′ĭ-ă). Undue length of the eyebrows.

hypertrichosis (hi″per-tri-ko′sis). Abnormal growth of hair. SYN: *hypertrichiasis*.

hypertrophia (hi-per-tro′fĭ-ă). Increased size of an organ, or of the body, due to growth. SYN: *hypertrophy*.

hypertrophic (hi-per-trof′ik). Pert. to hypertrophy.

hypertrophy (hi-per′tro-fĭ). Increased size of an organ or part, or of the body, due to growth, rather than to the formation of tumorous conditions. SYN: *hypertrophia*.

  h., ***compensatory.*** Hypertrophy resulting from increased function of an organ due to a defect.

  h., ***concentric.*** Hypertrophy in which the walls of an organ become thickened, with no enlargement, but with diminished capacity.

  h., ***eccentric.*** Hypertrophy of an organ with dilatation.

  h., ***false.*** Hypertrophy with degeneration of 1 constituent of an organ and its replacement by another.

  h., ***Marie's.*** Chronic arthral enlargement subsequent to chronic periostitis.

  h., ***numerical.*** Hypertrophy caused by increase in structural elements.

  h., ***physiological.*** SEE: *compensatory hypertrophy*.

  h., ***pseudomuscular.*** A disease usually of childhood, characterized by paralysis, depending upon degeneration of the muscles which, however, become enlarged from a deposition of fat and connective tissue.

  h., ***simple.*** Hypertrophy due to increase in size of structural parts.

  h., ***true.*** Hypertrophy caused by increase in size in all the different tissues composing a part.

  h., ***vicarious.*** Hypertrophy of an organ when another organ of allied function is disabled or destroyed.

hypertro′pia. Vertical strabismus upward.

hyperuresis (hi-per-ū-re′sis). Excess of urinary secretion. SYN: *enuresis, polyuria*.

hyperuricemia (hi″per-ū-ris-e′mĭ-ă). Abnormal amt. of uric acid in the blood.

hyperuricu′ria. Undue amt. of uric acid in the urine.

hypervas′cular. Excessively vascular.

hypervenosity (hi″per-ve-nos′ĭ-tĭ). Excessive development of the venous system. SYN: *supervenosity*.

hy″perventila′tion. Treatment by exposing the body to air.

hyperviscos′ity. Excessive viscosity or exaggeration of adhesive properties. Seen in anemias and inflammatory diseases.

hypervitaminosis (hi″per-vī-tăm-ĭn-o′sis). A condition caused by an excessive amount of vitamin. [of blood.

hypervolemia (hi″per-vol-e′mĭ-ă). Plethora

hypesthesia (hi-pes-the′zĭ-ă). Lessened sensibility to touch.

hypha (hi′fa). A filament or mold, or part of a mold mycelium.

hyphedonia (hip-he-dō′nĭ-ă). Abnormal diminution in gratification of desires.

hyphemia (hi-fe′mĭ-ă). 1. Blood in the ant. chamber of the eye in front of iris. 2. Anemia.

hyphidrosis (hip-hid-ro′sis). Diminished secretion of sweat.

Hyphomycetes (hi″fo-mi-se′tēs). Filamentous fungi with branched or unbranched threads. SYN: *molds*.

hypinosis (hip-in-o′sis). Deficiency of fibrin in the blood.

hypnagogic (hip-nag-oj′ĭk). 1. Inducing sleep or induced by sleep. SYN: *hypnotic*. 2. PSY: Pert. to hallucinations or dreams just before loss of consciousness. SEE: *hypnogenic zones*.

  h. ***state.*** A transitional state bet. sleeping and awaking and delusions which may result therefrom.

hypnalgia (hip-nal′jĭ-ă). False sense of pain experienced in a dream.

hyp′nic. Causing sleep. SYN: *somnifacient, somniferous*.

hyp′nocyst. A quiescent cyst or 1 whose activity is in abeyance.

hyp″nogenet′ic. Producing sleep.

  h. ***spots.*** Areas which, on being stimulated, produce sleep. SYN: *hypnogenic zones*.

hypnogenic zones (hip-no-jen′ik). Areas on the body which, when stimulated, produce sleep, esp. a sleep resembling somnabulism.

  The area may be the elbow or the popliteal spaces. SEE: *hypnagogic*.

hypnoidal (hip-noy′dal). Pert. to a condition between sleep and waking, resembling sleep.

hypnoidiza′tion. Induction of hypnosis.

hypnolepsy (hip′no-lep-sĭ). Irresistible sleepiness. SYN: *narcolepsy*.

hypnology (hip-nol′o-jĭ). Scientific study of sleep.

hypnopompic (hip-no-pom′pic). Dreams persisting after return of consciousness.

hypnosis (hip-no′sis). A subconscious condition in which the objective manifestations of mind are more or less, inactive, accompanied by abnormal sensibility to impressions, the subject responding to these impressions, unrestrained by the reasoning faculties. SEE: *autohypnosis, braidism, hypnotism, sleepwalking, somniloquy*.   [sleep.

hypnosophy (hip-nos′o-fĭ). The study of

hypnother′apy. Treatment by hypnotism, or by inducing prolonged sleep.

hypnot′ic. 1. Pert. to sleep or hypnosis. 2. An agent that induces sleep or which dulls the senses. EX: *chloral hydrate, sulfonethylmethane*.

hypnot′ics. Drugs which cause insensibility to pain by inhibiting afferent impulses, or the cortical centers of the brain receiving sensory impressions, and thus causing partial or complete unconsciousness.

hypnotism (hip'no-tizm). An induced sleep-like state during which patient is peculiarly susceptible to the suggestions of the hypnotist.

hyp'notist. One who practices hypnotism.

hypnotize (hip'no-tīz). To put under hypnotism.

hy'po. 1. A hypochondriac. 2. Popular name for hypodermic injection.

hypo-. Prefix: Less than, below.

hy'poacid'ity. A condition caused by lowered hydrochloric secretion.
TREATMENT: Dilute HCl by mouth.

hypoade'nia. Defective activity of the glands.   [insufficiency.

hypoadre'nalism, hypoadre'nia. Adrenal

hypoalimenta'tion. Insufficient nourishment. SYN: subalimentation.

hypoalonemia (hi"po-al-o-ne'mĭ-ă). Lack of salts in the blood.

hypoazoturia (hi"po-az-ot-ū'rĭ-ă). Diminished urea in the urine.

hypobaropathy (hi"po-bar-op'ă-thĭ). Symptoms produced by diminished air pressure, mountain sickness, aviator's sickness.

hyp'oblast. Internal layer of blastoderm. The external layer is called the epiblast.

hypoblastic (hi-po-blas'tik). Pert. to the inner layer of the blastoderm.

hypobulia (hi-po-bu'lĭ-ă). Lack of will power.

hypocalcemia (hi"po-kal-se'mĭ-ă). Abnormally low blood calcium.

hypocalcia (hi-po-kal'sĭ-ă). Lack of calcium in the system.

hypocap'nia. Lack of carbon dioxide in the blood.

hypochloremia (hi"po-klo-re'mĭ-ă). Having deficiency of the chloride contents of the blood.

hypochlorhydria (hi-po-klor-hi'drĭ-ă). Diminished secretion of hydrochloric acid.

hy'pochloriza'tion. Reduction of sodium chloride in the diet in nephritis and epilepsy.

hypochloruria (hi-po-klo-ru'rĭ-ă). Diminution of chlorides in the urine.

hypocholesteremia (hi"po-ko-les-ter-e'-mĭ-ă). Lowered cholesterin in the blood.

hypochon'dria. Abnormal concern about health with false belief of suffering from some disease. SYN: hypochondriasis.

hypochon'driac. 1. Pert. to the region of the hypochondrium,* or upper lateral region on each side of the body and below the thorax; beneath the ribs.
2. One having a morbid fear of disease.
h. region. Part of abdomen beneath lower ribs on both sides of epigastrium. SYN: hypochondrium.

hypochondriacal (hi"po-kon-dri'ă-kal). Affected with a morbid interest in health and disease.

hypochondrial reflex (hĭ-pō-kon'drĭ-ăl). A sudden inspiratory act resulting from sudden pressure below costal border.

hypochondriasis (hi"po-kon-dri'ă-sĭs). Morbid anxiety about one's health; a frequent symptom of depressed states. SYN: hypochondria.

hypochon'drium. That part of the abdomen beneath the lower ribs on each side of the epigastrium.

hypochromasia (hi"po-kro-ma'sĭ-ă). Lack of hemoglobin in the red blood cells.

hypochromatosis (hi"po-kro-mă-to'sis). Disappearance of the chromatin or nucleus in a cell. SYN: chromatolysis.

hypochro'mia. Disappearance of cellular chromatin.

hypochromic (hĭ-pō-krōm'ĭk). Pert. to hypochromia.

hypochro'sis. Lack of color in the blood because of low hemoglobin.

hypochylia (hi-po-ki'lĭ-ă). Lack of normal secretion of gastric juice.

hypocinesia (hi-po-sin-e'sĭ-ă). Diminished power of movement.

hypocolasia (hi-po-ko-la'zĭ-ă). Functional weakness of the inhibiting mechanism.

hypocondylar (hi-po-kon'dĭ-lar). Below a condyle.

hypocrinism (hi-po-kri'nizm). Deficient secretion of any gland, esp. an endocrine.

hypocyclosis (hi"po-si-klo'sis). Deficient accommodation.
h., ciliary. Weakness of ciliary muscle.
h., lenticular. Lack of elasticity in crystalline lens.
Both forms interfere with accommodation.

hypocystotomy (hi-po-sis-tot'o-mĭ). Perineal opening of the bladder.

hypocytosis (hi-po-si-to'sis). Lack of normal number of blood corpuscles.

hypodermatomy (hi-po-der-mat'o-mĭ). Subcutaneous incision or section, as of a muscle or tendon.

hypoder'mic. Under, or inserted under the skin, as a hypodermic injection.
h., antitoxin, serum, and vaccine. Subcutaneously in infrascapular region, infraclavicular region, or post. portion of axilla. May also be adm. intramuscularly or intravenously, all by a physician.   [physician.
h., intracutaneous. Usually adm. by a
h., intramuscular. Given in gluteal or in lumbar region. Used when a drug is not easily absorbed or when it is irritating and when large quantity of liquid is to be used.
h., intravenous. SITE: Median basilic, or median cephalic vein. To be adm. by a physician.
h., subcutaneous. Given in front of thighs, or outer surface of arms and forearm.

hypodermoclysis, hypodermatoclysis (hi"po-der-mok'lis-is, -mat-ok'lis-is). The injection of fluids into the subcutaneous tissues to supply the body with liquids quickly, as after shock or hemorrhage, diarrhea, or when the blood coagulation time is too long; in fact, it may be given in any condition in which it is impossible to give sufficient water by mouth or by rectum.

hypodynamia (hi"po-di-na'mĭ-ă). Vital debility. SYN: adynamia.

hypoeccrisia (hi-po-ek-ris'ĭ-ă). Imperfect excretion.

hypoeccritic (hi″po-ek-krit′ik). 1. Retarding normal excretion. 2. Pert. to insufficient or defective excretion.

hypoendocrinism (hi″po-en-dok′rĭ-nizm). Insufficiency of internal secretion in 1 or more glands.

hypoendocrisia (hi″po-en-do-kriz′ĭ-ă). Insufficiency of endocrine secretion. SYN: *hypoendocrinism*.

hypoeosinophilia (hi″po-e″o-sin-o-fil′ĭ-ă). Diminished quantity of eosinophil leukocytes of the blood.

hypoepinephria (hi-po-ep-ĭ-nef′rĭ-ă). Insufficiency of the adrenal secretion.

hypoesophoria (hi″po-es-o-fo′rĭ-ă). Downward and inward deviation of the eye.

hypoesthe′sia. Dulled sensitivity to touch.

hypoexophoria (hi″po-eks-o-fo′rĭ-ă). Downward and outward deviation of the eye.

hypogas′tric. Pert. to lower middle of the abdomen or hypogastrium.

h. artery. Arteria iliaca interna.

h. plexus. Sympathetic nerve plexus in the pelvis.

h. region. The hypogastrium. SEE: *abdominal region.*

hypogas′trium. Region below the umbilicus, or navel, between the right and left inguinal regions.

hypogen′esis. Cessation of growth or development at an early stage, causing defective structure. SYN: *ateliosis.*

hypogenitalism (hi-po-jen′it-al-izm). Decreased activity of the internal secretion of the genital glands resulting in poor development of the genital organs.

hypogeusia (hi-po-gū′sĭ-ă). Blunting of sense of taste.

hypoglobu′lia. Lack of cellular elements of the blood. SYN: *cytopenia, hypocytosis.*

hypoglos′sal. Situated under the tongue.

h. nerve. Twelfth cranial nerve. Exclusively motor supplying the tongue muscle. ORIG: Floor 4th ventricle. DIST: Hypoglossus and subhyoid muscles. BRS: Descendens noni (hypoglossi), muscular, thyrohyoid, geniohyoid, meningeal. SEE: *cranial nerves in Appendix.*

h. alternating hemiplegia. Medulla lesion paralyzing the tongue by involving the 12 fibers as they course through the uncrossed pyramid. The pathology may extend across the midline or dorsally, involving the medial fillet, causing contralateral anesthesia.

hypoglot′tis. 1. Undersurface of tongue. 2. Cystic tumor of floor of mouth. SYN: *ranula.*

hypoglyce′mia. Deficiency of sugar in the blood.

A condition in which there is less than 80 mg. of sugar per 100 cc. of blood.

SEE: *coma, hyperglycemia.*

hypoglycemic (hi-po-gli-se′mik). Pert. to or causing hypoglycemia.

h. shock. Production of shock by artificial production of hypoglycemia by intramuscular adm. of insulin in the treatment of schizophrenia.

hypoglycogenolysis (hi″po-gli-ko-jen-ol′ĭ-

sis). Defective hydrolysis of glycogen (glycogenolysis).

hypognathous (hi-pog′na-thus). Having a lower jaw longer than the upper one.

hypogonadism (hi-po-go′nad-izm). Defective internal secretion of the gonads.

hypohepatia (hi″po-he-pă′tĭ-ă). Deficient liver function.

hypohidrosis (hi-po-hi-dro′sis). Diminished perspiration. SYN: *hyphidrosis.*

hy″pohydrochlo′ria diet. (a) Avoid excessive quantities of fats and salts. (b) Avoid overeating. (c) Avoid much liquid. 1. Potato. 2. Dextrinized cereals. 3. Nuts. 4. Egg yolk. 5. Fruits. 6. Jellies. (d) Small amts. of broth or meat stimulate activity of the stomach.

hypohyloma (hi″po-hi-lo′mă). A tumor formed by hyperplasia of hylic tissue.

hypohypophysism (hi″po-hi-pof′ĭs-izm). Diminished activity of ant. lobe of the hypophysis. SYN: *hypopituitarism.*

hypoinosemia (hi-po-in-o-se′mĭ-ă). Decreased formation of fibrin in the blood.

hypoin′sulinism. Insufficient secretion of insulin. SYN: *diabetes mellitus.*

hypoisotonic (hi″po-is-o-ton′ĭk). Denoting a solution having lesser osmotic pressure than another solution.

hypokinesia (hi-po-kin-e′zĭ-ă). Defective motor reaction to stimulus.

hypokinet′ic. Pert. to hypokinesia.

hypokolasia (hi″po-kol-a′sĭ-ă). Imperfect inhibitory power.

hypolepidoma (hi-po-lep-id-o′mă). A hypoblastic tissue tumor.

hypoleukocytosis (hi″po-lŭ″ko-si-to′sis). A lessening of leukocytes in blood.

hypoliposis (hi-po-lip-o′sis). Deficiency of fat in the blood serum.

hypologia (hi-po-lo′jĭ-ă). A cerebral symptom marked by inadequate speech.

hypolymphemia (hi-po-lim-fe′mĭ-ă). Decreased lymphocytes in the blood with normal number of leukocytes.

hypomania (hi-po-ma′nĭ-ă). Mild mania without much change in behavior, but accompanied by sound associations and distractibility.

hypoma′niac. Pert. to maniacal exaltation, or one so affected.

hypomastia, hypomazia (hi-po-mas′tĭ-ă, -ma′zĭ-ă). Condition of having abnormally small breasts.

hy″pomelanchol′ia. Melancholia without delusions.

hypomenorrhea (hi″po-men-or-re′ă). Deficient menstrual flow.

hypomere (hi′po-mēr). That portion of the mesoderm that later forms the pleuroperitoneal walls.

hypometabolism (hi″po-me-tab′o-lizm). Lowered metabolism.

hypometria (hi-po-met′rĭ-ă). Shortened range of movement.

hypomnesia, hypomnesis (hi-pom-ne′zĭ-ă, -ne′sĭs). Impaired memory.

hypomorph (hi′po-morf). One with snort limbs who is short when standing in proportion to when sitting. The opposite of *hypermorph, q.v.* SEE: *mesomorph.*

hypomyotonia (hi″po-mi-o-to′nĭ-ă). Lacking in muscular tonus.

hypomyxia (hi-po-miks′ĭ-ă). Diminished secretion of mucus.

hyponeocytosis (hi″po-ne″o-si-to′sis). Decreased number of leukocytes (leukopenia) with immature cells in the blood.

hyponoia (hi-po-noy′ă). Sluggish mental activity or imagination. SYN: *hypopsychosis.*

hyponychium (hi-po-nik′ĭ-ŭm). The nail bed. SYN: *matrix unguis.*

hypoörchidia (hi″po-or-kid′ĭ-ă). Defective testicular secretion.

hypopancreatism (hi″po-pan′kre-ă-tizm). Diminished activity of the pancreas.

hypoparathyreosis (hi″po-par-ă-thĭ-rē-o′sis). A condition due to lessened or absent secretion of the parathyroids. SYN: *hypoparathyroidism.*

hypoparathyroidism (hi″po-păr-ă-thĭ′royd-izm). Insufficient secretion of the parathyroid glands.

hypopep′sia. Impaired digestion due to lack of pepsin.

hypopepsinia (hi-po-pep-sin′ĭ-ă). Deficient pepsin in the gastric juice.

hypoph′amine. The active principles of secretion of the post. lobe of the hypophysis cerebri.

    h., alpha. The pituitary hormone causing contractions of the uterus. SYN: *oxytocin.*

    h., beta. Postpituitary blood pressure-raising hormone. SEE: *vasopressin.*

hypophar′ynx. That part of pharynx below the laryngeal aperture.

hypophonesis (hi-po-fō-ne′sis). A diminished sound in auscultation or in percussion fainter than usual.

hypophonia (hi-po-fo′nĭ-ă). Abnormally weak voice due to incoördination of speech muscles.

hypophoria (hi-po-fo′rĭ-ă). Tendency of one visual axis to fall below the other one.

hypophosphatemia (hi″po-fos-fă-te′mĭ-ă). Phosphates below normal in the blood.

hypophrenia (hi-po-fre′nĭ-ă). Subnormal mentality.

hypophren′ic. 1. Pert. to subnormal mentality. 2. A feebleminded person.

hypophrenosis (hi-po-fre-no′sis). Feeblemindedness.

hypophyseal (hi-po-fiz′e-al). Pert. to the hypophysis.

hypophysectomy (hi″po-fĭ-sek′to-mĭ). Excision of the hypophysis cerebri.

hypophyseoprivic, hypophyseoprivous (hi″-po-fiz″e-o-priv′ĭk, -priv′ŭs). Noting a deficiency of internal secretion of the pituitary body.

hypophysioprivic, hypophysioprivous (hi-po-fiz″ĭ-o-priv′ik, -ō-pri′vŭs).Concerning a deficiency of the internal secretion of the hypophysis. SEE: *dyspituitarism, hypophyseoprivus.*

hypophysis (hi-pof′ĭ-sis) (pl. *hypophyses*). 1. Any undergrowth. 2. BNA. The pituitary body. SEE: *acidophilism, pituitary gland.*

    h. cerebri. Tiny organ situated in a sphenoid bone depression and attached to the brain by a pedicle.

    It is composed of 2 lobes, the ant. and the post. SYN: *pituitary gland.*

    h., pharyngeal. A body with a structure somewhat like the hypophysis, situated in the pharyngeal wall.

hypophysitis (hi-pof-is-i′tis). Inflammation of the pituitary body.

hypopiesis (hi-po-pi-e′sis). Subnormal arterial pressure.

hypopinealism (hi-po-pin′e-al-izm). Diminished secretion of the pineal body.

hypopituitarism (hi-po-pit-u′ĭ-tă-rizm). Diminished action of the pituitary body.

hypoplasia (hi-po-pla′zĭ-ă). Defective development of tissue.

hypop′nea. Infrequent respiration. SYN: *oligopnea.*

hypoproteinemia (hĭ″pō-prō-tē-ĭn-ē′mĭ-ă). Decrease in the normal quantity of protein in the blood.

hy″propro′teinism. Abnormal lack of protein in body causing or a symptom of kidney disease.

hypopselaphesia (hi-po-psel-af-e′zĭ-ă). Blunted tactile sense.

hypopsychosis (hi-po-sĭ-ko′sis). Weakness of the function of thought.

hypoptyalism (hi-po-ti′al-izm). Decreased salivary secretion.

hypopyesis (hi-po-pi-e′sis). Low blood pressure.

hypopyon (hi-po′pĭ-on). Pus in ant. chamber of the eye in front of iris but behind cornea, seen in corneal ulcer.

hyporeflex′ia. Diminished function of the reflexes.

hyposalemia (hi-po-sal-e′mĭ-ă). Decreased amt. of salts in the blood. SYN: *hypochloremia.*

hyposar′ca. Extreme dropsy (anasarca) of subcutaneous connective tissue.

hyposecre′tion. Lowered amt. of secretion.

hyposen′sitive. Having blunted hypersensitiveness.

hy″posensitiza′tion. Production of hyposensitiveness.

hyposialadenitis (hi″po-si″al-ad-en-i′tis). Submaxillary salivary gland inflammation.   [of smell.

hyposmia (hi-poz′mĭ-ă). Defect in sense

hyposmo′sis. Reduced osmotic rapidity.

hypospadia, hypospadias (hi-po-spa′dĭ-ă, -as). Congenital opening of the male urethra upon the undersurface of the penis; also an urethral opening into vagina.

hyposphyxia (hi-po-sfik′sĭ-ă). Sluggish circulation due to abnormally low blood pressure.

hypostasis (hi-pos′tas-is). 1. Deposit; sediment. 2. Feces. 3. Passive congestion. Opposite of *epistasis.**

hypostatic (hi-po-stat′ik). 1. Sedimentary; due to dependent position of parts of body. 2. A sediment or settling. 3. Deposit. SEE: *hypostatic pneumonia.*

hyposteatolysis (hi-po-ste-at-ol′is-is). Diminished emulsification of fats during digestion.

hyposthenia (hi-po-sthe'nĭ-ă). Subnormal strength; an enfeebled state; weakness.

hypostheniant (hi-pos-the'nĭ-ant). Reducing vital forces; debilitant.

hyposthenic (hi-pos-then'ĭk). Debilitant.

hyposthenuria (hi-pos-then-u'rĭ-ă). The secretion of urine of low specific gravity, chiefly in chronic nephritis.

    h., tubular. Hyposthenuria resulting from trauma of renal tubule epithelial cells.

    h., vascular. Hyposthenuria from renal vessel sensitiveness due to oversensitiveness of the renal blood vessels.

hypostypsis (hi-po-stip'sis). State of being slightly astringent.

hypostyptic (hi-po-stip'tĭk). Slightly astringent.

hy″posuprare′nalism. Suprarenal inactivity.

hyposynergia (hi″po-sin-er'jĭ-ă). Poor coordination.

hyposystole (hi-po-sis'to-le). A weak or lowered systolic rate.

hypotaxia (hi-po-taks'ĭ-ă). An imperfect coördination.

hypoten′sion. 1. Decrease of systolic and diastolic blood pressure below normal. 2. Deficiency in tonus or tension.

hypoten′sive. Denoting low blood pressure.

hypotensor (hi-po-ten'sor). Agent that lowers blood pressure.

hypothalamus (hi-po-thal'am-us). 1. Ganglionic substances beneath the thalamus on ventral side. 2. The region in which these ganglia are situated: (a) The *pars optica;* (b) the *pars mamillaris,* and (c) the *lamina cinerea.*

hypothenar (hi-poth'en-ar). The fleshy prominence on inner side of the palm next to the little finger.

    h. eminence. Prominence on palm below little finger.

hypother′mal. 1. Tepid. 2. Subnormal temperature below 98.6° F.

hypother′mia. 1. Having a body temperature below normal. 2. Frozen sleep. Refrigeration treatment for schizophrenia and cancer. 32° F. externally and 75° F. internally for 24 to 72 hours.

hypothesis (hi-poth'é-sis). A supposition; an assumption.

    h., cardionecteurs. Hypothesis that heart has 2 pacemakers or cardionecteurs; one, the atrionecteur, controls the atria, and the other, the ventriculonecteur, the ventricles.

    h., Harrower's. Hormone hunger.

    h., insular. The supposition that diabetes is caused by disordered function of the pancreatic islands of Langerhans.

    h., Makeham's. The assumption that death is due to 2 coexisting causes: 1. Chance, which is constant. 2. Inability to withstand destruction, which progresses geometrically.

    h., Planck's quantum. That energy is radiated or absorbed only in integral units equal to hn, in which h is Planck's constant, *q.v.,* and n is the frequency of vibration.

hypothrombinemia (hi″po-throm-bin-e'-mĭ-ă). Deficiency of thrombin in the blood, making hemophilia possible.

hypothymergasia (hi″po-thi″mer-ga'sĭ-ă). A condition of physical and mental depression.

hypothymergastic reaction (hi″po-thi-mer-gas'tik). Psychic disorder producing a sense of lonesomeness, sadness, and depression. Opp. of *hyperthymergastic reaction, q.v.*

hypothymia (hi-po-thi'mĭ-ă). Decreased emotional response to stimuli.

hypothymism (hi-po-thi'mizm). Thymus inactivity.

hypothyrea (hi-po-thi're-ă). Thyroid insufficiency. SYN: *hypothyreosis.*

hypothyreosis (hi″po-thi-re-o'sis). 1. Thyroid insufficiency. 2. Condition resulting from lack of thyroid secretion. SYN: *myxedema.*

hypothyroid (hi-po-thi'royd). Marked by insufficiency of thyroid secretion.

hypothyroida′tion. Condition causing insufficient thyroid secretion.

hypothyroidea (hi″po-thi-roi'de-ă). Diminished thyroid secretion. SYN: *hypothyreosis.*

hypothyroidism (hi-po-thi'roid-izm). A condition due to deficiency of the thyroid secretion, resulting in a lowered basal metabolism. A lesser degree of cretinism.

hypothyrosis (hi-po-thi-ro'sis). Insufficiency of thyroid secretion. SYN: *hypothyreosis.*

hypotonia (hi-po-to'nĭ-ă). 1. Reduced tension; relaxation of arteries. 2. Loss of tonicity of the muscles or intraocular pressure.

hypotonic (hi-po-ton'ik). 1. Pert. to defective muscular tone or tension. 2. A solution of lower osmotic pressure than another.

hypotoxicity (hi″po-toks-is'ĭ-tĭ). A reduced toxic quality; only slightly poisonous.

hypotrichosis (hi″po-tri-ko'sis). Abnormal deficiency of hair.

hypotrophy (hi-pot'ro-fĭ). Progressive degeneration and functional loss of cells and tissues. SYN: *abiotrophy.*

hypotropia (hi-po-tro'pĭ-ă). Ventrical strabismus downward.

hypouresis (hi″po-u-re'sis). Insufficient urination.

hypouricuria (hi″po-u-rĭ-ku'rĭ-ă). Deficient uric acid in the urine.   [tion.

hypourocrin′ia. Deficient urinary secre-

hypovaria (hi-po-va'rĭ-ă). Deficient internal secretion of the ovary and consequent retardation of puberty in girls.

hypovenosity (hi″po-ven-os'ĭ-tĭ). Incomplete development of the venous system in an area, resulting in atrophy, or degeneration.

hy″poventila′tion. Subnormal amt. of air in the lungs.

hypovitaminosis (hi″po-vĭ-tam-in-ō'sĭs). A condition due to a lack of vitamins in the diet.   .

hypovolemia (hi″po-vo-le'mĭ-ă). Diminished blood supply. SYN: *oligemia, oligohemia.*

hypoxanthine (hī"pō-zan'thin). A leuko-maine, $C_5H_4N_4O$; in muscles and tissues in a stage of urea and uric acid formation. It is formed during protein decomposition. In small amts. it is normal in urine.

hypoxemia (hi-poks-e'mĭ-ă). Insufficient oxygenation of the blood.

hypsibrachycephalic (hip"se-brak-e-sef-al'ĭk). Having a broad and high skull.

hypsicephalic (hip"si-sef-al'ĭk). Having a skull with a cranial index above 75.1°.

hypsicephaly (hip-si-sef'al-ĭ). The condition of having a skull with a cranial index over 75.1°.

hypsiconchous (hip-si-kong'kus). Having an orbital index above 85°.

hypsiloid (hip'sil-oid). U- or Y-shaped. SYN: *hyoid*.

　　h. cartilage. Y-cartilage.

　　h. ligament. Ligamentum iliofemorale.

hypsistaphylia (hip-si-staf-il'ĭ-ă). Having a narrow, high palatal arch.

hypsistenocephalic (hip-sist-en-o-sef-al'ĭk). Having a cranial index over 75.1°. SYN: *hypsicephalic.*

hypsoceph'alous. Having a cranial index over 75.1°. SYN: *hypsicephalic.*

hypsokine'sis. Tendency to fall backward when standing; seen in paralysis agitans.

hypsonosus (hip-son'o-sus). Mountain sickness; balloon sickness.

　　SYM: Epistaxis, headache, nausea.

hypsophobia (hip-so-fo'bĭ-ă). Fear of being at great heights. SYN: *aerophobia.*

hypurgia (hi-pur'jĭ-ă). Any minor factors which change the course of the disease, esp. for the better.

hys'tera. The uterus.

hysteral'gia. Neuralgia of the uterus.

hysterectomy (his-ter-ek'to-mĭ). Removal of body of uterus for cancer or myoma, usually by the abdominal route.

　　h., abdominal. Removal of the uterus through an abdominal incision.

　　h., chemical. Destruction of the endometrium by strong caustic substances.

　　h., Porro. Subtotal hysterectomy following cesarean section.

　　h., subtotal. Removal of the uterus, leaving the cervix uteri in place.

　　h., supracervical. Same as subtotal.

　　h., supravaginal. Same as subtotal.

　　h., total. Removal of body and cervix.

　　h., vaginal. Removal of the uterus through the vagina.

hystere'sis. Failure of related phenomena to keep pace with each other.

hystereurynter (his-ter-ū-rin'ter). An instrument for dilating the os uteri.

hysteria (his-te'rĭ-ă). A condition presenting somatic symptoms, simulating almost every type of physical disease, and a series of mental manifestations.

　　h. major. Very severe hysteria accompanied by epileptiform convulsions.

　　h. minor. Mild form of hysteria without loss of consciousness.

hyste'riac. A hysterical person.

hyster'ic, hyster'ical. Pert. to hysteria.

　　h. ataxia. Loss of sensation in leg muscles and skin in hysteria.

　　h. chorea. A form of hysteria with choreiform movements.

hystericoneuralgic (his-ter-ĭk-o-nū-ral'-jĭk). Pert. to pain of hysterical origin, but resembling neuralgia.

hysteritis (his-ter-i'tis). Inflammation of the uterus.

hysterobubonocele (his"ter-o-bu-bon'o-sēl). Inguinal hernia surrounding the uterus.

hysterocat'alepsy. Major hysteria with cataleptic symptoms.

hysterocele (his'ter-o-sēl). Hernia of the uterus, esp. when gravid.

hysterocervicotomy (his"ter-o-ser-vĭ-kot'o-mĭ). Cesarean section through the vagina. SYN: *hysterotrachelotomy.*

hysterocleisis (his-ter-o-kli'sis). Surgical closure of the os uteri.

hysterocystocleisis (his"ter-o-sis"to-kli'-sis). Operation fastening the cervix uteri in the wall of the bladder.

hysterodynia (his"ter-o-din'ĭ-ă). Uterine pain. SYN: *hysteralgia.*

hysteroepilepsy (his"ter-o-e'pi-lep-sĭ) Major hysteria with violent epileptiform convulsions.

hysterofrenic (his"ter-o-fren'ĭk). Arresting an attack of hysteria, noting pressure areas having this effect.

hysterogastrorrhaphy (his"ter-o-gas-tror'-af-ĭ). Fixation of uterus to gastric wall. SYN: *hysteropexy.*

hysterogen'ic. Causing a hysterical attack.

hysteroid (his'ter-oid). 1. Resembling hysteria. 2. Pert. to hysteria.

hysterokataphraxis (his"ter-o-kat"ă-fraks'-is). The operation of supporting the uterus by metallic sutures.

hysterolaparotomy (his"ter-o-lap-ă-rot'-o-mĭ). Uterine incision through abdominal wall; abdominal hysterectomy.

hysterolith (his'ter-o-lith). A calculus in the uterus.

hysterology (his-ter-ol'o-jĭ). Sum of what is known about the uterus.

hysterolox'ia. Oblique flexion of the uterus.

hysterolysis (his-ter-ol'ĭ-sis). Operation of loosening the uterus from its adhesions.

hysteromalacia (his-ter-o-mal-a'sĭ-ă). Uterine softening.

hysteroma'nia. 1. Hysterical mania. 2. Nymphomania.*

hysterometer (his-ter-om'et-er). Device for measuring the uterus.

hysterom'etry. Measurement of the size of the uterus.

hysteromyoma (his-ter-o-mi-o'mă).Myoma or fibromyoma of the uterus.

hysteromyomectomy (his"ter-o-mi"o-mek'-to-mĭ). Excision of a uterine fibroid.

hysteromyotomy (his"ter-o-mĭ-ot'o-mĭ). Uterine incision for removal of a solid tumor.

hysteroneurosis (his"ter-o-nū-ro'sis). A reflex neurosis due to uterine irritation.

hystero-oöphorectomy (his"ter-o-o"of-o-rek'to-mĭ). Removal of the uterus and 1 or both ovaries.

hysteropathy (his-ter-op'ath-ĭ). Any uterine disorder.

hysteropexy (his'ter-o-peks''ĭ). Abdominal fixation of uterus.

hysterophore (his'ter-o-fōr). Uterine pessary.

hystero'pia. A hysterical visual defect.

hysteropsychosis (his''ter-o-si-ko'sis). Mental disorder due to uterine disease.

hysteroptosia, hysteroptosis (his-ter-op-to'sĭ-a, -sis). Prolapse of the uterus.

hysterorrhaphy (his-ter-or'ă-fĭ). Suture of womb.

hysterorrhexis (his-ter-o-reks'is). Rupture of the uterus, esp. when pregnant.

hysterosalpingography (his''ter-o-sal-pĭn-gog'ră-fĭ). X-ray of the uterus and oviducts.

hysterosalpingo-oöphorectomy (his''ter-o-sal''pĭn-go-o''o-for-ek'to-mĭ). Surgical removal of uterus, oviducts, and ovaries.

hysterosalpingostomy (his''ter-o-sal-ping-os'to-mĭ). Anastomosis of the uterus with the distal end of the fallopian tube after excision of a strictured portion of the tube.

hysteroscope (his'ter-o-skōp). Instrument for examining the uterine cavity.

hysteroscopy (his-ter-os'ko-pĭ). Inspection of the uterus by use of mirror.

hys'terospasm. Uterine spasm.

hysterostomatocleisis (his''ter-o-sto-mat''-o-kli'sis). Operation for vesicovaginal fistula.

Closure of the cervix uteri, making the vesical and uterine cavities into a common cavity by means of the opening between them.

hysterostomatomy (his''ter-o-sto-mat'o-

mĭ). Surgical enlargement of the os uteri; incision of the os or cervix uteri.

°hysterosyph'ilis. A hysterical manifestation due to syphilis.

hysterosystole (his''ter-o-sis'to-le). A delayed contraction of the heart after its normal time; opp. to *extrasystole.*

hysterotabetism (his''ter-o-ta'bet-izm). Condition of hysteria and tabes combined.

hysterotokotomy (his''ter-o-to-kot'o-mĭ). Cesarean operation.

hys'terotome. Instrument for incision of the uterus.

hysterotomotokia (his''ter-o-tom''o-to'-kĭ-ă). Cesarean section.

hysterotomy (his-ter-ot'o-mĭ). 1. Incision of the uterus. 2. Cesarean section, *q.v.*

hysterotrachelorrhaphy (his''ter-o-tra-kel-or'ă-fĭ). A plastic operation for a lacerated cervix by paring the edges and suturing them together.

hysterotrachelotomy (his''ter-o-trak-el-ot'o-mĭ). Surgical incision of neck of uterus.

hysterotraumatic (his''ter-o-traw-mat'ik). Pert. to traumatic hysteria.

hysterotraumatism (his''ter-o-traw'mă-tizm). Hysteric symptoms due to or following traumatism.

hysterotris'mus. Uterine spasm.

hysterovagino-enterocele (his''ter-o-vaj''-in-o-en'ter-o-sél). Hernia surrounding uterus, vagina, and intestines.

hystriciasis, hystricism (his-trĭ-si'a-sis, his'trĭ-sizm). 1. Erection of hairs like the spines of a hedgehog. 2. A skin disease.

hyther (hi'ther). The combined effect of humidity and temperature of atmosphere upon the body.

I

i. Abbr. for *optically inactive.*

I Chem. symb for *ampere* and *iodine.*

ianthinopia (ī-ăn-thī-nō'pī-ă). Violet vision.

-iasis. Suffix: Same as *-osis*, meaning the state or condition of, as *psoriasis.*

iatraliptics (i-ă-tră-lip'tĭks). Treatment by inunction.

iatric (i-at'rik). Medical.

iatrochem′istry. Seventeenth century opinion that chemistry is the basis of all physiological phenomena.

iatrology (i-at-rol'o-jĭ). Medical science.

iatrotechnics (i-at-ro-tek'nĭks). The art and technic of medicine and surgery.

ice (īs) Water frozen at temperature below 32° F. (0° C.).

  i. bag, i. cap, i. collar. Devices for holding ice to be applied to a patient to obtain the effect of continuous cold in a circumscribed area.

  i. cravat. Ice pack applied around the neck.

  i., dry. Carbon dioxide in a solid form. Snow is a form of dry ice. Used as a commercial refrigerant; also used for therapeutic refrigeration in such skin diseases as *lupus erythematosus.*

Iceland moss (īs'land). A lichen. It contains a form of starch; a slightly tonic demulcent. Syn: *Cetraria.*

ichnogram (ik'no-gram). A footprint taken standing.

ichor (i'kor). Thin, fetid discharge from an ulcer or from a wound.

ichoremia (i-kor-e'mĭ-ă). Septic or toxic blood poisoning due to presence of ichorous matter. Syn: *ichorrhemia.*

ichorous (i'kor-us). Resembling ichor or watery pus.

ichorrhea, ichorrhoea (i-ko-re'ă). Profuse discharge of ichorous fluid.

ichorrhemia (i-kor-re'mĭ-ă). Toxic or septic blood poisoning due to presence of ichorous matter. Syn: *ichoremia.*

ichthammol (ik'tha-mol). A reddish brown, viscous fluid obtained by the destructive distillation of certain bituminous shale.

  Dosage: Externally, 5-10% ointment or solution.

ichthyism (ĭk'thĭ-ĭzm). Poisoning from eating stale or unfit fish.

ichthyo-. Combining form meaning *fish.*

ichthyoid (ik'thĭ-oyd). Fishlike. [mol.

ichthyol (ĭk'thĭ-ŏl). A brand of ichtham-

  Dosage: 5-10 gr. (0.3-0.6 Gm.).

ichthyophobia (ik-thĭ-o-fo'bĭ-ă). Aversion to fish.

ichthyosis (ik-thi-o'sis). Fish-skin disease. Congenital abnormality of the skin characterized by dryness, harshness, scaliness.

  i. follicularis. Ichthyosis in which sebaceous and epithelial material accumulate about the hair follicles.

  i. hystrix. A form with warts.

  i. sebacea. Functional disorder of the sebaceous glands. Syn: *seborrhea.*

  i. simplex. Ichthyosis with cutaneous roughening and dryness. Syn: *xeroderma.*

ichthyotic (ik-thĭ-ot'ik). Rel. to ichthyosis.

I. C. N. Abbr. for *International Council of Nurses.*

iconolagny (ī-kon'o-lag-nĭ). Sexual passion stimulated by pictures or statues or objects.

icterepatitis (ik-ter-ĕ-pă-tī'tis). Hepatitis associated with jaundice.

icteric (ik-ter'ik). Pert. to jaundice.

  i. fever. Jaundice combined with pernicious malaria.

  i. index. A number obtained by matching blood serum in a colorimeter against a standard solution of potassium dichromate (1:10,000), which gives a color approximately same as bilirubin.

icteritious (ik-ter-ish'us). Yellowish; resembling jaundice. Syn: *icteroid.*

icteroanemia. Icterus associated with anemia, hemolysis and splenic enlargement.

icterogenic, icterogenous (ik-ter-o-jen'ĭk, -oj'en-us). Causing jaundice.

icterohepatitis (ik″ter-o-hep-ă-tī'tis). Liver inflammation with jaundice.

icteroid (ik'ter-oyd). Resembling jaundice; yellow-hued.

icterus (ik'te-rus). Jaundice, *q.v.* Pigmentation of the tissues, membranes and secretions with bile pigments.

  i. castren′sis gravis. Serious camp jaundice. Syn: *Weil's disease.*

  i. castren′sis levis. Mild camp disease of catarrhal form.

  i. cythemoly′tic. A form caused by absorption of bile formed in excess quantities due to hemolysis.

  i. febri′lis. Weil's disease.

  i. gravis. Acute yellow atrophy of liver with cerebral disorders.

  i., hemolytic or **nonobstructive.** Rare chronic form, frequently congenital, with periodic attacks of intense hemolysis.

  i. index. A measurement of the color of blood serum, chiefly for the determination of color produced by bile pigments.

  i. me′las. Black jaundice.

  i. neonatorum. Jaundice of the newborn. A type of hemolytic jaundice. It may be benign or malignant.

  i., obstructive. Jaundice caused by obstruction to the flow of bile in the common or hepatic duct. [syphilis.

  i. precox. Jaundice of secondary

  i., suppression. Etiol: Caused by toxins in body which destroy the liver cells and red blood cells.

i. typhoides. Acute yellow atrophied condition of liver.

ictom'eter. An instrument for estimating the force of apex beat.

ic'tus. 1. A beat or stroke. 2. An attack.

i. cordis. A term applied to heartbeat.

i. epilepticus. Epileptic convulsion.
i. sanguinis. Apoplexy.
i. solis. Sunstroke.

id. BIOL: A biological germ structure carrying the heredity qualities; "an ancestral germ plasm."

PSY: The unconscious undominated by its ego, but by its own impulsions, which are of an instinctive nature, such as the pleasure urge. SYN: *microsome.**

idant (id'ant). A chromosome containing all the ids regarded as hereditary factors.

-ide. CHEM: An ending indicating a salt of a binary acid, as *sodium chloride.*

ide'a. A mental image; a concept.

i., autochthonous (aw-tok'thon-us). An unaccountable one.

i., compulsive. A persistent, obsessional impulse or thought.

i., dom'inant. One controlling all one's actions and thoughts.

i., fixed. One that completely dominates the mind, as a delusion.

i. of reference. An impression that the conversation or actions of others have reference to oneself.

idea, flight of. Rapid speech, often disconnected and incoherent, in certain mental diseases.

ideation (i-de-a'shun). The process of thinking; formation of ideas.

idée fixe (ē-dā fēks'). An obsession; a fixed idea. SEE: *idea.*

iden'tical. Exactly alike.

i. twins. Twins developed from 1 fertilized cell. SEE: *Hellin's law, twins.*

identifica'tion. A kind of daydream, as when one identifies himself with the hero of a book or play.

ideo-. Prefix: Pert. to mental images.

ideogenous (i-de-oj'en-us). Stimulated by an idea.

ideomo'tion. Muscular automatic movement activated by a dominant idea.

ideomo'tor. Pert. to ideomotion.

ideophrenic (id-e-o-fren'ik). Marked by abnormal ideas of a perverted nature.

idio-. Prefix: Individual, distinct, in compound words.

idioc'rasy. Peculiarity which renders one susceptible to certain habits or drugs.

idiocratic (ĭd"i-o-krat'ĭk). Pert. to idiocrasy.

id'iocy. Mental deficiency usually congenital. SEE: *idiot.*

i., amaurotic family. Form of idiocy seen in infants and small children in which there is increasing failure of vision and eventually death.

i., Aztec. Idiocy combined with microcephalia.

i., cretinoid. Endemic idiocy accompanied by stunted growth and frequently by goiter.

i., diplegic. Idiocy marked by paralysis of all extremities in infants.

i., epileptic. Idiocy accompanied by epilepsy.

i., genetous. Idiocy of congenital origin.

i., hemiplegic. Hemiplegic manifestations in infants.

i., hydrocephalic. Idiocy accompanied by chronic hydrocephalus.

i., intrasocial. Idiocy in which mentality permits some occupation.

i., microcephalic. SEE: *Aztec idiocy.*

i., Mongolian. Congenital form of idiocy in which person has Mongolian features, the nose being broad, the eyes slanting, and the skull flat.

i., paralytic. Idiocy combined with paralysis.

i., paraplegic. Idiocy combined with paraplegia.

i., sensorial. Mental deficiency caused by loss of 1 of the special senses.

i., traumatic. Idiocy caused by an injury received in infancy or in early childhood.

idiog'amist. One incapable of the sexual act with more than a few persons because of sexual discrimination.

idioglos'sia. Inability to articulate properly so that the sounds emitted are like those of an unknown language.

idioisolysin (id"ĭ-o-i-sol'ĭ-sin). A hemolysin active against the cells of an individual of the same species.

idiolysin (id-ĭ-ol'ĭ-sin). A lysin in the blood not formed in response to injection of an antigen.

idiometritis (id-ĭ-o-me-tri'tis). Inflammation of the uterine parenchyma.

idiomus'cular. Pert. to the muscles independent of nerve control.

i. contraction. Motion produced by degenerated muscles without nerve stimulus.

idioneurosis (id-ĭ-o-nū-ro'sis). Any functional neurosis arising without stimuli.

idiopathic (id-ĭ-o-path'ik). Pert. to conditions without clear pathogenesis, or disease without recognizable cause, as of spontaneous origin.

idiopathy (id-ĭ-op'ă-thĭ). A primary disease without apparent external cause. SYN: *autopathy.*

idiophrenic (id-i-o-fren'ik). Pert. to or originating in the mind alone.

i. psychosis. An organic disease of the brain producing a mental disorder.

idioplasm (id'ĭ-o-plazm). Inheritable substance in an ovum or germ cell.

idiosome (id'ĭ-o-sōm). 1. The indivisible element of living matter. 2. Spermatid's attraction sphere.

idiosyncrasy (ĭd-ĭ-o-sĭn'kră-sĭ). 1. Special characteristics by which persons differ from each other. 2. That which makes one react differently from others. A peculiar or individual reaction to an idea, an action, or some substance, an unusual susceptibility. SYN: *idiocrasy.*

i. of drug. When no effects are produced from large doses of a drug, or unusual effects from small doses or from certain drugs. Ex: *digitalis, hypnotics, mercury, potassium iodide,* and *salicylates.*

i. of effect. When small doses of a drug create a poisonous or opposite effect, an unusual or no effect.

i. to x-ray. Natural or an inherent tendency on the part of the skin to react vigorously to minute doses of x-rays.

idiosyncratic (id″ĭ-o-sin-krat′ĭk). Pert. to an idiosyncrasy. SYN: *idiocratic.*

id′iot. One with a congenital condition of feeblemindedness, or a serious intelligence defect, a mental age less than 3 years, or an intelligence quotient of less than 20. SEE: *idiocy.*

i., amaurotic. One born apparently normal but who, in a few months after birth, develops symptoms of idiocy, inability to hold the head up, imperfect vision, and sometimes the macula shows a cherry-red spot. Failure of vision, paralysis, and death follow.

i., Aztec. A microcephalic idiot.

i., complete or **profound.** One devoid of all primitive instincts, even that of self-preservation.

i., hydrocephalic. Idiot with chronic enlargement of head and atrophy of the brain.

i., microcephalic. One with skull too small for proportions of balance of body.

i., Mongolian. One who has a Mongolian cast of countenance, the nose being broad, the eyes slanting, and the skull flat.

idiot′ic. Like an idiot; said of an idea or action.

idiotrophic (id″ĭ-o-trof′ĭk). Capable of securing its own nourishment.

idiotrop′ic. Turning inward mentally. Individual.

i. type. An introvert type satisfied by his own emotions, and by inner contemplation and pursuits, who is content to live apart from social contacts.

idiotypic (id-ĭ-o-tip′ĭk). Rel. to heredity.

idioventricular (id-ĭ-o-ven-trĭk′ŭ-lar). Pert. to the cardiac ventricle alone when dissociated from the auricle.

id′organ. A unicellular organism supposedly capable of development into a metazoan.

idrosis (id-ro′sis). Excessive sweating. SYN: *hidrosis.*

ig″niextirpa′tion. Cautery excision.

ig″niopera′tion. An operation by cautery.

ignipuncture (ig″ni-punk′tur). The use of heated needles in cauterization by puncture.

ignis (ig′nis). Fire; cautery. SYN: *moxa.*

i. sa′cer. An inflammatory skin disease. SYN: *herpes zoster.*

i. Sanc′ti Anto′nii. Acute febrile disease with localized inflammation. SYN: *erysipelas; St. Anthony's fire.*

ileac (il′e-ak). Pert. to the ileum. SYN: *ileus.*

i. passion. Obstruction of the bowel.

ileëctomy (il-e-ek′to-mĭ). Excision of the ileum.

ileitis (il-e-i′tis). Inflammation of the ileum.

ileocecal (il-e-o-se′kăl). Rel. to the ileum and cecum.

i. valve. Sphincter muscles which guard the aperture of the ileum at the cecum, where the small intestines open into the ascending colon. It prevents food material from reëntering the small intestines. SEE: *Bauhin's valve.*

ileocecum (il-e-o-se′kum). The ileum and cecum combined.

ileocol′ic. Pert. to the ileum and colon. SEE: *ileocecal.*

i. valve. Passage where food is prevented from reëntering small intestines.

ileocolitis (il-e-o-ko-li′tis). Inflammation of mucous membrane of the ileum and colon.

ileocolostomy (il-e-o-ko-los′to-mĭ). Anastomosis between ileum and colon.

ileocolotomy (il-e-o-ko-lot′o-mĭ). Incision of ileum and colon.

ileoproctostomy (il″e-o-prok-tos′tō-mĭ). Establishment of opening bet. ileum and rectum.

ileorectostomy (il″e-o-rek-tos′tō-mĭ). Formation of passage bet. ileum and rectum. SYN: *ileoproctostomy.*

ileosigmoidostomy (il″e-o-sig-moid-os′to-mĭ). Surgical opening between the ileum and sigmoid flexure.

ileostomy (il-e-os′to-mĭ). Creation of a surgical passage through abdomen into ileum.

ileotomy (il-e-ot′o-mĭ). Incision into the ileum. SYN: *ileostomy.*

ileotransversostomy (il″e-o-trans-ver-sos′-to-mĭ). Connection of the ileum with the transverse colon.

iletin (i′le-tĭn). Insulin, *q.v.*

il′eum (pl. *ilea*). Lower 3rd portion of small intestines, from the jejunum to the ileocecal valve. It is about 12 ft. long.

ileus (il′e-us). Obstruction of small intestine.

i., adynamic. That caused by intestinal muscle paralysis.

i., dynamic; i., hyperdynamic. That caused by intestinal muscle contraction.

i., mechanical. That produced by an obstruction.

i., paralyticus. SEE: *adynamic ileus.*

il′iac. Rel. to the ilium.

i. crest. The hip. Upper free margin of the ilium. SYN: *crista iliaca.*

i. fascia. Transversalis fascia over ant. surface of the iliopsoas muscle.

i. fossa. Fossa iliaca, *q.v.*

i. region. Inguinal region on either side of hypogastrium.

i. roll. Sausage-shaped mass in left iliac fossa. Caused by induration of sigmoidal walls.

i. spine. Spina iliaca.

iliocolotomy (il-ĭ-o-kol-ot′o-mĭ). Opening into the colon in the iliac or inguinal region.

iliofemoral (il-ĭ-o-fem′or-al). Pert. to the ilium and femur.

ilioinguinal (il″ĭ-o-in′gwĭ-nal). Pert. to the groin and iliac regions.

iliolumbar (il-ĭ-o-lum′bar). Rel. to the iliac and lumbar regions.

iliometer (il-ĭ-om′e-ter). Device for measuring the iliac spines.

iliopectineal (il″ĭ-o-pek-tin′e-al). Rel. to the ilium and the pubes.

iliopsoas (il-ĭ-o-so′as). The compound iliacus and psoas magnus muscles.

   i. abscess. An abscess in the psoas and iliacus muscles.

iliosa′cral. Pert. to the sacrum and ilium.

iliotib′ial. Pert. to the ilium and tibia.

   i. band. A thick, wide fascial layer from the iliac crest to the knee joint.

il′ium. 1. The haunch bone. The wide upper portion of the innominate bone. 2. The flank. SYN: *os ilium.* SEE: *hip bone, Meckel's diverticulum, sacroiliac.*

ill (ĭl). Indisposed; not healthy; diseased.

illaqueation (il″ă-kwe-a′shun). Turning an inverted eyelash by drawing a loop of thread behind it.

illegal (ĭl-lē′găl). Contrary to authorized law.

illegitimate (ĭl″le-jĭt′ĭ-mĭt). 1. Not according to law; not authorized. 2. Born out of wedlock.

illness (ĭl′nĕs). 1. State of being sick. 2. Ailment.

illu′minating gas. This is a mixture of various combustible gases, including hydrogen and carbon monoxide.

illumination (il-lu-min-a′shun). 1. The lighting up of a part for examination or an object under a microscope. 2. Amt. of light thrown upon anything.

   i., axial. Light transmitted along the axis of a microscope.

   i., direct. Light thrown upon the object from a microscope.

   i., focal. Light upon the focus of a lens.

   i., oblique. Illumination of an object from 1 side.

illu′sion. PSY: Inaccurate perception; misinterpretation of sensory impressions, whereas a hallucination has no source in fact.

illu′sional. Pert. to, or of the nature of, an illusion.

image (ĭm′ĭj). A mental picture with a likeness of an objective reality.

   i., after. A retinal impression which persists after the stimulus is removed.

   i., direct; i., erect. Picture from rays not yet focused.

   i., false. The image formed by a deviating eye in strabismus, present in diplopia. SEE: *circle of diffusion.*

   i., inverted. Image that is turned upside down.

   i., real. Image formed by convergence of rays of light from an object.

   i., virtual. SEE: *direct image.*

imagery (ĭm′a-je-rĭ). Imagination; the calling up of events or mental pictures.

   Mental imagery may be of various types, *viz.*:

   i., auditory. When sounds can be recalled to mind, as thunder, wind, etc.

   i., motor. When movement only is recalled, as the passing of a train. Motor-mindedness is recognized in the mastery of spelling. The constant repetition of movements in writing make for automatic habit formation and fixation of the visual word-image.

   i., tactile. When the feel of an object can be readily recalled.

   i., taste and *i., smell.* Mental conception of taste or odor sensations previously experienced. Often very weak.

   i., visual. Mental conception of an object seen previously. This is probably the commonest type of imagery.

imagina′tion. The power of forming mental images.

imago (im-a′go). 1. An image or shadow. 2. A memory, esp. of a loved one, developed during childhood that has become clouded by idealism and imagination, and which is not always a correct one.

imbal′ance. Out of balance. Without equality in power between opposing forces.

   i., autonom′ic. Involuntary nervous system disturbance.

   i., sympathet′ic. Increased tonus of autonomic nervous system. SYN: *vagotonia.*

   i., vasomo′tor. Autonomic imbalance.

imbecile (im′be-sil). 1. One with defective mentality, but with intelligence greater than that of an idiot,* and with less than that of a moron. One with a mental age between 3 and 7 years, or a child with an intelligence quotient between 20 and 49, inclusive.

   2. Without strength of mind or body; esp. mentally weak. 3. Stupid.

imbecil′ity. Weakness of mind.

imbed′. To implant, as in a fixing substance.

imbibition (im″bi-bish′un). The absorption of fluid by a solid body without a chemical change in either.

imbricate, imbricated (im′bri-kāt). Overlapping, as tiles; overlapping aponeurotic layers.

imbrication (im-brĭ-ka′shun). 1. Overlapping, as tiles. 2. The overlapping of aponeurotic layers in abdominal surgery.

imida′zole or **imina′zole.** An organic compound characterized structurally by the presence of the heterocyclic ring

$$H - C - N - H$$
$$\| \qquad \|$$
$$H - C - N = C - H$$

which occurs in histidine and histamine.

imide-. Prefix: A compound with the bivalent atom group (NH).

immature (im-ma-tūr′). Not fully developed or ripened.

imme′diate. Direct without intervening steps.

   i. agglutination. Healing by first intention.

   i. auscultation. Auscultation by ear applied to the body. SEE: *auscultation.*

   i. cause. A cause directly originating a disease.

   i. contagion. Contagion by direct contact.

i. union. Healing by first intention.

immedicable (im-med'i-ka-bl). Incurable.

immersion (im-er'shun). Placing a body under water, or another fluid.

i., homogeneous. Immersion in which the stratum of air between objective and cover glass is replaced by a medium which deflects as little as possible the rays of light passing through the cover glass.

i. lens, oil. A special lens used with cedar oil and producing a high magnification; useful in studying bacteria.

immiscible (im-mis'i-bl). Pert. to that which cannot be mixed, as oil and water.

immobiliza'tion. The making of a part or limb immovable.

immune (ĭm-ūn'). 1. Protected or exempt from contagion. 2. Exempt from a certain disease by vaccination or inoculation.

i. bodies. Substances in those afflicted with an infectious disease formed by the tissues and possessing power to destroy or injure the disease-producing agent, or to neutralize its poisons.

immunifacient (im-u-ni-fa'shent). Making immune.

immun'ity. The state of being resistant to injury, particularly by poisons, foreign proteins, and invading parasites.

i., acquired. Secured by having had an attack by pathogenic organism and having overcome it, or by injection of bacteria.

i., active or actual. Can be produced by vaccination or by recovery from the disease itself.

i., congenital or natural. The condition ensuing when defensive substances, or antibodies,* are present in normal and untreated subjects.

i., passive. Produced by actual injection of sera containing the antibodies into the subject to be protected.

i., Profeta's. That of some children of syphilitic parents against syphilis.

immuniza'tion. Becoming immune or the process of rendering a patient immune. SEE: *autoimmunization, immunity.*

immunizing unit. A unit which expresses an antitoxin's strength. It varies with different antitoxins. SYN: *antitoxic unit.*

immunochemistry (im-mu''no-kem'is-tri). The chemistry of immunization.

immunogenic (im-u-no-jen'ĭk). Inducing immunity.

immunologic (im-mu-no-loj'ik). Pert. to immunology.

i. diseases. These are due to the action of antibodies, as in allergic hypersensitiveness to antigens, or to specific reactivity of the tissues.

immunol'ogy. The study of immunity to diseases, as: 1. Immunity to microbic diseases. 2. Serology. 3. Immunologic diseases.   [*cination.* SEE: *serology, serum, toxins, vac-*

immunopro'tein. Antitoxin; a bacteriolytic protein injected to produce immunity.

immunotherapy (im-mu-no-ther'ă-pi). The production of immunity.

immunotox'in. Antitoxin; substance injected to produce immunity.

immunotransfusion (im-mu-no-trans-fu'-zhun). Transfusion of blood from one who has been immunized by an autogenous vaccine.

immunpro'tein. A bacteriolytic substance formed by the injection of attenuated bacterial cultures.

impac'ted. Pressed firmly together so as to be immovable.

impaction (im-pak'shun). 1. Condition of being tightly wedged into a part; overloading of an organ, as the feces in the bowels. 2. Concussion.

impal'pable. Felt with difficulty; hardly perceptible to the touch.

impal'udism. Malaria. SYN: *paludism.*

im'par. Unpaired. SYN: *azygous.*

imparidigitate (im-par-i-dij'i-tāt). Having unequal number of fingers or toes. SYN: *perissodactylous.*

impe'dance. Resistance due to self induction, as that met by alternating currents in passing through a conductor; virtual as distinguished from ohmic resistance.

imper'ative. Obligatory; not controlled by the will; involuntary.

i. concept. An idea which dominates one, as a fear or doubt.

impercep'tion. Inability to form a mental picture; lack of perception.

imper'forate. Without an opening.

i. hymen. A hymen without an opening. Seldom discovered before puberty. Menstruation is interfered with and incision of hymen becomes necessary. SEE: *hymen.*

imperfora'tion. State of being closed or occluded. SYN: *atresia.*

imperious acts. Tics and motions not under control of the will. Urges of compulsion states. SEE: *impulsion.*

imper'meable. Impervious to fluids. Impenetrable.

imper'vious. Unable to be penetrated.

impetiginous (im-pe-tij'in-us). Rel. to impetigo.

impetigo (im-pe-ti'go). Inflammatory skin disease marked by isolated pustules which become crusted and rupture. Occurs principally around mouth and nostrils. SYN: *scrumpox.*

i. contagiosa. A contagious form. Children esp. afflicted.

i. herpetiformis. Rare form occurring usually in puerperal women and accompanied by serious systemic disturbance.

i. syphilit'ica. A pustular syphilide.

i. variolo'sa. Pustules in late stage of smallpox. SYN: *melitagra* (2).

implantation (im-plan-ta'shun). 1. Grafting. 2. Artificial impregnation of a substance under the skin into the blood, into the uterine canal, etc.

i., hypodermic. Introduction of solid medicine under the skin.

i., parenchymatous. Introduction of medicinal substance into a neoplasm.

i., teratic. Union of a fetal monster with a perfect fetus.

im'plants. Capillary tubes of glass, gold,

or platinum, containing radon for insertion into tissue.

impon′derable. Having little weight.

im′potence, im′potency. Weakness. Inability to copulate. Failure of sexual power.

    i., anatomic; i., organic. Impotence caused by a defect in the genitalia.

    i., atonic. Due to spinal exhaustion.

    i., paretic. Failure of impulse.

    i., psychic. Due to mental disturbance.

    i., symptomatic. Due to poor health, drugs, presence of disease, etc.

impotent (ĭm′pō-tĕnt). 1. Unable to copulate. 2. Sterile; barren.

impoten′tia. Impotence.

    i. coeun′di. Inability on part of the male to engage in the sexual act.

    i. erigen′di. Loss of power of erection.

impregnate (im-preg′nāt). 1. To render pregnant. To fertilize an ovum. 2. To saturate.

impreg′nated. 1. Rendered pregnant. 2. Saturated.

    i. carbon. Electrode having a carbon shell with core of various metals or salts of metals for use in a carbon arc lamp.

impregnation (im-preg-na′shun). Fertilization of an ovum; fecundation.

    i., artificial. Artificial implantation* of semen in the uterine canal.

    i., ovarian. Transmission of peculiarities not prevailing in the family of either parent but possessed by a male by whom the mother had previously been impregnated; the transmission of the peculiarities of a woman's first husband to her children by a succeeding husband. SYN: *adosculation, implantation, indirect atavism.*

impres′sio. A mark, as of 1 part upon another.

    i. cardi′aca. Depression on surface of liver for the heart. BNA.

    i. col′ica. Depression on undersurface of right lobe of liver. BNA.

    i. digitata. A depression on the inner cranial surface.

    i. duodena′lis. Depression on undersurface of liver beside the gallbladder indicating position of duodenum. BNA.

    i. gas′trica. Hollow under left lobe of liver indicating position of stomach. BNA.

    i. rena′lis. Hollow on undersurface of right lobe of liver adjacent to the right kidney. BNA.

impres′sion. 1. A hollow or depression in a surface. 2. Effect produced upon the mind by external stimuli. 3. Plastic imprint of the jaw and teeth for making a denture. SEE: *reflex center.*

impulse (im′puls). 1. Act of driving onward with sudden force. 2. An incitement of the mind, prompting an unpremeditated act. 3. PHYS: A change transmitted through certain tissues, esp. nerve fibers and muscles, resulting in physiological activity or inhibition.

    i., cardiac. The heartbeat felt at the left side of the chest at the 5th intercostal space.

    i., excitatory. One which stimulates activity.   [tivity.

    i., inhibitory. One which lessens ac-

    i., morbid. An uncontrollable desire to perform an abnormal act.

    i., nervous. Driving force or wave traversing a nerve fiber. SEE: *nervous impulse.*

impul′sion. Idea to do something or commit some act or crime suddenly imposed upon the subject which tortures him until the act is accomplished.

in-. Prefix: *Not, in, inside, within;* also *intensive action,* and denoting *fibrous tissue* or *fibrin.*

inac′tivate. To make inactive.

inactiva′tion. Rendering anything inert by using heat or other means.

    i. of complement. Loss of activity caused by heating serum to about 55° C. (131° F.) for half an hour.

inadequacy (in-ad′e-kwa-sĭ). Insufficiency; incompetence.

    i., renal. Inability of kidney to produce normal amt. of urine with proper proportion of solids and of a sp. gr. more than 1.014.

inalimental (in-al-im-en′tal). Unfit as food; not nutritious.

inan′imate. 1. Not alive; not animate. 2. Dull, lifeless.

inani′tion. A condition due to lack of any food material essential to the body, such as general underfeeding, undernutrition, or caloric insufficiency.

inappetence (in-ap′pe-tens). Lack of craving or desire, esp. for food.

inartic′ulate. 1. Not jointed; without joints. 2. Unable to pronounce distinct syllables or express oneself intelligibly. 3. Not given to expressing oneself verbally.

in artic′ulo mor′tis. At the time of death.

inassim′ilable. Not capable of being utilized by the body for nutrition.

inaxon (in-aks′on). An axis cylinder that gives off no dendrites until some distance from the neuron.

in′breeding. Producing offspring from those closely related.

incandes′cent. Glowing with light; white hot.

incar′cerated. Imprisoned, confined, constricted, as an irreducible hernia.

incarcera′tion. Legal confinement; imprisonment of a part; constriction.

inca′rial bone. Os incae; interparietal bone.

In′ca's bone. The interparietal bone.

incep′tion. 1. The beginning of anything. 2. Ingestion. 3. Intussusception.

incest (in′sest). Coitus between those of near relationship, a pathological phenomenon found in acquired or congenital states of mental weakness.

in′cidence. The range of occurrence of a disease.

in′cident. Happening, falling on, afferent.

    i. nerve. An afferent nerve.

incineration (in-sin-er-a'shun). Destruction by fire. Syn: *cremation.*

incipient (in-sip'i-ent). Beginning.

incise'. To cut, as with a sharp instrument.

incised (in-sizd'). Cut with a knife.
  i. wound. One clearly cut.

incision (in-sizh'un). A cut made with a knife, esp. for surgical purposes.

incisive (in-si'siv). 1. Cutting; having the power of cutting. 2. Rel. to the incisor teeth.
  i. bone. Ant. or medial part of the sup. maxilla.

incisor (in-si'zor). 1. That which cuts. 2. That which applies to the incisor teeth. 3. One of the cutting teeth, 4 in each jaw between the cuspids. See: *dentition.*
  i., prostatic. Surgical knife for incision of an enlarged prostate.

incisu'ra (pl. *incisurae*). An incision or notch.
  i. card'iaca. Notch in ant. border of left lung.
  i. cerebelli. The notch or sulcus separating the cerebellar hemispheres.

incisure (in-siz'ūr). A notch or slit.
  i's. of Schmidt and Lantermann. Oblique lines on medullated nerve fiber sheaths.

inclina'tion. Leaning from the normal, or from the vertical, as a tooth.

inclinometer (in-kli-nom'et-er). Device for measuring ocular diameter from vertical and horizontal lines.

inclu'sion. Being enclosed or included.

incoercible (in-ko-er'sib-l). Uncontrollable; not able to be held in check.
  i. vomiting. Uncontrollable vomiting.

incoherence (in-ko-her'ens). Inability to express oneself coherently, or to present ideas in a related order; sometimes due to interruption of one's thought processes.

incoherent (in-ko-he'rent). Not coherent or understandable.

incombus'tible. Incapable of being burnt.

incompatibil'ity. State which renders admixture of remedies unsuitable through chemical action, insolubility, formation of poisonous or explosive compounds; difference in solubility; or opposite action.
  i., physiological. A condition in which 1 or more substances in a mixture have a different physiological action than other substances in the mixture.

incompat'ible. 1. Not capable of uniting in solution. 2. Antagonistic in action, said of some drugs.

incom'petence, incom'petency. Inadequate ability to perform the function or action normal to an organ or part.
  i., aortic. Regurgitation of blood through the aortic valves.
  i. of cardiac valves. Condition in which heart valves permit the return of blood beyond them when closed.
  i., ileocecal. Inability of ileocecal valve to stop the return of the material from the colon to the ileum.

i., mental. Mental inability to retain charge of oneself or possessions.
  i., muscular. Imperfect closure of the cardiac valve due to weak action of papillary muscles.
  i., pyloric. Weakness of pyloric aperture which permits undigested food to leave the stomach and enter the duodenum.
  i., relative. Excessive dilatation of a cardiac cavity which makes perfect closure of opposite cardiac valve impossible.   [more cardiac valves.
  i., valvular. Leaky condition of 1 or

incom'petent. 1. One legally unable to execute a contract, such as a feebleminded or insane person. 2. Incapable.

incompres'sible. Compact; not compressible.

incon'tinence. 1. Inability to retain urine, semen, or feces, through loss of sphincter control, cerebral or spinal lesions. 2. Lack of sexual restraint.
  i., active. Discharge of feces and urine in the normal way at regulated intervals but involuntarily.
  i., intermittent. Loss of control of bladder on sudden pressure or movement, because of interruption of voluntary path above the lumbar center.
  i. of milk. Excessive milk flow. Syn: *galactorrhea.*
  i., overflow. Incontinence caused by pressure of urine retained in the bladder.
  i., paralytic. Constant voiding of small amt. of urine and feces due to relaxation of sphincters from lumbar center destruction.
  i., passive. Urinary incontinence of a form in which there is a full bladder that doesn't empty normally, but urine drips away upon pressure.
  i. of urine. Inability to control urination. Sphincter muscle always relaxed. See: *enuresis, scatacratia.*

incontinen'tia. Incontinence.
  i. alvi. Fecal incontinence.
  i. urinae. Involuntary continual dripping of urine.

incoör'dinate. 1. Not able to make coordinate muscular movements. 2. Unable to adjust one's work harmoniously with others.

incoördination (in-co-or-di-na'shun). Inability to produce harmonious, rhythmic, muscular action, but not due to weakness.

increment (in'kre-ment). 1. Increase or addition. 2. To increase or add to.

incre'tion. 1. Internal secretion. 2. Function activity of an endocrine gland. Syn: *chalone, hormone.*

incretogenous (in-kre-toj'en-us). Pert. to the internal secretions.

incretol'ogy. The science of the endocrine glands.

incretopathy (in-kre-top'ă-thI). Any disease of the endocrine glands.

in'cretory. Rel. to the internal secretion.

incretotherapy (in-kre-to-ther'ă-pĬ). Organotherapy; adm. of endocrine products.

incrusta'tion. Formation of crusts or scabs.

incubation (in-ku-ba'shun). 1. The interval between exposure to infection and the appearance of the first symptom. 2. BACT: The period of culture development. 3. The care of a premature infant in an incubator. 4. The development of an impregnated ovum. SYN: *latent period.*

in'cubator. 1. Apparatus for rearing premature babies in which the temperature may be regulated. 2. Apparatus for cultivating bacteria.   [nightmare.

incubus (in'ku-bus). 1. A burden. 2. A

in'cudal. Rel. to the incus.

incudectomy (in-ku-dek'to-mĭ). Surgical removal of the incus.

incudiform (in-ku'dĭ-form). Like an anvil in shape.

in"cudomal'leal. Rel. to the incus and malleus and articulation of the anvil and hammer in the tympanum.

incudostapedial (in-kŭ-do-stā-pe'dĭ-ăl). Pert. to the incus and stapes and articulation bet. anvil and stirrup in the tympanum.

incu'rable. Not capable of being cured. SYN: *immedicable.*

in'cus (pl. *inci*). The middle of the 3 ossicles in the tympanum; the anvil.

indagation (in-da-ga'shun). An investigation, esp. examination of the genitalia at termination of puerperium.

indenization (in-den-ĭ-za'shun). Arrest and development of cells in a part to which they have been carried by metastasis. SYN: *innidiation.*

indenta'tion. A depression or hollow.

index (in'deks) (pl. *indices*). 1. The forefinger. 2. The ratio between the measurement of a given substance compared with that of a fixed standard.

 i., alveolar. Degree of jaw prominence.

 i., cephalic. Skull breadth multiplied by 100 and divided by its length.

 i., cerebral. Ratio of greatest transverse to the greatest anteroposterior diameter of the cranium.

 i., color. The proportion of hemoglobin to each red blood corpuscle, the normal being regarded as 100. SYN: *blood quotient.*

 i., gnathic. Degree of jaw prominence expressed by a number.

 i., gonoöpsonic. Opsonic index in gonococcal infection.

 i., hemorenal. Ratio of blood's electrical resistance to urine's.

 i., opsonic. The ratio of number of bacteria which are ingested by leukocytes contained in normal serum, compared with the number ingested by leukocytes in the patient's own blood serum.

 i., pelvic. Ratio of pelvic conjugate and transverse diameters.

 i., phagocytic. Average of bacteria ingested per leukocyte of blood.

 i., refractive. Refraction coefficient.

 i., thoracic. Ratio of thoracic anteroposterior diameter to transverse diameter.

indican (in'dĭ-kăn). Potassium salt of indoxyl-sulfate, found in sweat and urine, and formed from indol.

indicanemia (in"dĭ-kan-e'mĭ-ă). Indican in the blood.

indicanu'ria. Excess of indoxyl-sulfate of potassium, a derivative of indol, in urine.

 In normal urine it is found in small quantities.

indica'tion. That which indicates the proper treatment.

 i., causal. That shown by a knowledge of the cause of a disease.

 i., morbid. That shown by diagnosis.

 i., symptomatic. That shown by symptoms.

in'dicator. A substance which can be used to distinguish acid from alkali. (In a more general sense, any substance which can be used to determine the completeness of a chemical reaction, as in volumetric analysis.)

indif'ferent. Neutral; tending in no specific direction.

indigenous (in-dij'en-us). Native to a country or region.

indigestible (in-dij-es'tĭ-bl). Not digestible.

indiges'tion. A complexus of symptoms affecting the digestive process but not an entity or a disease in itself. SYN: *dyspepsia.*

indigitation (in-dĭj-ĭ-ta'shun). Displacement of intestines by intussusception.* SYN: *invagination.*

indiguria (in"dĭ-gu'rĭ-ă). Indigo in the urine.

indirect'. Not direct.

 i. atavism. Phenomenon of transmission of characteristics not shown by, or prevailing in, the family of either parent, but possessed by a male by whom the mother had previously been impregnated. SYN: *ovarian impregnation.*

 i. cell division. Indirect changes in cell division. SEE: *karyokinesis.*

 i. reflexes. 1. Passive flexion of 1 part following flexion of another. 2. Passive flexion of 1 leg causing similar movement of opposite leg.

indirubin (in-dĭ-ru'bĭn). A reddish pigment sometimes seen in urine.

indirubinuria (in-dĭ-rū-bĭn-u'rĭ-ă). Indirubin in the urine.

indisposi'tion. Disorder; any slight or temporary illness.

indol(e. A solid, crystalline substance, C_8H_7N, found in feces, and interesting because of its presence among decomposition products of proteins and its relation to tryptophan. SYN: *ketol.*

indolaceturia (in-dol-as-ē-tu'rĭ-ă). Excretion of a considerable amt. of indolacetic acid in the urine.

in'dolent. 1. Indisposed to action. 2. Inactive; not developing; sluggish.

 i. ulcer. One that is sluggish but not painful.

indologenous (in-dol-oj'en-us). Causing the production of indol.

indoxyl (in-dok'sil). An oily substance,

C_8H_7NO, sometimes found in urine of the apparently healthy.

indoxylemia (in-doks-ĭ-le'mĭ-ă). Indoxyl in the blood.

indoxyluria (in-doks-il-u'rĭ-ă). Excretion of indoxyl in urine.

induced (in-dūsed'). Produced; caused.

  i., abortion. One brought about intentionally.

induc'tance. That property of an electric circuit by virtue of which a varying current induces an electromotive force in that circuit or a neighboring circuit.

induction (in-duk'shun). 1. The process of causing or producing, as an abortion. 2. The generation of electric current in a body by electricity in another body near it.

  i., coil. A transformer with open magnetic circuit, excited by an interrupted or variable current.

inductotherm (in-duk'to-therm). Device for producing pyrexia by electricity.

in'durate. 1. To harden. 2. Hardened.

in'durated. Hardened.

indura'tion. 1. The act of hardening. 2. An area of hardened tissue.

  i., cyanotic. An induration from long continued venous hyperemia, pressure on vessels causing transudation of blood and serum and formation of a dark, hard mass.

  i., fibrous, of the lung. A form of interstitial pneumonia. Hardened pigment forms red points on the lung.

  i., specific. The initial lesion of syphilis.

in'durative. Pert. to induration.

inebriant (in-e'brĭ-ant). 1. Any intoxicant. 2. Making drunk. [intoxicated.

ine'briate. To make drunk or to become

inebriation (in-e-bri-a'shun). State of intoxication, *q.v.* SYN: *drunkenness, intoxication.*

inelas'tic. Not elastic.

inemia (in-e'mĭ-ă). Excess fibrin or presence of inosite (muscle sugar) in the blood. SYN: *inosemia.*

inert'. Not active; sluggish.

inertia (in-er'shĭ-ă). 1. Tendency of a body to remain in repose. 2. Sluggishness; lack of activity.

  i., uterine. Absence or weakness of uterine contractions in labor.

in extremis (in-eks-tre'mis). At the point of death.

in'fant. 1. A babe. 2. A child not over 2 years of age. 3. In law, a minor, or one under legal age.

  i. development. For 3 days after birth a baby loses weight; in the next 4 days, however, it should regain its loss and weigh as much as it weighed at birth. From 1 year old to 10 years the yearly gain in the child should be 4 or 5 pounds; from 10 to 16 years the yearly gain should be about 8 pounds. Should hold up head by 4th month, sit up before 7th month, walk by 12th to 15th month, talk before 18th month.

  i., immature. One born near term, but underweight and poorly developed.

  i., mature. One born at the end of 270-290 days.

  i., premature. One born before term but viable, having a birth weight of 5½ lb. (2500 Gm.) or less, with a "crown-heel" length of 47 cm. or less; the birth weight being the most important factor.

  i. pulse. At birth, 120-150 per min.; at the end of 1st year, 120-110; 3rd-4th yr., 100; at puberty, pulse is that of an adult.

  i. respiration. At birth, 30-60 per min.; 1st yr., 25-30; 5th yr., 22-25; 14th yr., 20. SEE: *pulse, respiration, temperature.*

  i. temperature. Normal (rectal), 98°-99° F. Subnormal more important than in adults.

infanticide (in-fan'tis-īd). 1. The killing of an infant. 2. One who takes the life of an infant.

infantile (in'fan-tīl). Pert. to infancy.

  i. hernia. Oblique inguinal hernia back of the peritoneal funicular process.

  i. liver. Biliary cirrhosis* of children.

  i. paralysis. Acute ant. poliomyelitis.*

  i. tet'anus. Tetanus which begins with stiffening of jaw muscles. SYN: *trismus nascentium* or *neonatorum.*

infantilism (in-fan'til-izm). A condition in which the mind and body make slow development. Failure to attain adult characteristics, physical or psychic.

  i., angioplastic. Infantilism due to defective development of vascular system.

  i., Brissaud's. Infantile myxedema.

  i., cachectic. Infantilism caused by chronic infection or poisoning.

  i., celiac. Infantilism caused by celiac disease.

  i., dysthyroidal. Infantilism caused by defective thyroid.

  i., hepatic. Infantilism combined with cirrhosis of liver.

  i., Herter's. Infantilism of the intestines.

  i., idiopathic. Variety of arrested physical development, of unknown cause.

  i., intestinal. Infantilism associated with chronic intestinal disorder, causing the child to gain no weight nor to grow.

  i., Lorain. SEE: *idiopathic infantilism.*

  i., lymphatic. A form of infantilism associated with lymphatism.

  i., myxedematous. SYN: *cretinism.* SEE: *Brissaud's infantilism.*

  i., pancreatic. Infantilism caused by defect in pancreatic function.

  i., partial. Arrest in development of a lone tissue or part.

  i., renal. Infantilism caused by defect in renal function.

  i., reversive. Infantilism commencing subsequent to completion of bodily growth.

  i., symptomatic. Infantilism caused by poor tissue development.

  i., tardy. SEE: *reversive infantilism.*

i., toxemic. SEE: *intestinal infantilism.*

i., universal. Dwarfed stature, otherwise fairly normal development, except for absence of secondary sexual characteristics.

in'farct. 1. Extravasated matter, esp. in a vessel, causing coagulation and interference of circulation. 2. Infiltration with foreign particles.

infarc'tion. 1. Formation of an infarct. 2. Stoppage of a canal or passage, esp. by engorgement.

infec'tion. 1. Communication of a disease, as by entrance of pathogenic germs into an organism in any manner. 2. Agent which produces infection. 3. State of being infected by pathogenic microörganisms.

i., acute. Appears suddenly and runs a short course.

i., a. exacerbation. Recurrence after a period of quiescence.

i., chronic. One having a protracted course.

i., droplet. Acquired by inhalation.

i.-exhaustion psychosis. PSY: Mental disorder marked by delirium and mental confusion, occurring in connection with exhausted states.

i., focal. One occurring in a focus or cavity, and acting as a focus for dissemination of infectious material to other parts of the body. Ex: Apical tooth abscess causing infection of heart or joints.

i., local. Infection caused by germs lodging and multiplying at one point in a tissue and remaining there, as a boil.

i., low grade. Loosely used term for a subacute or chronic infection with only mild inflammation and without pus formation.

i., metastatic. Local infection caused by germs circulated from a focus of infection.

i., mixed. Caused by 2 or more organisms.

i., secondary. One in which the organisms implant themselves upon an existing primary infection in tissues.

i., simple. Due to a single species of organism.

i., subacute. Intermediate bet. acute and chronic.

i., terminal. One occurring in the late stage of a disease. Generally acute and septic.

infectious (in-fek'shus). 1. Able to be transmitted with or without contact. 2. Pert. to a disease due to a microörganism. 3. Producing infection. SEE: *eruptive.*

i. disease. Any disease caused by growth of pathogenic microörganisms in the body. May or may not be contagious.

infecundity (in-fe-kun'dĭ-tĭ). Barrenness; sterility in women.

inferior (in-fe'rĭ-or). Beneath; lower.

inferiority complex. PSY: A repressed state of mind in which one feels himself inferior to others. Such a group

of ideas may be manifested by the assumption of superiority, often resulting in over-compensation. OPP: *superiority complex.* RS: *complex.*

infest'. To infect by a parasite.

infesta'tion. Invasion by a parasite. SEE: *autoecic.*

infibulation (in-fĭb-u-la'shun). 1. Fastening the labia of the vagina together, or the prepuce over the glans penis. 2. Joining the lips of wounds by clasps.

infiltrate (in-fĭl'trāt). Diffused by or affected with infiltration.

infiltration (in-fĭl-tra'shun). Fluid or solid foreign substances deposited in and diffused through a tissue, organ, or cell. Ex: Infiltration of a tissue or organ with blood corpuscles, or a cell by fatty particles.

i., amyloid. Infiltration of tissue or viscera with a glycoprotein.

i. anesthesia. Injection of a cocaine or similar solution. SEE: *anesthesia.*

i., calcareous. Deposits of salts within a tissue.

i., cellular. Infiltration of round cells into tissues.

i., fatty. Deposit of fat in the tissues, or oil or fat globules in the cells.

i., glycogenic. Glycogen deposit in cells.

i., pigmentary. Of pigments.

i., purulent. Pus cells in a tissue.

i., serous. With diluted lymph.

i., urinous. With urine.

i., waxy. Amyloid degeneration.

in'finite distance. 1. Infinity. 2. Inner limit of vision, about 20 feet. The rays of light from that point are practically parallel.

infir'mary. A small hospital.

inflamma'tion. Morbid tissue reaction to injury, either direct or referred.

i., acute. One in which active processes are manifested.

i., adhesive. One conducive to the healing of wounds.

i., alterative. One in which the degenerative change predominates.

i., catarrhal. One affecting a mucous membrane which gives off epithelium.

i., chronic. One that makes the formation of connective tissue possible.

i., exudative. One in which there is a large accumulation of blood cells and serum.

i., reactive. One about a foreign body or a focus of infection.

i., specific. One caused by a specific microörganism.

i., suppurative. One that forms pus.

i., toxic. This is one due to toxin or poison.   [flammation.

inflam'matory. Rel. to or marked by inflation.

inflation (in-fla'shun). Distention of a part by air, gas, or liquid.

inflection (in-flek'shun). 1. An inward bending. 2. Change of tone or pitch of the voice; nuance.

influence machine. A particular type of "static machine." Probably the only type used in physical therapy.

influenza (in-flu-en'za). Grip, an acute infectious disease characterized by fever, extreme prostration, pain in head and back, and generally by catarrh of respiratory or gastrointestinal tract. SYN: *la grippe*.

influenzal (in-flu-en'zal). Relating to influenza.

infra-. Prefix: *Below*.

infraäxillary (in"fră-aks'il-a-rĭ). Below the axilla.

in"fraclavic'ular. Below the clavicle.

infracostal (in-fră-kos'tal). Below a rib.

infraglenoid (in"fră-glē'noyd). Beneath the glenoid fossa. SYN: *subglenoid*.

infrahyoid (in-fră-hi'oid). Below the hyoid bone.

inframam'mary. Below the mammary gland.

inframar'ginal. Below any edge or margin.
  l. convolution. The sup. temporal one.

inframax'illary. Below the jaw; submaxillary.

infranu'clear. Below the nucleus.

infraocclu'sion. Location of a tooth below the line of occlusion.

infraorbital (in-fră-or'bĭ-tal). Beneath the orbit.

infrapatellar (in"fră-pă-tel'ăr). Below the patella.

infrapsychic (in-fră-si'kik). Automatic; subconscious.

infrapu'bic. Below the pubis.

in'frared rays. Invisible heat rays beyond red end of spectrum.

infrascap'ular. Beneath the shoulder blade.

infraspi'nous. Beneath the scapular spine.

infraster'nal. Beneath the sternum.

infratrochlear (in"fră-trok'le-ăr). Beneath the trochlea.

infric'tion. Rubbing of ointments into the skin. SYN: *inunction*.

infundibuliform (in-fun-dib'u-lĭ-form). Funnel-shaped.
  l. fascia, l. process. The membranous layer investing the spermatic cord.

infundib'ulin. A 20% solution of an extract of the post. lobe of the hypophysis.

infundibulum (in-fun-dib'u-lum). 1. Funnel-shaped passage or body. 2. Tube connecting the frontal sinus with the middle nasal meatus. 3. Stalk of the pituitary gland. 4. Any renal pelvis division. 5. Cavity formed by fallopian fimbriae. 6. Terminus of a bronchiole. 7. Terminus at upper end of cochlear canal. 8. Conelike upper ant. angle of right cardiac ventricle, from which the pulmonary artery arises. SYN: *conus arteriosus*.

infu'sible. 1. Not capable of being fused or melted. 2. Capable of being made into an infusion.

infusion (in-fu'zhun). 1. Steeping a substance in cold or hot water below boiling point to obtain its active principles. 2. Product obtained by such a process. SYN: *infusum*. 3. Introduction of a liquid into a vein.
  l., intravenous. Injection of a solution directly into a vein, usually the cephalic

or median basilic vein. Normal saline intravenous solutions are usually temporary in effect due to loss of water in tissues.

infusodecoction (in-fu"zo-de-kok'shun). 1. Infusion followed by decoction. 2. A medicine made from a crude drug steeped in cold water and then in boiling water.

infusor (in-fu'zor). Instrument for injecting a liquid slowly into a vein.

Infusoria (in-fu-so'rĭ-ă). Microscopic unicellular animalcules; the highest type of *Protozoa*.

infu'sum. Liquid preparations made by treating vegetable substances with hot or cold water.

ingesta (in-jes'tă). Food and drink received into the body through the mouth.

inges'tion. The process of taking material (particularly food) into the gastrointestinal tract, or by which a cell takes in foreign particles.

Ingras'sias' apoph'yses. The lesser wings of the sphenoid.

ingravescent (in-grav-es'ent). Becoming more severe.

ingre'dient. Any part of a compound; a unit of a more complex substance.

in'growing. Growing inward.
  l. nail. One growing into the flesh. SYN: *onyxia*.

inguen (in'gwen). The groin.

inguinal (in'gwi-nal). Pert. to the region of the groin.
  l. canal. The one carrying the spermatic cord in the male, and the round ligament in the female. It is 1½ in. long; a potential source of weakness and may be the site of a hernia.
  l. glands. Those of the groin.
  l. hernia. Hernia in inguinal region.
  l. ligament. Fibrous l. bet. ant. sup. spine of ileum and the pubic spine and the pectineal line. SYN: *Poupart's ligament*.
  l. reflex. One in females resembling cremasteric* reflex in males.
  l. region. The groin. The iliac region on either side of the pubes.
  l. ring. Int. opening of the inguinal canal (abdominal inguinal ring), and the end of the inguinal canal (subcutaneous inguinal ring).

inhal'ant. That which may be inhaled.

inhalation (in-ha-la'shun). 1. Act of drawing in of breath, vapor, or gas into the lungs; inspiration. 2. Introduction of dry or moist air or vapor into the lungs for therapeutic purposes, such as *amyl nitrite* to relieve attack of angina pectoris, *aromatic spirits of ammonia* used to overcome fainting.

inhale'. To draw in the breath; to inspire.

inhaler (in-ha'ler). Device for inhaling medicinal vapors or steam.

inhe'rent. Intrinsic; belonging to anything naturally, originally, not as result of circumstances.
  l. cauterization. Deep cauterization.

inhibition (ĭn-hĭb-ĭsh'ŭn). 1. Act of repressing or state of being repressed; restraint. 2. PHYS: A stopping of an action or function of an organ. 3. PSY: Restraint of 1 mental process almost simultaneously by another opposed mental process; an inner impediment to free activity.

i., psychic. Arrest of an impulse, thought, action, or speech. The term is commonly applied to the denial of the sex instinct. SYN: *suppression.*

inhib'itor. That which inhibits.

inhibitory (in-hib'ĭ-to-rĭ). Checking or arresting any function or action.

inhibitrope (in-hib'ĭ-trōp). One in whom certain stimuli cause partial arrest of function.

iniac, inial (in'ĭ-ak, -ăl). Pert. to the inion.

inion (in'ĭ-on). 1. Occiput. 2. Back portion of neck. 3. External occipital protuberance.

initial (in-ish'al). Incipient; rel. to the beginning, or commencing.

initis (in-i'tis). 1. Inflammation of fibrous tissue. 2. Inflammation of a tendon. 3. Inflamed condition of a muscle. SYN: *myositis.*

inject'. To introduce fluid into the body or its parts artifically.

injec'ted. Filled by injection of fluid; congested.

injection (in-jeck'shun). 1. Forcing of a fluid into a vessel or cavity or under the skin. 2. Substance introduced in this manner. 3. State of being injected; congestion.

i., air. Spinal injection of air to locate a growth, degree of central atrophy in general paresis, and to find cause of epilepsy.

i., colonic. Into the colon.

i., epidural. Spinal injection given to relieve pain in limbs in tabes dorsalis or tabes paresis and in gastric crisis.

i., hypodermic. A subcutaneous one, generally in front of thighs, or outer part of arms or forearms.

i., intracutaneous. Injections into the skin, a method employed in giving of serums and vaccines when a local reaction is desired.

i., intramuscular. Into intramuscular tissue, usually in front of thigh or in 1 of the buttocks.

i., intravenous.* Into a vein.

i., lipiodol. Spinal injection to locate spinal cord block or tumor.

i., rectal. Into the rectum; an enema.

i., subcutaneous. Injection beneath the skin. SYN: *hypodermic injection.*

i., vaginal. A douche.

inject'ors. Various instruments for injecting medicinal fluids, making hypodermic injections and for transfusion of blood and intravenous injection.

in'jury. A hurt or damage.

ink poisoning. Many of the poisonings ascribed to ink are in the form of dermatitis. Several types of materials may be responsible. Ordinary ink may cause irritation, either because of irritating nature, or because of susceptibility of

particular skins. Sometimes cleaning materials used in removing ink stains have been found to be causative agents.

F. A. TREATMENT: Wash with alcohol, soap and water. Rinse carefully, apply a bland dressing, as calomel, cold cream, etc.

in'lay. A solid filling made to the shape of a cavity of a tooth and cemented into it.

in'let. Passage leading to a cavity.

i. of the pel'vis. The upper opening into the pelvic cavity.

innate'. Inborn; congenital.

innervate (ĭn-nur'văt). To stimulate a part.

innervation (in-er-va'shun). 1. Stimulation of a part through the action of nerves. 2. The distribution and function of the nervous system. 3. The nerve supply of a part.

i., collateral. Supply of nervous force through an adjacent nerve tract to a part of which original nerve supply has been injured or destroyed.

innidiation (in-nid-I-a'shun). Multiplication of cells in a part to which they have been carried by metastasis.

innocent (in'o-sent). Benign; not malignant. SYN: *innocuous.*

innoc'uous. Harmless.

innominate (in-nom'ĭ-năt). Nameless.

i. artery. Right artery arising from the arch of the aorta, dividing into the right subclavian and right common carotid arteries.

i. bone. Os innominata. The hip bone, composed of the *ilium, ischium,* and *pubis;* united to form the pelvis by the sacrum and coccyx.

SEE: *ischium, pubes.*

i. veins. Right and left vein formed by union of internal jugular with subclavian veins.

innoxious (in-ok'shus). Not harmful.

inoblast (in'o-blast). Connective tissue cell in embryonic form.

inochondritis (in''o-kon-dri'tis). Inflammation of a fibrocartilage.

inochondroma (in''o-kon-dro'mă). A chondroma or tumor with much fibrous tissue; fibrochondroma.

inoculability (in-ok-u-lă-bil'ĭ-tĭ). Quality of being susceptible to transmission of infection by inoculation.

inoc'ulable. 1. Transmissible by inoculation. 2. Susceptible to a transmissible disease. 3. Capable of being inoculated.

inoc'ulate. To inject the virus of a disease into the body.

inoculation (in-ok-u-la'shun). Intentional introduction of a virus into the system as a preventive against the acquisition of certain diseases; it may be antidiphtheritic, antirabic, antitetanic, or antityphoid.

inoc'ulum. A substance or virus introduced by inoculation.

inocyst (in'o-sĭst). A fibrous capsule.

inocystoma (in''o-sis-to'mă). Fibrous tumor undergoing cystic degeneration.

inocyte (in'o-sĭt). A fiber cell.

inoepithelioma (in″o-ep-ĭ-the-lĭ-o′mă). Epithelioma containing fibrous tissue.

inogen (in′o-jen). The hypothetical contractile substance of muscle supposed to become decomposed during contraction, and during rest of the muscle, to be re-formed.

inogenesis (in-o-jen′e-sis). The development of fibrous or muscular tissue.

ino′genous. Forming tissue or produced from it.

inoglia (in-og′lĭ-ă). The basement substance of connective tissue cells. SYN: *fibroglia.*

inohymenitis (in-o-hĭ-men-i′tis). Inflammation of any fibrous membrane or of an aponeurosis.

inoliomyoma (in″o-li-o-mĭ-o′mă). A smooth muscle tissue tumor.

in′olith. A concretion formed from fibrous tissue.

inoma (in-o′mă). A fibrous tumor. SYN: *fibroma.*

inomyoma (in-o-mi-o′mă). A fibrous tissue myoma. SYN: *fibromyoma.*

inomyositis (in-o-mi-o-si′tis). Chronic muscular inflammation with connective tissue hyperplasia. SYN: *fibromyositis.*

inomyxo′ma. A mixed myxoma and fibroma. SYN: *fibromyxoma.*

inoneuroma (in″o-nu-ro′ma). A mixed neuroma and inoma. SYN: *fibroneuroma.*

inop′erable. Unsuitable for being operated upon without danger of death.

inopex′ia. Tendency of the blood to spontaneous coagulation in the vessels.

inorgan′ic. 1. In chemistry, occurring in nature independently of living things. 2. Not pert. to living organisms. 3. Pert. to a functional disorder.
  i. acid. An acid composed of inorganic constituents. SYN: *acid, mineral.*
  i. chemistry. Chemistry dealing only with inorganic compounds.
  i. compound. One without carbon.

inosclerosis (in-o-skle-ro′sis). Increased fibrous tissue density.

inos′copy. Diagnosis by examining fibrinous deposits in body fluids.

inos′culating. Directly communicating; anastomosing.

inosculation (in-os-ku-la′shun). Union of two vessels; anastomosis.*

inosemia (in-o-se′mĭ-ă). Inosite in the blood.

inosin′ic acid. A muscle tissue acid.

inosite (in′o-sīt). A saccharine substance, $C_6H_{12}O_6 + 2H_2O$ in the human body as in the muscular substance of the heart, the brain, the kidneys), and in peas, beans, and other plants.

inositis (in-o-si′tis). Inflammation of fibrous tissue.

inosituria (in″o-si-tu′rĭ-ă). Inosite in the urine.

inosteotoma (in″os-te-ă-to′mă). Fatty tumor with fibroma.

inosto′sis. Bony tissue that re-forms to replace bony tissue that has been destroyed.

inosuria (in-o-su′rĭ-ă). Inosite in the urine. SYN: *inosituria.*

inotag′ma. A contractile element found in living protoplasm.

inotropic (in-o-trop′ik). Pert. to whatever modifies the contractility of the muscular tissue.
  i. nerves. Fibers of cardiac nerves which affect the force of combustion in a negative or positive manner.

in′quest. 1. A legal medical examination of a corpse to ascertain the cause of death. 2. The act of inquiring.

insaliva′tion. The process of mixing saliva with food, as in chewing.

insalu′brious. Not healthy or contributing to health.

insane (in-sān′). Mentally deranged; pert. to insanity.

insan′itary. Not conducive to health; unhealthful, esp. pert. to filth.

insan′ity. Legal term for mental derangement; a psychosis.*
  i., alcoholic-delusional. A degenerative process marked by delusions.
  i., circular. Returning in cycles.
  i., climacteric. Occurring at the menopause.
  i., concurrent. Caused by disease.
  i., confusional. Temporary, due to nervous shock.
  i., congenital. From birth.
  i., depressive. Melancholia.
  i., deuteropathic. Secondary to some other disease.
  i., diathetic. Inherited.
  i., homicidal. Desire to kill.
  i., manic depressive. Ordinarily a series of periods of psychotic depression or excessive well-being, appearing in any sequence and alternating with longer periods of relative normalcy.
  i., paroxysmal. Temporary attacks.
  i., perceptional. Illusions and hallucinations.
  i., recurrent. Occurring at intervals.
  i., senile. Due to old age.

insatiable (in-sā′shĭ-a-bl). Incapable of being satisfied or appeased.

inscriptio (in-skrip′shyo). Inscription.
  i. tendin′ea. Tendinous band traversing a muscle. BNA.

inscription (in-skrip′shun). Body of a prescription which gives the names of the drugs prescribed and dosage.

in′sect. Common name for any of the class *Insecta*, of the phylum *Arthropoda*, such as flies, mosquitoes, and ticks.

insecticide (in-sek′tĭ-sīd). 1. An agent used to exterminate insects. 2. Destructive to insects.

insemination (in-sem-in-a′shun). 1. Discharge of semen from the penis into the vagina during coitus. 2. Fertilization of an ovum.
  i., artificial. Artificial injection of semen into the uterine canal. Sometimes resorted to in sterility of the husband. Legal complications as to heritage and inheritance may arise and psychological results may be disastrous to all concerned. SEE: *impregnation.*

insen′sible. 1. Unconscious; without feeling or consciousness. 2. Not perceptible.

inser'tion. 1. The manner or place of attachment of a muscle to the bone that it moves. 2. A putting into.

insidious (in-sid'i-us). Stealthy, treacherous, hidden; not apparent, as a disease that does not exhibit early symptoms of its advent.

in'sight. PSY. Understanding of oneself or of any nervous or mental difficulties one may have.

in si'tu. In position.

insolation (in-so-la'shun). 1. Any exposure to the rays of the sun. 2. Heat- or sunstroke.

insoluble (in-sol'u-bl). Incapable of solution or of being dissolved.

insomnia (in-som'nĭ-ă). Chronic inability to sleep, or sleep prematurely ended or interrupted by periods of wakefulness.

inspect'. To examine visually.

inspec'tion. The ocular examination of the external surface of the body. SEE: *abdominal, chest, and circulatory system.*

inspersion (in-sper'shun). Sprinkling with powder or a fluid.

inspiration (in-spir-a'shun). Inhalation; drawing air into the lungs. Opp. of *expiration, q.v.*

  i., crowing. Peculiar noise in laryngismus stridulus* or spasmodic croup.*

  i., external. Interchange of gases in the lungs.

  i., forcible, difficult, labored. In which the muscles of inspiration are assisted by inspiratory auxiliaries (*i. e.,* muscles attached to chest which by contraction increase the thoracic cavity directly or indirectly by furnishing fixed support whereby other muscles may act more advantageously). If movements become excessively labored, there is brought into coördinate action every muscle in the body which can either directly or indirectly increase the cavity of the thorax.

  i., full. In which lungs are filled as completely as possible (voluntarily, as in determining the amount of complemental air, or involuntarily, as in cardiac dyspnea).

  i., internal. Interchange of gases in the tissues.

inspiratory (in-spi'ră-tor-ĭ). Pert. to inspiration.

inspissate (in-spis'ăt). To thicken by evaporation or absorption of fluid.

inspissated (in'spis-să-ted). Thickened by absorption, evaporation, or dehydration.

inspissation (in-spis-sa'shun). 1. Thickening by evaporation or absorption of fluid. 2. Diminished fluidity or increased thickness.

in'step. Arch on upper surface of foot in the middle, in front of ankle.

  Breaking down of this arch constitutes *flatfoot.* SEE: *cuboid bone.*

instillation (in-stil-a'shun). Pouring in a liquid, drop by drop.

instinct (in'stinkt). 1. Inherent (racial) patterns of expression normally manifested under suitable conditions, usually heavily loaded with emotional value (libido in its widest sense). Innate

urges, principally voluntary, with which one is born and which are necessary for the preservation of life.

  2. An urge, uncontrolled by reason, to react to stimuli of an emotional nature.

instinct'ive. Determined by instinct.

instrument (in'stru-ment). A tool or piece of apparatus.

instrumental (in-stru-men'tal). 1. Pert. to instruments. 2. Being the cause of anything.

  i. delivery. Delivery of a fetus with forceps.

instrumenta'tion. The use of instruments, and their care.

insufficiency (in-suf-fish'en-sĭ). The condition of being inadequate for its purpose.

  i., absolute. Insufficiency due to thickening, induration, or other change in cardiac valves.

  i., aortic. An imperfect closure of the aortic valves.

  i., cardiac. Inability of heart to function normally.

  i., functional mitral. Due to deficient muscular contractility in the heart.

  i., gastric. Inability of the stomach to empty itself.

  i., hepatic. Inability of the liver to function properly.

  i., mitral. In which the mitral valve inefficiently closes with rhythmic action of the heart.

  i., muscular. Condition of a relatively weak muscle compared with its antagonist.

  i. of the ocular muscles. An absence of dynamical equilibrium of the ocular muscles.

  i., relative. The dilatation of a valvular orifice of the heart because of general enlargement.

  i., valvular. Inability of cardiac valves to close perfectly, permitting leakage of blood.

insuf'flate. 1. To blow in, as in the lungs of a newborn infant. 2. To blow a medicated powder or medicinal vapor into a cavity.

insuffla'tion. The act of blowing a vapor or powder into a cavity, as the lungs.

insufflator (in'suf-fla-tor). Device for blowing powders into a cavity.

in'sula. 1. BNA. The island of Reil within the lateral cerebral fissure. 2. The islands of Langerhans in the pancreas, *q.v.* 3. Any round cutaneous body or patch.

insular (ins'u-lar). Rel. to any insula, esp. the islands of Langerhans.

  i. hypothesis. Theory that loss of function or destruction of islands of Langerhans is the cause of diabetes.

insula'tion. 1. Protection of an electrical conductor with some nonconducting medium, so as to prevent the escape of electricity. 2. The material or substance which insulates.

in'sulator. That which insulates; specifically, a substance or body that interrupts the transmission of electricity to surrounding objects by conduction; anything that exerts great resistance to the passage of an electric current by conduction. SEE: *nonconductor*.

in'sulin. A hormone of the internal secretion of the islets* of Langerhans in the pancreas, which aids the oxidation and utilization of blood sugar by the tissues, and controls the level of the blood sugar.

i., globin. New insulin combination being tried in cases not controlled by protamine zinc. It is said to have a number of advantages and easily controls all mild and moderately severe cases of diabetes.

i., protamine zinc. A preparation of insulin, modified by the addition of protamine and a zinc salt.

DOSAGE: Regulated by the physician.

i. shock. Circulatory insufficiency from overdose of insulin, causing too rapid blood sugar reduction.

i. s. treatment. Spinal injection of insulin for schizophrenia* to stimulate general metabolism, liver function, and to eliminate toxins. It has a specific vagotropic action and revives strong primitive normal responses and eliminates recent abnormal ones.

insulinemia (in-su-lin-e'mĭ-ă). An undue amt. of insulin in the blood.

insuliniza'tion. Insulin therapy.

insulinogenic (in-su-lin-o-jen'ĭk). Caused by hyperinsulinism.

insulinoid (in'su-lin-oid). Resembling or having the properties of insulin.

insulogenic (in-su-lo-jen'ĭk). Produced by overproduction or overadministration of insulin. SYN: *insulinogenic*.

insulo'ma. A tumor of the island of Reil or of the islands of Langerhans.

insulopath'ic. Rel. to or caused by abnormal insulin secretion.

insusceptibility (in"sus-sep"tĭ-bil'ĭ-tĭ). Incapability of becoming infected with a germ disease. SYN: *immunity*.

integration (in-te-gra'shun). 1. Assimilation. 2. A harmonious relationship of the parts constituting the whole of anything.

i., primary. Early recognition of the body and its psyche as apart from one's environment.

i., secondary. The process involved in developing the adult personality, through sublimation of the sex instinct and its components.

Integrator (in'te-gra-tor). Device for measuring body surfaces.

integument (in-teg'u-ment). 1. A covering. 2. The skin, consisting of the *corium* or *dermis*, and *epidermis*.

integumentary (in-teg-ū-men'tă-rĭ). Rel. to the integument. SYN: *cutaneous, dermal*.

in'tellect. The mind, or understanding; conscious brain function.

intellec'tual. 1. Pert. to the mind. 2. Possessing intellect.

intel'ligence. The capacity to comprehend relationships.

i. classification. Estimation of degree of intelligence possessed by different mental types.

i. quotient (I. Q.). An index of mental age or intelligence determined through the subject's answers to arbitrarily chosen questions, obtained by dividing the mental age by the chronological age, or 16 years, which is the arbitrary figure chosen for those 16 years or over, the divisor never exceeding this figure.

intem'perance. Excess in the use of anything; lack of moderation.

inten'sifying. Making intense.

i. screen. A thin sheet of celluloid or other substance coated with a finely divided substance which fluoresces under the influence of roentgen rays and is intended to be used in close contact with the emulsion of a photographic plate or film for the purpose of reinforcing the image. A fluorescent screen.

inten'simeter. An instrument, often a selenium cell or ionization chamber, designed to measure the intensity of a beam to about 14,000 Angstrom units.

intensity (in-ten'sĭ-tĭ). A high degree of activity; marked by tension.

i. of electric field. The intensity of an electric field is measured by the force exerted on unit charge. Unit field intensity is the field which exerts the force of one dyne on unit positive charge.

i. of roentgen rays. The attribute of a beam of roentgen rays which determines the rate of ionization of air at a given point, under the conditions stipulated in the definition of roentgen. It is expressed in roentgens per unit of time. SEE: *rays*.   [by intensity.

intensive (in-ten'sĭv). Rel. to or marked

intention (ĭn-tĕn'shŭn). 1. A natural process of healing. 2. Goal or purpose.

i., first. Healing without granulation or suppuration.

i., second. Healing by adhesion of two granulated surfaces with suppuration.

i., third. Healing of an ulcer, wound, or cavity by filling by granulation and followed by cicatrization. SEE: *first intention, granulation, resolution, second intention, third intention*.

i. tremor. One exhibited or intensified when attempting coördinated movements.

inter-. Prefix: In the midst, between.

interartic'ular. 1. Bet. two joints. 2. Situated bet. two articulating surfaces.

interatrial (ĭn"ter-at'rĭ-ăl). Located bet. the atria of the heart. SYN: *interauricular*.

interauricular (in"ter-aw-rik'u-lar). 1. Situated bet. the auricles or pinnae. 2. Interatrial.

in'terbrain. The hinder original part of the forebrain including the *thalamus*, pineal body (*epithalamus*) and geniculate bodies (*metathalamus*). SYN: *diencephalon, thalamencephalon*.

intercadence (in-ter-ka'dens). A supernumerary pulse wave bet. two regular beats.

intercalary (in-ter'kal-a-rĭ). 1. Inserted between as something in addition; extraneous. 2. Pert. to an upstroke on a pulse tracing which comes bet. two pulse beats, intercalated.

intercarot'ic. Bet. the ext. and int. carotid arteries.
> **i. body.** Small oval body in bifurcation of the common carotid artery; function unknown. SYN: *glomus caroticum.*

in"tercartilag'inous. Connecting or bet. cartilages.

intercellular (in-ter-sel'u-lar). Bet. the cells of a structure.

intercen'tral. Connecting or bet. two or more centers.

interchondral (in-ter-kon'dral). Bet. cartilages. SYN: *intercartilaginous.*

intercilium (in-ter-sil'ĭ-um). The space bet. the eyebrows. SYN: *glabella.*

interclavic'ular. Bet. the clavicles.

intercolumnar (in-ter-kŏ-lum'nar). Bet. columns.
> **i. fascia.** A membrane bet. pillars of the abdominal ring, enclosing the spermatic cord.
> **i. fibers.** Intercrural fibers.

intercon'dylar, intercon'dyloid, intercon'dylous. Bet. two condyles (the rounded eminence at the articular end of a bone).

intercos'tal. Bet. the ribs.

intercos"tohumera'lis. 1. The post. lateral branch of second intercostal nerve supplying the skin of the arm. 2. Similar branch of the third intercostal nerve.

in'tercourse. 1. Social contacts. 2. The sexual act. SYN: *coition, coitus, copulation.*

intercris'tal. Bet. two crests of a bone, organ, or process.

intercrural (ĭn"ter-kru'răl). Bet. the legs or 2 stalks.

intercur'rent. 1. Intervening. 2. Pert. to a disease attacking a patient with another malady.

interden'tal. Bet. the teeth.

interdentium (in-ter-den'shĭ-um). The space bet. any two contiguous teeth.

interdigita'tion. 1. Interlocking of toothed or fingerlike processes. 2. Processes so interlocked.

interfascicular (in-ter-fas-ik'u-lar). Bet. fasciculi.

interfemoral (in-ter-fem'or-ăl). Bet. the thighs.

interfib'rillar, interfib'rillary. Bet. fibrils.

interfi'lar. Bet. the fibrils of a reticulum.

interganglion'ic. Bet. ganglions.

interglob'ular. Bet. globules.
> **i. spaces.** Gaps in dentin due to failure of calcification. SYN: *Czermak's spaces.*

interlo'bar. Bet. lobes.

interlobi'tis. Inflammation of the pleura separating the pulmonary lobes.

interlob'ular. Bet. lobules of an organ.
> **i. emphysema.** Air bet. the lobes of the lung.

intermar'riage. 1. Marriage bet. persons of two different races or tribes. SYN: *miscegenation.* 2. Marriage bet. blood relations.

intermax'illary. Bet. the jaws or maxillae.

intermediary (in-ter-me'dĭ-ă-rĭ). 1. Situated bet. two bodies. 2. Occurring bet. two periods of time.
> **i. amputation.** One performed during the stage of inflammatory fever.
> **i. body.** An amboceptor; an immune body. SEE: *Ehrlich's side-chain theory.*
> **i. metabolism.** The series of intermediate compounds formed during digestion before the final excretion or oxidation products are eliminated from the body.

intermedin (in-ter-me'din). A pituitary hormone from pars intermedia of hypophysis. SEE: *hormone.*

intermediolat'eral. Intermediate but not central.
> **i. tract of spinal cord.** A lateral tract bet. the dorsal and ventral horns.

intermeningeal (in-ter-men-in'je-ăl). Bet. the meninges.

intermis'sion. 1. Interval bet. two paroxysms of a disease. 2. Temporary cessation of symptoms.

intermit'tence. 1. Condition marked by intermissions in the course of a disease or of a process. 2. A loss of one or more pulse beats.   [intervals.

intermittent (in-ter-mit'ent). Ceasing at
> **i. fever.** One in which there is complete absence of symptoms bet. paroxysms of the fever. SEE: *malaria, undulant fever, remittent fever.*
> **i. pulse.** One in which a beat is dropped at intervals; significant of cardiac exhaustion; serious in pneumonia.
> **i. temperature.** One that reaches the normal line at intervals during the course of a fever.

intermus'cular. Bet. muscles.

intern (in'tern). An assistant resident physician or surgeon on a hospital staff, usually a recent graduate. Cf. *externe.*

inter'nal. Within the body.
> **i. bleeding.** Internal hemorrhage, *q.v.*
> **i. capsule.** Nerve fiber leading into lenticular nucleus.
> **i. ear.** The *vestibule, semicircular canals,* and *cochlea.*
> **i. injury.** Injury of the large abdominal cavities in which important viscera or blood vessels are injured.
> **i. medicine.** Medicine as opposed to surgery.
> **i. secretion.** That of the ductless glands which, entering the blood stream, activates other glands and organs. SYN: *hormones, q.v.*
> SEE: *secretion, ductless gland, endocrine.*

internation (in-ter-na'shun). The act of incarcerating, as a mental patient.

international x-ray unit of intensity. Quantity of x-radiation, which, when secondary electrons are fully utilized and wall effect of chamber is avoided, produces in 1 cc. of atmospheric air at 0.0° C. and 76 cm. mercury pressure, such a degree of conductivity that one electrostatic unit of charge is measured at saturation current. Designated by r.

interne (in'tern). An assistant resident physician or surgeon on a hospital staff, usually a recent graduate. SYN: *intern.* SEE: *externe.*

intern'ist. One who treats internal diseases; not a surgeon.

in'ternode. Space bet. adjacent nodes.

internun'cial. Acting as a connecting medium.

   i. **fibers.** Fibers connecting nerve cells.

inter'nus. 1. Internal rectus muscle of the eye. 2. Internal.

interocep'tive. In nerve physiology, concerned with sensations arising within the body itself, as distinguished from those (as, for instance, sight) arising outside the body.

interoceptor (in"ter-o-sep'tor). A ceptor activated by stimuli within the body.

   i., **general.** An end organ carrying sensations of hunger, thirst, visceral pain, nausea, sexual and circulatory sensations.

   i., **special.** One for smell and taste.

interofec'tive. 1. Pert. to that which concerns the interior of an organism. 2. Cannon's term concerning the autonomic nervous system.

in"tero-infe'rior. Pert. to an inward and downward position.

interol'ivary. Bet. the olivary bodies.

interor'bital. Bet. the orbits.

inteross'eous. Situated or occurring bet. bones, as some muscles and ligaments.

interpalpebral (in-ter-pal'pe-bral). Bet. the eyelids.

interpari'etal. Bet. parietal bones.

   i. **bone.** Upper squamous portion of occipital bone. SYN: *os interparietale.*

   i. **suture.** Sagittal suture.

interparoxys'mal. Bet. paroxysms.

interpeduncular (in"ter-pe-dunk'u-lar). Bet. peduncles.

interphalangeal (in"ter-fă-lan'jē-ăl). In a joint bet. two phalanges.

interpolar (in"ter-po'lar). Bet. two poles.

   i. **path.** Path of galvanic current through tissues bet. poles.

interprox'imal. Bet. two adjoining surfaces.

   i. **space.** Triangular space bet. two adjacent teeth.

interpu'bic. Bet. the pubic bones.

interpu'pillary. Bet. the pupils.

interre'nal. Bet. the kidneys.

   i. **system.** The cortex of the adrenal gland.

interrenalin (in-ter-ren'al-in). Hormone of the adrenal cortex prepared for adm. orally.

interrenotropic (in-ter-re"no-trop'ik). Pert. to a dominating influence of the adrenals. SYN: *adrenotropic.*

interrupt'er. A mechanical or electrolytic device for making and breaking (closing and opening alternately) an electrical circuit. Such a device is ordinarily employed in low voltage, direct current circuits.

interscapil'ium. Area bet. the shoulders or scapulae.

interscap'ular. Bet. the scapulae.

   i. **reflex.** Scapular muscular contraction following percussion or stimulus bet. the scapulae.

intersca'pulum. Section of back bet. shoulder blades. SYN: *interscapilium.*

inter'stice. A space or gap in a tissue or structure of an organ.

interstitial (in-ter-stish'al). 1. Placed or lying bet.; pert. to interstices or spaces. 2. Occupying space bet. essential parts of an organ which comprises its proper tissue; opp. to *parenchymatous.*

   SEE: *cell, gland, irradiation, keratitis, pregnancy, tissue.*

intersystole (in-ter-sis'to-le). The period bet. the end of the auricular systole and the commencement of the ventricular systole.

intertrigo (in-ter-tri'go). A superficial dermatitis in the folds of the skin. SEE: *erythema intertrigo.* SYN: *paratrimma.*

intertrochanteric (in"ter-tro-kăn-ter'ĭk). Bet. the femur's two trochanters.

   i. **line.** The ridge bet. the greater and lesser trochanters of femur on post. aspect of the bone.

intertubular (in-ter-tu'bu-lar). Bet. or among tubules.

interureteral (in"ter-u-re'ter-al). Bet. the two ureters. SYN: *interureteric.*

interureteric (in"ter-u-re-ter'ik). Bet. the ureters. SYN: *interureteral.*

intervaginal (in-ter-vaj'in-al). 1. Bet. sheaths. 2. Within the vagina.

interval (in'ter-val). 1. The space or time bet. two objects or periods. 2. Break in the course of a disease or bet. paroxysms.

   i., **a.-c.;** *i.,* **atriocarotid;** *i.,* **auriculocarotid.** The interval bet. the auricular and carotid waves; the intersystolic period.

   i., **c.-a.;** *i.,* **cardio-arterial.** The time bet. apex beat and radial pulsation.

   i., **focal.** Distance bet. ant. and post. focal point.

   i., **lucid.** Brief remission of symptoms in a psychosis. [heart.

   i., **passive.** The rest period of the

   i., **postsphygmic.** The period bet. ventricular dilatation and opening of the auriculoventricular valves.

   i., **presphygmic.** Brief period bet. the ventricular systole and opening of the semilunar valves.

intervalvular (in-ter-val'vu-lar). Among valves.

intervascular (in-ter-vas'ku-lar). Situated bet. blood vessels.

interventric'ular. Bet. the ventricles.

interver'tebral. Situated bet. two adjacent vertebrae.

   i. **disc.** Broad and flattened disc of fibrocartilage bet. the bodies of vertebrae, as in *symphysis.**

intes'tin. Commercial preparation used as an intestinal antiseptic.

intes'tinal. Pert. to the intestines.

   i. **digestion.** The mixture of food and secretions described under *duodenal** digestion moves on rapidly through the jejunum and is then detained for some hours in the lone remaining part of the small intestine, the ileum.

i. d., chemical. The hydrolysis of starches and sugars to monosaccharides is accomplished by enzymes provided by the pancreatic and intestinal juices. The fats are emulsified by the bile, and then hydrolyzed by the action of the lipase (steapsin) of the pancreatic juice.

i. d., mechanical. Both digestion and absorption are accelerated by a continual mixing and moving of the intestinal contents.

i. flora. Bacteria in intestines of which *Bacillus acidophilus* is the most favorable.

i. gases. Carbon dioxide, hydrogen, methane, methylmercaptan, and sulfureted hydrogen.

i. juice. A secretion of the crypts of Lieberkühn and the simple follicles in the small intestines.

i. obstruction. *Acute*: Small intestine usually involved. Due to intussusception, strangulation, volvulus (twists), foreign bodies, knots, adhesions, tumors, stricture, and gallstones in intestines.
Chronic: Involves large intestine. Due to stricture, inflammation, abscesses, tumors, fecal matter or chronic peritonitis, and gallstones may obstruct feces. Gradual constipation, pain becoming more severe in few days followed by acute symptoms.

i. putrefaction. The chemical changes by bacteria in the intestine, forming the following: Indol, skatol, paracresol, phenol, phenylpropionic acid, phenylacetic acid, paraoxyphenylacetic acid, hydroparacumaric acid, fatty acids, carbon dioxide, hydrogen, methane, methylmercaptan and sulfureted hydrogen.

i. reflex. Intestinal contraction and relaxation above a portion of bowel which is stimulated.

intestine (in-tes′tin). The alimentary canal extending from the pylorus to the anus.

i., large. The large intestine extends from the ileum to the anus, and consists of cecum with vermiform appendix, colon, and rectum.

i., small. This begins with the *duodenum*, 8-10 inches long, which receives the food mass from the stomach through the pylorus, the bile from the liver and gallbladder, and the pancreatic juice from the pancreas. It connects with the *jejunum*, about 8 ft. long, which is usually empty after death. The jejunum, in turn, joins the *ileum* or twisted intestine, about 12 ft. long, which is attached to the large intestine by the *ileocecal* or *colic valve* that controls passage of food into large intestine.

intestinum (in-tĕs-tī′nŭm). Intestine.

i. rectum. BNA. The rectum.

in′tima. Innermost coat of a structure, as a blood vessel. SYN: *tunica intima*.

i. unguis. Root of the nail.

i. vasorum. Lining membrane of blood vessels.

intimal (in′tim-al). Pert. to the inner coat of a blood vessel, the intima.

intimi′tis. Inflammation of an intima.

intol′erance. Inability to endure or incapacity for bearing, as pain, or the effects of a drug or other substance.

intoxica′tion. The state of being poisoned; usually interpreted as being due to ethyl alcohol, but may be caused by numerous drugs and various diseases. SEE: *alcoholism, autointoxication.*

intra-. Prefix meaning *within.*

in″traäbdom′inal. Within the abdomen.

i. pressure. Pressure within the abdomen.   [teries.

intraärte′rial. Within an artery or arteries.

intraärticular (in-trä-ar-tik′u-lar). Within a joint.

intracap′sular. Within a capsule.

i. fracture. One occurring within the capsule of a joint.

intracartilaginous (in″tra-kar-tĭ-laj′in-us). Within a cartilage or cartilaginous tissue.

intracellular (in-tra-sel′u-lar). Within a cell or cells.

intracra′nial. Within the cranium or skull.

intracuta′neous. Within the substance of the skin. SYN: *intradermal.*

i. reaction. One following injection of tuberculin into the skin.

intracys′tic. Inside a bladder or cyst.

intrad (in′trad). Inwardly; toward the inner part.

intrader′mal. Within the skin. SYN: *intracutaneous.*

intradermoreaction (in″trä-derm″o-re-ak′-shun). One resulting from the injection of a reagent into substance of the skin.

in″traduode′nal. Within the duodenum.

intraduct′ (in′trä-dukt). Inside a duct.

intradu′ral. Within or enclosed by the dura mater.

intrafeb′rile. During the febrile stage.

intrafi′lar. Within a network.

i. mass. The fluid portion of protoplasm. SYN: *hyaloplasm, paramitome, paraplasm.*

intraligamen′tary. Within the leaves of a ligament.

intraligamentous (in″tra-lig-ă-men′tus). Within a ligament.

intralob′ular. Within a lobule.

intraloc′ular. Within the cavity of any structure.

intralum′bar. Within the lumbar region or portion of the spinal cord.

intraluminal (in-trä-lu′mĭ-nal). Within interior of any tubular structure. SYN: *intratubal.*

intramastoiditis (in-tra-mas-toid-i′tis). Inflammation of the antrum and mastoid process. SYN: *endomastoiditis.*

intramu′ral. Within the walls of a hollow organ or cavity.

intramus′cular. Inside a muscle.

i. injection. Hypodermic injection of drugs into a muscle.

intraoc′ular. Within the eyeball.

intraparietal (in-tra-pă-ri′e-tal). 1. Within the parietal lobe of the cerebrum. 2. Intramural.

intraperitone'al. Within the sac of the peritoneum.

intrapleu'ral. Within the pleural cavity.

intrapo'lar. Bet. two poles.

intrapon'tine. Within the *pons Varolii.*

intrapsychic, intrapsychical (ĭn-tra-sī'kĭk, kī-kăl). Having a mental origin or basis, such as conflicts and complexes.

intrapul'monary. Within the lung cavity.

intrapyretic (in-tră-pi-ret'ik). During the period of fever. SYN: *intrafebrile.*

intraspi'nal. 1. Ensheathed, within a sheath. 2. Within the spinal canal. SYN: *intrathecal.*

intrathecal (in-tra-the'kal). Intraspinal; within spinal canal.

intrathoracic (in-tră-tho-ras'ĭk). Within the thoracic area.

intratracheal (in"tră-trak'e-ăl). Introduced into, or inside, the trachea.

   i. anesthesia. Anesthesia administered through a catheter passed down the trachea.

in"tratu'bal. Within a tube, esp. the fallopian tube.   [cavity.

in"tratympan'ic. Within the tympanic

intrau'terine. Within the uterus.

   i. douche. Douche for washing out interior of the uterus. SEE: *douche.*

intravasation (in-trav-a-sa'shun). Passage into the blood vessels of matter formed outside of them through traumatic or pathological lesions.

intravenous (in-tra-ve'nus). Within or into a vein.

   i. infusion. Injection into a vein of an isotonic solution to secure an immediate result as in hemorrhage, to stimulate in shock or collapse and to dilute poisons in toxemia.

   i. injection. Surface over skin is sterilized, tourniquet or bandage applied to middle of arm, the median cephalic or median basilic vein at front of elbow being used. Hypodermic needle is inserted in the vein, pointing upward. Pressure should be loosed before injection, which should be given very slowly.

   i. medication. The injecion of a sterile solution of a drug or an infusion into a vein.

   i. treatment. This may consist of (*a*) intravenous injection or (*b*) intravenous infusion. The *injection* is usually known as the introduction of a solution into a vein with a hypodermic syringe. The *infusion* is usually known as the introduction of a solution in a larger quantity—250-500 cc. by means of a burette, needle, and rubber tubing.

intraventricular (in-tra-ven-trik'u-lar). Within a ventricle.

intravi'tal. During period of living.

in'tra vi'tam. During life.

intrin'sic. Inherent; belonging to a part.

   i. muscle. A muscle of the extremities, the origin and insertion of which are in the same limb.

intro-. Prefix meaning *in* or *into.*

introdu'cer. Device for controlling, directing and placing an intubation tube within the trachea. SYN: *intubator.*

introitus (in-tro'it-us). Any aperture in the body.

   i. canalis sacralis. Terminal opening of spinal canal at end of sacrum.

   i. laryngis. Upper opening of larynx.

   i. vaginae. Ext. orifice of vagina.

introjec'tion. PSY: Identification of the self with another, or with some object, the victim assuming the supposed feelings of the other personality.

intromission (in-tro-mish'un). An insertion or placing of one part into another, as the entry of the penis into the vagina.

intromittent (in-tro-mit'ent). Conveying or injecting into a cavity or body, as the ejaculation of semen into the vaginal canal.

   i. organ. Penis, which carries seminal fluid into body of the female.

introsusception (in-tro-sus-sep'shun). Invagination. The enfolding of one segment of intestine within another segment. SYN: *intussusception.*

introversion (in-tro-ver'shun). 1. Turning inside out of a part or organ. 2. PSY: The condition of an introvert, *q.v.* Invertism; dwelling within one's self and withdrawal from the external environment, as characterized in such pathological states as hypochondriasis,* melancholia,* and schizophrenia.*

in'trovert. 1. PSY: A personality reaction type characterized by the withdrawal from reality, fantasy formation, and stress on the subjective side of life adjustments, seen pathologically in extreme form in schizophrenia. OPP: *extrovert, q.v.* 2. *v.* To invaginate.

intubate (in'tū-bāt). To insert a tube in a part, esp. the larynx. SYN: *invaginate.*

intubation (in-tu-ba'shun). Insertion of a tube into the larynx through the glottis for entrance of air, or to dilate a stricture.

in'tubator. Device used in inserting a tube into the larynx.

intumesce (in-tū-mes'). To enlarge or swell.

intumes'cence. A swelling or the process of enlarging. SYN: *tumefaction.*

intumescent (in-tu-mes'ent). Swelling or becoming enlarged.

intussusception (in-tus-sus-sep'shun). 1. Growth of cells by deposit of particles bet. those already existing. 2. Invagination. The slipping of one part of an intestine into another part just below it.

intussuscep'tum. The inner segment of intestine which has been pushed into another segment.

intussuscipiens (in"tus-sus-sip'ī-ens). That portion of intestine which receives the intussusceptum.

inulase (in'u-lās). An enzyme that converts inulin into levulose.

in'ulin. 1. A polysaccharide found in plants yielding levulose. 2. An expectorant.

inunction (in-unk'shun). Ointment or medicated substance rubbed into the skin, to secure a local or a more general or systemic effect.

inus'tion. Cauterization; burning.

in u'tero. Within the uterus.

invaginate (in-vaj'ĭn-āt). To ensheath; to insert one part into another part.

invag'inated. Enclosed in a sheath; ensheathed.

invagina'tion. 1. The process of becoming ensheathed. Syn: *intussusception.* See: *evagination.* 2. Operation, of obliterative variety, for treatment of hernia.

in'valid. 1. Not well; weak. 2. A sickly person.

inva'sion. 1. The onset or beginning of a disease. 2. Process by which one becomes affected with disease due to parasites.

invermina'tion. Infestation by intestinal worms. Syn: *helminthiasis.*

inverse-square law. The intensity of radiation at any distance is inversely proportional to the square of the distance bet. the irradiated surface and a point source.

inversion (in-ver'shun). 1. Turning inside out of an organ, *e. g.,* the uterus. 2. In chemistry, the process of converting sucrose (which rotates the plane of polarized light to the right) into a mixture of dextrose and levulose, which mixture rotates the plane to the left.

   i., psychic. Lack of harmony bet. the physical and psychic self or sex.

   i., sexual. Deviation from normal sex relationship, diametrically opposite, *i. e.,* sexual interest in one of the same sex. Syn: *homosexuality.*

   i., uterine. A condition in which the fundus of the uterus protrudes through the cervix, and in some cases through the vaginal introitus.

in'vert. 1. One who, or that which is opposite the normal. See: *homosexual.*[*] 2. (in-vert'). To turn inside or upside down.

   i. sugar. A term usually applied to a mixture of levulose and dextrose, formed by inversion of sucrose by enzyme, invertase. See: *carbohydrate, inversion, sugar.*

invertase (in-ver'tās). A sugar-splitting ferment or enzyme found in the intestinal juice.

   It causes the inversion of sugar.

   See: *enzyme, sucrose, dextrose, levulose.*

invertin (in-ver'tin). An intestinal ferment which converts cane sugar into invert sugar. Syn: *invertase.*

invest'ing. Ensheathing, encircling with a sheath or coating, as tissue; surrounding.

invet'erate. Chronic; firmly seated, as a disease or a wound.

in vit'ro. In a glass, as in a test tube.

in vi'vo. In the living body.

in'volucre, involu'crum. 1. A sheath or covering. 2. The covering of newly formed bone enveloping sequestrum in infection of bone.

invol'untary. Independent of or even contrary to volition.

involution (in-vo-lu'shun). 1. A turning or rolling inward. 2. The reduction in size

of the uterus following delivery. 3. The retrogressive change in vital processes or in an organ after fulfilling their functions, such as that which follows the menopause. 4. A backward change. 5. Diminishing of an organ in vital power or in size.

   i. senile. Shriveling of an organ or part from old age.

   i., sexual. Cessation of menstrual function. Syn: *climacteric, menopause.*[*]

   i. of uterus. Return of uterus by absorption to normal size after childbirth.

involutional (ĭn-vō-lu'shŭn-ăl). Concerning involution or a turning inward.

   i. melancholia. Melancholia associated with senile and presenile types and manic-depressive group.

iodalbin (ī-ō-dal'bin). A compound of iodine and albumen containing approximately 21.5% iodine.

   Dosage: Average, 5 gr. (0.3 Gm.).

iodeikon (i-ō'de-kon). Brand of soluble iodophthalein.

iodide (i'o-dīd). A compound of iodine with another element.

iodine (ī'ō-dĕn, i'o-dĭn, or -dīn). A member of the halogen group. Symb: I. At. wt. 126.92; a solid, nonmetallic element first used in medicine in 1819.

   i. number. In chemistry, the number of grams of iodine that can be taken up by 100 Gm. of a fat or oil; a measure of the degree of unsaturation. Thus the unsaturated drying linseed oil has an iodine number of about 200; the nondrying cocoanut oil has one of 8 or 9.

iodism (i'o-dizm). Condition induced by prolonged use of iodine or its compounds. See: *iodine poisoning.*

i'odize. To administer or impregnate with iodine.

i'odized. Impregnated with iodine.

   i. salt. Salt containing 1 part sodium or potassium iodide to 5000 parts of sodium chloride. See: *salt.*

io'doform. USP: Yellow powder made by the action of iodine on acetone in the presence of an alkali.

   Dosage: Externally in the form of a dusting powder, or as a surgical dressing in the form of gauze impregnated with the drug.

io'doformism. Poisoning caused by iodoform.

iodother'apy. Use of iodine medication.

i'odum. Iodine.

i'on. Molecular constituent, *i. e.,* one or more atoms, carrying an electric charge.

ion'ic. Pert. to ions.

   i. medication. The introduction of chemical ions into the superficial tissues for medicinal purposes by means of a direct current.

ioniza'tion. 1. The process by which atoms or molecules emit their charges either positively or negatively, dissociating into ions. 2. Medication by introducing ions into superficial tissues.

   i. chamber. An enclosure containing two or more electrodes bet. which an electric current may be passed when the enclosed gas is ionized by any radiation. It is commonly used for determining the intensity of roentgen rays and other ionizing rays.

i. current. The movement of electric charges produced by the action of an applied electric field upon an ionized medium.

i., zinc. Therapeutic use of driving zinc ions into superficial tissues by the positive pole of the galvanic current.

i'onize. To separate into ions, breaking molecules into atomic particles, charging the larger with positive electricity, the smaller with negative electricity.

i''onom'eter. An instrument consisting of an ionization chamber, an electroscope, and an electric charging current designed to measure the amount of radiation used by roentgen rays or radium and to measure the intensity of the rays themselves. SEE: *roentgenometer.*

ionotherapy (i''on-o-ther'ă-pĭ). 1. Introduction of ions into the body. 2. Treatment of disease with violet rays. SYN: *iontophoresis,* 1.

iontophoresis (i-on''to-fo-re'sis). 1. Process of electrical current traveling through salt solution causing migration of metal ion to negative pole and radical ion to positive pole. 2. Introduction of various ions into tissues through the skin by means of electricity. SYN: *ionic medication.*

iontoquantimeter (i-on''to-kwon-tim'e-ter). Instrument used to measure the amount of radiation used by, and the intensity of, roentgen rays. SEE: *roentgenometer.*

iontoradiometer (i-on''to-ra-dĭ-om'e-ter). Instrument for measuring the amount and intensity of roentgen rays. SEE: *roentgenometer.*

iontotherapy (i-on''to-ther'ă-pĭ). Treatment by forcing ions into the body electrically.

iophobia (i-o-fo'bĭ-ă). 1. Fear of being poisoned. SYN: *toxicophobia.* 2. Fear of touching any rusty object.

iotacism (i-o'ta-sizm). Defective utterance marked by constant substitution of an *e* sound (Greek iota) for other vowels.

ipecac (ip'e-kak). USP. A dried root of a plant (*ipecacuanha*), grown in Brazil.
DOSAGE: As expectorant, 1 gr. (0.06 Gm.); as emetic, 15 gr. (1.0 Gm.). SEE: *emetine*

ipral sodium (ip'ral). A proprietary derivative of barbital; a persistent acting hypnotic.
DOSAGE: 2-4 gr. (0.12-0.25 Gm.).

ipsation (ip-sa'shun). Practice of masturbation.

ipsilateral, ipsolateral (ip-si-lat'er-al). On the same side. Affecting the same side of the body.

I. Q. Abbr. for *intelligence quotient.**

ir. Abbr. for *internal resistance.*

iral'gia. Pain felt in the iris. SYN: *iridalgia.*

iridal (ir'ĭd-al). Rel. to the iris.

iridalgia (ir-id-al'jĭ-ă). Pain felt in the iris. SYN: *iralgia.*

iridauxesis (ir''ĭ-dawk-se'sis). Increase in size of the iris. SYN: *iridoncus.*

iridectome (ir-id-ek'tōm). Instrument for cutting the iris.

iridectomesodialysis (ir-ĭ-dek''to-mes''o-dĭ-al'ĭ-sis). Formation of an artificial pupil, by separating adhesions on inner margin of iris.

iridectomize (ir-id-ek'to-mīz). To excise a portion of the iris.

iridec'tomy. Surgical removal of a portion of iris.
i., optical. Iridectomy done for purpose of making an artificial pupil.

iridectropium (ir-ĭ-dek-tro'pĭ-um). Partial eversion of the iris.

iride'mia. Bleeding from the iris.

iridencleisis (ir''id-en-kli'sis). Iris inclusion operation; the iris being incarcerated in the wound, thereby forming a fistula lined with iris tissue. Performed in glaucoma.

iridentropium (ir''ĭ-den-tro'pĭ-um). Partial inversion of the iris.

irideremia (ir-id-er-e'mĭ-ă). Partial or total absence of the iris. SEE: *aniridia.*

iridesis (i-rid'ē-sis). Formation of an iris artificially, by ligation.

iridic (ir-id'ik). Rel. to the iris. SYN: *iridal.*

ir'ido-. Combining form, pert. to the *iris.*

iridoavulsion (ir''ĭ-do-av-ul'shun). Tearing away (avulsion) of the iris.

iridocapsulitis (ir''ĭd-o-kap-sŭ-li'tis). Iritis with inflammation of the capsule of the lens.

iridocele (i-rid'o-sēl). Protrusion of a portion of the iris through a defect in the cornea.

iridochorioiditis, iridochoroiditis (ir''ĭ-do-ko''ri-oy-di'tis) (ir''ĭ-do-ko-roy-di'tis). Inflamed condition of both iris and choroid.

ir''idocolobo'ma. Congenital defect or fissure of the iris.

iridocyclectomy (ir''ĭ-do-si-klek'to-mĭ). Surgical removal of iris and ciliary body.

iridocyclitis (ir''id-o-si-kli'tis). Inflammation of iris and ciliary body.

iridocystectomy (ir''ĭ-do-sis-tek'to-mĭ). Plastic formation of an artificial pupil.

iridodesis (ir-id-od'es-is). Ligature of part of iris to form an artificial one. SYN: *iridesis.*

ir''idodiagno'sis. Diagnosis of disease by changes in color and form of the iris.

iridodialysis (ir''id-o-di-al'is-is). The separation of the outer margin of the iris from its ciliary attachment, usually due to trauma, forming an artificial pupil.

iridodila'tor. Substance causing dilatation of the pupil.

iridodonesis (ir''id-o-do-ne'sis). Tremulousness of iris, seen in an aphakik eye or one with subluxated lens. SYN: *hippus.*

iridokinesis (ir''id-o-kĭn-e'sis). The contracting and expanding movements of the iris.

iridology (ir-ĭ-dol'o-jĭ). The study of changes in the iris during course of a disease.

iridomalacia (ir″id-o-ma-la′sĭ-ă). Softening of the iris.

iridomedialysis (ir″id-o-med-ĭ-al′ĭ-sis). Separation of inner marginal adhesions of iris. SYN: *iridomesodialysis*.

iridomesodialysis (ir″id-o-mes″o-dĭ-al′ĭ-sis). Separation of adhesions around the inner border of iris.

iridomo′tor. Rel. to movements of the iris.

iridon′cus. Tumefaction of the iris or development of a tumor.

ir″idoparal′ysis. Paralysis of the pupil. SYN: *iridoplegia*.

iridoparelkysis (ir″ĭ-do-par-el′kĭ-sis). Dislocation of pupil due to prolapse of the iris.

iridoperiphacitis, iridoperiphakitis (ir″ĭ-do-per″ĭ-fă-si′tĭs, -per″ĭ-fă-ki′tĭs). Inflammation of the iris and ant. portion of capsule of the lens.

iridoplegia (ir″id-o-ple′jĭ-ă). Paralysis of sphincter of iris.

   i., **accommodative.** Inability of iris to contract when stimulated by accommodation.

   i., **complete.** Iridoplegia in which the iris fails to respond to any stimulation.

   i., **reflex.** Absence of light reflex with retention of accommodation reflex (Argyll-Robertson pupil*).

iridoptosis (ir-ĭ-dop-to′sis). Prolapse of the iris.

iridorrhexis (ir″id-or-reks′is). Rupture of or a tearing of the iris away from its attachment.

iridosclerotomy (ir″id-o-skle-rot′o-mĭ). Piercing of the sclera and of the border of the iris.

iridosis (ir-ĭ-do′sis). Portion of iris brought out through an incision in the cornea, to form an artificial iris. SYN: *iridesis, iridodesis*.

iridosteresis (ir″ĭ-do-stĕ-re′sis). Removal of the iris or a portion of it.

iridot′asis. Stretching the iris for glaucoma.

iridotomy (ir-ĭ-dot′o-mĭ). Incision of iris without excising a piece, done for the purpose of making a new aperture in the iris when the pupil is closed.

i′ris. The colored contractile membrane suspended between the lens and the cornea in the aqueous humor of the eye, separating the ant. and post. chambers of the ball and perforated in the center by the pupil. It regulates by contraction and dilatation the entrance of light.

   i. **bombé.** Seen in annular post. synechia (seclusio pupillae). The iris is bulged forward by the pressure of the aqueous humor which cannot reach the ant. chamber.

   i., **chromatic asymmetry of.** Difference in color of the two irides. One may be blue or gray and the other brown. May occur in early iritis or cyclitis. A normal condition except in those of neuropathic tendencies.

   i. **contraction reflex.** Normal contraction on exposure to light.

   i., **piebald.** Dark discoloration in irregularly shaped area. May be in one or both eyes.

I′rish moss. A genus of seaweeds; *chondrus crispus*.

iritic (i-rit′ik). Rel. to the iris.

iri′tis. Inflammation of the iris.

   i., **plastic.** Iritis in which the fibrinous exudate forms new tissue.

   i., **primary.** When the process develops in the iris itself. Seen in general diseases as syphilis, tuberculosis; metastatic in infectious diseases, gonorrhea and focal infections; also occurs in trauma and sympathetic ophthalmia.

   i., **purulent.** One with a purulent exudate.

   i., **secondary.** When the inflammation spreads from neighboring parts as diseases of cornea and sclera.

   i., **serous.** Serum forming the exudate.

iritomy (i-rit′o-mĭ). Formation of an artificial pupil. SYN: *iridotomy*.

i′ron. SYMB: *Fe*. A metallic element. In its natural state, iron is of no use to organic life. In combination with oxygen, it is absorbed by plant life as an inorganic oxide. It serves as a carrier of oxygen and in the production of chlorophyll, the coloring matter of plants.

   i. **arc.** One of the commonly employed sources of ultraviolet radiation for therapeutic purposes.

   i., **high diet.** Foods rich in iron and blood building substances are emphasized, *i. e.*, liver, beef heart, kidney, red meats, green leafy vegetables (esp. spinach); apricots, peaches, raisins, apples, prunes, molasses.

irot′omy. Formation of an artificial pupil. SYN: *iridotomy, iritomy*.

irra′diate. To administer x-rays or other forms of radiation.

irra′diating. Diverging or spreading out from a common center.

irradia′tion. 1. Therapeutic application of roentgen rays, radium rays, ultraviolet rays or other radiation to a patient. 2. Application of form of radiation to an object or substance to give it therapeutic value, or increase that which it already has.

   i., **interstitial.** Therapeutic irradiation by the insertion into the tissues of capillary tubes containing radon.

irreducible (ĭr-re-du′sĭ-bl). Not capable of being reduced, or made smaller.

irrel′evance. PSY: Giving an answer not in harmony with question.

irrespirable (ir″rĕ-spi′ra-bl). Unfit for breathing as a gas, or incapable of being breathed.

ir′rigate. To wash out with a fluid.

ir″riga′tion. The cleansing of a canal by the injection of water or other fluids, as an enema, or the washing of a wound. From 2-3 pt. of saline or antiseptic solution at 103° F. are used for wounds.

   i., **bladder.** Washing out of bladder for treatment of inflammation.

i., colonic. The flushing of the colon with water. SEE: *colonic irrigation, enema.*

ir"riga'tor. Device with hose attachment used for purpose of flushing or washing a part or cavity with fluids.

i., Hyam's. Instrument for applying prolonged irrigation to the urethra, cervix, and vagina, with hot solutions at an exact temperature under accurate control.

ir"ritabil'ity. 1. Inherent reaction to a stimulus. 2. Impatience.

i., electric. Response by a nerve or muscle to a current of electricity.

i., muscular. Normal response of muscle to a stimulus.

i., nervous. Response of a nerve to stimulus.

ir'ritable. 1. Reacting to a stimulus. 2. Sensitive to stimuli.

i. heart. A condition marked by nervous and cardiocirculatory disturbances with increased susceptibility to fatigue.

i. joint. A condition sometimes following a sprain, marked by recurring attacks of acute or subacute inflammation.

ir'ritant. An agent which, when used locally, produces more or less local inflammatory reactions. Ex: *iodine.*

i. poisons. These include a large number of poisons of great variety, not including the corrosive acids or alkalies.

irrita'tion. 1. Reaction to that which is irritating. 2. Extreme reaction to pain or pathological conditions. 3. Normal response to stimulus of a nerve or muscle.

ir'ritative. Pert. to that which causes irritation.

irrumation (ir-ru-ma'shun). Form of perversion marked by intromission of the penis into another individual's mouth. SYN: *fellatio.*

isacen (īs'a-sen). A compound somewhat resembling phenolphthalein.

DOSAGE: 1/12–1/8 gr. (0.005–0.02 Gm.).

Isambert's disease (e-zahm-bairz'). Ulcerated mucous membranes of mouth and fauces, usually tuberculous.

isarol (iz'a-rol). Ammonium sulfoichthiolate.

ischemia (is-ke'mĭ-ă). Local and temporary anemia due to obstruction of the circulation to a part.

ischesis (is-ke'sis). Suppression of a discharge, esp. a normal one.

ischiac, ischiadic (is'kĭ-ăk, is-kĭ-ad'Ĭk). Pert. to the hipbone. SYN: *ischiatic.*

ischial (is'kĭ-al). Pert. to the ischium.

ischialgia (is-kĭ-al'jĭ-ă). Neuralgic pain in the hip. SYN: *sciatica.*

ischiatic (is-ki-at'Ĭk). Pert. to the ischium or hipbone. SYN: *sciatic.*

ischiatitis (is-ki-ă-ti'tis). Sciatic nerve inflammation.

ischidrosis (is-kĭ-dro'sis). Suppression of perspiration.

ischio-. Prefix: pert. to the *ischium.*

ischiobulbar (is"kĭ-o-bul'bar). Rel. to the ischium and urethral bulb.

ischiocele (is'kĭ-o-sĕl). Hernia through the sciatic notch.

ischiococcygeus (is"kĭ-o-kok-sĭj'e-us). 1. Musculus coccygeus. 2. Post. portion of the levator ani.

ischiofemoral (is"kĭ-o-fem'or-al). Rel. to the ischium and femur.

ischiofib'ular. Rel. to the ischium and fibula.

ischiohebotomy (is"kĭ-o-he-bot'o-mĭ). Division of ascending ramus of the pubes, and of the ischiopubic ramus. SYN: *ischiopubiotomy.*

ischiomenia (is-ki-o-me'nĭ-ă). Suppression of the menses. SYN: *ischomenia.*

ischioneuralgia (is-ki-o-nu-ral'jĭ-ă). Neuralgic pain in the hip. SYN: *sciatica.*

ischiopubic (is-kĭ-o-pu'bĭk). Rel. to the ischium and pubes.

ischiopubiotomy (is"kĭ-o-pu-bĭ-ot'o-mĭ). Division of the ischiopubic ramus and ascending ramus of the pubes. SYN: *ischiohebotomy.*

is"chiorec'tal. Pert. to the ischium and rectum.

i. abscess.* Collection of pus in fatty cavity on either side of rectum.

If it breaks internally into the rectum an anal fistula may result.

ischium (is'kĭ-um) (pl. *is'chia*). Post. and inferior parts forming the lower portion of innominate or hipbone.

ischochymia (is-ko-ki'mĭ-ă). Retention of food in dilatation of the stomach.

ischogalactic (is-ko-gal-ak'tik). 1. Causing suppression of breast milk. 2. Agent which checks milk secretion. SYN: *antigalactic, lactifuge.*

ischomenia (is-ko-me'nĭ-ă). Menstrual suppression or retention.

ischuretic (is-ku-ret'ik). 1. Relieving or pert. to ischuria. 2. That which relieves urinary retention or suppression.

ischuria (is-ku'rĭ-ă). Suppression or retention of the urine.

island (i'land). A structure detached from surrounding tissues, or characterized by difference in structure.

i.'s of Langerhans (lang'er-hans). Cellular masses in interstitial tissue of the pancreas which secrete insulin.

i. of Reil. The *insula* within the lat. cerebral fossa, at beginning of sylvian fissure.

islet (i'lĕt). A tiny isolated mass of 1 kind of tissue within another type.

i. cells or tissue. The islands of Langerhans.

-ism. Suffix: Condition, or theory of, principle or method.

iso-. Combining form meaning equal.

isoagglutinin (i-so-ag-glu'tin-in). Antibody in a serum which agglutinates the blood cells of those of the same species from which it is derived.

isobare (i'so-bār). One of two or more chemical bodies having same atomic weight, and which may have similar or unlike properties.

i'sobody. An antibody acting on animals of the same species, from which it is derived.

isob'olism. Motor nerve fiber tendency to undergo maximal excitation on being subjected to a stimulus.

isocel'lular. Composed of equal and similar cells.

isochromatic (i-so-kro-mat'ik). Having the same color.

isochromatophil(e (i"so-kro-mat'o-fĭl or fĭl). Having same affinity for a dye.

isochronal (i-so-kro'nal). Acting in uniform time, or taking place at regular intervals.

isochron'ic. Performed in uniform time or at regular intervals. SYN: *isochronal*.

isochronous (i-sok'ro-nus). Performed in equal time. SYN: *isochronal*.

isochroous (ī-sok'ro-us). Of uniform color. SYN: *isochromatic*.

isocolloid (ī-so-kol'oyd). A colloid having the same composition in every transformation.

isocom'plement. One from the same individual or species which provides the amboceptor.

isocom'pounds. Any chemical compounds with same number but different arrangement of atoms in the molecule.

isocoria (i-so-ko'rĭ-ă). Equality of diameter of pupils.

isocytotoxin (i"so-si"to-tok'sĭn). A cytotoxin destructive to cells of the same species from which it is derived.

isodactylism (i-so-dak'til-izm). Condition of having fingers and toes of equal length.

isodiametric (i"so-di-a-met'rik). Having equal diameters.

isoelectric (i-so-e-lek'trik). Having equal electric potentials.

i"soenerget'ic. Showing equal force.

isogam'ete. A cell which, through conjugation or fusion with a similar cell, reproduces.

isogenesis (i-so-jen'es-is). Similarity in morphological development.

i'sograft. A graft taken from another individual or animal of the same species. OPP: *autograft*. SEE: *heterograft*.

isohemagglutinin (i"so-hem-ag-glu'tin-in). Substance normally present in most human blood serum and responsible for the clumping of corpuscles observed when incompatible bloods are mixed.

i"sohemol'ysin. Substance destroying red blood corpuscles of animals of same species from which it is obtained. SEE: *hemolysin*.

i"sohemol'ysis. Action of an isohemolysin.

isohypercytosis (i"so-hi"per-si-to'sis). Increase of leukocytes, the proportion of varieties being unchanged.

isohypocytosis (i"so-hi"po-si-to'sis). Decrease in number of leukocytes with proportion of varieties unchanged.

isoiconia (i"so-i-ko'nĭ-ă). Equality in size of two retinal images.

isoiconic (i"so-i-kon'ĭk). Having equal retinal images.

i'solate. 1. To separate or detach from other persons, as during an infectious disease. 2. To free from a chemical combination.

isola'tion. Limitation of movement and social contacts of patient suffering from, or a known carrier of communicable disease, in contradistinction to *quarantine*, which limits the movements of exposed or contact persons. SYN: *sequestration* 2. SEE: *quarantine*.

   l. ward. Hospital ward where patients suffering from communicable diseases may be kept apart from the rest of the patients.

isoleucine (i-so-lu'sēn). An amino-acid formed during hydrolysis of fibrin and other proteins.

isolophobia (i-so-lo-fo'bĭ-ă). Fear of being alone.

isolysin (i-sol'is-in). Substance which dissolves red corpuscles of animals of the same species from which it is obtained. SYN: *isohemolysin*.

isol'ysis. Destruction of red blood corpuscles produced by an isolysin. SYN: *isohemolysis*. SEE: *hemolysis*.

isolyt'ic. Rel. to isolysins.

isomer (i'so-mer). One of a set of chemical substances having an equal number of atoms, but different order of atomic arrangement in the molecule. SEE: *metamer, polymer*.

isomeric (i-so-mer'ĭk). Pert. to compounds of the same number of atoms but having different arrangement of atoms in the molecule. SEE: *metameric, polymeric*.

isomerism (i-som'er-izm). State of being composed of compounds of the same number of atoms, but having different atomic arrangement in the molecule. SEE: *metamerism, polymerism*.

isomet'ric. Having equal dimensions. OPP: *isotonic*.

   i. muscle. PHYS: Contraction in which a muscle increases its tension without shortening. [eyes.

isometro'pia. Same refraction of the two

isomor'phism. Condition marked by possession of the same form.

isomorphous (i-so-mor'fus). Possessing the same shape.

isonormocytosis (i"so-nor"mo-si-to'sis). State of having leukocytes normal in number and proportion of varities.

isop'athy. Therapeutic administration of the virus that caused the disease.

isophoria (i-so-fo'rĭ-ă). Equal tension of vertical muscles of the eyes with visual lines in same horizontal plane, both hyperphoria* and hypophoria* absent.

i"sose"rother'apy. Treatment with serum from one having had the same disease as the patient.

isose'rum. A serum from one having the disease for which a patient is to receive treatment.

i'sospore. A spore which, without conjugation, develops into an adult.

isosthenuria (i-sos-the-nu'rĭ-ă). The decreased variation in specific gravity of nephritic urinary specimens.

isostimula'tion. Cell stimulation by injection of the same cell substance.

isother'apy. Treatment by active causal agent of a disease. SYN: *isopathy.*

isother'mal. Of an equal degree of heat.

isothermognosis (i"so-ther-mog-no'sis). Abnormal perception in which stimulation by pain, heat, and cold are all felt as heat.

isoto'nia. The maintenance of equal tension in two solutions or substances.

isoton'ic. Having the same tension or tone. OPP: *isometric.*

   i. muscle. Muscle, with unchanged tension whicn contracts on stimulation.

   i. solutions. Those having the same osmotic pressure.

isotonicity (i-so-to-nis'i-ti). Maintaining and possessing a uniform tension or tone of solutions or substances.

isotope (i'so-tōp). Either of two bodies, identical chemically, but differing in at. wt.

isotropic (i-so-tro'pĭk). 1. Possessing similar qualities in every direction. 2. Having equal refraction.

isotyp'ical. Belonging to the same variety or classification.

issue (is'shu). 1. Offspring. 2. A suppurating sore maintained by a foreign body in the tissue and acting as a counter-irritant.

   i. pea. Small round foreign body used in tissues as a counterirritant.

-ist. Suffix: One who or an agent that does.

isthmectomy (is-mek'to-mĭ). Excision of an enlarged isthmus, esp. of the thyroid gland. SYN: *median strumectomy.*

isthmian (is'mĭ-an). Rel. to an isthmus.

isthmitis (is-mi'tis). Inflammation of the throat or fauces.

is"thmocholo'sis. Catarrh of fauces accompanied by bilious disturbances.

isthmoparalysis (is"mo-par-al'ĭ-sis). Paralysis of the muscles of the fauces. SYN: *isthmoplegia.*

isthmoplegia (is"mo-ple'jĭ-ă). Faucial paralysis.

isth'mospasm. Isthmian spasm, as of the fauces or of the fallopian tubes.

isthmus (is'mus). 1. A narrow passage connecting two cavities. 2. A constriction bet. two larger parts of an organ, or anatomical structure.

   i. of eustachian tube. Narrow portion of eustachian tube.

   i. faucium. Path bet. fauces and mouth.

   i. of thyroid. Band joining thyroid lobes.

isu'ria. Excretion of urine at a uniform rate, hour by hour.

itch. 1. Irritation of skin, inducing desire to scratch. SYN: *pruritus.* 2. Scabies. SEE: Names in alphabetical order.

   i. mite. *Sarcoptes scabiei.*

itch'ing. Pruritus; irritation of the skin, causing desire to rub or scratch the part.

-ite. Suffix denoting *of the nature of.* In chemistry a salt of an acid having the termination *-ous.*

i'ter. Passageway bet. two anatomical parts.

i'teral. Pert. to an iter.

ithycyphosis, ithyokyphosis (ith"ĭ-si-fo'sis, ith"ĭ-o-ki-fō'sis). Kyphosis with backward projection.

ithylordosis (ith"ĭ-lor-do'sis). Lordosis without lateral curvature of the spine.

-itis. (i'tis). Suffix: *inflammation of.*

I. U. Abbr. for *immunizing unit.*

i'vy poisoning. Dermatitis caused by contact with poison ivy.

Ixo'des. A genus of ticks, many of which are parasitic on man and animals.

ixodiasis (iks-o-di'a-sis). 1. Lesions of the skin caused by tick bites. 2. Any disease caused by ticks, as Rocky Mountain fever.

ixodic (iks-od'ik). Pert. to or caused by ticks.

ixomyelitis (iks-ō-mĭ-e-li'tis). Inflammation of the spinal cord in the lumbar region.

J

J. Symb. for the *joule* and for *Joule's equivalent.*

Jaboulay's button (zhab-oo-lā'). Two cylinders which may be screwed together for lateral intestinal anastomosis.

Jaccoud's sign (zhǎ-koo'). 1. Movement of chest wall in adherent pericardium, indicating leukemia. 2. Irregular and low pulse with raised temperature in adult tuberculous meningitis.

jack'et. A plaster of Paris or leather bandage applied to the trunk to immobilize spine or correct deformities.

   j., Sayre's. Plaster of Paris jacket used as a support for deformity of the spinal column.

   j., strait. Device for restraining the arms of a violently insane person. SYN: *camisole.*

   j., Willock's respiratory. A type of jacket for strengthening the respiratory movements in emphysema of the lungs.

jack-knife or **reclining position.** The patient lies on the back with shoulders elevated, thighs flexed on abdomen, legs on thighs, the thighs being at right angles to the abdomen. Employed when passing a urethral sound.

jack'screw. A threaded screw to expand the arch in regulating teeth.

jackson'ian epi'lepsy. A localized form with spasms confined to one part or one group of muscles. SEE: *epilepsy.*

Ja'cob's mem'brane. Retinal layer of rods and cones.

   J.'s ulcer. Epithelioma, usually of the face, which slowly eats away soft tissue and bones. SYN: *rodent ulcer.*

Ja'cobson's car'tilage. Hyaline cartilage supporting rudimentary sac in nasal septum.

   J.'s nerve. Nervus tympanicus.

   J.'s organ. Rudimentary sac in nasal septum.

   J.'s sulcus. Portion of middle ear containing branches of tympanic plexus.

Jacquemier's sign (zhak-me-āz'). Blue or purplish color of the vaginal mucosa, indicating pregnancy.

Jacquet's disease (zhǎ-kaz'). Reflex alopecia connected with dental anomalies.

jactitation (jak-ti-ta'shun). Convulsive movements. Restless tossing. Changing from one posture to another, usually characteristic of severe mental and febrile affections.

   j., periodic. Chorea.

Jadelot's lines, furrows, or **traits** (zhad-loz'). Three lines on the face, said to indicate disease in children.

   J.'s labial l. Down from corner of mouth; seen in respiratory diseases.

   J.'s nasal l. From lower border of ala nasi about outer side of orbicularis oris muscle; seen in abdominal disorders.

   J.'s ocular l. From inner canthus toward glenoid fossa; observed in cerebral disease.

Jaeger's test types (ya'gerz). Lines of type of various sizes, printed on a card for testing close visual acuteness.

jail fever. Typhus fever, *q.v.*

Jaksch's anemia or **disease** (yakshs). Infantile anemia with lymphatic enlargement and changes in spleen. SYN: *infantile pseudoleukemia.*

jal'ap, USP. The dried tuberous root of the plant of the same name.

   DOSAGE: 30 gr. (2 Gm.).

James' pow'der. Official antimonial powder.   [anodyne.

James'town weed. Antispasmodic and local

Janet's disease (zhǎ-nez'). A neurosis characterized by obsessions and phobias. SYN: *psychasthenia.*

jan'itor. The pylorus.

jan'itrix. The portal vein.

jar'gon. Unintelligible speech. SYN: *paraphasia.*

jar"gonapha'sia. A form of aphasia* in which words are jumbled so that speech is unintelligible. SYN: *paraphasia.*

Jarjavay's muscle (zhar-zhǎ-vāz'). The depressor urethrae muscle.

Jar'vis' snare. A snare for removing growths.

jaundice (jawn'dis). A disease marked by yellow skin and eye whites, due to changes in the liver cells or obstructions, which cause the bile pigment, bilirubin, to be diffused into the blood.

   j., acathectic. Form caused by functional hepatic cell disorder.

   j., acholuric. Jaundice without bile pigment in the urine.

   j., hematogenous. Due to rapid destruction of liver cells or red blood cells; yellow discoloration not so pronounced.

   j., hepatogenous. ETIOL: Due to catarrh of bile duct and duodenum, pressure from tumors or blood vessels, parasites, stricture of gallduct or obstruction by gallstones.

   j., malignant. Acute yellow atrophied condition of the liver.

   j. of newborn. Jaundice affecting newborn infants. SYN: *icterus neonatorum.*

   j., obstructive. That due to a mechanical impediment to the bile flow.

   j., simple catarrhal. ETIOL: Due to an infectious agent, extension of duodenal catarrh to common bile duct, or certain other diseases.

   j., xanthochromic. Jaundice without bile pigment in the urine, but with yellowish discoloration of soles and palms.

jaw. Either or both the maxillary and mandibular bones, bearing the teeth and forming mouth framework.

j. jerk reflex. Clonic movement resulting from percussing or stroking lower jaw.

j., lock. Tonic spasm of jaw muscles preventing opening of mouth. SYN: *tetanus, trismus.*

j., lumpy. Fungous disease affecting the jaw, brain, lungs, and gastrointestinal tract. SYN: *actinomycosis, q.v.*

j., swelling of. LOWER: May be due to alveolar abscess, a cyst, gumma, sarcoma, or actinomycosis. UPPER: Occurs in alveolar abscess, parotid tumor, parotitis, carcinoma, sarcoma, and necrosis of bone or disease of antrum.

jaw winking. Elevation of the upper eyelid when there is depression of the lower jaw.   [stitute.

jec'orin. Commercial cod liver oil sub-

jecur (je'kur). The liver.

jejunal (je-jū'nal). Rel. to the jejunum.

jejunectomy (jej-ū-nek'to-mǐ). Excision of part or all of the jejunum.

jejunitas (jej-ū'nĭt-as). Fasting.

jejunitis (jej-ū-ni'tis). Inflammation of the jejunum.

jejuno-. Combining form referring to the jejunum.

jeju'nocolos'tomy. Formation of artificial passage bet. jejunum and colon.

jejunoileostomy (je-ju"no-il-e-os'to-mǐ). Formation of a passage bet. jejunum and ileum.

jejunoileitis (jě-jun"o-il-e-i'tis). Inflamed condition of jejunum and ileum.

jejunojejunostomy (je-ju"no-je-ju-nos'to-mǐ). Formation of a passage bet. two parts of the jejunum.

jejunostomy (jě-ju-nos'to-mǐ). Surgical creation of a permanent opening into the jejunum.

jejunotomy (je-ju-not'o-mǐ). Surgical incision into the jejunum.

jejunum (je-ju'num). Two-fifths of small intestine siutated bet. duodenum and ileum.

Said to be empty after death; about 8 feet long.

j., inflammation of. SYM: Absence of diarrhea; colic, distention of abdomen, borborygmus, flocculent or semisolid stools, containing undigested food, unchanged bile, and some mucus. Tenderness over midabdomen relieved by pressure.

jell. 1. Precipitate of a colloid solution. 2. Jelly.

jel'ly. A thick, semisolid, gelatinous mass.

j., Wharton's. Soft, gelatinous connective tissue that constitutes the matrix of the umbilical cord.

jenne'rian vaccina'tion. Inoculation against smallpox. SEE: *vaccination.*

Jen'ner's stain. Eosin methylene blue stain.

jerk (jerk). A sudden muscular movement.

Innervation of a part is indicated, jerk resulting from stroke over a tendon or region. A reflex.

j., elbow. External stimulation of triceps when stretched, produces involuntary extension of forearm.

j., finger. Jerk responding to extension or flexion of a finger.

j., knee. Forward jerk of foot upon striking patellar tendon, when knee is flexed at right angles.

j., jaw. Result of striking lower jaw with mouth open. Indicative of cerebral lesion.

j., wrist. When hand is held down at arm's length, the hand being in extreme extension, lateral clonic movements of the hand occur; normal phenomenon.

jig'ger (*Dermatophilus penetrans*). A genus of insects. The sand flea. It burrows into the toes, causing irritation and inflammation. SYN: *chigo.*

jim'son weed. Stramonium, *q.v.*

jocasta complex (jo-kas'tă). A term implying a mother and son complex from part taken by Jocasta, mother in the Oedipus complex, who was the wife and mother of Oedipus.

jodum (yo'doom). Iodine.

Joffroy's reflex (jof'roy). Twitching of gluteal muscles when pressure is made against buttocks.

J.'s sign. 1. Absence of facial muscle contraction when eyes turn upward in exophthalmic goiter. 2. Inability to do simple sums in arithmetic. An early sign of general paralysis.

johim'bine. Alkaloid aphrodisiac.*

joint. An articulation. The point of juncture bet. two bones.

j., amphidiarthrodial. Joint both ginglymoid and arthrodial.

j., arthrodial. SEE: *gliding joint.*

j., ball and socket. Joint in which round end of one bone fits into cavity of another bone. SYN: *enarthrosis.*

j., biaxial. Joint possessing two chief movement axes at right angles to each other.

j., bilocular. Joint separated into two sections by interarticular cartilage.

j., bleeders'. Joint hemorrhage in hemophiliacs.

j., Brodie's. Arthrodial neuralgia due to hysteria.

j., Budin's. Congenital cartilaginous band bet. squamous and condylar parts of the occipital bone.

j. capsule. Capsular ligament or other body in a joint.

j., Charcot's. A disease in advanced syphilis. Wasting away of muscles below the joint.

j., Chopart's. Union of remainder of tarsal bones with os calcis and astragalus.

j., cochlear. Hinge joint permitting lateral motion.

j., compound. Joint made up of several bones.

j., condyloid. Joint permitting all forms of angular movements except axial rotation.   [joint.

j., Cruveilhier's. Atlanto-odontoid

j., diarthrodial. Joint having mobility in every direction.

j., dry. Arthritis of chronic villous type.

j., ellipsoid. Joint having two axes of motion through the same bone.

j., enarthrodial. SEE: *ball and socket joint.*

j., false. False joint formation subsequent to a fracture.

j., flail. Joint which is extremely relaxed, the distal portion of limb being almost beyond the control of the will.

j., ginglymoid. Joint having only forward and backward motion, like a hinge.

j., gliding. Diarthrosis permitting a gliding motion.

j., hemophiliac. SEE: *bleeders' joint.*

j., hinge. SEE: *ginglymoid joint.*

j., hysteric. Condition simulating arthritis caused by hysteria.

j., immovable. Joint without tissue bet. bones, rendering it immovable. SYN: *synarthrosis.*

j's, intercarpal. Articulations which the carpal bones form in relation to one another.

j., irritable. Inflamed spasmodic condition of joint of unknown cause.

j., Lisfranc's. Tarsometatarsal joint.

j., midcarpal. Joint dividing the carpal bones and the scaphoid, semilunar, and cuneiform bones.

j., mixed. Joint with surfaces joined by fibrocartilaginous disks.

j. mouse. Loose cartilage or other body in a joint.

j., movable. SEE: *diarthrodial joint.* SYN: *diarthrosis.*

j., m., slightly. One formed by interosseous ligaments or disks of cartilage, as bet. bodies of vertebrae, symphysis pubis, etc. SYN: *amphiarthrosis.*

j. movement. May be gliding; angular, including adduction, extension, abduction, flexion; circumduction, and rotatory.

j., multiaxial. SEE: *ball and socket joint.*

j., pisocuneiform. Joint of the pisiform and cuneiform carpal bones.

j., pivot. SEE: *rotary joint.*

j., polyaxial. SEE: *ball and socket joint.*

j., receptive or **reciprocal.** Saddle joint, *q.v.*

j., rotary. Rotating diarthrodial joint. SYN: *trochoides.*

j., saddle. Joint composed of two surfaces resembling saddles at right angles to each other.

j., simple. Joint composed of two bones.

j., spheroid. Multiaxial joint with spheroid surfaces.

j., spiral. SEE: *cochlear joint.*

j., synarthrodial. SEE: *immovable joint.*

j., tomato. Pain in the joints wrongly attributed to eating too many tomatoes.

j., trochoid. SEE: *rotary joint.*

j., uniaxial. Joint moving on a single axis.

j., unilocular. Joint with a single cavity.

Jolles' test (yŏl'es). Test for biliary pigments in urine.

joule (jool). Work done in one second by current of one ampere against a resistance of one ohm.

Joule's equivalent (jools). Amt. of work which, if converted into heat, will raise temperature of one pound of water 1° F.

J.'s law. 1. Rate of heat production in a part of a circuit is equal to the resistance of that part of the circuit multiplied by the square of the current. 2. In gas expansion, with no change in the amount of heat in a given quantity of gas, and no external work performed, there is no change in temperature.

ju'gal. Pert. to the cheek bone.

j. bone. Malar bone.

j. process. Temporal bone process forming zygomatic arch. SYN: *zygomatic process.*

juga'le. The point at the margin of zygomatic process.

jugate (jŭ'gāt). 1. Coupled, yoked. 2. Having ridges.

ju'gular. Pert. to the throat.

j. foramen. Opening caused by jugular notches of the occipital and temporal bones.

j. fossa. Depression in the petrosal portion of the temporal bone for the jugular vein.

j. ganglion. Nodes of vagus root and glossopharyngeal nerve in jugular foramen.

j. process. Projection from occipital bone toward the temporal bone.

j. veins. *External,* receives the blood from the ext. of the cranium and the deep parts of the face. It lies superficial to the sternocleidomastoid muscle as it passes down the neck to join the subclavian vein. *Internal,* receives blood from the brain and superficial parts of the face and neck. It is directly continuous with the transverse sinus, accompanying the internal carotid as it passes down the neck, and joins with the subclavian vein to form the innominate vein.

jugulate (jug'u-lāt). To arrest quickly a process or disease by therapeutic measures.

jugula'tion. Sudden arrest of a disease by therapeutic means.

jug'ulum. Neck or throat.

ju'gum. Ridge or furrow connecting two points.

j. penis. Forceps for temporarily compressing the penis.

j. petrosum. Eminence on petrous section of temporal bone showing the position of sup. semicircular canal. SYN: *arcuate eminence.*

juice. Liquid that exudes or is expressed from any part of an organism.

j., alimentary. The digestive juices.

j. canals. Connective tissue spaces forming origin of lymphatic vessels.

j., gastric. Secretions of the stomach consisting of water, salts, pepsin, rennin, and free hydrochloric acid.

j., intestinal. A clear, yellowish, viscid fluid; alkaline in reaction, secreted by

Lieberkühn's crypts. Syn: *succus entericus.* See: *intestinal juice.*

j., joint. A tenacious, colorless, stringy secretion that lubricates a joint. Syn: *synovia.*

j., pancreatic. A clear, viscid, alkaline digestive juice of the pancreas poured into the duodenum. It contains the enzymes *trypsin, amylase,* and *lipase* or *steapsin.*

jumentous (jū-men'tus). Like that of a horse; said of odor of urine.

jum'per. One with nervous disorder who is startled easily or who jumps at sound of a loud noise. See: *palmus.*

jump'ing disease'. Jumping spasmodic movements and feeble will. Syn: *palmus.*

junction (junk'shun). The place of union or coming together of two parts.

j., myoneural. Meeting point of a nerve with the muscle to which it is distributed.

j., sclerocorneal. Meeting point bet. the sclera and the cornea marked on the external surface of the eyeball by the outer scleral sulcus.

junctura (junk-tu'rā). Suture of bones. Articulation.

junk. Cushion utilized in fracture dressing.

junk'et. Flavored curds and whey.

Junod's arm or **boot** (zhu-nōz'). Airtight casing into which limb is placed and air exhausted, to relieve congestion.

jurymast (ju'rĭ-mast). Apparatus for support of head in disease of the spine.

jusculum (jus'ku-lum). Broth or soup.

Juster's reflex. Finger extension instead of flexion when palm of hand is irritated.

jus'to ma'jor. Bigger than normal, as a *pelvis.*

j., mi'nor. Smaller than normal, as a *pelvis.*

Jus'tus' test. A test for syphilis determined by the reaction on hemoglobin of a dose of mercury.

jute (jūt). Fiber used in dressings.

juvantia (ju-van'shĭ-ā). Adjuvant medicines which intensify action of other drugs or assist them.

juxta-. Prefix: Close proximity.

jux"taärtic'ular. Situated close to a joint.

juxtangi'na. Inflamed condition of pharyngeal muscles.

juxtaposition (juks"ta-po-zish'un). Position that is adjacent or side by side. Syn: *apposition, contiguity.*

juxtapylor'ic. Near the pylorus or pyloric orifice.

juxtaspi'nal. Near the spinal column.

K

K Chem. symb. for *kalium*, potassium.

Ka. Abbr. for *cathode*.

Ka'der's opera'tion. Surgical formation of a gastric fistula with feeding tube inserted through valvelike flap.

Kaes' feltwork. Nerve fiber network in cerebral cortex.

kaf'fir pox. Modified smallpox with pustules not umbilicated and without a secondary rise in temperature. SYN: *alastrim.*

Kahl'baum's disease. Cyclic dementia with marked muscular tension. SYN: *katatonia, q.v.*

Kahl'er's disease. Destructive bone marrow disease. SYN: *multiple myeloma, q.v.*

Kahn test. 1. A syphilitic test used as a control on the complement fixation test. 2. Test for presence of carcinoma.

kaif (kīf). A dreamy, tranquil state induced by drugs.

kainophobia (ki-no-fo'bĭ-ă). Abnormal aversion to new situations and things. SYN: *neophobia.*

kais'erling, Kais'erling's solution. Liquid used in preserving pathological specimens.

kakergasia (kak-er-gas'ĭ-ă). 1. Minor psychosis; a term used in place of "neurosis" and "psychoneurosis" when psychodynamic and not primarily nervous. 2. Poor mental functioning. SYN: *merergasia.*

kakergastic (kak-er-gas'tik). Pert. to minor psychoses.
  Applied to those still relatively normal, afflicted with vagaries but of a holergastic* nature. SYN: *merergastic.*

kakasthe'sia. 1. Any disorder of sensibility. 2. Malaise.

kakidro'sis. Unpleasant odor of the sweat. SYN: *bromidrosis.*

kak'ke. Endemic form of polyneuritis. SYN: *beriberi.*

kakosmia (kak-oz'mĭ-ă). Perception of bad odors which do not exist. SYN: *cacosmia, parosmia.*

kakotrophy (kak-ot'rof-i). Malnutrition. SYN: *cacotrophy.*

kala azar (kä'la-a'zar). Infectious disease of the East, from which thousands die annually.

kaliemia (kal-ĭ-e'mĭ-ă). Potassium in the blood.

kaligenous (ka-lij'en-us). Forming potash.

kalimeter (kal-im'e-ter). Device for determining degree of alkalinity of a substance. SYN: *alkalimeter.*

ka'lium. (K) Potassium. A mineral element necessary to the growth of cells, esp. those of the muscles and blood.

kallikrein (kăl-ĭk'rē-ĭn). Urinary extract, probably of pancreatic origin, used in disorders of the circulatory system.

kaolin (kā'o-lin). A yellowish white powder, occurring as a decomposition product of feldspar.

kaolinosis (kā"o-lin-o'sis). Pneumokoniosis caused by inhaling kaolin particles.

kaomagma (kā'ō-mag'ma). A 20% suspension of colloidal kaolin in 2½% aluminum hydroxide.
  DOSAGE: ½ oz. (15 cc.).
  k. with mineral oil. Kaomagma with 20% mineral oil.
  DOSAGE: ½ oz. (15 cc.).

Kapo'si's disease. Diffuse atrophic skin condition. SYN: *xeroderma pigmentosum, q.v.*

Karell cure (ka'rel). Rest in bed, milk sipped in small amounts (not over a quart a day for 5 or 6 days), for treatment of cardiac disease, high blood pressure, and renal insufficiency.
  K. diet. A saltless diet constituting a fraction of usual normal diet, given in small quantities at definite intervals, gradually increased by adding other foods; intended to relieve the vital organs.
  K. d., modified. Found useful when milk is not well tolerated. Food value, water, and salt content only slightly changed.   [cleus.

karyo-. Prefix: Referring to a cell's nucleus.

kar'yochromat'ophil. Having nucleus which stains.

karyochrome (kar'i-o-krōm). The cell of a nerve with an easily staining nucleus.

karyoc'lasis. The fragmentation of a cell nucleus.

karyogamy (kar-ĭ-og'ă-mĭ). Union of nuclei in cell conjugation.

karyogen (kar'ĭ-o-jen). A compound of iron in certain cell nuclei.

karyogenesis (kar'ĭ-ō-jĕn'ĕ-sĭs). Formation and development of a cell nucleus.

karyokinesis (kar'ĭ-o-kin-e'sis). 1. Changes taking place in a nucleus during indirect cell division. SYN: *mitosis.* 2. In a narrower sense, nuclear division only.

karyokinetic (ka"rĭ-o-kĭ-net'ĭk). 1. Pert. to karyokinesis. 2. Ameboid.

karyolobic (kar"ĭ-ō-lō'bĭk). Possessing a nucleus shaped like a lobe.

karyolobism (kar"ĭ-o-lo'bizm). A lobed condition of the nucleus of a leukocyte, as the polymorphonuclear neutrophiles.

kar'yolymph. Fluid in meshes of the nucleus. SYN: *nuclear sap.*

karyolysis (kar-ĭ-ol'ĭ-sis). 1. The destruction of a nucleus or loss of affinity for basic dyes. SYN: *chromatolysis.* 2. The nuclear changes in cell division. SYN: *karyokinesis.*

Karyol'ysus. A genus of Hemosporidia destructive to cells.

karyolyt'ic. Producing or rel. to karyolysis.

kar'yomit. Chromatin thread in a cell nucleus. SYN: *chromosome.*

karyomitome (kar-ĭ-om′ĭ-tōm). Network of the cell nucleus.

karyomitosis (kar″ĭ-o-mit-o′sis). Nuclear changes in cell division. Syn: *karyokinesis.*

karyomorphism (kar″ĭ-o-mōr′fizm). The form of a cell nucleus.

karyon (kar′ĭ-on). The cell nucleus.

karyophage (kar′ĭ-o-fāj). An intracellular protozoan parasite.

karyoplasm (kar′ĭ-o-plazm). Nuclear material of a cell as distinguished from cytoplasm or the protoplasm of a cell body.

karyorrhexis (kar″ĭ-o-rek′sis). Fragmentation of the chromatin in nuclear disintegration.

karyosome (kar′ĭ-o-sōm). Chromatin mass at nodes of nuclear network. Syn: *netknot, nucleolus.*

karyotheca (kar″ĭ-o-the′kă). The enveloping membrane of a cell nucleus.

kata-. Prefix: Down.

katab′olism. The breaking down process in metabolism. Syn: *catabolism.*

kataphrax′is. Surgical formation of metallic supports for an organ.

kataplasia (kat-ă-pla′sĭ-ă). Reversion of a degenerating or atrophied cell to the form of a developing or embryonic cell.

katastalsis (kat-ă-stal′sis). Term for gastric downward moving wave of contraction which occurs without a preceding wave of inhibition.

katathermometer (ka″ta-ther-mom′e-ter). A thermometer for measuring the efficiency of ventilation and cooling and drying processes.

katatonia (kat-a-tō′ni-a). A psychosis with marked muscular tension. It constitutes 10% of all cases of schizophrenia. Insanity ending in imbecility.

katelectrotonus (kat″el-ek-trot′o-nus). Increased excitability in a muscle or nerve in area near cathode during passage of a current. Syn: *catelectrotonus, q.v.*

katharom′eter. Electrical device to measure basal metabolic rates.

kathisophobia (kath-i-so-fo′bi-a). Fear of sitting down, and subsequent inability to sit still.

kation (kat′i-on). Element appearing at the cathode or negative pole in electrochemical decomposition. Syn: *cation.*

katolysis (kă-tol′ĭ-sis). Partial breaking down of chemical bodies into simpler compounds.

katophoria (ka-to-fo′rĭ-ă). Inclination of the eyeball downward. Syn: *katotropia.*

katotro′pia. Tendency of the eyeball to drop too far downward. Syn: *katophoria.*

kava, kava-kava (kă′vă). 1. Root of *Piper methysticum* used in wasting diseases, gout, and cystitis. 2. Intoxicating beverage prepared from the root.

K.B. Abbr. of Weltmann for normal coagulation band applied to reaction if flocculation is up to and including 6 tubes out of 10 used in the test showing flocculation, the tubes containing Weltmann's solution. Later experience shows flocculation in the 7th tube to be normal.

KBr. Potassium bromide.

KC₂H₃O₂. Potassium acetate.

KCl. Potassium chloride.

KClO. Potassium hypochlorite.

KClO₃. Potassium chlorate.

K₂CO₃. Potassium carbonate.

kefir, kefyr (ke′fer). A preparation of curdled milk.

kelectome (ke′lek-tōm). Instrument for removing specimen of tumor tissue.

kelis (ke′lis). 1. Skin disease with pigmented pink and purple patches and lesions leaving scars. Syn: *morphea.* 2. Skin tumor of dense tissue. Syn: *keloid.*

Kel′log's inspiratory lift-exercise. Abdominal exercise for the puerperium.

Kel′ly pad. A drainage pad for the operating table or bed made by wrapping one end of a rubber sheet over a rolled small blanket, forming a bolster; the bolster is twisted round like a horseshoe to form the pad, the free part of the sheet forming the apron. Also commercial inflatable rubber pad of horseshoe shape used in same way.

keloid (ke′loid). 1. Scar tissue. 2. A new growth of the skin consisting of dense tissue; most common in the colored race.

   k., acne. Hypertrophic scars on nape of neck at border of scalp. Etiol: *Suppurative folliculitis.*

   k., Addison's. Skin disease with pigmented patches and lesions. Syn: *morphea, q.v.*

   k., Alibert's. Growth of fibrous tissue usually at the site of a scar resembling a true keloid.

   k. en plaque. Circumscribed hard plate elevated a little over surface and imbedded in the skin.

keloidosis (ke-loi-do′sis). The formation of keloids.

kelotomy (ke-lot′o-mĭ). Operation for strangulated hernia through tissues of the constricting neck.

kenogenesis (ken-o-jen′ĕ-sis). Deviation from the normal in course of development. [spaces.]

kenophobia (ken-o-fo′bĭ-ă). Fear of empty

kenotox′in. Fatigue toxin due to muscular exercise.

kephalin (kef′a-lĭn). 1. A phospholipin found in brain tissue, and related to the lecithins with hematostatic action. 2. Commercial headache remedy. Syn: *cephalin.*

kephyr (ke′fer). Curdled milk preparation.

keratalgia (ker-a-tal′jĭ-ă). Neuralgia of the cornea.

keratectasia (ker-a-tek-ta′sĭ-ă). Conical protrusion of the cornea.

keratectomy (ker-ă-tek′to-mĭ). Excision of portion of cornea.

keratiasis (ker-ă-ti′a-sis). Horny wart formation.

kerat′ic. Rel. to horn. Syn: *corneous, horny.*

ker′atin. A scleroprotein substance in hair, nails, and horny tissue, insoluble in gastric juice.

keratinous (ker-at′in-us). Pert. to or composed of keratin.

keratitis (ker-a-ti'tis). Inflammation of cornea.

Ingestion of foods containing riboflavin or synthetic forms of it clear up the condition rapidly.

k., aspergillar. Keratitis of cornea due to infection from a mold.

k., band-shaped. Whitish or grayish band extending across the cornea.

k. bullosa. The formation of large, quite resistant blebs in the cornea of blind trachomatous eyes with increased tension.

k., deep. SEE: *interstitial keratitis.*

k., dendritic. Superficial branching corneal ulcers.

k. disciformis. Gray disk-shaped opacity in middle of cornea.

k., fascicular. Corneal ulcer resulting from phlyctenules which spread from limbus to center of cornea accompanied by fascicle of blood vessels.

k., herpetic. Vesicular keratitis in herpes zoster.

k., hypopyon. Serpiginous ulcer with pus in ant. chamber.

k., interstitial. Deep form of nonsuppurative keratitis with vascularization, occurring usually in syphilis and rarely in tuberculosis. Commonly found between 5th and 15th years.

k., lagophthalmic. Desiccation of cornea due to defective closure of lids.

k., mycotic. Produced by mold fungi.

k., neuroparalytic. Dull and slightly cloudy insensitive cornea seen in lesions of fifth nerve.

k., parenchymatous. SEE: *interstitial keratitis.*

k., phlyctenular. Circumscribed inflammation of conjunctiva and cornea accompanied by formation of small projections called phlyctenules which consist of accumulations of lymphoid cells. The phlyctenules soften at the apices, forming ulcers.

k., punctate. Cellular deposits on post. surface of cornea seen in diseases of uveal tract.

k., purulent. Keratitis with formation of pus.

k., sclerosing. Triangular opacity in deeper layers of cornea, complicating scleritis.

k., superficial punctate. Small gray spots in superficial layers of cornea, beneath Bowman's membrane, occurring in young persons.

k., trachomatous. Keratitis with abnormal membrane on cornea. SYN: *pannus.*

k., traumatic. Keratitis caused by wound of the cornea.

k., tuberculous. Infiltrating or interstitial keratitis with vascularization, due to *B. tuberculosis.*

k., vasculonebulous. SEE: *trachomatous keratitis.*

k., xerotic. Softening, desiccation, and ulceration of cornea. SYN: *keratomalacia.*

kerato-, kerat-. Combining form: Rel. to horny substances or to the cornea.

keratocele (ker-at'o-sēl). 1. Protrusion or herniation of Descemet's membrane through the floor of corneal ulcer. 2. Horny tumor.

keratoconus (ker-at-o-ko'nus). Conical protrusion of center of cornea without inflammation.

keratoderma (ker-ă-to-der'mă). 1. Superficial horny layer of the epidermis. 2. The cornea.

keratodermatitis (ker″ă-to-der-mă-ti'tis). Inflammation of the horny layer of the skin with proliferation.

ker″atoder'mia. 1. Superficial epidermal horny layer. 2. Cornea.

keratogenous (ker-ă-toj'en-us). Causing horny tissue development.

ker″atoglo'bus. Globular protrusion and enlargement of cornea seen in congenital glaucoma.

keratohelcosis (ker″a-to-hel-ko'sis). Corneal ulceration.   [corneal tissue.

ker'atoid. Horny or resembling horn or

keratoiditis (ker″ă-toid-i'tis). Inflammation of the cornea.

keratoiritis (ker″a-to-i-ri'tis). Inflammation of the cornea and iris.

keratoleptynsis (ker″ă-to-lep-tin'sis). Removal of the corneal surface, then covering the area with bulbar conjunctiva.

keratoleukoma (ker″ă-to-lu-ko'mă). White corneal opacity.

keratolysis (ker-ă-tol'is-is). 1. Loosening of horny layer of the skin. 2. Shedding of the skin at regular intervals.

keratolyt'ic. Rel. to or causing keratolysis. SYN: *desquamative.*

kerato'ma. 1. A callosity. 2. A horny growth. SYN: *keratosis.*

keratomalacia (ker″at-o-ma-la'sĭ-ă). Softening of the cornea seen in early childhood due to deficiencies of vitamin A.

keratome (ker'at-ōm). Knife for incising the cornea.

keratometer (ker-at-om'et-er). An instrument for measuring the curves of the cornea.

keratomycosis (ker″at-o-mī-ko'sis). Fungous growth on the cornea.

ker″atono'sis. Any noninflammatory disease of the horny layer of the skin.

keratonyxis (ker″ă-to-niks'is). Corneal puncture, esp. surgical puncture.

keratoplasty (ker'ă-to-plas″tĭ). Plastic operation on the cornea.

ker″atopro'tein. The protein of the hair, nails, epidermis, etc.

keratorrhexis (ker″a-to-rek'sĭs). Corneal rupture.

keratoscleritis (ker″ă-to-skle-ri'tis). Inflammation of both cornea and sclera.

keratoscope (ker'at-o-skōp). An instrument for examination of the cornea.

keratos'copy. Examination of the cornea and its reflection of light.

keratose (ker'ă-tōs). Horny.

keratosis (ker-at-o'sis). Horny growth.

k. follicularis. Skin disease in which papules contain scabby crusts which can be expressed.

k. palmaris et plantaris. Chronic disorder showing thickening of horny layer of palms and soles.

k. pilaris. Inflammatory disorder, chronic in course. Accumulation of horny material at follicular orifices, giving to affected surfaces a nutmeg-grater-like appearance, commonly in those with rough, dry skin.

k. seborrheica. Flat, rough, crusted or scaly keratic lesion.

k. seni'lis. Dry, harsh skin of the aged.

keratotome (ker-at'o-tōm). A knife for incising the cornea. SYN: *keratome*.

keratotomy (ker-at-ot'o-mĭ). Incision of cornea.

keraunoneurosis (kĕ-raw"no-nŭ-ro'sĭs). A neurosis from fear of a thunderstorm or from lightning stroke.

keraunophobia (kĕ-raw"no-fo'bĭ-ă). Dread of thunder and lightning.

kerectomy (ke-rek'to-mĭ). Excision of a portion of the cornea.

kerion (ke'rĭ-on). A form of *tinea tonsurans* with swollen discharging lesions.

kerither'apy. Treatment of burns and denuded surfaces with liquid paraffin.

Kerk'ring's folds or **valves.** Transverse folds of intestinal mucous membranes. SYN: *plicae circulares, valvulae conniventes*.

Ker'nig's sign. A symptom of meningitis, evidenced by reflex contraction and pain in the hamstring muscles when attempting to extend the leg after flexing the thigh upon the body.

ketogenesis (ke-to-jen'ĕ-sĭs). Production of ketones or acetone substances.

ketogenic diet (ke-to-jen'ĭk). One that produces acetone or ketone bodies, or mild acidosis. Highly beneficial in epilepsy.

ketol'ysis. The dissolution of acetone or ketone bodies.

ketolyt'ic. Pert. to ketolysis.

ke'tol. Crystalline substance formed in intestine and pancreas during putrefaction and digestion.

ketone (ke'tōn). Oxidation product of a secondary alcohol. Organic chemical substance of the general formula $\begin{smallmatrix} R \\ R \end{smallmatrix}\!\!>\!\!CO$.

The simplest example is *acetone*. The ketone acids in the body are the end products of fat metabolism.

k. bodies. Acetone bodies.

ketonemia (ke-to-ne'mĭ-ă). Acetone bodies in the blood. SYN: *acidosis*.

ketonuria (ke-ton-u'rĭ-ă). Acetone bodies in the urine.

ketopla'sia. The formation or excretion of ketones.

ketoplas'tic. Pert. to ketoplasia or formation of ketones.   [ketones.

ke'tose. A carbohydrate containing the

ketosis (kĕ-tō'sĭs). The accumulation in the body of the ketone bodies: Acetone, betahydroxybutyric acid, and aceto-acetic acid.

Key-Ret'zius foram'ina. Passages in the pia mater carrying the choroid plexus to the fourth ventricle.

Kg. Abbr. for *kilogram*.

KHCO₃. Potassium bicarbonate.

KHSO₄. Potassium bisulfate.

KI. Potassium iodide.

kibe (kīb). Inflamed patch on hands or feet caused by exposure to cold. SYN: *chilblain, q.v.*

kid'ney. One of two glandular, bean-shaped bodies, purplish-brown in color, situated at the back of the abdominal cavity, one on each side of the spinal column, which excrete waste matter in the form of urine.

k., amyloid. Kidney which is the seat of amyloid degeneration.

k., branny. Kidney in which spots of fatty degeneration give it the appearance of containing bran.

k., contracted. The small kidney of chronic interstitial or diffuse nephritis.

k., cystic. One that has undergone cystic degeneration.

k., embolic contracted. A contracted kidney in which embolic infarction of the renal arterioles produces degeneration of renal tissue, and hyperplasia of fibrous tissues produces irregular contraction.

k., fatty. One with fatty infiltration or degeneration of tubular, glomerular, or capsular epithelium, or of vascular connective tissue.

k., floating. One which is displaced and movable.

k., gouty. One with necrosis of renal connective tissue.

k., granular. A slow form of chronic nephritis, in which the size is diminished, and color is red with hard, fibrous, and granular texture.

k., hobnail. Granular kidney.

k., hog-back. That of chronic parenchymatous nephritis.

k., horseshoe. Congenital malformation with sup. or inf. extremities united by an isthmus of renal or fibrous tissue, in the form of a horseshoe.

k., lardaceous. Chronic nephritis, often secondary to syphilis, with infiltration with lardaceous matter of the malpighian bodies, arteries, tubes, and epithelium.

k., large mottled. A type of chronic parenchymatous nephritis.

k., large red. One resembling that of acute parenchymatous nephritis.

k., large white. A chronic parenchymatous nephritis, resulting from an acute inflammation, the organ exceeding 12 oz. in weight.

k., movable. Displaced or loosened. SYN: *nephroptosis*.

k., pigback. Congested kidney of alcoholic subjects.

k., red contracted. Gouty kidney.

k., sacculated. A condition in which the organ has been absorbed and only the distended capsule remains.

k., senile. One with atrophy of the glomeruli and tubules seen in old age.

k., small red granular. Granular kidney.

k., surgical. Suppurative pyelonephritis following operation upon urinary tract.

k., syphilitic. One with fibrous bands running across it, also caseating gummata, due to syphilis.

k., wandering. A floating kidney.

k., waxy. SEE: _lardaceous kidney._

Xienböck unit. Measurement of x-ray dosage; 1/10 of erythema dose.

Kier'nan's spaces. The spaces bet. the lobes of the liver.

Kiesselbach's area (ke'sel-bahks). An area on the ant. inferior part of the septum. The commonest site for septal bleeding.

Kil'ian's pelvis. Pelvis affected with osteomalacia. SYN: _pelvis spinosa._

kilo-. One thousand.

kil'ogram. One thousand grams.

kiloliter (kil'o-lē-ter). One thousand liters.

kil'ometer. One thousand meters.

kil'ovolt. One thousand volt unit.

kilovoltmeter (kil-o-volt'me-ter). A voltmeter calibrated in kilovolts.

kinanesthesia (kin″an-es-the'zĭ-ă). Inability to see extent of movement, or direction resulting in ataxia.

kinase (kĭn'ās). A colloidal substance in the intestines and some other organs which is necessary to activate enzymes.

kinemat'ics. Science of motion.

kineplas'tic. Pert. to laying down of primitive trace of muscle tissue.

kin'eplasty. A form of amputation so that motion is imparted to an artificial limb.

kinergety (kin-er'jet-ĭ). The potential capacity for kinetic energy.

kinesalgia (kin-es-al'jĭ-ă). Pain attending muscular movement.

kinesia (kin-e'sĭ-ă). 1. Sickness caused by motion, as seasickness, car sickness. 2. Active or passive hygienic exercises.

kinesialgia (ki-ne-sĭ-al'jĭ-ă). Pain caused by muscular movements. SYN: _kinesalgia._

kinesiatrics (ki-ne-sĭ-at'riks). Treatment involving active and passive movements. SYN: _kinesitherapy._

kinesiodic (ki-ne-sĭ-od'ik). Pert. to paths through which motor impulses pass.

kinesiology (kin-es-ĭ-ol'o-jĭ). The study of muscular movements.

kinesioneurosis (ki-ne″sĭ-o-nū-ro'sis). Functional disorder marked by tics and spasms.

k., external. Kinesioneurosis affecting external muscles.

k., vascular. Kinesioneurosis of the vasomotor system.

k., visceral. Kinesioneurosis affecting muscles of internal organs.

kinesipathy (ki-ne-sip'a-thĭ). 1. Treatment by movement. SYN: _kinesitherapy._ 2. Motor disturbance.

kinesis (kin-e'sis). Motion.

kinesither'apy. Treatment by movements.

kinesod'ic. Rel. to the conveyance of motor impulses.

kinesthesia (kin-es-the'zĭ-ă). 1. Ability to perceive extent or direction, or weight of movement. 2. Illusion of gliding through space.

kinesthesiometer (ki″nes-the-zĭ-om'ĕ-tĕr). Instrument for testing the muscular reaction.

kinesthet'ic. Rel. to kinesthesia.

kinetic (ki-net'ĭk). Pert. to or consisting of motion.

k. system. The endocrine glands.

kinetism (ki-net'izm). Ability to have muscular functioning.

kinetocyte (ki-net'o-sit). An egg-shaped, wandering cell in the blood, the others being _erythrocytes, leukocytes,_ and _platelets._

kinetocythemia (ki-ne″to-si-the'mĭ-ă). An abnormally large number of kinetocytes in the blood. SYN: _kinetocytosis._

kinetocytopenia (ki-ne″to-si″to-pe'nĭ-a). Lack of kinetocytes in the blood.

kinetocytosis (ki-ne″to-si-to'sis). More than normal number of kinetocytes in the blood.   [movement.

kinetogenic (ki-net-o-jen'ĭk). Causing

kinetoplasm (ki-ne'to-plazm). The chromophilic substance in nerve cells.

kinetosis (ki-ne-to'sis). Any disorder caused by motion, such as seasickness, car sickness, etc. SYN: _kinesia._

kinetotherapy (kĭ-net″o-ther'ă-pĭ). Treatment that employs active and passive movements. SYN: _kinesitherapy._

king's evil. Constitutional condition characterized by glandular swellings in neck and inflammation of joints and mucosa. So called, because it was thought curable by touch of a king. SYN: _scrofula._

kinom'eter. Instrument which measures displacements of the uterus.

kinomom'eter. Device which measures degree of motion of fingers and toes.

kinone (kĭ'nōn). 1. Substance derived from quinic acid. 2. Any benzene derivative in which 2 oxygen atoms replace 2 hydrogen atoms. SYN: _quinone._

ki'noplasm. That part of protoplasm upon which cellular motivity depends. SYN: _ergoplasm._

kinoplas'tic. Rel. to kinoplasm.

kin'osphere. One of the figures formed by division of the centrosome. SYN: _aster._

kinotox'in. Fatigue toxin. SYN: _cinotoxin._

ki'otome. Instrument for amputating the uvula.

kiotomy (ki-ot'o-mĭ). Use of the kiotome in amputating the uvula.

Kisch's reflex (kĭsh). Closure of an eye resulting from stimulation by heat or some tactile irritant on the ext. auditory meatus or deeper portions of canal up to tympanum.

Kite apparatus. Apparatus for reëducation of weak muscles and for assistance in overcoming contractures of forearm, wrist and fingers.

Klaus'ner's reaction or test. Serum of an assumed syphilitic is covered with distilled water in a test tube. Turbidity at plane of contact will show if syphilis is present.

Klebsiella (kleb-sĭ-el'ă). A genus of the family Bacteriaceae causing respiratory affections.

K. capsulatus. Encapsulated rods, singly or in chains in catarrhal inflammations of respiratory tract.

K. granulomatis. Found in granuloma inguinale.

K. ozaenae. A species causing ozena.

K. pneumoniae. Friedländer's bacillus, in certain pneumonias.

K. rhinoscleromatis. The cause of rhinoscleroma.

Klebs-Loeffler bacil'lus (klebs-lef'ler). The bacillus of diphtheria. SYN: *corynebacterium diphtheriae.* SEE: *diphtheria.*

Klem'perer's test meal. Milk, 500 cc.; 2 rolls, 70 Gm. This is given on an empty stomach and aspirated 2 hr. later.

kleptolagnia (klep″to-lag'nĭ-ă). Sexual gratification derived from stealing.

kleptomania (klep-to-ma'nĭ-ă). Impulsive stealing, the motive not being in the intrinsic value of the article to the patient. There is often deep regret following the act.

kleptoma'niac. 1. A psychopathic personality suffering from impulsive stealing. 2. Pert. to kleptomania.

kleptophobia (klep-to-fo'bĭ-ă). Morbid fear of stealing.

Klieg eye (klēg). Conjunctivitis, lacrimation and photophobia from exposure to the intense lights used in making moving pictures.

Kline test, Kline-Young test. A microscope slide precipitation test for presence of syphilis.

Klon'dike bed. Outdoor sleeping bed that protects patient from draughts.

klotogen (klot'o-jen). A standardized concentrate of vitamin K in peanut oil.

DOSAGE: *Prophylactic:* 1000 units given with 10 gr. bile salts, during meals, 3 times daily for 4 days. *Therapeutic:* 10,000 units by duodenal tube, followed by sufficient amount of bile salts dissolved in warm water.

Klumpke's paralysis (kloomp'kez). Atrophic paralysis of forearm.

Knapp's forceps. A forceps with blades like rollers for expressing trachomatous granulations on the palpebral conjunctiva.

knead'ing. A form of massage, consisting of grasping, wringing, lifting, rolling, or pressing part of a muscle or group of muscles. SYN: *pétrissage.*

knee. The ant. aspect of the leg at the articulation of the femur and tibia; also the articulation itself, covered anteriorly with the patella or kneecap. Formed by the femur, tibia, and patella.

k., Brodie's. A chronic, fungoid synovitis of the knee joint in which the affected parts become soft and pulpy.

k. chest position. Resting upon the knees and chest with forearms supporting the head. SEE: *position.*

k., game. A lay term for internal derangement of knee joint.

k., housemaid's. Inflamed condition of the bursa in front of the patella, with accumulation of fluid therein, frequently seen in scrubwomen.

k., in-. The condition in which the knees come together while the ankles are far apart, caused by an outward distortion of the leg throwing knee inside the normal line. SYN: *genu valgum, knock-knee.*

k. of the internal capsule. The curve at the meeting place of the ant. and post. limbs of the internal capsule.

k. jerk reflex. The reflex contraction or clonic spasm of the quadriceps muscle, produced by sharply striking the ligamentum patellae when the leg hangs loosely flexed at right angles.

k. joint. The articulation of the femur and tibia.

k. knock-. An outward distortion of the leg, throwing knee inside the normal line. SYN: *genu valgum, in-knee.*

k., lawn tennis. A sprain of int. semilunar cartilage of knee joint.

k., out-. Bowleg. SYN: *genu varum.*

knee'cap. The patella.

kneel'ing-squat'ting posi'tion. The patient stoops with knees pressed against the abdomen, and with trunk erect; employed in childbirth in difficult cases.

Kneipp cure (nīp). Application of water in various forms and degrees of temperature in the cure of disease, esp. wading in cold, dewy grass. SYN: *hydrotherapy.*

kneippism (nīp'izm). Walking barefoot in dewy grass, bathing in cold water, etc., as a cure of disease.

knife (nīf). A cutting instrument.

k., electric. A knife carrying a high frequency cutting current.

knit'ting. The union of pieces of a fractured bone.

KNO₃. Potassium nitrate, niter, saltpeter.

knock-knee. Condition of having the knees turned inward. SYN: *genu valgum, in-knee.*

knockout drops. Colloquial name for chloral hydrate given in alcoholic beverages to produce rapid coma.

Koag'amin. Commercial preparation of blood coagulant.

K. O. C. Abbr. of *cathodal opening contraction.* SYN: COC.

Kocher's reflex (kō'kĕr). Contraction of abdominal muscles following moderate compression of testicle.

Koch's bacil'lus (kōks). The bacillus of tuberculosis.

k.'s law or **postulate.** To prove an organism the cause of a disease or lesion: 1st, microörganism in question must appear in lesion at all times; 2nd, pure cultures must be obtained from it; 3rd, cultures must reproduce disease in animals and pure cultures be again obtained from these lesions.

K.'s lymph. Tuberculin.

KOH. Potassium hydroxide.

Kohlrausch's fold or **valve** (kōhl'rowshs). Fold of mucous membrane extending into rectum; rectal valve. SYN: *plica transversales recti.*

koilonychia (koy-lo-nik'ĭ-ă). Malformation of the fingernails; outer surface is concave.

koinotropic type (kroin'o-trop-ĭk). Term applied to one who can give and take, as the "good mixer."

ko'la. Cardiac and nerve stimulant derived from *Sterculia acuminata.*

Kol'mer test. 1. A modification of the Wassermann test. 2. Complement fixation test for some infectious diseases.

kolp-. Prefix: Vagina.

kolpi'tis. Inflammation of vaginal mucous membrane. SYN: *colpitis.*

kolpot'omy. A vaginal operation. SYN: *colpotomy, elytrotomy.*

kol'yone. 1. An antacid opposing action of a hormone. 2. An endocrine that diminishes activity of cells. SYN: *chalone, colyone.*

kolypeptic (ko-lĭ-pep'tĭk). Retarding digestion.

kolyphrenia (kol-ĭ-fre'nĭ-ă). Exaggerated mental inhibition.

kolyseptic (ko-lĭ-sep'tĭk). Antiseptic.

kolytic (ko-lit'ĭk). Hindering or presenting or checking, as a reaction to a stimulus.

Kondoleon's operation (kŏn-dō'lē-ŏn). Surgical removal of layers of subcutaneous tissue to relieve elephantiasis.

koniol'ogy. Science of dust and its effects. SYN: *coniology.*

koniometer (ko-nĭ-om'ĕ-ter). Device for estimating amt. of dust in the air.

koniosis (ko-nĭ-o'sĭs). Any morbid condition caused by dust. SYN: *coniosis.*

kopf-tet'anus. Tetanus developing subsequent to head wounds.

kopiopia (ko-pĭ-o'pĭ-ă). Eyestrain. SYN: *copiopia.*

Kop'lik's spots. Small red spots with bluish white centers on the oral mucosa, particularly in the region opposite the line of juncture of the molar teeth.

Kopp's asth'ma. Spasm of the glottis in infants not over two years of age.

koronion (ko-ro'nĭ-on). Apex of coronoid process of the mandible.

koroscopy (kor-os'ko-pĭ). Shadow test for refraction of the eye.

Korsakoff's psychosis or syndrome (kor'sak-ofs). One characterized by a psychosis with a polyneuritis, disorientation, muttering delirium, insomnia, illusions and hallucinations, painful extremities, rarely a bilateral wrist drop, more frequently bilateral foot drop with pain or pressure over the lower nerves.

Kott'mann's reaction or test. A blood serum reaction test to indicate whether or not the thyroid gland is functioning.

koumiss (koo'mĭs). Fermented milk beverage. SYN: *kumyss.*

kraurosis (kraw-rō'sĭs). Atrophy and dryness of the skin and mucous membranes of a part, esp. of the vulva.

    k. vul'vae. An atrophy of the skin and mucosa, seen in elderly women which pathologically consists of a marked atrophy of the vulvar skin, and which is characterized clinically by severe itching.

Krause's cells or corpuscles. Bodies in mucous membranes analogous to pacinian corpuscles.

    K.'s end bud or bulb. Expanded termination of a sensory nerve.

    K.'s glands. Mucous acinous glands of middle portion of conjunctiva.

    K.'s membrane. Thin, dark disk transversely crossing through and bisecting clear zone of a striated muscle.

    K.'s valve. Mucous membrane fold at juncture where lacrimal sac narrows into nasal duct. SYN: *Béraud's valve.*

kreatine (kre'at-in). Creatine, q.v.

kreatinine (kre-at'in-in). Creatinine, q.v.

kreotox'in. A poison in flesh due to a microörganism.

kreotox'ism. Meat poisoning.

kresep'tol. A cresol disinfectant more active than the solution cresol compound, USP, made with a specially purified cresol and free from the objectionable impurities present in ordinary official cresol.

kresol (kre'sol). USP: Brownish yellow fluid from coal tar, used as a germicide. SYN: *cresol, q.v.*

Krishaber's disease (krēs-ă-bairs'). Neurosis marked by dizziness, sleeplessness, palpitation and syncope.

Kromayer lamp (kro'mi-er). Water cooled, mercury quartz lamp for local ultraviolet treatments.

Krompecher's tumor (krŏm'pekh-ers). Rodent ulcer. SYN: *Jacob's ulcer.*

Kronecker's center (krŏn'ek-ers). The inhibitory cardiac center.

Krönig's area or field (kra'nĭg). Resonant region in the thorax over the apices of the lungs.

Kruk'enberg's tumor. A malignant tumor of the ovary, usually bilateral, and secondary to malignancies, esp. of the gastrointestinal tract.

kryp'ton. A gaseous element found in small amts. in the atmosphere. SYMB: *Kr.*

kry'ofin. Crystalline antipyretic and antineuralgic.

K_2SO_4. Potassium sulfate.

kumiss, kumyss (koo'mĭs). 1. Cow's milk with sugar and yeast after fermentation. 2. Fermented mare's milk. SYN: *koumiss.*

Kund'rat's lymphosarco'ma. Lymphosarcoma which affects adjacent glands, but does not invade neighboring organs.

Kussmaul's coma (koos'mawls). Diabetic coma.*

kyestein, kyesthein (ki-es'te-in). A scum which floats on the standing urine of pregnant women.

kyllosis (ki-lo'sĭs). Clubfoot.

ky'matism. Twitching of isolated segments of muscle. SYN: *myokymia.*

kymograph (ki'mo-graf). Instrument for recording wavelike motions, esp. in blood pressure.

ky'moscope. Device for measuring variations in blood pressure.

kyogenic (ki-o-jen'ĭk). Inducing pregnancy.

ypho-. Prefix: Humped.

yphoscoliosis (ki"fo-sko-lI-o'sis). Angular and lateral spinal curvature.

yphosis (ki-fo'sis). A convex backward curvature of the spine; humpback, usually resulting from tuberculosis or fracture of the body of a vertebra. SYN: *humpback, spinal curvature.*

yphotic (ki-fot'ik). Affected by or pert. to kyphosis.

ky'rin. A protein resisting tryptic digestion, which yields amino acids when treated with an acid.

kyrtorrhachic (kir-to-rak'ik). Spinal curvature with concavity backward.

kysthitis (kis-thi'tis). Inflammation of the vagina. SYN: *colpitis, vaginitis.*

kysthoptosis (kis-thop-to'sis). Prolapse of the vagina.

kyto-. Prefix: Denoting cell.

L

L. Abbr. for *Latin, Lactobacillus, left, length, lithium, light sense, liter.*

lab, lab ferment. Milk-curdling ferment in rennet. SYN: *zymogen.**

    l. **zymogen.** Preparatory substance from which a ferment or enzyme is formed.

Labarraque's solution (lăb-ar-ăk'). Chlorinated soda solution; a disinfectant.

Labbe's vein (lă-bā'). Vein connecting lateral to sup. longitudinal sinus.

la'bia (sing. *labium*). 1. Lips. 2. The lips of the vulva.

    l. **majora.** The 2 folds of cellular adipose tissue extending from the *mons veneris** to the perineum, lying on either side of the vulva, lozenge shaped, and having an outer and an inner surface, the inner surface resembling the mucous membrane of the vagina, and the outer part being skin covered by pubic hair.

    l. **minora.** The two mucocutaneous folds of membrane within the labia majora lying on the inner and upper portion of the labia majora, the upper portion ensheathing the clitoris.

labial (la'bĭ-al). 1. Pert. to the lips. 2. Letter formed by the lips.

    l. **glands.** Many racemose glands bet. labial mucosa and orbicularis muscle opening on lip's inner surface.

labialism (la'bĭ-al-izm). Defective speech in which labial sounds are stressed.

labidometer (la-bĭ-dom'et-er). Forceps for measuring fetal head in pelvis.

labile (lab'ĭl). Not fixed; unsteady; easily disarranged.

    l. **elements.** Tissue cells which multiply by indirect nuclear division. SEE: *mitosis.*

lability (lab-ĭl'ĭt-ĭ). State of being unstable or changeable.

labimeter (lab-im'et-er). Forceps (or attachment to) for measuring fetal head. SYN: *labidometer.*

labioalveolar (lab"ĭ-ō-ăl-ve'ol-ar). Pert. to lips and tooth sockets.

labiocervical (lab"ĭ-ō-ser'vĭ-kăl). Pert. to lips, and the neck of a tooth.

labioglossolaryngeal (la"bĭ"o-glos"o-lar-in'je-ăl). Pert. to lips, tongue, and larynx.

    l. **paralysis.** A neurosis characterized by progressive paralysis of the parts mentioned.

labioglossopharyngeal (la"bĭ-o-glos"o-far-in'je-ăl). Pert. to the lips, tongue, and pharynx.

labiograph (la'bĭ-o-grăf). Device for registering the lip movements in speaking.

labiology (lă-bĭ-ol'o-jĭ). Study of the lip movements in speaking or singing.

labiomancy (la'bĭ-o-man"sĭ). Interpreting speech by reading lip movements.

labiomental (la-bĭ-ō-men'tal). Pert. to the lower lip and chin.

labiomycosis (la"bĭ-o-mī-ko'sĭs). Any disease of the lips due to presence of a fungus.

labiopalatine (la"bĭ-ō-pal'ă-tĭn). Relating to the lips and palate.

labioplasty (la'bĭ-o-plas"tĭ). Plastic surgery of the lips. SYN: *cheiloplasty.*

labiotenaculum (la"bĭ-o-ten-ak'u-lum). Instrument for holding lips during an operation.

la'bium (pl. *labia*). A lip or a structure like one. SEE: *labia.*

    l. **cerebri.** Margin of the cerebral hemispheres overlapping the corpus callosum.

    l. **inferius.** Lower lip.

    l. **majus** (pl. *labia majora**). One of 2 lateral boundaries of the vulva with adipose tissue and hair.

    l. **majus pudendi.** Fold of integument forming lateral boundary of the vulva.

    l. **minus** (pl. *labia minora**). One of 2 inner lips of vulva within the labia majora.

    l. **minus pudendi.** Lesser, inner lip of vulva. SYN: *nympha.*

    l. **superius.** The upper lip.

    l. **tympanicum.** Outer edge of organ of Corti.

    l. **urethrae.** Lateral margin of meatus urinarius externus.

    l. **uteri.** Thickened margin of the cervix uteri.

    l. **vestibulare.** Vestibular or inner edge of organ of Corti.

la'bor. The physiological process by which the fetus is expelled from the uterus at term. Normal appearance 280 days after last menstruation.

    l., **artificial.** Labor brought on by the use of ecbolics or hydrostatic bags.

    l., **complicated.** Any complication occurring during the course of labor.

    l., **dry.** Labor after most of the amniotic fluid has been drained away.

    l., **false.** Uterine contractions coming on before the onset of actual labor.

    l., **induced.** Labor brought on by the use of ecbolic hydrostatic bags, or any other method that may be used.

    l., **instrumental.** Labor completed by mechanical means, such as the use of forceps.

    l., **missed.** The patient goes through actual labor but the fetus dies and is not expelled. [fetuses.

    l., **multiple.** Labor with 2 or more

    l., **precipitate.** Rapidly completed labor that occurs without the aid of an accoucheur.

    l., **premature.** Labor coming on between the 7th month of gestation and full term.

l., spontaneous. Labor that is completed without external aid.

laboratory (lab'or-a-to-rĭ). A place equipped for analytical or experimental work.

labrocyte (lab'ro-sīt). Large leukocyte containing basophil granules.
Seen in normal blood and in leukemia. SYN: *mast cell.*

la'brum (pl. *labra*). Lip.

labyrinth (lab'ĭ-rinth). 1. Intricate communicating passages. 2. The internal ear consisting of osseous and membranous labyrinths.

l., bony. Osseous labyrinth, *q.v.*

l., ethmoidal. Membranous labyrinth, *q.v.*

l. of kidney cortex. Cortical substance of that part of kidney arranged around the uriniferous tubules of medullary rays in the cortex.

l., Ludwig's. Spaces bet. the cortical arches and Bertin's columns.

l., membranous. Structure in osseous labyrinth consisting of utricle and saccule of vestibule; 3 membranous, semicircular canals, and membranous portion of cochlea.

l., olfactory. Membranous labyrinth, *q.v.*

l., osseous. Consists of vestibule, 3 semicircular canals, and cochlea. Channeled out of substance of petrous bone.

labyrinthectomy (lab-ĭ-rin-thek'tō-mĭ). Excision of the labyrinth.

labyrinthine (lab-ĭ-rĭn'thĭn). 1. Pert. to a labyrinth. 2. Intricate or involved, as a labyrinth.

labyrinthitis (lab-ĭ-rĭn-thi'tis). Inflammation (acute or chronic) of labyrinth.

labyrinthotomy (lab-ĭ-rin-thot'o-mĭ). Incision of the labyrinth.

lac (lak). 1. Milk. 2. Milky medicinal substance.

lacerate (las'er-āt). To tear, as into irregular segments.

lacerated (las'er-a-ted). Torn; broken.

lacera'tion. A wound or irregular tear of the flesh.

l. of cervix. Bilateral, stellate, or unilateral tear of the cervix uteri caused by childbirth.

l. of perineum. Injury to perineum caused by childbirth. If extending through sphincter ani muscle it is *complete.*

lacertus (lă-ser'tus). 1. Muscular part of the arm. 2. A muscular or fibrous band.

l. cordis. Muscular tissue bands on inner cardiac surface. SYN: *trabecula carneae.*

l. fibro'sus. Aponeurotic band from the biceps tendon to the bicipital or semilunar fascia of forearm.

lacrimal (lak'rim-ăl). Pert. to the tears.

l. bone. One at inner side of the orbital cavity.

l. duct. Duct which conveys the secretion from the glands to the conjunctival sac.

l. gland. The gland which secretes the tears.

l. reflex. Secretion of fluid resulting from irritation of corneal conjunctiva.

l. sac. Upper dilated portion of nasolacrimal duct situated in groove of lacrimal bone. Upper part is behind internal tarsal ligament. Measures 12 mm. in vertical and 6 mm. in transverse diameter.

lacrimalin (lak-rim'a-lĭn). Lacrimal substance supposed to induce a flow of tears.

lacrimase (lak'rim-ās). Enzyme from tears.

lacrima'tion. Secretion and discharge of tears.

lacrimotomy (lak-rim-ot'o-mĭ). Incision of lacrimal duct.   [teria.

lactac'idase. Enzyme in lactic acid bac-

lactacidemia (lakt-as-id-e'mĭ-ă). Lactic acid in the blood. SYN: *lacticemia.*

lactacidogen (lak-ta-sid'o-jen). The assumed intermediary substance in the transformation of glycogen to lactic acid during muscular contraction.

lactaciduria (lakt-a-sid-ū'rĭ-ă). Lactic acid excreted in the urine.

lactagogue (lak'tă-gog). Agent which induces secretion of milk.

lactalase (lak'tă-lās). Ferment converting dextrose into lactic acid.

lactalbu'min. The albumin of milk and cheese; a soluble simple protein.

lac'tase. An intestinal sugar splitting enzyme converting lactose into dextrose and galactose; found in intestinal juice.
SEE: *enzyme, maltase, sucrase, sugar.*

lactate (lakt'āt). A salt derived from lactic acid.

lactation (lak-ta'shun). 1. The period of suckling in mammals. 2. The function of secreting milk.

lacteal (lak'te-al). 1. Pert. to milk. 2. An intestinal lymphatic that takes up chyle and passes it to the lymph circulation, and by way of the thoracic duct to the blood vascular system.
SEE: *absorption, lymphatic.*

lactescence (lak-tes'ens). Condition of becoming, or resembling milk.

lac'tic. Pert. to milk.

l. acid. $CH_3CH(OH).COOH$. An acid formed when milk sours through the action of sugar on certain microörganisms in the air.

l. fermentation. The fermentation of milk and milk products.

lacticemia (lakt-ĭ-se'mĭ-ă). Lactic acid in the blood. SYN: *lactacidemia.*

lactiferous (lakt-if'er-us). Secreting and conveying milk.

l. ducts. Ducts of the mammary gland.

l. glands. 1. The mammary glands. 2. Montgomery's glands consisting of 20 to 24 glands in the areola of the nipples.

lactification (lak"tĭ-fĭ-ka'shun). Lactic acid production.

lactifuge (lak'tĭ-fuj). 1. Stopping milk secretion. 2. Agent stopping milk secretion. SYN: *ischogalactic.*

lactigenous (lak-tij'en-us). Producing milk.

lactigerous (lak-tij'er-us). Secreting or conveying milk.

lac'tin. Lactose, sugar of milk.

lactinated (lakt'in-āt-ed). Containing or prepared with milk sugar.

lactivorous (lakt-iv'or-us). Living upon milk.

lactobacillin(e (lakt-o-bas'il-īn). A preparation of lactic acid bacilli (1) to counteract intestinal putrefaction, (2) to cause lactic acid fermentation.

Lactobacillus (lakt-o-bă-sil'us). A genus of bacteria producing acid in milk and other substances.

    L. acidophilus. A lactic acid forming organism found in the intestinal contents of infants. It produces lactic acid fermentation of milk.

    L. boasoppleri. Nonmotile Grampositive rods found in gastric contents especially in cancer of stomach.

    L. bulgaricus. Forms the sour milk known as yoghurt.

    L. caucasicus. Kephir-producing ferment.

    L. helveticus. Type found in Swiss cheese.

    L. odontolyticus. Thought to be a cause of dental caries.

    L. panis. Type occurring in sour dough.

lactobutyrometer (lakt"o-bu-tĭ-rom'et-er). Instrument for estimating the butter fat content of milk.

lactocele (lakt'o-sēl). Cystic tumor of breast due to occlusion of a milk duct. SYN: *galactocele.*

lactocrit (lakt'o-krĭt). Instrument for determining the amt. of fatty substance in milk.

lactodensimeter (lakt-o-den-sim'et-er). Instrument for determining specific gravity of milk.

lactoglobulin (lak"tō-glob'ū-lĭn). A protein found in milk.

lactolase (lak'to-lās). An enzyme forming lactic acid. SYN: *lactacidase.*

lactolin (lakt'o-lin). Condensed or evaporated milk.

lactometer (lak-tom'et-er). Device for determining the specific gravity of milk.

lactophosphate (lakt'o-fos''făt). A salt derived jointly from lactic and phosphoric acid.

lactorrhea (lakt-or-re'ă). Discharge of milk between nursings and after weaning of offspring. SYN: *galactorrhea.*

lactoscope (lak'to-skōp). Device for determining quality of milk.

lac'tose. $C_{12}H_{22}O_{11} + H_2O$. A disaccharide which on hydrolysis yields glucose and galactose.

    DOSAGE: 1-6 oz. (30.0-180.0 Gm.) per day.

lactoserum (lakt-o-sēr'um). 1. Blood serum of an animal inoculated with milk; used to precipitate specific caseins from milk. 2. The whey of milk.

lacto'sum. USP. Term for lactose.

lactosuria (lak-to-su'rĭ-ă). Occurrence of milk sugar (lactose) in the urine.

    Frequent during pregnancy and lactation. Identified by osazone crystals.

lactotherapy (lakt-o-ther'ă-pī). 1. Treatment with milk diet. 2. Medicinal treatment of nursing infant with drugs given to mother to be excreted in milk. SYN: *galactotherapy.*

lac"totox'in. A milk ptomaine.

lacuna (la-ku'na) (pl. *lacunae*). 1. A small, hollow space, such as that found in bones, in which lie the osteoblasts. 2. A gap or hiatus.

    l., absorption. Howship's lacuna, *q.v.*

    l., bone. One of the isolated ovoid spaces bet. osseous lamellae, connected by canaliculi, containing a protoplasmic body or bone cell.

    l. cerebri. Cerebral infundibulum.

    l., haversian. One of those bet. the haversian lamellae.

    l., Henle's. One of those separating the muscular fasciculi of the heart.

    l., Howship's. 1. An absorption pit next to the periosteum. 2. A recess in bone filled with granulation tissue resulting from caries.

    l., intervillous. Sinus of maternal portion of placenta from which are suspended fetal placental villi.

    l. magna. Largest of orifices in Littre's glands.

    l. Morgagni. Recess in mucous membrane of male urethra.

    l. of the cornea. One of those bet. laminae of the cornea.

    l. pharyngis. Pit at pharyngeal end of eustachian tube.

    l. of the urethra. One of those in mucous membrane of the urethra, esp. along the floor and in the bulb.

    l. vasorum. Internal aperture of femoral canal.

lacunar (la-kū'nar). Pert. to lacunae.

lacunula (la-kū'nu-lă). Small or minute lacuna.

lacus (la'kus). Collection of fluid in small hollow or cavity.

    l. derivitionis. Venous space in tentorium cerebelli.

    l. lacrimalis. Space at inner canthus of eye where tears collect.

    l. sanguineus. Uteroplacental sinus.

    l. seminalis. Vault of vagina after insemination.

Laënnec's cirrhosis (lan-eks'). Atrophic cirrhosis of liver. SYN: *hobnail liver.*

    L.'s pearls. Round gelatinous masses in asthmatic sputum.

    L.'s râle. Modified subcrepitant râle due to mucus in bronchioles.

    L.'s thrombus. Globular thrombus in heart.

lag. 1. Period of time bet. application of stimulus and resulting reaction. SYN: *lag phase.* 2. Early period following bacterial inoculation into culture medium.

lagena (laj-ē'nă). Upper extremity of ductus cochlearis.

lageniform (laj-en'ĭ-form). Flask-shaped.

lagging (lăg'ĭng). Retarded movement of chest in pulmonary tuberculosis.

lagophthalmos, lagophthalmus (lag-of-thal'mos, -mus). Incomplete closure of palpebral fissure when lids are shut, resulting in exposure and injury to bulbar conjunctiva and cornea.

ag phase. The period after a stimulus is administered to the time of its response. See: *lag.*

a grippe (la grip'). Acute infectious disease of respiratory or gastrointestinal tract. Syn: *influenza, q.v.*

aity (lā'ĭ-tĭ). Portion of public nonprofessional in field of special professions.

aked. Said of the blood in hemolysis* or disintegration of the red blood corpuscles, freeing the hemoglobin into the blood plasma.

ak'ing. Freeing of hemoglobin from red blood corpuscles.

aky (lāk'ĭ). Resembling a lake, as (1) postcoital collection in vagina below cervix in normal conditions, (2) color of lake pigment, or (3) red transparency following hemolysis of blood serum.

aliatry (lal-i'a-trĭ). Study and treatment of speech disorders and defects.

alla'tion, lal'ling. A babbling form of stammering. Infantile form of speech. The constant use of "l" instead of "r."

alognosis (lal-og-no'sis). Understanding of prattle or speech.

aloneurosis (lal-o-nū-rō'sis). Speech impairment of neurotic origin.

alop'athy. Any disorder affecting the speech.

alophobia (lal-ō-fō'bĭ-ă). Morbid reluctance to speak due to fear of stammering or committing errors.

aloplegia (lal-o-ple'jĭ-ă). A paralysis of speech muscles without affecting action of tongue.

alorrhea (la-lor-re'ă). Abnormal flow of speech.

amarckism or **Lamarck's theory** (lam-ark'ism). Theory that structural changes are due to innate needs, and that these acquired characteristics may be transmitted to descendants.

ambda (lam'dă). Point or angle of junction of lambdoid and sagittal sutures.

ambdacism (lam'dă-sizm). 1. Stammering of *l* sound. 2. Inability to pronounce *l* sound properly.

ambdoid, lambdoidal (lam'doid, lam-doid'al). Shaped like Greek letter L.

l. ligament. Ligamentum fundiforme pedis.

l. suture. Suture bet. the occipital and 2 parietal bones.

Lamblia intestinalis (lam'blĭ-ă in-test-ĭ-nal'is). Flagellate protozoan parasite found in intestine.

lambliasis (lăm'blĭ'ă-sĭs). Condition of infection with Lamblia intestinalis, marked frequently by symptoms of dysentery.

lamella (lam-el'a) (pl. *lamellae*). 1. A medicated disc of gelatin inserted under lower eyelid and against the eyeball used as a local application to eye. 2. A thin plate or scale.

l., bone. Thin layer of ground substance of osseous tissue.

l., concentric. Plate of bone surrounding a haversian canal.

l., fundamental. A general name for all periosteal, intermediate, and medullary bone lamellae.

l., intermediate. Bone lamella filling irregular spaces bet. concentric lamellae.

l., medullary. The osseous lamella surrounding and forming wall of medullary cavity of tubular bones.

l., periosteal. Bone lamella next to and parallel with the periosteum, forming ext. portion of bone.

l., triangular. Small fibrous lamina bet. choroid plexuses of 3rd ventricle of the brain.

l., vitreous. Inner boundary of the choroid.

Syn: *Bruck's membrane, lamina basalis.*

lamellar (lam-el'lar). Arranged in thin plates or scales.

lam'ina (pl. *laminae*). 1. A thin, flat layer or membrane. 2. The flattened part of either side of the arch of a vertebra.

l. basalis. Layer of chorioid touching retinal pigmented layer.

l., Bowman's. Basement membrane beneath epithelium of cornea.

l. cartilaginis cricoideae. Flat, platelike, post. portion of cricoid cartilage.

l. c. thyroideae. One of the alae of the thyroid cartilage.

l. choriocapillaris. BNA. Choroid's middle layer containing close mesh of capillaries. Syn: *membrane, Ruysch's.*

l. choroidea inferior. Choroid plexus of the 4th ventricle.

l. cinerea. Gray substance bet. optic chiasm and callosum.

l. conchae. Surface of lateral mass of ethmoid bones.

l. cribrosa. Cribriform plate ot the ethmoid bone.

l. c. ant. inferior. Ant. portion of inferior fossula containing openings for passage of divisions of cochlear branch of auditory nerve.

l. c. sclerae. Innermost lamella of sclera which stretches over the foramen sclerae, forming a diaphragm which is perforated by numerous openings for passageway of optic nerve fibers.

l. lentis. Concentric layer forming the crystalline lens.

l. mastoidea. Basal plate of mastoid process.

l. medullaris. Layer of medullated nerve fibers, the thickened ext. layer of the typical cerebral cortex.

l., medullary, external. Outer of 2 white laminae in nucleus lentiformis.

l., medullary, inner. Internal medullary. Layer of fibers passing from thalamus to the red nucleus.

l. propria of the membrana tympani. Middle fibrous layer of tympanic membrane.

l. quadrigemina. Layer of gray matter forming roof of aqueduct of Sylvius and supporting the corpora quadrigemina.

l. spiralis. One which divides the int. of spiral canal of cochlea into 2 scalae and divides into lamina spiralis ossea, and lamina spiralis membrana.

l. suprachoroidea. Outermost layer of the choroid.

l. vitreous. Smooth, transparent membrane covering inner surface of choroid.

laminated (lam'in-āt-ed). Arranged in layers or laminae.

lamination (lam-in-ā'shun). 1. Layerlike arrangement. 2. In embryotomy, the slicing of the skull.

laminec'tomy. The excision of a vertebral post. arch.   [a lamina.

laminitis (lă-mĭn-i'tis). Inflammation of

lamp, therapeutic. Device for producing and applying light, heat, radiation, and various forms of radioactivity for the treatment of disease.

l., Birch-Hirschfeld. Carbon arc lamp with a filter of uviol glass and a quartz lens system for phototherapy in ophthalmology.

l., carbon arc. A lamp for the passage of electric current through 2 carbon rods, the ends of which are opp. each. other but a little distance apart, varying according to kinds of carbons employed. Carbon may be plain or cored with metals or impregnated with metallic salts. Comparatively little energy shorter than 2900 A° is emitted.

l., cold quartz. A low vapor pressure, low amperage, high potential, glow discharge similar to the Geissler tube. Power consumed is small, consequently no great rise in temperature of burner. About 95% of the radiation of wave lengths less than and including 3130 A° is emitted in the resonance line at 2537 A°.

l., cold red light. Is emitted by neon glow discharge tube like the neon signs.

l., colored. Colored bulbs absorb some radiation emitted, reduce the efficacy of the lamps for heating, and become hotter for the same output of radiant energy than clear bulbs; are more likely to burst.

l., Cooper Hewitt vapor. Commercial illuminant in long tube of flint glass; is a low vapor pressure glow discharge tube.

l., Duke-Elder. Mercury vapor arc slit lamp apparatus with quartz lens system for ultraviolet radiation therapy in eye conditions.

l., electrodeless high frequency induction. One in which bulb is evacuated and contains a globule of mercury, whose vapor is excited to luminescence through high frequency from 5000 volt secondary of the transformer, passing through the helix surrounding the bulb.

l., Finsen. A carbon arc lamp operating at 50 volts and 50 amperes so constructed that radiation is concentrated on an area 1 inch square; a water-cooled quartz system to remove infrared radiation and a compression quartz piece to dehematize the skin.

l., hot quartz. Quartz mercury arc lamp for ultraviolet radiation.

l., induced ultraviolet glow. Glow discharge is produced through an inductive effect. The quartz burner has the form of a sphere and a high frequency coil is wound around this sphere. This coil forms the primary winding of a high frequency transformer and the secondary winding is represented by the mercury vapor arc inside the sphere.

l., Kromayer. A water-cooled mercury quartz lamp, q.v., named after its inventor, Dr. Kromayer.

l., Mazda. A trade name for sun lamps which are known as Mazda S-1 and S-2, differing only in size. The globe is of special size which absorbs radiation of wave lengths shorter than 2800 A°.

l., mercury glow. A lamp producing suitable ionization by means of electrons emitted from a hot cathode.

l., mercury quartz. Burner containing in quartz tube fluid mercury. One type has 2 columns of mercury representing 2 electrodes, and some burners have a pure tungsten anode and a mercury cathode. Cooling may be by air or water.

l., mercury vapor. Operates at a high vapor pressure, and relatively high temperature and low voltage. SEE: hot quartz lamp.

l., neon glow. One that emits cold red light. Same as neon signs. Little therapeutic effect. SEE: cold red light lamp.

l., quartz mercury. SEE: mercury quartz.

l., S-1 and S-2 ultraviolet. It consists of a special ultraviolet transmitting glass bulb of same shape as an ordinary light bulb. In this are a tungsten filament, 2 tungsten electrodes, and a drop of mercury. Electric current forms a mercury vapor arc between the highly incandescent tungsten electrodes. A satisfactory source of ultraviolet lamp for home use. A source of ultraviolet radiation.

l., sky light. Radiation from the whole sky in summer has more ultraviolet shorter than 3660 A° than direct sunlight.

l., sun. SEE: Mazda lamp.

l., tungsten filament. A gas-filled tungsten lamp is useful as a source of visible and short infrared radiations, but even when enclosed in a bulb that transmits ultraviolet rays from 2800 to 3100 A° it emits but little ultraviolet of these wave lengths, although recognized as effective in preventing rickets.

l., uviol. An electric lamp with a globe of uviol glass. SEE: Ulilampe.

l., ultraviolet. SEE: carbon arc, Duke-Elder, mercury quartz, cold quartz, Finsen, Mazda, mercury glow, neon glow, S-1 and S-2, tungsten filament lamp, and uviarc.

l., violet ray. 1. Helical-shaped carbon filament, incandescent lamp in bulb of blue glass. It has no therapeutic effect, excepting that of heat. 2. A glass tube attached to a spark coil which emits a blue glow when it touches the body. It should not be used as a source of ultraviolet rays.

l., water-cooled carbon arc. A carbon arc of 20-30 amperes with concentration apparatus of quartz lenses and watery solution of cobalt and copper sulfates.

l., water-cooled quartz mercury vapor arc. A small quartz mercury vapor arc lamp enclosed in a double-walled metal box with a quartz window for generation and application of ultraviolet rays. Water is circulated between the walls to conduct away the intense heat. SYN: *Kromayer lamp.*

lamprophonia (lam-pro-fō'nĭ-ă). Marked distinctness or clearness of voice.

lamprophonic (lam-prŏ-fōn'ĭk). Possessing a clear voice.

lance (lans). 1. Two-edged surgical knife. 2. To incise with a lancet.

lancet (lan'sĕt). Pointed surgical knife with 2 edges.

lancinating (lăn'sĭ-nāt-ing). Sharp or cutting, as pain.

Lancisi's nerves (lan-che'zĭ). Striae in corpus callosum. SYN: *striae longitudinales, q.v.*

Landouzy-Dejerine atrophy (lan-dŭ-ze'da-zhē-rēn'). Atrophy of muscles of face and scapulohumeral group.

Landry's paralysis (lăn-drē'). A form of paralysis in which loss of motor power in lower extremities gradually extends to upper extremities and to circulatory and respiratory centers without sensory manifestations, trophic changes, etc. SYN: *acute ascending paralysis.*

land scurvy. Severe variety of purpura with hemorrhage of the mucosa. SYN: *purpura hemorrhagica.*

Lane's disease (lān). Chronic intestinal stasis.

    L.'s kinks. Bending or twisting of intestine at various points as result of upright position of body.

    L.'s operation. Short circuiting of the colon for chronic constipation, colitis, or obstruction.

Langerhans' islands (lahng'er-hahns). Cellular masses in interstitial tissue of pancreas, from which insulin is secreted.
    SEE: *diabetes, insulin, pancreas.*

Lange's test (lăng'ĕ). Diagnosis of cerebrospinal syphilis by degree of gold precipitation in varying concentrations of colloidal gold solution and spinal fluid—4/10% salt solution.

Lang'hans layer. Deep layer of chorionic villi, composed of cells.

lanolin, anhydrous (lan'o-lin), USP. The purified, fatlike substance obtained from the wool of sheep.
    l., hydrous, USP. Wool fat containing about 25% water.

lanugo (lan-oo'go). 1. Downy hair covering the body. 2. Fine downy hairs that cover the body of the fetus, esp. when premature.
    l. pudendarum. The pubic hair.

laparectomy (lap''ă-rĕk'tō-mĭ). Excision of strips or gores in abdominal wall. SYN: *enterectomy.*

laparo-. Combining form pert. to the *flank* and to operations *through the abdominal wall.*

laparocholecystotomy (lap''ar-o-kol''e-sis-tot'o-mĭ). Incision into gallbladder through abdomen.

laparocolostomy (lap''ar-o-kō-lŏs'tō-mĭ). Formation of permanent opening into colon through abdominal wall.

laparocolotomy (lap''ar-ō-kō-lot'ō-mĭ). Incision of colon through abdominal wall, forming an artificial opening. SYN: *laparocolostomy.*

laparocolpotomy (lap''ar-ō-kol-pot'ō-mĭ). Incision over Poupart's ligament dissecting peritoneum to vagina which is incised transversely, enabling dilation of cervix and extraction of child through os uteri. SYN: *celioelytrotomy, laparo-elytrotomy.*

laparocystectomy (la''pa-ro-sis-tek'to-mĭ). Removal of an extrauterine fetus or of contents of a cyst through an abdominal incision.

laparocystidotomy (lap''ar-o-sĭst-ĭ-dŏt'ō-mĭ). Bladder incision through the abdominal wall.

laparocystotomy (lap''ar-o-sis-tot'o-mĭ). Incision of abdomen to remove contents of a cyst or an extrauterine fetus.

laparoelytrotomy (lap''ar-o-el-ĭ-trot'o-mĭ). Abdominal incision to aid in removal of fetus. SEE: *cesarean operation.*

laparoenterostomy (lăp''ă-rō-ĕn-tĕr-ŏs'tō-mĭ). Formation of aperture into intestine through abdominal wall.

laparoenterotomy (lap''ar-o-en-ter-ot'o-mĭ). Opening into intestinal cavity by incision through the loins.

laparogastrostomy (lăp''ar-ō-găs-trŏs'tō-mĭ). Formation of permanent gastric fistula through abdominal wall. SYN: *celiogastrostomy.*

laparogastrotomy (lap''a-ro-gas-trot'o-mĭ). Abdominal incision into stomach.

laparohepatotomy (lăp''ar-ō-hĕp-ă-tŏt'ō-mĭ). Incision of the liver through abdominal wall from side.

laparohysterectomy (lap''ar-o-his-ter-ek'-to-mĭ). Abdominal removal of uterus.

laparohystero-oöphorectomy (lap''ar-o-his''ter-o-o''o-for-ek'to-mĭ). Removal of uterus and ovaries through an abdominal incision.

laparohysteropexy (lap''ar-o-his'ter-o-peks-ĭ). Abdominal fixation of the uterus.

laparohysterosalpingo-oöphorectomy (lăp''ar-ō-hĭs''tĕr-ō-săl-pĭn''gō-ō''of''or-ek'tō-mĭ). Removal of uterus, fallopian tubes, and ovaries through an abdominal incision. SYN: *celiohysterosalpingo-oöthecectomy.*

laparohysterotomy (lap''ar-o-his-ter-ot'o-mĭ). Abdominal incision into uterus. SEE: *cesarean section.*

laparoileotomy (lap''ar-o-il-e-ot'o-mĭ). Abdominal incision into ileum.

laparokelyphotomy (lăp''ăr-ō-kĕl-ĭ-fŏt'ō-mĭ). 1. Removal of an extrauterine fetus by laparotomy. 2. Suprapubic cystotomy. Syn: *laparocystotomy.*

laparomyitis (lăp″ăr-ō-mī-ī′tĭs). Inflammation of muscular portion of abdominal wall.

laparomyomectomy (lap″ar-o-mi-o-mek′to-mĭ). Abdominal excision of a muscular tumor.

laparonephreutomy (lăp″ar-o-ne-frek′to-mĭ). Renal excision abdominally.

laparorrhaphy (lăp-ăr-or′ră-fĭ). Abdominal wall suture. Syn: *celiorrhaphy.*

laparosalpingectomy (lăp″ar-o-săl-pin-jek′to-mĭ). Abdominal excision of a fallopian tube.

laparosalpingo-oöphorectomy (lăp″ăr-ō-săl-pĭn″gō-ō″ŏf-ō-rek′tō-mĭ). Removal of fallopian tubes and ovaries through abdominal incision. Syn: *celiosalpingo-oöthecectomy.*

laparosalpingotomy (lăp″ăr-ō-săl-pĭn-got′-ō-mĭ). Incision of oviduct through abdominal wall. Syn: *celiosalpingotomy.*

laparoscopy (lăp-ăr-os′kō-pĭ). Abdominal exploration employing instruments. Syn: *celioscopy.*

laparosplenectomy (lap″ar-o-splen-ek′to-mĭ). Abdominal excision of the spleen.

laparosplenotomy (lăp″ăr-ō-splĕn-ŏt′ō-mĭ). Incision of the spleen through abdominal wall.

laparotomy (lap-ar-ot′o-mĭ). Abdominal incision for any operation on internal organs.

laparotrachelotomy (lap″ar-o-tra-kĕl-ot′o-mĭ). Cesarean section with the incision through the lower segment of the uterus.

laparotyphlotomy (lăp″ăr-ō-tĭ-flŏt′ō-mĭ). Incision of cecum through lateral abdominal incision.

laparouterotomy (lăp″ăr-ō-ū-tĕr-ŏt′ō-mĭ). Incision of uterus through abdominal wall. Syn: *laparohysterotomy.*

lapis (la′pĭs). Stone.

laqueus (lak′we-us). A noose-shaped band, fillet, or cord.

l. umbilicalis. The umbilical cord.

lardaceous (lar-dā′shus). Resembling lard; waxy, fatty.

l. disease. Amyloid degeneration. The organs affected present a white waxy appearance due to the deposit of a firm, translucent substance called *lardacein* or *amyloid* which when treated with iodine produces a dark mahogany-brown color.

larocraine hydrochloride (lar′o-kān). A white, crystalline powder, of the procaine type, said to act more quickly and for a longer period of time than either cocaine or procaine.

Dosage: Varies according to its use, from ¼-5% solutions.

larva (lar′vă). The stage in insect life during which the "grub" emerges from its egg.

l. migrans. An extensive skin eruption due to a parasitic larva which burrows under the epidermis. Syn: *cercaria.*

laryngalgia (lăr-ĭn-găl′jĭ-ă). Neuralgia of the larynx.

laryngeal (lar-in′je-al). Pert. to the larynx.

l. reflex. Cough as result of irritation of larynx or fauces.

laryngectomy (lar-in-jek′to-mĭ). Excision of larynx.

laryngismal (lar-ĭn-jĭs′măl). Concerning or resembling affection with laryngeal spasm.   [larynx.

laryngismus (lar-in-jis′mus). Spasm of the

l., infantile. One occurring in children less than one year old, who are poorly nourished.

l. stridulus. A paroxysmal neurosis characterized by spasm of the adductors of the larynx and not excited by any local inflammation.

laryngitic (lar-ĭn-jĭt′ĭk). 1. Resulting from laryngitis. 2. Rel. to laryngitis.

laryngitis (lar-in-ji′tis). Inflammation of larynx.

l., acute catarrhal. Acute congestive laryngitis; catarrhal inflammation of laryngeal mucosa and the vocal cords.

l., atrophic. Laryngitis leading to diminished secretion and glandular atrophy of the mucous membrane.

l., chronic. A type due to a recurrent irritation, or following the acute form. Often secondary to sinus or nasal pathology, improper use of voice, excessive smoking or drinking.

l., c. hypertrophic. Hypertrophy of tissues accompanying chronic laryngitis.

l., diphtheritic. Invasion of larynx by diphtheria bacilli, usually with formation of membrane.

l., membranous. Characterized by inflammation of larynx with the formation of a false membrane of nondiphtheritic origin.

l., phlegmonous. Inflamed larynx with purulent infiltration or abscesses.

l., tuberculous. Secondary to pulmonary tuberculosis.

l., ulcerative. Chronic laryngitis with ulceration of the mucous membrane.

laryn′go-. Prefix: Pert. to the *larynx.*

laryngocele (lar-in′go-sēl). 1. Dilatation of larynx. 2. Protrusion of laryngeal mucosa.

laryngocentesis (lăr-ĭn″gō-sĕn-tē′sĭs). Incision or puncture of the larynx.

laryngofissure (lar-ing″go-fish′ur). The operation of opening the larynx by a median line incision through the thyroid cartilage.

laryngograph (lar-ing′o-grăf). Device for making a record of laryngeal movements.

laryngography (lăr-ĭn-gŏg′ră-fĭ). Description of larynx.

laryngologist (lar-ĭn-gol′o-jĭst). Specialist in laryngology.

laryngol′ogy. The practice of medicine dealing with the treatment of diseases of the larynx.

laryngometry (lăr-ĭn-gŏm′ĕ-trĭ). Systematic measurement of larynx.

laryngoparalysis (lăr-ĭn″gō-par-ăl-ĭ-sĭs). Paralysis of muscles of larynx.

laryngopathy (lăr-ĭn-gop′ă-thĭ). Any disease of the larynx.

laryngophantom (lăr-ĭn-gō-fan′tŏm). Plastic model of the larynx.

ryngopharyngeal (lar-ĭn″gō-far-ĭn′jē-ăl). Rel. jointly to larynx and pharynx.

ryngopharyngectomy (lăr-ĭn″gō-făr-ĭn-jek′tō-mĭ). Removal of the larynx and pharynx.

ryngopharyngitis (lăr-ĭn″gō-făr-ĭn-jī′tĭs). Inflammation of the larynx and pharynx.

ryngopharynx (lăr-ĭn-gō-făr′ĭnks). Lower portion of the pharynx that extends from the cornua of the hyoid bone or vestibule of the larynx to the lower border of the cricoid cartilage.

ryngophony (lăr-ĭn-gof′ō-nĭ). Voice sounds heard in auscultating the pharynx.

ryngoplasty (lăr-ĭn′gō-plăs-tĭ). Plastic reparative surgery of larynx.

ryngoplegia (la-ring″go-plē′jĭ-ă). Paralysis of laryngeal muscles.

ryngorhinology (lăr-ĭn″gō-rīn-ŏl′ō-jĭ). Science treating with diseases of the larynx and nose.

ryngorrhagia (lăr-ĭn-gor-ră′jĭ-ă). Laryngeal hemorrhage.

ryngorrhea (lăr-ĭn-gor-rē′ă). Excessive discharge of laryngeal mucus. SYN: *blennorrhea*.

ryngoscleroma (lăr-ĭn-gō-sklē-rō′mă). Scleroma affecting the larynx.

ryngoscope (lar-ĭn′go-skōp). Instrument for examining the larynx.

   l., solar. Two mirrors, one reflecting sun rays into mouth, again reflected into larynx by laryngeal mirror. Newer modifications use an alloy of aluminum and magnesium in reflecting mirrors.

ryngoscopic (lar-ĭn-gō-skŏp′ĭk). Pert. to observation with aid of small, long-handled mirror for reflecting interior of larynx.

ryngoscopy (lar-ĭn-gos′kō-pĭ). Examination of interior of larynx.

   l., direct. That done with laryngeal speculum or laryngoscope.

   l., indirect. That done with a mirror.

ryngospasm (lăr-ĭn′gō-spazm). Spasm of laryngeal muscles.

ryngostenosis (lar-ing″go-ste-nō′sis). Stricture of larynx.

   l., compression. From causes outside the larynx as result of abscesses, tumors, goiter, etc.

   l., occlusion. ETIOL: May be due to congenital bands or membranes, foreign bodies, tumors, cicatricial contraction following ulceration as in diphtheria and tertiary syphilis, penetrating wounds or corrosive fluid.

ryngostomy (lăr-ĭn-gos′tō-mĭ). Establishing permanent opening through neck into larynx.

ryngotracheitis (lăr-ĭn″gō-tra-kē-ī′tĭs). Inflamed condition of the larynx and trachea.

ryngostroboscope (lar-in-go-stro′bo-skōp). Instrument for inspection of vibration of vocal cords.

ryngotomy (lar-in-got′o-mĭ). Incision of larynx.

ryngotracheotomy (lar-in′go-tra-ke-ot′o-mĭ). Incision of larynx with section of upper tracheal rings.

laryngozerosis (lăr-ĭn″gō-zēr-ō′sĭs). Abnormal dryness of the larynx.

larynx (lar′inks) (pl. *larynges*). The organ of voice, the enlarged upper end of trachea; musculocartilaginous structure lined with mucous membrane.

lasciv′ia. Abnormal sexual desire. SYN: *nymphomania,* * *satyriasis.* *

lassitude (las′i-tūd). Weariness; exhaustion.

latency (lā′těn-sĭ). State of being concealed or hidden.

   l. period. 1. Interval bet. stimulation and response to it. SYN: *lag phase.* 2. Period bet. pregenital or infantile sexuality and onset of puberty or genital sexuality, occurring bet. ages of about 4 to 11 years. 3. Period of incubation in which a disease exists without manifesting itself.

la′tent. 1. Lying hidden. 2. Quiet; not active.

   l. content. PSY: That part of a dream that cannot be brought into the objective consciousness through any effort of will to remember.

   l. heat. Heat that disappears during evaporation or melting.

   l. period. 1. Time bet. a stimulus and its response. SYN: *lag phase.* 2. PSY: Time bet. ages of 4 to about 11 years separating infantile sexuality from onset of puberty or genital sexuality. SYN: *latency period,* 2. 3. Time during which a disease is supposed to be existent without manifesting itself; period of incubation.

laterad (lat′ěr-ăd). Toward a side or lateral aspect.

lateral (lat′er-al). Pert. to the side.

   l. sinus. Transverse and sigmoid portion of two cranial venous sinuses. Extends from occipital protuberance to jugular bulb.

latericeous, lateritious (lat-ěr-ĭ′shŭs). Resembling brick dust.

lateroflexion (lăt″ěr-ō-flek′shun). Bending or curvature toward a side.

lateroprone, laterosemiprone position (lăt″-ěr-ō-prōn′, -sěm′ĭ-prōn). Patient on left side leaning on chest, right knee and thigh drawn up, left arm back of patient. SYN: *Sims′ position, q.v.*

lateropulsion (lat-er-o-pul′shun). Involuntary tendency in cerebellar and labyrinthine disease to fall to one side.

lateroversion (lăt-ěr-ō-věr′shun). Tendency or a turning toward one side.

lathyrism (lath′ĭr-izm). Chick-pea poisoning. SYN: *lupinosis.*

latrine (la-trēn′). A public privy.

la′tus. The flank or side.

laud′able. Healthy; normal; said of *pus.*

laudanum (law′dan-um). Tincture of opium.

laugh (lăf). Sound produced by laughing. SYN: *risus.*

   l., sardonic. Spasm of facial muscle producing a grinning effect. SYN: *risus sardonicus.*

laughing gas (laf′ing). Nitrous oxide gas.

laughter reflex (lăf′těr). Uncontrollable

laughter resulting from tickling or pretense of tickling.

lavage (la-vazh'). Washing out of a cavity.

l., gastric. Washing out of the stomach. A stomach tube or catheter is used with solution of sterile water, or normal saline, or 2% boracic acid, or 1-5% sodium bicarbonate.

law. In the scientific sense, a statement which is found to hold true uniformly for a whole class of natural occurrences.

l., Ampère's. The directing force of electric currents on mobile magnets causes the latter's austral pole to deviate to the left of current.

l., Avoga'dro's. If temperature and ext. pressure are the same, all gases contain same number of molecules in equal volumes.

l., Behring's. Blood and serum of an immunized subject confers immunity when injected into another.

l., Bell-Magendie's. In spinal nerves the ant. roots contain only motor fibers and post. roots sensory fibers.

l., Bell's. Ant. spinal nerve roots are motor, and post. roots are sensory.

l's., Berthollet's. 1. When two salts react because of a solvent, if a new salt can be produced less soluble, this salt will be produced. 2. When dry heat is applied to "two salts, if a new salt can be produced more volatile, this salt will be produced."

l., Boudin's. There is an antagonism existing bet. malarial and tuberculous disease.

l., Boyle's. The volume occupied by a fixed quantity of every gas is inversely proportional, and density directly proportional, to pressure applied to the gas.

l., Brew'ster's. For any substance the polarizing angle is equal to that angle of incidence at which the portion of light that is reflected is at right angles to the portion refracted.

l's., Bunsen's. Chemical principles governing reactions occurring bet. compound bodies when one of them is present in considerable excess.

l., Charles'. When pressure is constant, volume of a gas varies as the absolute temperature.

l., Colles'. A syphilitic father may beget a syphilitic child without apparently infecting the mother, and this mother cannot be infected by nursing the child.

l. of conservation of energy. Energy can be neither created nor destroyed.

l., Coulomb's (koo'looms). 1. Electrified particles attract or repel each other with a force directly proportionate to the quantity of electricity acting, and inversely proportional to the square of the distance between the particles. 2. The force of torsion is proportional to the angle of torsion.

l., Courvoisier's. When the common bile duct is obstructed by a calculus, dilatation of gallbladder is rare; when otherwise obstructed, dilatation is common.

l., Dalton's. 1. The tension of a mixture of several gases or of a gas and a vapor equals the sum of tensions which each would separately possess. 2. The tension and amount of vapor which will saturate a given space at a given temperature are the same whether the space is empty or filled with a gas.

l. of definite proportions. Two or more chemicals when united to form a new substance do so in a constant and fixed proportion by weight.

l., Delboeuf's. If in any species a number of individuals, bearing a ratio not infinitely small to the entire number of births, are in every generation born with a particular variation neither beneficial nor injurious, and if not counteracted by reversion, the proportion of the new variety to the original form will increase till it approaches indefinitely near to equality.

l., Donders'. SEE: *Listing's law.*

l., Du Bois-Reymond's. A nerve through which a galvanic current is passed is stimulated by the making or breaking of the current or by any sudden change in its intensity.

l., Dulong and Petit's. The specific heat of any solid elementary body is in inverse ratio to its atomic weight.

l. of eccentricity of sensation. A sensation is referred to the termination or end organ of the stimulated nerve and not to the nerve center.

l's. of electrolysis, Faraday's. 1. Electrolysis cannot take place unless the electrolyte is a conductor. 2. The electrolytic action is same in all parts of the electrolyte. 3. The same electric current decomposes quantities of the electrolytes directly proportional to their chemical equivalents. 4. The quantity of an electrolyte decomposed is directly proportional to quantity of electricity passing through it.

l., Fechner's. The intensity of sensation is proportional to the logarithm of the strength of the stimulus.

l., Gay-Lussac's. 1. The tension of a gas varies directly with temperature if volume remains the same. 2. When gases or vapors react on each other the volumes both of the factors and of the products of the reaction always bear to each other some very simple numerical ratio. 3. Air and all of less liquefiable gases have a coefficient of expansion of $\frac{1}{273}$.

l., Godélier's. Tuberculous disease of the peritoneum is always accompanied by similar disease of the pleura.

l., Graham's. The rate at which a gas diffuses through a porous membrane is inversely proportional to the square root of the density of the gas.

l., Haeckel's fundamental biological. The ontogeny is a short repetition of the phylogeny of a species.

l. of the heart. Other things being equal, the stroke volume of the heart varies as the extent of diastolic filling; or, the energy of contraction is a function of the initial length of the muscle fibers.

l., Henry's. Dalton's law, *q.v.*

l., Hilton's. A nerve trunk supplying any joint supplies the muscles which move the joint and skin over insertion of such muscles.

l., Hooke's. If a body is distorted within limits of perfect elasticity, the force with which it reacts it proportional to amount of distortion.

l. of the intestine. Moderate distention of the intestine at a point causes relaxation below (aborally to the point) and contraction above.

l., Kirchoff's. When a beam of light is passed through a transparent body the latter absorbs those luminous rays which it is capable of emitting when heated to incandescence.

l., Koch's, Koch's postulate. To prove an organism to be the cause of a given disease or lesion: 1st, the microörganism in question must appear in the lesion at all times; 2nd, pure cultures must be obtained from it; 3rd, cultures must reproduce the disease in animals and pure cultures must be again obtained from these lesions.

l., Lambert's cosine. The intensity of radiation received by an absorbing surface varies as the cosine of the angle of incidence for parallel rays.

l., Listing's. If, with normal eyes and parallel visual lines, the visual line passes from the primary position into any other position, the rotatory movement of the eyeball in this secondary position is of such a kind as if it had been turned round a fixed axis, lying perpendicular to the first and second direction of the visual line.

l. of Magendie. Same as law of Bell.

l., Malaguti's. When solutions of two different salts are mixed, "metathesis occurs and 4 salts result, the proportions of salts to each other being dependent on strength or intensity of force with which the respective basic and acid radicles are united."

l., Mariotte's. Boyle's law, *q.v.*

l. of mass action. In chemical reactions the amount of change taking place is proportional to action mass of the reacting substance.

l., Mendel's. Offspring do not inherit characteristics from parents in equal or intermediate proportions, certain characteristics of 1 parent predominating and being transmitted to offspring in full measure.

These characteristics are termed *dominant.* Those of the other parent are called *recessive.* In second generation ¾ of offspring will inherit dominant characteristics, the remaining ¼ recessive traits.

l., Metchnikoff's. Phagocytes attack and destroy invading bacteria by intracellular digestion.

l., Mikulicz's. Anesthetic is not to be administered to an individual whose hemoglobin is below 30%.

l. of molecular weights. The weight of a molecule is the sum of the weights of its atoms and the relative molecular weight of a compound is equal to sum of the atomic weights of its components divided by two.

l. of multiple proportions. When two substances unite into form a series of chemical compounds the proportions in which they unite are simple multiples of one another or of one common proportion.

l., Nysten's. Rigor mortis travels progressively from muscles of mastication, through the face, neck, trunk, and arms, reaching the legs and feet last.

l., Ohm's. The relations bet. resistances, amount of current and electromotive force as $C = \dfrac{E}{R}$, in which $C =$ current, $E =$ electromotive force, and $R =$ resistance.

l., periodic. The physical and chemical properties of chemical elements are periodic functions of their at. wt.

Natural classification of elements according to their at. wt.; when arranged in order of their at. wt. or atomic numbers, elements show regular variations in most of their physical and chemical properties.

l., Pfeiffer's. The blood serum of an animal immunized against bacteria will destroy bacteria used for immunization by bacteriolysis.

l., Pflüger's, of contraction and stimulation. A law expressing relation of strength and direction of a galvanic current to its stimulating action upon a nerve.

l., Profeta's. The nonsyphilitic child of a syphilitic mother is immune against the acquired disease.

l. of projection. Stimulation of any point on the retina gives a visual sensation, projected outward along secondary axes from point stimulated through the nodal point.

l., psychophysical. To increase the intensity of a sensation in arithmetical progression one must increase the strength of stimulus in geometric progression.

l. of reciprocal proportions. In chemistry, the law that the proportions in which two elementary bodies unite with a third one are simple multiples or simple fractions of the proportions in which these two bodies unite with each other.

l., Ritter and Valli's. The law of increased inherent (*e. g.,* electric) excitability in a nerve when separated from its center. The heightened irritability begins at proximal and extends toward distal end, eventually disappearing in same order.

l., Rubner's. 1. *Law of constant energy consumption:* Rapidity of growth is proportional to intensity of the metabolic processes. **2.** *Law of constant growth quotient:* The same proportional part, or growth quotient, of total energy is utilized for growth.

l. of sines. Sine of angle of incidence equals the sine of angle of refraction multiplied by a constant quantity.

l., Stokes'. Muscles beneath an inflamed serous or mucous membrane are paralyzed.

l., Van't Hoff's, of temperature coefficient. In chemical reactions the intensity of reaction is doubled for each rise of 10° in temperature.

l., Virchow's. The cell elements of tumors are derived from preëxisting tissue cells.

l. of volumes. SEE: *Gay-Lussac's law.*

l., Waller's, of degeneration. If a spinal nerve is completely divided, the peripheral portion undergoes fatty degeneration, while the proximal part preserves its original character.

l., Weber's. When a stimulus is continually increased the smallest increase of sensation which we can appreciate remains the same, if the proportion of the increase of stimulus to the whole stimulus remains the same.

l., Wolff's. Changes in form and function of bones result in definite changes in their internal structure.

lax (lăks). Without tension.

laxative (lak'să-tĭv). A mildly purgative medicine; an aperient or mild cathartic producing one or two evacuations without pain or tenesmus. Ex: *Olive oil, liquid petrolatum, etc.*

layer (lā'ẽr). A sheetlike section.
SYN: *stratum.*

l., ambiguous. Second layer of cerebral cortex.   [retina.

l., bacillar. Rod and cone layer of

l., claustral. Layer of gray matter bet. external capsule and insula.

l., ganglionic. A layer of angular cells in cerebral cortex.

l., horny. Outer layer of the skin; stratum corneum.

l., osteogenetic. The innermost or bone-forming layer of the periosteum.

lazaret'to. 1. A quarantine station. **2.** Hospital for treatment of contagious diseases. SYN: *pesthouse.*

leaching (lēch'ing). Extraction of a substance from a mixture by washing the mixture with a solvent in which only the desired substance is soluble. SYN: *lixiviation.*

lead (lĕd). SYMB: *Pb.* A metallic element. At. wt. 206.9. Its compounds are poisonous.

l. acetate. USP. Sugar of lead.
DOSAGE: AV: Internally, 1 gr. (0.6 Gm.).

l. colic. That due to lead poisoning.

l. encephalopathy. Disease of brain caused by lead poisoning.

l. line. Bluish line on gums in lead poisoning.

l. pipe contraction. Cataleptic condition during which limbs remain in any position in which placed.

lead (lĕd). An electrocardiograph record.
The 3 common leads are: Lead I, right arm to left arm; lead II, right arm to left leg; lead III, left arm to left leg.

leaf (lēf). A plant organ usually shooting out from the side of a stem or branch; somewhat flattened and oval in shape, and green in color. Ex: *Belladonna, hyoscyamus, digitalis.*

leaflet (lēflĕt). One of the subdivisions of a compound leaf. Ex: *Senna, pilocarpus.*

lean (lēn). Without much fat or flesh, emaciated.

Leber's disease (lā'bĕr). Congenital atrophy of the optic nerve that is inherited.

L.'s plexus. Plexus of venules in eye bet. Schlemm's canal and Fontana's spaces.

Lecat's gulf (lă-kăts'). Bulbous portion of the urethra.

lechery (letch'er-i). Lewdness; sensualism.

lechopyra (lek-o-pī'ra). Puerperal fever.

lecithin (les'ĭth-ĭn). A fatty substance, of the group called phospholipins, found in blood, bile, brain, egg yolk, nerves, and other animal tissues, and yielding stearic acid, glycerol, phosphoric acid, and choline on hydrolysis. They are all derivatives of glycerin.
DOSAGE: 3-8 gr. (0.2-0.5 Gm.).

lectual (lekt'ū-ăl). Pert. to a bed or couch.

l. disease. Bed-confining disease.

Lederer's anemia (lĕd'ẽr-ẽrs). Acute hemolytic anemia.

leech (lētch). A blood-sucking water worm.

l., artificial. Cup and exhaust pump or syringe for drawing blood.

Lee's ganglion (lē). Cervical ganglion formed from 3rd and 4th sacral nerves and hypogastric and ovarian plexuses.

left"-hand'edness. Condition of being more adept in use of left hand. SYN: *sinistrality.*

left lateral recumbent position. The English or obstetrical position. Patient on left side, right knee and thigh drawn up. Used in rectal operations and obstetrics.

leg (lĕg). One of the 2 lower extremities including the femur, tibia, fibula, and patella; spec. the part between the knee and ankle.

l., Anglesey. A form of jointed artificial leg.

l., badger. Inequality in the length of the legs.

l., baker. Genu valbum, or knock-knee.

l., bandy. Same as bowleg.

l., Barbadoes. Elephantiasis of the legs.

l., bayonet. Uncorrected backward displacement of the knee bones, followed by ankylosis at the joint.

l., bird. Reduction in size of the leg from atrophy of the muscles.

l., boomerang. A disease of the leg bones occurring among Australian natives, causing a curvature of the leg resembling a boomerang.

l., bow-. *Genu varum;* an outward curving of the legs at the knees.

l., lawn tennis. Rupture of plantaris muscle accompanied by excruciating disabling pain in the posterior region of the knee.

l., milk. Phlebitis of the femoral vein occasionally following parturition and typhoid fever. Called also white leg. SYN: *phlegmasia alba dolens.*

l., scissor. Cross leg deformity; a result of double hip disease, in which the patient walks with the legs crossed.

l. type. Inherited progressive muscular atrophy.

l., white. SEE: *milk leg.*

leggings (lĕg'gĭngs). Sterile leg coverings used on patient while in operating room.

legitimacy (lē-jĭt'ĭm-ă-sĭ). 1. Condition of being legal. 2. Condition of being born in wedlock.

legumelin (leg-u'mel-in). An albumin present in many leguminous seeds, as in peas.

leiodermia (lī-ō-dĕr'mĭ-ă). Skin disease characterized by abnormal glossiness and atrophy.

leiomyofibroma (lī″ō-mī″ō-fī-brō′mă). Tumor containing leiomatous, myomatous, and fibromatous elements.

leiomyoma (lī″ō-mī-ō′mă). Myoma of unstriped muscle fibers.

leiomyosarcoma (lī″ō-mī″ō-săr-kō′mă). Combined leiomyoma and sarcoma.

leiphemia (lī-fē′mĭ-ă). Thinness, impoverishment, or depravity of the blood.

Leishmania (lēsh-man′ĭ-ă). A genus of organisms, one of which, *Leishmania donovani,* causes kala-azar.

Leiter's coil (lī′tĕr). Coil of flexible, metallic tubing used in warming or cooling a part.

lememia (lem-ē′mĭ-ă). The presence of plague bacilli in the blood.

lemic (lē′mĭk). Rel. to plague or epidemic disease.

lemmocyte (lem′mō-sīt). A cell which becomes a neurilemma cell.

lemniscus (lem-nis′kŭs). A bundle of sensory fibers (lateral or ext. and median or int.) in the medulla, and pons. SYN: *fillet, laqueus.* [eases.

lemoid (le′moyd). Pert. to contagious dis-

lemol′ogy. Study of contagious diseases.

lemoparalysis (le′mo-par-al′ĭs-ĭs). Paralysis of esophagus.

lemosteno′sis. Stricture of esophagus.

lenigallol (len-ĭ-gal′ŏl). A derivative of pyrogallic acid (triacetyl pyrogallol).

DOSAGE: In 1-6% ointment, usually with zinc oxide.

lenitive (len′ĭ-tiv). 1. Demulcent, soothing, slightly laxative. 2. A palliative.

lens (lĕnz) (pl. *lentēs*). A transparent refracting medium; usually made of glass.

l., achromatic. One for correction of aberration of refrangibility, or chromatic aberration.

l., bifocal. Having a double focus.

l., concave spherical. Formed of prisms with their apices together, therefore, thin at the center and thick at the edge. Used in myopia.

l., convex spherical. Formed of prisms with their bases together, therefore, thick at the center and thin at the edge. Used in hyperopia.

l., crystalline. Transparent, colorless stricture in eye; biconvex in shape, enclosed in a capsule and held in place just behind the pupil by the suspensory ligament. Consists of cortex and nucleus. Function is to focus rays so they form a perfect image on the retina.

l., cylindrical. Segment of a cylinder parallel to its axis, used in correcting astigmatism.

lenticonus (len-ti-ko′nus). Conical protrusion of ant. or post. surface of lens.

lentic′ular. 1. Lens shaped. SYN: *lentiform.* 2. Pert. to a lens.

l. fossa. Depression in ant. surface of vitreous for reception of the crystalline lens.

l. glands. Glands of the gastric mucosa.

lenticulostriate (len-tĭk″ū-lō-strī′āt). Rel. to the lenticular nucleus and corpus striatum.

lentiform (lent′ĭ-form). Lentil or lens shaped. SYN: *lenticular.*

lentiginous (lĕn-tĭj′ĭn-ŭs). 1. Affected by lentigo. 2. Covered with very small dots.

len′tigo (pl. *lentigines*). Small brown macules or yellow-brown pigmented areas on skin sometimes caused by exposure to sun and weather. SYN: *ephelis, freckle.*

lentitis (lĕn-tī′tĭs). Inflammation of the optic lens. SYN: *phakitis.*

leontiasis (lē-ōn-tī′ă-sĭs). Lionlike expression about face, accompanying certain diseases.

l. ossea. Enlargement and distortion of facial bones, giving one the appearance of a lion. The condition is rare and not fatal. SYN: *leontiasis.*

leotropic (lē-ō-trop′ĭk). Running from right to left in a spiral form. OPP: *dexiotropic.*

leper (lĕp′ĕr). Person afflicted with leprosy.

lepidic (lep-ĭd′ĭk). Indicating absence of definite stroma between cells, especially in tissue of lining membrane.

l. tissue. Lining membrane tissue.

l. tumor. Rind tumor. SYN: *lepidoma.*

lep′ido-. Combining form: Referring to *scales.*

lepidoma (lep-ĭ-dō′mă). Neoplasm originating from a lepidic tissue. SYN: *lepidic tumor, rind tumor.*

lepidosis (lĕp-ĭd-ō′sĭs). Any scaly or desquamating eruption. SYN: *lepra, 2, pityriasis.*

lepocyte (lep′ō-sīt). Nucleated cell with cell wall.

lepothrix (lep′o-thriks). Condition in which shaft of the hair is incased in hardened, scaly, sebaceous matter.

lepra (lĕp′rȧ). 1. Leprosy, but commonly used only in conjunction with other words to denote types of leprosy. 2. A dermatosis with desquamation.

l. alba. Skin is anesthetic and white, and different forms of paralysis follow.

l. anesthetica. Leprosy with anesthetic areas on body.

l. Arabum. Tubercular leprosy.

l. maculosa. Form with pigmented cutaneous areas.

l. mutilans. Final stage of true leprosy, or mutilation stage.

lepride (lĕp′rēd). Leprous cutaneous lesion.

leprology (lĕp-rŏl′ō-jĭ). The study of leprosy and methods of treating it.

leproma (lĕp-rō′mȧ). Tubercular lesion of leprosy.

leprosy (lep′ro-sĭ). A chronic, infectious disease in which there may be lesions of skin, membranes, or nerve tissue. Due to *Bacillus leprae,* or Hansen's bacillus. May occur at practically any age. Not easily transmissible, though considered contagious.

l., Italian. SEE: *Lombardy leprosy.*

l., Lombardy. Deficiency disease caused by lack of Vitamin B_2. SYN: *pellegra, q.v.*

l., nodular. Leprosy with granulation of tissues. SYN: *leproma.*

l., trophoneurotic. Anesthetic leprosy.

l., tubercular. Spots of erythema appear on body, become pigmented and hyperanesthetic and develop into tubercles from size of pea to walnut. Face, extremities, and genitals are the parts most commonly affected — occasionally mucous membranes, esp. of nose and throat, are invaded. Hair, eyebrows, and lashes drop out, eyes become inflamed, features distorted, voice husky. Disease may last years. Both the anesthetic and tubercular varieties are frequently seen in same patient.

leprotic (lĕp-rot′ĭk). 1. Rel. to leprosy. 2. Affected with leprosy. SYN: *leprous.*

leprous (lĕp′rŭs). 1. Pert. to leprosy. 2. Affected by leprosy. SYN: *leprotic.*

leptodermic (lep-tō-dĕr′mĭk). Possessing a thin skin.

leptomeninges (lep″to-men-ĭn′jēs). Pia mater and arachnoid as distinct from dura mater, because of their thinner and more delicate structure.

leptomeningitis (lep″to-men-in-ji′tis). Inflammation of the pia and arachnoid membranes.

leptopellic (lep-tō-pel′ĭk). Having an abnormally narrow pelvis.

leptophonia (lĕp-tō-fō′nĭ-ȧ). Weakness or feebleness of voice.

leptorrhine, leptorrhine (lep′tor-rīn). Having a very thin or slender nose.

leptosome (lĕp′tō-sōm). Person of thin, slight stature.

Leptospira (lĕp-tō-spī′rȧ). Genus of spirochetes; thin, spiral, and hookended.

L. icterohaemorrha′glae. Species causing acute infectious jaundice.

L. icteroi′des. Species causing yellow fever.

leptospirosis (lĕp″tō-spī-rō′sĭs). Condition resulting from Leptospira infection.

leptothricosis (lep″tō-thri-kō′sĭs). Disease from Leptothrix infection.

Leptothrix (lĕp′tō-thrĭks). A genus of bacteria often with long filaments.

Leptotrich′ia bucca′lis. An organism inhabiting the buccal cavity normally.

Leptus autumnalis (lep′tŭs). Parasitic mite larvae causing itch and sometimes wheals.

les′bian. 1. Pert. to lesbianism, or perverted sexual desire in women for those of their own sex only. 2. One who practices lesbianism.

les′bianism. Perversion in which sexual desire of women is only for one of their own sex.

lesion (le′zhun). 1. Morbid change in tissue formation locally. 2. An injury or wound. 3. Single infected patch in a skin disease.

l., degenerative. Lesion caused by or showing degeneration.

l., diffuse. Lesion spreading over a large area.

l., discharging. 1. Brain lesion discharging nervous impulses. 2. Lesion discharging an exudate.

l., focal. Lesion of small definite area.

l., indiscriminate. Lesion affecting separate systems of the body.

l., initial, of syphilis. Hard chancre.

l., irritative. Lesion stimulating or exciting activity in part of body where it is situated.

l., local. Lesion of nervous origin giving rise to local symptoms.

l., peripheral. One of nerve endings.

l., primary. First lesion of a disease, esp. used in referring to chancre of syphilis.

l., structural. One causing change in tissue.

l., systematic. One confined to organs of common function.

l., toxic. One resulting from sepsis.

l., vascular. One of a blood vessel.

le′thal. Pert. to or that which causes death.

lethargic (leth-ar′jĭk). 1. Affected with lethargy. 2. Rel. to lethargy. 3. Sluggish.

lethargy (leth′ar-jĭ). 1. A condition of functional torpor or sluggishness; stupor. 2. A state analogous to hypnotism, or the first stage of hypnotism.

l., African. Sleeping sickness.

l., hysteric. The sleep of hypnotic lethargy, the state in which many cases of apparent death and resurrection are found.

l., lucid. Retention of intellect but loss of will power with a consequent total lack of muscular response.

lethologica (lĕth-ō-loj′ĭk-ȧ). Temporary inability to remember a word or name, or an intended action.

leuc-. For words beginning thus, see *leuk-* words.

leucine (lū'sēn). Alpha-amino-isobutyl acetic acid, $CH_3.(CH_2)_3.CH(NH_2).COOH$, an amino acid found among the products of the digestion of proteins.

leucinosis (lū-sin-ō'sĭs). Excess of leucine in the body.

leucinuria (lū-sin-ū'rĭ-ă). Presence of leucine in urine.

leucitis (lū-sī'tĭs). Inflammation of the sclera. SYN: scleritis.

leukanemia (lū-kă-ne'mĭ-ă). Leukemia with marked anemia.

leukasmus (lū-kas'mŭs). Congenital absence of pigment in bands or patches of the skin. SYN: leukoderma.

leukemia (lū-ke'mĭ-ă). Disease characterized by a great excess of the white corpuscles with hyperplasia of the spleen or of the lymphatics or changes in the bone marrow.
SYN: leukocythemia.
    l., lymphatic. That in which the lymphatic glands are the seat of hyperplasia, with a marked increase in lymphocytes in blood; acute form occurs in children and young adults; spleen is slightly enlarged.
    l., myelogenous. That in which the medulla, esp. of the ribs, sternum and vertebrae, is converted into a pulpy material.
    l., pseudo-. A disease characterized by hyperplasia of the lymphatic structures, and by progressive anemia, without a marked increase of the white corpuscles.
    l., splenic. That in which spleen is enlarged from congestion and hyperplasia.

leukemic (lū-kēm'ĭk). 1. Rel. to leukemia. 2. Affected with leukemia.

leukemoid (lū-kē'moid). Having symptoms of leukemia.

leu'ko-, leuk-. Combining forms signifying deficiency of color.

leu'koblast. 1. Immature cell in red marrow of bones supposed to develop into erythrocyte. 2. Undeveloped leukocyte. SYN: myeloblast.

leukocidin (lū-ko-sid'in). An exotoxin that attacks leukocytes. SYN: leukotoxin, q.v.

leukocytal (lū-kō-sī'tăl). Rel. to leukocytes.

leukocyte (lū'ko-sīt). 1. White blood corpuscle. 2. Any unpigmented ameboid cellular mass in blood, lymph, or pus, or a wandering connective tissue cell.
    l., alpha. One of those disintegrating during coagulation of the blood.
    l., beta. One of those which do not disintegrate during coagulation.
    l., endothelial. Large wandering cell with phagocytic properties.
    l., hyaline. Large mononuclear leukocyte. SYN: monocyte.
    l., polymorphonuclear. Leukocyte with irregularly-shaped nucleus and fine granular cell. They predominate in purulent fluids due to pneumo-, strepto-, and staphylococcus, and sometimes in acute tuberculous fluids.

leukocythemia (lū-kō-sī-thē'mĭ-ă). Blood disease characterized by excess of white blood corpuscles and enlargement of spleen, lymphatic glands and bone marrow. SYN: leukemia, q.v.

leukocytic (lū-kō-sit'ĭk). Pert. to leukocytes.

leukocytoblast (lū-kō-sīt'ō-blast). Leukocyte mother cell.

leukocytogenesis (lū''kō-sīt''ō-jen'ĕ-sĭs). Leukocyte formation. SYN: leukopoiesis.

leukocytoid (lū'kō-sī-toid). Resembling a leukocyte.

leukocytol'ogy. The study of leukocytes and their function.

leukocytolysis (lū-kō-sī-tol'ĭ-sĭs). Destruction of leukocytes.

leukocytoma (lū-kō-sī-tō'mă). 1. Tumor composed of cells resembling leukocytes. 2. Tumorlike mass of leukocytes.

leukocytometer (lū''kō-sī-tom'et-er). Device for counting white blood corpuscles.

leukocytopenia (lū''kō-sīt''ō-pē'nĭ-ă). Subnormal number of leukocytes in peripheral blood. SYN: leukopenia.

leukocytoplania (lū''kō-sīt''ō-plā'nĭ-ă). Wandering of leukocytes through blood vessel walls. SYN: leukopedesis.

leukocytosis (lū''ko-sī-to'sĭs). Increase in the number of leukocytes (above 10,-000 per cu. mm.) in the blood, generally caused by presence of infection.

leukocytotherapy (lū''kō-sī''tō-thĕr'ă-pĭ). Treatment with leukocytic extracts.

leukocyturia (lū''ko-sī-tu'rĭ-ă). Leukocytes in the urine.

leukoderma (lū-ko-der'mă). Deficiency of pigmentation of the skin, esp. in patches. SYN: leukopathia.
    Classed as congenital, acquired and syphilitic.

leukodiagnosis (lū-ko-dī-ag-nō'sĭs). Diagnosis by observance of number, variety, or reaction of leukocytes.

leukokeratosis (lū''kō-kĕr-ă-tō'sĭs). White patch formation on the surface of mucosa of tongue, cheek and gums. SYN: leukoplakia.

leukolysin (lū-kol'ĭ-sĭn). Serum constituent destructive to leukocytes.

leukolysis (lū-kol'ĭ-sis). Destruction of leukocytes. SYN: leukocytolysis.

leuko'ma. A white, opaque corneal opacity.
    l. adherens. Corneal scar with incarcerated iris tissue.

leukomaine (lū-kō'ma-ēn, -ma-ĭn). Nitrogenous alkaloid developed in living tissue as distinguished from one in dead tissue, or one of vegetable origin.

leukomainemia (lū-kō-mă-ĭn-e'mĭ-ă). 1. Excess of leukomaines in blood. 2. Retention of excretory products in the blood.

leukomatous (lū-kōm'ă-tŭs). 1. Pert. to leukoma. 2. Suffering from leukoma.

leukomyelitis (lū''ko-mī-ĕ-li'tis). Inflammation of spinal cord's marrow or white substance.

leukomyelopathy (lū''kō-mī-ĕl-ŏp'ăth-ĭ). Disease involving white matter of spinal cord or myelon.

leukonecrosis (lū''ko-nĕ-krō'sĭs). Dry, light colored or white gangrene.*

leukonychia (lū-kō-nik'ĭ-ă). "Gift spots," white spots or streaks on the nails, due probably to air in interstitial corneal spaces, with local trauma as cause of production.

leukopathia (lū-kō-păth'ĭ-ă). 1. Absence of pigment in skin. SYN: *leukoderma.* 2. Disease involving leukocytes.

leukopedesis (lū-kō-ped-ē'sĭs). Passage of leukocytes through walls of blood vessels. SYN: *leukocytoplania.*

leukopenia (lū-kō-pe'nĭ-ă). Abnormal decrease of white blood corpuscles usually below 5000 per cu. mm.

   l., malignant. An acute infection with extreme leukopenia. SYN: *agranulocytosis.*

leukophlegmasia (lū-kō-flĕg-mā'zĭ-ă). Dropsical tendency with general edema and pale, flabby skin.

leukoplakia (lū-kō-plā'kĭ-ă). Formation of white spots or patches on the mucous membrane of the tongue or cheek.

   l. buccalis. Leukoplakia of the mucosa of the cheek. [tongue.

   l. lingualis. Leukoplakia of the

leukoplasia (lū-kō-pla'zĭ-ă). White patch formation on buccal mucosa. SYN: *leukoplakia, q.v.*

leukopoiesis (lū''kō-poi-ē'sĭs). Leukocyte production. SYN: *leukocytogenesis.*

leukopoietic (lū''kō-poi-et'ĭk). Forming leukocytes.

leukoprotease (lū-kō-pro'te-ās). An enzyme in polynuclear leukocytes that digests protein.

leukorrhagia (lū-ko-ra'jĭ-ă). Profuse white vaginal discharge. SYN: *leukorrhea, q.v.*

leukorrhea (lū-kōr-e'ă). An abnormal, white or yellowish mucous discharge from the cervical canal or the vagina.

   l., uterine. May affect mucous surface of cervix only, or fundus.
   SYN: *uterine catarrh.*

leukosarcoma (lū-kō-sar-kō'mă). An unpigmented sarcoma.

leukosis (lū-kō'sis). 1. Unnatural pallor. 2. Presence of an abnormal number of leukocytes in blood. 3. Increase in leukocyte forming tissue.

leukothrombin (lū''ko-throm'bin). A fibrin factor derived from leukocytes in the blood which helps to form thrombin.

leukotoxic (lū-kō-toks'ĭk). Destroying leukocytes.

leukotoxin (lū-kō-toks'ĭn). An exotoxin that attacks white blood cells. SYN: *leukocidin, leukolysin.* SEE: *erythrotoxin.*

leukous (lū'kŭs). White, esp. rel. to the skin.

leukotrichia (lū-kō-trik'ĭ-ă). Whiteness of the hair. SYN: *canities.*

levator (le-va'tor). 1. A muscle that raises a part; opposed to *depressor.* 2. An instrument which lifts depressed portions.

   l. ani. A broad muscle helping to form the floor of the pelvis.

   l. palpebrae superioris. A muscle which elevates the upper eyelid.

level of activities. Connector neurons are grouped into "levels" corresponding to different stages of development: (a) spinal cord level; (b) medullary level; (c) midbrain level; (d) basal ganglial level; (e) cortical level. Each level is responsible for certain activities but yet controlled by the one above it.

lever. Rigid bar used to modify direction, force, and motion.

   l., Davy's. A rigid rod for compressing the common iliac artery.

levocardiogram (lev-ō-kar'dĭ-ō-grăm). Part of cardiogram representing effect or action of left ventricle.

levoduction (lev-ō-dŭk'shun). Movement or drawing toward the left, esp. of an eye.

levogyrous (lev-ō-jī'rŭs). Causing to turn toward the left, applied esp. to substances that turn polarized light rays to the left. SYN: *levorotatory.*

levophobia (lev-ō-fō'bĭ-ă). Morbid dread of objects on the left side of the body.

levorotation (lev''ō-rō-tā'shun). Twisting or turning to the left.

levorotatory (lev''ō-rō'tă-tō-rĭ). Causing to turn toward the left, applied esp. to substances that turn polarized light rays to the left. SYN: *levogyrous.*

levotorsion (lev-ō-tor'shun). A twisting to the left. SYN: *levorotation.*

levoversion (lev-ō-vĕr'shun). A turning to the left. SYN: *levotorsion, levorotation.*

levulose. Fructose, or fruit sugar, a monosaccharide and a hexose, having the same empirical formula as dextrose, $C_6H_{12}O_6$.

   DOSAGE: 1-2 oz. (30.0-60.0 Gm.).

levulosemia (lev-ū-lō-sē'mĭ-ă). Presence of levulose in the blood.

levulosuria (lev-ū-lō-sū'rĭ-ă). Presence of levulose in the urine, usually in a form of diabetes.

Leyden jar (li'den). A glass jar coated partially, inside and out, with metal or tinfoil, or coated outside with metal and having salt solution inside; it is used as a capacitor.

Leydig's cells (li'dig). Interstitial tissue cells in the testicles, believed to be responsible for internal secretion of the testicles.

Li. Symbol for *lithium.*

liberomotor (lĭb''ĕr-ō-mō'tōr). 1. Pert. to voluntary movement. 2. Free from motor energy.

libidinous (lĭ-bĭd'ĭ-nŭs). Characterized by lust or lewdness. SYN: *lascivious, salacious.*

libido (lĭ-bī'dō, -bē'dō). 1. The sexual drive, conscious or unconscious. 2. The emotional craving activating human behavior.

lichen (li'ken). Any form of papular skin disease; usually noting *lichen planus.*

   l. acuminatus. A form of lichen ruber with papulosquamous type of eruption.

   l. agrius. Eczema of acute papular type.

   l. disseminatus. Form in which the eruption is placed unevenly.

   l. pilaris. Form affecting hair follicles. SYN: *keratosis pilaris.*

l. planus. Inflammatory skin disease of many varieties.

l. ruber. Form with red, papular lesions and constitutional symptoms. Extremely rare. Most common in poorly nourished, middle aged males.

l. scrofulosus. Form with red papules occurring chiefly in children of strumous diathesis.

l. spinulosus. Form with spine developing in each follicle. SYN: *keratosis pilaris, q.v.*

l. tropicus. Form with redness and inflammatory reaction of the skin. SYN: *miliaria rubra, prickly heat.*

lichenification (lī-ken″ĭ-fĭ-kā′shun). 1. Cutaneous thickening and hardening from continued irritation. 2. Changing of an eruption into resemblance to lichen.

lichenoid (lī′ken-oid). Resembling lichen.

lid reflex. Closure of eyelids resulting from direct corneal irritation.

Lieben's test (lē′ben). A test for acetone in the urine by caustic and iodine.

Yellow phosphate precipitates and iodoform indicates presence of acetone.

Lieberkuhn's crypts (lī′ber-kün, lē′ber-kün). Tubular glands on the intestinal mucosa surface.

Liebig's extract (lē′big). Variety of beef extract.

lie detector. An instrument for determining such minor but definite physical changes under the stress of lying (or any other emotion) as variations in respiratory rhythm and sweating of the hands. Increased perspiration lessens resistance to passage of electrical current.

lien (lī′en). The spleen.

lienal (lī′en-ăl). Rel. to the spleen. SYN: *splenic.*

lienculus (lī-en′kū-lŭs). An accessory spleen.

lienitis (lī-en-ī′tis). Inflammation of the spleen. SYN: *splenitis.*

lienocele (lī-en-ō-sēl). Splenic hernia. SYN: *splenocele.*

lienomalacia (lī″en-ō-mal-a′sĭ-ă). Softening of the spleen.

lienomedullary (lī″en-ō-med′ū-la-rĭ). Rel. to both spleen and bone marrow.

lienomyelogenous (lī″en-ō-mī-ĕl-oj′ĕ-nŭs). Derived from both the spleen and bone marrow.

lienomyelomalacia (lī″en-ō-mī″el-ō-mă-lā′sĭ-ă). Softening of the spleen and bone marrow.

lienopancreatic (lī″en-ō-păn-krē-at′ĭk). Rel. to the spleen and pancreas.

lienopathy (lī-en-op′ă-thī). Any disorder of the spleen. SYN: *splenopathy.*

lienorenal (lī″en-ō-rē′nal). Rel. to the spleen and kidney.

lienotoxin (lī″en-ō-toks′ĭn). Cytotoxin having specific action on splenic cells. SYN: *splenotoxin.*

lienteric (lī-en-ter′ĭk). 1. Pert. to diarrhea with stools containing undigested food. 2. Affected with lientery.

lientery (lī′en-ter-ĭ). Diarrhea with undigested foods in the stools.

lienunculus (li-en-un′kū-lŭs). 1. Detached mass of splenic tissue. 2. Detached part of spleen.

life (līf). 1. State of being alive; quality manifested by metabolism, growth, reproduction, and internal adaptation to environment; state in which the organs of an animal or plant are capable of performing all or any of their functions. 2. Time bet. birth and death.

ligament (lĭg′a-ment). A band of flexible connective tissue connecting the articular ends of bones, or supporting viscera, fasciae, or muscles.

l., accessory. A ligament which supplements another one, esp. one on lateral surface of a joint.

l., acromioclavicular. One extending from clavicle to the acromial process of the scapula.

l., adipose. Mucous ligament of the knee joint.

l.'s, alar. Two crescentic folds of synovial membrane extending upward on each side of the mucous ligament of the knee joint.

l., annular. A circular ligament.

l., appendiculoövarian. The ligament that runs from the broad ligament to the vermiform appendix.

l., arterial. A fibrous cord constituting the remains of the ductus arteriosus of the fetus.

l., atloaxoid. One uniting the atlas and axis.

l.'s, atloöccipital. Those uniting atlas and occipital bone.

l.'s, auricular. The ant., post., and sup. auricular ligaments uniting external ear to side of head.

l., Barkow's. Ant. and post. ligaments of elbow joint.

l., Béraud's. Suspensory ligament of the pericardium.

l., Bertin's. Iliofemoral ligament.

l., Bigelow's. Iliofemoral ligament. SYN: *Bertin's ligament.*

l., broad, of the liver. A wide, sickle-shaped fold of peritoneum, attached to lower surface of diaphragm and internal surface of right rectus abdominis muscle, and to the convex surface of liver.

l., broad, of uterus. Folds of peritoneum attached to lateral borders of uterus from insertion of fallopian tube above to the pelvic wall. It consists of 2 leaves between which are found the remnants of the wolffian ducts, cellular tissues, and the major blood vessels of the pelvis.

l., Burn's. Falciform process of fascia lata.

l., calcaneoastragaloid interosseous. A strong bundle of fibers extending from furrow on upper surface of os calcis, bet. its surfaces of articulation with the astragalus.

l., calcaneofibular. A thick, flattened, cylindrical ligament, bet. the apex of ext. malleolus and outer surface of os calcis.

l., Camper's. Deep perineal fascia.

l.'s, capsular. Heavy fibrous structures, lined with synovial membrane, surrounding articulations.

l., Carcassonne's. Triangular ligament of urethra. [bones.

l.'s, carpal. Those uniting carpal

l., caudal. Bundles of fibrous tissue uniting dorsal surfaces of the 2 lower coccygeal vertebrae and superjacent skin.

l., central. Thin distal portion of spinal cord. SYN: *filum terminale.*

l., check. One that restrains motion of a joint, esp. the lateral odontoid ligaments.

l., ciliary. One joining iris to corneosclera.

l., conoid. Post. portion of coracoclavicular ligament.

l., coracoacromial. Broad triangular one attached to the outer edge of coracoid process of the scapula, and to tip of acromion.

l., coracoclavicular. One uniting clavicle and the coracoid process of the scapula.

l., coracohumeral. Broad ligament attached to outer margin of coracoid process of the scapula and attached to the clavicle.

l., corniculopharyngeal. Fibrous tissue connecting cartilage of Santorini and cricoid cartilage.

l., coronary, of liver. A fold of peritoneum extending from post. edge of liver to diaphragm.

l.'s, costocentral. Ones uniting head of a rib with bodies of its vertebrae.

l., costocolic. One attaching splenic flexure of colon to diaphragm.

l., costocoracoid. One joining first rib and coracoid process of the scapula.

l.'s, costotransverse. One uniting ribs with transverse processes of vertebrae.

l., costotransverse, middle. One consisting of parallel fibers extending bet. a vertebra and its adjacent rib.

l.'s, costovertebral. Those uniting the ribs and vertebrae.

l., cotyloid. A fibrocartilaginous ring attached to margin of acetabulum.

l.'s, craniovertebral. Those extending bet. cranium and the vertebrae.

l., cricopharyngeal. A ligamentous bundle bet. upper and post. border of cricoid cartilage and ant. wall of pharynx.

l., cricosantorinian. Ligamentous bands uniting cartilages of Santorini with the cricoid cartilage.

l.'s, cricothyroid. Ones uniting cricoid and thyroid cartilages.

l., cricotracheal. The ligamentous structure uniting upper ring of trachea and the cricoid cartilage.

l., crucial. Cruciform ligament.

l., cruciform. A structure consisting of one ligament crossing another.

l. crural. Poupart's ligament.

l., deltoid. Int. lateral ligament of ankle.

l., dentate. Processes of pia mater extending across the subdural space on either side of spinal cord.

l., falciform. SEE: *great sacroischiadic ligament.*

l., falciform, of the liver. SEE: *broad ligament of the liver.*

l., gastrophrenic. SEE: *phrenicogastric ligament.*

l., gastrosplenic. Fold of peritoneum extending bet. the cul-de-sac of stomach and hilum of spleen. SYN: *gastrosplenic epiploön.*

l., Gimbernat's. Triangular flat expansion of aponeurosis of abdominal ext. oblique muscle.

l., glenohumeral. Fibers of the coracohumeral ligament passing into the joint, and inserted into inner and upper part of bicipital groove.

l., glenoid. 1. Fibrocartilaginous ring attached to margin of glenoid fossa of the scapula. 2. One which extends bet. palmar surfaces of phalanges and corresponding metacarpal bone.

l., glenoideobrachial. Thickened area of the shoulder's capsular ligament which is inserted into the lesser tuberosity of the humerus.

l., hepaticoduodenal. A fold of peritoneum from transverse fissure of liver to vicinity of the duodenum and right flexure of colon, forming ant. boundary of foramen of Winslow.

l., Hunter's. Round ligament of the uterus.

l., ileofemoral. Bundle of fibers forming the upper and ant. portion of the capsular ligament of the hip joint.

l., ileopectineal. A portion of the pelvic fascia attached to the ileopectineal line and to capsular ligament of hip joint. [ligament of hip joint.

l., iliotrochanteric. Part of capsular

l., infundibulopelvic. The upper free edge of the broad ligament in which the ovarian artery is found.

l., inguinal. SEE: *Poupart's ligament.*

l., interclavicular. Bundle of fibers bet. sternal ends of the clavicles, attached to interclavicular notch of sternum.

l.'s, interspinal, interspinous. Those extending from sup. margin of a spinous process of one vertebra to lower margin of one above.

l.'s, intervertebral. Fibrocartilaginous disks bet. vertebra.

l., lateral. One on side of a joint or on ext. side of a structure.

l.'s, lateral, of the liver. Folds of peritoneum extending from lower surface of diaphragm to adjacent borders of right and left lobes of the liver.

l., lateral occipitoatlantal. A ligament on each side bet. transverse processes of atlas and jugular process of the occipital bone.

l.'s, lateral odontoid. Strong ligaments extending bet. sides of odontoid process of the axis and inner sides of condyles of the occipital bone.

l.'s, lateral patellar. Membranous triangular ones extending on each side from condyle of femur and lateral margin of patella to inf. patellar ligament and extensor tendons of the leg.

l., odontoid, middle. One extending bet. apex of odontoid process of the axis and ant. margin of foramen magnum.

l., palpebral. Ligament bet. ext. border of orbit and eyelid tissue and bet. nasal process of sup. maxilla and margins of the tarsi.

l., phrenicogastric. A fold of peritoneum bet. esophageal end of stomach and the diaphragm.

l., posterior crucial. One arising from behind spine of the tibia and ext. semilunar fibrocartilage and connecting with the inner femoral condyle.

l., posterior, of knee joint. A flat thickening of the capsule ligament of the knee.

l., Poupart's. The lower portion of the aponeurosis of the ext. oblique muscle of the abdomen. SYN: *crural arch, femoral arch.*

l., pterygomaxillary. Band of fiber extending bet. apex of internal pterygoid plate of sphenoid bone and the post. extremity of internal oblique line of inferior maxilla.

l., pubic. The post. margin of sup. crus of the falciform process of the fascia lata.

l., reticular. One holding a muscle to a bone.

l., rhomboid. A strong structure extending from tuberosity of clavicle to outer surface of the cartilage of the first rib.

l., round. One resembling a round cord.

l., round, of the forearm. A small one bet. the coronoid process of ulna and a point below tuberosity of the radius.

l., round, of uterus. A long, round, fibrous band passing from fundal side of uterus, to be inserted into connective tissue of mons Veneris.

l., sacroischiadic, -ischiatic, or **-sciatic, great.** Triangular ligament attached by its base to sides of sacrum and coccyx and to post. inf. spine of ilium, and by its apex to tuberosity of the ischium.

l., sacroischiadic, lesser; sacrosciatic, lesser. Short ligament arising from the lateral margin of lower portion of sacrum and of upper portion of coccyx, in front of and blended with the great sacroischiadic ligament.

l.'s, stomach. The lesser omentum and the phrenicogastric ligament.

l., stylohyoid. A thin fibroelastic cord bet. lesser cornu of hyoid bone and apex of styloid process of the temporal bone.

l., stylomaxillary, stylomyloid. A broad fibrous band of tissue extending bet. styloid process of temporal bone and lower part of post. border of ramus of the inferior maxilla.

l., suprascapular. A thin fibrous band of tissue extending from base of coracoid process of scapula to inner margin of suprascapular notch.

l., supraspinal, supraspinous. One uniting apices of spinous processes of vertebrae.   [organ.

l., suspensory. One suspending an **l.'s, suspensory, of mamma.** Fibrous processes of layer of fascia covering ant. surface of the mamma.

l., suspensory, of mesentery. The root of the mesentery.

l., suspensory, of the penis. A triangular bundle of fibrous tissue extending from ant. surface of the symphysis pubis and adjacent structures to dorsum of the penis.

l.'s, suspensory, of the uterus. The broad ligaments, the round ones, and the rectouterine folds of the uterus.

l.'s, sutural. Thin, fibrous layers interposed bet. articulating surfaces of bones united by suture.

l., tarsal. The tarsoörbital fascia.

l., transverse, of atlas. A strong ligament passing over odontoid process of the axis.

l., transverse, of hip joint. A ligamentous band extending across cotyloid notch of the acetabulum.

l., transverse, of knee joint. A fibrous band extending from ant. margin of external semilunar fibrocartilage of knee to extremity of the internal semilunar fibrocartilage.

l., trapezoid. Ant. ext. portion of the coracoclavicular ligament.

l. of Treitz. Fold of peritoneum from duodenojejunal junction to left crus of diaphragm.

l., triangular. Triangular portion of the aponeurosis of ext. oblique muscle.

l., uteroövarian. Attaches the inner surface of the ovary to the uterine horn.

l., uterorectosacral. Arises from the sides of the cervix and passes upwards and backwards, passing around the rectum, to the second sacral vertebra.

l., vaginal, of the testicle. Obliterated portion of the tunica vaginalis.

l., vesicoumbilical. Ligament connecting bladder and umbilicus. SYN: *Urachus.*

l., vesicouterine. The fold of peritoneum that attaches the bladder to the ant. wall of the uterus.

l., Winslow's. Posterior ligament of the knee joint.

l., Y-shaped, of Bigelow. Iliofemoral ligament.

l. of Zinn. Membranous structure forming common tendon of origin for ext., inf., and int. recti muscles of the eye.

ligamentopexis (lĭg-ă-mĕn″tō-peks'ĭs). Suspension of uterus on the round ligaments.

ligamentous (lig-ă-men'tŭs). 1. Rel. to a ligament. 2. Like a ligament.

ligamentum (lĭg-a-men'tum (pl. *ligamenta*). Ligament. ·

l. arcuatum. The ligamentous part of the diaphragm, external and internal.

l. arteriosum. A fibrous cord, from pulmonary artery to arch of aorta, the remains of the ductus arteriosus of the fetus.

l. cruciatum atlantis. Cruciform ligament.

l. cruciatum cruris. An X-shaped process of the deep fascia of the leg.

l. dentatum, denticulatum. A delicate band of connective tissue on each side of the myelon.

l. nuchae. A thin, fibrous membrane connecting the trapezial muscles.

l. palpebrale. Ligamentous band, external and internal, bet. outer margin of the orbit and tissues of eyelids.

l. patellae. A strong, flat band securing the patella to the tibia.

l. pectinatum. The spongy tissue filling up sinus of ant. chamber of eye at junction of cornea and sclera, forming the root of the iris.

l. spirale. A projecting band attached to wall of the cochlea, upon which is inserted the lamina spiralis membranacea.

l. subflavum. Yellow elastic tissue connecting the lamina of the vertebrae from axis downward.

l. suspensorium. Suspensory ligament, q.v.

l. teres. 1. A triangular band of fibers arising from the margins of the cotyloid notch at bottom of the acetabulum. 2. Round ligament of the forearm. 3. Middle costotransverse ligament.

ligate (lī'gāt). To apply a ligature.

ligation (li-gā'shun). The application of a ligature. Syn: *cirsodesis*.

ligature (lĭg'a-tūr). 1. Process of binding or tying. 2. A band or bandage. 3. A ligament. 4. A thread or wire for tying blood vessels.

light (līt). The sensation produced by electromagnetic radiation which falls on the retina.

l., axial. Light with rays parallel to each other and to optic axis.

l., diffused. Rays broken by refraction.

l., polarized. Light in which waves vibrate in one direction only.

l., red. Cold, red light is emitted by neon glow discharge tube. Intensity of total radiation is low.

l. reflex. Reflection of light from normal eardrum membrane.

l., refracted. Rays bent from original course.

l., sun-. Radiation from the sun.

l. therapy. A limited term used by some physicians to designate the therapeutic application of radiation in the visible spectrum; some include also ultraviolet radiation.

l., transmitted. That which passes through an object.

l. unit. A foot candle. This is the amt. of light measured one foot from a standard candle. The light intensity of the average room is from 3 to 10 foot candles, whereas 25-100 would be better.

At noon, on a clear day, the sun gives 10,000 candle ft. of light; under a tree we get 1,000; on a porch, 500; on a fairly cloudy day, 200. The term foot candle takes the place of "candle power."

light (līt). 1. Not heavy. 2. Pale.

l. diet. All foods allowed in soft diet* plus whole grained cereals, easily digested raw fruits and vegetables. Foods not pureed or ground.

light'ening. Uterine descent into pelvis during primary stage of labor.

ligula (lĭg'ū-lä). Strip of white substance on the margin of the fourth ventricle.

limb (lĭm). 1. An arm or leg. 2. Appendage resembling an arm or leg. 3. An extremity.

l., pelvic. A lower extremity.

l., thoracic. An upper extremity.

limbic (lĭm'bĭk). Pert. to a limbus or border. Syn: *marginal*.

limbus (lĭm'bŭs). The edge or border of a part.

l. conjunctivae. The edge of conjunctiva overlapping the cornea.

lime (līm). CaO. A substance obtained from limestone.

l. water. Solution of lime and distilled water.

limen (lī'mĕn). Edge, threshold.

liminal (lĭm'ĭ-năl). Hardly perceptible; rel. to the threshold of consciousness.

limitans (lĭm'ĭ-tăns). 1. Used in conjunction with other words to denote limiting. 2. Used synonymously to indicate membrana limitans.

limo'sis. Abnormal hunger; depraved appetite.

limotherapy (lim-ō-ther'ă-pĭ). Treatment by restriction of diet, or fasting.

lincture (lĭnk'tūr), **linctus** (-tŭs). Medicine to be taken by licking.

line (līn). Boundary mark or narrow mark.

l., abdominal. Line indicating abdominal muscle boundaries.

l., adrenal. In defective adrenal activity, white line seen on abdomen following drawing of fingernail across it.

l., alveobasilar. One from nasion to alveolar point.

l., alveolonasal. From alveolar to nasion.

l. of anus, inferior sinuous. Convoluted line at junction of mucous membrane of rectum with integument at anus.

l., auriculobregmatic. From auricular point to bregma.

l., axillary (ant., post. and mid-). Downward from axilla.

l., base. From infraorbital ridge through middle of external auditory meatus to midline of occiput.

l., basiobregmatic. From basion to bregma.

l., Baudelocque's. Ext. conjugate diameter of pelvis.

l.'s, Beau's. Transverse lines on the fingernails.

l., biauricular. From one auditory meatus over vertex to other.

l., blue. One on gums in chronic lead poisoning.

l., Borsieri's. White line made by fingernail in early stages of scarlet fever.

l., Burton's. See: *blue line.*

l., Camper's. One from ext. auditory meatus to just below nasal spine.

l., Clapton's. Green line on gums in copper poisoning.

l., Corrigan's. Purplish line on gums in copper poisoning.

l., costoarticular. From sternoclavicular joint to point on 11th rib.

l., costoclavicular. Line midway bet. nipple and sternum border.

l. of demarcation. Division bet. healthy and diseased tissue.

l., Douglas'. Curved lower edge of post. sheath of rectus abdominis muscle just below level of iliac crest.

l. of Douglas, semicircular. Curved lower edge of int. layer of aponeurosis of the obliquus abdominis internus.

l., ectental. Bet. ectoderm and entoderm on embryo.

l., Ellis'. Curved line at upper border of a pleuritic effusion.

l., facial. Straight line touching glabella and point at lower border of face.

l. of femur, internal supracondylar. Inner of 2 ridges into which linea aspera of femur divides.

l. of fibula, oblique. Prominent ridge on int. surface of shaft of fibula.

l. of fixation. Imaginary line drawn from subject viewed to the fovea centralis.

l., gingival. 1. Line of junction of cementum and enamel of a tooth. 2. One on neck of tooth where gum is attached.

l., iliopectineal. Bony ridge marking brim of pelvis.

l. of ilium, curved (sup., inf., and mid-). Prominent lines of iliac region.

l. of ilium, intermediate. Ridge upon crest of ilium bet. inner and outer lip.

l. of inferior maxilla, internal oblique. Ridge on int. surface of lower jaw.

l., interauricular. One joining the 2 auricular points.

l.'s, intercellular. The narrow intervals bet. contiguous cells of epithelium or endothelium.

l., intercondylar, intercondylean. Transverse ridge joining condyles of femur above the intercondyloid fossa.

l., interjugal. One joining the jugal points.

l., intermalar. One joining nalar points.

l., intertrochanteric. Ridge upon post. surface of femur ext. bet. greater and lesser trochanters.

l., intertuberal. One joining inner borders of ischial tuberosities below small sciatic notch.

l., mammary. From one nipple to other.

l., mammillary. Vertical line through center of nipple.

l., median. One joining any 2 points in the periphery of the median plane of the body, or one of its parts.

l., nasobasilar. Through basion and nasion.

l., nuchal (sup., inf., and mid-). Inf. and sup. curved lines of occiput and ext. occipital protuberance.

l.'s of occipital bone, curved. Two lines on either half of outer surface of occipital bone.

l. of occipital bone, superior curved. Semicircular line passing outward and forward from ext. occipital protuberance.

l., parasternal. Line midway bet. nipple and sternum border.

l. of parietal bone, superior curved. Ridge upon outer surface of parietal bone.

l., parturient. Axis of the birth canal.

l., pectineal. That portion of iliopectineal line formed by the os pubis.

l. of radius, oblique. Prominent ridge from lower part of bicipital tuberosity downward and outward to form ant. border of the bone.

l., scapular. Downward from lower angle of scapula.

l., semilunar. Curved tendinous condensation of aponeurosis of obliquus abdominis externus.

l., sight. From center of pupil to viewed object, imaginary.

l., spinoumbilical. Imaginary line drawn from ant. sup. spine of ilium to umbilicus.

l., sternal. Median line of sternum.

l., sternomastoid. From bet. heads of sternomastoid muscle to mastoid process.

l., supraorbital. Across forehead above root of ext. angular process of frontal bone.

l., temporal. Curved line on outer surface of parietal bone just below parietal eminence.

l.'s, test. Those for detecting fracture or shortening of neck of femur.

l. of tibia, oblique. Rough ridge crossing post. surface of tibia obliquely downward.

l., umbilicopubic. That portion of median line extending from umbilicus to symphysis pubis.

l., visual. One that extends from object to macula lutea passing through the nodal point. [cal line.

linea (lin'e-ă) (pl. *lineae*). An anatomi-

l. alba. The white line of connective tissue in middle of abdomen from sternum to the pubis.

l. albicans. Line on abdomen in advanced pregnancy, in dropsy or tumor.

l. aspera. A longitudinal ridge on sup. surface of middle third of the femur.

l. costoarticularis. A line bet. the sternoclavicular articulation and point of the 11th rib.

l. cruciatae. The 4 ridges upon inner surface of the occipital bone.

l. directionis pelvis. The axis of pelvic canal.

l. eminens. A ridge on post. surface of the patella.

l. eminens cartilaginis cricoideae. Vertical ridge in middle line of post. half of the cricoid cartilage.

l. eminens transversa ossis hyoidei. Horizontal ridge crossing ant. surface of body of hyoid bone.

l. eminentes. Ridges upon ant. surface of scapula in subscapular fossa.

l. ni'gra. Black line or discoloration of the abdomen seen in pregnant women during latter part of term. It runs from above the umbilicus to the pubes.

l. obliqua cartilaginea. An oblique line extending downward and outward from tubercle of thyroid cartilage.

l. quadrati. An eminence commencing about middle of post. intertrochanteric line, and descending vertically for about 2 inches along post. surface of shaft of femur.

l. sternalis. Median line of the sternum.

l. terminalis. BNA. Bony ridge on inner surface of ilium continued on to pubis which divides true and false pelvis.

l. transversae ossis sacralis. Ridges formed by lines of union of the 4 sacral vertebrae.

linear (lĭn'ē-ar). Pert. to, or resembling, a line.

l. measure. Measure of length.

lingism (lĭng'ĭzm). Exercise cure or treatment, esp. without the aid of apparatus. Syn: *kinesitherapy.*

Ling's cure, L.'s system (ling). Treatment by movements.

lingua (lĭng'gwă). Tongue, or tonguelike structure.

lingual (lĭn'gwal). 1. Pert. to the tongue. 2. Tongue-shaped.

lingula (lĭn'gū-lă). Tongue-shaped process, esp. lingula cerebelli.

l. cerebelli. Tongue of cerebellum prolonged forward on upper surface of sup. medullary velum.

l. of sphenoid. Ridge between the body and ala magna of the sphenoid.

l. Wrisbergi. Connecting fibers of motor and sensory roots of the trifacial nerve.

lin'iment. A liquid containing a medicament and oil, alcohol or water for use externally, applied by friction method.

linimentum (lĭn-ĭm-en'tŭm). Liquid preparation for external use and usually applied with rubbing. Four are official.

li'nin. An achromatic, threadlike substance which forms the nuclear network of a cell; the nucleoplasm is found in its reticulum, in the form of granules.

linitis (lĭn-ī'tĭs). Inflamed condition of gastric cellular tissue.

l., plastic. Linitis with hypertrophy of connective tissue about the stomach.

lin'seed. Seeds of the common flax.

l. poultice. One made from crushed linseed which is heated. Test for heat with hand before applying.

l. tea. A soothing demulcent drink for colds. Add 1 tablespoonful of linseed to 1 pint of water. The juice of a lemon may be added and sugar. Some use ¼ oz. of liquorice and ¼ oz. of candy. It is then simmered in a saucepan for half an hour, strained, and served hot.

lint (lĭnt). 1. Linen scraped until soft and woolly for dressing wounds. 2. Cotton fiber.

lintin (lĭn'tĭn). Prepared absorbent cotton; fabric used in dressings.

liomyofibroma (lī-ō-mī-o-fī-brō'mă). Tumor in which lioma, myoma, and fibroma are characterized.

lip. 1. Soft structure around the oral cavity, externally. 2. One of the lips of the pudendum (*labium majus* or *minus*).

l., bluish or purplish. May appear in the aged, in those exposed to great cold, and in carbon monoxide poisoning.

l., dry. May be seen in fevers, or be caused by drugs such as atropine, by thirst, or exhaustion.

l., fissured. May occur after exposure to cold, in certain forms of indigestion, and in children in congenital syphilis. The dribbling of saliva, and a toothless condition may cause fissures in the corners of the mouth.

l., hare. Slit appearance of upper lip due to developmental failure of continuity.

l., pale. May be seen in anemia and wasting diseases, in prolonged fever, and after a hemorrhage.

l. rashes. These may be manifestations of typhoid fever, meningitis, or pneumonia. In secondary syphilis, chancre, cancer, and epithelioma, mucous patches may appear.

l. reading. Catching meaning of a speaker by watching movements of his lips without hearing his words.

l. reflex. Reflex movement of lips when angle of mouth is suddenly and lightly tapped during sleep.

lipacidemia (lĭp"ă-sĭ-dē'mĭ-ă). Fatty acid in the blood.

lipaciduria (lĭp"ă-sĭ-dū'rĭ-ă). Fatty acids in the urine.

liparocele (lĭp'ă-ro-sēl). 1. Scrotal hernia containing fat. 2. A fatty tumor.

liparous (lĭp'ăr-ŭs). Obese; fat.

liparomphalus (lĭp-ă-rom'fă-lŭs). Fatty tumor located at, or involving, the umbilical cord.

lipase (lī'pās, lī'pās). A lipolytic or fat splitting enzyme found in the blood, pancreatic secretion and tissues.

Emulsified fats of cream and egg yolk are changed in the stomach to fatty acids and glycerol by gastric lipase.

lipasuria (lĭp-ăs-u'rĭ-ă). Lipase in the urine.   [tissues.

lipectomy (lĭ-pek'to-mĭ). Excision of fatty

lipemia (lĭ-pē'mĭ-ă). Fat in the blood.

l. retinalis. Condition in which retinal vessels appear reddish white, or white; found in cases of lipemia.

lipid(e (lĭp'ĭd, lĭp'ĭd). A comprehensive term for fats and soaps. SYN: *lipin, lipoid, q.v.*

lipin (lĭp'ĭn). Term for fat and fatlike substances.

They may be simple, compound, or derived. SEE: *fat, lipoid.*

lipiodine (lĭp-ī'ō-dĭn). Solid form of iodipin.

lipiodol (lĭp-ī'ō-dōl). An iodized oil obtained by fixation of iodine in poppyseed oil.

l. injection. May be cisternal, lumbar, or both, depending upon whether the suspected block is near the cisterna magna or below it.

lipo-, lip-. Combining forms pert. to fat.

lipoarthritis (lip-ō-arth-rī'tĭs). Inflammation of fatty tissues of joints.

lipoblast (lĭp'ō-blast). Immature fat cell.

lipoblastoma (lĭp-ō-blast-ō'mă). Tumor of fatty tissue. SYN: *adipoma, lipoma.*

lipocaic (lĭp-ō-kā'ĭk). Pancreatic hormone controlling hepatic fat supply.

Recently, it has been used successfully to clear up psoriasis.

lipocardiac (lĭp"ō-kar'dĭ-ăk). 1. Pert. to fatty heart degeneration. 2. Sufferer from fatty degeneration of heart.

lipocele (lĭp'ō-sēl). Presence of fatty tissue in a hernial sac. SYN: *adipocele, liparocele.*

lipocere (lĭp'ō-sēr). Waxy substance resulting from exposure of fleshy tissue to moisture with the exclusion of air. SYN: *adipocere.*

lipochondroma (lĭp"ō-kŏn-drō'mă). Tumor both fatty and cartilaginous.

lipochrome (lĭp'ō-krōm). Colored substance of fatty nature.

lipoclasis (lĭp-ok'lā-sĭs). Splitting up of fat. SYN: *lipolysis, lipodieresis.*

lipoclastic (lĭp-ō-klas'tĭk). Fat splitting. SYN: *lipolytic.*

lipocyte (lĭp'ō-sīt). Fat cell.

lipodieresis (lĭp-ō-dī-er'ē-sĭs). Splitting or destruction of fat. SYN: *lipoclasis.*

lipodystrophy (lĭp-ō-dĭs'trō-fĭ). Disturbance or defectiveness of fat metabolism.

l., intestinal. Disease characterized principally by fat deposits in intestinal and mesenteric lymphatic tissue and by fatty dirrhea, loss of weight and strength, and arthritis.

lipoferous (lĭp-ŏf'ĕr-ŭs). Causing or carrying fat.

lipofibroma (lĭp"ō-fī-brō'mă). Tumor indicating lipoma and fibroma.

lipogenesis (lĭp-ō-jĕn'ē-sĭs). Fat formation.

lipogenetic (lĭp-ō-jĕn-ĕt'ĭk). Fat producing. SYN: *lipogenic, lipogenous.*

lipogenic (lĭp-ō-jĕn'ĭk). Fat producing. SYN: *lipogenetic, lipogenous.*

lipogenous (lĭp-ŏj'ĕn-ŭs). Producing fat. SYN: *lipogenetic, lipogenic.*

lipogranuloma (lĭp"ō-gran-ŭ-lo'mă). Inflammation of fatty tissue with granulation and development of oily cysts.

lipoid (lĭp'oid). 1. Substance resembling fats in appearance and solubility, but containing other groups than the glycerol and fatty acids which make up the true fats. 2. Similar to fat.

lipoidemia (lĭp-oi-dē'mĭ-ă). Lipoids in the blood.

lipoidosis (lĭp-oi-do'sĭs). Presence of anisotropic lipoids in tissue.

lipoiduria (lĭp-oi-dū'rĭ-ă). Lipoids in the urine.

lipolipoidosis (lĭp"ō-lĭp-oi-dō'sĭs). Infiltration of fats and lipoids into a tissue.

lipolysis (lĭp-ol'ĭs-ĭs). The decomposition of fat. [hydrolyze fats.

lipolytic (lĭp-ō-lĭ'tĭk). Having ability to

l. digestion. The conversion of neutral fats by hydrolysis into fatty acids and glycerol; fat splitting.

l. enzyme. Fat splitting ferment. SYN: *lipase.* SEE: *enzymes.*

lipoma (lĭ-po'mă). A fatty tumor. SEE: *chondrolipoma.*

They are frequently multiple, but not metastatic.

l. arborescens. Excrescence of fatty tissue within a tendon sheath.

l. colloides. A myxolipoma.

l., cystic. One containing cysts.

l., diffuse. One not definitely circumscribed.

l. diffusum renis. Condition in which fat displaces parenchyma of the kidney.

l. durum. One in which there is marked hypertrophy of the fibrous stroma and capsule.

l., hernial. A lipocele.

l. myxomatodes. A lipomyxoma.

l., nasal. A fibrous growth of the subcutaneous tissue of the nostrils.

l., osseous. One in which the connective tissue has undergone calcareous degeneration.

l. telangiectodes. A rare form containing a large number of blood vessels.

lipomatosis (lĭp-ō-mă-to'sĭs). Excessive deposit of fat in the tissues. SYN: *liposis, obesity.*

l. renis. Fatty infiltration of renal parenchyma. SYN: *lipoma diffusum renis.*

lipomatous (lĭp-ō'mă-tŭs). 1. Of the nature of lipoma. 2. Affected with lipoma.

lipometabolic (lĭp"ō-met-ă-bol'ĭk). Rel. to metabolism of fat.

lipometabolism (lĭp-ō-mĕ-tab'ol-ĭzm). Fat metabolism.

lipomyxoma (lĭp"ō-miks-ō'mă). Tumor indicating lipoma and myxoma.

lipopectic (lĭp-ō-pek'tĭk). Characterized by lipopexia.

lipopexia (lĭp-ō-pek'sĭ-ă). Accumulation of fat in the body. SYN: *adipopexia.*

lipophage (lĭp'o-fāg). Cell absorbing fat.

lipophagic (lĭp-ō-fā'jĭk). Consuming, destroying, or absorbing fat. SYN: *lipolytic.*

lipophil (lĭp'ō-fĭl). 1. A fat absorber or solvent. 2. Absorbing fat.

lipophrenia (lĭp-ō-frē'nĭ-ă). Mental failure or collapse.

liposarcoma (lĭp-ō-sar-kō'mă). Sarcoma with fatty elements.

lipo′sis. Accumulation of fat in a part.

lipothymia (lĭ-po-thī′mĭ-ă). Faintness; syncope.*

lipotropic (lĭp-ō-trŏp′ĭk). Said of a basic dye having an affinity for fat.

lipotropy (lĭp-ot′rō-pĭ). The affinity of a basic dye for fat.

lipoxeny (lĭp-oks′ĕ-nĭ). Desertion of host by parasitic organism.

Lipschuetz cell (lĭp′shŭtz). Cell with single and double granules in its protoplasm, which are stainable with hematoxylin. Syn: *centrocyte.*

lipuria (lĭ-pu′rĭ-ă). Fat in the urine.

liquefacient (lĭk-we-fa′shent). 1. Agent which produces a conversion into liquid. 2. Converting into liquid.

liquefaction (lĭk-we-fak′shun). The conversion of a solid into a liquid.

liquescent (lĭk-wes′sent). Becoming liquescent. Syn: *deliquescent.*

liqueur (lĭ-ker′). Alcoholic spirit. Aromatically flavored, often colored, and sweetened. A cordial.

liquid (lĭk′wĭd). 1. Flowing easily. 2. Substance which flows without being melted. See: *emulsion, liquefacient, liquefaction.*

   l. air therapy. Therapeutic application of low temperatures. See: *refrigeration.*

   l. measure. Measure of liquid capacity.

li′quid di′et. Coffee with hot milk, tea, water, albumin water, milk in all forms, milk and cream mixtures, cocoa, cream soups strained, fruit juices, meat juices, beef tea, clear broths, gruels, meat soups strained, eggnogs. See: *fluid diet.*

   l. d., full. Restricted liquid diet plus gruels, strained fruit juice, tomato juice, strained cream soups, milk and cream beverages, albumins, plain gelatin, custard, plain ice cream, junket. coffee, tea.

   l. d., high caloric. Full liquid diet reinforced with lactose, glucose, dextrimaltose, ice cream, ices, coffee, tea, etc.

   l. d., or fluid, without milk. Cereal water, strained fruit and strained vegetable juices, albumins, plain gelatin, water ices, ginger ale, clear fat-free broth, beef juice, coffee, tea, etc.

   l. d., restricted. Fat-free broth tea (no cream), ginger ale, bland fruit juice, such as pear, white cherry, or peach juice.

   l. d., surgical. Strained fruit juices, ginger ale, fat-free broth, strained cream soup, milk and cream beverages, albuminized fruit juices, tea, coffee, gelatin beverage if ordered.

liquor (lĭk′er). 1. Any liquid or fluid. 2. An alcoholic beverage. 3. Pharm: Solution of medicinal substance in water.

   l. amnii. The fluid in the amniotic sac in which the fetus floats.

   l. folliculi. The fluid contained in the graafian follicle.

   l. lymphae. Fluid portion of lymph.

   l. puris. Liquid portion of pus.

   l. sanguinis. Blood serum or plasma.

   l. solutions. Aqueous solutions of nonvolatile substances presenting the greatest variety in strength, character, and method of preparation. They are usually very active medicinal preparations. There are 21 official solutions.

lisping (lĭsp′ing). Substitution of sounds due to defect in speech, as of *th* sound for *s* and *z*.

lissotrichy (lĭs-sot′rĭ-kĭ). Condition of having straight hair.

lis′terism. Theory and practice of antisepsis.

liter (lē′tĕr). Metric fluid measure; 1000 cc., 270 fl. drams, 61 cu. in., 33.8 fl. oz., 1.056 qt. See: *metric system.*

lithagogue (lĭth′ă-gŏg). 1. Agent which expels calculi. 2. Expelling calculi.

lithectasy (lĭth-ek′ta-sĭ). Removal of a stone from bladder by dilation of the urethra.

lithemia (lĭth-e′mĭ-ă). Excess of lithic or uric acid in the blood due to imperfect metabolism of the nitrogenous substances. Syn: *uricemia.* See: *oxypathy.*

lithiasis (lĭth-ĭ′ă-sĭs). 1. Formation of calculi and concretions. 2. Uric acid diathesis.

   l. biliaris. Gallstones.

   l. nephritica. Stone formation in the kidneys. Syn: *nephrolithiasis.*

   l. renalis. Kidney stones.

lithiatry (lĭth-ĭ′ă-trĭ). Medical treatment of calculus.

lithic acid (lĭth′ĭk). Acid found in urine. Syn: *uric acid.* [*calculus.*

litho-, lith-. Prefixes: Pert. to *stone* or

lithocenosis (lĭth-ō-sĕn-ō′sĭs). Removal of crushed fragments of calculi. Syn: *litholapaxy, lithotrity.*

lithoclast (lĭth-o-klăst). Forceps for breaking up large calculi. Syn: *lithotrite.*

lithoclasty (lĭth′ō-klăs-tĭ). The crushing of a stone into fragments that it may pass through natural channels.

lithoclysma (lĭth-ō-klĭs′mă). Injection of calculary solvents into urinary bladder.

lithocystotomy (lĭth″ō-sĭs-tot′ō-mĭ). Incision of bladder to remove calculus.

lithodialysis (lĭth″ō-dĭ-al′ĭ-sĭs). Fragmentation or solution of calculi. Syn: *litholysis.*

lithogenesis (lĭth-ō-jen′ĕ-sĭs). Formation of concretions.

lithokonion (lĭth-ō-kō′nĭ-on). Instrument for pulverizing vesical calculi.

litholapaxy (lĭth-ol′a-păks-ĭ). The operation of crushing a stone in the bladder followed by immediate washing out of the crushed fragments through a catheter.

lithology (lĭth-ol′ō-jĭ). The science dealing with calculi.

litholysis (lĭth-ol′ĭ-sĭs). Dissolving of calculi. Syn: *lithodialysis.*

lithometer (lĭth-om′ĕ-tĕr). Instrument for estimating size of calculi.

lithometra (lĭth-ō-me′tră). Uterine tissue ossification.

lithomyl (lĭth′ō-mĭl). Instrument for crushing a vesical stone. Syn: *lithokonion.*

lithonephrotomy (lĭth″o-nĕ-frot′ō-mĭ). Incision of kidney for removal of renal calculus.

lithontriptic (lĭth-ŏn-trĭp′tĭk). An agent that tends to dissolve calculi.

lithopedion (lĭth″ō-pe′dĭ-ŏn). A fetus which has died and become petrified.

lithophone (lĭth′o-fōn). Instrument for determining by sound the presence of calculi in the bladder.

lithoscope (lĭth′o-skōp). Instrument for examining stone in bladder.

lithotome (lĭth′o-tōm). Instrument for performing lithotomy.

lithotomy (lith-ot′o-mĭ). Incision into bladder for removing a stone.

   l., bilateral. Incision across perineum.

   l., high. Suprapubic incision.

   l., lateral. Front of rectum to one side of raphe.

   l., median. In median line in front of anus.

   l., position. Upon the back with thighs flexed upon abdomen and legs upon thighs, which are abducted. SYN: *dorsosacral.*

   l., rectal. Through the rectum.

   l., vaginal. Through vaginal wall.

lithotony (lĭth-ot′ō-nĭ). Removal of a calculus through small incision instrumentally dilated.

lithotresis (lĭth-ō-trē′sĭs). Drilling or boring of holes in a calculus to facilitate crushing.

lithotripsy (lĭth′ō-trĭp-sĭ). Crushing of a calculus in bladder or urethra.

lithotriptic (lĭth-o-trĭp′tĭk). 1. An agent that dissolves calculi. 2. Pert. to lithotripsy. SYN: *lithontriptic.*

lithotrite (lĭth′o-trīt). Instrument for crushing stone in the bladder. SEE: *lithotrity.*

lithotrity (lith-ot′rĭ-tĭ). Crushing of a stone to small fragments in the bladder. SEE: *litholapaxy.*

lithous (lĭth′ŭs). Rel. to a calculus or stone. SYN: *calculous.*

lithoxiduria (lĭth″oks-ĭ-dū′rĭ-ă). Presence of xanthic oxide in the urine.

lithuresis (lĭth-u-re′sĭs). Passage of calculus through the urethra during urination.

lithureteria (lĭth″ŭ-re-tē′rĭ-ă). Disease of the ureter due to presence of calculi.

lithuria (lĭth-u′rĭ-ă). Excess of uric acid and urates in the urine.

litmus (lĭt′mus). A blue dyestuff made by fermenting certain coarsely powdered lichens.

   l. paper. Chemically prepared blue paper which is turned red by acids, and remains blue in alkali solutions; used as test for acid in urine. SEE: *indicator.*

litter (lĭt′ter). A stretcher for carrying the wounded or the sick.

Little's disease (lĭt′tls). Congenital spastic paralysis on both sides (diplegia), although it may be *paraplegic* or *hemiplegic* in form.

livedo (lĭv-ē′dō). Patchy or general dark discoloration of the skin. SYN: *lividity.*

liver (lĭv′er). Large gland in the body,
30x15x8 cm., 1500 to 1800 Gm. in wt., situated on right side beneath the diaphragm; right hypochondriac epigastric, and part of left hypochondriac regions, level with bottom of sternum, undersurface, concave, covers stomach, duodenum, hepatic flexure of colon, right kidney and suprarenal capsule, secretes bile and aids metabolism.

   l., abscess of. Temperature up in evening, low in morning; sweats and chills; liver enlarged, painful, tender, may be bulging and fluctuation. Pus may be detected by aspirating needle.

   l., acute yellow atrophy of. A rare and grave disease, characterized anatomically by a rapid destruction of the liver tissues, and manifested by jaundice and hemorrhages, a reduction in size of liver and marked cerebral phenomena.

   l., amyloid. An enlargement of liver, due to the deposition of an albuminoid substance.

   l., cancer of. Male sex, heredity and traumatism predisposing factors.

   l., cirrhosis of, atrophic. A chronic disease characterized anatomically by a hyperplasia of the connective tissue and destruction of the secreting cells shown chiefly by symptoms of portal obstruction.

   l., c. of, hypertrophic. In which the connective tissue hyperplasia starts from the periphery of the capillary bile ducts instead of from ramifications of portal vein as in atrophic form.

   l., fatty. Infiltration of liver with fat.

   l., hyperemia of. Liver enlarged and filled with blood.

   l., h. of, active. Commonly due to dietetic indiscretions (billiousness), may result from overindulgence in alcohol— hot climates.

   l., h. of, passive. SYM: Same, though less marked. Liver often quite large and in extreme cases such as follow tricuspid regurgitation it may pulsate.

   l., inflammation of. SYM: (1) Symptoms of gastroduodenal catarrh usually precede, *i. e.,* coated tongue, anorexia, fetid breath, epigastric distress, vomiting and perhaps diarrhea; (2) obstructive jaundice indicated by yellow skin and conjunctivae, light stools and dark urine; (3) in acute cases slight fever and swelling of the liver, which is tender to touch.

   l., nutmeg. That of amyloid and heart disease, and fatty infiltrations. It has a peculiar mottled appearance and dilatation of capillaries.

   l. spots. Yellowish-brown spots on skin following some digestive disturbances.

liver extract. A standardized concentrate of the antianemic principles of fresh liver.

   DOSAGE: According to the red cell count, from 200 to 500 Gm. of fresh liver equivalent, daily.

livid (lĭv'ĭd). 1. Ashen, cyanotic. 2. Discolored, as a bruise.

lividity (lĭv-ĭd'ĭ-tĭ). 1. Skin discoloration, as from a bruise or venous congestion. 2. State of being livid.

Livierato's reflex (lĭv-yăr-ä'tō). Reduction of area of cardiac dullness resulting from manual friction of precordial and epigastric areas.

livor (lī'vor). 1. Lividity, q.v. 2. Cutaneous dark spot on dependent portion of a cadaver.

lixiviation (lĭks"ĭv-ĭ-ā'shŭn). Separation of soluble from insoluble substances by washing and filtration.

lobar (lō'bar). Pert. to a lobe.

l. pneumonia. Inflammation of 1 or more lobes of the lungs. SEE: *pneumonia, lobar.*

lobate (lō'bāt). 1. Pert. to a lobe. 2. Having a deeply undulated border. 3. Producing lobes.

lobe (lōb). A globular part of an organ separated by boundaries.

l., caudate. Elevation of hepatic tissue extending bet. spigelian lobe and right lobe.

l., central. Island of Reil, which forms floor of lateral cerebral fossa.

l.'s of the cerebrum. Ant., middle and post. lobes of brain.

l., crescentric. One of 2 lobes on upper surface of a cerebellar hemisphere.

l., cuneate. A convolution on int. surface of cerebral hemisphere.

l., digastric. A lobe of the lower surface of cerebellum.

l. of the ear. Lower portion of auricle having no cartilage.

l., floating. A projecting portion of right lobe of liver which may extend below crest of the ilium.

l., frontal. That part of a cerebral hemisphere in front of central and sylvian fissures.

l., Home's. Pedunculated median lobe of prostate gland, frequently hypertrophied in old age.

l., insular. SEE: *central lobe.*

l.'s, lateral, of the prostate. The portions on each side of the urethra.

l.'s, lateral, of thyroid gland. The 2 main portions, 1 on each side of trachea, united below by thyroid isthmus.

l., limbic. Marginal section of cerebral hemisphere on medial aspect. SYN: *gyrus fornicatus.*

l., linguiform. Riedel's lobe.

l.'s of the lung. Small divisions containing terminal ramification of a bronchial tube and pulmonary vessels.

l.'s of the mamma. The glandular tissues of mammary gland divided by fibrous or areolar tissue.

l., marginal. First frontal convolution of the cerebrum.

l., median. Sup. vermiform process of the cerebrum.

l. of the nose. A rounded eminence at extremity of dorsum of nose.

l., occipital. Caudal region of either hemicerebrum.

l., olfactory. A series of convolutions below horizontal portion of the intraparietal fissure of cerebrum, containing olfactory bulb.

l.'s, optic. Upper pair of corpora quadrigemina.

l.'s, orbital. The convolutions above the orbit.

l.'s of the pancreas. Roundish aggregations of glandular tissue separated by connective tissue.

l., parietal. Upper and lateral portion of hemisphere of cerebrum.

l.'s of the prostate. The lateral lobes and the middle lobe of the gland.

l., quadrate, of cerebellum. Large lobe on upper surface of cerebellum.

l., quadrate, of liver. An oblong elevation on lower surface of liver.

l., Riedel's. Floating lobe, q.v.

l., rolandic. Operculum of the insula.

l., semilunar. Post. lobe of upper surface of each hemisphere of the cerebellum.

l., spigelian. Irregular quadrangular portion of liver behind fissure for portal vein and bet. fissure for vena cava and ductus venosus.

lobectomy (lō-bĕk'tō-mĭ). Surgical removal of a lobe of any organ or gland.

lobengulism (lō-ben'gŭ-lizm). Condition marked by increase of subcutaneous fat and decrease or complete abeyance of the sexual function.

lob'ular. Composed of small lobes.

lobulate, lobulated (lŏb'ū-lāt, -lāt-ed). 1. Consisting of lobes or lobules. 2. Pert. to lobes or lobules. 3. Resembling lobes. SYN: *lobular.*

lobule (lŏb'ūl). A small lobe.

l., fusiform. Inf. temporoöccipital convolution.

l., paracentral. Sup. convolution of ascending frontal and parietal convolutions forming a union of both.

lobulus (lŏb'ū-lŭs). A lobule. SYN: *lobule.*

l. centralis vermis superior. A small lobe at ant. part of sup. vermiform process.

l. epididymidis. Segments into which the epididymis is divided by transverse septa from its tunica albuginea.

l., parietalis. One of 2 portions of the parietal lobe.

l. testiculi. Conical lobules, from 250 to 400, which make up glandular structure of the testicle.

lobulet, lobulette (lŏb-ū-lĕt'). A very small lobule or a part of one.

lobus (lō'bŭs). Lobe.

l. cerebelli anteriores. The lobes forming ant. and sup. portion of hemisphere of the cerebellum.

l. pulmonales. Lobes of the lung.

l. reniculi. Lobes in fetal kidney which later form the malpighian pyramids.

local (lō'kăl). Limited to one place or part.

localization (lō-kăl-ĭ-zā'shun). 1. Limitation to a definite area. 2. Determination of the seat of an infection. 3.

Relation of a sensation to its point of origin.

l., cerebral. Determination of centers of various faculties in particular parts of the brain.

localized (lō'kăl-īzd). Restricted to a limited region.

lochia (lō'kĭ-ă). The discharge from the uterus of blood, mucus and tissue, during the puerperal period.

lochial (lo'kĭ-al). Pert. to the lochia.

lochiocolpos (lō″kĭ-ō-kŏl'pŏs). Retention of lochia in the vagina.

lochiometra (lō″kĭ-ō-mē'tră). Retention of lochia in the uterus.

lochiometritis (lō″kĭ-ō-mē-trī'tis). Puerperal inflammation of the uterus.

lochiopyra (lō-kĭ-op'ĭr-ă). Puerperal fever. [flow of lochia.]

lochiorrhagia (lo-kĭ-or-ra'jĭ-ă). Excessive

lochiorrhea (lō″kĭ-or-rē'ă). Abnormal flow of lochia.

lochioschesis (lō-kĭ-os'kē-sĭs). Retention or suppression of the lochia.

lochometritis (lō″kŏ-mē-trī'tĭs). Puerperal inflammation of uterus.

lockjaw. Tonic spasm of muscles of jaw. SEE: *tetanus, trismus.*

locomotion (lō-kō-mō'shun). Movement of a body from one place to another.

locomotor (lō-kō-mō'tor). Pert. to or concerning locomotion.

l. ataxia. A sclerosis affecting the post. columns of the spinal cord. SYN: *tabes dorsalis.* SEE: *ataxia, Charcot's arthropathy.*

locular (lŏk'ū-lăr). Divided into small cavities.

loculated (lŏk'ū-lāt-ĕd). Containing or divided into loculi. SYN: *locular.*

loc'ulus (pl. *loculi*). 1. A cell. 2. A small cavity.

lo'cum ten'ens. A substitute. Physician who substitutes for another temporarily.

lo'cus. A spot or place.

l. caeruleus, l. cinereus, l. ferrugineus. A dark-colored depression in floor of 4th ventricle at its upper part.

l. luteus. The true olfactory area of the nose. It has yellow granules in its epithelium.

l. niger. Gray matter separating the crusta and tegmentum of the crura cerebri. SYN: *substantia nigra.*

Loeffler's bacillus (lĕf'lĕr). The bacillus of diphtheria.

logaditis (lō-gă-dī'tĭs). Inflammation of the scleroric coat of the eye. SYN: *scleritis.*

logagnosia (lŏg-ăg-nō'sĭ-ă). Word blindness. SYN: *aphasia.*

logagraphia (lŏg-ă-grăf'ĭ-ă). Loss of ability to express ideas in writing. SYN: *agraphia.*

logamnesia (lŏg-ăm-nē'zĭ-ă). Aphasia of a sensory character. Inability to recognize spoken or written words.

logomania (lŏg-ō-mā'nĭ-ă). Repetitious, continuous, and excessive flow of speech seen in monomania.

logoneurosis (lŏg″ō-nū-rō'sĭs). Any neurosis marked by speech disorders.

logopathia (lŏg-ō-păth'ĭ-ă). Any disorder of speech.

logopedia (lŏg-ō-pē'dĭ-ă). Science dealing with speech defects, and their correction.

logoplegia (lŏg-ō-plē'jĭ-ă). Paralysis of the speech organs.

logorrhea (lŏg-or-ē'ă). Unusual loquacity seen in insanity. SYN: *garrulousness, logomania.*

logospasm (lŏg'ō-spazm). Spasmodic word enunciation.

-logy. Suffix meaning *discourse, science* or *study of.*

loimic (loi'mĭk). Pert. to pestilence or plague.

loimology (loi-mŏl'ō-jĭ). Science concerned with contagious diseases, esp. plague.

loin (loyn). Lower part of back and sides bet. the ribs and pelvis.

longevity (lŏn-jĕv'ĭ-tĭ). Unusual length of life.

long-. Prefix meaning *long.*

long flame arc lamp. According to distance bet. electrodes, carbon arc lamps are either short or long flame.

longsightedness (lawng-sī'tĕd-nĕs). Farsightedness. SYN: *hyperopia, q.v.*

Lophotrichea (lō-fō-trĭk'ē-ă). Microörganisms possessing flagella in tufts.

lophotrichous (lō-fŏt'rĭk-ūs). Having bunches of flagella at one end.

lordoma (lŏr-dō'mă). Forward incurvation of the spine. SYN: *lordosis.*

lordoscoliosis (lŏr″dō-skō-lĭ-ō'sis). Lordosis and scoliosis combined.

lordosis (lor-dō'sĭs). Abnormal ant. convexity of the spine.

lotion (lō'shun). Liquid medicinal preparation for local bathing of a part.

loupe (lūp). A magnifying lens.

louse (lows). Animal parasite infesting hairy parts. SYN: *pediculus, Phthirius.* SEE: *nit.*

l., body. Pediculus corporis.

l., crab. Phthirius inguinalis.

l., head. Pediculus capitis.

lous'iness. State of being infested with lice.

Loven's reflex (lōv'en). Vasodilation with corresponding increase in size of organ resulting from stimulation of afferent nerve of organ.

Low'man bal'ance board. Tilted board for walking with feet inverted to restore proper muscle balance and to correct static faults.

low protein diet. Breakfast, 413 calories; lunch, 695; supper, 704. Total daily, 1812. No salt except what is used in cooking, which will equal 3 or 4 Gm. per day.

loxarthron (lŏks-ar'thron). Oblique deformity of a joint without dislocation.

loxia (loks'ĭ-ă). Wry neck. SYN: *torticollis.*

loxotic (lŏks-ot'ĭk). Distorted in an awry manner.

loxotomy (lŏks-ot'ō-mĭ). Amputation by oblique section.

lozenge (loz'ĕnj). Small, dry, medicinal

solid to be held in mouth until it dissolves. SYN: *troche.*

lubb (lŭb). Word denoting 1st cardiac sound in auscultation.

lubb-dupp (lŭb-dŭp). The 2 sounds heard in auscultation marking a complete cycle of the heart.
Pause following the cycle is slightly longer than that bet. the 2 sounds.

lubricant (lŭb'rĭ-kănt). 1. Agent which makes smooth. 2. Making smooth.

lub'ricating en'ema. One given to soften feces and lubricate anal canal after hemorrhoidectomy, or to soften fecal impaction. SEE: *enema.*

Lucas-Championniere disease (lŭ-ka"-shawn-pē-ōn-yair"). Pseudomembranous affection of the bronchi.
L.-C. method. Early massage and mobilization in treating fractures.

lucid (lū'sĭd). Clear, esp. applied to clarity of the mind.
l. interval. Period of normal mentality bet. psychiatric attacks.

lucidity (lū-sĭd'ĭ-tĭ). Quality of clearness or brightness, most especially with regard to mental conditions. SEE: *lucid.*

lucotherapy (lŭ-kō-ther'ă-pĭ). Therapeutic use of light rays. SYN: *phototherapy.*

Ludwig's angi'na (lŭd'wĭg). A suppurative inflammation of subcutaneous connective tissue adjacent to a maxillary gland. SEE: *angina.*

Luer's syringe. One made of glass for intravenous and hypodermic use.

lues (lū'ēz). Any pestilential disease; the plague, esp. syphilis.
l. venerea. Syphilis.

luetic (lū-et'ĭk). 1. Pert. to syphilis. 2. Affected with syphilis. SYN: *syphilitic.*

luetin (lū'et-ĭn). A killed culture of Treponema pallidum for the Noguchi skin test for syphilis.

Lugol's caustic (lŭ'gol). Aqueous solution of 25% each of iodine and potassium iodide.
L.'s solution. Iodine, 5%; potassium iodide, 10%, and water to make 100 cc. DOSAGE: 3 ℆ (0.2 cc.).

lumbago (lŭm-bā'gō). Dull, aching pain across loins due to sudden cooling of overheated lumbar muscles, or turning body or rising from sitting posture causes an exacerbation which is sometimes so severe patient cries out.

lumbar (lŭm'băr). Pert. to the loins. SEE: *lumbago.*
l. nerves. Five pairs, corresponding with the lumbar vertebrae.
l. puncture. One made into the subarachnoid space of the spinal cord bet. the 2nd and 5th lumbar vertebrae (or more approximately in the 4th lumbar interspace, the middle of the line connecting the iliac crests).
l. reflex. Irritation of the skin over the erector spinal muscles causing contraction of muscles of the back.
l. region. Each side of umbilical region above the iliac, below the hypochondriac.

l. vertebrae. Five bones of spinal column between sacrum and dorsal vertebrae.

lumbarization (lŭm-băr-ĭ-zā'shŭn). Coalescence of the 1st sacral vertebra with the last lumbar vertebra.

lumbo-. Combining form pert. to the *loins.*

lumbocolostomy (lŭm"bō-kō-los'tō-mĭ). Colostomy by lumbar incision.

lumbocolotomy (lŭm-bō-kō-lot'ō-mĭ). Incision into the colon through lumbar region.

lumbocostal (lŭm-bō-kos'tăl). Rel. to the loins and ribs.

lumbodynia (lŭm-bō-dĭn'ĭ-ă). Pain and rigidity in the loins. SYN: *lumbago.*

lumbrical (lŭm'brĭ-kăl). Like a worm. SYN: *vermiform.*

lumbrica'lis. One of the muscles of the hand or foot which are wormlike in shape.

lumbricide (lum'brĭ-sīd). Destructive to, or an agent which destroys lumbricoid worms.

lumbricoid (lum'brĭ-koid). 1. Resembling an earthworm. 2. Worm parasitic in the intestines.

lubricosis (lum-brĭ-kō'sis). Condition resulting from being infected with lumbricoids.

lumbri'cus. An earthworm parasitic in intestines.

lumen (lū'měn) (pl. *lumina*). 1. The space within an artery, vein, intestine, or tube. 2. Unit of light, the amt. of light emitted in a unit solid angle by a uniform point source of 1 international candle.

luminal (lū'mĭ-năl). Rel. to lumen of tubular structure, such as a blood vessel.

luminal (lu'min-al). A brand of phenobarbital.*
DOSAGE: ½ gr. (0.03 Gm.).
l. sodium. A brand of soluble phenobarbital.*

lunacy (lū'nă-sĭ). Mental derangement. SYN: *insanity, psychosis.*

lu'nar. Pert. to the moon, a month, or silver.
l. caustic. Silver nitrate.

lunaria (lūn-ar'ĭ-ă). Menstruation.

lunatic (lū'nă-tĭk). 1. An insane person. 2. Insane, mad.

lunet, lunette (lū-nět'). A concavo-convex lens for spectacles.

lung (lung). ANAT: One of 2 cone-shaped, spongy organs of respiration.
l., apoplexy of. An effusion of blood into the pulmonary tissues.
l., cirrhosis of. A chronic disease of the lung, characterized by an overgrowth of fibrous tissue.
l. collapse. Absence of air from portion of lung. May be congenital and result from deficient respiration.
l. congestion, active. This results from increased afflux of blood to the lungs.
l. c., hypostatic. Congestion of dependent portions of the lungs occurring in asthenic diseases which necessitate a protracted recumbent position.

l. c., passive. Results from obstruction to the flow of blood from the lungs to the heart.

l., edema of. Effusion of serous fluid into air vesicles and into interstitial tissue of lungs.

l., gangrene of. A putrefactive necrosis of lung. Secondary condition to some inflammatory disease of the lung. It is excited by the entrance of bacteria of putrefaction—but unless system is considerably reduced in vitality the tissues, even though diseased, show wonderful resistance and escape putrefaction.

l., hemorrhage from. Hemoptysis.*

l. inflammation. Pneumonia.*

l., iron. Device for inducing respiration artificially.

lung motor. Apparatus designed to give artificial respiration. Inferior to prone pressure method.

lunula (lu″nu-lă). The semilunar white arch or area near the root of the nail.

l. lacrimalis. Small ridge of bone separating antrum of Highmore from the lacrimal groove.

l. of valves of heart. One of 2 narrow portions of flaps of the semilunar and mitral valves.

l. scapulae. Notch behind coracoid process in upper border of the scapula through which passes the suprascapular nerve.

lupiform (lu″pĭ-form). Resembling lupus.

lupoma (lū-pō′mă). Nodule of lupus, esp. a primary one.

lupous (lū′pŭs). 1. Pert. to lupus. 2. Affected with lupus.

lupus (lū′pŭs). Tuberculous skin disease, acute or subacute.

l., disseminated follicular. Lupus of face with small and large papules.

l. erythematosus. Superficial inflammation of skin with scaling patches.

l. hypertrophicus. Lupus with vegetations.

l. maculo′sus. Lupus with maculae.

l. nonex′edens. Lupus without ulcerations.

l. serpigino′sus. Lupus spreading with creeping ulcerations.

l. tu′midus. Lupus with edematous infiltrations.

l. verrucosus. Lesion consisting of an elevated plaque with indolent inflammatory base and a warty papillary surface.

l. vulgaris. Patches on skin which break down and ulcerate, leaving scars on healing. Most common form of lupus.

Luschka's gland (loosh′kä). The coccygeal gland, a tiny organ near tip of coccyx.

L.'s tonsil. Pharyngeal tonsil bet. nasopharyngeal openings of eustachian tubes. SEE: adenoids.

Lust's reflex (lŭst). Dorsal flexion and abduction of foot resulting from percussion of ext. branch of sciatic nerve.

lu′teal. Pert. to luteum.

l. hormone. A secretion of the corpus luteum.

lutein (lū′tē-ĭn). 1. Yellow pigment derived from corpus luteum, egg yolk, and fat cells or lipochromes. 2. Internal ovarian secretion.

DOSAGE: 2-10 gr. (0.12-0.6 Gm.).

luteolipoid (lu″tē-ō-lĭp′oyd). Substance found in corpus luteum which seems to have hemostatic action during the menstrual period.

luteoma (lū-tē-ō′mă). Tumor arising from the corpus luteum.

luteum (lu′tē-ŭm). Yellow.

l., corpus. Yellow cellular mass which forms in position of ruptured graafian follicles in ovary. It persists and enlarges in pregnancy.

lutin (lū′tin). Hormone of corpus luteum which aids in preparation of endometrium for fertilized ovum. SYN: progestin.

luxation (lŭks-ā′shŭn). Displacement of organs or articular surfaces; dislocation of a joint.

lux′us. Excess of anything.

Luy's body. Small ganglion under the optic layer. SYN: subthalamic nucleus.

lycanthropy (lī-kan′thrō-pĭ). Mania in which patient believes himself a wild beast, esp. a wolf. SYN: lycomania.

lycomania (lī-kō-mā′nĭ-ă). Delusion of being a wild animal, esp. a wolf. SYN: lycanthropy.

lye (lī). Liquid from leaching of wood ashes. SEE: alkalies, sodium hydroxide.

l. burns. Treat with hydrosulfosol,* which is safe for use around eyes, nose, and mouth. Spray with hydrosulfosol solution every hr. first 24 hr.

ly′ing-in. 1. The puerperal state. 2. Being in confinement.

lymph (lĭmf). The lymph is a body alkaline fluid found in the lymphatic vessels and cisterna chyli.

l., animal. Vaccine lymph from an animal.

l. cell or corpuscle. A lymph leukocyte.

l. channels. Irregular open spaces in lymph structures.

l., inflammatory. Exudate due to inflammation.

l., intercellular. Tissue fluid.

l., intravascular. Chyle; that of the lymph vessels.

l., Koch's. Tuberculin.

l. nodes. Glands scattered along the path of the lymphatics, esp. in the neck, armpits, and at bend of the elbow and knee.

l. scrotum. Scrotal lymphatic dilatation.

l. sinuses. Same as lymph channels.

l. spaces. Those esp. in connective tissue filled with lymph.

lymphadenectasis (lĭmf″ă-den-ĕkt′ă-sĭs). Dilatation or distention of a lymphatic gland.

lymphade′nia. Hyperplasia affecting lymphatic tissue.

l. ossea. Bone marrow hyperplasia accompanied by Bence-Jones protein in urine.

lymphadenitis (lĭmf″ad-en-i′tĭs). Inflammation of a lymphatic gland.
  l., tuberculous. ETIOL: Infection.
lymphadenoma (lĭmf″ă-den-ō′mă). Hyperplasia of the lymphatic glands. SYN: *lymphoma.*
lymphadenomatosis (lĭmf″ă-den-ō″mă-tō′sĭs). Condition of general lymphatic engorgement. SYN: *lymphomatosis.*
lymphagogue (lĭmf′ă-gŏg). An agent which stimulates the production or flow of lymph.
lymphangiectasis (lĭmf″ăn-jĭ-ek′tă-sĭs). Dilatation of lymphatic vessels. SYN: *lymphectasia.*
lymphangioendothelioma (lĭmf-ăn″jĭ-ō-en″dō-thēl-ĭ-ō′mă). Endothelioma originating from lymph vessels. SYN: *lymphendothelioma.*
lymphangiofibroma (lĭmf-an″jĭ-ō-fī-brō′mă). Fibroma and lymphangioma combined.
lymphangioma (lĭmf″ăn-jĭ-ō′mă). Tumor composed of lymphatic vessels.
lymphangiophlebitis (lĭmf-ăn″jĭ-ō-flē-bī′tĭs). Inflammation of lymphatic vessels and veins.
lymphangioplasty (lĭmf-an′jĭ-ō-plăs-tĭ). Formation of artificial lymphatics.
lymphangiosarcoma (lĭmf-an″jĭ-ō-săr-kō′mă). Lymphangioma and sarcoma combined.
lymphangiotomy (lĭmf″an-jĭ-ot′ō-mĭ). 1. Dissection of the lymphatics. 2. Anatomy of the lymphatics. SYN: *lymphotomy.*   [tion of the lymphatics.
lymphangitis (lĭmf-an-ji′tĭs). Inflammation.
lymphatic (lĭm-fat′ĭk). Small, transparent vessel that carries lymph.
lymphaticostomy (lĭmf″ăt-ĭ-kos′tō-mĭ). Making of a permanent aperture into a lymphatic duct.
lymphatism (lĭmf′ă-tĭzm). 1. The lymphatic temperament. 2. Sluggishness in the vital processes. 3. Excess in lymphoid structures. SYN: *status lymphaticus, q.v.*
lymphatitis (lĭmf-ă-tī′tĭs). Inflammation of lymphatic vessel. SYN: *lymphangitis.*
lymphatolysis (lĭmf-ă-tol′ĭ-sĭs). Destruction of tissue of lymphatics.
lymphatolytic (lim-fat-ō-lit′ĭk). Destructive to lymphatics.
lymphectasia (lĭmf-ĕk-tă′zĭ-ă). Dilatation of the lymphatics. SYN: *lymphangiectasis.*
lymphedema (lĭmf-ĕ-dē′mă). Edema due to obstruction of lymphatics. SYN: *serous edema.*
lympheduct (lĭm′fe-dŭkt). Duct or vessel for carrying lymph.
lymphemia (lĭmf-ē′mĭ-ă). Hypertrophy of lymphatics with lymphocytes in blood.
lymphendothelioma (lĭmf-ĕn″dō-thēl-ĭ-ō′mă). Tumor from proliferation and dilatation of lymphatics with overgrowth of myxomatous tissue.
lymphenteritis (lĭmf″ĕn-tĕr-i′tĭs). Serous infiltration accompanying inflammation of bowels.
lympherythrocyte (lĭmf-ĕr-ĭth′rō-sīt). Erythrocyte lacking in hemoglobin.

lymphization (lĭmf-ĭ-zā′shŭn). Formation of lymph.
lymphnoditis (lĭmf-nōd-ī′tĭs). Inflamed condition of a lymph node.
lymphoadenoma (lĭmf″ō-ad-en-ō′mă). 1. A tumor of lymphoid tissue. 2. Hypertrophied condition of the lymphatics. SYN: *lymphadenoma.*
lymphoblast (lĭmf′ō-blast). A leukocyte of lymphatic origin.
lymphoblastoma (lĭmf-ō-blast-ō′mă). Tumor composed of lymphocytes. SYN: *lymphosarcoma.*
lymphoblasto′sis. Excessive number of lymphoblasts in the blood.
lymphocele (lĭmf′ō-sēl). Tumor containing lymph. SYN: *lymphocyst.*
lymphocerastism (lĭmf-ō-ser′ăs-tĭzm). Formation of lymph cells.
lymphocyst (lĭmf′ō-sĭst). Tumor containing lymph. SYN: *lymphocele.*
lymphocyte (lĭmf′ō-sīt). Lymph cell or white blood corpuscle without cytoplasmic granules. They normally number from 25-30% compared with white cells. May increase to 90% in lymphatic leukemia.
  l., large. Frequently difficult to classify; characterized by irregular shape, easily indented by any other cell.
  l., small. Characterized by deeply staining, compact nucleus taking a dark blue.
lymphocythemia (lĭmf″ō-sī-the′mĭ-ă). Excess of lymph cells in the blood.
lymphocytopenia (lĭmf″ō-sīt″ō-pē′nĭ-ă). Less than normal number of lymphocytes in the blood.
lymphocytopoiesis (lĭmf″ō-sīt″ō-poi-ē′sĭs). Lymphocyte production.
lymphocyto′sis. Excess of lymph cells. SYN: *lymphocythemia.*
lymphocytotoxin (lĭmf″ō-sīt″ō-toks′ĭn). A toxin destructive to lymphocytes.
lymphodermia (lĭmf-ō-dĕr′mĭ-ă). Disease of cutaneous lymphatics.
lymphoduct (lĭmf′ō-dŭkt). A lymphatic vessel or duct. SYN: *lympheduct.*
lymphogenous (lĭmf-oj′en-ŭs). Forming lymph.   [lymph node.
lymphoglandula (lĭmf-ō-glăn-dū′lă). A
lymphogonia (lĭmf″ō-go′nĭ-ă). Large lymphocytes with large nuclei appearing in lymphatic leukemia.
lymphogranuloma (lĭmf″ō-grăn-ū-lō′mă). Venereal disease marked by inflammation of lymph glands with enlargement and ulceration. SYN: *lymphogranuloma inguinale.*
  l. inguinale, l. venerea. Venereal granuloma of the pudenda with ulcerations.
lymphogranulomatosis (lĭmf″ō-grăn-ū-lō″mă-tō′sĭs). 1. Infectious granuloma of the lymphatics. 2. Hodgkin's disease.
lymphoid (lĭmf′oid). Resembling lymph. SYN: *adenoid.*
lymphoidectomy (lĭmf-oid-ek′tō-mĭ). Surgical removal of lymphoid tissue.
lymphoidocyte (lĭmf-oid′ō-sīt). Embryonic blood cell bet. a lymphocyte and a lymphoblast.

lymphokinesis (lĭmf″ō-kĭn-ē′sĭs). Endolymphic movement in the semicircular canals.

lympholeukocyte (lĭmf″ō-lū′kō-sīt). One of the type of white corpuscles containing no granules and being mononuclear.

lymphology (lĭmf-ol′ō-jĭ). Science of the lymphatics.

lymphoma (lĭmf-o′mă). A lymphoid tissue tumor.

   l. granulomatosum. Small, white lymphatic nodule in liver in Hodgkin's disease.

lymphomatosis (lĭmf″ō-mă-tō′sĭs). General lymphatic engorgement; general deposition of lymphomata throughout the body.

   l. granulomato′sa. Malignant granuloma. SYN: *Hodgkin's disease.*

lymphomatous (lĭmf-ō′mă-tŭs). 1. Pert. to a lymphoma. 2. Affected with lymphomata.

lymphopath′ia vene′rea. Venereal disease marked by ulceration and enlargement of lymph nodes in inguinal area. SYN: *lymphogranuloma inguinale.*

lymphopathy (lĭmf-op′ă-thĭ). Any lymphatic disease.

lymphopenia (lĭmf-ō-pē′nĭ-ă). Deficiency of lymphocytes in the blood.

lymphoplasm (lĭmf′ō-plăzm). The elastic protoplasmic supporting threads or fibrillar network of cells.

lymphoplasmia (lĭmf-ō-plaz′mĭ-ă). Lack of hemoglobin in red blood corpuscles.

lymphopoiesis (lĭmf-ō-poi-ē′sĭs). Formation of lymphocytes.

lymphopoietic (lĭmf-ō-poi-et′ĭk). Forming lymphocytes.

lymphorrhagia (lĭmf-or-rā′jĭ-ă). Flow of lymph from ruptured lymph vessels. SYN: *lymphorrhea.*

lymphorrhea (lĭmf-or-rē′ă). Internal or external discharge of lymph through a wound. SYN: *lymphorrhagia.*

lymphosarcoma (limf-ō-sar-kō′mă). Sarcoma of lymph tissue; lymphatic sarcoma.

lymphostasis (lĭmf-os′tă-sĭs). Stoppage of flow of lymph.

lymphotome (lĭmf′o-tōm). Instrument for removing glandular growths from tonsils.

lymphotomy (lĭmf-ot′ō-mĭ). 1. Excision of adenoid growths. 2. Anatomy of lymphatics. SYN: *lymphoidectomy, adenoidectomy.*

lymphotrophy (lĭmf-ot′rō-fĭ). Lymph nourishment of cells in regions devoid of blood vessels.

lymphuria (lĭmf-ū′rĭ-ă). Lymph in the urine.

lymphvascular (lĭmf-vas′kū-lar). Rel. to the lymphatic vessels.

lypemania (lī-pē-mā′nĭ-ă). Dementia with extreme mental depression. SYN: *melancholia.*

lypothymia (lī-pō-thī′mĭ-ă). Great mental depression or despondency.

lyra (lī′ră). Triangular space on ventral surface of corpus callosum bet. post. columns of the fornix.

lysemia (lī-sē′mĭ-ă). Disintegration of blood.

lysimeter (lī-sĭm′ĕ-ter). Apparatus for determining solubilities.

lysin (lī′sĭn). A specific antibody acting destructively upon cells and tissues.
   SEE: *immune body.*

lysine (lī′sēn). An amino acid which is a hydrolytic cleavage product of protein through digestion.
   It is essential for growth and repair.

lysis (lī′sĭs). 1. The gradual decline of a fever or disease. The opp. of *crisis.* 2. Destruction of blood cells, etc., by a lysin, as when rabbit's red corpuscles are dissolved by dog's serum. SEE: *crisis, hemolysis.*

lysogenesis (lī-sō-jen′ĕ-sĭs). The production of cell-dissolving substance known as lysin.

lysogenic (lī-sō-jen′ĭk). Producing lysins.

lysozyme (lī′sō-zĭm). A bacteria-destructive substance present in tears, and other body secretions, and tissues.

lyssa (lĭs′să). An acute infectious disease, transferable by inoculation, which particularly attacks the nervous system. SYN: *hydrophobia, rabies.*

lyssin (lĭs′sĭn). Virus of lyssa. SYN: *hydrophobia.*

lyssodexis (lĭs-sō-deks′ĭs). Inoculation or infection with lyssin.

lyssoid (lĭs′soid). Resembling lyssa or rabies.

lyssophobia (lĭs-sō-fō′bĭ-ă). 1. Hysteria resembling rabies. 2. Fear of rabies.

lyterian (lī-tēr′ĭ-an). Indicative of lysis.

lytic (lĭt′ĭk). Rel. to lysis or a lysin.

lyze (līz). To bring about lysis.

M

M. Abbr. for *mille*, a thousand; *misce*, mix.

m. Abbr. for *meter* and *minim*; in chemistry, for *meta-*.

M. A. Abbr. for *meter angle*.

ma. Abbr. for *milliampère*.

M + Am. Abbr. for *compound myopic astigmatism*.

Macdowel's frenum (măk-dow'ĕl). Part of post. layer of pectoralis major which extends into muscular substance.

mace (mās). A spice from the nutmeg tree, employed as flavoring similarly to nutmeg.

maceration (măs-ĕr-a'shŭn). 1. Process of softening a solid by steeping in a fluid. 2. State of emaciation.

Mache unit (mä'kĕ). The unit of measurement of concentration of radium emanation. Abbr. *M. u.*, or German, *M. E.* SEE: *unit*.

machonnement (mash-shŏn-mon'). Movement of jaws resembling chewing.

macies (mā'shĭ-ēz). Atrophy, wasting, emaciation.

MacKenzie exercise apparatus. Mechanical device, devised by Tait MacKenzie for exercise.

macrencephalia, macrencephaly (mak-ren-sĕ-fa'lĭ-ă, -sef'a-lĭ). Abnormal size of brain. SYN: *macrocephalia*.

macro-, macr-. Combining forms meaning *large, long*.

macrobiosis (măk"rō-bī-ō'sĭs). State of surpassing normal span; longevity.

macroblast (mak'rō-blast). A large, nucleated red blood cell. SYN: *megaloblast*.

macrocephalia (măk-rō-sĕ-fa'lĭ-ă). Abnormal largeness of head. SYN: *macrencephalia*.

macrocephalous (măk-ro-sef'ă-lŭs). Pert. to or having an excessively large head.

macrocephaly (măk-rō-sĕf'al-ĭ). Abnormal size of head. SYN: *macrocephalia*.

macrocheilia (mak-rō-ki'lĭ-ă). Abnormal size of lip caused by permanently dilated lymphatic spaces, as in cavernous lymphangioma of the lip. SYN: *macrolabia*.

macrocheiria (mak-rō-kī'rĭ-ă). Excessive size of the hands. SYN: *macrochiria*.

macrochilia (mak-rō-kī'lĭ-ă). Excessive size of the lip, caused by permanently dilated lymphatic spaces. SYN: *macrocheilia*.

macrochiria (mak-rō-kī'rĭ-ă). Large size of hands.

macrococcus (măk-rō-kok'ŭs). A bacterial microörganism, of the largest type recognized. SYN: *megacoccus*.

macrocornea (măk-rō-kor'nē-ă). Abnormal size or projection of the cornea. SYN: *keratoglobus, megalocornea*.

macrocytase (mak-rō-sī'tās). Enzyme in leukocytes capable of digesting organic substance.

mac'rocyte. 1. Erythrocyte larger than normal. 2. Large lymphocyte found in pernicious anemia.

macrocythemia (măk"rō-sī-thē'mĭ-ă). Abnormal number of macrocytes in the blood.

macrocytosis (măk"rō-sī-tō'sĭs). Development of macrocytes, esp. in greater numbers than normal.

macrodactylia (mak"rō-dak-til'ĭ-ă). Excessive size of 1 or more of the digits.

macrodont (mak'rō-dont). Having abnormally large teeth. SYN: *megadont*.

macroesthesia (măk"rō-ĕs-thē'zĭ-ă). A state in which objects seen or felt appear to be greatly magnified.

macrogenitosomia (mak"rō-jen"i-to-sō'mĭ-ă). Precocious body development in general, with unusually large genitalia.

macroglia (mak-rog'lĭ-ă). A neuroglia with large multipolar cells. SEE: *glia cell, spider cell*.

macroglos'sia. Hypertrophied condition of the tongue.

macrognathia (mak-rō-nā'thĭ-ă). Abnormal size of jaw.

macrolabia (măk-rō-lā'bĭ-ă). Abnormal size of lip. SYN: *macrocheilia*.

macrolymphocyte (mak"rō-limf'ō-sīt). A huge lymphocyte.

macromastia (măk-rō-mas'tĭ-ă). Abnormal size of the breasts.

macromazia (măk-rō-mā'zĭ-ă). Abnormal development of breasts. SYN: *macromastia*.

macromere (măk'rō-mēr). Blastomere of large size.

mac"ronor'moblast. Large, nucleated red blood corpuscle.

mac"ronor'mocyte. Huge red blood corpuscle.

mac"ronu'cleus (pl. *macronuclei*). Main nucleus of a cell.

macrophage, macrophagus (măk'rō-fāj, -rof'a-gus). A large mononuclear leukocyte which ingests other cells.

macrophallus (măk"rō-făl'ŭs). Abnormally large penis.

macropodia (măk-rō-pō'dĭ-ă). Abnormally large feet.

macroprosopia (măk"rō-prō-sō'pĭ-ă). Large facial features.

macropsia (mak-rop'sĭ-ă). Condition in which objects look larger than they really are.

macrorhinia (măk-rō-rīn'ĭ-ă). Excessive size of the nose, either congenital or pathological.

macroscelia (mak-rō-sēl'ĭ-ă). Abnormal size of the legs.

macroscopic (mak-rō-skop'ĭk). Large enough to be seen by the naked eye. OPP: *microscopic*. SYN: *megascopic*.

macroscopy (mak-ros'ko-pĭ). Examination of an object with the naked eye.

macrosomatia (mak"rō-sō-mă'shĭ-ă). Abnormally large size of body. SYN: *macrosomia*.

macrosomia (măk-rō-sō'mĭ-ă). Abnormal size of body. SYN: *macrosomatia*.

macrostomia (măk-rō-stō'mĭ-ă). Excessively large mouth.

macrotia (mak-ro'shĭ-ă). Abnormal size of ears.

macula (mak'u-lă) (pl. *maculae*). A blemish, spot, or stain on the skin. SYN: *macule*. SEE: *roseola, vibices*.

   m. acustica. Acoustic nerve termination in both sacculus and utriculus, about 3 mm. in length.

   m. albida. White mark found on liver in some contagious diseases. SYN: *tache blanche*.

   m. atrophica. Glistening white spot on skin following a circumscribed hemorrhage.

   m. caerulea. Steel gray or blue stain of epidermis, without elevation, which does not disappear on pressure, occurring esp. with pediculosis pubis or bites from fleas.

   m., cerebral. Reddened line, becoming deeper and persisting for some time, esp. in tubercular meningitis, by drawing the fingernail across the skin.

   m. corneae. Opaque spot in cornea.

   m., germinal. A nucleolus in an ovular nucleus.

   m. gonorrhoeica. Red spot at orifice of vulvovaginal gland. Seen in gonorrheal vulvitis.

   m. lutea. The yellow spot on the retina, about 1/12 in. (2.08 mm.) to outer side of the optic nerve's exit, the exact center of the retina. Area of acute or central vision. SEE: *choroiditis, areolar and central*.

   m. solaris. A freckle.

macular (măk'u-lar). 1. Rel. to macules. 2. Having macules.

maculate(d (măk'u-lāt, -lāt-ĕd). Spotted, as with macules.

maculation (măk-ū-lā'shun). Process of becoming maculate. Development of macules.

macule (mak'ūl). Discolored spot or patch on the skin, neither elevated nor depressed, of various colors, sizes and shapes.

mad. 1. Not rational. 2. Suffering from infection with rabies. SYN: *insane, rabid*.

madarosis (mad-ă-ro'sis). Loss of cilia or eyelashes and eyebrows.

madescent (mad-es'ent). Slightly moist, or becoming so.

madidans (mad'ĭd-ăns). Exuding, moist, as in some skin lesions.

mador (ma'dor). A dripping sweat.

Madura foot. Fungous disease of the foot. SYN: *mycetoma*.

Magendie's foramen (mă-zhan-de'). The median of 3 openings in the roof of the 4th ventricle which is in front of the cerebellum and behind the *pons varolii*, connecting the ventricle with the subarachnoid space.

   M.'s law. The post. spinal roots are *sensory;* the anterior ones *motor*.

   M.'s solution. Aqueous solution of morphine sulfate, 16 gr. to 1 oz. of water.

   M.'s spaces. Those bet. the arachnoid and pia at level of fissures of brain.

maggot. Larva of an insect.

   m. treatment. A method of treating septic wounds. Meat maggots, introduced into a sloughing septic wound, ingest the necrotic material, leaving the wound with a clean granulating surface. The maggots are then removed and destroyed. SEE: *osteomyelitis*.

magistery (maj'ĭs-tĕr-ĭ). 1. Specially compounded remedy. 2. A precipitate.

magistral (măj'ĭs-trăl). Concerning medicines prescribed by a physician for a particular case. SEE: *officinal*.

magma (mag'mă). 1. Mass left after extraction of principle. 2. Salve.

magnesia (măg-nē'zĭ-ă). Magnesium oxide.

   m., milk of. An aperient composed of magnesium hydroxide and water.

magnesium. SYMB: *Mg*. At. wt. 24.32. Sp. gr. 1.74. A white mineral element found in soft tissue, muscles, bones, and to some extent in the body fluids.

   m. carbonate ($MgCO_3.3H_2O$). USP. A bulky, white, odorless powder.

   DOSAGE: As antacid, 10 gr. (0.6 Gm.); as a laxative, 2 drams (8 Gm.).

   m. citrate solution. USP. A solution containing an amount of magnesium citrate corresponding to approximately 1.6% magnesium oxide.

   DOSAGE: 12 fl. oz. (350 cc.).

   m. oxide (MgO). USP. Calcined magnesia. *Light* magnesia. A white, very bulky, fine powder.

   DOSAGE: As an antacid, 4 gr. (0.25 Gm.); as a laxative, 45 gr. (3 Gm.).

   Heavy. USP. magnesii oxidum ponderosum.

   DOSAGE: Same as magnesium, light.

   m. phosphate tribasic. A white, odorless powder.

   DOSAGE: 15-75 gr. (1.0-5.0 Gm.).

   m. sulfate (epsom salt) ($MgSO_4.7H_2O$). USP. Small, colorless crystals. Saline bitter taste.

   DOSAGE: As cathartic, ½ oz. (15 Gm.).

magnet. Iron made magnetic by an electric current. [horseshoe.

   m., horseshoe. One in shape of a

   m., operation. Removal of metal particles with a magnet.

magnetic. Pert. to a magnet or having magnetism.

   m. field. The space permeated by the magnetic lines of force surrounding a permanent magnet or coil of wire carrying electric current.

   m. induction. The production of magnetic properties in iron or other magnetic metals by the influence of a magnetic field or of a magnet.

m. lines of force. The lines indicating the direction of the magnetic force in the space surrounding a magnet or constituting a magnetic field.

magnetism (măg'nĕ-tĭzm). The property of repulsion and attraction of certain substances.

magnetotherapy (mag″nĕt-ō-ther'ă-pĭ). Application of magnets or magnetism in treating diseases.

magnification (mag-nĭ-fĭ-kā'shun). Process of increasing apparent size of an object, esp. under microscope.

mag′num. Largest of the carpal bones.

maidenhead (măd'en-hĕd). Thin, crescentic fold partly closing vaginal opening and once considered a sign of virginity. SYN: hymen.

maidism, maidismus (mā'ĭ-dĭzm, -dĭz'mŭs). 1. Another name for pellagra. 2. Poisoning from imperfect maize.

maieusiomania (mī-ū-sĭ-ō-mā'nĭ-ă). Insanity following childbirth.

maieusiophobia (mī-ū-sĭ-ō-fō'bĭ-ă). Extreme fear of childbirth.

maieutics (mī-u'tĭks). Obstetrics.

maim (mām). 1. To injure seriously; to disable. 2. An injury or hurt.

main or main line (mān). P. T. The conductor that delivers the current as it comes in from the street supply or from a motor generator, if one is used.

main (măn). Hand.

m. en griffe (ahn-grēf'). Flexion and atrophy of the hand in a claw shape.

m. succulente (sŭk-ŭ-lahnt'). Edema of a hand.

Majocchi's disease (mah-yok'ē). Ringform, purplish eruption of lower limbs; purpura annularis telangiectodes, q.v.

makro-. For words beginning thus, see under macro-. [order.

mal (mahl). An evil, a sickness or a disorder.

m. de mer. Seasickness.

m., grand. A major epileptic attack with convulsions.

m., petit. A minor attack of epilepsy without convulsions.

mala (ma'lă). 1. The cheek. 2. The cheekbone.

malachite green (mal'ă-kīt). Dye sometimes used in treating trypanosomiasis and as an indicator.

malacia (măl-ā'sĭ-ă). 1. Softening of tissues of an organ, or of a part of them. 2. A morbid appetite for some specific food, esp. condiments.

malacoma (măl-ă-kō'mă). Softening of an organ or part of the body. SYN: malacia, malacosis.

malacoplakia (mal-ă-kō-plā'kĭ-ă). Existence of soft patches in mucous membrane of a hollow organ.

m., vesical. Soft, funguslike patches on mucosa of the bladder.

malacosarcosis (măl-ă-kō-sar-kō'sĭs). Softness of tissue, especially muscular.

malacosis (măl-ă-kō'sĭs). Softening of an organ or part of the body, abnormally. SYN: malacia, malacoma.

malacosteon (mal-ă-kos'tē-ŏn). Softening of the bones. SYN: osteomalacia.

malacotic (mal-ă-kot'ĭk). 1. Soft. 2. Affected with malacia. 3. Rel. to malacia.

m. teeth. Those of soft texture easily affected by caries.

malacotomy (măl-ă-kot'ō-mĭ). Incision of soft areas of the body, esp. of the abdominal wall.

malady (mal'ă-dĭ). A condition of ill health. SYN: disease.

malaise (mă-lāz'). Discomfort, uneasiness, indisposition, often indicative of infection.

malar (mā'lar). Pert. to cheekbones.

m. bone. A 4-pointed bone on each side of the face, uniting the frontal and sup. maxillary bones with the zygomatic process of the temporal. SYN: cheekbone. SEE: skeleton.

malaria (ma-lā'rĭ-ă). A disease due to circulation and multiplication in the blood of certain parasites (Plasmodium).

m., algid. Vomiting and diarrhea, marked prostration, Hippocratic facies, shallow and irregular respiration. Thready, rapid and intermittent pulse.

m., bilious. Abdominal pain, nausea, vomiting of bile-stained or blood-flecked mucus, feeling of thoracic oppression.

m., cephalgic. Unusually severe headache, nausea, vomiting, etc.

m., choleriform. Resembles Asiatic cholera. Seizures occur with nausea, vomiting, severe abdominal pain, diarrhea, dehydration.

m., delirious. Delusions, hallucinations, maniacal excitement.

m., eclamptic. Chill, fever, severe headache; sometimes nausea and vomiting. Convulsions resembling eclampsia. More common in children.

m., latent. Parasites exist within blood stream, but give rise to no recognizable symptoms. Individuals having this form constitute portion of carriers.

m., masked. Symptoms atypical. Cerebral derangement may be main complaint.

m., pernicious. Onset may be sudden, resembling apoplexy; coma usually comes, however, after obvious, severe, and intense symptoms.

m., pleuritic and pulmonic. Fever, thoracic pain, cough, dyspnea, sometimes hemoptysis, râles. Periodicity of symptoms may aid diagnosis. Blood findings are conclusive.

m., quartan. Short and less severe paroxysms. Sporulation occurs each 72 hours, causing seizures with that interval.

m., quotidian estivoautumnal. Paroxysms occur with daily periodicity due to 24-hour sporulation. Abrupt rise and fall of temperature.

m., sudoriferous. Sweating is excessive and leads to collapse.

m., syncopal. Characterized by collapse on slightest exertion

m., tertian. Sporulation each 48 hours. Symptoms more common during the day. Paroxysms divided into chill, fever and sweating stages. Cold stage is usually 10-15 minutes, but may last an hour or more. Febrile stage varies from 4-6 hours.

m., t. estivoautumnal. Indistinct chill, usually only a chilly sensation. Intense headache, profound weakness, marked muscular aching. Marked mental depression. Coated tongue, feeble and accelerated pulse, rapid respiration. Febrile stages may be 36 hours long.

malarial (mă-lar'ĭ-ăl). 1. Affected with malaria. 2. Causing malaria. 3. Resembling malaria. 4. Pert. to malaria. SYN: *malarious.*

malarialize (ma-lar'ĭ-al-īz). To treat paresis and parasyphilitic conditions by injecting malaria organisms into the body.

malarious (ma-lar'ĭ-ŭs). Of the nature of, or afflicted with malaria.

malariology (mă-lar-ĭ-ol'ō-jĭ). The scientific study of malaria.

malariotherapy (mă-lar-ĭ-ō-ther'ă-pĭ). Method of treating paresis and parasyphilitic conditions by injecting malarial organisms into the body.

Malasse'zia. A genus of fungi.

M. fur'fur. The cause of tinea versicolor.

M. trop'ica. Cause of tinea flava.

malassimilation (mal"ăs-sĭm-ĭ-lā'shŭn). Defective, incomplete, or faulty assimilation, esp. of nutritive material.

malaxation (mal-aks-a'shun). Kneading movement used in massage.

male (māl). 1. Masculine. 2. One of the sex that fertilizes; one potentially capable of producing sperm.

m. sex hormone. Hormone found in urine and secreted by the testicles, which regulates development at puberty of male characteristics. SYN: *androsterone.***

malemission (mal-ē-mĭs'shŭn). Failure of semen to be ejaculated from the urethra during coitus.

malformation (măl-for-mā'shŭn). Deformity; abnormal shape or structure.

malic (ma'lĭk). Pert. to apples.

m. acid. An acid found in some fruits, such as apples. SEE: *acid.*

malign (mă-līn'). Malignant.

malignancy (mă-lĭg'năn-sĭ). 1. Opposition to treatment. 2. Severe form of occurrence, tending to grow worse. SYN: *virulence.*

malignant (mă-lĭg'nănt). Virulent. Growing worse; resisting treatment, said of cancerous growths.

malinger (mă-lĭng'er). To feign illness, usually to arouse sympathy.

malingerer (mă-lĭng'ger-er). 1. One who pretends to be ill or to be suffering from a nonexistent disorder to arouse sympathy. 2. One who pretends slow recuperation from a disease once suffered in order to continue to receive benefits of sick insurance.

malis (ma'lĭs). A cutaneous, parasitic disease.

malleation (măl-lē-ā'shŭn). Spasmodic ac-

tion of the hands in which they seem drawn to strike any near object, as spasmodic rapping against thighs, furniture, etc. SEE: *tic.*

malleoincudal (măl"lē-ō-ĭn'kū-dăl). Concerning or pert. to the malleus and incus.

malleolar (măl-le'ō-lar). Concerning the malleolus.

malleolus (mă-le'o-lus). (pl. *malleoli*). The protuberance on both sides of the ankle joint, the lower extremity of the fibula being known as the *lateral malleolus,* and the lower end of the tibia as the *medial malleolus.*

m., ext., lateral, outer. Process on outer edge of fibula at lower end.

m., int., inner, medial. Round process on inner edge of tibia at lower end.

malleotomy (măl-lē-ot'ō-mĭ). 1. Division of the malleus. 2. Division of ligaments to permit separation of the malleoli.

mallet finger (mal'let). Loss of power extension in a finger, causing permanent flexion. SYN: *drop-finger.*

m. toe. Abnormal flexion or loss of power of extension of a toe. SYN: *hammer toe.*

malleus (mal'ē-ŭs). (pl. *mallei*). 1. The largest of the 3 auditory ossicles in the middle ear, attached to the eardrum, and articulating with the incus. 2. Glanders, an acute febrile disease with suppuration and necrosis of cartilage and bone.

malnutrition (mal-nū-trĭ'shŭn). Lack of necessary food substances in the body or improper absorption and distribution of them.

maloplasty (mal'ō-plas-tĭ). Plastic surgery of the cheek.

malpighian (măl-pĭg'ĭ-ăn). Concerning or described by Marcello Malpighi.

m. bodies. 1. Small, round bodies which commence in the cortex near the uriniferous tubules, forming the malpighian corpuscle of the kidney and a glomerulus packed into Bowman's capsule. 2. Small glandular patches throughout the spleen. SEE: *rete.*

m. capsule. Envelop. of a malpighian body resembling a pouch.

m. cones. Conical protuberances in the renal medulla, containing the tubules and secreting mechanism.

m. corpuscles. The capsula glomeruli and capillaries in the kidneys. The water of the urine is secreted therein. SYN: *corpusculum renis.*

m. glomer'ulus. The blood vessels and coil of capillaries surrounded by the malpighian corpuscle.

m. layer. Germinative, mucous and granular layers of the epidermis.

m. tuft. Capillary inner portion of a malpighian body.

malposition (măl-pō-zĭ'shŭn). Faulty or abnormal position or placement, esp. of the body or one of its parts.

malpractice (măl-prak'tĭs). Wrong or injurious treatment, esp. applied to performing illegal abortions.

malpresentation (mal-prē-zen-tā'shun). Abnormal position of fetus rendering natural delivery difficult or impossible.

malt (mawlt). Germinated grain, usually barley, used in fermentation of ale and beer. [by *Brucella melitensis*.

Malta fever. An infectious disease caused

maltase (mawlt'ās). A salivary and pancreatic enzyme which acts on sugar.

maltose (mawl'tōs). Malt sugar ($C_{12}H_{22}O_{11}$). A disaccharide converted from starch by hydrolysis, through the action of the intestinal enzyme, *maltase*.

It is found in malt, its products, and in sprouting seeds. SEE: *disaccharose*.

malum (ma'lŭm). A disease.

   m. perforans pedis. Ulcer of the foot of perforating type. It begins with thickening of the epidermis.

malunion (măl-ūn'yŭn). Growth of the fragments of a fractured bone in a faulty position, forming an imperfect union.

mamelonation (mam-el-ō-nā'shun). Nipplelike prominences on a part or organ.

mamma (măm'ă) (pl. *mammae*). One of 2 glands and structures in the female secreting milk; situated between the 3rd and 6th ribs when not pendulous. SYN: *breast*. SEE: *anisomastia, areolitis*.

mammalgia (mam-al'jĭ-ă). Pain in the breast. SYN: *mastalgia*.

mammary (măm'ă-rĭ). Pert. to the breast.

   m. glands. Two compound glands of the female breast secreting milk. They are made up of lobes and lobules bound together by areolar tissue.

mammectomy (măm-mek'to-mĭ). Removal of the breast. SYN: *mastectomy*.

mammilla (măm-ĭl'lă). 1. Nipple. 2. Any structure resembling a nipple.

mammillary (mam'ĭl-lar-ĭ). Like or concerning a nipple.

mammillated (mam'mĭl-lā-tĕd). Having protuberances like a nipple.

mammillation (măm-ĭl-la'shŭn). 1. Condition of having a granulated appearance or nipplelike projections. 2. A nipplelike protuberance.

mammilliform (mam-mĭl'ĭ-form). Shaped like a nipple.

mammilliplasty (măm-mĭl'ĭ-plăs-tĭ). Plastic operation on a nipple. SYN: *thelyplasty*.

mammillitis (măm-mĭl-ī'tĭs). Inflammation of a nipple. SYN: *thelitis*.

mam'min. Mammary gland hormone causing cessation of the menses.

mammitis (măm-ī'tĭs). Inflamed condition of the breast. SYN: *mastitis*.

mammose (mam'ōs). 1. Having unusually large breasts. 2. Shaped like a breast.

mammotomy (măm-ot'ō-mĭ). Surgery of a breast. SYN: *mastotomy*.

mammotropin (măm-ōt'rō-pĭn). Name of lactogenic principle of the ant. pituitary lobe. SYN: *prolactin*.

man (măn). 1. Member of the human race; a human being. 2. Male member of the species. SEE: "*anthrop-*" words.

mancinism (man'sĭn-ĭzm). State of being left-handed.

mandelic acid (man'-del'ik). A crystalline compound derived from benzaldehyde.

DOSAGE: Usually in the form of the sodium or ammonium salt, averages 12 Gm. per day.

mandible (man'dĭ-bl). A jawbone, esp. the lower one. The inferior maxilla.

mandibular (măn-dib'ū-lar). Rel. to the lower jaw.

   m. reflex. Clonic movement resulting from percussing or stroking lower jaw.

m. and m. enema. One given because its ingredients form gases and distend the bowel, thus causing frequent and copious bowel movements. SEE: *enema*.

mandrin (man'drĭn). A guide for a flexible catheter.

manducation (măn-dū-ka'shŭn). The chewing of food. SYN: *mastication*.

maneuver (măn-ōō'ver). OBS: Manipulation of the fetus and placenta to aid in delivery. SEE: *labor*.

   m., Crede's. Method of expressing the placenta first described by Crede, in which the hand is placed on the fundus of the uterus with the thumb on the ant. wall and the fingers on the post. wall, the placenta being pushed out by pressure in the direction of the birth canal.

   m., Leopold's. Method of abdominal palpation for the diagnosis of presentation and position of the fetus in utero.

   m., Mauriceau - Smellie - Veit. Method employed to deliver the aftercoming head in breech presentation.

   m., Muller's. Similar in import and method to that of Munro Kerr.

   m., Munro Kerr. A method for determining the presence of disproportion bet. the fetal head and the maternal pelvis.

   m., Pinard's. Fingers behind knee and push it toward and past the body, causing flexion of knee. Foot is then grasped and brought down in breech presentation.

   m., Prague. A method for the delivery of the aftercoming head in a breech delivery when the occiput is post.

   m., Scanzoni. Double application of forceps in post. position of the occiput.

Man'fan's disease. Spastic paraplegia found in children with hereditary syphilis.

manganese (man'gă-nēz). SYMB: *Mn*. AT. WT.: 54.93. SP. GR.: 7.2. A metal element found in many foods, and in some plants, and in the tissues of the higher animals.

mania (mā'nĭ-ă). Insanity characterized by exaltation or delirium.

   m. à pótu. Delirium tremens.

   m., Bell's. Periencephalitis in acute form.

   m., puerperal. A form of mental derangement occurring occasionally during the puerperium.

   m., religious. Mania resulting from excessive religious fervor.

   m., transitory. Short attacks of frenzy.

m., unproductive. Behavior characteristic of mania by lack of spontaneity in speech or muteness sometimes seen in manic-depressive psychosis. SEE: *alcoholism.*

maniac (mā'nĭ-ăk). An insane person.

maniacal (mă-nī'ăk-ăl). 1. Like a maniac. 2. Affected with mania.

man'ic-depres'sive insan'ity. Cyclic or circular insanity in which there are alternating moods of depression and mania. SEE: *insanity, manic-depressive.*

man'ikin. 1. A model of the human body or its parts. 2. A dwarf.

manipulation (măn-ĭp-ū-la'shŭn). Any treatment or procedure involving use of the hands.

manipula'tive surgery. Use of manipulation in surgery, bonesetting, etc.

Man'naberg's symptom. Accent of 2nd pulmonic sound in diseases of the abdomen.

man'nerism. Acts which are in keeping with the personality. A peculiar modification of an ordinary movement.

mannite (man'ĭt). Manna sugar, $C_6H_{14}O_6$, exuded from manna. It is a laxative.

Mann'kopf's sign. Pulse acceleration exhibited on pressing a painful point, seen in neurasthenia.

manometer (măn-om'et-er). Instrument for determining liquid or gaseous pressure.

m., aural. Instrument for ascertaining mobility of membrane during inflation.

mantle (man'tl). The cerebral cortex. SYN: *brain mantle, pallium.*

manual (man'ū-al). 1. Pert. to the hands. 2. Performed by or with the hands.

manubrium (man-u'brĭ-um). 1. The upper bone of the sternum articulating with the clavicle and first pair of costal cartilages. 2. That portion of the malleus* resembling a handle. SEE: *umbo.*

m. sterni. Same as *manubrium, 1.*

manus (ma'nus). The hand.

manustupration (man"u-stu-pra'shun). Masturbation.

mapharsen (mă-far'sen). A compound containing 29% trivalent arsenic.

DOSAGE: Initially, for women 0.02 Gm. and for men 0.04 Gm. intravenously; second injection, which is usually given from 5-7 days, slightly increased. Maximum dose is regarded as 0.06 Gm. and advised not to be given any patient at the first injection.

marantic (mă-răn'tĭk). 1. Pert. to marasmus. 2. Wasting away.

marasmic (mă-raz'mĭk). Affected with marasmus; wasting away. SYN: *marantic.*

marasmopyra (mar-az-mo-pi'ră). Hectic fever.

marasmus (mar-az'mus). Emaciation, wasting. Infantile atrophy which occurs almost wholly as a sequel to acute diseases, esp. diarrheic diseases of infancy.

marble bones. Abnormally calcified bones with spotted appearance in a roentgeno-

gram. SYN: *Albers-Schönberg disease, osteosclerosis* fragilis generalisata.*

mareo (mar-a'ō). Seasickness.

m. de la Cordillera. Mountain sickness.

marginal (mar'jĭn-ăl). Concerning a margin or border.

margination (mar-jĭ-nā'shŭn). Cleavage of leukocytes to walls of blood vessel in first stages of inflammation.

margin'oplasty. Plastic surgery of a border, as of an eyelid.

margo (mar'go). A border.

Marienbad (mah-re'ĕn-baht). A spa in Czechoslovakia for cardiovascular disease, urinary disorders, anemia, dyspepsia.

Marie's disease (mă-rē'). Chronic condition of enlargement of bones and soft tissues of hands, feet, and face. SYN: *acromegaly, hypertrophic pulmonary osteoarthropathy.*

M.'s sign. Hand tremor seen in exophthalmic goiter.

marine' treat'ment. Routine bathing of the tuberculous patient in sea water; is of tonic value, esp. when combined with heliotherapy.

Mariotte's law (mar-ē-ot'). Boyle's* law.

M.'s spot. The blind spot of the eye. SYN: *optic papilla.*

maritonucleus (măr"ĭ-tō-nŭ'klē-ŭs). Nucleus of ovum after being entered by the sperm cell. SYN: *genoblast.*

mark. A nevus, bruise, cut, or spot on the surface of a body.

m., birth-. Blemish on the skin at birth.

m., mother's. Birthmark.

marriage (mar'rĭj). State of being united to one of the opposite sex as husband and wife; wedlock. SEE: *misogamy, polyandry, polygamy.*

mar'row. The medulla or soft tissues in the hollow of long bones, and medullary cavities, and in the extremities of the long bones.

m., red. That in cancellous tissue of bone. Concerned with the production, maintenance and disposal of red blood cells and hemoglobin.

m., spinal. Spinal cord.

m., yellow. That in the medullary canal of long bones.

marsh fever. Malarial fever.

m. gas. Methane, *q.v.*

Marsh's test. A test to detect the presence of arsenic.

marsupialization (mar-sū"pī-al-ĭ-za'shun). Process of raising the borders of an evacuated tumor sac to the edges of the abdominal wound, and stitching them there to form a pouch.

marsupia patellaris (mar-sū"pī-ă pă-tel-lā'rĭs). The knee joint's alar ligaments.

martial (mar'shal). Pert. to or containing iron. SYN: *ferruginous.*

Martin's bandage. Rubber bandage for varicose veins, ulcers, and other similar conditions.

maschaladenitis (mas-kal-ă-den-ī'tĭs). Inflammation of axillary glands.

maschaliatry (mas-kal-ĭ-at'rĭ). Treatment by axillary inunctions.

masculation (măs-kŭ-lā'shŭn). Male sex characteristics formation.

mas'culin. Male sex hormone.

masculine (măs'kŭ-lĭn). Having male characteristics.

masculonucleus (mas″kŭ-lō-nū'klē-ŭs). Male pronucleus. SYN: *arsenoblast*.

mask. A covering for the face, as the gauze mask of a surgeon or nurse.

　m., ecchymotic. Traumatic asphyxia.

　m., Fontana's. Fold transversely on a nerve trunk when it has been severed.

　m., Hutchinson's. A feeling of compression over face as though one is wearing a mask. A symptom of tabes dorsalis.

　m., luetic. Blotchy brown pigmentation of cheeks, forehead, and temples, seen in tertiary syphilis.

　m., Parkinson's. Immobile facial appearance as a result of encephalitis lethargica. The face is devoid of expression, the skin smooth and without a wrinkle.

　m. of pregnancy. Pigmented spots on the face seen in some pregnant women.

　m., uterine. Mask of pregnancy or uterine disease.

masked (măskd). Covered from view.

masochism (mas'o-kĭzm). A psychopathic condition due to weakness and glandular insufficiency, esp. of the gonads and adrenals, which condition demands the stimulation of pain (generally whipping), before the subject is able to react to the sexual stimulus.

masochist (mas'ō-kĭst). A person addicted to masochism.*

mass (măs). Soft, solid preparation for internal use, and of such consistency that it may be molded into pills.

mas'sa. Mass, *q.v.*

　m. innominata. Tubular body on spermatic cord above the epididymis, the remains of post. part of the wolffian body. SYN: *paradidymis*.

massage (mas-săzh'). Manipulation; methodical pressure, friction, and kneading of the body. Must always be applied upon the bare skin.

　m., auditory. Massage of the eardrum membrane.

　m., douche. Massage resulting from the application of a douche.

　m., electrovibratory. Massage by means of an electric vibrator.

　m., general. Consists of centripetal stroking in connection with some muscular kneading from the toes upward.

　m., hydropneumatic. Massage by means of air forced through a tube at the end of which is a chamber containing water, the water chamber being applied to the part massaged.

　m., introductory. Consists of centripetal strokings around the affected part.

　m., local. Consists in treatment confined to particular parts.

　m., tremolo. A variety of mechanic massage.

　m., vapor. A treatment of a cavity by a medicated and nebulized vapor under interrupted pressure.

　m., vibratory. Massage by rapidly repeated light percussion with a vibrating hammer or sound.

masseter (mas-sē'tĕr). The muscle which closes the mouth and is the principal muscle in mastication.

masseur (ma-sur'). 1. A man who gives massages. 2. An instrument for massaging.

masseuse (ma-suz'). A woman who gives massages.

massive (măs'sĭv). Bulky; consisting of a large mass; huge.

　m. collapse of the lung. Dyspnea and pain in chest, esp. in patients who have suffered severe shock and collapse after abdominal operation or thyroidectomy. Patient's condition resembles that of postoperative pneumonia, but the collapsed lung expands in 2-3 days. The condition is a dangerous one.

massotherapy (măs-ō-ther'ă-pĭ). Use of massage in treatment of disease.

mastadenitis (măst-ă-den-ĭ'tĭs). A mammary gland inflammation.

mastalgia (mast-al'jĭ-ă). Pain in the breast. SYN: *mastodynia*.

mastatrophia (mast-ă-trō'fĭ-ă). Atrophy of breasts. SYN: *mastatrophy*.

mastatrophy (mast-at'rō-fĭ). Atrophy of breasts. SYN: *mastatrophia*.

mastauxe (mas-tawk'se). Excessive size of the breast.

mast cell. A mononuclear leukocyte with basophil granules found in the blood, esp. in leukemia.

mastectomy (mas-tek'to-mĭ). Excision of the breast.

masthelcosis (măs-thĕl-kō'sĭs). Ulcerated condition of breast.

mastication (măs-tĭ-kā'shŭn). Chewing. The comminution and insalivation of the food in the mouth is the first stage of digestion.

masticatory (măs'tĭk-ă-tō-rĭ). 1. Pert. to mastication. 2. Any substance chewed to stimulate secretion of saliva.

mas'tigote. A member of the family Mastigophora, or protozoa with flagella.

mastitis (măs-tī'tĭs). Inflammation of the breast.

　m., interstitial. Inflammation of glandular substance of the breast.

　m., stagnation. Caked breast.

mastocarcinoma (măst″ō-kăr-sĭn-ō'mă). Carcinoma of the breast.

mastochondroma (mast″ō-kon-drō'mă). Cartilaginous breast tumor.

mastodynia (măst-ō-dĭn'ĭ-ă). Neuralgia of the breast.

mastoid (mas'toid). 1. Pert. to mastoid process of the temporal bone. 2. The mastoid process of temporal bone. 3. Formed like a nipple.

　m. antrum. Hollow air space in the mastoid process.

　m. bone. Mastoid process of temporal bone.

　m. cells. Mastoid sinuses.

m. *disease*. Inflammation of mastoid.
m. *operation*. Outward drainage of mastoid cells.

m. *process*. Part of temporal bone; contains antrum, mastoid cells, portion of transverse and sigmoid sinus, facial nerve. SEE: *tegmen*.

mastoidal (măs-toi'dăl). Rel. to mastoid process.

mastoida'le. The mastoid process' lowest point.

mastoidalgia (mas-toid-al'jĭ-ă). Pain in the region of the mastoid.

mastoidec'tomy. Excision of mastoid cells. Simple and radical.

mastoideocentesis (măs-toid-ē-ō-sen-tē'-sĭs). Surgical puncture of the mastoid process.

mastoidotomy (mas-toid-ot'ō-mĭ). Incision into mastoid process.

mastology (mast-ol'ō-jĭ). Science or study of the breasts.

mastoiditis (măs-toid-ī'tĭs). Inflammation of the mastoid process.

m., *Bezold's*. Abscess underneath insertion of sternocleidomastoid muscle due to pus breaking through the tip cell.

m., *zygomatic*. Suppuration of cells in root of zygoma with swelling over the zygoma.

mastomenia (mas-to-me'nĭ-ă). Vicarious menstruation from the mammary glands.

mastoncus (mas-ton'kŭs). Any tumor of the breast.

mastoöccipital (mas"tō-ok-sĭp'ĭ-tăl). Rel. to mastoid process and occipital bone.

mastopathy (măs-top'ă-thĭ). A disease of the mammary glands.

mastopexy (mas'tō-pĕks-ĭ). Surgical correction of a pendulous breast by fixation. SYN: *mazopexy*.

mastoplasia (măst-ō-plā'zĭ-ă). Hyperplasia of mammary gland tissue. SYN: *mazoplasia*.

mastorrhagia (măs-tōr-ā'jĭ-ă). Hemorrhage from the breast.

mastoscirrhus (măs-tō-skĭr'ŭs). A hard cancer of breast.

mastotomy (măst-ot'ō-mĭ). Surgical incision of a breast.

masturbate (mas'ter-bāt). To arouse self-excitement through titillation of the genital organs.

masturbation (măs-ter-bā'shŭn). Self-production of an orgasm by titillating the genitals either by hand or some mechanical means.

m., *psychic*. When the orgasm ensues through psychic processes such as phantasy and without physical contacts.

match'es. Lucifer matches are usually made of phosphorus, *q.v.*, and potassium chlorate and may be lit by friction.

maté (mah'ta). Paraguay tea made from the leaves of *Ilex paraguayensis*.

materia medica (mă-tē'rĭ-ă mĕd'ĭ-kă). That branch of science dealing with all drugs used in treatment of diseases, their source, preparation, dosage, and use.

materies morbi (mă-te'rĭ-ēs mor'bĭ). The matter or substance which is the cause of disease.   [a mother.

mater'nal. 1. Rel. to the mother. 2. From

maternity (mă-ter'nĭ-tĭ). 1. The condition of motherhood. 2. Lying-in hospital. SEE: *accouchée*.

maternology (ma-ter-nol'ō-jĭ). The scientific study of motherhood.

matrix (mā'trĭks) (pl. *matricēs*). 1. The womb. 2. The formative portion of a tooth or nail. 3. The intercellular substance of a tissue. 4. Mold for casting.

m. *unguis*. Nail bed.

matrixitis (mā-trĭks-ī'tĭs). Inflammation of the bed of a nail. SYN: *onychia*.

mattoid (mat'oid). Person not in full control of mental faculties, but not to extent of insanity. SYN: *paranoiac*.

maturate (ma'tūr-āt). 1. To ripen. 2. To suppurate. SYN: *suppurate*.

maturation (măt-ū-rā'shŭn). 1. Maturing; ripening, as a *graafian follicle*. 2. Suppuration. 3. Last stage in sex cell formation.

matu'rity. State of being mature or fully developed; time when a person becomes capable of reproducing; puberty.

mature (ma-tūr'). Fully developed or ripened.

matutinal (ma-tū'tĭ-năl). Occurring early in the day, as *morning sickness;* in the morning.

matzoon (măt-zūn'). Milk with a ferment containing lactic acid, bacilli, and other organisms.

maxill'a (pl. *maxillae*). BNA. A jawbone, esp. the upper one; the superior maxilla. SEE: *skeleton*.

m., *inferior*. The lower jawbone, or mandible.

m., *superior*. Upper jawbone.

maxillary (măk'sĭ-la-rĭ). Pert. to the jaw, esp. the upper.

m. *bones*. Maxilla sup. and inf., upper and lower jawbones.

m. *sinus*. The antrum of Highmore; air cavity in sup. maxilla opening into middle meatus of nose.

maxillitis (măks'ĭl-ī'tĭs). Inflammation of maxilla or maxillary gland.

maximal (maks'ĭ-mal). Greatest possible; highest.

maximum (maks'ĭ-mum). 1. The greatest quantity. 2. Height of a disease.

mayidism (mā'ĭd-ĭzm). Deficiency disease due to lack of Vitamin B. SYN: *pellagra, q.v.*

Mayo enema. One which causes gas to form in the intestine, inflating the bowel and producing bowel action. SEE: *enema*.

Mayo-Robson's point. A point just above and to right of the umbilicus, where pressure causes tenderness in pancreatic disease.

"Mazda" lamp. Tungsten filament lamp enclosed in a bulb of special glass that transmits ultraviolet rays at wave lengths extending from 280-310 millimicrons. Types C X, S-1, and S-2.

mazopexy (mā'zō-pĕks-ĭ). Correction of a pendulous breast by surgical fixation. SYN: *mastopexy*.

mazoplasia (mă-zo-plā′zĭ-ă). Hyperplasia of mammary gland tissue. SYN: *mastoplasia*.

McBurney's incision. Abdominal incision employed in appendectomy.

An incision is made parallel to the path of external oblique muscle, about 1-2 inches away from ant. sup. spine of right ilium, cutting through the external oblique to the internal oblique and transversalis, separating their fibers.

McB.'s point. Point of tenderness in acute appendicitis, situated on a line bet. the umbilicus and the right ant. sup. iliac spine, about 1 or 2 inches above the latter.

McCarthy's reflex. Contraction of orbicularis palpebrarum with closure of lids resulting from percussion above supraorbital nerve.

McCormac's reflex. Adduction of 1 leg resulting from percussion of patella tendon of opposite leg.

meal (mēl). Portion of food eaten at a particular time to satisfy the appetite. SEE: *test meal, Von Leube motor test meal, -test meal.*

mean (mēn). In statistics, a number derived from a series of other numbers by a prescribed method of computation. SEE: *median.*

m. deviation. In statistics, a number representing the degree of variation found in a series of observations. The mean is first found; next, by subtraction, the differences bet. the mean and each observation; then the sum of all the differences, treated as positive; then the quotient of this sum by the total number of observations. Thus the mean deviation of the series 5, 6, 7 is $(1+0+1)/3 = 0.67$; the mean deviation for the series 4, 6, 8 is $(2+0+2)/3 = 1.33$.

measles (mē′zls). A highly contagious disease characterized by catarrhal symptoms and the presence of maculopapular eruption.

measure (mĕ′zhŭr). 1. A determined extent or quantity. 2. To determine the extent or amount of an area or substance. [passage.

meatal (mē-ā′tăl). Pert. to a meatus or

meatometer (mē-ā-tom′ĕt-ĕr). Device for measuring a passage or opening.

meat poisoning. Poisoning from eating diseased or putrified animal flesh.

meatorrhaphy (mē-ăt-or′af-ĭ). Suture of the severed end of a meatus, usually the *meatus urinarius.*

meatoscopy (mē-ăt-os′kō-pĭ). Instrumental examination of a meatus.

meatotome (mē-at′ō-tōm). Knife with probe or guarded point for enlarging meatus by direct incision.

meatotomy (mē-ā-tot′ō-mĭ). Incision of urinary meatus to enlarge the opening. SYN: *porotomy.*

meatus (mē-ā′tŭs) (pl. *meatūs*). A passage or opening.

m. acusticus externus. [BNA.] External auditory canal from tympanum to pinna.

m. acusticus internus. [BNA.] Canal in the petrous portion of temporal bone, containing facial and auditory nerves and vessels.

m. audito′rius. Ext. and int. passages of the ear.

m. nasi communis. Common nasal cavity on either side of septum.

m. nasi inferior. Space beneath inf. turbinate.

m. nasi medius. Space beneath middle turbinate.

m. nasi superior. Space beneath sup. turbinate.

m. urinarius. External opening of the urethra; usually said of the male.

mechanical rectifier. A device which, by changing contacts at the proper moment in a cycle, changes alternating current into pulsating direct current.

mechanics (mē-kăn′ĭks). Science of force and matter.

mech′anism. PSY: Combination of mental processes by which a result is obtained.

m., mental. PSY: Method of utilizing energy from instinctive drives with their accompanying emotions to deal with internal and external pressures upon the personality.

mechanology (mĕk-ăn-ŏl′ō-jĭ). Study of force and matter.

mechanotherapy (mĕk″an-ō-thĕr′ă-pĭ). Use of various types of mechanical apparatus to perform passive movements and to exercise various parts of the body. Ex: MacKenzie and Zander apparatus.

mecholyl (mĕk′ō-lĭl). Commercial name for acetyl-beta-methylcholine chloride. DOSAGE: 3-7½ gr. (0.2-0.5 Gm.).

meckelectomy (mek-el-ek′tō-mĭ). Excision of Meckel's ganglion.

Meck'el's cartilage. A vestigial cecal appendage of the ileum.

M.'s divertic′ulum. A congenital sac or blind pouch sometimes found in lower portion of the ileum. Strangulation may cause intestinal obstruction. SEE: *diverticulum, diverticulitis.*

M.'s ganglion. Ganglion located in the sphenomaxillary fossa giving off nerves to eyes, nose, and palate. SYN: *sphenopalatine ganglion.*

M.'s space. Area in dura holding the gasserian ganglion.

mecometer (mē-kom′ĕt-ĕr). Device for measuring an infant's length.

meconism (mek′ō-nizm). 1. Opium poisoning. 2. The opium habit.

meconium (me-kō′nĭ-um). 1. Opium; poppy juice.
2. First feces of a newborn infant, made up of salts, liquor amnii, mucus, bile, and epithelial cells; greenish black to light brown almost odorless and of a tarry consistency.

medi-. Prefix: The *middle.*

media (me′dĭ-ă). 1. Middle or muscular coat of an artery. SYN: *tunica media.* 2. Plural of *medium.*

me′dial. 1. Pert. to middle. 2. Internal.

me′dian. 1. Middle; central. 2. In statistics, a number obtained by arranging the given series in order of size and taking the middle number; one then has as many greater as there are less. Thus, in the series 5, 7, 8, 9, 10 the median is 8. See: *mean*.

m. artery. An interosseous branch.

m. line. The sagittal line, an imaginary line from the top and middle of the head through the sagittal suture to the floor. The parts nearest to it are called mesial, and those farthest from it lateral.

m. nerve. One of motion and sensation having its origin in the brachial plexus.

mediastinal (mē-dǐ-ǎs-tī′nǎl). Rel. to the mediastinum.

mediastinitis (mē-dǐ-as-tǐ-nī′tis). Inflammation of tissue of the mediastinum.

mediastinopericarditis (mē-dǐ-ǎs″tǐ-nō-pěr″ǐ-kär-dī′tǐs). Inflammatory condition of mediastinum and pericardium.

mediastinum (mē-dǐ-ǎs-tī′nŭm). 1. A septum of cavity bet. 2 principal portions of an organ. 2. The folds of the pleura and intervening space bet. right and left lung. The interpleural space. It contains the thoracic viscera. See: *chylomediastinum*.

m. testis. Partial testicular septum.

mediate (me′dǐ-āt). 1. Accomplished by indirect means. 2. Intermediate.

medicable (med′ǐ-kǎ-bl). Amenable to cure.

medical (měd′ǐ-kal). Pert. to medicine.

m. jurisprudence. Principles of medicine in their application to questions of law.

med′icament. A medicine or remedy.

medicate (měd′ǐ-kāt). 1. To treat a disease with drugs. 2. To impregnate with medical substances.

medication (měd-ǐ-kā′shŭn). 1. Treatment with remedies. 2. Impregnation with medicine.

m., hypodermic. Treatment by injection of remedies beneath the skin.

m., ionic. Introduction of ions of drugs into the body by cataphoresis.

m., substitutive. Medical therapy to cause a nonspecific inflammation to counteract a specific one.

medicinal (mē-dǐ′sǐn-ǎl). Pert. to medicine.

m., enema. One to which some drug or medication has been added, for retention or absorption, particularly in cases where medication cannot be adm. by mouth. See: *enema*.

medicine (měd′ǐ-sǐn). 1. A drug. 2. The art of preventing, caring for, and assisting in the cure of disease, and the care of the injured. 3. Treatment of disease medically as distinguished from surgery.

m., clinical. Observation and treatment at the bedside.

m., eclectic. Selection from all systems of medicine.

m., forensic. Application of medical knowledge to legal affairs.

m., patent. A medicine for which a patent has been granted. See: *patent* *medicine*. [venting disease.

m., preventive. The practice of pre-

m., proprietary. Medicine in which proprietary interests have been secured by patent, copyright of labels, or secrecy of composition. See: *proprietary* *medicine*.

medicine, rectal administration of. In diseases of the rectum and adjacent parts, medication is often applied by way of the anus, esp. if medication cannot be adm. by mouth, as in persistent nausea or emesis, during unconsciousness or delirium, or on account of the bad taste of the medication.

medicinerea (měd″ǐ-sǐn-ē′rē-a). Internal gray matter of the claustrum and lenticula of the brain.

medicochirurgical (měd″ǐ-kō-kī-rur′jǐ-kǎl). Concerning both medicine and surgery.

medicolegal (měd″ǐ-kō-lē′gǎl). Rel. to medical jurisprudence or forensic medicine.

med′icus. A physician.

medinal (med′ǐ-nal). Soluble barbital, barbital sodium.

    Dosage: 5-15 gr. (0.3-1.0 Gm.).

medio-. Prefix meaning *the middle*.

mediopontine (mē″dǐ-ō-pon′tǐn). Rel. to center of the pons Varolii.

mediotarsal (mē″dǐ-ō-tar′sǎl). Rel. to the middle of the tarsus.

medipeduncle (mē″dǐ-pē-dun′kl). Cerebellar middle peduncle.

medium (mēd′ǐ-ŭm) (pl. *media*). 1. An agent through which an effect is obtained. 2. Substance used for the cultivation of microörganisms. Syn: *culture medium*. 3. Substance through which impulses are transmitted.

medulla (mē-dul′lǎ). 1. The marrow. 2. Substance in the kidneys below the cortex. 3. Medulla oblongata. 4. Spinal cord. See: *accelerating center, cardioinhibitory center*.

m. of kidneys. Renal pyramids.

m. nephrica. Pyramids of kidneys.

m. oblongata. Enlarged portion of spinal cord in cranium after it enters the foramen magnum of the occipital bone; the lower portion of the brain stem.

m. ossium. Marrow in bone.

m. spinalis. Spinal cord.

medullary (med′ū-lar-ǐ). Concerning marrow, or any medulla.

medullated (med′ū-lāt-ěd). Covered by or containing marrow or medulla.

m. nerve fiber. A white nerve fiber.

medullispinal (me-dŭl′ǐ-spī′nǎl). Rel. to the spinal cord.

medullitis (měd-ū-lī′tǐs). Inflammation of marrow. Syn: *myelitis*.

medullization (měd-ū-lǐ-zā′shŭn). Conversion to marrow abnormally.

medulloarthritis (měd″ū-lō-ar-thrī′tǐs). Inflammation of marrow elements of bone ends.

medulloblastoma (měd″ū-lō-blas-tō′mǎ). Malignant nerve tissue tumor.

medullocell (mĕd-ū'lō-sĕl). Marrow cell. SYN: *myelocyte*.

medulloepithelioma (mĕd"ū-lō-ep"'ĭ-thēl-ĭ-ō'mă). Tumor composed of retina epithelium and of neuroepithelium. SYN: *neuroepithelioma, glioma*.

mega-, meg-. Combining forms meaning *great, large*.

megabacterium (mĕg"ă-băk-tēr'ĭ-ŭm). One of the largest bacterium.

megabladder (mĕg'ă-blăd-ĕr). Permanent abnormal distention of the urinary bladder. SYN: *megalocystis*.

megacephalic (mĕg-ă-sĕf-al'ĭk). Having an abnormally large head. SYN: *macrocephalous*.

megacoccus (mĕg-ă-kok'ŭs). A large size coccus. SYN: *macrococcus*.

megacolon (meg-ă-ko'lon). Extremely dilated colon.

megacoly (meg'ă'kol-ĭ). Dilatation of the colon.

megadont (mĕg'ă-dont). Possessing very large teeth. SYN: *macrodont*.

megadyne (meg'ă-dīn). A unit equal to one million dynes.*

megakaryocyte (mĕg'ă-kar'ĭ-ō-sīt). Large bone marrow cell with large or multiple nuclei. SYN: *megaloblast, myeloplax*.

megalakria (mĕg-ă-lak'rĭ-ă). Trophic disorder marked by progressive enlargement of head, hands, feet, and thorax. SYN: *acromegaly*.

megalgia (mĕg-al'jĭ-ă). Very severe pain.

megalo-. Combining form meaning *large, great*.

megaloblast (mĕg'ă-lō-blăst). A large size nucleated red blood corpuscle, from 11-20 microns in diameter, oval and slightly irregular. SYN: *macroblast*.

megalocardia (mĕg-ă-lō-kar'dĭ-ă). Cardiac hypertrophy. SYN: *cardiomegaly*.

megalocephalic (mĕg-ă-lō-sef-al'ĭk). Having an abnormally large skull. SYN: *megacephalic, macrocephalic*.

megalocephaly (meg"ă-lō-sef'ă-lĭ). Abnormal size of the head. SYN: *macrocephaly*.

megalocornea (mĕg"ă-lō-kor'nē-ă). An enlarged cornea.

megalocystis (mĕg"ă-lō-sĭs'tĭs). Abnormal, permanent enlargement of the bladder. SYN: *megabladder*.

megalocyte (mĕg'ăl-ō-sīt). Red blood corpuscle larger than average.

megalodactylous (mĕg"ă-lō-dak'tĭl-ŭs). Having very large digits.

megalodontia (mĕg"ă-lō-don'shĭ-ă). Abnormal size of teeth.

megaloenteron (mĕg"ă-lō-ĕn'tĕr-on). Excessive size of the intestine. SYN: *enteromegaly*.

megalogastria (mĕg"ă-lō-gas'trĭ-ă). Excessive size of stomach. SYN: *gastromegaly*.

megaloglossia (mĕg"ă-lō-glos|sĭ-ă). Enlargement of the tongue. SYN: *macroglossia*.

megalohepatia (mĕg"ă-lō-hĕ-pat'ĭ-ă). Abnormal enlargement of the liver. SYN: *hepatomegaly*.

megalokaryocyte (mĕg-ă-lō-kar'ĭ-ō-sīt). A large bone marrow cell with multiple nuclei. SYN: *megakaryocyte*.

megalomania (meg"a-lo-mā'nĭ-ă). A psychosis characterized by ideas of personal exaltation and delusions of grandeur.

megalomelia (mĕg"ă-lō-mēl'ĭ-ă). Abnormally large size of the limbs. SYN: *macromelia*.

megalonychosis (mĕg"ă-lō-nĭ-kō'sĭs). Hypertrophy of the nails.

megalopenis (mĕg"ă-lō-pē'nis). Abnormally large penis. SYN: *macrophallus*.

megalophthalmus (mĕg-ă-lŏf-thal'mus). Abnormally large eyes.

megalopsia (meg-a-lop'sĭ-ă). An affection of the eyes in which objects appear enlarged. SYN: *macropsia*.

megaloscope (meg'a-lo-skŏp). A speculum that magnifies.

megalosplenia (mĕg"ă-lō-splēn'ĭ-ă). Hypertrophy of the spleen. SYN: *splenomegaly*.

megalosyndactyly (mĕg"ă-lō-sin-dak'til-ĭ). A condition of large and webbed digits.

megaloureter (mĕg-ă-lō-ūr'ĕ-tĕr). Increase in diameter of the ureter.

megarectum (mĕg-ă-rek'tŭm). Excessive dilatation of the rectum.

megaseme (mĕg'ă-sēm). 1. Having an orbital aperture with an index exceeding 89, said of a skull. 2. A megaseme aperture.

Megas'toma. A protozoan.

   M. intestinale. A protozoan inhabiting the intestine.

megophthalmus (mĕg-of-thal'mŭs). Abnormally large eyes. SYN: *buphthalmus, megalophthalmus*.

megrim (mē'grĭm). 1. Sick headache. SYN: *migraine, q.v.* 2. A whim. 3. Vertigo.

meibomian cyst (mī-bō'mĭ-ăn). Small tumor on eyelid, the result of inflammation of a meibomian gland. SYN: *chalazion*.*

   m. gland. One of the sebaceous follicles bet. the tarsi and conjunctiva of eyelids.

Meinicke reaction or **test** (mi'nĭk-e). Tests for syphilis. 1. Floccular reaction. 2. Turbidity reaction. 3. Clearing reaction.

meiocardia (mī'ō-kar'dĭ-ă). Systole; heart contraction.

Meissner's corpuscles (mīs'nĕr). Laminated, ovoid corpuscles attached to nerve fibers; found at tips of fingers and toes, in skin over lips, the mammary glands and genitals.

   M.'s plexus. One in submucosa of small intestine. Derived from the myenteric plexus.

mel. Honey.

melaena (mel-e'na). 1. Black vomit. 2. Ta~ry evacuations. SEE: *melena*.

melagra (mĕl-a'gră). Pain in the limbs. SYN: *melalgia*.

melalgia (mĕl-a)'jĭ-ă). Neuralgia of the limbs. SEE: *meraigia*.

melancholia (mĕl-an-ko'lĭ-ă). Depression of mental condition, with or without delusions or violent mania, characterized by great apathy.

m., affective. Involving or due to the emotions.

m. agita'ta. Melancholia with much motor excitement.

m. attonita. Characterized by mental and physical stupor.

m., climacteric. Occurring at the menopause.

m., convulsive. Occurring in connection with packsonian epilepsy.

m., involution. Despondency, suicidal tendencies, feelings of unworthiness and mental agitation occurring between 45 and 60 years of age.

m., panphobic. Characterized with dread of everything.

m., paretic. Preceding paresis.

m., puberty. Melancholia with feelings of inferiority.

m., sexual. Melancholia associated with fear of impotence, venereal disease, unsatisfied sexual desires.

m., simplex. Without delusions, a mild form.

m. stuporo'sa. SEE: *melancholia attonita.*

m., suicidal. Having impulse to commit suicide combined with melancholia.

melanedema (měl-an-e-dē'mǎ). Black deposit in the lungs; melanosis of the lungs. SYN: *anthracosis.*

melanemia (měl-an-e'mǐ-ǎ). Unnaturally dark color of blood, due to pressure of melanin or free, dark pigment.
Seen mainly in pernicious anemia.

melanephidrosis (měl-ăn-ěf-ǐ-drō'sǐs). Black sweat. SYN: *melanidrosis.*

mélangeur (mǎ-lon-jher'). Apparatus for drawing and diluting blood specimens for microscopic examination.

melanidrosis (měl-an-ǐd-rō'sǐs). Black sweat. SYN: *melanephidrosis.*

melaniferous (měl-ăn-if'ěr-ūs). Containing melanin or some other black pigment.

mel'anin. The pigment which gives color to hair, skin and the choroid of the eye, and is present in some cancers, as in *melanoma.*
Melan can be prepared chemically.

melanism (měl'ăn-ĭzm). Excessively black pigmentation of the organs and tissues.

melano-. Prefix meaning *black* or *darkness.*

melanoblastoma (měl'ǎ-nō-blǎs-tō'mǎ). A tumor containing melanin.

melanocarcinoma (měl'ǎ-nō-kar-sǐn-ō'mǎ). A cancer which is darkly pigmented.

melanocyte (měl'an-ō'sǐt). Pigmented leukocyte.

melanoderma (měl'an-ō-der'mǎ). A dark skin discoloration.

melanogenesis (mel'an-ō-jěn'ě-sǐs). Formation of melanin.

melanoglossia (měl'ăn-ō-glŏs'sǐ-ǎ). Black tongue. SYN: *glossophytia.*

melanoid (měl'ǎ-noid). 1. Concerning or resembling melanosis. 2. Melanin which is chemically prepared.

melanoleukoderma (mel'an-ō-lū-kō-der'mǎ). Mottled skin.

m. col'li. Mottled skin of neck sometimes seen in syphilis. SYN: *collar of Venus, venereal collar.*

melano'ma. A pigmented mole or tumor. SYN: *nevus pigmentosus.*

melanomatosis (měl-an-ō-mat-ō'sǐs). Formation of melanomas on or beneath the skin.

melanonychia (měl-ǎ-nō-nik'ǐ-ǎ). Black pigmentation of the nails.

melanopathy (mel-an-op'ǎ-thǐ). 1. Dark pigmentation of skin. 2. Disease with dark pigmentation of the skin. SYN: *melanoderma, melasma.*

melanophore (mel'an-ō-fōr). Cell carrying dark pigment.

melanoplakia (měl'an-ō-plā'kǐ-ǎ). Condition marked by pigmented patches on the buccal mucosa.

mel"anorrhag'ia. Black feces. SYN: *melanorrhea.*

melanorrhea (měl-an-or-re'ǎ). Black stools. SYN: *melena,* 2.

melanosarcoma (měl"ǎ-nō-sar-kō'mǎ). Sarcoma containing melanin.

melanoscirrhus (měl-ǎ-nō-skir'rūs). Black pigmented cancer. SYN: *melanocarcinoma.*

melanosis (měl-an-ō'sǐs). Unusual deposit of black pigments in different parts of body.

m. lenticularis. Rare skin disease, beginning in early youth, characterized by scattered pigment discolorations, ulcers, atrophy, etc. SYN: *xeroderma pigmentosum.*

melanot'ic. 1. Blackish in color. 2. Pert. to melanosis.

melanuria (měl-an-u'rǐ-ǎ). Dark pigments in urine.

melasma (měl-az'mǎ). Any discoloration of the skin. SYN: *nigredo cutis.*

m. gravidarum. Discoloration of the skin during pregnancy.

m. suprarenale. Hypofunction of the suprarenals with cutaneous pigmentation and severe anemia. SYN: *Addison's disease,* q.v.

melena (měl-ē'nǎ). 1. Black vomit. 2. Evacuations resembling tar, due to action of intestinal juices on free blood. Common in the newly born.

melenemesis (mel-e-nem'ě-sǐs). Black vomit caused by blood that has been acted upon by the gastric juice. SYN: *melena,* 1.

melicera, meliceris (měl-ǐ-sēr'ǎ, -ǐs). Cyst containing matter of honeylike consistency.

melissopho'bia. Insane fear of bee or wasp stings.

melitagra (měl-ǐ-tag'rǎ). A form of eczema with soft crusts resembling honey.

melitemia (mel-ǐ-te'mǐ-ǎ). Sugar in the blood. SYN: *glycemia.*

melitis (měl-ǐ'tǐs). Inflammation of cheek.

melitoptyalism (měl'ǐt-ō-tǐ'al-ǐzm). Saliva containing glucose. SYN: *glycoptyalism.*

melituria (mel-ǐ-tu'rǐ-ǎ). Diabetes mellitus; excretion of sugar in urine.

mellite (mel'ǐt). Any medicated preparation of honey.

melodiotherapy (mel-ō″dĭ-ō-ther′a-pĭ). Treatment by music. SYN: *musicotherapy.*

melomania (mel-ō-mā′nĭ-ă). Insane love for music.

meloncus (mĕl-on′kŭs). Tumor of the cheek.

meloplasty (mel′ō-plas-tĭ). Reparative surgery of a cheek or limb.

melosis (mel-ō′sĭs). 1. Act of probing, as in a wound or ulcer. 2. Act of using a catheter.

melt′ing point. Temperature at which conversion of a solid to a liquid begins.

mem′ber. An organ or part of the body, esp. a limb.

membrana (mem-brā′na). Membrane.

   m. adventitia. Any covering membrane not made up of the tissues of organ so covered.

   m. basila′ris. Membrane forming floor of ductus cochlearis.

   m. basilaris of the cochlea. Portion of lamina spiralis membranacea of cochlea into which bases of Corti's and Deiter's cells are inserted.

   m. caduca vera. SEE: *membrana decidua.*

   m. capsularis genu. Capsular ligament of knee.

   m. cellulosa. SEE: *membrana decidua.*

   m. chorii. The chorion.

   m. communis. Membrane common to 2 structures.

   m. decidua. BNA. Membrane lining the uterus during pregnancy and cast off in parturition. SYN: *decidua.*

   m. eboris. Layer of odontoblasts bet. tooth pulp and wall of pulp cavity.

   m. elastica laryngis. Layer of yellow elastic tissue subjacent to mucosa of larynx helping to form the true vocal cords.

   m. flaccida. Shrapnell's membrane.

   m. germinativa. The blastoderm.

   m. granulosa. Layer of granular cells forming lining of maturing graafian vesicle.

   m. humoris aquei. Membrane of Descemet.

   m. intercipientes. Membranes separating one space from another, as the diaphragm.

   m. limitans externa retinae. A very delicate membrane in the retina bet. outer granular layer and layer of rods and cones.

   m. limitans interna retinae. The hyaloid capsule.

   m. pituito′sa. Schneiderian membrane lining the nasal fossa.

   m. prolifera. The blastoderm.

   m. propria. A thin layer of connective tissue upon which rests the epithelium.

   m. pupillaris. Thin, vascular, transparent membrane closing the fetal pupil during the development of the eye.

   m. ruyschiana. Middle layer of the choroid, bet. the vitreous lamina and the layer of larger blood vessels.

   m. succingens. Visceral layer of the pleura.

   m. tectoria. Corti's membrane covering organ of Corti in the ear.

   m. tympani. The drum membrane, or tympanic membrane.

   m. tympani reflex. Reflection of light from normal eardrum membrane.

   m. tympani secundaria. A membrana closing the fenestra ovalis.

   m. vestibularis Reissneri. Membrane separating cochlear canal from the scala vestibuli.

   m. vi′brans. Tenser part of membrane of eardrum.

   m. vocalis. Mucous membrana covering the vocal bands.

membrane (mem′brăn). A pliable layer of substance lining, separating, or enveloping the internal parts of the body.

   m., arachnoid. Middle layer of membranes covering brain and spinal cord.

   m., basement. Delicate membrane underlying epithelium of mucous surfaces, and serving as a support for delicate structures.   [brane.

   m. bone. Bone originating in a mem-

   m., Bowman's. Thin homogeneous membrane separating corneal epithelium from proper substance of the cornea.

   m., brain and spinal cord. Pia mater, inner membrane; dura mater, outer membrane, and arachnoid, middle membrane.

   m., Bruch's. The lamina basalis constituting the inner layer of the choroid.

   m., Corti's. Membrane covering organ of Corti in ear.

   m., costocoracoid. Dense fascia bet. the pectoralis minor and subclavius muscles.

   m., cricothyroid. Membrane connecting thyroid and cricoid cartilages of the larynx.

   m., croupous. False yellowish-white membrane in the larynx during croup.

   m., Débove's. Layer bet. epithelium and basement membrane of mucosa of the bronchi, trachea, and intestinal tract.

   m., decidual. Membrane covering the fetal envelope.

   m., Descemet's. Elastic membrane forming lining surface of the cornea.

   m., diphtheritic. Fibrinous false membrane on mucous surfaces in diphtheria.

   m., drum. The tympanic membrane.

   m., elastic. One formed by elastic tissue fibers, as in the coats of arteries, etc.

   m., false. Fibrinous exudate on a mucous surface of a membrane, as in diphtheria.

   m., fenestrated. The tunica intima of an artery.

   m., fetal. The chorion, amnion, or allantois.

   m., germinal. The blastoderm.

   m., homogeneous. A fine membrane covering villi of the placenta.

   m., hyaline. 1. Basement* membrane. 2. Membrane bet. outer root sheath of a hair follicle and inner fibrous layer.

m., hyaloid. One investing the vitreous humor of the eye, seen on longitudinal section.

m., Krause's. Dark membranous band limiting the sarcomere in striated muscle.

m., meconic. A membrane forming a layer in rectum of the fetus.

m., medullary. Endosteum.*

m., mucous. Membrane lining cavities and canals communicating with the air and kept moist by secretion of mucus.

m., Nasmyth's. Epithelial membrane covering enamel of teeth in the fetus; also for a short time after birth.

m., obturator. Fibrous membrane closing the obturator foramen.

m., palatine. One covering buccal roof.

m., periodontal. One covering roots of teeth.   [bling serous membrane.

m., pseudoserous. Membrane resem-

m., pupillary. Transparent membrane closing the fetal pupil. If it persists after birth it is known as persistent pupillary membrane.

m., pyogenic. Granular lining of an abscess or fistula.

m., pyophylactic. Protective lining of an abscess that prevents reabsorption.

m., Reissner's. Membrane separating the cochlear canal from the scala vestibuli. SYN: *membrana vestibularis Reissneri.*

m., Ruysch's. Choroid's middle layer composed of a close capillary network.

m., schneiderian. Mucosa of the nasal fossae. SYN: *membrana pituitosa.*

m., semipermeable. Membrane allowing passage of water but not substances in solution.

m., serous. One covered with endothelial cells lining closed cavities and forming inner coat of a blood vessel.

m., Shrapnell's. That portion of the tympanic membrane filling the notch of Rivinus.

m., synovial. Membrane lining a joint and secreting synovia.

m., tectorial. Corti's membrane.

m., Tenon's. Fibroelastic membrane surrounding the eyeball. SYN: *Tenon's capsule.*

m., thyrohyoid. One joining the hyoid bone and the thyroid cartilage.

m., tympanic. The drum membrane.

m., virginal. The hymen.

m., vitreous. Descemet's membrane.

m., yolk. Ext. capsule of the ovum.

membraniform (mem-bran'ĭ-form). Resembling or of the nature of a membrane. SYN: *membranoid, membranous.*

membranocartilaginous (mĕm″brăn-ō-kăr-tĭl-aj'ĭ-nŭs). 1. Pert. to membrane and cartilage. 2. Derived from both membrane and cartilage.

membranoid (mĕm'brā-noid). Resembling a membrane. SYN: *membraniform, membranous.*

membranous (mem'bran-ŭs). 1. Rel. to a membrane. 2. Resembling a membrane. SYN: *membraniform, membranoid.*

membrum virile (mĕm'brŭm vĭr-il'e). The penis.

memory. The mental registration of past experience.

menacme (mĕn-ăk'mē). The menstrual period of a woman's life. SEE: *menstruation.*

menarche (mĕn-ar'kē). Beginning of menstruation.

In a group of 100 subjects it was found that the menarche occurred:
In 8 between ages 11 and 11.99 years
In 22 between ages 12 and 12.99 years
In 32 between ages 13 and 13.99 years
In 23 between ages 14 and 14.99 years
In 11 between ages 15 and 15.99 years
In 4 between ages 16 and 16.99 years

Mendel's law. Offspring do not inherit characteristics of parents in equal or intermediate proportions, but certain characteristics of 1 parent are predominant, and are therefore transmitted to the offspring in full measure, being termed *dominant.* The characteristics of the other parent are termed *recessive.*

In the 2nd generation, ¾ of the offspring will have dominant characteristics, the remaining ¼ recessive characteristics.

M.'s reflex. Dorsal flexion of 2nd to 5th toes.

menhidrosis (mĕn-hī-drō'sĭs). Vicarious menstruation through sweat glands.

Ménière's disease (mā-nē-ārs'). Disturbance in labyrinth seen in great variety of conditions, as drug poisoning, circulatory disturbances, infectious diseases, as in the exanthemata, and chancre of syphilis, blood dyscrasias, neuritis of vestibular branch of 8th nerve, and tumors of cerebellopontine angle.

meningeal (men-in'jē-ăl). Rel. to the meninges.

meningeorrhaphy (mē-nĭn-jē-or'ră-fĭ). Suture of any membranes, esp. those of brain and spinal cord.

meninges (mĕn-ĭn'jēz) (sing. *meninx*). 1. Membranes. 2. The 3 membranes investing the spinal cord and brain; the *dura mater,* external; the *arachnoid,* middle, and *pia mater,* internal.

meningina (me-nĭn-jī'nă). The pia mater and adjacent layer of the arachnoid combined. SYN: *pia-arachnoid.*

meninginitis (me-nĭn-jī-nī'tis). Inflammation of the pia-arachnoid membrane. SYN: *leptomeningitis, piarachnitis.*

meningioma (me-nĭn-jī-ō'mă). Tumor of the meninges.

meningism (men-ĭn'jĭzm). Irritation of the brain and spinal cord with simulation of meningitis, but without actual inflammation.   [gitis.

meningitic (me-nin-jit'ĭk). Pert. to menin-

meningitis (men-in-ji'tis). Inflammation of the membranes of spinal cord or brain.

SEE: *choriomeningitis, Kernig's sign, leptomeningitis, pachymeningitis.*

m., basilar. Inflammation at base of brain of the meninges.

m., cerebral. Acute or chronic meningitis of brain membranes.

m., cerebrospinal. Meningitis of brain and cord.

m., c., epidemic. A specific infectious disease caused by invasion of meningococci, characterized anatomically by inflammation of the cerebrospinal meninges, and clinically by intense pain in head, back, and limbs; convulsions; irregular fever, and frequently by a petechial eruption.

m., chronic. ETIOL: Generally results from injury, syphilis, sunstroke, or caries of the bone.

m., otitic. Meningitis as a complication of otitis.

m., septicemic. Meningitis due to septic blood poisoning.

m., serous. Serous exudation in meningitis into cerebral ventricles.

m., spinal. Meningitis of spinal cord membranes.

m., tuberculous. An acute inflammation of the cerebral meninges excited by the tubercle bacillus.

meningitophobia (men-nin-jit-ō-fō'bĭ-ă). Meningism due to fear of brain disease.

meningoarteritis (me-nĭn-gō-ăr-tĕr-īt'ĭs). Inflammatory condition of the meningeal arteries.

meningocele (men-ĭn'gō-sēl). Congenital hernia, the meninges protruding through an opening of the skull or spinal column.

meningocerebritis (me-nĭn-gō-ser-e-brī'tĭs). Inflamed condition of brain and meninges. SYN: *meningoencephalitis.*

meningococcemia (me-nĭn-gō-kŏk-sē'mĭ-ă). Meningococci in the blood.

meningococcus (men-in-go-kok'us) (pl. *meningococci*). The microörganism responsible for cerebrospinal meningitis. SEE: *coccus, Neisseria meningitidis.*

meningoencephalitis (men-in"go-en-sef-al-ī'tĭs). Inflammation of meninges and cerebral cortex of the brain.

meningocortical (me-nĭn-gō-kor'tĭ-kal). Pert. to the meninges and the cortex.

meningoencephalocele (me-nĭn"gō-en-sĕf'ăl-ō-sēl). Hernia of brain and meninges.

meningoencephalomyelitis (me-nĭn"gō-ĕn-sĕf"ăl-ō-mī-ĕl-ī'tĭs). Inflammation of the brain, spinal cord, and their meninges. [Softening of any membrane.

meningomalacia (me-nĭn-gō-mă-lā'sĭ-ă).

meningomyelitis (men-ĭn"gō-mī-ĕl-ī'tĭs). Inflammation of spinal cord and its membranes; less commonly of the dura mater, also.

meningomyelocele (me-nĭn"gō-mī'ĕl-ō-sēl). Hernia of spinal cord and membranes.

meningopathy (me-nĭn-gop'ă-thĭ). Any pathological condition of the meninges.

meningorrhachidian (me-nĭn"gor-ră-kid'ĭ-an). Concerning the spinal cord and meninges.

meningorrhagia (me-nĭn"gor-ra'jĭ-ă). Meningeal hemorrhage. SYN: *meningorrhea.*

meningorrhea (me-nĭn-gor-rē'ă). Meningeal hemorrhage. SYN: *meningorrhagia.*

meningosis (men-ĭn-gō'sĭs). Membranous joining of bones, as in the infant.

meningotyphoid (me-nĭn"gō-tī'foid). Typhoid fever with symptoms of meningitis.

meninguria (me-nĭn-gū'rĭ-ă). Presence of membraniform shreds in urine.

meninx (me'ninks) (pl. *meninges*). Any membrane, but esp. one of the coverings of the brain or spinal cord.

meniscitis (men-ĭs-kī'tĭs). Inflamed condition of an interarticular cartilage.

meniscocyte (men-ĭs'kō-sīt). A crescent-shaped red blood cell.

meniscocytosis (men-ĭs"ko-sīt-ō'sĭs). Crescent cells in the blood; sickle cell anemia.

meniscus (men-ĭs'kus). 1. Concavo-convex lens. 2. Interarticular fibrocartilage of crescent shape, found in certain joints. SYN: *meniscus articularis.*

m. articularis. [BNA]. SEE: *meniscus, 2.*

menocelis (men-ō-sē'lĭs). Spotted cutaneous condition sometimes seen in women failing to menstruate. [mone.

menofor'mon. A commercial ovarian hormone.

menolipsis (men-ō-lip'sĭs). Temporary absence or retention of menses.

menolysin (mĕn-ol'ĭs-ĭn). Commercial preparation for treating amenorrhea and dysmenorrhea.

menometrorrhagia (mĕn"ō-mĕt-ror-rā'jĭ-ă). Abnormal hemorrhagic condition of uterus, esp. bet. menstrual periods.

menopause (mĕn'ō-pawz). That period which marks the permanent cessation of menstrual activity.

Average Age of Women at Menopause

Per Cent	Age
12	36-40
26	41-45
41	46-50
15	51-55

Six per cent had their menopause before 35 or after 55.

menophania (men-ō-fa'nĭ-ă). First appearance of the menses at puberty.

menoplania (men-ō-plā'nĭ-ă). Vicarious menstruation; menstruation through other than the normal outlet, as through the nose.

menorrhagia (men-ō-ra'jĭ-ă). Excessive bleeding at the time of a menstrual period, either in number of days or amount of blood, or both.

menorrhalgia (men-or-ral'jĭ-ă). Painful menstruation. SYN: *dysmenorrhea.*

menorrhea (men-or-ē'ă). 1. Normal menstruation. 2. Free or profuse menstruation. SYN: *menorrhagia.*

menoschesis (men-os'kĕ-sis). Suppression of menses.

menosepsis (men-o-sep'sĭs). Septic poisoning from retained menstrual discharge.

menostasis (men-os'tă-sĭs). Suppression of menses. SYN: *amenorrhea.**

menostaxis (men-ō-stak'sĭs). Prolonged menstruation.

menotox'in. A toxin which develops in women during menstruation.

menoxenia (men-ok-se'nĭ-ă). Abnormal menstruation.

menses (men'sĕz). Monthly flow of bloody fluid from the uterus; catamenial flow.

menstrua (men'strŭ-ă) (pl. of *menstruum*). The menses.

menstrual (men'strŭ-ăl). Pert. to menstruation. SYN: *catamenial*.

m. cycle. Interval, averaging about 28 days, from 1 menstrual period to another in which uterus undergoes changes.

menstruant (men'strŭ-ănt). 1. In the condition of menstruating. 2. One who menstruates.

menstruate (men'strŭ-āt). To discharge menses.

menstruation (měn-strŭ-ā'shŭn). Periodic flow of blood from the uterus, containing disintegrated structural elements of the endometrium at more or less regular intervals throughout the active sexual life of women.

menstruous (men'strŭ-ŭs). Rel. to menstruation.

menstruum (men'strŭ-um). A solvent; a medium. SEE: *vehicle*.

mensuration (men-sū-rā'shŭn). The process of measuring. SEE: *chest, measure*.

mentagra (men-tag'ra). Inflammation of the hair follicles, esp. of the beard, with pustular eruptions. SYN: *sycosis*.

mentagrophyton (men-tag-rof'ĭ-ton). The fungus which is the cause of sycosis.

men'tal. 1. Rel. to the mind. 2. Rel. to the chin.

m. age. Age of a person mentally, determined by a group of mental tests. SEE: *age, mental; Binet*.

m. apparatus. A term that includes the ego, the id, and the super ego.

m. deficiency. May be due to following causes: Postinfectional, posttraumatic (natal and postnatal), epilepsy, endocrine disorders, growths, prenatal influences, undiagnosed causes.

m. fog. Clouding of consciousness.

m. hygiene. Science of maintaining healthy mental and emotional responses and preventing development of insanity and neurosis.

men'tha. Mint.

m. piperita. Peppermint.

m. pulegium. Pennyroyal.

m. viridis. Spearmint.

men'thol. USP. Colorless crystals obtained from oil of peppermint or other mint oils.

DOSAGE: 1 gr. (0.06 Gm.).

mentim'eter. Measurement of mental capacity.

ment'ism. Involuntary creation of mental images.

mentula (men'tū-lă). The penis.

mentulagra (men-tū-lag'ră). Painful involuntary erection of the penis, sometimes curved. SYN: *chordee, priapism*.

mentulate (men'tū-lāt). Possessing a large penis.

mentulomania (měn'tū-lō-mā'nĭ-ă). Mental state characterized by addiction to masturbation.

men'tum. The chin. SYN: *genion*.

mephit'ic. Noxious, foul, as a poisonous odor.

m. air or gas. Carbon dioxide.

meralgia (mer-al'jĭ-ă). Neuralgia of the thigh. SEE: *sciatica*.

m. paresthet'ica. Affection of nerves of the thigh causing itching, tingling, pain, burning, and sometimes numbness.

merbaphen (měr'băf-ĕn). USP. A compound of mercury containing about 33% mercury.

DOSAGE: From 1-2 cc. of a 10% solution, intramuscularly, or intravenously. Give first a tolerance test of ½ cc.

Mercier's bar or **barrier** (mer-se-ā'). A curved fold at the neck of the bladder, forming post. margin of the trigonum vesicae.

mercurial (mer-kū'rĭ-al). 1. Pert. to mercury. 2. A substance containing mercury.

m. palsy. Paralysis induced by mercurial poisoning.

m. rash. Rash caused by application of mercurial preparations locally.

mercurialism (mer-kū'rĭ-al-ĭzm). Chronic poisoning by mercury seen as a result of continuous administration of mercury for medical purposes.

mercurialization (mer-kū'rĭ-al-ĭ-zā'shŭn). Condition of influencing with mercury.

mercurialized (měr-kū'rĭ-ă-līzd). 1. Impregnated with mercury. 2. Influenced by or treated with mercury.

mercuric (mer-ku'rik). Rel. to bivalent mercury.

m. chloride ($HgCl_2$). A common compound of mercury formerly used in the household as an antiseptic, as a douche, and to destroy household pests.

m. oxide (HgO). A powder, usually yellow in color. Used in ointments. When red, it is used to dress sores in syphilis.

mercurin (mer'ku-rĭn). The sodium salt of an organic mercurial compound, containing about 40% mercury.

DOSAGE: In the form of cocoa butter suppository, containing 0.5 Gm.

mercurochrome (mer-kū'ro-krōm). A compound containing about 23% mercury, used as a germicide in 1 to 4% solution.

mer'curol. A mercuric acid compound used in infections of the genitourinary tract and the conjunctiva.

DOSAGE: ½-2 gr. (0.03-0.12 Gm.).

mercurous (mer-kū'rus, mer'ku-rus). Rel. to monovalent mercury.

m. chloride (HgCl) (Calomel). USP. This is a heavy white powder used in small doses in medicine as a laxative.

DOSAGE: Mild, as laxative, in fractional doses, 2½ gr. (0.15 Gm.).

mercury (mer'ku-rĭ) (quicksilver). SYMB: Hg. A silvery liquid element most commonly used in thermometers, barometers, dentistry, and medicine. When heated, gives off poisonous fumes.

m., ammoniated. USP. White precipitate.

DOSAGE: Externally, 5 to 10% ointment.

m. bichloride. USP. Corrosive sublimate.

SEE: *mercuric chloride, nephrosis*.

m. iodide, red. USP. Mercury biniodide.
DOSAGE: Average, 1/15 gr. (0.004 Gm.).
m. iodide, yellow. USP. Protiodide of mercury.
DOSAGE: Average, 1/6 gr. (0.01 Gm.).
m. mass. USP. Blue mass.
DOSAGE: 5 gr. (0.3 Gm.).
m. salicylate. USP.
DOSAGE: Average, 1 gr. (0.06 Gm.), intramuscularly.
m. succinimide.
DOSAGE: Subcutaneously, mainly, 1/6 gr. (0.01 Gm.).
m. vapor arc. An electric discharge through mercury vapor.

mere (mēr). One of the sections into which a zygote splits.

meridrosis (mer-id-rō′sĭs). Local perspiration.

merinthophobia (mĕr-ĭn-thō-fō′bĭ-ă). Morbid fear of being tied.

Merismopedia (mer-is-mō-pē′dĭ-ă). A genus of bacteria including all micrococci which divide into 2 planes.

merispore (mer′ĭ-spōr). A secondary spore resulting from the division of another spore.

mero-. Combining form meaning *the thigh.*

meroblastic (mer-ō-blast′ĭk). Pert. to a yolk in an ovum which contains nutritive material as well as the germinal protoplasm with cleavage taking place only in the protoplasm. OPP: *holoblastic.*

merocele (mer′ō-sēl). Hernia of the thigh.

merocoxalgia (mer″ō-koks-al′jĭ-ă). Painful condition of the thigh and hip.

merocrine (mer′o-krĭn). Pert. to a secretory gland, part of whose cells produce secretions without injury to the balance of the cells. OPP: *holocrine, q.v.*

meroergasia (mĕr″ō-ĕr-gā′zĭ-ă). Partial mental disorder with symptoms of emotional instability. SEE: *holergastic.*

merogenesis (mĕr″ō-jen′ĕ-sĭs). Multiplication or reproduction by segmentation.

merology (mer-ol′ō-jĭ). Anatomy of the elementary tissues.

meromicrosomia (mĕr″ō-mĭ″krō-sō′mĭ-ă). Abnormal smallness of some part or structure of the body.

meronecrosis (mer″ō-nĕk-rō′sĭs). Necrosis of cells.

meroparesthesia (mer″ō-păr-ĕs-thē′sĭ-ă). Change in the extremities' tactile reactions.

meropia (mer-o′pĭ-ă). Partial blindness.

merorrhachischisis (mĕr-ōr-ră-kis′kĭ-sis). Fissure of a portion of the spinal cord.

meroscope (me′rō-skōp). Device used in performing meroscopy.

meroscopy (mĕr-os′kō-pĭ). Auscultation of the separate parts of the cardiac cycle.

merosmia (mĕr-os′mĭ-ă). Inability to detect certain odors.

merosystolic (mĕr-ō-sĭs-tol′ĭk). Rel. to a portion of the systole.

merotomy (mer-ot′o-mē). Division into sections or segments.

merozoite (mer-ō-zō′ĭt). A spore formed in schizogenous reproduction of protozoa.

mersalyl (mer′sal-ĭl). A complex mercurial preparation in the form of a white crystalline powder, containing 39.6% mercury.
DOSAGE: 8 ♏ (0.5 cc.) of a 10% solution, intravenously, or intramuscularly (never subcutaneously), at intervals of 3-5 days, as may be required. Initial dose should be 0.5 cc. as a tolerance test.

merthiolate (mer-thi′ō-lāt). An organic combination containing about 50% mercury, and less toxic than bichloride, used as a disinfectant in solutions of 1:5000 to 1:1000, aqueous, or in the form of a tincture, as an ointment, 1:2000. *For ophthalmic use,* 1:5000 ointment, or 1:10,000 aqueous.

Méry's glands (ma-rē′). Two bulbourethral glands. SYN: *Cowper's glands.*

mesad (mes′ăd). Toward a median point.

mesal (mes′ăl). In a middle line or plane.

mesameboid (mes-ă-mē′boid). A wandering cell of the mesoderm.

mesaortitis (mĕs-ā-or-tī′tĭs). Inflammation of the middle aortic coat.

mesaraic, mesareic (mes-ar-ā′ĭk, -e′ĭk). Rel. to the mesentery. SYN: *mesenteric.*

mesarteritis (mĕs-ar-tĕr-ī′tĭs). Inflammation of the tunica media or middle coat of an artery.

mesaticephalic (mĕs-ăt″ĭ-sef-al′ik). Having a skull with a length-breadth index of 75-80 degrees, or of medium length.

mesatipellic, mesatipelvic (mĕs-ăt″ĭ-pĕl′lĭk, -pel′vĭk). Having a pelvis with an index bet. 90 and 95 degrees.

mesectic (mĕs-ek′tĭk). Using up a normal amount of oxygen. SEE: *mionectic, pleonectic.*

mesencephal (mĕs-ĕn′sĕf-ăl). Middle area of brain. SYN: *mesencephalon, midbrain.*

mesencephalon (mes-en-sef′al-on). The midbrain consisting of the corpora quadrigemina, the crura cerebri, and the aqueduct of Sylvius.

mesenchyma (mes-en′kim-ă). Portion of embryonic mesoderm that produces connective tissue.

mesenter′ic. Pert. to the mesentery.

mesenteriolum (mes-en-ter-ĭ-ō′lum). A small mesentery, as that of a diverticulum of the intestine.

mesenteriopexy (mes-en-ter′ĭ-ō-peks-ĭ). Fixation of a torn mesentery.

mesenteriorrhaphy (mes″en-ter-ĭ-or′ra-fĭ). Suturing of the mesentery.

mesenteriplication (mĕs″ĕn-tĕr-ĭ-plĭ-kā′shun). Taking tucks in the mesentery surgically.

mesenteritis (mes″ĕn-tĕr-ī′tĭs). Inflamed condition of the mesentery.

mesenteron (mes-en′ter-on). Middle portion of the embryonic digestive tract.

mesentery (mes′en-ter-ĭ). A peritoneal fold, connecting the intestine with the post. abdominal wall.
m., proper. That of the small intestine.

mesiad (mes'ĭ-ad). Toward the middle line. SYN: *mesad.*

mesial (me'sĭ-ăl). Toward the middle line, esp. of the dental arch. SEE: *median line.*

mesion (mes'ĭ-on). The imaginary plane dividing the body into right and left symmetric halves. SYN: *meson.*

mesiris (mes-ĭ'ris). Middle portion of the iris.

mesmeric (mes-mer'ĭk). Rel. to or induced by hypnotism; fascinating.

mesmerism (mes'mer-izm). Originally the theory of Mesmer, it now means therapeutics employing hypnotism or hypnotic suggestion.

mesoaortitis (mes"o-ā-or-tī'tis). Inflamed condition of aortic middle coat. SYN: *mesaortitis.*

mesoappendicitis (mes-ō-ap-pen-dĭ-sī'tis). Inflamed condition of the mesoappendix.

mesoappendix (mes"ō-ap-pen'dĭks). Mesentery of the vermiform appendix.

mesoblast (mes'o-blast). Embryonic middle layer of the blastoderm, bet. the hypoblast and epiblast from which arise the bone, skin, connective tissue, muscles, internal genitalia, and excretory organs. SYN: *mesoderm.* SEE: *acroblast.*

mesobronchitis (mes"ō-bron-kī'tis). Inflammation of the middle layer of the bronchi.

mesocardia (mes-ō-kar'dĭ-ă). Location of the heart in the middle line of the thorax, being a normal position in fetal stage, but a malposition in life.

mesocardium (mes-ō-kar'dĭ-um). 1. Portion of mediastinal pleura attached to pericardium. 2. Embryonic membrane connecting the heart with the body wall and the intestine.

mesocecum (mes-ō-se'kŭm). Mesentery attaching the cecum.

mesocele (mes'ō-sēl). Sylvian aqueduct in the brain.

mesocephalic (mes-ō-sef-al'ĭk). 1. Pert. to the midbrain. 2. Having a medium-sized head.

mesocephalon (mes-ō-sef'ă-lon). The midbrain.

mesocolic (mes-ō-kol'ĭk). Concerning the mesocolon.

mesocolon (mes-ō-kō'lon). Mesentery connecting colon with post. abdominal wall.

mesocolopexy (mes"ō-kō'lō-peks-ĭ). The taking of tucks in the mesocolon and then suturing it to make it shorter. SYN: *mesocoloplication.*

mesocoloplication (mes"ō-kō"lō-plĭ-kā'-shun). The operation of shortening the mesocolon by taking a tuck in it.

mes'ocord. A portion of the umbilical cord attached to the placenta.

mesoderm (mes'ō-derm). The middle layer of cells in the germinal membrane of an embryo. SYN: *mesoblast, q.v.* SEE: *ectoderm, entoderm.*

mesodmitis (mes-od-mī'tis). Inflamed condition of the mediastinum. SYN: *mediastinitis.*

mesoduodenum (mes"ō-dū-ō-dē'nŭm). Mes-

entery connecting duodenum to abdominal wall.

mesogastric (mes-ō-gas'trĭk). 1. Pert. to umbilical region. 2. Pert. to the mesogastrium.

mesogastrium (mes"ō-gas'trĭ-um). 1. The umbilical region. 2. Embryonic mesentery from which the stomach develops.

mesoglia (mes-og'lĭ-ă). Neuroglia tissue cell of moderate size. SYN: *oligodendroglia.*

mesognathic (mes-og-nā'thĭk). Having a gnathic index bet. 98 and 103.

mesognathion (mes-og-nā'thĭ-on). The intermaxillary or premaxillary bone.

mesohyloma (mes-ō-hī-lō'mă). Tumor derived from the mesothelium.

mesoileum (mes-ō-il'ē-ŭm). Mesentery of the ileum.

mesojejunum (mes-ō-jĕ-jū'nŭm). Mesentery of the jejunum.

mesol'obus. Corpus callosum.

mesometritis (mes-o-me-tri'tis). Inflammation of the uterine musculature. SYN: *myometritis.*

mesometrium (mes-o-me'trĭ-um). 1. The uterine musculature. 2. BNA. The broad ligament below the mesovarium.

mesomorph (mes'ō-morf). A well-proportioned person of medium height. SEE: *hypermorph, hypomorph.*

mesom'ula. An early embryonic stage when there is a mass of mesenchyma enclosed in mesoderm and entoderm.

meson (mes'on). Imaginary plane dividing body into symmetric halves. SYN: *mesion.*

mesonephric (mes-ō-nef'rĭk). Rel. to the mesonephron.

m. duct. Embryonic duct which becomes *vas deferens* in the male and rudimentary in the female. SYN: *wolffian duct.*

mesonephron, mesonephros (mes-ō-nef'ron, -ros). Embryonic excretory organ. SYN: *wolffian body.*

mesoneuritis (me-sō-nū-ri'tis). Inflammation of the substance of a nerve or of its lymphatics.

mesoömentum (mes"ō-ō-men'tum). Mesentery of the omentum.

mesopexy (mes'ō-peks-ĭ). Operation of shortening the mesentery by taking a tuck in it.

mesophilic (mes-ō-fil'ĭk). Preferring moderate temperature, as some bacteria which develop best at body temperature.

mesophryon (mes-of'rĭ-on). Midpoint in smooth space bet. the eyebrows. SEE: *glabella.*

mesopneumon (mes-ō-nū'mŏn). Meeting point of 2 pleural layers at hilus of the lung.

mesorchium (mes-or'kĭ-um). Peritoneal fold which holds fetal testes in place.

mesorectum (mes-ō-rĕk'tŭm). Mesentery of the rectum.

mes''oret'ina. Middle or mosaic layer of retina.

mesoropter (mes-ō-rop'ter). Normal eye position with muscles at rest.

mesorrhachischisis (měs″or-ră-kĭs′kĭ-sĭs). Fissure of a portion of the spinal cord. SYN: *merorrhachischisis*.

mesorrhaphy (mes-o′ră-fĭ). Suture of the mesentery. SYN: *mesenteriorrhaphy*.

mesorrhine (mes′or-rīn). With a nasal index variously quoted to range anywhere bet. 47 and 53.

mesosalpinx (měs″ō-sal′pĭnks). BNA. The free margin of the upper division of the broad ligament, within which lies the oviduct.

mesoseme (mes′ō-sēm). Possessing an orbital index bet. 83 and 90.

mesosigmoid (měs-ō-sĭg′moid). Mesentery of the sigmoid flexure.

mesosternum (mes″ō-ster′nŭm). The middle or second section of the sternum. SYN: *gladiolus*.

mesothelium (měs-ō-thē′lĭ-ŭm). The layer of cells, derived from the mesoderm lining the primitive body cavity; in the adult it becomes the epithelium covering the serous membranes.

mesothenar (mes-ō-thē′nar). The adductor pollicis muscle.

mesotropic (mes-ō-trŏp′ik). Situated in or turned toward the median plane of a body, member, or organ.

mesoturbinate (měs-ō-tur′bĭ-nāt). Middle turbinate bone.

mesovarium (měs-ō-va′rĭ-ŭm). BNA. The portion of the peritoneal fold that connects the ant. border of the ovary to the post. layer of the broad ligament.

meta-, met-. Combining forms meaning *after, between, with*.

metabasis (mět-ab′ă-sĭs). Change of any kind in the progress of a disease.

metabiosis (mět-ă-bī-ō′sĭs). Dependence of an organism for its existence upon another and giving no recompense.

metabolic (met-a-bol′ĭk). Rel. to metabolism.

metabolimeter (mě-tab″ō-lĭm′e-těr). Device for measuring rate of basal metabolism.

metabolin (mě-tab′ō-lin). Any metabolism product.

metab′olism. The successive transformations to which a substance is subjected from the time it enters the body to the time it or its decomposition products are excreted, and by which function of nutrition is accomplished and energy and living substance are provided.

 m., basal. The number of calories per 24 hours per square meter of body surface liberated by a person in muscular relaxation (but not sleep) and in the postabsorptive state. It is usually calculated from the rate of oxygen consumption, since the utilization of 1 liter of oxygen under the above conditions by normal persons on a mixed diet is accompanied by the release of 4.825 cal. of heat. Also called basal metabolism rate.

 m., constructive. Transformation of matter into protoplasm. SYN: *anabolism, q.v.*

 m., destructive. Decomposition of protoplasm into waste products. SYN: *catabolism, q.v.*

 m. energy. Metabolism expressed in terms of energy.

metabolite (mě-tab′ō-līt). Any product of metabolism.

metacar′pal. Pert. to the bones of the metacarpus, or bones of the hand. SEE: *skeleton*.

metacarpus (met-ă-kar′pus). The 5 metacarpal bones of the palm of the hand. SEE: *carpometacarpal*.

metacele (met′ă-sēl). Caudal portion of 4th ventricle of brain.

metachromasia, metachromatism (mět-ă-krō-mā′zĭ-ă, -krom′a-tĭzm). Change of color, esp. one produced by staining.

metachromatic (met″ă-krō-mat′ĭk). Pert. to metachromatism.

 m. bodies or **granules.** Granules in protoplasm which stain deeply and differently from the surrounding ones; seen in various bacteria.

metachromatin (met-ă-krōm′ă-tin). Basophil portion of chromatin.

metachromophil (met-a-krōm′ō-fil). Not reacting normally to staining.

metachrosis (met-ă-krō′sĭs). Change of color in animal life.

metachysis (me-tak′is-is). 1. Blood transfusion. 2. The introduction of any substance directly into the blood stream by mechanical means.

metacoele (met′a-sēl). Post. part of 4th ventricle of brain.   [gestation.

metacyesis (met-ă-si-ē′sĭs). Extrauterine

metagaster (met-ă-gas′ter). Permanent embryonic intestinal canal derived from the protogaster.

metagen′esis. Alternation of generation.

metagglutinin (met-ag-glū′tĭn-in). An agglutinin in an antigen which acts on closely related organisms of the antigen.

metagrippal (met-ă-grip′al). Occurring as a consequence of influenza.

metaicteric (met″ă-ik-ter′ik). Occurring as a consequence of jaundice.

metainfective (mět-ă-ĭn-fek′tĭv). Occurring as a consequence of an infection.

metakinesis (mět″ă-kĭn-ē′sĭs). 1. Separation of new cells in cell division. 2. Stage in cell reproduction when chromatic loop divides into 2. SYN: *metaphase, q.v.*

metal fume fever (or braziers' chills). This results from absorbing the fumes in special occupations such as welding, metal founding, torch metal cutting, and galvanizing. Zinc commonest cause of these disturbances.

metallesthesia (mět″al-ĕs-thē′sĭ-ă). Recognition of metals by touching them.

metallic (mě-tal′ik). 1. Pert. to metal. 2. Composed of or resembling a metal.

 m. tinkling. A peculiar ringing or bell-like auscultatory sound in pneumothorax, and over large pulmonary cavities.

metallophobia (mě″tal-ō-fō′bĭ-ă). Psychiatric fear of metals and metallic objects and of touching them.

metalloscopy (mě-tăl-os'kō-pĭ). Determination of the effects of applying metals to the body, and its sensitivity to them.

metallotherapy (mě-tal-ō-ther'ă-pĭ). Treatment by applying metals to the affected part.

metallur'gy. Study and methods of using metals.

metameric (mět-ă-měr'ĭk). Rel. to metamerism. SYN: *isomeric.*

metamerid (met-am'er-id). A substance that is metameric.

metamerism (met-am'er-izm). Isomerism when the component elements are identical and in the same ratio, but their structural arrangement in the molecule is not the same.

metamorphopsia (mět"ă-mor-fop'sĭ-ă). OPHTH: Visual distortion of objects; found in refractive errors, esp. astigmatism, retinal disease, choroiditis, detachment of retina, and tumors of retina and choroid.

metamorphosis (met-ă-mor'fō-sĭs). A structural change during the life of an organism.

    m., fatty. Fatty degeneration.

    m., viscous. Collection of blood plates in thrombosis.

metanephron, metanephros (met-ă-něf'ron, -nef'ros). The post. segmental body or primitive embryonic kidney from which the kidney is developed.

metaneutrophil (met-ă-nū'trō-fĭl). Not reacting normally with neutral stains.

metanucleus (met-ă-nū'klē-us). The egg nucleus after expanding beyond the germinal vesicle.

metaphase (met'ă-fāz). The stage in cell division during which the chromatic loop divides in two.

metaphen (met'ă-fěn). A yellow, odorless powder containing about 56% mercury in organic combination.

    DOSAGE: As a tincture for skin sterilization, 1:200. For irrigations for delicate membranes, from 1:2500 to 1:10,000 aqueous solution.

metaphrenia (mět-a-frē'nĭ-ă). A condition in which the libido is withdrawn from its natural associations and directed to the more practical activities of life, such as gainful occupation.

metaphyllin (met"ă-fĭl'ĭn). Theophylline with ethylene diamine.

    DOSAGE: 1½ gr. (0.1 Gm.).

metaphysis (mě-taf'ĭ-sis). End of a long bone's diaphysis or shaft where it meets the epiphysis.

metaplasia (met-ă-plā'zĭ-ă). Conversion of 1 kind of tissue into another.

metaplasm (met'ă-plăzm). Reserve material present in protoplasm, esp. stored nutritive substance.

metaplastic (met-ă-plas'tik). Pert. to or formed by metaplasia.

metaplexus (met-ă-pleks'us). Choroid plexus of the brain's 4th ventricle.

metapneumonic (met-ă-nū-mon'ĭk). Succeeding or as a consequence of pneumonia.

metapophysis (met-ă-pof'ĭ-sis). Mammillary process on the superior articular processes of a vertebra.

metapore (met'ă-pōr). The aperture of Magendie.

metapro'tein. Derived protein resulting from the action of acids or alkalies, in which the molecule is changed to form protein insoluble in neutral solvents but soluble in alkalies and weak acids.

metapyretic (mět"ă-pĭ-rět'ĭk). Performed or occurring during fever.

metastable (met"ă-stā'bl). Changing from one condition to another; unstable.

    m. solutions. Those of supersaturation in relation to amt. of dissolved substance.

metastasis (mě-tas'tă-sĭs). 1. Movement of bacteria from one part of the body to another. 2. Change in location of a disease or of its manifestations or transfer from one organ or part to another.

metastasize (me-tas'tă-sīz). To invade by metastasis.

metastatic (met-ă-stat'ĭk). Pert. to metastasis.

metasternum (met-ă-ster'num). Last bone of sternum; the ensiform process.

metasyphilis (met-ă-sif'ĭ-lis). 1. Congenital syphilis with no local lesions but presenting general degeneration. 2. Condition due to syphilis. SYN: *parasyphilis.*

metatarsalgia (met-ă-tar-sal'jĭ-ă). Neuralgia of the metatarsus. SYN: *Morton's disease.*

metatarsectomy (met"ă-tar-sek'tō-mĭ). Removal of the metatarsus.

metatarsophalangeal (met"ă-tar"sō-fă-lan'jē-ăl). Concerning the metatarsus and phalanges.

metatarsus (mět-ă-tar'sŭs). The 5 bones bet. the instep and the phalanges. SEE: *skeleton.*

metathalamus (met-ă-thal'ă-mus). BNA. The post. part of the thalamus including the 2 geniculate bodies.

metathesis (mě-tath'ě-sis). 1. A changing of places. 2. Forcible transference of a disease process from one part to another where it will be more accessible for treatment. 3. Double decomposition chemically.

metatrophia (met-ă-trō'fĭ-ă). A condition due to disorder of nutrition.

metatro'phic. 1. Pert. to metatrophia. 2. Requiring lifeless organic matter for food. SYN: *saprophytic.*

metatropism (mět-ăt'rō-pĭzm). Masculine behavior in women and feminine behavior in men.

metatuberculosis (mět"ă-tū-ber-kū-lō'sĭs). A condition of tuberculous reactions with nontuberculous lesions.

metaxeny (mě-taks'ĕ-nĭ). Adoption of another host by a parasite when conditions are unfavorable to it with normal host. SYN: *metoxeny.*

Metch'nikoff's theory. Microörganisms are ingested by living cells, as by leukocytes and other phagocytes. SYN: *phagocytosis.*

metencephalon (met"ĕn-sěf'ă-lon). BNA.

1. Most caudal portion of the brain or primitive cerebral vesicle from which are developed the cerebellum, pons, and pontine portion of 4th ventricle. 2. The cerebellum and pons considered together. Syn: *afterbrain, hindbrain.*

metensomatosis (met″en-sō-mat-ō′sis). Incorporation with, or transformation into, another body.

meteorism (mē′tē-or-izm). Distention by gas in the abdomen. Syn: *tympanites.*

me′ter. A linear standard of measurement, 39.371 inches.

   m. angle. Angle of visual axis 1 meter distant.

   m. atom. An Angstrom* unit or 1.094 yd. See: *metric system.*

methane (CH₄). A combination of carbon with hydrogen; the same as the so-called "fire damp" in mines.

methanol (meth′an-ol). Methyl alcohol. Syn: *wood alcohol.*

methemoglobin (met″hĕm-ō-glo′bin). A compound closely related to oxyhemoglobin found in the blood following poisoning by certain substances.

   It gives blood a chocolate-brown color and is useless as a carrier of oxygen.

methemoglobinemia (met″hem″ō-glōb″ĭ-nē′mĭ-ă). Presence of methemoglobin in the blood.

methemoglobinuria (met″hem-ō-glōb″ĭ-nū′rĭ-ă). Presence of methemoglobin in the urine.

methenamine (mĕth″ĕn-a′mĕn). USP. Formin, hexamethylene, urotropin. Colorless crystals, with sweetish taste.

   Dosage: 5 gr. (0.3 Gm.). Best results obtained by giving alternate doses of an equal amount of sodium acid phosphate.

methomania (meth-ō-mā′nĭ-ă). Psychiatric craving for intoxicating drinks. Syn: *dipsomania.*

methyl (meth′ĭl). In organic chemistry, the radical CH₃, seen, for instance, in the formula for methyl alcohol, CH₃OH.

   m. alcohol. A colorless liquid with a peculiar alcoholic odor largely used as a solvent for paints, varnishes, etc.

   m. chloride. Gas obtained by distilling methyl alcohol.

   m. ether. An anesthetic gas without color.

   m. oxide. See: *methyl ether.*

   m. salicylate (sal-is′il-āt). USP. Oil of wintergreen, oil of gaultheria. Produced from distillation of leaves of sweet birch.

   Dosage: Internally, 5 to 20 ♏ (0.3-1.2 cc.).

   m. violet. Stain employed in histology and bacteriology. Syn: *pyoktanin.*

methylene blue (meth′ĭ-lēn). USP. Methylthionine chloride. A dark green crystalline powder, producing a distinct blue stain.

   Dosage: Average, 2½ gr. (0.15 Gm.). As an antidote, 50 cc. of a 1% solution, intravenously.

metopantralgia (met″ō-pan-tral′jĭ-ă). Pain in frontal sinuses.

metopantritis (met-ō-pan-trī′tis). Inflamed condition of frontal sinuses.

metopic (met-op′ĭk). Rel. to the forehead.

metopion (met-ō′pĭ-on). Craniometric point in forehead midway bet. frontal eminences.

metopism (met′ō-pĭzm). Persistence of the frontal sinus in an adult.

metopodynia (met-ō-pō-din′ĭ-ă). Headache in frontal area of head.

meto′pon. Cranial ant. lobule.

metoposcopy (met-ō-pos′kō-pĭ). The study of physiognomy.

metoxenous (mĕ-toks′ĕn-ŭs). Denoting a parasite spending each of its 2 cycles on a different host. Syn: *heterecious.*

metoxeny (mĕ-toks′ĕ-nĭ). Adoption of a new host in each cycle by a parasite having 2 cycles of existence. Syn: *heterecism.*

metra (mē′tra). The uterus.

metralgia (me-tral′jĭ-ă). Pain in the uterus.

metranemia (met-ră-nē′mĭ-ă). Local uterine anemia.

metranoikter (met-ră-nō-ĭk′ter). Instrument for dilating cervix uteri by means of 2 or 4 spring blades when a wide, prolonged dilation is necessary.

metrapectic (met-ră-pek′tĭk). Denoting a disease that is transmitted by the mother, who herself is unaffected by it.

metratome (met′ră-tōm). Instrument for incising the uterus.

metratomy (mĕt-răt′ō-mĭ). Surgical incision of the uterus. Syn: *metrotomy.*

metratonia (mĕ-tra-to′nĭ-ă). Uterine atony occurring after childbirth.

metratrophia (met-ra-tro′fĭ-ă). Atrophy of the uterus.

metrauxe (me-trawk′se). Hypertrophy of the uterus.

metrazol (met′ră-zōl). Pentamethylene tetrazol, cardiazol. A white powder, chemically neutral substance.

   Dosage: 1½ gr. (0.1 Gm.) orally or subcutaneously.

metre (mē′ter). Meter, *q.v.*

metrechoscopy (mĕt-rĕk-os′kō-pĭ). Mensuration and auscultation combined with inspection.

metrectasia (mĕt-rĕk-tā′zĭ-ă). Uterine dilatation.

metrectomy (mē-trek′to-mĭ). Surgical removal of the uterus. Syn: *hysterectomy.*

metrectopia (met-rek-to′pĭ-ă). Displacement of the uterus.

metrelcosis (mĕt-rĕl-kō′sĭs). Uterine ulceration.

metreurynter (met-rū-rin′ter). An inflatable bag which is inserted in the os uteri and distended to dilate the cervix.

metreurysis (me-trū′rĭ-sĭs). Dilatation of cervix uteri with the metreurynter.

met′ric sys′tem. One based upon the meter (39.371 inches) as the unit of measurement; the gram (15.432 gr.) the unit of weight; the liter (1.056 qt. liquid, or 0.908 qt. dry measure) as the unit of volume.

CONVERSION RULES: To change grams to grains multiply by 15, or divide by 0.064. To change grains to grams divide by 15, or multiply by 0.064. To change grams to ounces divide by 30. To change ounces to grams or cc. multiply by 30. SEE: *avoirdupois, household measures, Troy weight.*

metritis (me-trī'tis). Inflammation of the uterine musculature accompanied by an extensive increase in fibrous tissue.

metro-. 1. Combining form (*metron*) meaning rel. to measure or measurements. 2. From *metra,* the *uterus,* meaning *rel. to the uterus.*

metrocarcinoma (mĕt″rō-kăr-sĭ-nō'mă). Uterine carcinoma.

metrocele (met'rō-sēl). Uterine hernia.

metroclyst (met'ro-klĭst). Device for douching the uterus.

metrocolpocele (met″rō-kol'pō-sēl). Protrusion of uterus into the vagina which pushes the vaginal wall downward.

metrocystosis (met″rō-sĭs-tō'sĭs). Formation of uterine cysts.

metrocyte (me'trō-sīt). A mother cell.

metrodynia (met-rō-din'ĭ-ă). Uterine pain.

metrofibroma (me-trō-fī-brō'mă). Uterine fibroma.

metromalacosis (me″trō-mal-ă-kō'sĭs). Malacia or softening of uterine tissues.

metroma′nia. 1. Nymphomania. Insanity caused by uterine disease.
2. Insanity characterized by continuous writing of verses.

metroneuria (me-trō-nū'rĭ-ă). A uterine nervous affection.

metronome (met'ro-nōm). Apparatus for recording intervals or periods of time.

metroparalysis (met″rō-pă-ral'ĭ-sĭs). Uterine paralysis.

metropath′ia haemorrhag′ica. Condition of the uterus characterized by hemorrhage, usually accompanied by hypertrophy of the uterine mucous membranes and ovarian cystic disease. SEE: *fibrosis uteri.*

metropathic (me-tro-path'ĭk). Pert. to or caused by uterine disorders.

metropathy (me-trop'ă-thĭ). Any uterine disease.

metroperitonitis (me″trō-per-ĭ-tō-nī'tĭs). Inflamed condition of uterus and peritoneum.

metrophlebitis (me″trō-flē-bī'tĭs). Inflamed condition of uterine veins.

metroptosis (met-rop-tō'sĭs). Dropping of the uterus.

metrorrhagia (met-ror-ra'jĭ-ă). Bleeding from the uterus, esp. at any time other than during the menstrual period.

metrorrhea (met-ror-rē'ă). Any morbid discharge from the uterus.

metrorrhexis (met-ror-reks'is). A uterine rupture.

metrorthosis (me-tror-thō'sĭs). Correction of uterine displacement.

metrosalpingitis (met-rō-săl-pĭn-jī'tĭs). Inflamed condition of uterus and oviducts.

metroscope (met'ro-skōp). Instrument for examining the uterus.

metrostaxis (me-tro-stak'sĭs). Persistent but slight hemorrhage from the uterus.

metrostenosis (me-trō-stĕn-ō'sĭs). Contraction of the uterine cavity.

metrosteresis (me-trō-ster-ē'sĭs). Removal of the uterus. SYN: *hysterectomy, metrectomy.*

metrother′apy. Treatment of a condition by measurement, as in restoration of joint function following injury, measuring the angle of joint motion and recording the progress, has a psychologic effect on patient.

metrotome (mē'trō-tōm). Instrument used in incising the uterus.

metrotomy (me-trot'ō-mĭ). Incision of the uterus. SYN: *hysterotomy.*

metrourethrotome (met-ro-u-re'thrō-tōm). Device for incising the urethra and measuring depth to be incised.

metrypercinesis (met″ri-per-sin-ē'sis). Excessive contraction of the uterus causing abnormal labor pains.

metycaine (met'ĭ-ka″ĭn). A white crystalline substance formerly known as neothesin.
DOSAGE: As an application to the eye, 2% solution recommended; for infiltration, use ½-1%.

Meynert's commis′sure (mi′nerts). Fibrous tract extending from subthalamic body to base of 3rd ventricle.

M. F. D. Abbr. for *minimum fatal dose.*

Mg. Symb. for *magnesium.*

mg. Symb. for *milligram.*

miasm, miasma (mī′azm, mī-az′mă). A foul emanation or odor.

miasmatic (mī-az-mat′ĭk). Pert. to miasm.

mication (mi-ka′shun). 1. Rapid winking that is involuntary. 2. A quick motion.

micella (mī-sēl′ă). One of the ultramicroscopic units of organized bodies. SYN: *bioblast, tagma.*

mick′ey finn. Slang term for an alcoholic drink which is tampered with voluntarily, in order to produce ill effects in the drinker, as acute nausea or diarrhea. SEE: *knockout drops.*

micrencephalon (mĭk-rĕn-sef′ă-lon). 1. Cerebellum. 2. Smallness of brain; cretinism.

micrencephalous (mi-kren-sef′al-ŭs). Possessing a small brain.

micro-, micr-. Combining forms denoting *small size* or *extent.*

microaerophilic (mī″krō-a-er-ō-fil′ĭk). Growing at low oxygen tension.

mi″croanal′ysis. Analytical examination of tiny granules.

microbe (mī′krōb). 1. A minute one-celled form of life not distinguishable as to its vegetable or animal nature. 2. Bacteria, germs producing fermentation, putrefaction and disease; microörganism.

microbemia (mī-krō-bē′mĭ-ă). Diseased condition caused by presence of microorganisms in the blood. SYN: *microbiohemia.*

microbian (mī-krō′bĭ-an). Rel. to a microbe. SYN: *microbic.*

microbic (mī-krōb′ĭk). Concerning microbes. SYN: *microbian.*

microbicidal (mī-krōb-ĭs-ī′dal). Destructive to microbes.

microbicide (mī-krŏb′ĭs-īd). An agent which is destructive to microbes.

microbiohemia (mī″krŏb-ĭ-ō-hē′mĭ-ă). A condition resulting from microbes in the blood. SYN: *microbemia.*

microbiology (mī″krō-bī-ol′ō-jĭ). Scientific study of microbes.

microbiophobia (mī″krō-bī-ō-fō′bī-ă). An abnormal fear of microbes. SYN: *microphobia.* [microbes.

microbism (mī′krŏb-ĭzm). Infection with

microbioscope (mī-kro-bĭ′ō-skōp). Form of microscope for studying changes in living tissue.

microbiotic (mī-krō-bī-ot′ĭk). Of microbic life, or origin.

microblast (mī′krō-blăst). Minute red blood corpuscle. SYN: *microcyte.*

microblepharism, microblephary (mī-krō-blef′ar-izm, -ar-ĭ). Condition of having abnormally small eyelids.

microcalory (mī″krō-kal′ō-rĭ). A unit of heat, the amount required to raise the temperature of 1 cc. of distilled water from 0° to 1° C.

microcardia (mī″krō-kar′dĭ-ă). Unusually small heart.

microcaulia (mī″krō-kaw′lĭ-ă). Unusually small size of penis.

microcentrum (mī-krō-sĕn′trum). 1. A small nucleus. SYN: *micronucleus.* 2. Motor or dynamic center of a cell.

microcepha′lia. Abnormal smallness of the head.

microcephalic (mī-krō-sef-al′ĭk). Having or pert. to a small head; one below 1350 cc. capacity.

microcephalous (mī-kro-sef′al-us). Having an abnormally small head.

microcephalus (mik-rō-sef′a-lŭs). 1. Person with an exceptionally small head, esp. an idiot. 2. Fetus with a very small head.

microcephaly, microcephalism (mī-krō-sef′ă-lĭ, -lĭzm). Abnormal smallness of head often seen in idiocy; it is congenital.

microchemistry (mī-krō-kem′ĭs-trĭ). Chemical work in which the aid of the microscope is required.

Micrococcus (mī″krō-kŏk′ŭs). 1. A small coccus. 2. A genus of the Schizomycetes, of the family *Coccaceae.*

   M. a′cidi lactici. Micrococcus in milk; cause of lactic acid fermentation.

   M. ascofor′mans. Micrococcus occurring in bothriomycosis.

   M. bucca′lis. Nonpathogenic organism found in the mouth.

   M. capillo′rum. One of the scalp affecting color of hair.

   M. catarrha′lis. *Neisseria catarrhalis.*

   M. cereus. A species sometimes seen in pus; nonpathogenic.

   M. cit′reus. Micrococcus found in osteomyelitis and in water.

   M. endocardi′tidis ruga′tus. Form seen in ulcerative endocarditis.

   M. fla′vus conjuncti′vae. Form found in the conjunctiva.

   M. foetidus. Form found in caries and fetid cases of pharyngitis.

   M. gelatino′sus. Form found in milk.

   M. gingi′vae pyogenes. Nonmotile Micrococcus in alveolar abscess.

   M. gonorrhoeae. *Neisseria gonorrhoeae.*

   M. intracellularis meningitidis. *Diplococcus intracellularis.*

   M. lanceolatus. *Diplococcus pneumoniae.*

   M. liquefa′ciens conjuncti′vae. Seen in normal human conjunctiva.

   M. loewenber′gii. Seen in nose in ozena.

   M. melitensis. Cause of Malta fever.

   M. mucilaginosus. Cause of slimy milk.

   M. nasa′lis. Found in nasopharynx.

   M. neofor′mans. Found in various tumors.

   M. of osteomyelitis. Pathogenic in osteomyelitis.

   M. pasteu′ri. Found in saliva.

   m., pathogenic. Any micrococcus producing disease.

   M. pyo′genes ten′uis. Found in large abscesses.

   M. restit′uens. Converts peptone into albumin.

   M. rosenbach′ii. Derived from pus of abscesses.

   M. ro′seus. Found in sputum of influenza.

   M. saliva′rius sep′ticus. Found in sputum of puerperal septicemia.

   M. tetragenus. A species in sputum and walls of cavities in the lung.

   M. urea. A micrococcus decomposing urea into ammonia.

   M. urinal′bus. Found in urine in cystitis and pyelonephritis.

   M. vir′idis flaves′cens. Seen in lymph of varicella.

   M. xanthogen′icus. Seen in yellow fever.

   m., zymogenic, zymogenous. Any micrococcus causing fermentation.

microcor′nea. Abnormally small cornea.

microcoulomb (mī-krō-kū′lōm). One-millionth part of a coulomb.

microcrith (mī′kro-krith). Unit of weight equal to 1 atom of hydrogen.

microcrystalline (mī-krō-kris′tal-īn). Composed of microscopic crystals.

microcyst (mī′krō-sĭst). A very small cyst.

microcytase (mī-krō-sī′tās). Cytase acting on bacteria and formed by leukocytes.

mi′crocyte. 1. A small multinuclear leukocyte from 3½-6 microns in diameter. 2. Degenerating, small, nonnucleated, red blood corpuscle.

microcythemia (mī″krō-sī-the′mĭ-ă). Abnormally small erythrocytes in the blood.

microdactylia (mī″krō-dak-til′ĭ-ă). Abnormal smallness of the digits.

microdissection (mī″krō-dĭ-sek′shŭn). Dissection with aid of the microscope.

microdont (mī′krō-dont). Possessing very small teeth.

microdontism (mī-krō-don′tĭzm). Unusual smallness of the teeth.

microfarad (mī-krō-far′ăd). One-millionth

of a farad which is the capacity of a condenser which, when charged with 1 coulomb, gives a difference of potential of 1 volt.

microgamete (mī-krō-gam′ĕt). Male element in conjugation of protozoa.

microgametocyte (mī-krō-gam-ē′tō-sīt). Mother cell of the microgamete.

microgastria (mī-krō-gas′trĭ-ă). Unusual smallness of the stomach.

microgenitalism (mī″krō-jĕn′ĭt-ăl-ĭzm). Abnormal smallness of the external genitals.

microglia (mī-krog′lĭ-ă). Neuroglia tissue probably derived from the mesoderm, forming a portion of the adventitial structure of the central nervous system.

microgliacyte (mī″krō-glĭ′ă-sīt). Embryonic cell of a neuroglia.

microglos′sia. Small size of the tongue.

micrognathia (mī-krog-nā′thĭ-ă). Abnormal smallness of jaws.

microgram (mī′krō-gram). One-millionth part of a gram.

micrograph (mī′krō-graf). Apparatus for magnifying and recording minute movements.

micrography (mī-krog′ră-fĭ). 1. Study of physical appearance and characteristics of microbes. 2. Very minute writing, engraving, etc.

microgyria (mī-krō-jir′ĭ-ă). Smallness of cerebral convolutions.

microhepatia (mī-krō-hĕ-pat′ĭ-ă). Abnormally small size of the liver.

microhistology (mī-krō-his-tol′ō-jĭ). Histology with aid of a microscope.

microhm (mī′krōm). One-millionth of an ohm.

mi′croleuk′oblast. A nongranular bone marrow cell. SYN: *myeloblast.*

microliter (mī′krō-lē-ter). One-millionth part of a liter.

microlith (mī′krō-lith). A very tiny calculus.

microlithiasis (mī″krō-lĭ-thī′ă-sĭs). The development of very minute calculi.

micrology (mī-krol′ō-jĭ). Science of microscopic investigations.

microlymphoidocyte (mī″krō-lĭm-foid′ō-sīt). An immature, tiny lymphoidocyte.

micromania (mī-krō-mā′nĭ-ă). A delusion that one has become small or infantile or insignificant.

micromazia (mī-krō-mā′zĭ-ă). Abnormally small size of the breasts.

micrometer (mi-krom′et-er). Device for making microscopic measurements.

micromillimeter (mī-krō-mil′ĭ-mē-ter). One-millionth part of a millimeter. SYN: *micron.*

micromyces (mī-krom′ĭ-sēs) (pl. *micromycetes*). Minute fungus.

micromyelia (mī-krō-mī-ē′lĭ-ă). Abnormally small size of spinal cord.

micromyeloblast (mī-krō-mī′el-ō-blast). A nongranular bone marrow cell. SYN: *myeloblast.*

micron (mī′kron). SYMB: μ. The millionth part of a meter; the thousandth part of a millimeter; about 1/25,000 part of an inch.

microne (mī′krōn). A colloid particle that is distinguishable with the microscope.

micronucleus (mī-krō-nū′klē-us) (pl. *micronuclei*). 1. A small nucleus. 2. The smaller of the 2 nuclei of infusoria considered as containing the inheritable germ substance.

microörganism (mi-kro-or′gan-izm). Minute living body not perceptible to the naked eye, esp. a bacterium or protozoon.

micropathology (mī″krō-path-ol′ō-jĭ). Study of microörganismal diseases and their cell and tissue changes.

microphage, microphagus (mi′kro-fāj, -krof′ag-us). A small phagocyte; polymorphonuclear leukocyte; most active in attacking bacteria.

microphakia (mī″krō-fā′kĭ-ă). Abnormally small lens.

microphallus (mī-krō-fal′us). Abnormally small size of penis. SYN: *microcaulia.*

microphobia (mī-krō-fō′bĭ-ă). Psychopathic fear of microbes. SYN: *microbiophobia.*

microphone (mi′kro-fōn). Device for augmenting sound.

microphonia (mī-krō-fō′nĭ-ă). Weakness of voice.

microphonoscope (mī-krō-fō′nō-skōp). Form of biaural stethoscope for augmenting the sound.

microphotograph (mī″krō-fō′tō-graf). A photograph of microscopic substance, or substance viewed under a microscope. SYN: *photomicrograph.*

microphthalmia (mi-krof-thal′mĭ-ă). Abnormally small size of eyes.

microphthalmus (mī-krŏf-thal′mus). 1. Person with unusually small eyes. 2. Condition characterized by abnormally small eyes.

microphysics (mī-krō-fīz′ĭks). The branch of science dealing with the forces controlling ultimate structure of matter.

microphyte (mī′krō-fīt). Any microscopic plant, esp. if parasitic.

micropia (mi-kro′pĭ-ă). A condition in which objects seem diminished in size. SYN: *micropsia.*

micropodia (mī-krō-pō′dĭ-ă). Unusually small size of the feet

micropsia (mi-krop′sĭ-ă). Condition in which objects seem smaller than they usually are.

Seen in paralysis of accommodation, retinitis and choroiditis. SYN: *micropia.*

micropus (mī-krō′pus). One with unusually small feet.

micropyle (mi′kro-pīl). The opening in the ovum for entrance of the spermatozoon.

microscope (mī′krō-skōp). Instrument which greatly magnifies very minute objects.   [eyes.

   m., binocular. Microscope for both

   m., compound. One with 2 or more lenses or lens systems for use in observing the minutest bodies.

   m., simple. One with a simple or single lens.

microscopic, microscopical (mī-krō-skop'-ik, -ĭ-kal). 1. Pert. to the microscope. 2. Visible only by using the microscope.

microscopy (mī-krŏs'kōp-ĭ). Inspection with the microscope.

microseme (mi'krō-sēm). Possessing an orbital index less than 83.

microsoma (mi-kro-so'mă). 1. Chromatin granule of the cell nucleus. 2. Unusually small stature.

microsome (mi'krō-sōm). 1. Very minute granule in protoplasm. 2. Corpuscle.

microsomia (mi-kro-so'mĭ-ă). Abnormally small size of body.

microspectroscope (mi-kro-spek'trō-skōp). A combined spectroscope and microscope.

microsphygmia, microsphyxia (mi-kro-sfĭg'-mĭ-ă, -sfĭks'ĭ-ă). Smallness of the pulse.

microsplenia (mī-krō-splē'nĭ-ă). Abnormal smallness of the spleen.

Microsporon (mĭk-ros'por-on). A minute genus of fungi that may cause disease of the skin, hair, or nails.

  M. audouini. Species that causes head ringworm or *tinea tonsurans.*

microstat (mĭk'rō-stăt). The microscope's stage and finder.

microstomia (mī-krō-stō'mĭ-ă). Unusual smallness of the mouth.

microtia (mi-kro'shĭ-ă). Unusually small size of the auricle or external ear.

microtome (mi'kro-tōm). Instrument for preparing thin sections for microscope.

microtomy (mi-krot'o-mĭ). The process of cutting into sections.

microvolt (mi'krō-volt). One-millionth part of a volt.

microzyme (mi'krō-zīm). A microörganism causing fermentation.

micturate (mĭk'tū-rāt). To pass the urine. SYN: *urinate.*

micturition (mĭk-tū-rĭ'shŭn). The voiding of urine. SYN: *urination.*

mid'brain. The corpora quadrigemina, the crura cerebri and aqueduct of Sylvius which connect the pons and cerebellum with the hemispheres of the cerebrum. SYN: *mesencephalon, q.v.*

midgut (mid'gut). Embryonic source of liver, duodenum, pancreas, jejunum, and ileum.

midriff (mid'rĭf). The diaphragm.

mid'wife. A female who practices the art of aiding in the delivery of children.

midwifery (mid-wĭf'er-ĭ). The art of assisting at childbirth. SYN: *obstetrics.*

migraine (mi'grān). Periodic pain in 1 side of the head, principally along the course of the 5th cranial nerve, accompanied by disordered vision, nausea, languor, and chill.

migration (mī-grā'shun). Passage of cells, etc., from 1 position to another; *physiological,* as the migration of an ovum from the ovary into the fallopian tube, or *pathological,* as migration of leukocytes through the wall of a blood vessel into surrounding tissues.

  m., external, of the ovum. The entrance of an ovum into the oviduct of the opposite ovary.

  m., e., of the semen. Passage of semen from 1 oviduct to the opposite ovary.

  m., internal, of the ovum. Passage of an ovum (after going through the uterine horn on same side as its ovary) into the opp. horn of a *uterus bilocularis.*

  m. of the testicle. Descent of testicle into the scrotum. SYN: *descensus testis.*

  m. of white blood corpuscles. Passage of white blood corpuscles through walls of capillaries during acute inflammation.

migratory (mi'gră-tō-rĭ). 1. Pert. to migrate. 2. Changing or capable of changing positions. [*micro-*

mikro-. For words commencing thus, see

Mikulicz's disease (mĭk'ū-lĭts). Chronic hypertrophic enlargement of lacrimal and salivary glands.

  M. drain. A method for draining the abdominal cavity after operating.

  M.'s law. Patients with hemoglobin below 30% must not be given a general anesthetic.

  M.'s mask. Gauze-covered frame worn over nose and mouth during performance of operation.

  M.'s pad. Folded gauze pad for packing off the viscera in abdominal operations and used as a sponge in general.

  M.'s syndrome. Characteristics of Mikulicz's disease appearing as a complication of another disease.

mil. One-thousandth part of an inch or liter; equivalent to a cubic centimeter.

mil'dew. A parasitic fungus, and plant disease produced by it.

Miles' operation. One for carcinoma of the rectum.

miliaria (mil-ĭ-a'rĭ-ă). A form of vesicles due to obstruction of the sweat glands. Acute inflammation of the sweat glands.

  m. crystallina. Form with vesicles opaque and white.

  m. rubra. Same as miliaria crystallina with the addition of inflammation, lesions being on a slightly inflamed base. SYN: *lichen tropicus, prickly heat.*

miliary (mil'ĭ-ă-rĭ). Resembling millet seed.

  m. fever. An infectious disease accompanied by fever.

  m. tubercles. Small gray nodules in first stage of tuberculosis.

  m. tuberculosis. Acute, generalized tuberculosis with minute tubercles in the affected part or organ.

milieu (mēl-yew'). Environment.

milium (mĭl'ĭ-ŭm). Small pink and white nodule below the epidermis, caused by clogged sebaceous glands.

  m., colloid. Tiny papule formed beneath the epidermis due to colloid degeneration.

milk. A secretion of the mammary glands, density about 1.032, for feeding the young.

  m., acidophilus. Milk or soy bean oil inoculated with *B. acidophilus.*

  m., bacillary. Milk fermented by a *Lactobacillus.*

m., blue. Milk altered by the *B. cyanogenes.*

m., butter-. That left after removal of butter following churning.

m., casein. Milk prepared with a large quantity of casein and fat, but little sugar and salts.

m., certified. That certified by a Board of Health as pure.

m., condensed. Partly evaporated and sweetened milk.

m., diabetic. Milk with small amt. of lactose.

m. ferment. A diastatic ferment found in milk.

m., homog'enized. Milk with fats combined with the body of the milk.

m., lactobacillary. Milk with cultures of lactic acid bacteria.

m. leg. Acute edema of the leg. SYN: *phlegmasia alba dolens, q.v.*

m. of magnesia. Magnesium hydroxide in permanent suspension.

m., modified. Water and lactose mixed with cream of cow's milk.

m., mother's. That from the mammary glands of a woman. The protein, fat, carbohydrate, and mineral salts are exactly balanced to promote growth of the infant.

m., pasteurized. Milk heated for 30 minutes at 140 or 158° F. (60 or 70° C.) to kill the living bacteria. SEE: *pasteurization.*

m., peptonized. Milk partly digested with pepsin and hydrochloric acid, or pancreatic extract and sodium bicarbonate.

m. poisoning. SYM: Headache, vertigo, thirst, vomiting, indigestion, diarrhea, frequently skin eruptions, and possible collapse are the usual symptoms.

m., protein. Milk with high protein and low carbohydrate and fat content.

m., ropy. That which has become viscid.

m. sickness. Disease of cattle and sheep transmitted to man through milk and butter, characterized by vomiting, pain, constipation, and muscular tremors. SYN: *slows, trembles.*

m., skimmed. Milk after removal of cream.

m., sour. Milk with lactic acid caused by lactic acid bacteria.

m., sterilized. Milk boiled to kill bacteria.

m., sugar of. Lactose.

m. teeth. First or deciduous teeth.

m. tumor. Retention of milk in mammary gland.

m., uterine. White, milklike substance in the gravid uterus bet. villi of the placenta.

m., uviol. Milk sterilized by ultraviolet rays.

m., vegetable. The latex of plants.

m., witch's. 1. Colostrumlike fluid in mammary gland of a newborn child due to slight inflammations. 2. Milk secreted by the human male at birth and puberty.

milk'pox. Modified form of smallpox prevalent in South Africa. Called *alastrim* in America. SEE: *amaas.*

milli-. Prefix meaning *a thousandth part.*

milliam'meter. Ammeter registering in milliamperes. SEE: *ammeter.*

milliampere (mil''e-ahm-pair'). P.T. One one-thousandth of an ampere.

m. minute. An electrical unit of quantity, equivalent to that delivered by 1 milliampere in 1 minute.

millicurie (mil''ĭ-ku're). P.T. One-thousandth of a curie.

m.'s destroyed. A unit of the quantity of radiation furnished by a tube of radon. One millicurie in decaying gives 133.3 millicurie hours of radiation.

m. hour. A practical unit of dosage for radon. One millicurie of radon applied for 1 hour. The biologic effect depends on time, filtration, distance.

milligram (mil'ĭ-gram). One-thousandth of a gram.

milliliter (mil'ĭ-le-ter). One-thousandth of a liter. SYN: *1 cc.*

millimeter (mil'ĭ-mĕt-er). One-thousandth of a meter.

millimicron (mil-i-mi'kron). One-thousandth of a micron; one-millionth of a millimeter. SYMB: mμ.

mime'sis. Simulation of an organic disease, esp. of one that simulates another; most appropriately used of hysteria.

mimetic, mimic (mi-met'ĭk, mĭm'ĭk). Imitative.

m. convulsion. Facial convulsion.

m. labor. False labor.

m. spasm. Spasm of facial muscles.

min. Abbr. for *minim.*

mind (mīnd). Integration of functions of the brain resulting in intelligence.

No conclusive scientific definition of mind has yet been given.

m. blindness. A condition in which one does not recognize what is seen due to a brain lesion. A form of aphasia.

m. deafness. Inability to comprehend what is heard. A form of aphasia.

mineral (mĭn'er-ăl). 1. A chemical element or compound occurring in nature as a product of inorganic processes. 2. One of the 3 classifications of matter, the others being animal and vegetable.

m. elements. The human body is composed of the following chemical elements: Oxygen, 65%; carbon, 18%; hydrogen, 10%; nitrogen, 3.0%; calcium, 1.5%; phosphorus, 1.0%; potassium, 0.35%; sulfur, 0.15%; chlorine, 0.15%; magnesium, 0.05%; iron, 0.04%; iodine, 0.00004%, with traces of copper, manganese, zinc, fluorine, silicon, cobalt, aluminum, arsenic, and nickel. In the body they are found in the bones, teeth, nails, hair, tissues, fluids, and some of the body organs.

m. oil. Petroleum.

m. water. Water charged with inorganic salts.

minim (min'ĭm). One-sixtieth part of a fluidram. SYN: *drop.*

minimal (min'ĭ-mal). Least.

m. dose. Smallest dose producing an effect.

minimum (min'ĭ-mum). Least quantity or lowest limit. SEE: *threshold.*

m. lethal dose. Smallest quantity of a substance producing death.

m. wave length. The shortest wave length in a roentgen ray or gamma ray spectrum. It is definitely related to the maximum voltage applied to the roentgen ray tube in accordance with the Planck-Einstein quantum equation.

Minin light (min'ĭn). A lamp for the administration of violet and ultraviolet light, producing local anesthesia.

minor (mī'nor). Less important.

Minot-Murphy diet (mī'nŏt). Diet for pernicious anemia containing large quantities of liver.

minuthesis (min″ū-thē′sĭs). 1. Decrease in specific sensitivity resulting from continual stimulation to a sense organ; sense organ fatigue. 2. Decrease in symptoms of a disease. SYN: *miosis.*

miocardia (mī-ō-kar′dĭ-ă). Systolic lessening of heart's volume. SYN: *systole.*

mionectic (mī-ō-nek′tik). Pert. to having or using a subnormal amount of oxygen, esp. blood. SEE: *mesectic, pleonectic.*

mioplas′mia. Abnormal lessening of the amount of blood plasma.

miopragia (mī-ō-prā′jĭ-ă). Decrease of functional power.

miosis (mī-ō′sĭs). 1. Abnormal contraction of pupils. 2. Period of diminishing symptoms in a disease. 3. Reduction phase in chromosome development.

miot′ic. 1. An agent that causes the pupil to contract, such as eserine and pilocarpine. 2. Pert. to or causing contraction of the pupil. 3. Diminishing. 4. Pert. to chromosome reduction.

mire (mīr). OPHTH: An object used as a test, the images of which denote the amount of astigmatism.

mirror drill. Exercises before a mirror practicing control of convulsive tics.

m. speech. That which reverses the order of words in a sentence or pronounces words backward. SEE: *lalopathy.*

m. writing. Writing in which the words are reversed, as seen in a mirror.

mis-. Prefix implying *not, bad, wrong, improper,* etc.

miscar′riage. A term used synonymously with *abortion,* and referring to the interruption of pregnancy prior to the 7th month.

misce (mĭs′e). Abbr. **M.** Mix. A direction to the pharmacist placed upon a prescription for mixing the preparation.

miscegenation (mis″ej-en-a′shun). Sex relations or marriage bet. those of different races. [mixed.

miscible (mĭs′ĭ-bl). Capable of being

misemission (mĭs″ē-mĭs′shun). Failure of seminal emission in coitus.

misocainia (mis-o-ki′nĭ-ă). An aversion to new ideas. SYN: *misoneism.*

misog′amy. Abnormal aversion to marriage.

misogyny (mĭs-oj′ĭn-ĭ). Abnormal hatred of women.

misologia (mis-o-lo′jĭ-ă). Aversion to mental work.

misoneism (mĭ-sō-nē′izm). Aversion to new things or new ideas; conservatism.

misopedia (mĭ-sō-pe′dĭ-ă). Abnormal dislike for children or the young.

misophobia (mis-ō-fō′bĭ-ă). Morbid fear or dread of contamination or filth.

Mist, mist. Abbr. for *mistura, q.v.*

mistura (mĭs-tū′ră). Preparation intended for internal use, and containing suspended insoluble substances which do not unite chemically.

Should always be shaken before using. There are 2 official mixtures.

mite (mīt). A minute arachnid, a member of the order Acarina.

mithridatism (mĭth′rĭ-dăt″ĭzm). Immunity to a poison acquired by taking it in doses of increasing size.

mitigated (mit′ĭ-gāt-ed). Diminished in severity. SYN: *allayed, moderated.*

mitochondria (mĭt″ō-kon′drĭ-ă). Granular and filamentous structures in cell cytoplasm.

mito′ma, mi′tome. A fine network support or framework of protoplasm in a cell.

mitosin (mĭt′ō-sĭn). A hormone aiding in mitosis or maturation of follicles.

mito′sis (pl. *mitosēs*). Indirect nuclear division; the usual process of cell reproduction.

mitosome (mī′tō-sōm). 1. A body giving rise to the middle piece of the spermatozoon. 2. Chromatin mass in a cellular nucleus.

mitotic (mī-tot′ĭk). Pert. to mitosis.

mitral (mī′tral). Pert. to the bicuspid or mitral valve. SEE: *facies, mital.*

m. disease. That of the mitral valve. SEE: *heart.*

m. murmur. One produced at the mitral valve.

m. orifice. Left auriculoventricular aperture.

m. regurgitation. Due to failure of valve to close completely, allowing blood to flow back into the auricle.

m. stenosis. Narrowing orifice of the valve obstructing free flow from auricle to ventricle.

m. valve. Valve bet. left auricle and left ventricle. SYN: *bicuspidalis, valvula.*

mittelschmerz (mit′el-shmărts). Pain bet. menstrual periods.

mit′tor. A neuron terminal which transmits impulses to ceptors of the adjoining neuron.

mixed (mikst). Consisting of 2 or more intermingling substances.

m. diet. One consisting of all the food elements in proper proportion. There is no scientific validity to the theory that carbohydrates and proteins should not be eaten together. Over 6000 determinations have been made which proved that the acid response to carbohydrates, to proteins, and to both taken together, is the same and that a mixed diet does not interfere with gastric secretions or with any of the digestive functions. The presence of protein seems to prolong carbohydrate assimilation.

m. nerves. The spinal nerves containing sensory or afferent, and motor or efferent fibers.

mixture (mĭks'tŭr). A combination of 2 or more substances without chemical union. SEE: *mistura.*

mm. Abbr. for *millimeter.*

mmm. Abbr. for *micromillimeter.*

Mn. Symb. for *manganese.*

mnemic (nē'mĭk). Relating to memory.

m. hypothesis or **theory.** Stimuli leave engrams (definite traces) on protoplasm, which when frequently repeated set up a habit which persists after the stimuli cease; these engrams possibly may be transmitted to descendants. SYN: *mnemism.* [*q.v.*]

mnemism (nē'mĭzm). Mnemic hypothesis,

mnemonics (nē-mon'ĭks). The art of memory culture.

mobile (mo'bĭl). Movable.

m. spasm. Tonic spasm with irregular, slow movements of limbs following hemiplegia.

mobility (mō-bĭl'ĭ-tĭ). State or quality of being mobile; facility of movement.

mobilization (mo''bĭl-ĭ-zā'shŭn). 1. The making of a fixed or ankylosed part movable. 2. Restoration of motion to a joint.

mobilize (mō'bĭl-īz). 1. To incite to physiological action. 2. To render movable; to put in movement.

modal (mōd'al). Pert. to form without reference to substance.

modal'ity. 1. Quality of being modal. 2. A method of application or the employment of any therapeutic agent; limited usually to physical agents. The word is avoided by scholarly writers. 3. Any state that modifies the action of a drug. 4. PSY: Whole character of stimuli or sensations determined by the class to which they belong.

mode (mōd). Any class occurring most frequently; a series of variables. SEE: *mean, median.*

modiolus (mō-dī'ō-lŭs). BNA. Central pillar or axial part of cochlea extending from the base to the apex.

modulus (mod'ū-lŭs). A unit of physical effects, as a *calorific unit.*

modus (mo'dus). A method or a mode.

m. operandi. Method of performing an act.

Moebius' sign (mā'bĭ-ŭs). A symptom in Graves' disease in which one eye converges and the other diverges when looking at the tip of one's nose.

mogigraphia (mō-jĭ-grăf'ĭ-ă). Writers' cramp.

mogilalia (moj-ĭ-la'lĭ-ă). Any speech defect, as *stuttering.*

mogiphonia (mō-jĭ-fō'nĭ-ă). Difficulty in emitting vocal sounds due to strain.

mogitocia (moj-ĭ-tō'sĭ-ă). Difficult birth or parturition.

Mohrenheim's space (mor'en-hīm). Space bet. pectoralis major and deltoid just beneath the clavicle.

moist (moyst). Damp, wet.

m. chamber. A vessel for keeping microscopic objects moist.

mol(e (mōl). A gram-molecule, a quantity of a chemical compound whose weight in grams equals its molecular weight. Thus 18.016 Gm. of water would be 1 mol.

mo'lar. 1. Pert. to a mass; not molecular. 2. Pert. to a mole. 3. A grinding or back tooth, one of three on each side of the jaws.

m. solution. One in which there is 1 *mole* of the solute dissolved in each liter of the solution.

mold (mōld). 1. A fuzzy coating of · a fungous nature, on the surface of decaying vegetable matter. 2. A parasitic fungus causing mold. 3. A receptacle into which liquid plastic material is poured to shape it as it dries. 4. To shape a mass, as a *pill.* * 5. To shape the fetal head, adapting it to the plevic inlet.

mold'ing. 1. Shaping of the fetal head, adapting itself to pelvic inlet. 2. Manual shaping of infant's features following delivery. 3. A protective border, used in plastic surgery. 4. Casting of a reproduction.

mole (mōl). 1. A congenital discolored spot elevated above the surface of the skin. SYN: *nevus.*

2. A uterine mass arising from a poorly developed or degenerating ovum.

m., blood. A mass made up of blood clots, membranes, and placenta, retained following abortion.

m., Breus'. Malformation of the ovum, a decidual tuberous subchorional hematoma.

m., carneous. Blood mole which has assumed a fleshlike appearance, when retained in uterus for some time.

m., false. One formed from a tumor or polypus.

m., fleshy. SEE: *carneous mole.*

m., hydatid, hydatidiform. A polycystic mass in which the chorionic villi have undergone cystic degeneration.

m., stone. Calcareous degeneration in the uterus.

m., true. Mole representing the degenerated ovum itself.

m., vesicular. SEE: *hydatidiform mole.*

molecular (mō-lek'ū-lar). Pert. to a molecule.

m. layer. 1. Cortical layer of cerebellar or cerebral substance. 2. (Inner). Inner retinal plexiform layer. 3. (Outer). Outer retinal plexiform layer.

m. lesion. One not even visible through a microscope.

m. weight. Relative weight attained by totalling the weight of its constituent atoms, using the atomic weight of oxygen, 16, as a unit. SEE: *atomic weight.*

molecule (mŏl'ē-kūl). 1. The smallest quantity into which a substance may be

divided without loss of its characteristics. 2. Any small portion of a substance. 3. A chemical combination of
two or more atoms which form a specific
chemical compound; the chemical elements are formed by the combination
of atoms.

moli′men (pl. *molimina*). Effort to establish any normal function, esp. the
monthly effort to establish the menses
and disturbances experienced at the
time.

    m. climacterium virile. A neurasthe-
nia in men bet. 45-55 resulting from
change of the testicular secretion.

    m., men′strual. SEE: *molimen.*

Möllgaard treatment (mŭl′gahrd). Treatment of tuberculosis with sanocrysin
and sometimes with serum.

mollities (mol-ĭsh′ĭ-ēz). Abnormal softening of a part.

    m. ossium. Softening of the bones.
SYN: *osteomalacia.*

Moil's glands. Modified sweat glands at
border of eyelids. SYN: *ciliary glands.*

molluscous (mol-lŭs′kŭs). Concerning molluscum.

molluscum (mol-us′kum). A mildly infective skin disease characterized by tumor
formations on the skin.

    m. contagiosum. The usual mildly
contagious form of molluscum.

    m. fibrosum. A form showing masses
of fibrocellular tissue.

    m. simplex. SEE: *molluscum fibro-
sum.*

momentum (mō-měn′tum). 1. Quantity of
motion. 2. Force of motion acquired by
a moving object as a result of continuance of its motion; impetus.

mon′ad. 1. A univalent element. 2. A
unicellular organism.

monarthritis (mŏn-ar-thrī′tĭs). Arthritis
affecting a single joint.

monarticular (mŏn-ar-tĭk′ū-lăr). Concerning or affecting one joint.

monaster (mŏn-as′ter). Single starlike
figure formed in mitosis.

monathetosis (mŏn″ăth-e-tō′sĭs). Athetosis affecting a single part of the body.

Mondonesi's reflex (mon-dō-na′zĭ). Contraction of facial muscles following
pressure on eyeball.

monesthetic (mŏn-ĕs-the′ĭk). Affecting
only one of the senses.

Mongo′lian id′iocy. Congenital form with
resemblance to an Asiatic. SEE: *idiocy.*

Monil′ia. A genus of parasitic fungi or
molds.

monilethrix (mŏn-ĭl′ĕ-thrĭks). Disease in
which the hair becomes brittle and
nodulated so that it has a beaded appearance.

moniliform (mŏn-ĭl′ĭ-form). Resembling a
necklace or string of beads.

moniliosis (mŏn-ĭl-ĭ-ō′sĭs). Infection with
any species of Monilia.

mono, mon-. Prefixes: *One, single.*

monoanesthesia (mŏn-ō-ăn-ĕs-the′sĭ-ă).
Anesthesia of a single member or organ.

monobasic (mŏn-ō-bā′sĭk). Having but one
atom of hydrogen replaceable by a base.

monoblepsia (mŏn-ō-blĕp′sĭ-ă). 1. OPHTH:
Condition marked by a tendency to shut
one eye to see clearly.

    2. Color blindness in which only one
color can be seen.

monobrachius (mŏn″ō-brā′kĭ-us). 1. State
of having only one arm. 2. Fetus with
only one arm.

monobromated (mŏn″ō-brō′māt-ĕd). Pert.
to chemical compound with only one
atom of bromine in each molecule.

monocalcic (mŏn-ō-kal′sĭk). Pert. to a
chemical compound containing only one
atom of calcium in the molecule.

monocelled (mŏn′ō-sĕld). Composed of a
single cell.

monochord (mŏn′ō-kord). An instrument
for testing upper tone audition by means
of friction.

monochorea (mon″ō-kor-ē′ă). Chorea
which affects but a single part.

monochromatic (mŏn″ō-krō-măt′ĭk). 1.
Having but one color. 2. A color-blind
person to whom all colors appear to be
of one hue.

monochromator (mŏn-ō-krō′mă-tor). Instrument for selective transmission of
homogeneous radiant energy.

monococcus (mŏn-ō-kŏk′ŭs). A form of
coccus existing singly instead of as part
of the usual group or chain.

monocular (mŏn-ok′ū-lar). Concerning or
affecting but one eye.

monoculus (mŏn-ok′ū-lŭs). 1. A bandage
for shielding one eye. 2. A fetus with
only one eye.

monocyesis (mŏ-nō-sī-ē′sĭs). Average pregnancy with a single fetus.

monocyte (mŏn′ō-sīt). A large mononuclear leukocyte.

monocytic (mŏn-ō-si′tĭk). Concerning or
resembling monocytes.

monocytopenia (mŏn″ō-sīt″ō-pe′nĭ-ă). Diminished number of monocytes in the
blood.

monodactylism (mŏn-ō-dak′tĭl-ĭzm). Condition, usually congenital, of having
only one digit on a hand or foot.

monodal (mō-nod′ăl). Connected with one
terminal of a resonator so that the
patient acts as a capacitor for entrance
and exit of high frequency currents.

monodiplopia (mŏn″ō-dī-plō′pĭ-ă). Double
vision in one eye only.

monogenesis (mŏn-ō-jen′ĕ-sĭs). 1. Asexual
reproduction. SYN: *parthenogenesis.* 2.
Direct development of offspring resembling parent. 3. Theory that all living
things develop from a single cell. OPP:
polygenesis.

monogenous (mŏn-oj′en-us). Produced or
reproducing asexually.

monogerminal (mŏn-ō-jerm′ĭn-ăl). Rel. to
or developed from a single germ, as
twins.

monograph (mŏn′ō-grăf). A treatise dealing with a single subject.

monohemerous (mŏn-ō-hĕm′ĕr-ŭs). Continuing for only one day.

monohydrated (mŏn-ō-hī′drāt-ed). United
with only one molecule of water.

monoideaism, monoideism (mŏn-ō-ĭ-dē′ă-ĭzm, -dē′ĭzm). Domination by only one idea.

monolocular (mŏn″ō-lok′ū-lar). Having only 1 cell or cavity. Syn: *unilocular*.

monomania (mŏn-ō-mā′nĭ-ă). Insanity on one subject only, a term found in legal phraseology.

monoma′niac. One afflicted with monomania.

monomastigote (mŏn-ō-măs′tĭ-gōt). Possessing only one flagellum.

monomelic (mŏn-ō-mel′ĭk). Affecting a single limb.

monomeric (mŏn-ō-měr′ĭk). Consisting of, or affecting, a single piece or segment of a body.

monomicrobic (mŏn″ō-mī-krō′bĭk). Caused by one species of microbe.

monomorphic (mŏn-ō-mor′fĭk). Unchangeable in form.   [muscle.

monomyople′gia. Paralysis of only one

monomyositis (mŏn″ō-mī-ō-sī′tĭs). Inflamed condition of only one muscle.

mononeural (mŏn-ō-nū′răl). Supplied by or concerning a single nerve.

mononeuritis (mŏn″ō-nū-rī′tĭs). Inflamed condition of a single nerve.

mononuclear (mŏn-ō-nū′klē-ăr). Having one nucleus. Syn: *uninuclear*.

mononucleosis (mŏn-ō-nū-klē-ō′sĭs). Presence of more than normal number of mononuclear leukocytes in the blood.

   m. infections. Glandular fever with great increase of mononuclear leukocytes in the blood.

monoparesis (mŏn-ō-par′es-ĭs). Paralysis of a single part of body.

monoparesthesia (mŏn″ō-păr-ĕs-thē′sĭ-ă). Paresthesia of only one region or limb.

monopathy (mŏn-op′ăth-ĭ). 1. A disease attacking only one part of the body. 2. Mental suffering due to solitude or lack of sympathy.

monophagia (mŏn-ō-fā′jĭ-ă). 1. Appetite for only one kind of food. 2. The habit of eating of just one meal a day.

monophasia (mŏn-ō-fā′zĭ-ă). Inability to utter anything but one word or phrase repeatedly.

monophobia (mŏn-ō-fō′bĭ-ă). Abnormal fear of being alone.

monophyletic (mŏn″ō-fīl-ĕt′ĭk). Originating from a single source.

monoplasmatic (mŏn″ō-plăz-măt′ĭk). Composed of but one tissue or substance.

monoplast (mŏn′ō-plăst). An organism that is unicellular and which keeps the same form throughout its life.

monoplegia (mŏn-ō-plē′jĭ-ă). Paralysis of a single limb, or of one side of the face or body.

monopolar (mŏn-ō-pōl′ăr). Using 1 terminal only, the ground acting as the 2nd terminal. See: *monoterminal*.

monorchid (mŏn-or′kĭd). Person having only 1 testicle.

monorchidism, monorchism (mŏn-ôr′kĭd-ĭzm, mŏn′or-kĭzm). Condition in which there is only 1 descended testicle.

monorchis (mŏn-or′kis). A male having only 1 testicle or but 1 descended testicle.

monosaccharide (mŏn-ō-sak′ar-id). A sugar which cannot be decomposed into simpler sugars. Ex: *fructose, galactose, glucose.*

monosaccharoses (mŏn-ō-sak′ă-rōs-ĕs). A group name for *monosaccharides, q.v.* Simple sugars which cannot be split into sugars of lower molecular weight.

monosome (mŏn′ō-sōm). An accessory chromosome which, without dividing, goes into only 1 of the daughter cells.

monospasm (mŏn′ō-spazm). Spasm affecting a single part or organ.

monosymptomatic (mŏn″ō-sĭmp-tō-mat′-ĭk). Having only 1 dominant symptom.

monosyphilide (mŏn-ō-sĭf′il-ĭd). Characterized by only a single syphilitic lesion.

monoter′minal. Using 1 terminal only in the giving of treatments, the ground acting as the 2nd terminal for the completion of the electrical circuit.

monothermia (mŏn-ō-therm′ĭ-ă). Condition in which bodily temperature is stable.

Monotricha (mŏn-ot′rĭk-ă). Bacteria having a single flagellum at 1 pole.

monotrichous (mon-ot′rĭ-kus). Pert. to or having a single flagellum.

monovalent (mon-ō-va′lent). Having the combining power of a single hydrogen atom. Syn: *univalent*.

monoxide (mŏn-ŏk′sĭd). An oxide having only 1 atom of oxygen.

Monro's foramen (mŏn-rō′). Point of communication bet. 3rd and lateral ventricles of the brain.

   M.'s sulcus. Sulcus on 3rd ventricle's lateral wall from the foramen interventriculare to the aditus ad aquaeductum cerebri. Syn: *aulix*.

mons (mŏns) (pl. *montēs*). An anatomical eminence above the surface of the body.

   m. pubis. BNA. Pubic eminence. Syn: *mons Veneris*.

   m. Veneris. A pad of fatty tissue and coarse skin overlying the symphysis pubis in the woman. After puberty covered with short, curly hair called the *escutcheon.* Typically triangular in shape. See: *pubes*.

mon′ster. A malformed fetus. Syn: *teras, teratism.*   [ster.

monstripar′ity. The act of bearing a mon-

monstros′ity. 1. Monster. 2. Congenital malformation.

Montgom′ery's glands. Small prominences around the nipple of the breast which enlarge during pregnancy and lactation. See: *areola, mamma.*

monthlies (mŭnth′lēs). The menses.

monticulus (mon-tĭk′u-lus). A protuberance.

   m. cerebelli. BNA. Protuberance of the superior vermis whose ant. portion is called the *culmen,* the post. portion the *declive.*

mood (mōōd). Temporary state of mind in regard to or as result of emotion.

moogrol (moo′grōl). Ethyl chaulmoograte. An oily liquid of faint odor.

   Dosage: Intramuscularly, 1 cc. weekly.

morament (mōr-am′ent). A moron of low grade. A person who is mentally defective and without moral sense.

moramentia (mōr-ă-měn′shĭ-ă). State of being without moral sense.

Morand's disease (mor-anz′). Paresis affecting the lower extremities.

morbid (mor′bĭd). 1. Diseased. 2. Pert. to disease.

morbid′ity. 1. State of being diseased. 2. Prevalence of disease in proportion to the population of a given area.

morbific (mor-bĭf′ĭk). Causing or producing disease.

morbilli (mor-bil′ī). Measles.

mor′bus. Disease.

   m. caducus. Epilepsy.

   m. caeruleus. Cyanosis which is congenital.

   m. coxa′rius. Hip joint disease.

   m. miseriae. Condition due to neglect and want.

morcellation, morcellement (mor-sel-ā′-shŭn, -mon′). Method of removing a tumor or organ in pieces.

mordant (mor′dănt). A substance which fixes a stain or dye, as *alum* and *phenol*.

mordication (mor″dĭ-kā′shŭn). Gradual disintegration by chemical process. SYN: *corrosion*.

morgagnian (mor-gan′yē-ăn). Pert. to or described by Morgagni.

Morgagni's caruncle (mor-gan′yĕs). The middle prostatic lobe.

   M.'s cataract. One that is hypermature with a softened cortex and a hard nucleus. SEE: *cataract*.

   M.'s hy′datid. Remains of müllerian duct attached to testicle or oviduct.

   M.'s liquor. Fluid bet. lens of eye and capsule.

   M.'s ventricle. Ventriculus laryngis. SEE: *ventricle*.

morgue (morg). A public mortuary; a place for holding dead bodies before disposing of them.

moria (mo′rĭ-ă). 1. Simple dementia. 2. Foolishness.

moribund (mor′ĭ-bŭnd). In a dying condition; dying.

morioplasty (mo′rĭ-ō-plas-tĭ). Plastic surgery to restore portions of the body which have been lost through accident or disease.

morn′ing sickness. The nausea and vomiting that affect pregnant women during first few months of pregnancy, particularly in the morning.

mo′ron. A feebleminded person, not beyond the Binet age of 12, having the mentality ordinarily attained between 8 and 12; some authorities state 8 to 11 years. Of greater intelligence than an imbecile. The term implies no moral defect. SEE: *idiot, imbecile.*

moronic (mōr-on′ĭk). Feebleminded.

moronity (mōr-on′ĭ-tĭ). Feeblemindedness.

Moro's reaction or **test.** Test to determine the presence of tuberculosis, by application of an ointment of 5 cc. of old tuberculin and 5 Gm. of anhydrous wool fat to the thorax for 1 minute.

An eruption of red papules on the skin appears in 24-48 hours if tuberculosis is present.

   M.'s reflex. A variety of defensive reflexes. The throwing out of the arms in an attitude of embrace, in fearful response.

morosis (mo-rō′sĭs). The mental state of a moron. Feeblemindedness. SYN: *moronity.*

morphea (mor-fe′ă). Skin disease characterized by discrete, circumscribed, grayish or yellowish patches, firm but not hard, bordered by pinkish or purplish areolae on breasts, head, face, lower extremities, with telangiectases on the lesions.

mor′phia. Morphine, *q.v.*

morphi′na. Morphine, *q.v.*

morphine (mor′fēn). Main alkaloid found in opium, occurring in bitter, colorless crystals.

   Very satisfactory in combination with scopolamine in obstetrics.

   m. sul′fate. USP. The sulfate of an alkaloid obtained from opium and occurring as white, feathery crystals, incompatible with alkalies, tannic acid, and iodides.

   DOSAGE: 1/8-1/2 gr. (0.008-0.03 Gm.).

morphinism (mor′fĭn-ĭzm). Morbid condition due to habitual or excessive use of morphine. Morphine habit.

morphinomania, morphiomania (mor″fĭn-ō-mā′nĭ-ă, -fe-ō-mā′nĭ-ă). 1. Morbid desire for morphine. 2. Insanity resulting from use of morphine.

morphogenesis (mor″fō-jĕn′ĕ-sĭs). Stimulation of growth and development of form.

morphogenetic (mor″fō-jĕn-et′ĭk). Stimulating growth and development of form.

morphology (mor-fol′ō-jĭ). Science of external structure and form without regard to function.

morphometry (mor-fom′e-trĭ). The measurement of external portions of forms and organisms.

morphon (mor′fon). An individual elemental structure of an organism or person.

morphosis (mor-fō′sis). Formative process of an organ or part.

morphotic (mor-fot′ĭk). Pertaining to or concerning morphosis.

morpio, morpion (mor′pĭ-ō, -pĭ-on). The crab louse infesting the pubic area.

mors. Death.

mor′sus diab′oli. Fimbriae of a fallopian tube.

mor′tal. 1. Causing death. 2. Subject to death. 3. Human.

mortality (mor-tal′ĭ-tĭ). 1. State of being mortal. 2. The death rate.

mortar (mor′tar). Vessel, with a smooth interior, used for powdering or pulverizing drugs with a pestle.

mortification (mor″tĭ-fĭ-kā′shŭn). Death or failure of a tissue, organ, or part. SYN: *gangrene, necrosis.*

mortinatality (mor″tĭ-nă-tal′ĭ-tĭ). Ratio of stillbirths to normal births.

mort′ise joint. Ankle joint.

Mor′ton's disease. Neuralgia of the metatarsus.

mortuary (mor′tu-a-rĭ). 1. Temporary place for keeping dead bodies before burial. SYN: *morgue*. 2. Rel. to the dead or to death.

morula (mor′ū-lă). Solid mass of cells, resembling a mulberry, resulting from segmentation of vitellus of an ovum.

moruloid (mor′u-loid). 1. BACT: A colony made up of a mass resembling a mulberry. 2. Resembling a mulberry.

mosquito (mŏs-kē′tō). 1. A blood-sucking insect of several families, as *Anopheles, Stegomyia, Culex, Aedes*. 2. Laboratory device for withdrawing blood from a blood vessel.

mossy cell (maws′ĭ). A large neuroglia cell with multiple short processes. SEE: *neuroglia cell*.

moth′er. 1. Female parent. 2. A structure which gives rise to others.

    m. cell. A cell which, by fission or budding, gives rise to similar cells.

    m. cyst. An echinococcus cyst enveloping smaller ones.

    m. liquor. That left after removal of crystals from a solution.

    m.'s mark. A birthmark. SEE: *mark*.

    m.'s star. Single starlike figure in mitosis. SYN: *monaster*.

motile (mō′tĭl). Able to move spontaneously.

motiline (mo′tĭl-ĭn). A hormone stimulating contraction.

motility (mō-tĭl′ĭt-ĭ). Capability of moving spontaneously.

motion (mō′shun). 1. A change of place or position; movement. 2. Evacuation of the bowels. 3. (Pl.) Matter evacuated. SEE: *"cine-" words, efferent, "kine-" words, circus movements*.

    m., active. Movements caused by the patient's own intention.

    m., passive. Movements due to an attendant causing the part to be moved.

motor (mō′tor). 1. Causing motion. 2. A part or that which induces movements, as *nerves* or *muscles*.

    m. aphasia. A condition in which the patient understands but cannot express himself in words, or read aloud.

    m. area. Post. part of frontal lobe ant. to the central sulcus.

    m., electric. Apparatus for the conversion of electric energy into mechanical energy. The reverse of the dynamo.

    m. end plate. Flat expansion ending a motor nerve fiber where it connects with a muscle fiber.

    m. generator. A transforming device consisting of a motor mechanically connected to a generator.

    Such machines are designed to generate direct current when alternating alone is available, or *vice versa*.

    m. nerves. Those causing a muscle or part to move.

    m. oculi. Third cranial nerve.

    m. points. Points where the motor nerve enters the muscle, and where visible contraction can be elicited with a minimal amount of stimulation.

    m. reflex. Any reflex of motor origin; opposite of sensory reflex.

    m., universal. Motor activated by both types of current.

    m. zone. Area affected by stimulation of a motor nerve.

motorial (mō-tor′ĭ-ăl). Concerning motion or a motor center.

motoricity (mō-tor-ĭs′ĭt-ĭ). Capability of movement.

motorium (mō-tōr′ĭ-ŭm). Motor center of a body or organism.

motorius (mō-tōr′ĭ-ŭs). Any motor nerve.

    m. oculi communis. Third cranial nerve. SYN: *motor oculi*.

motorpathy (mō-tōr′păth-ĭ). Treatment of a condition by prescribed movements. SYN: *kinesitherapy, kinetotherapy*.

mottling (mŏt′lĭng). A condition which is marked by discolored areas.

moulage (moo-lahzh′). 1. A wax model or reproduction, as of a skin condition. 2. Molding of a wax model.

mould (mōld). SEE: *mold*.

moulding (mōld′ĭng). SEE: *molding*.

mounding. Lumping, as the mounding of a wasting muscle when struck a quick, firm blow.

mountain fever (mown′tĕn). 1. A short, remittent fever occurring in mountain regions. 2. SEE: *mountain sickness*. 3. Rocky Mountain spotted fever; tick fever; undulant fever.

    m. sickness. Condition characterezed by nausea, headache, increased pulse, etc., suffered by those unable to adjust themselves to high altitudes or rare atmosphere. SYN: *mareo de la Cordillera*.

mounting (mownt′ĭng). The arrangement of specimens on slides, frames, chart boards, display boards, or any background for study.

mouse unit (mows). Least amount of estrus-producing hormone which induces, in a spayed mouse, a characteristic desquamation of the vaginal epithelium.

mouth (mowth). 1. The opening of any cavity. 2. The cavity within the cheeks, containing the tongue and teeth, and communicating with the pharynx.

    m., digestion in. SEE: *salivary digestion*.

    m., examination of. Consider size, color, moisture of lips, rashes, abrasions, cysts, fissures, crusts, discoloration, odor of breath, etc. SEE: *mastication*.

movement (mōōv′měnt). 1. Act of passing from place to place or changing position of body or its parts. 2. Evacuation of feces.

    m., ameboid. Movements resembling that of the ameba by rapid projection or withdrawal from any part of the surface of a process, or change in position and form by flowing of all the protoplasm into 1 of the processes.

    m., autonomic. A spontaneous, involuntary movement, independent of ext. stimulation.

m., brownian. A peculiar rapid whirling and oscillating movement of minute particles seen under the microscope, as of the granular particles within the salivary corpuscles.

m., ciliary. That of the cilia of a ciliated cell or epithelium.

m., circus. A phenomenon in an animal after injury to 1 corpus striatum, optic thalamus, or crus cerebri, causing it to move about in a circle.

m., disorders of. May be due to injury or disease of (a) muscle, (b) nerve ending, (c) motor nerve, (d) spinal cord, or (e) of the brain.

m.'s, fetal. Muscular movements performed by the fetus in utero.

m., molecular. See: *brownian movement.*

m., pendular. Swaying movements of the intestine when exposed, due to rhythmic contractions of the circular layer of muscle.

m.'s, respiratory. All the movements caused by respiration. See: *inspiration, expiration, respiration.*

m. of restitution. A partial rotation of the fetal head, in cases of head presentation.

m., vermicular. Peristalsis.

m. vibratile. Ciliary movement.

moxa (mŏk'sa). Inflammable substance used as a cautery for the skin, or as a counterirritant.

moxibustion (mŏks-ĭ-bŭst'shŭn). Cauterization by means of a cylinder or cone of cotton wool, called a moxa, placed on the skin and fired at the top.

moxosophyra (moks-ō-sof-ĭ'rä). A hammer heated and used as a cautery.

mu (mū). A micron, 1/1000 of a millimeter or 1/25,000 of an inch.

M. u. Abbr. for Maché unit and mouse unit.

mucedin (mū'se-dĭn). A substance obtained from gluten.

Much-Holzmann reaction (mook-holts'-mahn). Inhibition of hemolysis of erythrocytes by cobra venom in manic-depressive insanity and dementia precox. Syn: *psychoreaction.*

muciferous (mū-sĭf'ĕr-ŭs). Secreting or producing mucus.

muciform (mū'sĭ-form). Appearing similar to mucus.

mucigen (mū'sĭ-jĕn). A substance in the mucous membranes that may be converted into mucin.

mucigenous (mū-sĭj'ĕn-ŭs). Producing mucus. Syn: *muciferous.*

mucilage (mū'sĭ-lăj). Vegetable preparation used in pharmaceuticals. See: *mucilagō.*

mucilaginous (mū-sĭl-aj'ĭn-ŭs). Resembling mucilage; slimy; sticky.

mucila'go. Thick, viscid, adhesive liquid, containing gum or mucilaginous principles dissolved in water, usually employed to hold insoluble substances in suspension in aqueous liquids or as a demulcent. There are 2 official mucilages.

mucin (mu'sin). 1. An albuminoid found in mucus and connective tissue, and various secretions such as saliva, bile, and the synovial fluid, formed from mucigen, and yielding a slimy solution in water.

2. A commercial preparation made from the gastric mucosa of the hog, used in the treatment of ulcers of the digestive tract.

Dosage: Daily, 80-100 Gm. (100 Gm.-1½ qt., ½ milk and cream, flavored to taste, and divided into 12 hourly doses.)

mucinemia (mū-sĭn-ē'mĭ-ă). Mucin in the blood.

mucinogen (mū-sĭn'ō-jĕn). A glycoprotein which forms mucin.

mucinoid (mū'sin-oid). Appearing similar to mucin.

mucinuria (mū-sĭn-ū'rĭ-ă). Presence of mucin in the urine.

muciparous (mū-sĭp'ăr-ŭs). Producing or secreting mucus. Syn: *muciferous, mucigenous.*

mucitis (mū-sī'tĭs). Inflammation of any mucosa.   [*to mucus.*

muco-. Combining form, *having relation*

mucocele (mū'kō-sēl). 1. Enlargement of the lacrimal sac. 2. A mucous cyst. 3. A mucous polypus.

mucocutaneous (mū″kō-kū-tā'nē-ŭs). Concerning a mucous membrane and the skin.

mucodermal (mū-kō-dĕr'măl). Pert. to a mucous membrane and the skin. Syn: *mucocutaneous.*

mucoenteritis (mū″kō-ĕn-tĕr-ī'tĭs). Inflammation of intestinal mucosa.

mucofibrous (mū-kō-fī'brŭs). Made up of mucous and fibrous tissues.

mucoglobulin (mū″kō-glŏb'ū-lĭn). Any protein group to which plastin belongs.

mucoid (mū'koyd). 1. Glycoprotein similar to mucin. 2. Muciform similar to mucus.

mucomembranous (mū″kō-mem'bran-ŭs). Composed of or rel. to mucosa. Syn: *mucosal.*

mucopurulent (mū-kō-pur'ū-lĕnt). Consisting of mucus and pus.

mucopus (mū'kō-pŭs). Mucus combined with or resembling pus.

mucor (mū'kor). 1. Animal mucus. 2. Mold. 3. (M-). A genus of mold fungi seen on dead and decaying matter.

mucoriferous (mū-kor-ĭf'ĕr-ŭs). Covered with mold or a moldlike substance.

mucorin (mū'kor-ĭn). An albuminoid substance derived from molds.

mucormycosis (mū-kor-mĭ-kō'sĭs). A fungous disease due to Mucor.

mucosa (mū-kō'să) (pl. *mucosae*). Mucous membrane.

mucosal (mū-kō'săl). Concerning any mucous membrane.

mucosanguineous (mū″kō-san-gwĭn'ē-ŭs). Containing mucus and blood.

mucosedative (mū″kō-sĕd'ă-tĭv). Soothing to mucosae of the body. Syn: *demulcent.*

mucoserous (mū″kō-sēr'ŭs). Composed of mucus and serum.

mucosin (mū'kō-sĭn). Mucin found in thick, sticky mucus.

mucous (mū'kŭs). Having the nature of or resembling mucus.

   m. colitis. Inflammation of the mucosa of the colon. SEE: *colitis.*

   m. membrane. That lining passages and cavities communicating with the air, and which secretes mucus.

   m. polypus. Small growth from mucous lining of the cervix or uterus.

   m. rashes in mouth. Stomatitis, measles, scarlet fever. ON LIPS: Typhoid fever, meningitis, pneumonia. In secondary syphilis, chancre, cancer, and epithelioma mucous patches appear.

mucus (mū'kŭs). A viscid fluid secreted by mucous membranes and glands, consisting of mucin, leukocytes, inorganic salts, water, and epithelial cells.

mulatto (mū-lăt'tō). First generation born of pure negro and white parentage; popularly anyone of white and negro blood mixed.

Müller's ducts. Embryonic tubes from which the oviducts, uterus, and vagina develop in the female; in the male they become atrophied.

   M.'s dust bodies. Blood fragments or dust. SEE: *hemokonia.*

   M.'s fibers. Finely striated circular fibers of the retina.

   M.'s fluid. Solution of 1 part sodium sulfate, 2 parts potassium bichromate in 100 parts of distilled water; used for hardening objects for microscopic examination.

   M.'s ganglion. Jugular ganglion.

   M.'s muscle. 1. Ciliary circular fibers. 2. Inf. and sup. palpebral muscles. 3. Muscular covering over sphenomaxillary fissure.

   M.'s reaction. A sphincterlike muscular reaction at the point where the canal of the cervix uteri joins the cavity of the body of the uterus at an advanced stage of pregnancy.

   M.'s ring. Muscular ring at junction of cervical canal and the gravid uterus.

   M.'s trigone. Portion of *tuber cinereum* folding over the optic chiasm.

mult-, multi-. Prefixes meaning *many, much.*

multiarticular (mŭl''tĭ-ar-tĭk'ū-lar). Concerning, having, or affecting many joints.

multicapsular (mŭl''tĭ-kap'sū-lar). Composed of many capsules.

multicellular (mŭl''tĭ-sĕl'ū-lar). Consisting of many cells.

multicuspid, multicuspidate (mul-tĭ-kus'-pĭd, -pĭ-dāt). Having several cusps.

multifid (mŭl'tĭf-ĭd). Divided into many sections.

multiform (mŭl'tĭ-form). Having many forms or shapes. SYN: *polymorphous.*

multiglandular (mŭl''tĭ-glănd'ū-lar). Concerning several glands.

multigrav'ida. A woman who has borne children 2 or more times. SYN: *multipara.*

multiinfection (mŭl''tĭ-ĭn-fek'shŭn). A mixed infection with several organisms developing at the same time.

multilobular (mŭl''tĭ-lōb'ū-lar). Formed of, or possessing many lobules.

multilocular (mŭl''tĭ-lok'ū-lar). Having many cells or compartments. SYN: *multicellular.*

multimammae (mul''tĭ-mam'mē). Condition of possessing more than the normal number of breasts. SYN: *polymastia.*

multinodal (mul-tĭ-nō'dăl). Having many nodes or knots.

multinodular (mŭl-tĭ-nod'ū-lar). Possessing many nodules or small knots.

multinuclear, multinucleate (mul-tĭ-nū'klē-ar, -āt). Possessing several nuclei.

multipara (mul-tĭp'ă-ră). A woman who has borne more than 1 child.

multiparity (mul-tĭ-par'ĭ-tĭ). 1. Condition of having borne more than 1 child. 2. Production of more than 1 child at birth.

multiparous (mŭl-tĭp'ăr-ŭs). 1. Having borne more than 1 child. 2. Producing more than 1 child at birth.

multiple (mul'tĭ-pl). 1. Consisting of, or containing more than 1; manifold. 2. Occurring simultaneously in various parts of the body.

   m. personality. Condition in which the subject may develop more than 2 personalities. SEE: *dual personality, vigilambulism.*

multipolar (mul-tĭ-pōl'ar). Possessing more than 2 poles.

multiter'minal. Providing several sets of terminals, making possible the use of several electrodes.

multivalent (mul-tĭ-vā'lent). Having ability to combine with more than 2 atoms of a univalent element or radical.

mummification (mum''mĭ-fĭ-kā'shun). 1. Mortification producing a hard, dry mass. SYN: *dry gangrene.* 2. Drying and shriveling of a body, as a dead *fetus.*

mumps (mŭmps). An acute, contagious, febrile disease characterized by inflammation of the parotid gland and other salivary glands.

mural (mū'ral). Pert. to a wall of an organ or part.

muriate (mūr'ĭ-āt). 1. An old synonym for *chloride.* 2. To charge with chlorine or certain chlorine compounds.

muriated (mūr'ĭ-āt-ĕd). Charged with or containing chlorine or certain chlorine compounds.   [acid', *q.v.*

muriat'ic acid. Commercial hydrochloric

mur'mur. Sound heard in auscultation* due to the more or less forcible closure of the heart's valves.

   m., aneurysmal. Whizzing systolic sound heard over an aneurysm.

   m., aortic obstructive. Harsh systolic one heard with and after the 1st heart sound. Loudest at the base.

   m., a. regurgitant. Blowing, hissing following 2nd heart sound.

   m., apex. Inorganic murmur over apex of heart.

   m., arterial. Soft flowing one, synchronous with pulse.

m., bronchial. Murmur heard over large bronchi, resembling respiratory laryngal murmur.

m., cardiac pulmonary. Murmur caused by movement of heart against lungs.

m., diastolic. Murmur during dilation of heart.

m., direct. Murmur caused by obstruction of blood in normal course.

m., dynamic. Murmur due to irregular action.

m., friction. Murmur caused by rubbing of 2 inflamed mucous surfaces.

m., functional. May be due to changes in the blood and the type of contraction of the heart muscle. They do not indicate organic disease of the heart. They may disappear upon a return to health. They must not be mistaken for true pathological murmurs.

m., hemic. Sound heard on auscultation of anemic persons without a valvular lesion.

m., indirect. Murmur heard when blood flows in abnormal directions.

m., inorganic. Murmur not due to structural changes.

m., organic. Murmur due to structural changes.

m., regurgitant. Murmur due to backward flow of blood current.

m., systolic. Murmur heard during contraction of heart, due to obstruction.

m., tricuspid. One caused by disease of tricuspid valves.

m., vesicular. One heard in normal breathing.

Murphy's button. Mechanical device used to connect visceral ends of a divided intestine in anastomosis.

M.'s drip or **treatment.** Continuous slow passage of normal saline solution into the rectum; usually used in treating peritonitis.

muscae volitantes (mus'sē vol-ĭ-tan'tēz). Black specks seen floating in the vitreous humor of the eye and visible to the patient; often seen in myopia.

muscle (mus'el). Organ composed of contractile tissue which effects the movement of any organ or part of the body.

m., abductor. Muscle which draws away from the midline.

m., adductor. Muscle which draws toward the midline.

m., antagonistic. Muscle which neutralizes the function of another.

m.'s, antigravity. Muscles which pull against the force of gravity to maintain posture.

m., appendicular. One of the skeletal muscles of the limbs.

m., articular. A joint muscle.

m., axial. A skeletal muscle of the head or trunk.

m., bipennate. Muscle in which the fibers converge toward a central tendon on both sides.

m. bound. Condition caused by overuse in which muscles are less elastic and bulkier.

m., constrictor. A muscle which compresses a part.

m., corrugator. Muscle drawing the skin up and causing it to wrinkle.

m. curve. A tracing of muscular contraction.

m., digastric. Muscle with a fibrous insertion bet. 2 fleshy bellies.

m., extensor. Muscle which straightens a part.

m., extrinsic. Muscle with origin and insertion in different parts.

m. fatigue. Contraction of a muscle represents *latency, contraction,* and *relaxation.* During contraction the muscle is shortened. The contraction is more or less modified by fatigue, the height of contraction is lowered, the relaxation delayed, lengthening the period of latency. Stimuli occurring in too rapid succession may prevent relaxation. Overexertion spreads the body's lactic acid to muscles not being used which, with a deficiency of oxygen intake, brings about fatigue.

m.'s, fixation. Accessory muscles which aid in steadying a part.

m., flexor. Muscle which bends a part.

m., fusiform. A muscle resembling a spindle.

m., intrinsic. Muscle with origin and insertion on the same limb.

m., involuntary. Muscle not controlled by the will; mainly smooth.

m., joint. Muscle which produces motion in a joint.

m., nonstriated; m., organic. Muscle without markings on its fibers; mainly involuntary.

m., pennate. Muscle with central or lateral tendon toward which fibers converge on 1 or both sides.

m. plasma. Fluid found in muscular tissue.   [myosin.

m. serum. Muscle plasma without

m., skeletal. Muscle which is connected with a bone; mainly striated.

m., skew. Muscle which pulls a part obliquely.

m., smooth. Nonstriated muscle.

m., somatic. Skeletal muscle.

m., sphincter. Muscle controlling an opening.

m., striated; m., striped. Muscle with bands dividing its fibers; mainly voluntary.

m. sugar. Sugar found in muscular tissue. SYN: *inosite.*

m.'s, synergistic. Muscles aiding one another in function.

m., unipennate. Muscle whose fibers converge on only 1 side of a tendon.

m., unstriated; m., unstriped. Muscle without markings; mainly involuntary.

m., visceral. Nonstriated, involuntary muscle in structure of an internal organ.

m., voluntary. Muscle whose action is controlled by will; excepting the cardiac muscle; all striated muscles are voluntary.

mus'cular. 1. Pert. to muscles. 2. Possessing well developed muscles.

m. contractions, graduated. Accomplished by gradually sheathing the core of specially designed faradic coil with operator's right hand which slowly increases the current, while the operator's left hand applies small, active electrode to muscles under treatment.

m. reflex. Muscle contraction, either or both isotonic and isometric.

m. rheumatism. That affecting the muscles.

muscularis (mŭs-kū-la′rĭs). Muscular coat of a hollow organ or tubule.

m. mucosae. Unstriated muscular tissue layer of mucous membrane.

musculation (mŭs-kū-lā′shŭn). 1. Muscular arrangement in the body. 2. Muscular action. SYN: *musculature.*

mus′culature. The arrangement of muscles in the body or its parts.

mus′culin. Muscle tissue globulin or protein.   [cle.

musculo-. Combining form *pert. to a mus-*

musculocutaneous (mŭs″kū-lō-kū-tān′ē-ŭs). 1. Pert. to the muscles and skin. 2. Supplying or affecting the muscles and skin.

musculomembranous (mŭs″kū-lō-mĕm′brăn-ŭs). Pert. to or consisting of muscle and membrane.

mus′culus (pl. *musculi*). Muscle, *q.v.*

mu″sicoma′nia. Insane love of music.

mu″sicother′apy. Treatment of mental diseases with music.

musk (mŭsk). Dried secretion of the preputial follicles of male musk deer. Used as a stimulant and sedative.

DOSAGE: 1-10 gr. (0.06-0.6 Gm.).

mussitation (mŭs-sĭ-tā′shŭn). The muttering of delirium or the moving of the lips without sound.

must. Unfermented grape juice.

mutacism (mū′tă-sĭzm). Excessive or improper pronunciation and use of letter m or its sound. SYN: *mytacism.*

mutant (mū′tănt). In heredity, a sport or variation which breeds true.

mutase (mū′tās). 1. Enzyme which accelerates oxidation reduction reactions through activation of oxygen and hydrogen. 2. A food preparation made from leguminous plants high in protein content.

mutation (mū-tā′shŭn). 1. Change; transformation; instance of such change. 2. Sudden, permanent variation with offspring differing from parents in a marked characteristic as differentiated from gradual variation through many generations, so called by De Vries. Also person showing such change.

mute (mūt). 1. One who is unable to speak. 2. Dumb; without ability to speak.

m., deaf. Individual who is unable to hear or to speak.

mutism (mū′tĭzm). 1. Condition of being unable to speak. 2. PSY: Persistent inhibition to speech; seen in *dementia precox.*

mutualism (mū′tū-ăl-ĭzm). Relationship of 2 organisms living together, both benefiting. SYN: *symbiosis, 2.*

myalgia (mī-al′jĭ-ă). Tenderness or pain in the muscles; muscular rheumatism.

myameba (mī-ăm-ē′bă). A muscle cell considered as an organism.

myasis (mī-ā′sĭs). Condition which arises from larvae of flies or maggots in the body or upon mucous membranes. SYN: *myiasis.*

myasthenia (mī-ăs-thē′nĭ-ă). Muscular weakness.

m., angiosclerotic. Vascular changes producing excessive muscular fatigue.

m. gastrica. Loss of muscular tone in coats of the stomach.

m. gravis. Great muscular weakness without atrophy.

m. pseudoparalytica. Muscular weakness simulating paralysis due to myasthenia.

myasthe′nic. Marked by muscular weakness.

m. face. A type of myasthenia, in which 1 side of the face will have a normal smile, and the other side a sneer, when attempting to smile.

myatonia (mī-ă-tō′nī-ă). Deficiency or loss of muscular power.

m. congenita. Myatonia of early childhood; it is not hereditary. SYN: *Oppenheim's disease.*

myatrophy (mī-at′rō-fī). Muscular wasting away.

mycelium (mī-se′lĭ-ŭm). Mass of vegetative portion of fungus consisting of hyphae forming molds.

mycelioid (my-se′lĭ-oid). Appearing like molds and yeast colonies having filaments radiating from the center.

mycethemia (mī-se-thē′mĭ-ă). Fungi in the blood. SYN: *mycohemia.*

mycetism, mycetismus (mī′se-tĭzm, -tĭz′mŭs). Poisoning from eating mushrooms.

mycetogenetic, mycetogenic, mycetogenous (mī-sē″tō-jĕn-ĕt′ĭk, -jĕn′ĭk, -toj′ĕn-ŭs). Induced by fungi.

mycetoma (mī-se-tō′mă). A disease induced by fungi, seen in India, which attacks the foot. SYN: *Madura foot.*

Myco. Abbr. for *Mycobacterium.*

Mycobacte′rium. A genus of bacillary organisms, including those of leprosy and tuberculosis.

mycocyte (mī′kō-sīt). A cell found in mucous tissue.

Mycoderma (mī-kō-der′mă). Genus of fungi forming membranes in fermenting liquids.

M. ace′ti. Mother of vinegar.

mycoder′ma. Mucous membrane.

mycodermatitis (mī″kō-der-mă-tī′tĭs). Inflamed condition of a mucous membrane. SYN: *catarrh.*

mycogastritis (mī-kō-gas-trī′tĭs). Inflamed condition of mucosa of stomach.

mycoid (mī′koyd). Funguslike.

m. degeneration. Excessive formation of mucus in catarrhal conditions, or in tumors.

mycohemia (mī-kō-hē′mĭ-ă). Fungi present in the blood.

mycology (mī-kol′ō-jī). Science of fungi.

mycomyringitis (mī″kō-mi-rin-jī′tĭs). Fungous inflammation of membrana tympani.

mycophylaxin (mī″kō-fĭl-ăks′ĭn). A phylaxin which destroys microörganisms.

mycosis (mī-kō′sĭs). Any disease induced by a fungus.

　　m. favosa. Formation of honeycomblike crusts over hair follicles with itching and unpleasant odor. SYN: *favus, q.v.*

　　m. fungoides. A rare chronic inflammatory malignant disease probably of septic origin that affects the superficial and deep layers of the skin, and occasionally the mucous membrane.

　　m. leptothrica. Disease caused by *Leptothrix buccalis,* consisting of gray or black deposits on tongue and buccal mucosa usually with constitutional symptoms.

　　m. tonsillaris benigna. A name applied by Frankel to a peculiar form of pharyngeal disease induced by undue accumulations of Leptothrix upon pharyngeal tissue.

mycosozin (mī-kō-sō′zĭn). A sozin that destroys microörganisms.

mycotic (mī-kŏt′ĭk). Caused by or affected with microörganisms.

mydaleine (mĭd-ā′le-ēn). A poisonous ptomaine from putrefied visceral organs, acting mainly on the heart.

mydriasis (mid-rī′ăs-ĭs). Abnormal dilation of the pupil.

mydriatic (mid-rī-at′ĭk). 1. Causing pupillary dilatation. 2. Any drug which dilates the pupil.　　　　　　[cation.

myectopia (mī-ĕk-tō′pĭ-ă). Muscle dislo-

myelalgia (mī-el-al′jĭ-ă). Pain of the spinal cord or its membranes.

myelanalosis (mī″el-ă-nal-ō′sĭs). Gradual wasting of spinal cord. SYN: *tabes dorsalis.*

myelapoplexy (mī-el-ap′ō-plĕks-ĭ). Hemorrhagic effusion into the spinal cord.

myelasthenia (mī-ĕl-ăs-thē′nĭ-ă). Spinal exhaustion; neurasthenia arising from spinal causes.

myelatelia (mī-ĕl-ă-tē′lĭ-ă). Defective development of spinal cord.

myelatrophy (mī-el-at′rof-ĭ). Wasting of the spinal cord.

myelauxe (mī-ĕl-awks′ē). Abnormal enlargement of spinal cord and marrow.

myelemia (mī-ĕl-ē′mĭ-ă). Abnormal number of marrow cells in the blood. SYN: *myelocytosis.*

myelencephalon (mī″ĕl-ĕn-sef′ă-lon). 1. The cerebrospinal axis, composed of the spinal cord and brain. 2. Afterbrain; portion of embryo from which arise the medulla oblongata and the bulbar area of the 4th ventricle.

my′elin. 1. Fatlike white material composing sheath of a medullated nerve fiber. SYN: *white substance of Schwann.* 2. A lipoid substance seen in animal tissues, as the brain.

myelination (mī-ĕl-ĭn-ā′shŭn). Process of acquiring a myelin sheath. SYN: *myelinization.*

myelinic (mī-ĕl-ĭn′ĭk). Concerning or composed of myelin.

myelinization (mī″ĕl-ĭn-ĭ-zā′shŭn). Acquirement of myelin sheath for nerve fibers. SYN: *myelination.*

myelinogenetic (mī″ĕl-ĭn-ō-jĕn-et′ĭk). Producing myelin or a myelin sheath.

myelinosis (mī″ĕl-ĭn-ō′sĭs). Fatty degeneration during which myelin is produced.　　　　　　　　　　　　[tis.

mye.itic (mī-el-it′ĭk). Concerning myeli-

myelitis (mi-el-i′tis). 1. Inflammation of the spinal cord. 2. Inflammation of bone marrow.

　　m., acute. Simple acute form which develops following injury.

　　m., bulbar. Myelitis involving the oblongata.

　　m., central. Myelitis in which the gray matter is esp. involved.

　　m., c., acute. Resembles acute transverse myelitis, but the trophic disturbances are more marked and duration shorter. Usually fatal in 1 to 2 weeks.

　　m., chronic. Form progressing slowly but steadily.

　　m., compression. Myelitis caused by pressure on the cord, as by a hemorrhage.

　　m., cornual. Myelitis affecting the spinal cord's horns of gray matter.

　　m., descending. Myelitis affecting successively lower areas of the spinal cord.

　　m., diffuse. Myelitis involving large sections of the cord.

　　m., disseminated. Myelitis with several separated foci on the cord.

　　m., hemorrhagic. Myelitis with hemorrhage.

　　m., parenchymatous. Myelitis of nerve substance.

　　m., sclerosing. Myelitis with hardening of cord, and interstitial tissue growth.

　　m., systemic. Myelitis affecting only certain tracts of the cord.

　　m., transverse. Myelitis involving the whole thickness of the cord.

　　m., t., acute. Acute form of myelitis involving entire thickness of cord, developing subsequent injury to spinal cord.

　　m., traumatic. Myelitis due to cord injury.

myelo-. Prefix denoting the *spinal cord,* or *bone marrow.*

myeloblast (mī′ĕl-ō-blăst). Bone marrow cell which develops into a myelocyte.

myeloblastemia (mī″ĕl-ō-blăst-ē′mĭ-ă). Occurrence of myeloblasts in the blood.

myeloblastoma (mī″ĕl-ō-blăst-ō′mă). 1. Tumor containing myeloblasts. 2. Myelogenic form of leukemia.

myelobrachium (mī″ĕl-ō-brā′kĭ-ŭm). The cerebellar inferior tubercle.

myelocele (mi′ĕl-ō-sēl). 1. A form of spina bifida with spinal cord protrusion. 2. Central canal of spinal cord.

myelocyst (mī′ĕl-ō-sĭst). Cyst arising from the spinal cord.

myelocystocele (mī″ĕl-ō-sĭst′ō-sēl). Cystic tumor of spinal cord.

myelocystomeningocele (mī″ĕl-ō-sĭst″ō-men-ĭn′gō-sēl). Combined myelocystocele and meningocele.

myelocyte (mī′el-ō-sīt). 1. A large cell in red bone marrow, from which leukocytes are derived. 2. Any gray matter nerve cell.

myelocythemia (mī″ĕl-ō-sī-thē′mĭ-ă). Presence of an excess number of myelocytes in the blood. SYN: *myelocytosis*.

myelocytic (mī″ĕl-ō-sit′ĭk). Characterized by presence of, or pert. to, myelocytes.

myelocytoma (mī″ĕl-ō-sīt-ō′mă). Leukemia with leukocytes arising from both myeloid and lymphoid substance. SYN: *chronic myelogenous leukemia*.

myelocytosis (mī″ĕl-ō-sī-tō′sĭs). Myelocytes in large quantities in the blood. SYN: *myelocythemia*.

myelodiastasis (mī″ĕl-ō-dī-as′tă-sĭs). Destruction and disintegration of spinal cord.

myelodysplasia (mī″ĕl-ō-dĭs-plā′zĭ-ă). Defective formation of the spinal cord.

myeloencephalic (mī″ĕl-ō-ĕn-sĕf-al′ĭk). Concerning the spinal cord and brain.

myeloencephalitis (mī″ĕl-ō-ĕn-sĕf-ă-lī′tis). Inflamed condition of spinal cord and brain.

myelogangliitis (mī″ĕl-ō-găng-lĭ-ī′tĭs). Severe choleraic condition due to gangliitis of solar and hepatic plexus.

myelogenesis (mī″ĕl-ō-jen′ē-sĭs). 1. The development of brain and spinal cord. 2. Development of myelin.

myelogenic, myelogenous (mī-ĕ-lō-jen′ĭk, -lŏj′ĕn-ŭs). Producing or originating in marrow, or in the spinal column.

myelogeny (mī-ĕl-oj′ĕn-ĭ). Production of myelin sheaths by bone marrow.

myelogone, myelogonium (mī′ĕl-ō-gōn, mī″ĕl-ō-gōn′ĭ-ŭm). 1. Myeloblast. 2. Myeloid white blood cell with a deeply stained nucleus and a reticulate nucleus stained with eosin.

myelography (mī-ĕl-og′ră-fĭ). Roentgenographical inspection of the spinal cord.

myeloid (mī′el-oid). 1. Medullary; like marrow. 2. Pert. to the spinal cord. 3. Resembling a myelocyte, but not necessarily originating from bone marrow.

myeloidosis (mī″ĕl-oid-ō′sĭs). Formation of myeloid tissue, esp. abnormal tissue formation.

myelolymphocyte (mī″ĕl-ō-lĭmf′ō-sīt). Tiny lymphocyte formed abnormally in bone marrow.

myeloma (mī-ĕl-o′mă). 1. Soft growth from medullary cavity of ends of long bones.
2. Encephaloid tumor. 3. Giant cell sarcoma.
   m., multiple. Diffuse hyperplasia of bone marrow with painful swellings on ribs and skull. SYN: *Kahler's disease, lymphadenia ossea*.

myelomalacia (mī″ĕl-ō-mă-lā′sĭ-ă). Abnormal softening of spinal cord.

myelomatosis (mī″ĕl-ō-mă-tō′sĭs). Disease marked by multiple tumors of the bone marrow, pernicious anemia, and albumosuria. SYN: *multiple myeloma*.

myelomenia (mī-ĕl-ō-mē′nĭ-ă). Vicarious menstrual discharge in the spinal cord.

myelomeningitis (mī″ĕl-ō-men-ĭn-jī′tĭs). Inflamed spinal cord and membranes; spinal meningitis.

myelomeningocele (mī″el-ō-men-ĭn′gō-sēl). Spina bifida with portion of cord and membranes protruding.

myelomyces (mī-el-ō-mī′sēs). Malignant growth resembling brain substance. SYN: *encephaloma*.

myelon (mī′el-on). The spinal cord.

myeloneuritis (mī″ĕl-ō-nū-rī′tĭs). Multiple neuritis and myelitis combined.

myelonic (mī-ĕl-on′ĭk). Pert. to the spinal cord.

myeloparalysis (mī″ĕl-ō-pă-ral′ĭ-sĭs). Paralysis of the spine.

myelopathy (mī-ĕl-op′ă-thĭ). Any pathological condition of the spinal cord.

myelopetal (mī-ĕl-op′et-ăl). Proceeding toward the spinal cord.

myelophage (mī′ĕl-ō-fāj). A myelin ingesting macrophage.

myelophthisis (mī-ĕl-of′thĭ-sĭs). Atrophy of the spinal cord. SYN: *myelanalosis*.

my′eloplast. A bone marrow cell similar to a leukocyte.

my′eloplax. Large, multinuclear, bone marrow cell.

myeloplaxoma (mī″ĕl-ō-plăks-ō′mă). Tumor composed of myeloplaxes.

myeloplegia (mī″ĕl-ō-plē′jĭ-ă). Paralysis of spinal origin.

myelopoiesis (mī″ĕl-ō-poy-ē′sĭs). The development of marrow or myelocytes.

myelorrhagia (mī-ĕl-ōr-rā′jĭ-ă). Hemorrhage into myelon.

myelorrhaphy (mī-ĕl-or′ra-fĭ). Suture of a cut or wound of the spinal cord.

myelosarcoma (mī″ĕl-ō-săr-kō′mă). Sarcoma of bone marrow cells and tissue. SYN: *osteosarcoma*.

myelosclerosis (mī″ĕl-ō-sklĕr-ō′sĭs). Sclerosis of the spinal cord. SYN: *spinal sclerosis*.

myelosis (mī-ĕl-ō′sĭs). Formation of a myeloma or medullary tumor.

myelospongium (mī″ĕl-ō-spon′jĭ-ŭm). Embryonic network from which the neuroglia arises.

my″elother′apy. Treatment of disease with extract of spinal cord or bone marrow.

myelotome (mī′ĕl-ō-tōm). Instrument used to dissect the spinal cord.

myelotomy (mī-ĕl-ot′ō-mĭ). Dissection of the spinal cord.

myelotoxic (mī-ĕl-ō-toks′ĭk). 1. Destroying bone marrow. 2. Pert. to or arising from diseased bone marrow.

myelotoxin (mī-ĕl-ō-toks′ĭn). Toxin which destroys marrow cells.

myenergia (mī-ĕn-er′jĭ-ă). Muscular energy.

myenteric (mī-ĕn-ter′ĭk). Concerning the myenteron.
   m. reflex. Intestinal contraction and relaxation above a portion of bowel which is stimulated.

myenteron (mī-en′tĕr-ŏn). Muscular layer of the intestine.

myesthesia (mĭ-ĕs-thē'zĭ-ă). Muscle sensitivity.

myiasis (mĭ-ī'ă-sis). A disease caused by infestation with the larger pestiferous organisms, such as the larvae of maggots, flies, etc.

myiodesopsia (mĭ″i-ō-dĕs-op'sĭ-ă). Condition in which spots are seen before the eyes. SEE: *muscae volitantes.*

myitis (mĭ-i'tĭs). Inflamed condition of a muscle. SYN: *myositis.*

mylohyoid (mĭ″lō-hī'oid). Pert. to the hyoid bone and the molar teeth.

myo-. Combining form pert. to *muscle.*

myoalbumin (mĭ″ō-al-bū'mĭn). Albumin found in muscular tissue.

myoalbumose (mĭ-ō-al'bū-mōs). A protein derived from muscle plasma.

myoarchitectonic (mĭ″ō-ar″kĭ-tĕk-ton'ĭk). Pert. to or resembling structural arrangement of muscle of of fibers.

myoatrophy (mĭ-ō-ăt'rō-fĭ). Muscular wasting.

myoblast (mĭ'ō-blast). An embryonic cell which develops into muscle fiber cell.

myobra'dia. Slow muscular reaction to stimulation.

myocardia (mĭ-ō-kar'dĭ-ă). Noninflammatory cardiac failure.

myocardiac, myocardial (mĭ-ō-kar'dĭ-ăk, -ăl). Concerning the myocardium.

myocardiograph (mĭ″ō-kar'dĭ-ō-grăf). Instrument for recording heart movements.

myocardiosis (mĭ-ō-kăr-dĭ-ō'sĭs). Noninflammatory cardiac disorder. SYN: *myocardia.*

myocard'ism. Tendency toward development of myocardial disorders.

myocarditis (mĭ-ō-kar-dī'tĭs). Inflammation of the cardiac muscular tissue.

   m., acute, primary. Acute interstitial inflammation of the myocardium.

   m., a., secondary. Acute inflammation of the heart muscle.

   m., a., septic. Localized, suppurative inflammation of the heart muscle.

   m., chronic. Characterized by round cell infiltration of interstitial tissue, followed by parenchymatous changes of muscle fibers.

   m., Fiedler's. Myocardial progressive failure without infection.

   m., fragmentation. Fragmentation of the myocardium.

   m., indurative. Chronic myocarditis causing hardening of muscular walls of the heart.

   m. scarlatinosa. Myocarditis associated with scarlet fever.

myocardium (mĭ-ō-kar'dĭ-ŭm). Muscular mass of the heart made up of striated muscular tissue. SEE: *Aschoff's bodies.*

myocardosis (mĭ″ō-kăr-dō'sĭs). 1. Cardiac disorder without known pathological lesion. 2. Any degenerative condition (except myofibrosis) of the heart muscle.

myocele (mĭ'ō-sēl). 1. Muscular protrusion through a muscle sheath. 2. Cavity in a muscular segment.

myocelialgia (mĭ″ō-sē-lĭ-al'jĭ-ă). Abdominal muscle pain.

myocelitis (mĭ-ō-sē-lī'tĭs). Inflamed condition of abdominal muscles.

myocellulitis (mĭ″ō-sĕl-ū-lī'tĭs). Myositis combined with cellulitis.

myocerosis (mĭ″ō-sē-ro'sĭs). Waxy degeneration of a muscle.

myochorditis (mĭ″ō-kor-dī'tĭs). Inflammation of the muscles of the larynx.

myochrome (mĭ'ō-krōm). Reddish pigment derived from hemoglobin and found in muscle. SYN: *myohematin.*

myochronoscope (mĭ″ō-krō'nō-skōp). Device for determining time for producing a muscular contraction.

myoclonia (mĭ-ō-klo'nĭ-ă). Condition of intermittent, clonic spasm or twitching of a muscle or muscles.

myoclonus (mĭ-ok'lō-nŭs). Twitching or clonic spasm of a muscle or group of muscles. SYN: *paramyoclonus.*

   m. multiplex. Condition marked by persistent and continuous muscular spasms.

myocoele (mi'o-sēl). The hollow portion of a myotome; muscle chamber.

myocolpitis (mĭ″ō-kol-pī'tis). Muscular tissue inflammation of the vagina.

myocomma (mĭ-ō-kŏm'mă). 1. A segment of embryonic muscle along neural tube. SYN: *myotome.* 2. Septum dividing the myotomes.

myocrismus (mĭ-ō-kris'mŭs). A peculiar crackling sound sometimes heard in auscultation resulting from contraction of a muscle. [cell.

myocyte (mĭ'ō-sīt). A muscular tissue

myocytoma (mĭ″ō-sĭ-tō'mă). Tumor containing muscle cells.

myodemia (mĭ-ō-de'mĭ-ă). Fatty degeneration of muscular tissue.

myodesopsia (mĭ″ō-des-op'sĭ-ă). Vision of muscae volitantes or specks before the eyes. SYN: *myiodesopsia.*

myodiastasis (mĭ″ō-dĭ-as'tă-sĭs). Division or rupture of a muscle.

myodynamia (mĭ″ō-dĭ-nam'ĭ-ă). Muscular force or strength.

myodynamometer (mĭ″ō-dī-nă-mom'ĕt-ĕr). Device for measurement of muscular strength.

myodynia (mĭ-ō-dīn'ĭ-ă). Any muscle pain. SYN: *myalgia.**

myoedema (mĭ″ō-ē-dē'mă). 1. Lumping in a wasting muscle when struck. SYN: *mounding.* 2. Muscular edema.

myoelectric (mĭ″ō-ē-lĕk'trĭk). Pert. to muscular electrical properties.

myoendocarditis (mĭ″ō-ĕn″dō-kar-dī'tĭs). Inflammation of the cardiac muscular wall and membranous lining.

myoepithelial (mĭ″ō-ĕp-ĭ-thē'lĭ-ăl). Containing muscular and epithelial cells.

myoepithelium (mĭ″ō-ĕp-ĭ-thē'lĭ-ŭm). Epithelium combined with muscular cells; muscle epithelium.

myofascitis (mĭ″ō-făs-ĭ'tĭs). Inflamed condition of a muscle and its fascia.

myofibril, myofibrilla (mĭ-ō-fī'brĭl, -fĭ-brĭl'lă) (pl. *myofibrillae*). A tiny fibril found in muscular tissue, running parallel to the cellular long axis, from 1 cell to another,

myofibroma (mī″ō-fī-brō′mă). Tumor containing muscular and fibrous tissue.

myofibrosis (mī″ō-fī-brō′sĭs). Increase of connective or fibrous tissue with degeneration of muscular tissue.

myogelosis (mī-ō-jel-ō′sĭs). Hardening of a portion of muscle.

myogen (mī′ō-jĕn). A protein found in muscle plasma, which is spontaneously coagulable.

myogenesis (mī-ō-jĕn′ē-sĭs). Formation of muscular tissue.

myogenetic (mī″ō-jĕn-et′ĭk). Having origin in muscle. SYN: *myogenic*.

myogen′ic, myog′enous. Arising from muscle.

m. theory. The cardiac movements start in the heart muscle itself and not in nerve centers in or near the heart; opposed to the neurogenic* theory.

myoglia (mī-og′lĭ-ă). A fibrous network in muscular tissue resembling neuroglia in appearance.

myoglobulin (mī″ō-glob′ū-lĭn). A coagulable globulin seen in muscular tissue.

my′ogram. A tracing made by the myograph of muscular contractions.

myograph (mī′ō-grăf). Instrument for tracing movements caused by muscular contractions.

myographic (mī-ō-graf′ĭk). Pert. to a myograph, or the tracings made by it.

m. tracing. A myogram or muscular tracing.

myography (mī-og′ră-fī). 1. Recording of muscular contractions by a myograph. 2. Description of the muscles and their action.

myohematin (mī″ō-hem′ăt-ĭn). Red pigment from hemoglobin found in muscles. SYN: *histohematin*.

myohysterectomy (mī″ō-hĭs-tĕr-ek′tō-mī). Excision of the body of the uterus, leaving the cervix in place. SYN: *subtotal hysterectomy*.

my′oid. Resembling muscle.

myoidema (mī-oi-dē′mă). 1. The mounding of a muscle. 2. Muscular edema. SYN: *myoedema*.

myoideum (mī-oid′ē-ŭm). Muscle tissue.

my′oidism. Muscular contraction responding to a direct stimulus without nervous control. [mia in a muscle.

myoischemia (mī″ō-ĭs-kē′mĭ-ă). Local anemia.

myokerosis (mī″ō-kĕ-rō′sĭs). Waxy degeneration of muscle or muscular tissue.

myokinesis (mī″ō-kĭn-ē′sĭs). 1. Muscular activity. 2. Surgical displacement of muscular fibers.

myokinetic (mī″ō-kĭn-et′ĭk). Pert. to motile muscular element as contrasted with the myotonic* element.

myokymia (mī-ō-kĭm′ĭ-ă). Twitching of fibers of a muscle.

It may be functional and is also seen in organic affections and general paresis.

myolemma (mī-ō-lĕm′ă). Sheath investing a muscle fiber. SYN: *sarcolemma*.

myolin (mī′ō-lĭn). Substance supposedly found in muscular fibrils.

myolipoma (mī″ō-lĭ-pō′mă). Muscle tissue tumor containing fatty elements.

myology (mī-ol′ō-jī). The science or study of the muscles and their parts.

myolysis (mī-ol′ĭ-sĭs). Fatty degeneration and infiltration with destruction of muscular tissue accompanied by separation and disappearance of muscle cells.

myoma (mī-ō′mă). A tumor containing muscle tissue. SEE: *chondromyoma*.

m. cysticum. A sarcoma containing groups of muscular tissue.

m., eccentric. Myoma in muscular wall of a hollow organ projecting externally.

m. lymphangiectodes. Myoma containing dilated lymphatic vessels.

m., nonstriated. A tumor of unmarked muscle tissue. SYN: *leiomyoma*.

m. striocellulare. Fibroma with striated muscular fibers. SYN: *rhabdomyoma*.

m. telangiectodes. Coiled blood vessel tumor in muscular fibers.

myomalacia (mī″ō-mă-lā′sĭ-ă). Softening of muscular tissue.

m. cordis. Softening of the heart muscle.

myomatosis (mī-ō-mă-tō′sĭs). The development of myomas.

myomatous (mī-ō′mă-tŭs). Pert. to or resembling a myoma.

myomectomy (mī-ō-mek′tō-mī). 1. Removal of a portion of muscle or muscular tissue. 2. Removal of a myomatous tumor, generally uterine, usually by abdominal section, leaving the uterus in place.

myomelanosis (mī″ō-mĕl-ă-nō′sĭs). Darkening of muscle tissue.

myomere (mī′ō-mēr). Embryonic muscular segment along the neural tube. SYN: *myocomma, myotome*.

myometer (mī-om′ĕt-ēr). Device for measurement of muscular contractions.

myometritis (mī″ō-me-trī′tĭs). Inflamed condition of the muscular part of the uterus.

myometrium (mī″ō-me′trĭ-ŭm). Muscular structure of the uterus.

myomohysterectomy (mī-ō″mō-hĭs-tĕr-ĕk′tō-mī). Hysterectomy performed to remove a myomatous uterus.

myomotomy (mī-ō-mot′ō-mī). Excision of a myoma, usually uterine. SYN: *myomectomy*.

my′on. A muscle.

myonarcosis (mī″ō-năr-kō′sĭs). Muscular numbness.

myonephropexy (mī″ō-nef′rō-pĕk″sī). Fixation of a movable kidney by attaching it to a portion of muscular tissue with sutures.

myoneuralgia (mī″ō-nū-răl′jī-ă). Neuralgia in a muscle.

myoneurasthenia (mī″ō-nūr-ăs-thē′nĭ-ă). Neurasthenic muscular relaxation.

myoneure (mī′ō-nūr). A nerve cell which aids muscular action.

myoneuroma (mī″ō-nū-rō′mă). A neuroma partially composed of muscular elements.

myoneuro′sis. Any muscular neurosis.

myonicity (mī-ō-nĭs′ĭt-ĭ). Contraction and relaxation of living muscular tissue.

myonosus (mī-on'ō-sŭs). A disease of muscular tissue. SYN: *myopathy*.

myopachynsis (mī″ō-păk-in'sĭs). Abnormal thickening of muscle tissue.

myopalmus (mī-o-pal'mŭs). Twitching of muscles. [sis in a muscle.

myoparalysis (mī″ō-pă-ral'ĭ-sĭs). Paraly-

myopathic (mī-ō-path'ĭk). 1. Pert. to muscular disease. 2. One suffering from a muscular disease.

  m. facies. Facial expression caused by relaxation of facial muscles.

myopathy (mī-op'ă-thĭ). Any diseased condition of a muscle.

  m., facial. Atrophy of facial muscles.

  m., pseudohypertrophic. A progressive disease occurring bet. the ages of 5 to 10 in which development of muscles becomes deranged.

  m., spinal. Myopathy caused by disease or injury of the spinal cord.

myope (mi'ōp). One afflicted with myopia or nearsightedness.

myopericarditis (mī″ō-per-ĭ-kar-dī'tis).Inflammation of the pericardium and cardiac muscular wall.

myoperitonitis (mī″ō-pĕr-ĭ-tō-nī'tĭs). Inflammation of muscular peritoneal tissue.

myophage (mī'ō-fāj). A phagocyte that devours muscle tissue.

myophone (mī'ō-fōn). Device for conveying sound of muscular contractions.

myo'pia. Defect in vision so that objects can only be seen distinctly when very close to the eyes; nearsightedness.

  Light rays come to a focus in front of the retina.

  m., axial. Myopia due to elongation of the axis of the eye.

  m., chromic. Color blindness when viewing distant objects.

  m. of curvature. Myopia due to curvature of the eye's refracting surfaces.

  m., index. Myopia resulting from abnormal refractivity of the media.

  m., malignant. Pernicious myopia.

  m., pernicious. Myopia with progressive disease of the choroid, terminating in blindness.

  m., prodromal. Myopia in which reading is possible without glasses; seen in incipient cataract.

  m., progressive. Myopia that increases steadily during adult life.

  m., stationary. Myopia that comes to a stop after adult growth is attained.

  m., transient. Myopia seen in spasm of accommodation, as in acute iritis or iridocyclitis.

myopic (mī-op'ĭk). Pert. to or affected with myopia.

  m. crescent. Post. crescentic protrusion seen in myopia.

myoplasm (mī'ō-plazm). The contractile part of the muscle cell, as differentiated from the sarcoplasm.*

myoplastic (mī-ō-plăst'ĭk). Pert. to plastic use of muscle tissue or plastic surgery on muscles.

myoplasty (mī'ō-plas-tĭ). Plastic surgery of muscle tissue.

myoplegia (mī″ō-plē'jĭ-ă). Muscular paralysis.

myoprotein (mī″ō-prō'tē-ĭn). A protein found in muscle tissue.

myoproteose (mī″ō-pro'te-ōs). A protein found in muscle plasma. SYN: *myoalbumose*.

myop'sin. A proteolytic ferment in the pancreatic juice.

myopsychosis (mī″ō-sī-kō'sĭs). A muscular affection connected with a mental disorder.

myorrhaphy (mī-or'ă-fĭ). Suture of a muscle wound.

myorrhexis (mī-or-eks'ĭs). Rupture of a muscle.

myosalgia (mī-ō-sal'jĭ-ă). Pain in a muscle. SYN: *myalgia*.

myosalpingitis (mī″ō-săl-pĭn-jī'tĭs). Inflamed condition of muscular tissue of a fallopian tube.

myosarcoma (mī″ō-sar-kō'mă). Tumor containing both muscular tissue and connective tissue cells.

myosclerosis (mī″ō-sklĕr-ō'sĭs). Hardening of muscle.

myoseism (mī'ō-sīzm). Muscular contraction of a jerky nature.

my'osin. A protein derivative of myosinogen found in the muscle plasma, the coagulation of which produces rigor mortis.

  m. ferment. A coagulating enzyme in muscle plasma. It converts myosinogen into myosin.

myosinogen (mī″ō-sĭn'ō-jĕn). One of 2 main (globulin) proteins in muscular tissue.

myosinose (mī-os'ĭn-ōs). A proteose resulting from the hydrolysis of myosin.

myosinuria (mī″ō-sĭn-ū'rĭ-ă). Myosin in the urine.

myo'sis. Contraction of the pupil.

myositis (mī-ō-sī'tĭs). Inflammation of muscle tissue, generally due to traumatism, to contiguous inflammation, diathetic states, or to parasites. SEE: *fibrositis*.

  m. a frigore. Muscular rheumatism affecting muscles of back, chest, or neck attributed to sudden chilling of part.

  m. fibrosa. SEE: *interstitial myositis*.

  m., interstitial. Myositis with hyperplasia of connective tissue.

  m. ossificans. Myositis marked by ossification of muscles.

  m., parenchymatous. Myositis of substance of a muscle.

  m. purulenta. Suppurative myositis.

  m., rheumatic. A common form which may affect muscle tissue, fascia, or connective tissue.

  m., traumatic. May be simple, with pain and swelling, or suppurative.

  m. trichinosa, m., trichinous. Myositis due to infestation with trichinae.

myospasm (mī'ō-spăzm). Spasmodic contraction of a muscle.

myosteo'ma. A bony growth found in muscle tissue.

myostroma (mī-ō-strō'mă). Framework or basement substance of muscle tissue.

myostromin (mĭ-ō'strō'mĭn). Protein found in muscle framework.

myostypsis (mĭ''ō-stĭp'sĭs). 1. A contraction of muscles. 2. Obstruction of any functional movement.

myosuria (mĭ-ō-sū'rĭ-ă). Presence of myosin in the urine. SYN: *myosinuria.*

myosuture (mĭ''ō-sū'chŭr). Stitching of a muscle.

myosynizesis (mĭ-ō-sin-ĭ-zē'sis). Adhesion of muscular layers of tissue.

myotactic (mĭ''ō-tăk'tĭk). Pert. to the muscular sensitivity.

myotasis (mĭ-ot'ă-sĭs). Stretching of a muscle. [cles.

myotat'ic. Pert. to the stretching of mus-

myotenontoplasty (mĭ''ō-ten-on'tō-plast-ĭ). Plastic operation involving muscles and tendons. SYN: *tenontomyoplasty.*

myotenositis (mĭ''ō-tĕn-ō-sī'tĭs). Inflamed condition of a muscle and its tendon.

myotenotomy (mĭ''ō-tĕn-ot'ō-mĭ). Division of the tendon of a muscle.

myotherapy (mĭ''ō-ther'ă-pĭ). Treatment by administration of muscular tissue extract.

myothermic (mĭ''ō-therm'ĭk). Pert. to rise in muscle temperature due to its activity.

myot'ic. 1. An agent that will contract the pupil of the eye. Ex: *physostigmine, pilocarpine.* 2. Producing contraction of a pupil.

myotility (mĭ-ō-til'ĭ-tĭ). Contractility of a muscle.

myotome (mĭ'ō-tōm). 1. Knife for cutting muscles. 2. Muscular portion of primitive segment of the body. SYN: *myocomma, somite.*

myotomy (mĭ-ot'ō-mĭ). Division or anatomical dissection of muscles.

myotonia (mĭ-ō-tō'nĭ-ă). Tonic spasm of a muscle, or temporary rigidity. SYN: *Thomsen's disease.*

  m. congenita. A disease characterized by tonic spasms of the muscles induced by voluntary movements; usually congenital and transmitted from 1 generation to another.

myoton'ic. 1. Pert. to tonic muscular spasm. 2. Pert. to the tonic muscular element as compared with the myokinetic* or motile element of a muscle.

myotonometer (mĭ''ō-tō-nom'ĕt-ēr). Instrument used to measure muscular tonus.

myot'onus. A tonic muscle spasm with temporary rigidity.

myot'rophy. Nutrition of the tissues of muscle.

myovas'cular. Pert. to blood vessels and cardiac muscle.

Myriapoda (mĭr-ĭ-ap'ō-dă). Group of arthropods including millepedes and centipedes.

myriapodiasis (mir''ĭ-ăp-ō-dī'ă-sĭs). Infestation with 1 of the Myriapoda.

myringa (mĭr-ĭn'gă). The tympanic membrane or eardrum.

myringectomy (mĭr-ĭn-jĕk'tō-mĭ). Excision of the myringa or eardrum. SYN: *myringodectomy.*

myringitis (mĭr-ĭn-jī'tĭs). Inflammation of the tympanum or eardrum.

  m. bullosa. Myringitis with blebs or vesicular inflammation of the outer layer.

myringodectomy (mĭ-rĭn-gō-dĕk'tō-mĭ). Excision of the tympanum. SYN: *myringectomy.*

myringodermatitis (mĭr-ĭn'gō-dĕr-mă-tī'-tĭs). Inflamed condition of outer layer of the membrana tympani.

myringomycosis (mĭr-ĭn''gō-mī-kō'sĭs). Disease of eardrum due to parasitic fungi.

myringoplasty (mĭr-ĭn'gō-plăst-ĭ). Plastic operation on membrana tympani.

myringoscope (mĭr-ĭn'gō-skōp). Instrument used for examination of the eardrum.

myringotome (mĭ-rĭn'gō-tōm). Knife for incising the tympanic membrane.

myringotomy (mĭr-ĭn-got'ō-mĭ). Incision of tympanic membrane.

myrrh (mur). USP. A gum resinous substance of great antiquity, cherished as a constituent of incense and perfume; most important use today is as an aromatic, astringent mouthwash.

mysophobia (mĭ-sō-fō'bĭ-ă). Abnormal aversion to dirt or contamination.

mytacism (mĭ'tă-sĭzm). Excessive or incorrect use of the letter *m* or the *m* sound. SEE: *metacism, mutacism.*

mythomania (mĭth-ō-mā'nĭ-ă). Abnormal tendency to lie and exaggerate.

mythophobia (mĭth-ō-fō'bĭ-ă). Abnormal dread of making a false or incorrect statement.

myurous (mi-u'rŭs). Gradually diminishing or tapering; said of certain symptoms, as the heartbeat which, under certain conditions, grows feebler and then stronger.

myxadenitis (mĭks-ad-en-ī'tĭs). Inflamed condition of mucous glands.

myxadenoma (miks-ad-en-ō'mă). 1. A tumor with the structure of a mucous gland. 2. A tumor of glandular structure containing mucous elements. SYN: *myxoadenoma.*

myxangitis (miks-an-jī'tis). Inflammation of mucous gland ducts.

  m. fibrosa. Myxangitis accompanied by hyperplasia.

  m. hyalinosa. Myxangitis with hyaline degeneration about the ducts.

myxangoitis (miks''an-gō-ī'tis). Inflammation of vessels with mucous discharge.

myxasthenia (mĭks-ăs-thē'nĭ-ă). Imperfect or insufficient secretion of mucus.

myxedema (mĭks-ĕ-dē'mă). A trophic disease due to hypofunction of thyroid gland.

  m., congenital. Cretinism.
  The face is "moon-shaped," features coarse, nostrils thick, with thick lips and large mouth.

myxedematoid (mĭks-ĕ-dēm'ă-toid). Resembling myxedema.

myxedematous (mĭks-ĕ-dēm'ă-tŭs). Marked by or concerning myxedema.

myxemia (mĭks-ē'mĭ-ă). Accumulation of mucin in the blood. SYN: *mucinemia.*

myxidiotic (mĭks-ĭd-ĭ-otʹĭk). Myxedema with few physical symptoms, but marked mental defects.

myxiosis (mĭks-ĭ-oʹsĭs). A mucous discharge or secretion.

myxo-, myx-. Combining form meaning *of*, or *pert. to mucus.*

myxoadenoma (mĭks″ō-ăd-en-oʹmă). 1. Glandular tumor containing mucus. 2. Tumor of structure of a mucous gland. SYN: *myxadenoma.*

myxocystoma (mĭks″ō-sĭs-toʹmă). 1. A cystic tumor containing mucus. 2. Ovarian cyst with lining structure resembling mucous membrane.

myxocyte (mĭksʹō-sīt). A typical mucous tissue cell, usually polyhedral or stellate.

myxodermia (mĭks-ō-derʹmĭ-ă). 1. Edematous softening of the skin. 2. Disease marked by cutaneous discoloration and softening and muscular contraction.

myxoedema (mĭks-ē-dēʹmă). Condition due to deficiency of thyroid secretion or removal of the gland. Not congenital.

myxoenchondroma (mĭks″ō-ĕn-kŏn-droʹmă). A cartilaginous tissue tumor which has undergone partial mucous degeneration.

myxofibroma (mĭks″ō-fī-broʹmă). Tumor composed of mucous and fibrous elements.

myxoglioma (mĭks″ō-glī-oʹmă). Tumor composed of myxomatous and gliomatous elements.

myxoid (mĭksʹoid). Similar to or resembling mucus.

myxoidedema (miks-oid-e-deʹma). Severe form of influenza.

myxoinoma (mĭks″ō-ĭn-oʹmă). Tumor composed of mucous and fibrous elements.

myxolipoma (mĭks″ō-lĭ-poʹmă). Mucous tumor with fatty tissue elements in it.

myxoma (mĭks-oʹmă). A benign mucous tumor. SEE: *chondromyxoma.*

   m., cartilaginous. Myxoma with a firmer consistence than usual or with cells like those of cartilage.

   m., cystic, cystoid. One with parts fluid enough to resemble cysts.

   m., enchondromatous. One with nodules of hyaline cartilage.

   m., erectile. SEE: *telangiectatic myxoma.*

   m., fibrous. A myxoma composed mainly of fibrous tissues.

   m., intracanalicular, of the mamma. One developing in the interstitial connective tissue of the mamma.

   m. lipomatodes. SEE: *lipomatous myxoma.*

   m., lipomatous. One containing much fat.

   m., telangiectatic, vascular. One of highly vascular structure.

myxomatosis (mĭks″ō-mă-toʹsĭs). 1. Formation of multiple myxomas. 2. Degeneration of myxomatous type.

myxomycetes (mĭks″ō-mī-sēʹtēs). Certain species of fungoid organisms; slime molds.

myxomyoma (mĭks-ō-mī-oʹmă). Muscle tissue tumor that has undergone mucous degeneration.

myxoneuroma (mĭks″ō-nŭ-rōʹmă). Tumor composed of mucous and nerve tissue elements.

myxoneurosis (mĭks-ō-nŭ-roʹsĭs). Neurosis of mucous membranes.

myxopapilloma (mĭks″ō-păp-ĭl-oʹmă). Combination myxomatous and papillomatous tumor or tumors.

myxopod (mĭksʹō-pod). The earliest form of malarial parasite. SYN: *schizont.*

myxopoiesis (mĭks″ō-poy-ēʹsĭs). The production of mucus.

myxorrhea (mĭks-or-rēʹă). Free discharge from mucous surfaces. SYN: *blennorrhea.*

   m. gastrica. Excessive mucous secretion in the stomach.

   m. intestinalis. Secretion of mucus from the bowel in neurotic persons in times of mental stress.

myxosarcoma (mĭks″ō-săr-koʹmă). Mixed tumor, partly myxomatous and partly sarcomatous, having undergone partial degeneration.

myxosarcomatous (mĭks″ō-săr-koʹmăt-ŭs). Pert. to or of the nature of myxosarcoma.

myxospore (mĭksʹō-spor). Spore embedded in a gelatinous mass, seen in some fungi and protozoa.

Myxosporidia (mĭks-ō-spor-ĭdʹĭ-ă). Parasitic sporozoans, most commonly found in epithelial cells of lower vertebrates.

myzesis (mī-zēʹsĭs). Sucking.

N

N. Symb. for *nitrogen*.

n. Chemical symb. for *normal*.

Na. Symb. for *sodium*.

nabothian cysts (na-bō'thĭ-ăn). Retention cysts formed by the nabothian follicles at neck of uterus. SEE: *cyst*.

    n. follicles, n. glands. Mucous follicles of the external os uteri. They contain a glairy fluid.

    n. menorrhagia. Accumulated mucus in the pregnant uterus, the result of excessive secretion of the uterine glands.

NaBr. Sodium bromide.

N. A. C. G. N. National Association of Colored Graduate Nurses.

NaCl. Sodium chloride.

NaClO. Sodium hypochlorite.

Na₂CO₃. Sodium carbonate.

nacreous (na'kre-us). Having an iridescent, pearl-like luster, as bacterial colonies.

N. A. D. Abbr. for *no appreciable disease*.

Naegele's obliquity (na'ge-le). Inclination of fetal head, laterally in a flat pelvis.

    N.'s pelvis. An obliquely contracted pelvis, caused by disease in infancy.

NaHCO₃. Sodium bicarbonate.

nail (nāl). A horny cell structure of the epidermis forming flat plates upon the dorsal surface of the terminal phalanges. SYN: *unguis*.

    n. bed. The end of a finger or toe covered by the nail. SYN: *nail matrix*.

    n. culture. Test tube culture in which the culture grows in the shape of a nail.

    n., eggshell. Nail plate is soft, semi-transparent, bends easily, and splits at end. Associated with arthritis, peripheral neuritis, leprosy, and hemiplegia. May be the only visible sign of late syphilis.

    n. fold. Groove in the cutaneous tissue surrounding the margins and proximal edges of the nail.

    n., hang. Broken epidermis at edge of the nail. SYN: *agnail*, (1).

    n., ingrowing. Nail with tissue overgrowing its edges.

    n. matrix. The nail bed.

    n., reedy. One marked by longitudinal fissures.

    n. skin. The quick of the nail.

    n. wall. Epidermis covering edges of the nail. SYN: *vallum unguis*.

naked (nā'kĕd). Uncovered, exposed to view, nude, bare.

nanism (na'nizm). Condition of being dwarflike in build.

    n., symptomatic. Nanism with deficient dentition, sexual development, and ossification.

nanocephalism (nan-ō-sef'ăl-ĭzm). Condition of having an abnormally small head.

nanocephalous (nan-ō-sef'ă-lŭs). Having an abnormally small head.

nanocormia (na-nō-kor'mĭ-ă). Abnormally dwarfed thorax or body.

nanoid (na'noid). Dwarflike.

nanosomia (na-nō-so'mĭ-ă). State of being a dwarf. SEE: *nanism*.

nanous (nan'ŭs). Dwarfed or stunted.

na'nus. 1. A dwarf. 2. Stunted; dwarflike.

NaOH. Sodium hydroxide.

nap (năp). 1. To slumber. 2. A short sleep; a doze.

nape (nāp; năp). Upper back part of neck.

napex (na'peks). Scalp beneath the occipital protuberance.

naphtha (naf'thă). 1. A volatile inflammable liquid distilled from carbonaceous substances. 2. Petroleum, esp. more volatile varieties.

naphthalene (naf'thă-lēn). A hydrocarbon, one of principal constituents of coal tar.

naphthol (năf'thŏl). Coal tar substance used as an antiseptic and in certain dyes.

    Also prepared from naphthalene.

napiform (na'pĭ-form). BACT: Formed like a turnip, as gelatin liquefaction.

naprapathy (nap-răp'ăth-ĭ). Method of manipulation practiced by a certain school in the treatment of disease which is based upon the assumption that disease is due to faulty functioning of ligaments.

narcism, narcissism (nar'sĭzm, nar-sĭs'ĭzm). 1. Self-love or self-admiration, 2. Voluptuous pleasure derived from observing one's own naked body.

narcissistic (nar-sĭs-sĭst'ĭk). Pert. to narcissism.

    n. object choice. Selection of another like one's own self as the object of love, friendship or liking.

narco-. Prefix: *numbness, stupor*.

narcoanesthesia (nar″kō-ăn-ĕs-thē'zĭ-ă). Anesthesia produced by a narcotic, as scopolamine and morphine.

narcohypnia (nar″kō-hĭp'nĭ-ă). Numbness following sleep.

narcolepsy (nar″ko-lep-sĭ). Overwhelming attacks of sleep which the victim cannot inhibit. SYN: *sleep epilepsy; sleep, paroxysmal*.

narcoleptic (nar-kō-lĕp'tĭk). Pert. to or marked by an overwhelming desire to sleep.

narcoma (nar-kō'mă). Coma or stupor from use of a narcotic.

narcomania (nar-kō-mā'nĭ-ă). 1. Abnormal craving for alcohol or narcotics. 2. Insanity due to use of alcohol or narcotics.

narcomaniac (nar-kō-mā'nĭ-ăk). 1. Pert.

to narcomania. 2. One affected by narcomania.

narcomatous (nar-kō-mă′tus). Pert. to a state of stupor from use of narcotics.

nar′cose. In a stuporous state.

narco′sis. Unconscious state due to narcotics.

> **n., basal.** Narcosis produced prior to administration of ether or any general anesthetic.

> **n., insufflation.** General anesthesia produced by administering the anesthetic through a tube passed bet. the vocal cords into the trachea.

> **n., medullary.** General anesthesia induced by a local anesthetic injected in the sheath of the spinal cord in lumbar region. SYN: *spinal anesthesia.*

> **n. paralysis.** Paralysis induced by pressure on a nerve during surgical anesthesia.

narcosomania (nar-kō″sō-mā′nĭ-ă). Morbid craving for, or insanity produced by narcotics. SYN: *narcomania.*

narcot′ic. 1. Producing stupor or sleep. 2. Drug producing stupor, complete unconsciousness and allaying pain.
> Narcotics are more powerful than hypnotics.

narcotism (nar′kŏt-ĭzm). 1. State of stupor induced by a narcotic. SYN: *narcosis.* 2. An addiction to the use of narcotics.

nar′cotize. To render unconscious through the use of a narcotic.

naris (na′rĭs) (pl. *nares*). The nostril.

> **n., anterior.** BNA. External nostril.

> **n., posterior.** BNA. Either internal opening into pharynx.

nasal (nā′zl). 1. Pert. to the nose. 2. Uttered through the nose. 3. A nasal bone.

> **n. bones.** The 2 small bones forming the arch of the nose.

> **n. douche.** Injection of fluid into 1 nostril, with fluid passing into the other nostril, escaping by way of the nasopharynx out of the mouth.

> **n. feeding.** Nasal gavage, *q.v.*

> **n. fossae.** Post. nasal and nasopharyngeal cavities.

> **n. gavage.** Feeding through a tube in the nasal passage.

> **n. height.** Distance bet. lower border of nasal aperture and the nasion.

> **n. index.** The greatest width of the nasal aperture in relation to a line from the lower edge of the nasal aperture to the nasion.

> **n. line.** Line from lower edge of the ala nasi curving to outer side of the orbicularis oris muscle, seen in abdominal disorders. SYN: *Jadelot's furrow or line.*

> **n. obstruction.** Commonest causes: (a) Irregular septum; (b) enlarged turbinates; (c) nasal polypi. Many complications result. TREATMENT: Nasal douches, inhalations and operative care: (a) Resection of septum; (b) turbinectomy; (c) removal of polypi; (d) opening and draining sinuses.

> **n. reflex.** Contraction of facial muscles due to irritation of nasal mucosa.

> **n. width.** Maximum width of nasal aperture.

nascent (năs′ĕnt; nā′sĕnt). 1. Just born; incipient or beginning. 2. Pert. to a substance being set free from a compound.

nasion (nā′zĭ-ŏn). The point where the nasofrontal suture is cut across by the median anteroposterior plane.

nasitis (nā-zī′tĭs). Inflammation of the nose.

Nasmyth's membrane (naz′mĭth). Epithelial membrane enveloping enamel of a tooth for short period after birth.

naso-. Combining form, *rel. to the nose.*

nasoantritis (nā″zō-ăn-trī′tĭs). Inflammation of nose and antrum of Highmore with rhinitis.

nas″ofron′tal. Pert. to nasal and frontal bones.

nas″ola′bial. Connected with or rel. to the nose and lip.

nasolacrimal (nā″zō-lăk′rĭm-ăl). Pert. to nose and lacrimal mechanism.

nasology (nā-zol′ō-jĭ). Study of the nose and its diseases.

nasomental (nā″zō-měn′tăl). Pert. to the nose and chin.

> **n. reflex.** Contraction of mentalis muscle with elevation of lower lip and wrinkling of skin of chin resulting from percussion of side of nose.

nasopalatine (nā″zō-păl′ăt-ĭn). Pert. to both nose and palate.

nasopharyngeal (nā″zō-făr-ĭn′jē-ăl). Pert. to the pharynx and nose.

nasopharyngitis (nā″zō-făr-ĭn-jī′tĭs). Inflamed condition of the nasopharynx. SYN: *rhinopharyngitis.*

nasopharynx (nā″zō-far′ĭnks). Part of pharynx situated above the soft palate (postnasal space). SYN: *rhinopharynx.*

nasoscope (nā′zō-skōp). Electrical device for examination of the nasal cavity.

nasoseptitis (nā″zō-sěp-tī′tĭs). Inflamed condition of the nasal septum.

nasosinuitis, nasosinusitis (nā″zō-sĭn-ū-ī′tĭs, -sī-nū-sī′tĭs). Inflammation of the nasal accessory sinuses and cavities.

nas′tin. Oily substance from streptothrix of leprosy which, combined with benzoyl chloride, is said to produce active immunity against leprosy.

nasus (nā′sŭs). The nose.

nasute (nā′sūt). Having a large or long nose.

natal (nā′tăl). 1. Pert. to birth or the day of birth. 2. Pert. to the nates or buttocks.

natal′ity. The birth rate.

natant (nā′tănt). Floating; swimming.

nates (nā′tēz). 1. Gluteal region; fleshy prominences formed by the gluteal muscles and covering of fat and skin. SYN: *buttocks.* 2. The ant., sup. or upper 2 corpora quadrigemina.* SEE: *testes.*

natimortality (nā″tĭ-mor-tăl′ĭ-tĭ). Rate of stillbirths in proportion to the general birth rate.

native (nā′tĭv). 1. Born with; inherent.

2. Natural, normal. SYN: *indigenous*. 3. Belonging to, as place of one's birth.

n. albumin. A protein group found in tissues. SEE: *albumin*.

nativistic theory (nă-tĭv-ĭs'tĭk). The mind forms ideas and possesses an inherent knowledge not derived from sensations or experience.

natremia (na-trē'mĭ-ă). Sodium in the blood.

natrium (na'trĭ-um). SYMB: Na. Sodium.

na'tron. Sodium carbonate.

na'trum. Homeopathic name for soda or sodium.

natuary (nă'tū-ar-ĭ). A lying-in ward.

nat'ural. Not abnormal or artificial.

na'turopath. One who practices naturopathy.

naturopathy (nă-tūr-op'ă-thĭ). A system of healing by natural and physical methods other than drugs, surgery, radium or x-ray.

naupathia (naw-path'ĭ-ă). Seasickness.

nausea (naw'shē-ă; naw'sē-ă). Inclination to vomit; usually preceding emesis if of gastric origin.

n. gravidarum. Morning sickness of pregnancy.

n. navalis. Seasickness. SYN: *mal de mer, naupathia*.

nauseant (naw'shē-ănt; naw'sē-ănt). 1. Causing nausea. 2. That which causes nausea.

nauseate (naw'shē-āt; naw'sē-āt). To cause or affect with nausea.

nauseous (naw'shus; naw'shē-ŭs). Producing nausea, disgust or loathing.

navel (nā'vĕl). The depression or scar in center of abdomen, where the umbilical cord of fetus is attached. SYN: *umbilicus, q.v.*

n. string. Umbilical cord.

navicula (nă-vĭk'ū-lă). Fossa navicularis.*

navicular (nă-vĭk'ū-lar). 1. Shaped like a boat. 2. Scaphoid bones in the carpus and in the tarsus. SEE: *skeleton*.

N. D. A. National Dental Association.

near point. Closest point of distinct vision, with maximum accommodation.

It recedes with age, varying from 3 in. in 2 yr. to 40 in. at 60 yr.

n. p., absolute. For either eye.

n. p., relative. For both eyes taken together.

nearsight (nēr'sīt). Ability to see clearly only a short distance. SYN: *myopia*.

near'sight"ed. Able to see clearly only a short distance. SYN: *myopia*.

nearsight'edness. Ability to see distinctly only a short distance. SYN: *myopia*.

nearthrosis (nē-ar-thrō'sĭs). A false joint or abnormal articulation.

nebula (nĕb'ū-lă). 1. Slight haziness. 2. Clouds in urine. 3. Group of oily substances.

n. corneae. Grayish opacity of the cornea.

nebuliza'tion. 1. Treatment with spray method. 2. Conversion into a vapor. SYN: *vaporization*.

nebulizer (nĕb'ū-lī-zĕr). An atomizer or sprayer.

Neca'tor america'nus. The hookworm. SYN: *Ankylostoma americanum*.

neck (nĕk). 1. Part of body bet. head and shoulders. 2. The constricted portion of an organ, or that resembling a neck.

n., anatomical. Constriction just below the head of the humerus. SYN: *collum anatomicum*.

n., back of. Nape of the neck. SYN: *nucha, scruff*. [neck.

n., Madelung's. Diffuse lipoma of the

n., Nithsdale. Goiter.

n., surgical. Narrow part of humerus below the tuberosity. Fracture here is common.

n. of womb. The cervix uteri.

n., wry. Torsion of the neck caused by contracted muscles. SYN: *torticollis*.

necretomy (nĕ-krĕk'to-mĭ). Surgical removal of necrosed tissue.

necremia (nĕk-rē'mĭ-ă). Death of most of the erthrocytes in the blood; decomposition of the blood.

necro-. Combining form meaning *pertaining to death*.

necrobiosis (nĕk-rō-bĭ-ō'sĭs). Gradual degeneration and death of tissue. SEE: *necrosis*.

necrobiotic (nĕ"krō-bī-ŏt'ĭk). Pert. to or affected by necrosis. SYN: *necrotic*.

necrocytosis (nĕ"krō-sī-tō'sĭs). Cellular death or decomposition.

necrogenic, necrogenous (nĕ-krō-jĕn'ĭk, -krŏj'ĕn-ŭs). Caused by, pert. to, or originating in dead matter.

necrology (nĕk-rol'o-jĭ). The study of mortality statistics.

necrologist (nĕk-rol'ō-jĭst). A student of mortality statistics.

necromania (nĕk-rō-mā'nĭ-ă). 1. Abnormal interest in dead bodies or in death. 2. Mania with desire for death.

necrometer (nĕk-rom'ĕt-ĕr). Device for measurement of dead organs.

necronarcema (nĕ-krō-nar-sē'mă). Rigidity of a dead body. SYN: *rigor mortis*.

necronectomy (nĕk-rōn-ĕk'tō-mĭ). Excision of a necrotic part. esp. of necrotic ossicles.

necroparasite (nĕk-rō-par'ă-sīt). A vegetable organism which lives in dead organic matter. SYN: *saprophyte*.

necrophagous (nĕ-krŏf'ă-gŭs). Feeding or existing on dead bodies or matter.

necrophile (nĕk'rō-fīl). One who has a morbid interest in or violates dead bodies.

necrophilia (nĕk-rō-fīl'ĭ-ă). 1. Sexual perversion with desire for, or coitus with, dead bodies. 2. Strong desire for death. SYN: *necrophilism*.

necrophilism (nĕk-rŏf'ĭl-ĭzm). 1. Sexual perversion in which there is insane love for, or violation of, the dead. 2. Strong desire for death.

necrophilous (nĕk-rŏf'ĭl-ŭs). 1. Having a morbid fondness for, or feeding on, dead tissue. 2. Pert. to or affected with necrophilism.

necrophobia (nĕk-rō-fō'bĭ-ă). 1. Abnormal aversion to dead bodies. 2. Insane dread of death. SYN: *thanatophobia*.

necropneumonia (nĕk″rō-nû-mō′nĭ-ă). Pulmonary gangrene.

necropsy (nĕk′rŏp-sĭ). The scientific examination of a dead body to determine cause of death or pathological conditions. SYN: *autopsy, necroscopy, postmortem.*

necropyoculture (nĕk″rō-pī-ō-kŭl′tshŭr). A culture from pus in which the leukocytes are dead.

necrosadism (nĕk″rō-sā′dĭzm). Sexual gratification derived from the mutilation of dead bodies.

necroscopy (nĕ-krŏs′kō-pĭ). Scientific inspection of a dead body to find cause of death or pathological condition. SYN: *autopsy, necropsy.*

necrose (nĕk-rōs′). To cause or to undergo necrosis.

necrosis (nĕk-rō′sĭs). Death of areas of tissue or bone surrounded by healthy parts; death in mass as distinguished from *necrobiosis,* a gradual degeneration. SYN: *gangrene, mortification.*

   n., anemic. Necrosis caused by disturbed circulation in a part.

   n., Balser's fatty. Pancreatitis with grangrenous areas in the fatty tissues.

   n., caseous. SEE: *cheesy necrosis.*

   n., central. Necrosis which affects only the center of a part.

   n., cheesy. Necrosis of tuberculous type with cheeselike formation.

   n., coagulative. Necrosis due to embolic infection or exuding inflammations.

   n., colliquative. Necrosis caused by liquefaction of tissue due to autolysis or bacterial putrefaction.

   n., dry. Necrosis with dryness of the sequestrum.

   n., embolic. Necrosis resulting from an embolus which causes anemic necrosis.

   n., fat. Necrosis in small scattered areas in the fatty tissue.

   n., fibrinous. SEE: *coagulative necrosis.*

   n., focal. Coagulative necrosis in small scattered areas.

   n., moist. Necrosis with softening and moist condition of the dead bone.

   n., putrefactive. Necrosis caused by bacterial decomposition.

   n., superficial. Necrosis affecting only the bone surface.

   n., thrombotic. Necrosis due to thrombus formation.

   n., total. Necrosis affecting an entire part.

   n. ustilaginea. Dry necrosis due to ergot poisoning.

necrotic (nĕk-rŏt′ĭc). Rel. to death of a portion of tissue.

necrotomy (nĕk-rŏt′ō-mĭ). 1. Dissection of a cadaver. 2. Excision of a sequestrum or other necrotic tissue.

nectarine (nĕk″ter-ēn′). Av. SERVING: 125 Gm. Pro. 0.8, Carbo. 19.9. VITAMINS: A+, C+.

needle (nēd′l). A pointed instrument for stitching, ligaturing or puncturing.

   n., abdominal. Straight type with sharp point. SYN: *Keith's needle.*

   n., aneurysm. Needle with handle and hooked, curved point.

   n., aspirating. Long, hollow needle used in extracting fluids from cavities.

   n., Ferguson's. Full, curved, fine needle for intestinal operations.

   n., fistula. Needle with shorter curve than ordinary full curved needles, used also in suturing dense tissues.

   n., Hagedorn. 1. Straight, flat needle with round eye. 2. Curved, flat needle bent on edge instead of on the flat, with round eye.

   n. holder. Device similar to a scissors used to hold surgical needles.

   n., hypodermic. Needle of different lengths and bores of a hollow type, used in injecting or withdrawing fluid under the skin.

   n., Keith's. SEE: *abdominal needle.*

   n. spray. Spray bath through tiny horizontal jets of approximately needle size.

   n., staphylorrhaphy. Needle with handle and curved point.

need'ling. Treatment by puncturing with a needle. SYN: *discission.*

neëncephalon (nē-ĕn-sĕf′ă-lŏn). The higher nerve centers comprising the cerebral cortex and fibers of pyramidal tracts.

negative (neg′ă-tiv). 1. Without positive statement. 2. Lacking results. 3. PSY: Marked by resistance or retreat, as to a suggestion. 4. Directed away from a source of stimulation. 5. Not affirming presence of an organism, as a negative diagnosis.

   n. culture. One not revealing the suspected organism.

   n. electricity. Static electricity in which elementary unit is the electron, and which is produced by friction.

   n. electrode. The chemically active pole by which currents leave. SYN: *cathode, negative pole.*

   n. glow. The luminous glow that is adjacent to the cathode in a vacuum tube through which an electrical discharge is passing.

   n. reaction. Absence of a positive indication of disease, as a negative Wassermann reaction for syphilis.

   n. sensation. One caused by stimulus not perceived in consciousness.

   n. sign. Minus sign (—) used in subtraction and to indicate a lack.

negativism (nĕg′ă-tĭv-ĭzm). Behavior peculiarity marked by not performing suggested actions (*passive negativism*) or in doing the opposite (*active negativism*), as seen in dementia precox.

Ne'gri bodies. Very minute bodies formed in nerve cells of the brain of one affected by rabies.

Neisseria (nī′sĕ-rĭ-ă). A genus of Coccaceae, diplococci with flattened spherical shapes.

   They are arranged in pairs, nonmotile, gram-negative and parasitic.

N. catarrhalis. Species found in inflammation of the mucosa.

N. flava. Species seen in respiratory catarrhs.

N. gonorrhoeae. Species causing gonorrhea. SYN: *gonococcus.*

N. intracellularis. Intracellular organism causing cerebrospinal meningitis. SYN: *meningococcus.*

N. meningitidis. SEE: *Neisseria intracellularis.*

Nelaton's cath′eter. A flexible, soft rubber catheter.

N.'s line. One from ant. sup. spine of the ilium to tuberosity of the ischium.

nem. A food value unit, the value in calories of 1 Gm. of mother's milk, equalling about 2/3 calory.

Nemathel′minthes. A roundworm. SEE: *Platyhelminthes.*

nematoblast (nem′ă-tō-blast). Rudimentary spermatozoon from division of the spermatocyte. SYN: *spermatoblast.*

nematocide (nem′ă-tō-sīd). An agent that kills nematode worms.

Nematoda, Nematodes (něm-ăt-ō′dă, -dez). An order of threadlike worms, mostly parasitic.

nematode, nematoid (něm′ă-tōd, -ăt-oid). 1. Filamentous; threadlike. 2. A species of the Nematoda.

nematodiasis (něm″ăt-ō-dī′ă-sĭs). Infestation by a parasite belonging to the order Nematoda.

nembutal (něm′bū-tăl). Pentobarbital sodium. One of the newer barbiturates, believed to have a short hypnotic action, and pronounced sedative effect.

DOSAGE: As a hypnotic, 1½ gr. (0.1 Gm.).

SEE: *pentobarbital sodium.*

neo-. Combining form meaning *new* or *recent.*

neoarsphenamine (nē″o-ars-fěn-am′ēn). An arsenic compound containing about 20% arsenic.

DOSAGE: Average for man, 7-10 gr. (0.45-0.6 Gm.). For women of average weight, 5 gr. (0.3 Gm.) to 7 gr. (0.45 Gm.) maximum. Intravenous injections preferable.

neoarthrosis (nē″ō-ar-thrō′sĭs). A false joint. SYN: *nearthrosis.*

ne′oblast. Part of a mesoblastic element from which the vascular and connective structures originate. SYN: *parablast.*

neoblas′tic. Pert. to, or constituting, a new growth of tissue.

neocerebellum (nē″ō-sěr-ē-běl′ŭm). Lateral lobes of the cerebellum, the more recently developed part.

neocinchophen (nē-ō-sĭn′kō-fěn). USP. A tasteless preparation of cinchophen and less likely to cause gastric irritation.

DOSAGE: 8 gr. (0.5 Gm.).

neocinetic (nē-ō-sin-et′ĭk). Pert. to a division of the motor system of peripheral nerves. SYN: *neokinetic.*

neocyte (nē′ō-sīt). An immature white blood corpuscle.

neocytosis (nē″ō-sī-tō′sĭs). Presence of immature leukocytes in the blood. SYN: *skeocytosis.*

neoencephalon (nē″ō-ěn-sěf′ă-lŏn). The higher nerve centers. SYN: *neëncephalon.*

neofetus (nē-ō-fē′tŭs). Embryo during 8th and 9th week of intrauterine existence.

neoformation (nē″ō-for-mā′shŭn). 1. Regeneration. 2. A neoplasm or new growth.

neogala (nē-og′ăl-ă). The first milk following childbirth. SEE: *colostrum.*

neogenesis (nē-ō-jěn′ē-sĭs). Regeneration or re-formation, as of tissue.

neogenetic (nē″ō-jěn-ět′ĭk). Newly formed; relating to new formations.

neohymen (nē-ō-hī′měn). A false or new membrane. SYN: *pseudomembrane.*

neokinetic (nē″ō-kĭn-et′ĭk). Pert. to a division of the motor mechanism of peripheral nerves.

neologism (nē-ol′ō-jĭzm). 1. A new word or phrase, or a new meaning attached to an old word or phrase. 2. PSY: A mental condition in which the patient coins new words which are meaningless, or words to which he gives *special* significance without being aware of their normal significance. SEE: *lalopathy.*

neomembrane (nē-ō-měm′brān). A false or a new membrane. SYN: *neohymen.*

neomorph (nē′ō-mōrf). BIOL: A new formation or development which is not inherited from a similar structure in an ancestor.

neon (nē′ŏn). SYMB: Ne. An inert, gaseous element in the air derived from liquid argon. At. wt. 20.2.

neonal (nē′ō-năl). A compound of barbituric acid, considered more active.

DOSAGE: 1½ gr. (0.1 Gm.).

neonatal (nē-ō-nā′tăl). Concerning the newborn. SEE: *period.*

neopallium (nē″ō-pal′ĭ-ŭm). That portion of cerebral hemisphere not belonging to the rhinencephalon or corpus callosum, comprising most of the convoluted cortex and its associated white fibers.

neopathy (nē-ōp′ă-thĭ). 1. A newly found disease. 2. A new complication or new condition of a disease.

neophilism (nē-ōf′ĭl-ĭzm). Morbid love of novelty and new persons and scenes.

neophobia (nē″ō-fō′bĭ-ă). Fear of new scenes or novelties; aversion to all that is unknown or not understood. SYN: *cainotophobia.*

neophrenia (nē″ō-frē′nĭ-ă). Mental deterioration or primary psychical failure in early youth.

neoplasia (nē″ō-plā′zĭ-ă). The development of new tissues or neoplasms.

neoplasm (nē′ō-plăzm). A new formation of tissue, abnormally, as a tumor or growth. It serves no useful function, but grows at the expense of the healthy organism or part.

n., benign. A growth not spreading by metastases or infiltration of tissue.

n., histoid. A neoplasm in which structure resembles the tissues and elements which surround it.

n., malignant. A growth, such as cancer, that infiltrates tissue, metastasizes, and often recurs after removal.

n., mixed. A neoplasm composed of tissues from 2 of the germinal layers.

n., multicentric. A growth arising from a number of distinct groups of cells.

n., organoid. A neoplasm in which the structure is similar to some organ of the body.

n., unicentric. A growth having origin in 1 group of cells.

neoplastic (nē″ō-plas′tĭk). Pert. to, or of the nature of, new, abnormal tissue formation.

neoplasty (nē′ō-plăs-tĭ). Surgical formation or restoration of parts.

neoprontosil (nē″ō-pron′tō-sĭl). A sulfonamide compound, recently come into use and thought to be less severe in its effects than sulfanilamide.

DOSAGE: Orally, from 5 to 15 gr. at the discrimination of the physician, proportioned according to body weight of the patient and the condition. In pregnancy, 40 gr. daily in 5-day courses. Subcutaneously or intramuscularly, 15-20 cc. of a 2.5% solution are recommended in severe cases.

neosalvarsan (nē″ō-săl′var-săn). A compound of arsenic. SEE: neoarsphenamine.

DOSAGE: Intraven., 10 gr. (0.6 Gm.).

neosil′ver arsphenamine (ars″fĕn-ăm′ĕn). A silver derivative of arsphenamine, containing about 20% arsenic and 6% silver.

DOSAGE: For adults, 0.3-0.4 Gm. intravenously, at intervals of 5-7 days. Course of treatment recommended: 10 or 12 injections, with the same caution observed as in the use of neoarsphenamine.

neo-sil′vol. Colloidal silver iodide compound containing 18-22% silver iodide.

DOSAGE: In solutions of 5-40% strength.

neostomy (nē-os′tō-mĭ). Formation of opening into an organ or bet. 2 organs.

neostriatum (nē″ō-strī-ā′tŭm). The caudate nucleus and outer, darker part of the lenticular nucleus of the brain.

neo-synephrin hydrochloride (nē″ō-sĭn-ef′rin). A synthetic alkaloid, with therapeutic effects similar to, but more lasting than, those of ephedrine and adrenalin.

DOSAGE: ¼-1 cc. of a 1% solution.

neothalamus (nē″ō-thal′am-ŭs). The cortical part of the optic thalamus.

neothesin (nē-ō-thes′in). Local anesthetic, one of the cocaine group, used in 1-20% solution.

neothe′sol. A mixture of procaine, refined French almond oil and 2 other chemicals, said to produce local anesthesia lasting for 14 days.

nephelometer (nĕf-ĕl-om′ĕt-ĕr). Apparatus for measuring the turbidity of a fluid for the number of bacteria in a suspension.

nephelometry (nĕf-ĕl-ŏm′ĕt-rĭ). The employment of the nephelometer.

nephelopia (nĕf-el-ō′pĭ-ă). Dim or cloudy vision from lessened transparency of the ocular media.

nephradenoma (nĕf-răd-ĕn-ō′mă). Renal adenoma.

nephralgia (nĕf-ral′jĭ-ă). Renal pain.

nephralgic (nĕf-răl′jĭk). Pert. to renal pain.

n. crises. Ureteral paroxysmal pain in locomotor ataxia.

nephrapostasis (nĕf-ră-pos′tă-sĭs). Renal abscess or purulent inflammation of the kidney.

nephrasthenia (nē-frăs-thē′nĭ-ă). A slight nephrosis without actual disease of the renal tubules.

nephratony (nĕf-rat′ō-nĭ). Lack of normal renal tone.

nephrauxe (nĕf-rawks′ē). Renal hypertrophy.

nephrectasia, nephrectasis, nephrectasy (nĕf-rĕk-ta′zĭ-ă, -rĕk′tă-sĭs, -tă-sĭ). Renal distention.

nephrectomy (nĕf-rek′tō-mĭ). Removal of a kidney.

nephrelcosis (nĕf-rĕl-kō′sĭs). Ulceration of the mucosa of the kidney.

nephrelcus (nĕf-rel′kŭs). Renal ulcer.

nephremia (nĕf-rē′mĭ-ă). Congested state of kidney. SYN: nephrohemia.

nephremphraxis (nĕf″rem-fraks′is). Obstruction in the renal vessels.

nephric (nĕf′rĭk). Pert. to the kidney or kidneys. SYN: renal.

nephridium (nĕf-rĭd′ĭ-ŭm). An embryonic segment from which are developed part of the ovary or testis, and the excretory portion of the kidney.

nephrin (nef′rin). An amino acid derived from protein digestion. SYN: cystine.

nephrism (nĕf′rĭzm). Aggregate of symptoms produced by chronic kidney disease.

nephritic (nĕf-rĭt′ĭk). 1. Rel. to the kidney. 2. Pert. to nephritis. 3. An agent used in nephritis.

nephritis (nē-frī′tĭs or nĕf-rī′tĭs) (pl. nephritides). Inflammation of the kidney.

n., acute. An inflammatory form involving the glomeruli, the tubules, or the entire kidney. It is of various types, depending on the portion of the kidney involved, degenerative, diffuse, suppurative, hemorrhagic, interstitial, and parenchymatous.

n., arteriosclerotic. SEE: chronic interstitial nephritis.

n., catarrhal. Acute nephritis with stoppage of the tubules.

n., cheesy. A chronic form with caseous degeneration and suppuration.

n., chronic. Progressive form in which entire structure of kidney may be affected, or affection may be confined to the glomerular or tubular processes. One variety of nephritis may merge with another, causing a diffuse nephritis. Symptoms depend upon the tissues involved. [tis.

n., desquamative. SEE: acute nephri-

n., diffuse, acute. An inflammatory process involving more or less the entire kidney.

n., d., chronic. SEE: *interstitial nephritis, chronic.*

n. dolorosa. A form with hypertrophy of the capsule and pain in the kidney.

n., exudative. Form with blood serum exudation.

n., focal. Nephritis with foci of inflammation distributed throughout the kidney.

n., glomerular. A form involving the renal glomeruli. It may be acute or chronic. SEE: *glomerulonephritis.*

n., g., acute. Acute form in which the pulse is rapid, and hypertension, edema, and urine containing albumin, blood, and casts are present. There is retention of urea and salt.

n., g., chronic. Form almost always following acute glomerular nephritis. It is marked by hyalinization of the glomeruli, arteriosclerosis, hypertension, albuminuria, edema, and later uremic symptoms. Usually fatal. SEE: *glomerulonephritis, chronic.*

n., g., focal, embolic. Nephritis in which emboli lodge in the capillary loops of the glomeruli, occluding them.

n., g., f., nonembolic. Nephritis in which not all of the glomeruli are affected and those affected are not equally so.

n., hemorrhagic. Acute nephritis with tubular hemorrhage and subsequent hematuria.

n., idiopathic. Nephritis of unknown etiology.

• n., indurative. Chronic nephritis marked by atrophy of the renal secreting structure and enlargement of the connective tissue stroma.

n., interstitial, acute. Rare form of acute nephritis in which there occur areas of cellular infiltration irregularly distributed bet. the tubules and around the glomeruli. SEE: *nephritis, glomerular, focal, nonembolic,* for symptoms and treatment.

n., i., chronic. Glomeruli and interstitial tissue involved.

n., lipomatous. Fatty infiltration of the renal parenchyma. SYN: *lipomatosis renis.*

n., parenchymatous, acute. Acute form affecting the parenchyma.

n., p., chronic. Progressive form with loss of strength and flesh.

n., productive. Nephritis with blood serum exudation and dilatation of the connective tissue stroma.

n., saturnine. Nephritis from lead poisoning.

n., suppurative. Purulent form of nephritis.

n., s., acute. Purulent form with abscess formation.

n., s., chronic. Cheesy and tubercular form of nephritis.

n., tubal; n., tubular. Nephritis affecting the renal tubules.

n., tuberculous. Nephritis due to presence of tubercle bacilli.

nephro-. Prefix: Pert. to the kidney.

nephroabdominal (nĕf″rō-ăb-dom′ĭ-năl). Concerning the kidney and abdomen.

nephrocapsectomy (nĕf″rō-kap-sek′tō-mĭ). Renal decapsulation for relief of chronic nephritis.

nephrocardiac (nĕf″rō-kar′dĭ-ăk). Concerning the heart and kidney.

nephrocele (nĕf′rō-sēl). Renal hernia.

nephrocolic (nĕf″rō-kŏl′ĭk). 1. Severe, colicky pain in ureter due to passage of stone. 2. Concerning the colon and kidney.

neph″rocol′ica. Colicky cramp in ureter from passage of stone.

nephrocolopexy (nĕf″rō-kŏl′ō-pĕks″ĭ). Surgical suspension of kidney and colon using the nephrocolic ligament.

nephrocoloptosis (nĕf″rō-kō-lŏp-tō′sĭs). Condition in which the kidney and colon are displaced downward.

nephrocystanastomosis (nĕf″rō-sĭst-ăn-ăs″-to-mō′sĭs). Surgical formation of a connection bet. kidney and the bladder, in permanent ureteral obstruction.

nephrocystitis (nĕf″rō-sĭs-tĭ′tĭs). Inflamed condition of kidneys and bladder.

nephrocystosis (nĕf″rō-sĭs-tō′sĭs). Formation of cysts in the kidneys.

   n., bacterial. Nephrocystosis having a bacterial etiology.

   n., capsular. Nephrocystosis affecting Bowman's capsule.

   n., catarrhal. Nephrocystosis with the epithelium desquamated from the tubules.

   n., desquamative. SEE: *catarrhal nephrocystosis.*

   n., diffuse. A form, acute or chronic, affecting both the parenchyma and the stroma.

   n., fibrous. Nephrocystosis affecting the stroma.

   n., glomerular. Nephrocystosis especially affecting the glomeruli.

nephrogenetic, nephrogenic, nephrogenous (nĕf″rō-jĕn-ĕt′ĭk, -jĕn′ĭk, -rōj′ĕn-ŭs). Arising in or from the renal organs.

nephrohemia (nĕf″rō-hē′mĭ-ă). Renal congestion. SYN: *nephremia.*

nephrohydrosis (nĕf″rō-hĭ-drō′sĭs). Accumulation of renal fluid due to obstruction.

nephrohypertrophy (nĕf″rō-hĭ-pĕr′trō-fĭ). Overgrowth or dilatation of the kidneys.

nephroid (nĕf′roid). Resembling a kidney; kidney-shaped. SYN: *reniform.*

nephrolith (nĕf′rō-lĭth). Stone in the kidney.

nephrolithiasis (nĕf″rō-lĭth-ī′ă-sĭs). The formation of renal stones. SYN: *lithiasis nephritica, lithiasis renalis.* SEE: *calculus, renal.*

nephrolithotomy (nĕf″rō-lĭth-ot′ō-mĭ). Renal incision for removal of calculus.

nephrology (nĕf-rŏl′ō-jĭ). Science of the structure and function of the kidney.

nephrolysin (nĕf-rol′ĭs-ĭn). A toxic principle from animal serum that dissolves kidney cells. SYN: *nephrotoxin.*

nephrolysis (nĕf-rol′ĭs-ĭs). 1. Surgical detachment of an inflamed kidney from adhesions. 2. Destruction of kidney tissue by action of a nephrotoxin.

nephroma (nĕf-rō'mă). Renal tumor or 1 of renal tissue.

nephromalacia (nĕf″rō-mă-lā'sĭ-ă). Abnormal renal softness or softening.

nephromegaly (nĕf″rō-mĕg'ă-lĭ). Extreme enlargement of 1 or both kidneys.

nephromere (nĕf'rō-mēr). Segment in embryo from which kidney develops. SYN: *nephrotome*.

nephron (nĕf'ron). A unit in the kidney (said to be a million of them in each kidney) representing the excretory function of the organ.

nephroncus (nĕf-rŏn'kŭs). A renal tumor.

nephroparalysis (nĕf″rō-păr-ăl'ĭ-sis). Paralyzed renal function.

nephropathy (nĕf-rop'ă-thĭ). Disease of the kidney.

nephropexy (nĕf'rō-pĕks-ĭ). Surgical attachment of a floating kidney.

nephrophthisis (nĕf-rŏf'thĭs-ĭs). 1. Tuberculosis of the kidney, with caseous degeneration. 2. Suppurative nephritis with wasting of the kidney substance.

nephroptosis (nĕf-rŏp-tō'sĭs). Prolapse or downward kidney displacement.

nephropyelitis (nĕf″rō-pī-ĕl-ī'tĭs). Inflammation of the renal pelvis and substance. SYN: *pyelonephritis*.

nephropyosis (nĕf″rō-pī-o'sĭs). Purulence of a kidney.

nephrorrhagia (nĕf-ror-ā'jĭ-ă). Renal hemorrhage into pelvis and tubules.

nephrorrhaphy (nĕf-ror'ă-fĭ). Suture of a floating kidney to the post. wall of the abdomen.

nephrosclerosis (nĕf″rō-sklĕ-rō'sĭs). Renal sclerosis or hardening. SEE: *nephritis, chronic interstitial*.

nephrosis (nĕf-rō'sĭs). Condition in which there are degenerative changes in the kidneys without the occurrence of inflammation.

 n., amyloid. Nephrosis due to deposition of amyloid within the walls of the renal blood vessels and at the base of the cells of the tubules. Marked degeneration of kidney tissue results.

 n., dehydration. Condition arising in the absence of sufficient fluids in the body. These may be lost in vomiting, severe diarrheas, or the intake may be inadequate.

 n., Epstein's. A chronic metabolic form occurring with endocrine disturbances.

 n., febrile. Condition in which mild changes take place in the kidneys of patients with acute infectious diseases, manifested by traces of albumin in urine.

 n., larval. SEE: *febrile nephrosis*.

 n., lipoid. A chronic disease of unknown etiology in which large amounts of albumin are lost in urine, resulting in depletion of the plasma protein and development of nephrotic edema.

 n., necrotic or *necrotizing*. Condition in which there is extensive death of the kidney tubules.

 n. of pregnancy. Degenerative change in the kidney during pregnancy.

 n., true. SEE: *lipoid nephrosis*.

nephrostoma, nephrostome (nē-fros'tō-mă nĕf'ros-tōm). The internal orifice of a wolffian tubule, connected with the celom in the human embryo.

nephrostomy (nĕf-ros'to-mĭ). Formation of an artificial fistula into the renal pelvis.

nephrotic (nĕf-rot'ĭk). Rel. to, or caused by, nephrosis.

nephrotome (nĕf'rō-tōm). Embryonic bridge of cells, connecting primitive segments along neural tube to the somatopleure and splanchnopleure, from which arises the urogenital system.

nephrotomy (nĕf-rot'ō-mĭ). Incision (not exploratory) of the kidney.

nephrotoxin (nĕf″rō-tŏks'ĭn). A specific toxin which destroys renal cells.

nephrotresis (nĕf-rō-trē'sis). Formation of a permanent excretory opening in the kidney through the loin.

nephrotyphus (nĕf-rō-tī'fŭs). Typhus fever complicated by hemorrhage of the kidney.

nephroureterectomy (nef″rō-ū-rē″tĕr-ĕk'tō-mĭ). Surgical excision of kidney with the ureter or part of it.

nephrozymosis (nĕf″rō-zī-mō'sĭs). Condition in which there is an infectious, fermentative disease of the kidney. SEE: *zymosis*.

nephrydrosis (nĕf-ri-drō'sĭs). Water collected in the renal pelvis due to obstruction. SYN: *hydronephrosis, nephrohydrosis*.

nepiology (nē-pī-ol'ō-jĭ). Pediatrics concerned with young infants.

Neptune girdle. Compress of linen covered by flannel which encircles the trunk from lower end of sternum to the pubes. Used in applying wet packs, esp. cold. Used to reduce cerebral congestion, visceral irritation, and congestion of int. organs.

Nernst's law (nĕrnst). Current necessary to stimulate a muscle varies as the square root of its frequency.

nerval (ner'văl). Concerning nerves. SYN: *neural*.

nervation (ner-vā'shŭn). Arrangement of nerves in the body. SYN: *neuration*.

nerve (nerv). An association of filamentous or cordlike bands or fibers of nervous tissue which connect parts of the nervous system with other organs of the body, and conducting nervous impulses to and from these organs.

 n., afferent. One which transmits impulses from the periphery to a nerve center.

 n. block. The prevention of stimuli from reaching consciousness by infiltrating the nerve supply of the field with novocain or other regional anesthetic, or by pressure, as in surgical operations.

 n., calorific. Nerve increasing heat in a part upon stimulation.

n. cell. The essential component of nervous tissue, consisting of a cell body and processes. SYN: *neuron.* SEE: *nerve.*

n. center. A group of cells concerned with those impulses controlling or regulating a bodily function.

n., centrifugal. SEE: *efferent nerve.*

n., centripetal. SEE: *afferent nerve.*

n., compound. SEE: *mixed nerve.*

n., depressor. An afferent nerve, which, when stimulated, depresses the vasomotor centers.

n., efferent. One transmitting impulses from a nerve center to the periphery.

n. ending. Terminal point of a nerve.

n., excitatory. Nerve transmitting impulses which stimulate function.

n. fiber. A unit of a nerve trunk composed of an axis cylinder, a myelin sheath, and a neurilemma. SEE: *nerve.*

n. f., medullated. Nerve fiber with myelin sheath bet. the axis cylinder and the neurilemma.

n. f., nonmedullated. One consisting of only an axis cylinder and a neurilemma.

n. fibril. A fine fiber in the cytoplasm and cell processes of a neuron. SYN: *neurofibrilla.*

n., frigorific. A sympathetic nerve causing a lowering in temperature on stimulation.

n. grafting. Insertion of a piece of healthy nerve, usually from an animal, to replace a degenerated portion in the human. SYN: *neuroplasty.*

n. hillock. Small bulge where a nerve fiber enters a muscle.

n. impulse. Name for the excitatory process which travels along a nerve fiber when stimulated.

n., inhibitory. One which, upon stimulation, lessens activity in a part.

n., mixed. One containing both afferent (sensory) and efferent (motor) fibers.

n., motor. One containing motor fibers and conveying motor impulses. SYN: *efferent nerve.*

n. plexus. A group of nerves intertwined like a braid.

n., pressor. An afferent nerve, which, when stimulated, excites vasomotor activity, increasing its function.

n., secretory. Nerve whose stimulation excites secretion in a part.

n., sensory. Nerve which conducts impulses from a sensory organ to a nerve center.

n., somatic. A sensory or motor nerve.

n. storm. Sudden attack of nervousness or nervous disorder.

n. stretching. Stretching of a nerve or nerve trunk to relieve pain.

n., sympathetic. Nerve of the sympathetic system which supplies the internal viscera and coats of blood vessels.

n. tract. Group of nerve fibers connected by a sheath. SYN: *fasciculus.* SEE: *nerve.*

n., trophic. Nerve aiding in nutritional regulation of a part.

n. trunk. An aggregation of nerve fiber bundles or fasciculi, bound together by a sheath, the epineurium. SEE: *nerve.*

n., vasoconstrictor. One which contracts a blood vessel upon stimulation.

n., vasodilator. One which dilates blood vessels upon stimulation.

n., vasomotor. Nerve which controls the caliber of a blood vessel.

nervi (ner′vī). Nerves.

n. erigentes. Minute sacral nerve branches supplying rectum, bladder, and genitalia.

n. nervorum. Tiny nerves distributed to nerve trunks.

nervimotil′ity. Power of nerve motion.

nervimotor (ner-vim-ō′tor). Concerning a motor nerve.

nervimus′cular. Rel. to nerves and muscles, or to nerve supply of a muscle.

nervine (ner′vēn). 1. Acting as a nerve sedative. 2. An agent that lessens irritability of nerves and increases nerve energy.

nervo-. Combining form *pert. to a nerve.*

nervomus′cular. Rel. to nerve supply of muscles. SYN: *nervimuscular.*

ner′von. A cerebroside found in nervous tissue.

nervosism (ner′vō-sizm). 1. Neurasthenia or nervousness. 2. The idea that morbid conditions depend upon alterations of nerve force.

nervous (ner′vus). 1. Characterized by instability of nerve action; excitability. 2. Pert. to the nerves.

n. debility. Nervous fatigue with resultant physical exhaustion. SYN: *neurasthenia.*

n. exhaustion. SEE: *nervous debility.*

n. impulse. The excitatory process set up in nerve fibers by means of stimuli.

n. prostration. SEE: *nervous debility.*

n. system. A system of extremely delicate nerve cells, elaborately interlaced with each other, collectively consisting of the brain, cranial nerves, spinal cord, spinal nerves, autonomic ganglia, ganglionated trunks, and nerves, maintaining the vital function of reception and response to stimuli.

nervousness (ner′vus-nes). Morbid excitability of the nervous system associated with unrest.

nervule (ner′vul). A small nerve.

ner′vus (pl. *nervi*). Nerve, *q.v.*

nestiatria (nes-tī-a′trī-ă). Therapeutic use of hunger cure. SYN: *nestotherapy.*

nestiostomy (nes-tī-os′tō-mī). The surgical formation of a permanent jejunal fistula through the abdominal wall.

nes′tis. 1. Jejunum. 2. Fasting.

nestither′apy. Use of hunger cure therapeutically.

nestother′apy. Therapeutic use of fasting or reduced diet.

net knot. Chromatin mass in a cell nucleus forming a nucleolus. SYN: *karyosome.*

net'tle rash. Skin rash with intense itching, resembling condition produced by stinging with nettles. SYN: *hives, urticaria.*

net'work. Fiber arrangement in a structure resembling a net. SYN: *rete, reticulum.*

neu (nū). A nerve fiber sheath. SYN: *neurilemma.*

Neumann's disease (noi'mänz). Malignant form of pemphigus with growths. SYN: *pemphigus vegetans, q.v.*

neura (nū'rä) (sing. *neuron*). Nerves.

neurad (nū'răd). Toward the neural axis or aspect.

neuradynamia (nū-rä-dī-nä'mĭ-ä). Nervous disorder with extreme fatigue. SYN: *neurasthenia.*

neuragmia (nū-rag'mĭ-ä). The bruising or ripping of a nerve trunk above or below a ganglion.

neural (nū'răl). Pert. to nerves or connected with the nervous system.

n., spine. Spinous vertebral process.

neuralgia (nū-ral'jĭ-ä). Severe, lancinating pain along the course of a nerve.
   SEE: *geniculate, sciatica.*

n., cardiac. Angina pectoris.

n., degenerative. Neuralgia caused by degenerative changes in the nerves or nerve cells.

n., epileptiform. Spasmodic facial neuralgia. SYN: *tic douloureux.*

n., facialis vera. Geniculate neuralgia.

n., Fothergill's. Trigeminal neuralgia.

n., geniculate. Neuralgia with paroxysmal lancinating pain in the ear.

n., hallucinatory. Impression of local pain without actual peripheral pain.

n., Hunt's. Geniculate neuralgia.

n., idiopathic. Neuralgia without structural lesion or pressure from a lesion.

n., intercostal. Pain follows course of intercostal nerves; frequently associated with eruption of herpes zoster; spots of tenderness near vertebral column, in middle of nerve, and near sternum. May be dependent upon spinal caries, or thoracic aneurysm.

n., mammary. Neuralgia of the breast. SYN: *mastodynia.*

n., Morton's. Neuralgia of joint of 3rd and 4th toes.

n., nasociliary. Neuralgia of eyes, brows, and roof of nose.

n., occipital. Involves upper cervical nerves. A spot of tenderness found bet. mastoid process and upper cervical vertebrae. May be due to spinal caries.

n., otic. Geniculate neuralgia.

n., reminiscent. Continued mental impression of pain after neuralgia has ceased.

n., stump. Pressure on nerves in stump after amputation, causing pain.

n., symptomatic. Neuralgia not primarily involving the nerve structure.

n., trifacial. Neuralgia involving 1 or more branches of the trifacial nerve.

neuralgic (nū-ral'jĭk). Of, or concerning, neuralgia.

neuralgiform (nū-ral'jĭ-form). Resembling neuralgia.

neuramebimeter (nū"răm-ē-bĭm'ĕt-ēr). Device for determining time of response of a nerve to a stimulus.

neuranagenesis (nū"ran-a-jen'ĕ-sĭs). Regeneration or re-formation of nerve tissue.

neurangio'sis. A vascular neurosis.

neurapophysis (nū-rä-pof'ĭ-sĭs). 1. Either side of the neural arch in a vertebra. 2. Spinous process of a vertebrae.

neurarchy (nū'rar-kē). The dominancy of the nervous system over the body.

neurarthropathy (nū-rar-throp'ă-thĭ). Disease of the joints and nerves.

neurasthenia (nū-răs-thē'nĭ-ä). An ill-defined disease commonly following depressed states characterized by a sense of weakness or exhaustion, or by the symptoms of various types of organic disease without the existence of organic disease in a degree sufficient to justify the subjective complaints of the patient.

n., sexual. Disorder arising from excessive fear due to statements of quacks, associates, etc., concerning early masturbation as a cause of imbecility or insanity.

n., traumatic. Either the expression of actual brain change, too slight to be objectively demonstrable, or a true, latent neurasthenic reaction brought to light by injury or the hope of compensation for injury.

neurastheniac, neurasthenic (nū-răs-thē'nĭ-ăk, -nĭk). 1. Suffering from or concerning neurasthenia. 2. Individual suffering from neurasthenia.

neurataxia, neurataxy (nū-rä-tak'sĭ-ä, nū'rä-tak-sĭ). Functional nervous disorder. SYN: *neurasthenia, q.v.*

neuration (nū-rā'shŭn). Arrangement or distribution of nerves. SYN: *nervation.*

neuratrophia, neuratrophy (nū-rä-trō'fĭ-ä, -răt'rō-fĭ). Atrophy of the nervous tissue or deficient nutrition of the nervous system.

neuraxial (nū-răks'ĭ-ăl). Concerning a neuraxis.

neuraxis (nū-răks'ĭs). 1. An axis cylinder of a nerve cell. 2. The cerebrospinal axis.

neuraxitis (nū-răks-ĭ'tĭs). 1. Inflamed condition of a neuraxis. 2. Encephalitis.

n., epidemic. Epidemic encephalitis.

neuraxon(e (nū-răks'ōn). The axis cylinder process of a nerve cell. SYN: *axon.* SEE: *nerve.*

neure (nūr). A nerve cell. SYN: *neuron.*

neurectasy, neurectasia, neurectasis (nū-rĕk'ta-sĭ, -rĕk-tā'zĭ-ä, -rĕk'ta-sĭs). Surgical nerve stretching.

neurectomy (nū-rĕk'tō-mĭ). Partial or total excision or resection of a nerve.

neurectopia, neurectopy (nū-rĕk-tō'pĭ-ä, nūr-ek'tō-pĭ). Displacement or abnormal position of a nerve.

neurenergen (nū-ren'ẽr-jĕn). Substance said to supply energy to the neurons.

neurenteric (nū-rĕn-ter'ĭk). Rel. to the neural canal and intestinal tube of the embryo.

    n. canal. Temporary canal of the embryo bet. the medullary and intestinal tubes.

neurepithelium (nur″ep-ĭ-the'lĭ-ŭm). 1. Epithelial structures forming the terminations of nerves of special sense. 2. Embryonic layer from which arises the cerebrospinal axis. SYN: *neuroepithelium.*

neurergic (nū-rer'jĭk). Concerning the activity of a nerve.

neurexairesis (nū-rĕks-ĭ-rē'sĭs). Ripping or tearing out of a nerve to relieve neuralgia.

neuriatry (nū-rī'ă-trĭ). Study and treatment of diseases of nervous system. SYN: *neurology.*

neurilemma (nū″rĭ-lĕm'ă). An elastic nerve fiber sheath. SEE: *nerve, substance of Schwann.*

neurilemmitis (nū″rĭ-lĕm-mī'tĭs). Inflamed condition of a neurilemma.

neurility (nū-rĭl'ĭ-tĭ). Ability of nerve fibers to conduct stimuli.

neurimotility (nū-rĭ-mō-tĭl'ĭ-tĭ). Power of neural motion. SYN: *nervimotility.*

neurimo'tor. Concerning a motor nerve.

neurine (nū'rēn). 1. An albuminous substance in nerve tissue. 2. Poisonous ptomaine found in decomposition of protagon, fungi, and fish. 3. An extract of nerve tissue used therapeutically. 4. A name for nerve energy.

neurinoma (nū-rĭn-ō'mă). A tumor derived from connective tissue in a nerve fiber. SYN: *neurofibroma.*

neurinomatosis (nū″rĭn-ō-mă-tō'sĭs). Condition of having multiple neurinomas on nerve fibers. SYN: *neurofibromatosis.*

neurite (nu'rīt). The axis cylinder process of a neuron. SYN: *axon, neuraxon.*

neuritic (nū-rĭt'ĭk). Concerning, or suffering from, neuritis.

neuritis (nū-rī'tĭs). Inflammation of a nerve or nerves, usually associated with a degenerative process.

    n., adventitial. Inflammation of nerve sheath.

    n., ascending. Neuritis along a nerve trunk away from periphery.

    n., axial. Parenchymatous neuritis.

    n., degenerative. Neuritis with rapid degeneration of nerve.

    n., descending. Neuritis along nerve trunk toward the periphery.

    n., diphtheritic. Neuritis following diphtheria.

    n., disseminated. Segmental neuritis.

    n., endemic. Beriberi or multiple neuritis.

    n., interstitial. Neuritis of connective tissue of a nerve.

    n., intraocular. Neuritis of retinal region of optic nerve.

    n., migrans; n., migrating. A roving neuritis.

    n., multiple. Inflammation of many spinal nerves at the same time.

    SYN: *polyneuritis.* SEE: *beriberi.*

    n. nodosa. Neuritis with formation of nodes on nerves.

    n., optic. Neuritis of optic nerve.

    n., parenchymatous. Neuritis of nerve fiber substance.

    n., peripheral. Neuritis of terminal nerves or of end organs.

    n., retrobulbar. Neuritis of optic nerve behind eyeball.

    n., rheumatic. Neuritis with symptoms of rheumatism.

    n., segmental. Neuritis affecting segments of a nerve interspersed with healthy segments.

    n., senile. Neuritis in feet and legs of the elderly.

    n., simple. Inflammation of single nerve trunk.

    n., sympathetic. Neuritis of opposite nerve without attacking nerve center.

    n., tabetic. Neuritis in locomotor ataxia.

    n., toxic. Neuritis from alcohol.

    n., traumatic. Neuritis following an injury.

neuro-. Combining form *rel. to a nerve.*

neuroamebiasis (nū-rō-ă-mē-bī'ă-sĭs). Neuritis occurring as a sequela to amebic dysentery.

neu″roanat'omy. Study of structure of the nervous system.

neuroarthritism (nū″rō-ar'thrĭt-ĭzm). Tendency toward contraction of nervous and gouty disorders.

neuroarthropathy (nū″rō-ar-throp'ăth-ĭ). Disease of a joint combined with disease of the central nervous system.

neurobiology (nū″rō-bī-ol'ō-jĭ). Biological approach in studying the nervous system.

neurobion (nū-ro-bī'on). A hypothetical particle connected with renewal of nerve tissue.

neurobiotaxis (nū″rō-bī″ō-tak'sĭs). Migration of nerve cells during development toward source of nutrition and stimulation.

neuroblast (nū'rō-blăst). 1. An embryonic cell giving rise to a neuron. 2. Immature neuron.

neuroblastoma (nū″rō-blăs-tō'mă). A tumor composed of immature or embryonic neurons.

neurocanal (nū″rō-kă-năl'). The central canal of the spinal cord.

neurocardiac (nū″rō-kar'dĭ-ăk). 1. Pert. to the nerves supplying the heart or nervous system and the heart. 2. Concerning a cardiac neurosis.

neurocele (nū'rō-sēl). Ventricles and cavities in the cerebrospinal axis.

neurocentral (nū″rō-sĕn'trăl). Pert. to the centrum of a vertebra and the neural arch.

neurocentrum (nū″rō-sĕn'trŭm). A vertebral element which unites with another on opposite side to form a neural arch, from which vertebral spine develops.

neuroceptor (nū″rō-sep'tor). A dendritic terminus which receives a stimulus from an adjoining nerve process.

neurochemistry (nū″rō-kĕm'ĭs-trĭ). Physiological chemistry dealing with nervous tissue.

neurochitin (nū-rō-kī'tĭn). The substance supporting nerve fibers in nervous tissue.

neurochondrite (nū″rō-kon'drīt). One of the primordial cartilaginous elements from which arises the neural arch of a vertebra.

neurochorioretinitis (nū″rō-kō″rĭ-ō-rĕt-ĭn-ī'tĭs). Inflammation of choroid and retina combined with optic neuritis.

neurochoroiditis (nū″rō-kō-roi-dī'tĭs). Inflamed condition of the choroid coat and optic nerve.

neurocirculatory (nū″rō-sur'kū-lă-tō″rĭ). Pert. to circulation and the nervous system.

n. **asthenia.** A combination of nervous and circulatory disturbances with fatigue and precordial pain, usually seen in soldiers. SYN: *irritable heart, soldier's heart.* SEE: *asthenia.*

neurocity (nū-ros'ĭt-ĭ). Nerve force.

neurocladism (nū-rok'lăd-ĭzm). Reunion of ends of a divided nerve by attraction of processes of nerve cells. SYN: *odogenesis.*

neuroclonic (nū″rō-klon'ĭk). Marked by spasms of nervous origin.

neurocoele (nū'rō-sēl). System of cavities in cerebrospinal axis. SYN: *neurocele.*

neurocranium (nū″rō-krā'nĭ-ŭm). The part of the skull enclosing the brain.

neurocrine (nū'rō-krĭn). Concerning an endocrine influence on the nervous system.

neurocrinia (nū-rō-krĭn'ĭ-ă). Endocrine stimulus of nervous system.

neurocutaneous (nū″rō-kū-tā'nē-ŭs). Pert. to the nervous system and skin.

neurocyte (nū'rō-sīt). A nerve cell. SYN: *neuron.*

neurocytoma (nū″rō-sī-tō'mă). A tumor formed of cells, usually ganglionic, of nervous origin. SYN: *neuroma, 2.*

neurodealgia (nū″rō-dē-al'jĭ-ă). Pain in the retina.

neurodendrite, neurodendron (nū″rō-dĕn'drīt, -dron). Protoplasmic branched process of a nerve cell. SYN: *dendrite, dendron.*

neurodermatitis (nū″rō-dĕr-mă-tī'tĭs). Cutaneous inflammation of neural origin, or accompanied by nervous disorder, marked by itching.

neurodermatosis (nū″rō-dĕr-mă-tō'sĭs). Any skin disease of neural origin.

neurodiagnosis (nū″rō-dī-ăg-nō'sĭs). Diagnosis of nervous disorders.

neurodocitis (nū″rō-dō-sī'tĭs). Lesion of nerve roots due to pressure.

neurodynamia (nū″rō-dī-nam'ĭ-ă). Nervous energy or force.

neurodynamic (nū″rō-dī-nam'ĭk). Concerning nervous force or energy.

neurodynia (nū″rō-dĭn'ĭ-ă). Pain in a nerve or nerves. SYN: *neuralgia.*

neuroelectricity (nū″rō-ē-lĕk-trĭs'ĭ-tĭ). Electricity generated by the nervous system.

neuroelectrotherapeutics (nū″rō-ē-lĕk″trō-

ther-ă-pū'tĭks). Electricity in treatment of neural diseases.

neuroenteric (nū″rō-ĕn-ter'ĭk). Pert. to the embryonic intestinal tube and neural canal. SYN: *neurenteric.*

neuroepidermal (nū″rō-ĕp-ĭ-dŭr'măl). Pert. to or giving rise to nervous system and epidermis.

n. **layer.** Ext. or outermost layer of the blastoderm which gives rise to epidermis and nervous system. SYN: *ectoderm, epiblast.*

neuroepithelioma (nū″rō-ĕp″ĭ-thē-lĭ-ō'mă). A tumor of neuroepithelium in a nerve of special sense.

neuroepithelium (nū″rō-ĕp″ĭ-thē'lĭ-ŭm). 1. A specialized epithelial structure forming the termination of a nerve of special sense. 2. Embryonic layer of the epiblast from which the cerebrospinal axis is developed.

neuroequilibrium (nū″rō-ē″kwĭ-lĭb'rĭ-ŭm). Balance of neural tension.

neurofibril, neurofibrilla (nū-rō-fī'brĭl, -fī-brĭl'ă) (pl. *neurofibrils, neurofibrillae*). A tiny fiber in the cytoplasm of a neuron which continues on into the nerve processes. SEE: *nerve.*

neurofibroma (nū″rō-fī-brō'mă) (pl. *neurofibromata* or *-mas*). A tumor of connective tissue of a nerve including medullated layer of a nerve fiber. SYN: *neuroma, false; pseudoneuroma.*

neurofibromatosis (nū″rō-fī-brō″mă-tō'sĭs). Condition in which there are tumors of various sizes on peripheral nerves. They may be neuromas or fibromas.

neurofibrositis (nū″rō-fī″brō-sī'tĭs). Inflammation of nerve fibers and sensory nerve fibers in muscular tissue.

neurofil (nū'rō-fĭl). A mass of fibers arising at the beginning of the axis cylinder and enveloping the neuron.

neurogangliitis (nū″rō-gan-glī-ī'tĭs). Inflamed condition of a neuroganglion.

neuroganglion. A mass of neurons on a nerve trunk acting as a nerve center. SEE: *nerve.*

neurogen (nū'rō-jen). A substance which supposedly liberates nervous force at the synapse.

neurogenesis (nū″rō-jĕn'ĕ-sĭs). 1. Growth or development of nerves. 2. Development from nervous tissue.

neurogenetic (nūr″ō-jĕn-et'ĭk). 1. Pert. to nerve formation. 2. Pert. to origin in nerves.

neurogenic, neurogenous (nū-rō-jĕn'ĭk, -roj'ĕn-ŭs). Originating in nerve cells.

n. **theory.** Cardiac muscle fibers move only in response to neural stimuli. OPP: *myogenic theory.*

n. **tonus.** Tonic muscular contraction due to stimuli from nerve centers.

neurogeny (nū-roj'ĕn-ĭ). 1. Nerve development or growth. 2. Formation from nervous tissue.

neuroglia (nū-rōg'lĭ-ă). Connective tissue forming the supporting substance of the nerve cells of the cerebrospinal axis.

n. **cell.** Spider and mossy cell in the neuroglia. SYN: *glia cell.*

neurogliac (nū-rog'lĭ-ăk). Pert. to the supporting tissue of nerve cells.

neurogliacyte (nū-rŏg'lĭ-ă-sīt). Any one of the cells found in neuroglial tissue.

neurogliar, neuroglic (nū-rŏg'lĭ-ăr, -lĭk). Pert. to or resembling the supporting tissue of nerve cells.

neuroglioma (nū″rō-glĭ-o'mă). Tumor of neurogliar tissue. SYN: *glioma.*

   n., ganglionar; n., ganglionare. Glioma with ganglion cells.

neurogliosis (nū″rō-glĭ-ō'sĭs). Development of numerous neurogliomas.

neurogram (nū'rō-grăm). The impression left upon the physical brain following any cerebral experience which is retained as unconscious memory. SEE: *engram.*

neurography (nū-rog'ră-fĭ). 1. A study or description of the nervous system. 2. Formation of neurograms in the brain.

neurohematology (nū″rō-hem″at-ol'ō-jĭ). The study of hemic changes in neural diseases.

neurohistology (nū″rō-hĭs-tol'ō-jĭ). The study of nervous tissue.

neurohypophysis (nū″rō-hĭ-pof'ĭs-ĭs). Post. portion of the pituitary gland.

neuroid (nū'roid). 1. Resembling nervous substance or nerves. 2. Neurapophysis, *q.v.* [gestion.

neuroinduction (nū″rō-ĭn-dŭk'shŭn). Sug-

neuroinidia (nū″rō-ĭn-idʹī-ă). Insufficient nutrition of nerve cells.

neuroinoma (nū″rō-ĭn-ō'mă). A connective tissue tumor arising from a nerve fiber. SYN: *neurofibroma.*

neuroinomato'sis. Multiple tumors of the peripheral nerves, either fibromas or neuromas. SYN: *neurofibromatosis.*

neurokeratin (nū″rō-ker'ă-tĭn). The variety of keratin found in myelinated nerve fibers.

neurokinet (nū-rō-kin'ĕt). An apparatus for neural stimulation by mechanical percussion.

neurokyme (nū'rō-kĭm). Energy of the nerve impulse and of all nervous activity.

neurolabyrinthitis (nū″rō-lăb-ĭr-ĭn-thī'tĭs). Inflammation of the nerves of the labyrinth.

neurolemma (nū″rō-lem'ă). 1. Sheath of a nerve fiber. 2. Rarely used name for retina.

neurologic, neurological (nū-rō-loj'ĭk, -ĭ-kal). Pert. to the study of nervous diseases.

neurologist (nū-rol'ō-jĭst). A specialist in diseases of nervous system.

neurology (nū-rol'ō-jĭ). The branch of medicine that deals with the nervous system and its diseases.

neurolymph (nū'rō-lĭmf). The cerebrospinal fluid.

neurolysin (nū-rol'ĭs-ĭn). A substance which destroys nerve cells.

neurolysis (nū-rol'ĭs-ĭs). 1. Exhaustion of a nerve or nerves from prolonged stimulation. 2. Stretching of a nerve to relieve tension. 3. Loosening of adhesions surrounding a nerve. 4. Disintegration of nerve tissue.

neurolytic (nū-rō-lit'ĭk). Concerning neurolysis.

neuroma (nū-rō'mă). 1. A tumor of a nerve fiber. 2. A tumor composed of ganglion cells, or cells of nervous origin.

   n., amputation. Neuroma occurring on a stump after amputation.

   n., amyelinic. Neuroma of a nerve fiber that has no myelin sheath.

   n. cutis. Neuroma of the derma.

   n., cystic. Neuroma with cystic formations.

   n., false. Tumor arising from connective tissue of nerves, including the myelin sheath. SYN: *neurofibroma, pseudoneuroma.*

   n., ganglionated. Neuroma composed of nerve cells.

   n., multiple. Condition in which many neuromas develop in the body. SYN: *neuromatosis.*

   n., myelinic. Neuroma composed of medullated nerve fibers.

   n., plexiform. Congenital neuroma involving all branches of a nerve. Usually found around head and are painless.

   n. telangiectodes. Neuroma with an abundance of blood vessels contained within it.

   n., traumatic. Neuroma occurring in wounds or on an amputation stump.

   n., true. Tumor of nerve fibers or cells of nervous origin. SYN: *neuroma.* SEE: *ganglioneuroma.*

neuromalacia (nū″rō-mal-a'sĭ-ă). Pathological softening of neural tissue.

neuromast (nū'rō-măst). A clump of neuroepithelium composing a sense organ. SYN: *nerve hillock.*

neuromatosis (nū-rō″mă-tō'sĭs). Multiple neuromas occurring in the body.

neuromatous (nū-rō'mă-tŭs). Rel. to a neuroma.

neuromechanism (nū″rō-mĕk'ăn-ĭzm). The neural structure controlling organic and systemic function.

neuromelitococcosis (nū″rō-melʹī-tō-kok-kō'sĭs). Undulant fever with pronounced neural disturbances.

neuromere (nū'rō-mēr). 1. Embryonic segment from which a portion of the nervous system arises. 2. A segment of the cerebrospinal nervous system.

neuromimesis (nū-rō-mĭm-e'sĭs). Resemblance of hysteria to organic disease.

neuromittor (nū-rō-mit'or). Nerve terminus which sends a stimulus to the neuroceptor of an adjacent nerve.

neuromotor (nū-rō-mō'tor). Pert. to efferent nerve impulses.

neuromuscular (nū″rō-musʹkū-lăr). Concerning both nerves and muscles.

neuromyelitis (nū-rō-mi-ĕl-ī'tĭs). Inflamed condition of spinal neural and medullary substance.

neuromyon (nū-rō-mī'ŏn). The nerve elements of a muscle.

neuromyositis (nū″rō-mī″ō-sī'tĭs). Inflammation of both nerves and muscles of a part.

neuron(e (nū'rŏn). Basic unit of nervous

tissue, nerve cell and its processes, the dendrite and the axon. SYN: *nerve cell.*

n., central. Connecting or internuncial neuron interposed between other neurons.

neuronatrophy (nū-rŏn-at'rŏ-fĭ). Any nervous disease caused by sclerosing of the neurons.

neuronephric (nū'rŏ-nĕf'rĭk). Concerning the neural and renal systems.

neuroneuronitis (nū'rŏ-nū'rŏn-ī'tĭs). Inflammation of both nerve cells and roots of the spinal cord. SYN: *neuronitis.*

neuron'ic. Concerning a nerve cell.

neuronitis (nū-rŏn-ī'tĭs). Inflammation, or degenerative inflammation of nerve cells.

neuronophage (nū-rŏn'ŏ-fāj). A phagocyte which eats neurons.

neuronophagia, neuronophagy (nū-ron-ŏfā'jĭ-ă, -of'ă-jĭ). Destruction of nerve cells by phagocytes.

neuronosis (nū'rŏ-nō'sĭs). Any disease of neural origin.

neuronyxis (nū-rŏ-niks'ĭs). Neural puncture.

neuroparalysis (nū'rŏ-pă-ral'ĭs-ĭs). Paralysis due to a nervous disorder.

neuropath (nū'rŏ-păth). One predisposed to neural disorders.

neuropathic (nū-rŏ-păth'ĭk). Rel. to neural disorders.

neuropathogenesis (nū'rŏ-păth"ŏ-jĕn'ĕsĭs). Development of a neural disease.

neuropathology (nū'rŏ-pă-thol'ŏ-jĭ). The study of the diseases of the nervous system and the structural and functional changes occurring in them.

neuropathy (nū-rop'ă-thĭ). Any disease of the nerves.

neurophage (nū'rŏ-fāj). A phagocyte that absorbs cells. SYN: *neuronophage.*

neurophonia (nū'rŏ-fō'nĭ-ă). A tic or spasm of muscles of speech resulting in an involuntary cry or sound.

neurophthisis (nū-rof'thĭ-sĭs). Atrophy of nerve tissue.

neurophysiology (nū'rŏ-fĭz-ĭ-ol'ŏ-jĭ). Physiology of the nervous structure of the body.

neuropil, neuropile, neuropilem (nū'rŏ-pĭl, -pĭl, nū'rŏ-pī'lĕm). 1. Network of unmyelinated fibrils into which nerve processes of central nervous system divide. 2. Terminus of a nerve fiber.

neuroplasm (nū'rŏ-plăzm). Protoplasmic content of a neuron.

neuroplasmic (nū'rŏ-plaz'mĭk). Concerning the protoplasm of a neuron.

neuroplasty (nū'rŏ-plăs-tĭ). Reparative surgery of the nerves.

neuroplexus (nū'rŏ-plĕks'ŭs). An intertwined bundle of nerves.

neuropodium (nū'rŏ-pŏ'dĭ-ŭm). The delicate terminal fibril of an axis cylinder process.

neuropore (nū'rŏ-pōr). Embryonic opening from neural canal to exterior.

neuropsychiatry (nū'rŏ-sī-kī'ă-trĭ). Study and treatment of nervous and mental diseases.

neuropsychic (nū'rŏ-sī'kĭk). Pert. to neural phenomena from a psychic point of view.

neuropsychology (nū'rŏ-sī-kol'ŏ-jĭ). The science of connection of neurological and psychological facts.

neuropsychopathy (nū'rŏ-sī-kop'ăth-ĭ). A neurosis in combination with a mental disease.

neuropsychosis (nū-rŏ-sī-kō'sĭs). Neurosis complicated by mental symptoms.

neuropyra (nū-rŏ-pī'ră). Fever induced or accompanied by nervousness.

neuropyretic (nū'rŏ-pī-ret'ĭk). Rel. to nervous fever.

neurorecidive (nū'rŏ-rĕs'ĭ-dĭv). Nervous symptoms in syphilis following a salvarsan injection. SYN: *neurorelapse.*

neurorecurrence (nū'rŏ-rē-kŭr'ănz). Nervous manifestation as a sequel to salvarsan injection. SYN: *neurorelapse.*

neurorelapse (nū'rŏ-rē-lăps'). Nervous symptoms in syphilis subsequent to an injection of salvarsan. SYN: *neurorecidive, neurorecurrence.*

neuroretinitis (nū'rŏ-rĕt'ĭn-ī'tĭs). Inflamed condition of optic nerve and retina.

neurorrhaphy (nū-ror'ă-fĭ). Suturing of ends of a severed nerve.

Neurorrhyctes hydrophobiae (nū'rŏ-rĭk'tēs hī-drŏ-fō'bĭ-ē). Supposed microorganisms of rabies. SYN: *Negri bodies.*

neurosarcokleisis (nū'rŏ-săr"kŏ-klī'sĭs). Operation for relief of neuralgia by resection of a wall of the osseous canal carrying a nerve and transplanting the nerve to soft tissues.

neurosarcoma (nū"rŏ-săr-kō'mă). A sarcoma containing neuromatous components.

neurosclerosis (nū"rŏ-sklĕ-rō'sĭs). Hardening of nervous tissue.

neurosensory (nū"rŏ-sĕn'sō-rĭ). Concerning a sensory nerve.

neurosis (nū-rō'sĭs). Functional disorder of the nervous system without demonstrable physical lesion.

    n., accident. A nervous disorder caused by injury or an accident.

    n., anxiety. Neurosis in which fear or apprehension is the essential symptom. SEE: *anxiety neurosis.*

    n., association. Neurosis in which association of ideas causes mental repetition of an experience.

    n., compensation. Neurosis developing after an accident in people who think they can obtain compensation by being ill.

    n., compulsion. Neurosis marked by overpowering impulse to perform acts against the will.

    n., expectation. Condition in which anticipation of an occurrence produces nervous symptoms.

    n., fatigue. Neurasthenia, *q.v.*

    n., obsessional. Uncontrollable obsessions dominating the victim's behavior; a psychoneurosis.

    n., occupational; n., professional. Neurosis in a group of muscles caused by constant repetition of an act, as in playing the piano.

n., sexual. Disorder of sex function, as impotence.

n., traumatic. SEE: *accident neurosis.*

n., war. Disorder with or without physical cause brought on by conditions of war. SYN: *shellshock.*

neuroskeleton (nū″rō-skĕl′ĕt-ŏn). The true skeleton or internal bony framework which aids in protection of parts of central nervous system. SYN: *endoskeleton.*

neurosome (nū′rō-sōm). 1. The cell body of a neuron. 2. One of the tiny fragments in the ground substance of the nerve cell protoplasm.

neurospasm (nū′rō-spăzm). Spasmodic muscular twitching due to a nervous disorder.

neurosplanchnic (nū-rō-splank′nĭk). Concerning the cerebrospinal and sympathetic nervous systems.

neurospongioma (nū″rō-spŭn-jĭ-ō′mă). A tumor composed of neurogliar tissue. SYN: *neuroglioma.*

neurospongium (nū″rō-spŭn′jĭ-ŭm). 1. A meshwork of nerve fibrils in the cytoplasm of a neuron. 2. The reticular layer of the retina.

neurosthenia (nū″rō-sthē′nĭ-ă). Abnormal response of nerves to stimuli.

neurosurgery (nū″rō-sur′jē-rĭ). Surgery of the nerves and nerve structure.

neurosuture (nū″rō-sū′chŭr). Stitching of ends of a cut nerve. SYN: *neurorrhaphy.*

neurosyphilis (nū″rō-sĭf′ĭ-lĭs). Syphilis affecting the nervous structures. SEE: *dementia paralytica.*

neurotabes (nū″rō-ta′bēz). Multiple neuritis complicated by ataxic symptoms.

neurotagma (nū-rō-tag′mă). Linear arrangement of the neuron's structural elements.

neurotension (nū″rō-tĕn′shŭn). Operative stretching of a nerve. SYN: *neurectasis.*

neurothecitis (nū″rō-the-sī′tĭs). Inflamed condition of a nerve sheath.

neurotherapeutics (nū″rō-thĕr-ă-pū′tĭks). Treatment of disorders of the nervous system. SYN: *neurotherapy.*

neurotherapy (nū-rō-ther′ă-pĭ). Treatment of neural disorders. SEE: *psychotherapy.*

neurothlipsis (nū″rō-thlĭp′sĭs). Irritation or pressure on a nerve.

neurotic (nū-rot′ĭk). 1. One suffering from instability of the nervous system. 2. Nervous or pert. to a neurosis. 3. A nervine or sedative.

neuroticism (nū-rŏt′ĭ-sĭzm). A condition or trait of neurosis.

neurotization (nū-rot-ĭ-zā′shŭn). 1. Acquisition of nervous substance. 2. Renewal of a nerve after division. 3. Surgical introduction of a nerve into a paralyzed muscle.

neurotology (nū″rō-tol′ō-jĭ). The study of ear lesions in combination with neural complications.

neurotome (nū′rō-tōm). 1. Fine knife used in the division of a nerve. 2. An embryonic segment from which arises a part of the nervous system.

neurotomy (nū-rot′ō-mĭ). Division or dissection of a nerve.

neurotonia (nū″rō-tō′nĭ-ă). Nerve stretching.

neurotonic (nū″rō-ton′ĭk). 1. Concerning neural stretching. 2. Stimulating a disordered nervous system.

neurotony (nū-rot′ō-nĭ). Nerve stretching.

neurotoxic (nū″rō-toks′ĭk). Poisonous to the nerve cells.

neurotoxin (nū″rō-toks′ĭn). A toxin that attacks nerve cells. SYN: *neurolysin.*

neurotrauma (nū-rō-traw′mă). Nerve lesion. SYN: *neurotrosis.*

neurotripsy (nū′rō-trip-sĭ). Surgical crushing of a nerve.

neurotrophasthenia (nū″rō-trof-ăs-thē′-nĭ-ă). Malnutrition of the nervous system.

neurotrophy (nū-rot′rō-fĭ). Nutrition of the nerves.

neurotropic (nū″rō-trop′ĭk). 1. Pert. to, or having a chemical affinity for nervous tissue. 2. Pert. to neurotropism.

neurotropism (nū-rot′rō-pĭzm). Attraction which nutritive elements, basic dyes, and microörganisms have for nervous tissue.

neurotrosis (nū″rō-trō′sĭs). A lesion of a nerve. SYN: *neurotrauma.*

neurovaccine (nū″rō-văk′sēn). A standardized vaccine virus of specific strength secured by cultivation in a rabbit's brain.

neurovaricosis (nū″rō-văr-ĭ-kō′sĭs). Multiple swellings along the pathway of a nerve.

neurovascular (nū″rō-văs′kū-lăr). Concerning both the nervous and vascular systems.

neurovegetative (nū″rō-vĕj′ĕ-tā-tĭv). Noting the vegetative nervous system.

neutral (nū′trăl). 1. Neither alkaline nor acid. 2. Indifferent; having no positive properties.

n. diet. One in which total basic ash is equal to or exceeded by the total acid ash. A slight excess of acids is usually planned. Protein allowance, 0.65-1 Gm. per Kg. ideal body weight. All food prepared and served without salt.

n. principle. A proximate principle of neutral reaction, not otherwise classified. Ex: *aloin, elaterin.*

neutralization (nū-tral-ĭ-zā′shŭn). 1. The opposing of one force or condition with an opposite force or condition to such degree as to cause counteraction that permits neither to dominate. 2. The reaction in which the hydrogen ion of an acid and the hydroxyl ion of a base unite to form water, the other producing a salt.

neutralize (nū′tral-īz). 1. To counteract. 2. CHEM: To destroy peculiar properties of or effect of; to make inert.

neutroclusion (nū″trō-klū′zhŭn). State in which the anteroposterior occlusal positions of the teeth or the mesiodistal positions are normal, but malocclusion of the other positions exists.

neutron (nū′trŏn). Elementary particle

with approximately the mass of a hydrogen atom, but without any electric charge.

It is a constituent of the atomic nucleus.

neutropenia (nū-trō-pē'nĭ-ă). Abnormally small number of neutrophil cells in the peripheral blood stream.

neutrophile (nū'trō-fīl, -fĭl). 1. Staining easily with neutral dyes. 2. A leukocyte which stains easily with neutral dyes. SEE: *polymorphonuclear leukocyte.*

neutrophilia (nū"trō-fĭl'ĭ-ă). Increase in the number of neutrophile leukocytes.

neutrophilic, neutrophilous (nū-trō-fĭl'ĭk, -trof'ĭ-lŭs). Staining readily with neutral dyes. SYN: *neutrophil.*

neutrotaxis (nū"trō-taks'ĭs). The attracting or repelling power of neutrophil leukocytes.

nevoid (nē'voyd). Resembling a nevus.

   n. elephantiasis. Enlarged scrotum due to distention of lymphatics and hyperplasia of tissues. SYN: *lymph scrotum.*

nevolipoma (nē-vō-lip-ō'mă). Rare lipoma containing numerous blood vessels, probably a degenerated nevus.

nevose (nē'vōs). Spotted or marked with nevi. SEE: *nevus.*

nevus (nē'vŭs). 1. A congenital discoloration of a circumscribed area of the skin due to pigmentation. SYN: *birthmark, mole.* 2. Circumscribed vascular tumor of the skin, usually congenital, due to hyperplasia of the blood vessels. SEE: *angioma.*

   n. angiectodes. SEE: *nevus vascularis.*

   n. angiomatodes. Extensive diffuse angiomatous condition of the subcutaneous tissues.

   n. araneus. Acquired or congenital dilatation of the capillaries, marked by red lines radiating from a central red dot. SYN: *spider nevus.*

   n., capillary. Nevus of dilated capillary vessels, elevated above the skin.

   n., cutaneous. Nevus formation on the skin.

   n. flammeus. Reddish discoloration of the face or neck, usually not elevated above the skin. A serious deformity due to large size and color.

   n. lipomatodes. Fatty connective tissue tumor, probably a degenerated nevus, containing numerous blood vessels.

   n. maternus. A birthmark.

   n. pigmentosus. Congenital pigment spot varying in color from light yellow to blackish.

   n. pilosus. A nevus covered with hair.

   n., spider. SEE: *nevus araneus.*

   n. spilus. Pigmented nevus with smooth surface.

   n., strawberry. SEE: *nevus vascularis.*

   n., telangiectatic. Nevus containing dilated capillaries.

   n. vascularis, n. vasculosus. Nevus in which superficial blood vessels are enlarged.

   SYN: *strawberry nevus.*

   n. venosus, n. venous. Nevus formed of dilated venules.

   n. verrucosus. Nevus with a raised wartlike surface.

new growth. Any morbid new formation, as a tumor. SYN: *neoplasm.*

nexus (neks'us). A connection or link; a binding together.

N. F. Abbr. for *National Formulary.*

NH₃. Ammonia.

NH₄Cl. Ammonium chloride.

Ni. Symb. for nickel.

niccolum (nĭk'ō-lŭm). Nickel, *q.v.*

nickel (nĭk'el). SYMB: Ni. Metallic element with an at. wt. of 58.6, salts of which are used medicinally.

   n. arc. One that emits strongly at 230 and esp. at 350 millimicrons.

Nicolaier's bacillus (nik-ō-li'er). The *Bacillus tetani.*

Nicolas-Favre disease (nē"kō-lă făvr'). Venereal disease marked by involvement of inguinal lymph glands with an exuding lesion. SYN: *Frei's disease, lymphogranuloma venerea.*

Nicol'lia. A genus of parasitic protozoa found in the blood.

nicotine (nĭk'ō-tēn, -tĭn). A poisonous alkaloid found in all parts of the tobacco plant, but esp. in the leaves.

nicotinic acid (nĭk"ō-tĭn'ĭk). A white crystalline substance known for some time to chemists, but recently come into prominence in the medical field as a possible active constituent of vitamin B complex.

   DOSAGE: 5 gr. (0.3 Gm.) daily.

nicotinism (nĭk'ō-tēn-ĭzm, -tĭn-izm). Poisoning from excessive use of tobacco or nicotine.

nictitate (nĭk'tĭ-tāt). To wink.

nictitating (nĭk'tĭ-tāt-ĭng). Winking or blinking.

   n. spasm. Clonic spasm of eyelid with continuous winking.

nictation, nictitation (nĭk-tā'shun, nĭk-tĭ-tā'shun). The act of involuntary winking due to a nervous disorder.

nidal (nī'dal). Pert. to a nucleus or an implanted fertilized ovum.

nidation (nī-da'shun). 1. Periodic intramenstrual preparation of endometrial epithelium. 2. Implantation of fertilized ovum in the uterine endometrium. 3. Formation of a colony or nest.

nidulus (nĭd'ū-lŭs). Point of origin of a nerve.

nidus (nī'dŭs). 1. A cluster; nestlike structure. 2. Focus of infection. 3. A nucleus or origin of a nerve.

   n. avis. SEE: *nidus hirundinis.*

   n. hirundinis. Depression on each side of inf. surface of cerebellum in which is lodged the tonsil.

night blindness (nīt blĭnd'nĕs). Absence of or defective vision in the dark. SYN: *nyctalopia, nyctotyphlosis.*

Nightingale, Florence (nīt'ĭn-gāl). Originator of modern nursing.

   N. oath or pledge. "I solemnly pledge myself before God and in the presence of this assembly to pass my life in purity and to practice my profession faithfully. I will abstain from whatever is deleterious and mischievous, and will not take or knowingly administer any harmful drug. I will do all in my power to elevate the standard of my profession, and I will hold in confidence all personal matters committed to my keeping, and all family affairs coming to my knowledge in the practice of my calling. With loyalty will I endeavor to aid the physician in his work and devote myself to the welfare of those committed to my care."

nightmare (nīt'măr). A bad dream accompanied by great fear and a feeling of suffocation, once believed to be caused by a female monster or spirit that sat upon the dreamer. SYN: *oneirodynia*. SEE: *antephialtic*.

nightshade (nīt'shăd). Any of the species of *Solanum*. SEE: *atropine, belladonna*.

night sweat (nīt swĕt). Profuse sweating during sleep at night.

night terrors (nīt tĕr'ĕrs). Form of nightmare in children causing them to awaken in terror, screaming.

nightwalking (nīt''wauk'ĭng). State in which individual walks about habitually while sleeping. SYN: *somnambulism*.

nigra (nī'gră). Mass of gray matter bet. the dorsal and pedal parts of the crus cerebri. SYN: *substantia nigra*.

nigral (nī'grăl). Rel. to the substantia nigra.

nigredo (nī-grē'dō). Blackness.

   n. cutis. Nigredo of the skin. SYN: *melasma*.

   n. nativa. Natural dark dermal pigmentation.

nigrescence (nī-gres'ĕns). The process of becoming black or the blackness produced.

nigricans (nī'grĭ-kăns). Blackened.

nigri-, nigro-. Combining forms meaning *pert. to blackness*.

nigrismus (nī-grĭz'mŭs). Black pigmentation. SYN: *melasma, nigredo*.

nigrities (nī-grĭsh'ĭ-ēz). Blackness; black pigmentation.

   n. linguae. A black pigmentation of the tongue. SYN: *glossophytia*.

nihilism (nī'ĭ-lĭzm). 1. Disbelief in beneficial properties of medicine. 2. PSY: A delusion that everything is unreal.

Nikolsky's sign (nĭ-kol'skĭ). Condition of the external layer of the skin in which it can be rubbed off by slight friction or injury.

ninth cranial nerve. Glossopharyngeal nerves.

   n.-day erythema. A nontoxic erythema which sometimes appears on the 9th day in a course of medication.

niphablepsia (nĭf''ă-blĕp'sĭ-ă). Blindness caused by light glare on snow.

niphotyphlosis (nĭf''ō-tĭf-lō'sĭs). Snow blindness. SYN: *niphablepsia*.

nipple (nĭp'l). 1. The protuberance in each breast from which, in the female, the lactiferous ducts discharge. SYN: *mammilla, papilla, teat*. 2. Artificial substitute for female nipple to be used on a nursing bottle.

   n. shield. Mechanical device to protect the nipple during lactation period.

nirvanin (nĭr-van'ĕn). Colorless, soluble, crystalline local anesthetic, less toxic than cocaine.

Nissl's bodies or granules (nĭs'el). Granular bodies scattered throughout the cell body of a neuron or nerve cell, which stain with cytoplasm of the basic dyes and are supposed to represent a store of nervous energy.

   SYN: *chromophilic or tigroid bodies*.

   N.'s degeneration. Slow degeneration of a neuron following division of nerve fiber supplying it.

nisus (nī'sŭs) (pl. *nisūs*). 1. An effort or struggle. 2. The desire for coitus on the part of certain animals in the spring. 3. Contraction of the muscles of the abdomen and diaphragm in the expulsion of the feces or urine.

   n. formativus. The effort of fertilized ovum to take on the characteristics of the species from which it is derived.

nit (nĭt). The egg of a louse or any other parasitic insect. SEE: *pediculosis*.

niter (nī'ter). 1. Saltpeter, potassium nitrate. 2. A salt or ester of nitric acid.

   n., sweet spirit of. Spirit of nitrous ether; *spiritus aetheris nitrosi, U.S.P.*

niton (nī'tŏn). Inert gas in radium emanation. SYMB: Nt. AT. WT.: 222.4. SYN: *radon*.

nitrate (nī'trāt). A salt of nitric acid.

nitrated. Combined with nitric acid or a nitrate.

nitration. Combination with nitric acid or a nitrate.

nitrato (nī-trā'tō). Combining form denoting presence of nitrate group; NO_3.

nitre (nī'tĕr). 1. A salt or ester of nitric acid. 2. Potassium nitrate. SYN: *niter*.

nitremia (nī-trē'mĭ-ă). Abnormal quantity of nitrogen in the blood.

nitric acid. HNO_3. A colorless, corrosive, poisonous liquid in concentrated form, employed as a caustic and disinfectant in treatment of venereal ulcers, poisoned wounds, and esp. the bites of rabid animals. It is widely used in industries and in chemical laboratories.

   n. a., fuming. Combination of nitric acid which emits fumes of a choking nature. SEE: *fumes*.

nitrification (nī''trĭ-fĭ-ka'shun). Process brought about by bacteria, in which nitric acid and nitrates are liberated in the soil by oxidation of nitrogen in ammonium salts.

nitrifying (nī''trĭ-fī'ing). Liberating nitrous and nitric acid from ammonium salts; said of bacteria.

   n. bacteria. Those which liberate nitric and nitrous acids from free nitrogen and ammonia.

nitrile (nī'trĭl, nī'trĭl). An organic compound in which the nitrogen of ammonia exists with all 3 of the hydrogen atoms displaced.

nitrite (nī'trīt). A salt of nitrous acid.

nitritoid (nī'trĭ-toyd). Resembling a nitrite.

n. crisis. A syndrome resembling symptoms produced by the use of a nitrite, usually occurring after arsphenamine injection.

nitrituria (nī-trĭ-tū'rĭ-ă). Nitrites or nitrates present in the urine.

nitro-. Combining form denoting (a) presence of niter in some form, (b) presence of the group NO_2.

nitrobacteria (nī"trŏ-băk-tē'rĭ-ă). Bacteria in the soil which convert ammonium salts into nitric acid and nitrates by oxidation. SEE: *nitrogen cycle.*

nitrogen (nīt'rŏ-jen). SYMB: N. A colorless, odorless, tasteless, gaseous element occurring free in the atmosphere, forming 4/5 of its volume. Atomic weight, 14.008.

n. cycle. The return of nitrogen from animal life to the soil, from which plants derive their supply, and in turn its return to animal life through plants taken as food.

n. equilibrium. Condition during which nitrogen excreted in the urine equals amt. taken in by the body in the food.

n. lag. Time required after a given protein is ingested until an equal amt. of nitrogen is excreted in the urine as that ingested.

n., nonprotein. A nitrogenous component of the blood that is not a protein.

n. partition. Percentage of nitrogen in the urine shown by each nitrogenous constituent.

nitrogenization (nī"trŏ-jen-ĭz-ā'shŭn). The act of combining a substance with nitrogen or 1 of its compounds.

nitrogenous (nī-troj'ĕn-ŭs). Pert. to or containing nitrogen.

nitroglycerin (nī"trŏ-glĭs'ĕr-ĭn). Any nitrate of glycerol, specifically the trinitrate, a heavy, oily, explosive, colorless liquid obtained by treating glycerol with nitric and sulfuric acids.

nitromuriatic acid (nī"trŏ-mū-rĭ-at'ĭk). A mixture of 1 part nitric and 3 parts hydrochloric acid used in commercial industries because it dissolves all the metals including platinum and gold.

nitron (nī'tron). Molecular weight of a radium emanation.

nitrous (nī'trŭs). Containing nitrogen in its lowest valency.

n. oxide. N_2O. Colorless, sweet-tasting gas with pleasing smell causing temporary general anesthesia when inhaled.

niveau diagno'sis (nē-vo'). Determination of the exact level of a lesion.

N. L. N. E. Abbr. *National League of Nursing Education.*

N. N. R. Abbr. for *New and Nonofficial Remedies,* the title of a book published by the American Medical Association, listing and describing the articles that stand accepted by the Council on Pharmacy and Chemistry of the A. M. A.

No. Abbr. L. *numero,* to the number of.

N_2O. Nitrous oxide.

N_2O_3. Nitrogen trioxide.

N_2O_5. Nitrogen pentoxide.

noble cells. Those of the organs, muscles, and nerves as differentiated from wandering and connective tissue cells.

Noble's enema. One dram of turpentine mixed well with glycerin, 2 ounces; mix 3 ounces of magnesium sulfate with 4 ounces of water, and pour the 2 mixtures together.

nociassociation (nō"sĭ-ă-sō'sĭ-ā'shŭn). Discharge of nervous energy as exhibited in form of shock, exhaustion, etc., following stimuli of the nature of trauma and operations.

nociceptive (nō"sĭ-sept'ĭv). Having the ability to receive painful stimuli.

nociceptor (nō"sĭ-sĕp'tŏr). A peripheral mechanism for reception of stimuli of pain.

nociinfluence (nō"sĭ-ĭn'flōō-ĕns). Harmful or injurious influence.

nociperception (nō"sĭ-pĕr-sĕp'shŭn). The perception by the nerve centers of injurious influences or painful stimuli.

Noct. Abbr. for *night.*

noctalbuminuria (nok"tal-bŭ-mĭn-ū'rĭ-ă). Excess of albumin voided in urine at night. SYN: *nyctalbuminuria.*

noctambulism (nŏk-tăm'bŭ-lĭzm). Sleep walking. SYN: *somnambulism.*

noctiphobia (nŏk"tĭ-fō'bĭ-ă). Fear of the night and darkness. SYN: *nyctophobia.*

nocturia (nŏk-tū'rĭ-ă). Urination, esp. excessive, during the night. SYN: *nycturia.* SEE: *enuresis.*

noctur'nal. Pert. to or occurring in the night. OPP: *diurnal.* SEE: *"nyct-" words.*

n. enuresis.* Urinary incontinence during sleep at night. SYN: *bedwetting.*

nocuity (nŏk-ū'ĭt-ĭ). Injuriousness; harmfulness.

nodal (nō'dăl). Pert. to a protuberance.

n. points. One of 2 points situated on axis of a lens that any incident ray sent through 1 will produce a parallel emergent ray sent through the other.

n. rhythm. Cardiac rhythm with origin at auriculoventricular node.

nodding (nŏd'ĭng). Quick inclination of the head downward. SYN: *nutation.*

n. spasm. Nodding of the head due to spasm of the sternomastoid muscles. SYN: *salaam convulsion.*

node (nŏd). A knot, knob, protuberance, or swelling.

n., auriculoventricular. Commencement of bundle of His in right auricle of heart.

n's., Bouchard's. Nodes on 2nd joints of the fingers in gastric dilatation.

n's., Féréol's. Nodes that are subcutaneous and seen in acute rheumatism.

n's., gouty. Nodes seen in gout.

n's., Haygarth's. Swelling of joints in arthritis deformans.

n's., Heberden's. Nodes on fingers seen in hypertrophic arthritis.

n's., Hensen's. Cell proliferation in the impregnated ovum, the beginning of the primitive streak.   [node.

n., Keith and Flack's. Sinoauricular

n., lymph. Mass of lymphoid tissue along the course of lymphatic vessels.

n's., Meynet's. Those in capsules of joints and tendons in rheumatism.

n's., Parrot's. Osteophytes around ant. fontanel seen in hereditary syphilis.

n. piedric. Node on the hair shaft seen in piedra.*

n's. of Ranvier. Round constrictions of the myelinated nerve fibers.

n's., Schmidt's. The medullated interannular segments of a nerve fiber.

n., singer's. Trachoma of vocal cords.

n., sinoauricular. One at entrance of sup. vena cava into right auricle where cardiac rhythm originates. SYN: *pacemaker.*

n's., solitary lymph. Small lymph nodes over entire mucous membrane of the intestines.

n., syphilitic. Circumscribed swelling at end of long bones due to congenital syphilis. Sensitive and painful during inflammation, esp. at night. SEE: *Parrot's nodes.*

nodose (nō'dōs). Swollen or knotlike at intervals; marked by nodes or projections.

nodosity (nō-dōs'ĭ-tĭ). 1. A protuberance or knot. 2. Condition of having nodes.

nodular (nod'ū-lăr). Containing or resembling nodules.

nodule (nod'ūl). 1. A small node. 2. Tiny protuberance on inferior cerebellar vermiform process at its ant. extremity. SEE: *chalarosis, cladosporiosis.*

n., Albini's. Nodules on free edges of auriculoventricular valves in infants.

n's., apple jelly. Elevations on leprous ulcers. They are of reddish color.

n's., Arantius'. Central fibrous tubercles in segments of semilunar valves. SYN: *corpora Arantii.*

n's., Aschoff's. Those in myocardium, seen in rheumatism.

n's., Bianchi's. SEE: *Arantius' nodules.*

n's., Bouchard's. Nodules on finger joints in gastric dilatation.

n's., endolymphangeal. Small ones within lymphatic vessels formed by adenoid tissue.

n's., epicardial. Those over epicardial vessels.

n's., Gamna. Yellowish-brown ones in the spleen in certain enlargements. SYN: *tabac nodules.*

n's., Leishman's. Pinkish ones seen in certain types of Oriental sore.

n's., lymph. Lymph glands found throughout the lymphatics.

n's., lymphatic, lymphoid. Adenoid tissue localized in masses of nucleated corpuscles.

n's., Morgagni. SEE: *nodules of Arantius.*

n's., tabac. SEE: *Gamna nodules.*

nodulus (nod'ū-lŭs) (pl. *noduli*). Nodule.

n. lymphatici aggregati. BNA. Lymphoid tissue nodules on mucosa of small intestines. SYN: *Peyer's patches.*

nodus (nō'dŭs). Node.

noematachograph (nō-ē″mă-tak'ō-grăf).

Device for recording time taken in mental activity.

noematachometer (nō-ē″mă-tak-om'ĕt-ĕr). Device for measurement of the time taken in a simple perception. SYN: *noematachograph.*

Noguchi's test (no-goo'tshe). 1. Skin test for syphilis. A few drops of luetin are injected beneath the skin. A positive result appears within 1 day, increases in size, and lasts several days. This test is more constant in tertiary syphilis and in latent forms than the Wassermann reaction.

2. A modified Wassermann test for syphilis. Extracts of animal heart muscle, as antigen, human corpuscles, complement serum from guinea pigs, and hemolytic amboceptor from rabbits are materials used in it. Results are based on amt. of inhibition of hemolysis.

3. A test for general paresis as shown by the globulin content of spinal fluid when mixed with butyric acid and normal sodium hydroxide solution.

noise (noyz). Sound of any sort, usually a loud, harsh one. SEE: *odynacusis.*

noli-me-tangere (nō'lĭ-mē-tan'jĕ-rē). Cancerous ulcer, generally of the face, which eats away bone and soft tissue.

noma (nō'mă). A gangrenous progressive condition, generally found in children, spreading from the mucous membrane of the cheek or gum to the cutaneous surface. SYN: *cancrum oris, stomatitis, gangrenous.*

n. pudendi, n. vulvae. A similar condition affecting the labia majora.

no'madism. PSY: Impulse to wander.

nomenclature (nō'mĕn-klā″chur). System of technical or scientific names. SYN: *terminology.*

nomogram (nŏm'ō-gram). Representation by graphs, diagrams, or charts of the relationship bet. numerical variables.

nomography (nō-mog'ră-fĭ). A graphic representation of the relation bet. numerical variables. [normal site.

nomotopic (nŏm-ō-tŏp'ĭk). Occurring at the

non-. Prefix denoting *not, negation.*

nona-, non-. Prefix meaning *ninth.*

nona (nō'nă). Acute or chronic infectious disease of central nervous system. SYN: *encephalitis lethargica, sleeping sickness.*

nonan (nō'năn). Having increased symptoms or reappearing every 9th day, as the paroxysms of malaria.

non compos mentis (nŏn kŏm'pŏs mĕn'tĭs). Not of sound mind.

nonconductor (nŏn″kŏn-dŭk'tŏr). A substance that does not conduct or conducts with difficulty heat, sound, or electricity.

nonelectrolyte (nŏn″e-lek'tro-līt). A nonconducting solution.

nonipara (nō-nĭp'ăr-ă). A woman who has given birth 9 times.

nonlax'ative diet. Low residue diet* with boiled milk and toasted crackers. No strained oatmeal, vegetable juice, or fruit juice given. Fats and concentrated sweets are restricted.

nonpolar (nŏn-pō'lĕr). Not having separate poles; sharing electrons.

 n. compound. One formed by the sharing of electrons.

nonpro'tein. Any substance not a protein.

 n. nitrogen. 1. A nitrogenous constituent of blood that is not a protein. 2. Sum of all nonprotein nitrogen in the blood. SEE: *nitrogen.*

non repetat. Do not repeat.

nonrestraint (nŏn'rē-strănt'). Treatment of the insane without using mechanical restraint.

nonseptate (nŏn-sĕp'tāt). Having no dividing walls.

nonsexual (nŏn-sĕk'shū-ăl). Without sex. SYN: *asexual.*

nontoxic (nŏn-tŏks'ĭk). Not poisonous or productive of poison.

nonunion (nŏn-ūn'yŭn). Failure of bone fragments to knit together.

no'nus. 1. Ninth. 2. Hypoglossal or *ninth* cranial nerve.

nonviable (nŏn-vī'ă-bl). Incapable of life or of living.

noökleptia (nō-ō-klep'tĭ-ă). An obsession that one's thoughts are being stolen by others.

noöpsyche (no'o-sī-ke). Reasoning or intellectual processes.

N. O. P. H. N. Abbr. *National Organization for Public Health Nursing.*

norm (norm). A type or standard pattern.

nor'ma. A line used to define the various aspects of the cranium.

 n. frontalis. Cranial outline viewed from the front.

 n. inferior. Cranial outline of inferior aspect.

normal (nor'măl). 1. Standard; performing proper functions; natural; regular. 2. BIOL: Not affected by experimental treatment; occurring naturally and not because of a disease or experimentation. 3. PSY: (a) Free from mental disorder; (b) of average development or intelligence. 4. CHEM: A term used to describe a solution so made that 1 liter contains 1 gram equivalent of the solute.

 n. body temperature. 98.6° F.

 n. formula of response. PT: A condensed statement of the results of stimulating motor nerves with direct current. A large flat electrode (indifferent) is placed over a convenient surface (*e. g.,* the back of the neck) while a more pointed electrode (different) is held over the motor nerve to be studied.

 n. pulse. 72-80 beats per minute.

 n. respiration. 18-24 per minute.

 n. salt. An ionic compound containing no replaceable hydrogen or hydroxyl ions.

 n. solution. Solution containing 1 Gm., molecular weight, of dissolved substance divided by the hydrogen equivalent of the substance per liter of solution.

 n. s., saline. One of salt in distilled water. Bet. 0.6 and 0.9% salt solution, usually 8.5 Gm. to enough distilled water to make 1000 cc.

normalization (nŏr-măl-ĭ-zā'shŭn). Modification or reduction to normal.

normoblast (nor'mō-blăst). A nucleated red blood corpuscle similar in size to an ordinary erythrocyte.

normochromasia (nŏr''mō-krō-mā'zĭ-ă). Average staining capacity in a cell or tissue.

normocyte (nor'mō-sīt). An average-sized red blood corpuscle. SYN: *erythrocyte.*

normocytosis (nor''mō-sī-tō'sĭs). A normal state of the corpuscular elements of the blood.

normoglycemia (nor''mō-glī-sē'mĭ-ă). Normal state of sugar content of the blood.

normoglycemic (nor''mō-glī-se'mĭk). Having a normal amount of sugar in the blood.

normoörthocytosis (nor''mō-or''thō-sī-tō'sĭs). Increase in the blood of the number of leukocytes, but with normal proportion of the different varieties.

normoplasia (nor''mō-pla'zĭ-ă). A specific variation in the character of a cell within normal limits.

normoskeocytosis (nor''mō-skē''ō-sī-tō'sĭs). Normal number of the leukocytes of the blood with deviation* to the left, *i. e.,* with immature forms present.

normosthenuria (nor''mō-sthĕn-ū'rĭ-ă). Urination of normal amount and specific gravity.

normotonic (nor''mō-ton'ĭk). 1. Having normal muscular tonus. 2. One who has normal muscle tonus.

normotopia (nor''mō-tō'pĭ-ă). Situation in the regular place.

normotopic (nor''mō-top'ĭk). In the right location; pert. to the normal situation.

normovalemia (nor''mō-vō-lē'mĭ-ă). Normal state of blood volume.

Norris' corpuscles. Colorless red blood corpuscles not visible in the blood plasma.

Norwe'gian itch. Severe form of scabies marked by pustules and crusts, seen usually in leprosy.

nose (nōz). Projection in center of face; the organ of olfaction and the entrance which warms, moistens, and filters the air for the respiratory tract. SYN: *nasus, organon olfactus.*

nosebleed (nōz'blēd). Hemorrhage from nose. SYN: *epistaxis.*

nosema (no-sē'mă). 1. Ailment (nosema) or disease. 2. A genus of Microsporidia.

noso-. Combining form meaning *pert. to disease.*

nosochthonography (nos''ok-thon-og'ră-fĭ). Study of geography of diseases; medical geography. SYN: *nosogeography.*

nosocomium (nŏs''ō-kō'mĭ-ŭm). A hospital or infirmary.

nosode (nos'ōd). A bacterial vaccine used in treatment of the disease of which it is the causative agent.

nosogenesis, nosogeny (nos''ō-jĕn'ē-sĭs, nos-oj'en-ĭ). The development and progress of a disease.

nosogeography (nos''ō-jē-og'ră-fĭ). Study of medical geography. SYN: *nosochthonography.*   [tion of a disease.

nosography (no-sog'ră-fĭ). The descrip-

nosohemia (nŏs-ō-hē'mĭ-ă). Disease of the blood.

nosointoxication (nos"ō-ĭn-tok"sĭ-kā'shŭn). Pathological interference with metabolic processes resulting in autointoxication.

nosology (no-sol'o-jĭ). The science of description, or the classification of diseases.

nosomania (nos"ō-mā'nĭ-ă). 1. The delusion that one is diseased. 2. Morbid fear of disease.

nosomycosis (nos"ō-mĭ-kō'sĭs). Any disease caused by a parasitic fungus or Schizomycete.

nosonomy (nos-on'ō-mĭ). The science of disease classification.

nosoparasite (nos"ō-par'ă-sīt). A microorganism associated with a disease which it modifies but does not cause.

nosophobia (nō"sō-fō'bĭ-ă). Abnormal aversion to illness, or to a particular affection.

nosopoietic (nō"sō-poy-ĕt'ĭk). Producing or causing disease.

nosotherapy (nos"ō-ther'ă-pĭ). Treatment of 1 disease by voluntarily introducing another microörganism into the body.

nosotoxicosis (nos"ō-tok"sĭ-kō'sĭs). Disorder caused by toxic products of another disease.

nosotoxin (nos"ō-tok'sĭn). Any toxin productive of or associated with disease.

nosotrophy (nos-ot'rō-fĭ). Nursing care and feeding of the sick.

nostalgia (nos-tal'jĭ-ă). Homesickness. SEE: *cainotophobia.*

nostology (nŏs-tol'ō-jĭ). The study of physiological stages of senility.

nostomania (nos"tō-ma'nĭ-ă). Nostalgia* verging on insanity.

nos'tril. Apertures of the nose. SYN: *naris.* SEE: *nose.*

n. reflex. Reduction of opening of naris on affected side in lung disease in proportion to lessened alveolar air capacity on affected side.

nostrum (nŏs'trŭm). A patent or a quack remedy.

notal (nō'tăl). Concerning the back. SYN: *dorsal.*

notalgia (nō-tal'jĭ-ă). Painful condition of the back. SYN: *dorsalgia.*

notch (nŏtsh). A rather deep indentation or narrow gap in the edge of a part. SYN: *incisura.*

n., acetabular. Notch in the margin of the acetabulum opp. the obturator foramen.

n., aortic. One in sphygmogram from rebound at aortic valve closure.

n., clavicular. One at the upper angle of the sternum with which the clavicle articulates.

n., cotyloid. SEE: *acetabular notch.*

n., interclavicular. A rounded one at top of manubrium of sternum, bet. surfaces articulating with the clavicles.

n., interlobar. One in ant. margin of liver, separating left and right lobes.

n's., intervertebral. The ones constituting the intervertebral foramina.

n., ischiatic. Sacrosciatic, *q.v.*

n., jugular. One which forms the post. and middle portions of jugular foramen.

n., nasal. A deep gap at inner margin of facial surface of maxilla.

n., parotid. One bet. ramus of mandible and mastoid process of temporal bone.

n., popliteal. A shallow depression separating tuberosities of head of tibia posteriorly.

n. of Rivinus. The one in the upper and ant. portion of osseous ring attached to which is the tympanic membrane.

n's., sacrosciatic. Two notches on post. border of innominate bone.

n., sigmoid. One bet. the condyle and the coronoid process of ramus of mandible.

n., suprascapular. One sometimes converted into a foramen by a ligament or bony process, in upper border of scapula.

n., suprasternal. SEE: *interclavicular notch.*

note (nōt). A sound of definite pitch.

n. blindness. Inability to recognize musical notes, due to a central lesion.

notencephalocele (no"tĕn-sef'al-ō-sēl). Protrusion of brain substance at the back of the head.

notifʹable diseases. The laws of the various states require that certain diseases when existing shall be reported to the local health authorities, such as a Board of Health. A fine may be levied for not doing so. Among the diseases generally required to be reported are: All communicable or contagious diseases, such as smallpox, scarlet fever, relapsing fever; diphtheria or membranous croup; enteric fevers, such as typhoid fever; erysipelas; puerperal pyrexia and sepsis; cholera; typhus. cerebrospinal fever; acute anterior poliomyelitis; polioencephalitis; encephalitis lethargica; tuberculosis; dysentery; pneumonia; epidemic diarrhea; chickenpox; gonorrhea; syphilis. SEE: *quarantine, reportable diseases.*

notochord (nō'tō-kord). The embryonic spinal cord.

notomyelitis (nō"tō-mĭ-ĕ-lī'tĭs). Inflamed condition of the spinal cord.

noumenal (nū'mē-năl). Pert. to rational intuition opposed to sensual perception.

noumenon (nū'mē-nŏn). An object of rational apprehension as opposed to perception.

nourishment (nur'ĭsh-mĕnt). 1. Act of nourishing or of being nourished. 2. Sustenance; nutriment. SEE: *trophic, trophic center.*

novaspirin (nō-văs'pĭr-ĭn). A crystalline substance of the aspirin type, representing about 62% salicylic acid. Perhaps less powerful than aspirin, but believed to be tolerated better.

DOSAGE: 10-15 gr. (0.65-1 Gm.).

novasurol (nō-văs'ū-rōl). SEE: *merbaphen.*

novatropine (nov-at'rō-pēn). The methyl

bromide of the alkaloid homatropine, less active and less toxic than atropine.
  DOSAGE: 1/24 gr. (2.5 mg.).

novocain (nō'vō-kān). A commercial brand of procaine hydrochloride, USP.
  DOSAGE: *Infilt.*, 4 gr. (0.25 Gm.); *instill.*, 1½ gr. (0.1 Gm.).

noxa (noks'ă) (pl. *noxae*). Anything harmful to health.

noxious (nok'shus). Harmful; not wholesome.

N. P. N. Abbr. for *nonprotein nitrogen*.

n-rays. Rays discovered by Blondlot in 1903 making certain bodies luminous.

nubecula (nū-bek'ū-la). Cloudiness of the cornea or the urine.

nubile (nū'bĭl). Pert. to a girl who has attained puberty and who is thus able to marry.

nubility (nū-bĭl'ĭ-tĭ). Marriageableness, said of female at puberty, the final state of sex development.

nucha (nū'kă). Nape of neck.

nuchal (nū'kal). Pert. to the neck or *nucha*.

Nuck's canal or **diverticulum** (nook). Peritoneal pouch descending along round ligament of uterus.

nuclear (nū'klē-ăr). Resembling or concerning a nucleus.
  n. cell division. Changes occurring in a nucleus in indirect cell division. SYN: *karyokinesis.*
  n. fibril. Tiny fibril of chromatin in a cell nucleus.
  n. sap. Liquid of a cell nucleus found within the meshwork.

nuclease (nū'klē-ās). Any enzymes in animals and plants which facilitate hydrolysis of nuclein and nucleic acids.

nucleate (nū'klē-āt). 1. Having a nucleus. 2. To form a nucleus. 3. A salt or ester of nucleic acid.

nucleation (nū'klē-ā'shŭn). Nucleus formation.

nuclei (nū'klē-ī). Pl. of nucleus.

nucle'ic acid, nuclein'ic acid. Acid which, combined with proteins, forms nuclein.
  DOSAGE: 1-5 gr. (0.06-0.3 Gm.).

nuclein (nu'klē-ĭn). A normal chemical constituent of a cell nucleus, a colorless, shapeless substance obtained by hydrolysis of nucleoproteins or cells containing nucleic acid and proteins rich in phosphorus.
  DOSAGE: *Hypoderm.* of 0.5% solut., 8 ṃ (0.5 cc.).
  n. bases. Adenine, guanine, xanthine, hypoxanthine. SYN: *xanthine bases.*

nucleo-. Pertaining to a *nucleus*.

nucleoalbumin (nu''klē-ō-ăl-bū'mĭn). A protein compound composed of protein and an undefined phosphorus. Former name for phosphoprotein, *q.v.*

nucleoalbuminuria (nū''klē-ō-al-bu''mĭ-nū'rĭ-ă). Nucleoalbumin found in urine.

nucleoalbumose (nū''klē-ō-ăl'bū-mōs). Partly hydrated nucleoalbumin found in the urine of patients with osteomalacia.

nucleochylema (nū''klē-ō-kī-lē'mă). The chylema of the cell nucleus differentiated from that of the cytoplasm.

nucleofugal (nū-klē-of'ū-găl). Moving from a nucleus in the cell.

nucleohiston(e (nū''klē-ō-hĭs'ton, -tōn). A substance in leukocytes, lymph, and thymus glands, composed of nuclein and histone.

nucleoid (nū'klē-oyd). Resembling a nucleus. [cleolus.

nucleolar (nū-klē'ō-lăr). Pert. to a nucleolus.

nucleoliform (nū-klē'ō-lĭ-form). Like a nucleolus.

nucleolin (nū-klē'ō-lĭn). The substance composing the nucleolus. SYN: *plastin.*

nucleolus (nū-klē'ō-lŭs) (pl. *nucleoli*). A spherical body within the cell nucleus. SYN: *karyosome, plasmosome.*

nucleomicrosome (nū''klē-ō-mī'krō-sōm). Any 1 of the minute granules making up a nucleoplasmic fiber.

nucleon (nū'klē-ŏn). Acid substance found in muscle, blood, milk which is related to the nucleins and yields peptone.

nucleopetal (nū-klē-op'ĕt-ăl). Seeking or moving toward the nucleus.
  n. movement. The attraction of a male pronucleus toward the female pronucleus.

nucleoplasm (nū'klē-ō-plăzm). 1. Protoplasm of a nucleus. SYN: *karyoplasm.* 2. Reticular substance of a nucleus. 3. Ground substance of a nucleus.

nucleoprotein (nū''klē-ō-prō'tē-ĭn). The combination of 1 of the proteins with nucleic acid to form a conjugated protein found in cell nuclei.

nucleoreticulum (nū''klē-ō-rĕ-tĭk'ū-lŭm). Any mesh framework in a nucleus.

nucleospindle (nū''klē-ō-spĭn'dl). Spindle-shaped body occurring in karyokinesis.*

nucleotherapy (nū''klē-ō-thĕr'ă-pĭ). The use of nuclein in therapy.

nucleotide (nū'klē-ō-tĭd). Compound of nucleic acid and a base, formed by hydrolysis of nucleic acid.

nu''cleotox'in. A toxin acting upon or produced by cell nuclei.

nucleus (nū'klē-ŭs) (pl. *nuclei*). 1. A central point about which matter is gathered, as in a calculus. SYN: *core.*
  2. The vital body in the protoplasm of a cell, the essential agent in growth, metabolism, reproduction, and transmission of characteristics of a cell.
  3. A group of nerve cells or mass of gray matter in the central nervous system, esp. the brain.
  4. CHEM: Heavy central atomic particle in which most of the mass and total positive electric charge are concentrated.
  n., abducent. A gray nucleus, the origin of abducens nerve, on floor of 4th ventricle, behind trigeminal nerve.
  n., accessory auditory. A ganglionic mass at the convergence of the 2 roots or divisions of the auditory nerve.
  n. ambiguus. BNA. Nucleus of the glossopharyngeal and vagus nerves in oblongata.
  n. amygdaloid. A mass of gray matter forming the ant. extremity of descending cornu or lateral ventricle.

n., angular. SEE: *Bechterew's nucleus.*

n., arcuate. The largest of the masses of cinerea in the arciform fibers of the pyramids on the ventral side.

n., auditory. Nest of nerve cells where auditory nerves arise.

n., Bechterew's. Nucleus giving origin to roots of auditory nerve.

n., Burdach's. Upper part of cuneate fasciculus in oblongata.

n., caudate. Portion of striated body projecting into lateral ventricle.

n., chromatic. Principal nucleus of a cell.

n. cinereum. Gray matter of the restiform bodies.

n., cuneate. SEE: *Burdach's nucleus.*

n., daughter. Nucleus produced by the division of mother nucleus.

n., Deiter's. Main terminal nucleus of the vestibular nerve in oblongata.

n., dentate. Indented layer of gray matter in center of white substance of cerebellum. SYN: *corpus dentatum.*

n., ectoblastic. One in cells of the epiblast.

n., emboliform. A small mass of gray matter in central white substance of the cerebellum.

n. fasti'gii. BNA. Small mass of gray matter in white substance of vermis of the cerebellum.

n. funiculi gracilis. BNA. Elongated mass of gray matter in dorsal pyramid of medulla oblongata.

n., germinal. Nucleus resulting from union of male and female pronuclei.

n., gonad. Reproductive nucleus of a cell.

n., gray. Gray substance of spinal cord.

n., hypoglossal. Large multipolar nerve cells in inf. triangle of 4th ventricle.

n. hypothalamicus. BNA. A lenslike mass of gray matter in the subthalamic region of the hypothalamus.

n., intraventricular. SEE: *caudate nucleus.*

n., lenticular. In corpus striatum, gray matter of its extraventricular portion.

n. lentis. Nucleus of crystalline lens.

n., mother. One that divides into 2 or more parts called *daughter nuclei.*

n., motor. A ganglionic mass in the central nervous system giving origin to motor nerve fibers.

n., oculomotor. Nucleus of the oculo-motor nerve.

n., olivary. One of 2 bands of gray matter, 1 in the medulla below the olive, the other on inner side of facial nerve in the pons.

n. pulposus. Gelatinous mass in center of intervertebral disks.

n., pyramidal. Band of gray matter near olivary nucleus in the medulla.

n. quintus. Trigeminal nerve nucleus.

n. ruber. BNA. Mass of red colored gray matter in crus cerebri close to optic thalamus.

n., subthalamic. SEE: *nucleus hypothalamicus.*

n., vesicular. Nucleus having deeply staining membranes and pale center.

n. vestibularis. SEE: *Bechterew's nucleus.*

n., vitelline. One formed by union of male and female pronuclei within the vitellus.

n., white. Central white substance of corpus dentatum of olive.

nude (nūd). 1. Bare; naked; unclothed. 2. An unclothed body.

nudi-. Combining form denoting *uncovered, naked.*

nudomania (nŭ-dō-ma'nĭ-ă). Abnormal desire to be nude.

nudophobia (nŭ-dō-fō'bĭ-ă). Abnormal fear of being unclothed. SYN: *gymnophobia.*

Nuel's space (nū'ĕl). Space bet. outer rods of Corti and Deiter's cells and hair cells in organs of Corti.

Nuhn's gland (noon). Mucous gland on each side of frenum of the tongue. SYN: *Blandin's gland.*

nullipara (nŭl-ĭp'ă-ră). A woman who has borne no children.

nulliparity (nŭl-ĭ-par'ĭ-tĭ). Condition of not having given birth to a child.

nulliparous (nŭl-lĭp'ăr-ŭs). Never having borne a child.

numb (nŭm). 1. Insensible; lacking in sensation of power and motion, esp. from cold. 2. To render senseless or inert.

number (nŭm'bĕr). 1. A total of units. 2. A symbol graphically representing an arithmetical sum.

numbness (nŭm'nĕs). Lack of sensation in a part, esp. from cold. SEE: *narcohypnia.*

numeral (nū'mĕr-ăl). 1. Denoting or pert. to a number. 2. A word or figure expressing a number.

num'miform, num'mular. 1. Coin-shaped, said of some mucous sputum. 2. Arranged like a stack of coins.

num'mulation. The formation of a coin-shaped mass.

nunnation (nŭn-ā'shŭn). Frequent and abnormal use of the n sound.

nupercaine (nu'per-kăn). A white powder or crystals manufactured from cinchoninic acid.

nuptiality (nŭp"shĭ-ăl'ĭ-tĭ). 1. The number of marriages in proportion to the population. 2. Wedding. 3. Conjugal character.

nurse (ners). One who cares for the sick or wounded, esp. a registered nurse. SEE: *nutrix.*

n., charge. One in charge of a single hospital ward.

n., community; n., district. A visiting nurse.

n., dry. An infant's nurse who does not suckle the child.

n., general duty. One not specializing.

n., graduate. One who is a graduate of an accredited school of nursing.

n., head. A supervisor at the head of a hospital nursing staff.

n., health. A community nurse.

n., practical. One with experience in nursing but who is not a graduate of a school of nursing.

n., private. A nurse in charge of a single patient.

n., private duty. One not a member of a hospital staff who is called in to care for an individual patient in the hospital.

n., probationer. One under observation in a nursing school before being admitted as a student.

n., public health. A graduate nurse employed by a Board of Health.

n., registered. A graduate nurse who has been registered and legally licensed to practice by state authority.

n., school. A registered nurse whose duties are to supplement the work of the physician in medical inspection of pupils.

n., trained. A registered nurse.

n., visiting. A registered nurse, employed by an association to care for the sick poor in their homes.

n., wet. A woman who gives suck to infants of others.

nurse (ners). 1. To feed an infant at the breast. 2. To care for an invalid. 3. To care for a young child. 4. To suckle.

nur'ses' contracture. Tetany sometimes seen in nurses.

nur'sing. 1. Scientific care of the sick by a graduate, registered nurse. 2. Loosely applied to any care of the sick. 3. Suckling at the female breast, as an infant. 4. Lactation.

nutation (nŭ-tā'shŭn). Nodding, as of the head.

n. of sacrum. Partial rotation of the sacrum on its transverse axis to give greater space for passage of the fetus.

nutriceptor (nū'trĭ-sĕp'tor). One which reacts with nutritive matter to nourish a cell.

nutrient (nū'trĭ-ĕnt). 1. Food that supplies the body with its necessary elements. 2. Nourishing.

nutriment (nū'trĭ-mĕnt). That which nourishes; nutritious substance.

nutriology (nū'trĭ-ol'ō-jĭ). The science of use of foods in diet and therapy.

nutrition (nū-trĭ'shŭn). 1. Absorption of food elements and transformation into living tissue, the processes of which include *ingestion, digestion, absorption, assimilation,* and *excretion, q.v.* 2. Nourishing substance.

nutritional (nū-trĭsh'ŭn-ăl). Rel. to nutrition.

nutritious (nū-trish'ŭs). Affording nutriment. SYN: *nutritive.*

nutritive (nū'trĭ-tĭv). Pert. to the process of assimilating food; having the property of nourishing.

n. enema. One of predigested foods to give sustenance to a patient unable to take nourishment in the usual way. SEE: *enema.*

nutritorium (nū-trĭt-o'rĭ-ŭm). The entire body mechanism directly concerned with nutrition.

nutritory (nū'trĭ-tō''rĭ). Nutritive, nourishing.

nutrix (nū'trĭks). A woman nurse.

nux vomica (nŭks vom'ĭ-ka). A poisonous seed from an East Indian tree, containing several alkaloids, the principal ones being brucine and strychnine, *q.v.* USP.
DOSAGE: Of tincture, 15 ℳ (1 cc.).

nyctalbuminuria (nĭk''tăl-bū''min-ū'rĭ-ă). A cyclic albuminuria occurring at night. SYN: *noctalbuminuria.*

nyctalgia (nĭk-tal'jĭ-ă). Pain during the night.

nyctalopia (nĭk-tă-lō'pĭ-ă). 1. A condition in which person cannot see well in a faint light or at night. SYN: *night blindness.* 2. Incorrectly, having better sight at night or in semidarkness than by day; night vision. SEE: *hemeralopia.*

nyctamblyopia (nĭk''tam-blĭ-ō'pĭ-ă). Poor vision at night without visible eye changes.

nyctaphonia (nĭk-tă-fō'nĭ-ă). Hysterical loss of voice during the night.

nycthemerus (nĭk-them'ĕ-rŭs). 1. Space of a day and a night. 2. Pert. to a night and day. SYN: *ephemeral.*

nycterine (nĭk'tĕr-ĭn). 1. Taking place at night. 2. Obscure.

nyctohemeral (nĭk''to-hē'mer-al). Rel. to both day and night.

nyctophilia (nĭk''to-fĭl'ĭ-ă). A predilection for darkness or for night. SYN: *scotophilia.*

nyctophobia (nĭk''tō-fō'bĭ-ă). Abnormal dread of the night, or of darkness.

nyctophonia (nĭk''tō-fō'nĭ-ă). Hysterical loss of voice only during the day.

nyctotyphlosis (nĭk''tō-tĭf-lō'sĭs). Poor vision at night. SYN: *night blindness. nyctalopia.*

nycturia (nĭk-tū'rĭ-ă). Urination, esp. excessive, during the night. SYN: *nocturia.* SEE: *enuresis.*

nygma (nĭg'mă). A puncture wound.

nym'pha (pl. *nymphae*). One of the labia minora,* the small folds of mucous membrane forming the inner lips of the vulva.

n. pendulae. Stretched pendulous nymphae.

nymphectomy (nĭm-fĕk'tō-mĭ). Excision of hypertrophied nymphae.

nymphitis (nĭm-fĭ'tĭs). Inflamed condition of the nymphae.

nymphocaruncular sul'cus (nĭm''fō-kăr-ŭn'kū-lăr). The depression bet. the hymen and the labium minus, on either side.

nymphohymenal sul'cus (nĭm''fō-hī'mĕn-ăl). Trench bet. labium minus and the hymen on either side.

nympholepsy (nĭm'fō-lĕp-sĭ). 1. Frenzied ecstasy usually erotic in nature. 2. Operative removal of the nymphae.

nymphomania (nĭm''fō-mā'nĭ-ă). Abnormally excessive sexual desire in the female. SYN: *furor femininus, furor uterinus.* SEE: *satyriasis.*

nymphomaniac (nĭm''fō-ma'nĭ-ăk). 1. Woman who is afflicted with excessive sexual desire. 2. Marked by excessive sexual desire.

nymphoncus (nĭm-fon′kŭs). Swelling or tumor of the nymphae.

nymphotomy (nĭm-fot′ō-mĭ). 1. Removal of the nymphae. SYN: *nymphectomy*. 2. Incision into a nympha. 3. Removal of the clitoris.

nystagmic (nĭs-tag′mĭk). Rel. to or suffering from condition of involuntary eyeball movements.

nystagmiform (nĭs-tag′mĭ-form). Pert. to or suffering from involuntary eyeball motion.

nystagmograph (nĭs-tag′mō-grăf). Apparatus for recording the oscillations of the eyeball in nystagmus.

nystagmoid (nĭs-tag′moyd). Similar to, or resembling nystagmus.

nystagmus (nĭs-tag′mŭs). Constant involuntary movement of the eyeball.

  n., aural. Nystagmus due to disorder in the labyrinth of the ear.

  n., Cheyne's. Nystagmus with rhythmical movements of the eye.

  n., lateral. Horizontal movement of eyes from side to side.

  n., palatal. Spasm of levator palati muscle.

  n., rotatory. Rotation of the eyes about the visual axis.

  n., vertical. Up and down ocular movements.   [turbances.

  n., vestibular. That due to ear dis-

Nysten's law (nī′stĕn). Rigor mortis begins with muscles of mastication and progresses down the body affecting legs and feet last. SEE: *rigor mortis*.

nyxis (niks′ĭs). Puncture or piercing. SYN: *paracentesis*.

O

O. Symb. of *oxygen* and abbr. for various terms, as: *oculus*, eye; *octarius*, pint.

o-. Abbr. for *ortho-*, most commonly used in chemical terminology.

O₂. Symb. for the *two eyes*.

O₃. Symb. for *ozone*.

oakum (ō'kŭm). Loose fiber obtained by unravelling old hemp ropes, used occasionally as a surgical dressing.

oarialgia (ō"ăr-ĭ-ăl'jĭ-ă). Ovarian pain. Syn: *ovarialgia*.

oaric (ō-a'rĭk). Pert. to an ovary. Syn: *ovarian*.

oario-, oari-. Prefix *pert. to the ovary*.

oariopathy (ō"ăr-ĭ-op'ăth-ĭ). Any disease of the ovary.

oariotomy (ō"ă-rĭ-ot'ō-mĭ). Incision into an ovary or surgical removal of a tumor or the ovary itself. Syn: *ovariotomy*.

oaritis (ō-ă-ri'tĭs). Inflamed condition of an ovary. Syn: *ovaritis*.

oarium (ō-ā'rĭ-um) (pl. *oaria*). An ovary. Syn: *ovarium*.

oasis (ō-ā'sĭs) (pl. *oāsēs*). Area of healthy tissue surrounded by a diseased portion.

oat (ōt). Grain or seed of a cereal grass used as an article of diet.

ob-. Combining form meaning *towards, against, in the way of*.

O. B. Abbr. for *obstetrics*.

obcordate (ŏb-kor'dāt). Inversely heart-shaped.

obdormition (ŏb-dor-mĭsh'ŭn). Numbness followed by tingling in a limb produced by pressure of the nerve trunk supplying it.

Limb is commonly referred to as being asleep.

obduction (ŏb-duk'shŭn). Scientific inspection of a dead body to learn pathological conditions and cause of death. Syn: *autopsy, necropsy*.

obelion (ō-bē'lĭ-ŏn). A craniometric point on the sagittal suture bet. the 2 parietal foramina.

obese (ō-bēs'). Extremely fat. Syn: *corpulent*.

obesity (ō-bē'sĭ-tĭ). Abnormal amount of fat on the body. Syn: *adiposity, corpulence, polysarcia*.

  o., endogenous. Obesity caused by some abnormality within the body, endocrine, nervous, or due to faulty salt and water metabolism.

  o., exogenous. Obesity due to excessive intake of food.

  o., hyperplasmic. Obesity caused by increased quantity of body protoplasm.

  o., hypoplasmic. Obesity due to lowering of body protoplasm and increase in fat and water content.

obex (ō'bĕks). BNA. A thin, triangular band of nervous substance over the calamus scriptorius in roof of cranial 4th ventricle.

obfuscation (ŏb-fŭs-kā'shŭn). 1. Clouding or dimming, as of the cornea. 2. Mental confusion.

ob'ject. That which is visible or tangible to the senses.

  o. blindness. Affection in which brain fails to recognize things seen correctly by eyes. See: *apraxia*.

  o. choice. Selection of love object decided by a fixation developed in pregenital stage.

  o. glass, o. lens. Microscope lens closest to the object.

  o. libido. Love or interest expressed external to oneself upon persons, objects, causes. See: *anaclitic choice*.

  o. symbolism. A concept formed, or an emotion incited by seeing an object, as in ideas like *heart* of *stone*, the *brow* of a hill, the *lap* or *bosom* of *nature*, etc.

objective (ob-jek'tiv). 1. Perceptible to other persons, said of symptoms. 2. Directed toward external things. 3. The lens of a microscope which is closest to the object.

  o. symptoms. Those apparent to physical means of diagnosis.

obligate (ob'lĭ-gāt). 1. To make necessary or to require. 2. Compulsory, bound.

  o., aerobic. A microbe that must have oxygen in order to live.

  o., anaerobic. A microörganism that lives only without oxygen.

  o. parasite. One that can exist only at the expense of another plant or organism.

oblique (ŏb-lēk'). Slanting; diagonal.

  o. muscles. Two muscles of the eye; also 2 in the abdomen.

obliquimeter (ŏb-lĭk-wim'ĕt-ĕr). Apparatus for indicating the angle of the pelvic brim with the upright body.

obliquity (ŏb-lĭk'wĭ-tĭ). The state of being oblique.

  o., Litzmann's. Inclining of the fetal head until the post. parietal bone presents to the uterine canal.

  o., Nägele's. Presentation of the fetal head with ant. parietal bone toward the uterine canal with oblique biparietal diameter in relation to the pelvic brim.

  o., Roederer's. Presentation of fetal head with occiput at pelvic brim.

obliquus (ŏb-lĭk'wŭs). A name applied to several muscles.

  o. reflex. Contraction of ext. obliquus muscle in toto on application of stimulus to skin of thigh below Poupart's ligament.

obliteration (ŏb-lit"ĕr-ā'shŭn). Extinction or complete occlusion of a part by means of surgery, degeneration, or disease.

oblongata (ŏb"lon-ga'tă). The medulla oblongata; the cylindrical extension of the spinal cord as it enters the brain, about an inch long, reaching to the pons, and forming part of base of 4th ventricle.   [medulla oblongata.

oblongatal (ob″lon-gā′tal). Rel. to the

obmutescence (ŏb-mū-tes′ĕns). Loss of vocal power. SYN: *aphonia.*

obnubilation (ŏb-nū-bil-ā′shŭn). An impaired or confused state of mind.

obscure (ŏb-skūr′). Hidden, indistinct, as the cause of a condition.

obses′sion. An uncontrollable desire to dwell on an idea or an emotion, or to perform a specific act.

It is not uncommon among normal persons, but if not banished may become all compelling and developing into a "compulsion neurosis." A dominating condition in certain psychoses.

   o's., impulsive. Those accompanied by action. They sometimes become manias.

   o's., inhibitory. Obsessions accompanied by impediments to action. They represent the phobias, *q.v.*

   o's., intellectual. Recurring and persistent obsessions unaccompanied by action. Typical of the habitual worriers.

obses′sional neuro′sis. A psychoneurosis marked by obsessions controlling the behavior of the individual. SYN: *compulsion neurosis.*

obsolete (ŏb′sō-lēt). Indistinct or absent; noting an organ or characteristic having a functional counterpart in an earlier stage.

obstetric, obstetrical (ŏb-stet′rĭk, -rĭ-kăl). Pert. to obstetrics or midwifery.

   o. forceps. Instrument used to facilitate delivery of the fetus.

obstetrician (ŏb-stĕt-rĭsh′ăn). A physician or one who treats women during pregnancy and parturition.

obstetrics (ob-stet′rĭks). Scientific management of women during pregnancy, childbirth, and the puerperium.

obstipation (ŏb-stĭp-ā′shŭn). 1. The act or condition of obstructing. 2. Obstinate or extreme constipation due to an obstruction.

obstruction (ŏb-struk′shŭn). 1. Blocking of a structure that prevents it from functioning normally. 2. A thing that impedes; an obstacle.

   o., intestinal. Blockage of the lumen of the intestine. SEE: *intestinal obstruction.*

obstruent (ŏb′strū-ĕnt). 1. Blocking up. 2. That which closes a normal passage in the body; an astringent.

obtund (ŏb-tŭnd′). To dull or blunt, as sensitivity or pain.

obtundent (ŏb-tŭn′dĕnt). 1. Deadening sensibility of a part, or reducing irritability, soothing. 2. A soothing remedy.

obturation (ŏb-tū-rā′shŭn). Closure of a passage or opening.

   o. of teeth. Filling of a cavity.

obturator (ob′tū-rā″tor). 1. Anything that obstructs or closes a cavity or opening. 2. Rel. to the obturator membrane. 3. Bridge for spanning the gap in the cleft palate.

   o. foramen. The one in the anterior part of the os innominatum bet. pubis and ischium.

   o. membrane. The sturdy one occluding the obturator foramen.

   o. muscles. Two muscles on each side in the pelvic region which rotate the thighs outward.

obtuse (ŏb-tūs′). 1. Not pointed or acute; dull or blunt. 2. Stupid; dull mentally.

obtusion (ŏb-tū′zhŭn). Blunting or weakening of normal sensation, as in certain diseases.

occipital (ŏk-sĭp′ĭ-tăl). Concerning the back part of the head.

   o. bone. Bone in lower back part of skull bet. the parietal and temporal bones.

   o. lobe. Post. lobe of the cerebral hemisphere which is shaped like a 3-sided pyramid.

occipitalis (ŏk-sĭp″ĭ-tā′lĭs). The posterior portion of the occipitofrontalis muscle at back of the head.

occipito-. Combining form showing relationship bet. the occiput and another part.   [skull.

occiput (ok′sĭ-pŭt). The back part of the

occlude (ŏ-klūd′). To close up, obstruct or join together, as the masticatory surfaces of the teeth.

occlusio pupillae. Condition in which the pupil is closed by a membrane.

occlusion (ŏ-klū′zhŭn). 1. The closure, or state of being closed, of a passage. SYN: *imperforation.*

   2. Absorption of gas by a substance which doesn't thereby lose its characteristic property.

   3. Relation of the teeth when the jaws are closed.

oc′cult. Obscure; hidden, as a hemorrhage.

   o. blood. Blood in such minute quantity that it can only be recognized by microscope or chemical means.

occupa′tion neuro′sis. A functional disorder of a part, caused by certain occupations, as writer's cramp.

occupa′tional ther′apy. Use of any activity or occupation for purposes of treatment.

ochlesis (ŏk-lē′sĭs). Any disease caused by conditions of overcrowding.

ochlophobia (ŏk-lō-fō′bĭ-ă). Abnormal dread of crowds or populated places.

ochrodermia (ō″krō-der′mĭ-ă). A yellow state of the skin.

ochrometer (ō-krom′ĕt-ĕr). Device for estimating the capillary blood pressure by compression of a finger until its skin becomes blanched.

ochronosis, ochronosus (ō-krō-nō′sĭs, -sŭs). A rare condition marked by dark pigmentation of the ligaments, cartilage, fibrous tissues, skin, and urine.

octa-, octo-. Combining forms meaning *eight.*

octan (ŏk′tăn). Reappearing on every 8th day, as a fever.

octane (ŏk′tān). A hydrocarbon of the paraffin series. $CH_3(CH_2)_nCH_3$.

octarius (ŏk-ta'rĭ-ŭs). Pint.

octavalent (ok″tă-vā'lĕnt). Having a valence of 8.

octipara (ŏk-tĭp'ă-ră). A woman who has given birth to 8 children.

octoroon (ŏk-tō-roon'). One who has one-eighth negro blood and seven-eighths white blood; progeny of a white person and a quadroon.

ocular (ŏk'ū-lăr). 1. Concerning the eye or vision. 2. Eyepiece of a microscope.

oculist (ŏk'ū-lĭst). A specialist in diseases of the eye.

oculocephalogyric re′flex (ok″ū-lō-sĕf″-ă-lo-gi'rĭk). Associated movements of eye, head, and body in focalizing vision upon an object.

oculogyration (ok″ū-lō-jī-rā'shŭn). Motions of the eyeball.

oculogyric (ok″ū-lō-jĭ'rĭk). Producing or concerning movements of the eye.

oculomotor (ŏk″ū-lō-mō'tor). Rel. to eye movements. SYN: *oculogyric.*

 o. nerve. The 3rd cranial nerve.

oculomotorius (ok″ū-lō-mō-tor′ĭ-ŭs). The oculomotor or 3rd cranial nerve.

oculomycosis (ok″ū-lō-mĭ-kō'sĭs). Any disease of the eye or its parts caused by a fungus.

oculonasal (ŏk″ū-lō-nā'sal). Concerning both the eye and the nose.

oculoreaction (ok″ū-lō-rē-ak'shŭn). A reaction in the eye, upon the instillation of toxins of tuberculosis and typhoid.

oculozygomatic (ok″ū-lō-zī-gō-mat′ĭk). Pert. to the eye and zygoma.

 o. line. Line bet. inner canthus of eye and cheek supposedly indicating neural disorders.

oculus (ok'ū-lŭs). Eye.

O. D. Abbr. for *oculus dexter,* right eye.

od (ŏd). The supposed magnetic force which acts upon the nervous system to produce hypnotism.

odaxesmus (o-daks-ĕz'mŭs). 1. The biting of the tongue, lip, or cheek during an epileptic attack. 2. Itching or biting sensation, a paresthesia.

odaxetic (o-dăks-ĕt′ĭk). Producing a stinging or itching sensation.

Oddi's sphincter (ŏd'dĭ). A contraction at the opening of the common bile duct at the ampulla of Vater.

odogenesis (ō-dō-jĕn'ĕ-sĭs). The reëstablishment of connections bet. the divided ends of a nerve by nerve process attraction. SYN: *neurocladism.*

odontagra (ō-dŏn-tăg'ră). Toothache, esp. when originating from gout.

odontalgia (o-don-tal'jĭ-ă). Toothache. SYN: *odontodynia.*

 o., phantom. Pain felt in the area from which a tooth has been pulled.

odontatrophy (ō″don-tăt′rō-fĭ). 1. Decay of the teeth. 2. Imperfect development of the teeth.

odontectomy (ō-dŏn-tek'tō-mĭ). Surgical removal of a tooth. [the teeth.

odonterism (ō-don'tĕr-ĭzm). Chattering of

odontia (ō-dŏn'shĭ-ă). 1. Pain in a tooth. SYN: *odontalgia.* 2. Condition or abnormality of the teeth.

odontiasis (ō″dŏn-tī'ăs-ĭs). 1. Cutting of the teeth. SYN: *dentition, teething.* 2. Disease caused by teething.

odontitis (ō-dŏn-tī'tĭs). Inflammation of the pulp of a tooth.

odonto-, odont-. Combining form meaning *tooth.*

odontoblast (ō-don'tō-blăst). One of the cells which fill the pulp chamber of the teeth.

 They produce the dentine and deposit it in layers on inside of the teeth for years after they have erupted.

odontobothrion (ō-don″tō-both′rĭ-ŏn). Socket of a tooth.

odontodynia (ō-dŏn″tō-din′ĭ-ă). Toothache. SYN: *odontalgia.*

odontogen (ō-don'tō-jĕn). The substance from which dentine arises.

odontogenesis, odontogeny (ō-don″tō-jĕn′-ĕ-sĭs, -toj′ĕn-ĭ). The origin and formation of the teeth.

odontoid (ō-don'toyd). Toothlike.

 o. process. The toothlike projection from upper surface of the body of the 2nd cervical vertebrae.

odontology (ō-dŏn-tol'ō-jĭ). The science of dealing with the teeth and their care. SYN: *dentistry.*

odontoma (ō-dŏn-tō'mă). Tumor of a tooth or of the dental tissue.

 o., coronary. Bony tumor at crown of a tooth.

 o., follicular. Bony shell in gums below tooth margin, usually after 2nd dentition. [a tooth.

 o., radicular. Bony tumor at root of

odontonecrosis (ō-don″tō-nĕ-krō'sĭs). Decay or gangrene of a tooth.

odontopathy (ō-dŏn-top'ăth-ĭ). Any disease of the teeth.

odontophobia (ō-don″tō-fō'bĭ-ă). 1. Abnormal aversion to the sight of teeth. 2. Abnormal fear of dental surgery.

odontoplerosis (ō-don″tō-plē-rō'sĭs). The filling of a dental cavity.

odontoprisis (ō-don″tō-pri'sĭs). Grinding of the teeth.

odontorrhagia (ō-don″tō-rā'jĭ-ă). Hemorrhage from a tooth socket following extraction.

odontorthosis (ō-dŏn-tŏr-thō'sĭs). Operation of straightening irregular teeth.

odontosis (ō-dŏn-tō'sĭs). 1. Development of teeth. 2. Eruption of teeth.

odontotherapy (ō-don″tō-ther′ă-pĭ). Care of diseased teeth.

odontotripsis (ō-don″tō-trĭp'sĭs). Natural abrasion of the teeth.

odontotrypy (ō-dŏn-tot'rĭ-pĭ). 1. Drilling of a tooth. 2. Perforation of a tooth to draw off pus from an inner abscess.

 Different locations of abscess call for different treatment.

odor (ō'der). 1. That quality of a substance which renders it perceptible to sense of smell. 2. Any smell, esp. a sweet scent. 3. Any sensation of sense of smell.

odoriferous (ō″der-ĭf′ĕ-rŭs). Bearing scent, having an odor; fragrant; perfumed.

odorous (ō'dŏr-ŭs). Having an odor, scent, or fragrance.

odynacusis (ō-dĭn-ă-kū'sĭs). A condition in which noises cause pain in the ear.

odynometer (ō-dĭn-om'ĕt-ēr). Device for measuring pain.

odynophagia (ō-dĭn-ō-fā'jĭ-ă). Pain upon swallowing.

odynophobia (o''dĭn-ō-fō'bĭ-ă). Abnormal dread of pain. [labor pains.

odynopoeia (ō''dĭn-ō-pē'ă). Induction of

Oedipus com'plex (ē'dĭ-pŭs). Abnormally intense love of the child for parent of the opposite sex retained in adulthood.

Oertel's terrain cure (er'tel). Graduated exercise, mountain climbing, diet, and reduction of fluids for heart cases, obesity, circulatory diseases, etc.

offi'cial. Said of medicines authorized as standard in the U. S. Pharmacopeia, and in the National Formulary.

officinal (of-ĭs'in-al). Regularly kept in a druggist's stock. SEE: magistral.

-OH. Hydroxyl group.

ohm (ōm). Practical unit of resistance, the resistance through which a difference of potential of 1 volt will produce a current of 1 ampere.

　　O.'s law. The law determined experimentally by the physicist Ohm, which states that the strength of an electric current in a direct current circuit varies directly as the applied electromotive force, and inversely as the resistance of the circuit; or, the current i expressed in amperes equals the electromotive force E in volts, divided by the resistance R in ohms:

$$i = \frac{E}{R}$$

-oid. Suffix meaning having the form of, or likeness of, as ovoid.

oidiomycetes (ō-ĭd'ĭ-ō-mĭ-sē'tēs). A group of fungi including the Oidium.

oidiomycosis (ō-ĭd'ĭ-ō-mĭ-kō'sĭs). Disease due to infection by an Oidium.

Oidium (ō-ĭd'ĭ-ŭm). 1. A genus of fungi of the family Moniliaceae. 2. (oidium) A fungus of this genus.

　　O. albicans. A microscopic fungus that causes thrush.

　　O. lactis. White mold on bread and sour milk.

　　O. Schoenlein'ii. Fungus of favus. SYN: Achorion Schoenleinii.

　　O. tonsurans. Fungus of ringworm. Trichophyton tonsurans.

oikomania (oy-kō-mā'nĭ-ă). Nervous disorder induced by unhappy home surroundings.

oikophobia (oy''kō-fo'bĭ-ă). Morbid dislike of the home. SYN: ecomania.

oil (oyl). A greasy liquid not miscible with water, usually obtained from a mineral, vegetable, or animal source.

ointment (oynt'mĕnt). A fatty, soft substance having antiseptic or healing properties.

ol. Abbr. for oleum, oil.

O. L. A. Abbr. for L. occipito laevo anterior, fetal presentation with the occiput toward the maternal left acetabulum.

old age. Human life after 70 years.

　　o. sight. Defective changes in vision due to advancing old age.

olea (ō'lē-a). 1. L. for olive. 2. Pl. of oleum, oils.

oleaginous (ō-lē-ăj'ĭ-nŭs). Greasy; oily; unctuous.

oleate (ō'lē-āt). 1. Any salt of oleic acid. 2. Salt of oleic acid dissolved in an excess of the acid.

oleatum (ō-lē-at'ŭm). Preparation made by dissolving metallic salts or alkaloids in oleic acid. SYN: oleate, 2.

olecranal (ō-lĕk'răn-ăl). Concerning the olecranon.

olecranarthritis (ō-lek''răn-ar-thrī'tĭs) Inflamed condition of the elbow joint.

olecranarthrocace (ō-lĕk''răn-ar-throk'ă-sē). Tuberculous ulceration of the elbow joint.

olecranarthropathy (ō-lĕk''răn-ar-throp'-ăth-ĭ). Any disease of the elbow joint.

olecranoid (ō-lĕk'răn-oyd). Similar to the olecranon.

olecranon (ō-lek'răn-ŏn, ō''lē-krā'nŏn). BNA. A large process of the ulna projecting behind the elbow joint and forming the bony prominence of the elbow.

oleic (ō-lē'ĭk). Derived from or pert. to oil.

　　o. acid. A colorless, oily liquid prepared from fats, the salts of which are oleates.

olein (ō'lē-ĭn). An oleate of glyceryl found in nearly all fixed oils and fats; an important part of oils. SYN: triolein.

oleo-. Combining form meaning oil.

oleoarthrosis (ō''lē-ō-ar-thrō'sĭs). Therapeutic introduction of oil into a joint.

oleoinfusion (ō''lē-ō-ĭn-fū'zhŭn). Combination of a drug and oil.

oleomargarine (ō''lē-ō-mar'jă-rēn). Artificial butter from lard or tallow.

oleoresin (o''le-o-rez'in). Extract of plant containing resinous substance and oil, prepared by dissolving the crude drug in ether, acetone, or alcohol.

oleosaccharum (ō-lē-ō-sak'ăr-ŭm). A substance compounded of sugar and volatile oil.

oleotherapy (ō''lē-ō-ther'ă-pĭ). Therapeutic injection of oil. SYN: eleotherapy.

oleothorax (ō-lē-ō-thō'răks). Therapeutic injection of oil into the pleural cavity.

oleum (ō'lē-ŭm). Oil.

　　o. morrhuae. Cod liver oil.

　　o. percomorphum. Mixture of oils from livers of various members of order Percomorphi. More potent than cod liver oil in Vitamins A and D.

　　o. ricini. Castor oil.

olfactie (ōl-făk'tĭ). Unit of smell; the threshold of stimulation for an odor.

olfaction (ōl-fak'shŭn). The sense of smell. Smelling.

olfactive (ōl-fak'tĭv). Pert. to the sense of smell. SYN: olfactory.

olfactology (ōl-făk-tol'ō-jĭ). Scientific investigation of sense of smell.

olfactometer (ōl''fak-tom'et-ēr). Apparatus for testing the power of the sense of smell.

olfactory (ōl-fak'tō-rĭ). Pert. to smell.

o. area. Area in the hippocampal convolution. Ant. portion of the callosal gyrus and the uncus.

o. bulb. Enlarged ant. extremity of the olfactory nerve.

o. bundle. Mass of fibers in the fornix.

o. lobe. A cranial lobe projecting from ant. lower part of each cerebral hemisphere.

o. nerves. The nerves supplying the nasal organ.
First pair of cranial nerves. Differs from other nerves in being composed exclusively of nonmedullated fibers. FUNCT: Special sense of smell. ORIG: Olfactory bulb. DIST: Nasal mucous membrane. BRS: It has 20 brs.

o. organ. The nose.

oligemia (ol-ig-e′mĭ-ă). Deficient amount of blood in the body. SYN: *oligohemia.*

oligergasia (ol-ĭ-gĕr-ga′sĭ-ă). Psychic disorder from deficiency due to imperfect development.

olighydria (ol-ĭ-gĭd′rĭ-ă). Deficient perspiration.

oligo-, olig-. Combining form meaning *small* or, in the plural sense, *few.*

oligocholia (ol-ĭg-ō-kō′lĭ-ă). Lack of bile.

oligochromemia (ol″ĭg-ō-krō-mē′mĭ-ă). Lack of sufficient hemoglobin in the blood.

oligochylia (ol-ĭ-gō-ki′lĭ-ă). Deficiency of chyle.

oligochymia (ol-ĭg-ō-ki′mĭ-ă). Deficiency of chyme.

oligocystic (ol-ĭ-gō-sĭst′ĭk). Having just a few cysts, as a tumor.

oligocythemia (ol″ĭ-gō-sĭ-thē′mĭ-ă). Deficiency in number of red blood corpuscles.

oligocytosis (ol″ĭ-gō-sĭ-tō′sĭs). Deficiency of red blood corpuscles. SYN: *oligocythemia.*

oligodactylia (ol-ĭ-gō-dăk-tĭl′ĭ-ă). Subnormal number of fingers or toes.

oligodendroglia (ol″ĭ-gō-den-drog′lĭ-ă). Adventitial cells found in central nervous system, with characteristic vinelike processes. SYN: *mesoglia.*

oligodipsia (ol-ĭ-gō-dĭp′sĭ-ă). Abnormal lack of desire for fluids.

oligodynamic (ŏl″ĭ-gō-dĭ-năm′ĭk). Effective in a small quantity.

oligoerythrocythemia (ol″ĭ-gō-er″ith-rō-sĭ-thē′mĭ-ă). Deficiency of hemoglobin or red blood corpuscles.

oligogalactia (ol″ĭ-gō-gă-lak′tĭ-ă). Deficient milk secretion.

oligogenics (ol-ĭ-gō-jĕn′ĭks). Limitation of the number of offspring by artificial mediums such as contraceptives. SYN: *birth control.*

oligoglobulia (ol″ĭ-gō-glŏb-ū′lĭ-ă). Deficiency of red blood corpuscles. SYN: *oligocythemia.*

oligohemia (ol″ĭ-gō-hē′mĭ-ă). Insufficiency of blood in the body. SYN: *oligemia.*

oligohydramnios (ol″ĭg-ō-hĭ-dram′nĭ-ŏs). Abnormally small amount of amniotic fluid.

oligohydruria (ol″ĭ-gō-hĭ-drū′rĭ-ă). Highly concentrated urine.

oligoleukocythemia (ol″ĭ-gō-lū″kō-sī-thē′mĭ-ă). Reduction in leukocytic content of blood. SYN: *leukopenia.*

oligoleukocytosis (ol″ĭ-gō-lū″kō-sĭ-tō′sĭs). Decreased number of leukocytes in the blood. SYN: *leukopenia, oligoleukocythemia.*

oligomania (ol-ĭ-gō-mā′nĭ-ă). Insanity involving only a few mental faculties.

oligomastigate (ol-ĭ-gō-mas′tĭ-gāt). Characterized by 2 flagella.

oligomenorrhea (ol″ĭg-ō-měn-ō-rē′ă). Scanty or infrequent menstrual flow.

oligopepsia (ol-ĭ-gō-pĕp′sĭ-ă). Insufficient digestive tone.

oligophosphaturia (ol″ĭ-gō-fŏs-făt-ū′rĭ-ă). Scanty amount of phosphates in the urine.

oligophrenia (ol″ĭg-ō-frē′nĭ-ă). Mental deficiency due to faulty development. SYN: *imbecility.*

oligoplasmia (ŏl″ĭg-ō-plăz′mĭ-ă). Insufficient amt. of blood plasma.

oligopnea (ol-ĭg-op′nē-ă). Infrequent respiration. SYN: *hypopnea.*

oligoposia (ol-ĭ-gō-pō′sĭ-ă). Inadequate use of liquids in diet. SYN: *oligoposy.*

oligoposy (ol-ĭ-gop′ō-sĭ). Insufficient use of liquids in the diet. SYN: *oligoposia.*

oligoptyalism (ol-ĭ-gō-tī′ă-lĭzm). Insufficient secretion of saliva. SYN: *oligosialia.*

oligoria (ol-ĭ-gō′rĭ-ă). A form of melancholia in which there is apathy toward things and people.

oligosialia (ol″ĭ-gō-sĭ-a′lĭ-ă). Scanty salivary secretion. SYN: *oligoptyalism.*

oligospermia (ol″ĭ-gō-spĕr′mĭ-ă). Paucity of spermatozoa in seminal fluid.
It may be temporary or permanent. SEE: *aspermatism.*

oligotrophia (ŏl″ĭ-gō-trof′ĭ-ă). Insufficient nourishment.

oligotrophy (ol-ĭ-gō′trō-fĭ). Inadequate nutrition.

oliguresis (ol-ĭg-ū-rē′sĭs). Scantiness of urine; infrequent urination.

oliguria (ol-ĭg-ū′rĭ-ă). Diminished amt. and frequency of urination.

oliva (ō-lī′vă). BNA. An olive-shaped gray body behind the ant. pyramid of the medulla oblongata. SEE: *olivary body.*

ol′ivary. Shaped like an olive; oval.

o. body. One of 2 oval prominences on each side of the ant. surface of the medulla oblongata just below the pons.

olive oil enema. Mix 4 oz. of olive oil with 1 dr. of turpentine, beating the mixture well so as to break the oil globules.

olive (ŏl′ĭv). Oliva, BNA.

o., inferior. Olivary body.

o., superior. Layer of gray matter with a core in the cerebellar hemispheres. SYN: *nucleus dentatus.*

-ology. Suffix meaning *science of, knowledge, study of.*

olophonia (ol-ō-fōn′ĭ-ă). Malformation of vocal organs with resulting unnatural speech.

Olshausen's sign (ŏls′how-zĕn). If a tumor

ant. to uterus is found in an unmarried woman it will probably be a dermoid* cyst.

-oma. Suffix denoting *a tumor.*

omagra (ō-mag'ră). Attack of gout in the shoulder. [der.

omalgia (ō-mal'jĭ-ă). Neuralgia of shoulder.

omarthritis (ō-mar-thrī'tĭs). Inflamed condition of the shoulder joint.

Ombrédanne's mask (ŏm-brā-dăhn'). Mask for ether administration in exact dosage.

ombrophobia (ŏm-brō-fō'bĭ-ă). Fear and anxiety induced by storms, threatening clouds, or rain.

ombrophore (ŏm'brō-for). Portable apparatus for administering shower baths.

omental (ō-měn'tăl). Pert. to the omentum, the peritoneal fold supporting the viscera.

omentectomy (ō-měn-těk'tō-mĭ). Surgical removal of a portion of the omentum.

omentitis (ō-měn-tī'tĭs). Inflamed condition of omentum.

omentopexy (ō-měn'tō-pěks"ĭ). Fixation of the omentum to the abdominal wall.

omentorrhaphy (ō-měn-tor'ră-fĭ). Suture of the omentum.

omentosplenopexy (ō-men"tō-splē'no-pěks-ĭ). Fixation of the spleen and omentum. Omentopexy and splenopexy.

omentotomy (ō-měn-tot'ō-mĭ). Surgery of the omentum.

omentum (ō-měn'tŭm) (pl. *omenta*). A fold of peritoneal layers connecting and supporting the viscera.

o., great. It is suspended from the greater curvature of the stomach.

It contains fat and aids in keeping the intestines warm, and preventing friction. SYN: *epiploon majus.*

o., lesser. It passes from the lesser curvature of stomach to transverse fissure of the liver. SYN: *epiploon minus.*

omitis (ō-mī'tĭs). Inflamed condition of the shoulder.

omni- (om'nĭ). Prefix meaning *all.*

omnip'otence of thought. PSY: Infantile concept of reality whereby one expects his wishes to be instantly accomplished, as a child that gains its objectives through crying, comes to believe in his own omnipotence because of a parent's surrender to his demands.

omnivorous (ŏm-nĭv'ō-rŭs). Living on all kinds of food.

omo-. Combining form meaning *shoulder* or *pert. to the shoulder.*

omodynia (ō-mō-din'ĭ-ă). Pain of the shoulder.

omohyoid (ō-mō-hī'oyd). 1. Concerning the scapula and the hyoid bone. 2. Muscle attached to the hyoid bone and the scapula.

ɔmphal-, omphalo-. Combining form *relating to the navel.*

omophagia (ō-mō-fā'jĭ-ă). The custom of eating foods raw, esp. flesh.

omphalectomy (ŏm-făl-ek'tō-mĭ). Surgical removal of the umbilicus.

omphalic (om-fal'ĭk). Concerning the umbilicus.

omphalitis (ŏm-făl-ī'tĭs). Inflamed condition of the navel.

omphalocele (ŏm-făl'ō-sēl). Hernia of the navel. SEE: *hernia.*

omphalomesenteric (om"fal-ō-měs-ěn-ter"-ĭk). Concerning the umbilicus and mesentery.

omphaloncus (om-fal-on'kŭs). Umbilical tumor or swelling.

omphalophlebitis (ŏm"făl-ō-flē-bī'tĭs). Inflamed condition of umbilical veins.

omphalorrhagia (ŏm"făl-ŏr-rā'jĭ-ă). Umbilical hemorrhage.

omphalorrhea (om-fal-or-ē'ă). Discharge of lymph at the navel.

omphalorrhexis (om-fal-or-rěks'ĭs). Rupture of the navel.

omphalos (om'făl-ōs). Umbilicus. SYN: *navel.*

omphalosotor (om-fal-ō-sō'tór). Device used in replacing the prolapsed umbilical cord at childbirth.

omphalospinous (om-fal-ō-spī'nŭs). Concerning the navel and the ant. sup. spine of the ilium.

omphalotomy (om-făl-ot'ō-mĭ). Division of umbilical cord at birth.

omphalotripsy (om"făl-ō-trĭp"sĭ). Severing of the umbilical cord by a crushing method.

onanism (ō'năn-ĭzm). Coitus interruptus,* so named because it was practiced by the Biblical character Onan, but the term is used also, erroneously, to designate masturbation, *q.v.*

onanist (ō'năn-ĭst). One who practices coitus interruptus or, erroneously, masturbation.

Onanoff's reflex (ŏn-ăh-nŏf'). Contraction of bulbocavernous muscle resulting from compression of glans penis.

onchocerca (ŏng-kō-ser'kă). A genus of filarial worms.

onchocerciasis (ŏng-kō-ser-kī'ăs-ĭs). Condition produced by infestation with 1 of the species of Onchocerca.

oncogenesis (ong"kō-jěn'ē-sĭs). Tumor formation and development.

oncogenous (ŏng-koj'ē-nŭs). Forming or producing tumors.

oncograph (ŏng'kō-grăf). Device attached to oncometer for making record of the internal organs' size.

oncology (ŏng-kŏl'ō-jĭ). The branch of medicine dealing with tumors.

oncolysis (ŏng-kol'ĭ-sĭs). The absorption or dissolution of tumor cells.

oncolytic (ong-kō-lĭt'ĭk). Destructive to tumor cells.

oncoma (ong-kō'mă). A tumor or swelling. Term is no longer commonly used.

oncometer (ŏng-kom'ět-ēr). Apparatus for measurement of variations in size of the internal organs. SEE: *plethysmograph.*

oncosis (ŏng-kō'sĭs). 1. A condition characterized by the development of tumors. 2. A swelling or tumor.

oncosphere (ong'kō-sfēr). Embryonic stage of a tapeworm in which it has hooks.

oncothlipsis (ŏng-kō-thlĭp'sĭs). Pressure due to presence of a tumor.

oncotic (ŏng-kŏt-ĭk). Concerning, caused, or marked by swelling.

oncotomy (ŏng-kot′ō-mĭ). The operation of cutting into a tumor, abscess, or boil.

oncotropic (ong-kō-trop′ĭk). Possessing special attraction for tumor cells. SYN: *tumoraffin.*

oneiric (ō-nī′rĭk). Resembling, rel. to, or accompanied by dreams.

oneirism (ō-nī′rĭzm). A condition of cerebral automatism resembling the prolongation of a dream after waking.

oneirodynia (ō-nī-rō-dĭn′ĭ-ă). Painful dreaming; nightmare.*

   o. activa. Walking while sleeping. SYN: *somnambulism.*

   o. gravans. A bad dream. SYN: *nightmare.*   [aspect of dreams.

oneirology (ō-nī-rol′ō-jĭ). The scientific

oneiroscopy (o-nī-ros′kō-pĭ). Analysis of dreams in the diagnosis of the individual's mental state.

one-two-three enema. One consisting of *one* oz. magnesium sulfate, *two* oz. glycerin, and *three* oz. water. SEE: *enema.*

oniomania (ō-nĭ-ō-mā′nĭ-ă). A psychoneurotic symbolism evidenced by an abnormal urge to spend money.

oniric (ō-nī′rĭk). Concerning a dream. SYN: *oneiric.*

onirism (ō-nī′rĭzm). Dreamlike hallucination in a waking state. SYN: *oneirism.*

onkinocele (ŏng-kĭn′ō-sēl). Inflammation, with swelling, of a tendon sheath.

onomatology (ŏn-o-mă-tol′ō-jĭ). Science of names. SYN: *nomenclature, terminology.*

onomatomania (ŏn-ō-mă-tō-mā′nĭ-ă). An abnormal or morbid impulse to dwell upon and repeat certain words, their imagined hidden meanings and significance, or to try to recall frantically a particular word.

onomatophobia (ŏn-ō-mă-tō-fō′bĭ-ă). Condition in which there is abnormal fear of hearing a certain name or word, because of an imaginary dreadful meaning attached to it.

onomatopoiesis (ŏn-ō-mă-tō-poy-ē′sĭs). Imitation of natural sounds by the use of created, usually meaningless, imitative words and sounds.

onto-. Combining form, *being.*

ontogenesis (ŏn″tō-jĕn′ĕ-sĭs). Origin and development of the individual. SYN: *ontogeny.*

ontogeny (ŏn-toj′ĕn-ĭ). 1. The history of the development of an individual. 2. The belief that the human species was an act of special creation. SYN: *ontogenesis.* SEE: *phylogeny.*

onychatrophia (ŏn″ĭ-kă-trō′fĭ-ă). Wasting away of the nails.

onychauxis (ŏn″ĭ-kawk′sĭs). Hypertrophy of the nails.

onychia (on-ĭk′ĭ-ă). Inflammation of the nail bed with suppuration and, frequently, loss of the nail. SYN: *onychitis.* SEE: *paronychia.*

   o. lateralis. Suppuration of tissues in the area lateral to fingernail.

   o. maligna. Type in debilitated persons in which there is fetid ulceration and loss of the nail.

   o. parasitica. Any parasitic disease of the nails.

onychitis (on-ĭk-ī′tĭs). Inflammation of the nail bed. SYN: *onychia.*

onychocryptosis (ŏn″ĭ-kō-krĭp-tō′sĭs). Ingrowing of the toenail.

onychograph (ŏn-ĭk′ō-grăf). Device for making record of capillary blood pressure under the fingernails.

onychogryposis (on″ĭ-kō-grĭ-pō′sĭs). Abnormal growth of the nails with inward curvature.

onychoid (on′ĭ-koyd). Similar to a nail, esp. a fingernail.

onycholysis (ŏn-ĭ-kol′ĭ-sĭs). Loosening or detachment of the nail from the nail bed.

onychoma (on-ĭ-kō′mă). Tumor of the nail or the nail bed.

onychomalacia (ŏn″ĭ-kō-mă-lā′sĭ-ă). Unnatural softening of the nails. SEE: *hapalonychia.*

onychomycosis (on″ĭ-kō-mī-kō′sĭs). Disease of the nails due to a parasitic fungus.

onychonosus (ŏn-ĭ-kon′ō-sŭs). Any disease of the nails.

onychopathy (ŏn-ĭ-kop′ăth-ĭ). Any disease of the nails. SYN: *onychonosus.*

onychophagy (ŏn-ĭ-kof′ă-jĭ). The practice of biting the nails.

onychophosis (ŏn-ĭk-ō-fō′sĭs). Accumulation of horny layers of epidermis under the toenail.

onychophyma (ŏn″ĭ-kō-fī′mă). Painful degeneration of the nail with hypertrophy.

onychoptosis (ŏn-ĭk-ŏp-tō′sĭs). Dropping off of the nails.

onychorrhexis (ŏn″ĭ-kō-rĕk′sĭs). Nail splitting.

onychosis (ŏn-ĭ-kō′sĭs). Any diseased condition of the nails. SYN: *onychopathy.*

onychotomy (ŏn-ĭ-kot′ō-mĭ). Surgical incision of a fingernail or toenail.

onychotrophy (ŏn-ĭ-kŏt′rō-fĭ). Nourishment of the nails.

onyx (on′ĭks). 1. A finger- or toenail. 2. Pus collection bet. the corneal layers of the eye.

onyxis (ŏn-ĭk′sĭs). Ingrowing of the nails.

onyxitis (ŏn-ĭk-sī′tĭs). Inflamed condition of matrix of a nail, with suppuration and loss of the nail. SYN: *onychia.*

oö-. Combining form denoting an *egg*, or the *primordial cell* that develops into an ovule.

oöblast (ō′ō-blăst). A cell derived from the germinal epithelium which gives rise to an ovum.

oöcyesis (ō″ō-sī-ē′sĭs). Ectopic pregnancy in the ovary.

oöcyst (ō′ō-sĭst). 1. An encased oöspore, before or after cell division. 2. The membrane enclosing the oöspore.

oöcyte (ō′ō-sīt). The early or primitive ovum before it has developed completely.

oögenesis (ō″ō-jĕn′ĕ-sĭs). Formation and development of the ovum.

oögonium (ō″ō-gō′nĭ-ŭm) (pl. *oögonia*). 1.

The primordial cell from which an oöcyte originates. 2. Descendant of primordial cell from which the oöcyte arises. 3. Female element of a fungus, which forms the oöspore when fertilized.

oökinesis (ō″ō-kĭn-ē′sĭs). The movements of division taking place in an ovum during maturation, fertilization, and segmentation, esp. active changes of the vitellus.

oöphor-. Combining form indicating *ovary*.

oöphoralgia (ō″ŏf-ō-ral′jĭ-ă). Neuralgic pain in an ovary.

oöphorauxe (ō″ŏf-ō-rawks′ē). Ovarian enlargement.

oöphorectomy (ō″ŏf-ō-rĕk′tō-mĭ). Excision of an ovary. SYN: *ovariectomy*.

oöphorin (ō-ŏf′ō-rĭn). A commercial hormone preparation made from the ovaries of cows and swine.

oöphoritis (ō″ŏf-ō-rī′tĭs). Inflamed condition of the ovary. SYN: *ovaritis, q.v.*

　　o., follicular. Inflammation of the graafian follicles.

oöphorocystosis (ō-ŏf″ō-rō-sĭs-tō′sĭs). Development of an ovarian cyst.

oöphoroepilepsy (ō-ŏf″ō-rō-ĕp′ĭ-lĕp-sĭ). Epilepsy caused by irritation or disease of the ovary.

oöphorohysterectomy (ō-ŏf″ō-rō-hĭs-tĕr-ĕk′tō-mĭ). Surgical removal of the uterus and ovaries. SYN: *oöthecohysterectomy*.

oöphoroma (ō-ŏf-ō-rō′mă). Malignant ovarian tumor.

oöphoromania (ō-ŏf″ō-rō-mā′nĭ-ă). Insanity arising from an ovarian disease.

oöphoron (ō-ŏf′ō-rŏn). An ovary. SYN: *oötheca.*

oöphoropeliopexy (ō-ŏf″ō-rō-pe′lĭ-ō-pĕk-sĭ). Suture of a displaced ovary to the pelvic wall.

oöphoropexy (ō-ŏf″ō-rō-pĕk″sĭ). Fixation of a displaced ovary. SYN: *oöphoropeliopexy.*

oöphorosalpingectomy (ō-ŏf″ō-rō-săl-pĭn-jĕk′tō-mĭ). Excision of an oviduct and ovary.

oöphorostomy (ō-ŏf-ō-rŏs′tō-mĭ). Creation of an artificial opening into an ovarian cyst for drainage.

oöphorrhaphy (ō-ō-or′ă-fĭ). Suture of a displaced ovary to the pelvic wall.

oösperm (ō′ō-spĕrm). The cell formed by union of the spermatozoon with the ovum; the fertilized ovum.

oötheca (ō-o-thē′kă). An ovary.

oöthecohysterectomy (ō-o-thē″kō-hĭs-tĕr-ĕk′tō-mĭ). Excision of the uterus and ovaries.

oötherapy (ō″o-ther′ă-pĭ). Treatment with ovarian substance.

opacity (ō-păs′ĭ-tĭ). 1. Darkness; shading from light. 2. Lack of transparency. 3. Mental dullness.

opaque (ō-pāk′). 1. Dark. 2. Not transparent. 3. Stupid.

open (ō′pĕn). 1. Not shut. 2. Uncovered, exposed, as to air. 3. To make an aperture in, as to open a boil. 4. Interrupted, said of an electric circuit, when current cannot pass.

operable (ŏp′ĕr-ă-bl). 1. Practicable. 2. Admitting of treatment by operation with reasonable expectation of cure.

operate (ŏp′ĕr-āt). 1. To perform an excision or incision or to make a suture on the body or any of its organs or parts to restore health. 2. To produce an effect, as a drug.

operation (ŏp-ĕr-ā′shŭn). 1. The act of operating. 2. A surgical procedure to restore health. 3. Action of a drug.

　　o., major. One involving danger to life.

　　o., minor. Operation not serious or risking life.

　　o., radical. Operation performed to effect complete cure.

　　o., subtotal. One in which not quite all of the organ is removed, as subtotal removal of thyroid gland.

operative (op′ĕr-ă-tĭv). 1. Effective, active. 2. Pert. to or brought about by an operation. 3. A drug that is acting.

　　o. procedure. A surgical operation.

opercular (ō-pur′kū-lăr). Concerning a covering.

operculum (ō-pur′kū-lŭm) (pl. *opercula*). 1. Any covering. 2. Plug of mucus which fills up the opening of the cervix upon impregnation. 3. BNA. Convolutions covering the island of Reil.

ophiasis (ō-fī′ăs-ĭs). Baldness occurring in windy streaks upon the head.

ophidiophobia (ō-fĭd″ĭ-ō-fō′bĭ-ă). Abnormal fear of snakes.

ophidism (ō′fĭd-ĭzm). Poisoning from snake bite.

ophiotoxemia (ō″fĭ-ō-tŏk-sē′mĭ-ă). Poisoning due to venom injected by a snake.

ophiotoxin (ō-fĭ-ō-tŏk′sĭn). A poison in cobra venom.

ophritis, ophryitis (ŏf-rī′tĭs, -rē-ī′tĭs). Inflammation of the eyebrow.

ophryon (ō′frē-on). Meeting point of the facial median line with a transverse line across the forehead's narrowest portion.

ophthalmagra (ŏf-thăl-măg′ră). Gouty or rheumatic inflammation of the eye, with pain. [the eye.

ophthalmalgia (ŏf-thăl-măl′jĭ-ă). Pain in

ophthalmatrophy (ŏf-thăl-măt′rō-fĭ). Atrophy of eyeball.

ophthalmectomy (ŏf-thăl-mĕk′tō-mĭ). Excision of an eye.

ophthalmia (ŏf-thăl′mĭ-ă). Severe inflammation of the eye, usually including the conjunctiva.

　　o., catarrhal. Conjunctivitis of a severe, frequently purulent, form.

　　o., Egyptian. Granular conjunctivitis. SYN: *trachoma.*

　　o., gonorrheal. Severe, purulent form due to infection with gonococcus.

　　o., granular. Severe purulent conjunctivitis with formation of granules on the eyelids. SYN: *trachoma.*

　　o., metastatic. Sympathetic inflammation of the choroid due to pyemia or metastasis.

　　o., migratory. SEE: *sympathetic ophthalmia.*

o. neonatorum. Severe purulent conjunctivitis in the newborn.

o., neuroparalytic. Corneal inflammation due to a nerve lesion.

o., phlyctenular. Vesicular formations on epithelium of conjunctiva or cornea.

o., purulent. Purulent inflammation of eye, usually due to gonococcus.

o., scrofulous. SEE: *phlyctenular ophthalmia.*

o., spring. Conjunctivitis in the spring of the year.

o., sympathetic. Plastic or serous uveitis in one eye caused by some disorder in the other eye.

o., varicose. Ophthalmia seen in varicose veins of the conjunctiva.

ophthalmiatrics (ŏf-thăl-mĭ-at'rĭks). The treatment of eye diseases.

ophthalmic (ŏf-thăl'mĭk). Pert. to the eye.

o. nerve. A branch of the trigeminal or trifacial nerve (5th cranial nerve). It is sensory and its branches are the *lacrimal, frontal,* and *nasociliary,* etc.

ophthalmitis (ŏf-thăl-mī'tĭs). Inflamed condition of the eye.

ophthalmo-. Combining form *pert. to the eye.*

ophthalmoblennorrhea (ŏf-thăl"mō-blĕn-ŏr-rē'ä). Purulent inflammation of the eye or conjunctiva, usually due to the gonococcus.

ophthalmocele (ŏf-thăl'mō-sēl). Abnormal protrusion of the eyeballs. SYN: *exophthalmos.*

ophthalmocopia (ŏf-thăl-mō-kō'pĭ-ä). Ocular fatigue; eyestrain. SYN: *asthenopia, q.v.*

ophthalmodesmitis (ŏf-thăl"mō-dĕs-mī'tĭs). Inflammation of tendons of the eye.

ophthalmodiagnosis (ŏf-thăl"mō-dī-ăg-nō'sĭs). Diagnosis of eye conditions by means of the ophthalmoreaction.*

ophthalmodynia (ŏf-thăl-mō-dĭn'ĭ-ä). Pain in the eye. SYN: *ophthalmalgia.*

ophthalmofundoscope (ŏf-thăl"mō-fŭnd'ō-skōp). Apparatus used in examining the fundus of the eye.

ophthalmography (ŏf-thăl-mŏg'răf-ĭ). Description of the eye, and its disorders.

ophthalmogyric (ŏf-thăl-mō-jī'rĭk). Causing or concerning ocular movements. SYN: *oculogyric.*

ophthalmolith (ŏf-thăl'mō-lĭth). A calculus of the lacrimal duct.

ophthalmologist (ŏf-thăl-mol'ō-jĭst). One who treats the eye and its disorders.

ophthalmology (ŏf-thăl-mol'ō-jĭ). The science dealing with the eye and its diseases.

ophthalmomalacia (ŏf-thăl"mō-măl-a'sĭ-ä). Shrinkage or softness of eye.

ophthalmometer (ŏf-thăl-mŏm'ĕt-ĕr). Instrument for making measurements of corneal astigmatism.

ophthalmometry (ŏf-thăl-mom'ĕt-rĭ). Measurement of the ocular defects and refractive powers.

ophthalmomycosis (ŏf-thăl"mō-mī-kō'sĭs). Any fungous disease of the eye.

ophthalmomyitis (ŏf-thăl"mō-mī-ī'tĭs). Inflammation of the ocular muscles.

ophthalmomyositis (ŏf-thăl"mō-mī-ō-sī'tĭs). Inflamed condition of the eye muscles. SYN: *ophthalmomyitis.*

ophthalmomyotomy (ŏf-thăl"mō-mī-ot'ō-mĭ). Surgical section of the muscles of the eyes.

ophthalmoneuritis (ŏf-thăl"mō-nū-rī'tĭs). Inflamed condition of the optic nerve.

ophthalmopathy (ŏf-thăl-mop'ä-thĭ). Any eye disease.

ophthalmophlebotomy (ŏf-thăl"mō-flē-bŏt'ō-mĭ). Incision of the eye to overcome congestion of conjunctival veins.

ophthalmophthisis (ŏf-thăl-mŏf'thĭs-ĭs). Softening or shrinking of the eyeball. SYN: *phthisis bulbi.*

ophthalmoplasty (ŏf-thăl'mō-plăs"tĭ). Ocular plastic surgery.

ophthalmoplegia (ŏf-thăl"mō-plē'jĭ-ä). Paralysis of ocular muscles.

o. externa. Paralysis of extraocular muscles.

o. interna. Paralysis of intraocular muscles.

o., nuclear. Ophthalmoplegia due to lesion of nuclei of origin of the ocular motor nerves.

o. partialis. Paralysis of not all of ocular muscles.

o. progressiva. Form in which all muscles become involved slowly.

o. totalis. Paralysis of both internal and external ocular muscles.

ophthalmoptosis (ŏf-thăl-mŏp-tō'sĭs). Protrusion of the eyeball. SYN: *exophthalmos.*

ophthalmoreaction (ŏf-thăl"mō-rē-ăk'shŭn). Reaction of the conjunctiva resulting on instillation of a drop of tuberculin or typhoid fever toxin into the eye of persons suffering from the diseases.

ophthalmorrhagia (ŏf-thăl-mō-rā'jĭ-ä). Ocular hemorrhage.

ophthalmorrhea (ŏf-thăl-mō-rē'ä). Flow of blood from eye.

ophthalmorrhexis (ŏf-thăl-mō-rĕks'ĭs). Rupture of an eyeball.

ophthalmoscope (ŏf-thăl'mō-skōp). Instrument for examining interior of the eye.

ophthalmoscopy (ŏf-thăl-mŏs'kō-pĭ). The examination of the interior of the eye.

o., direct. Examination in which image in interior of eye is upright.

o., indirect. Examination in which image in interior of eye is inverted.

ophthalmostat (ŏf-thăl'mō-stăt). Instrument used to hold the eye still during an operation.

ophthalmostatometer (ŏf-thăl"mō-stăt-om'ĕt-ĕr). Instrument for ascertaining position of eyes.

ophthalmothermometer (ŏf-thăl"mō-thĕr-mom'ĕt-ĕr). Instrument for determining local temperature in eye diseases.

ophthalmotonometer (ŏf-thăl"mō-tō-nŏm'ĕt-ĕr). Instrument for determining tension within globe of eye.

ophthalmotoxin (ŏf-thăl"mō-toks'ĭn). Cytotoxin derived on injection of emulsions of the ciliary body.

ophthalmotrope (ŏf-thăl′mō-trōp). Instrument for showing the movements of the ocular muscles.

ophthalmotropometer (ŏf-thăl″mō-tro-pom′ĕt-ĕr). Instrument for measuring the eye movements.

opiate (ō′pī-āt). 1. A drug derived from opium. 2. A drug inducing sleep. 3. To deaden, to put to sleep.
   SEE: *depressant, narcotic, sedative, etc.*

opiomania (ō″pī-ō-mā′nĭ-ă). Morbid addiction to use of opium or its derivatives.

opiophagism (ō-pī-ŏf′ă-jizm). Addiction to the use of opium, esp. the eating of it.

opisthenar (ō-pīs′the-năr). Back of the hand.

opisthion (ō-pīs′thĭ-ŏn). Craniometric point at middle of lower border of foramen magnum.

opistho-, opisth-. Combining form meaning *backward, behind.*

opisthognathism (ŏp″ĭs-thŏg′nă-thĭzm). Skull abnormality marked by a retreating lower jaw.

opisthoporeia (ō-pĭs″thō-pō-rī′ă). Involuntary walking backward due to loss of motor control.

Opisthorchis (ō-pĭs-thor′kĭs). A genus of parasitic fluke worms with testicles near the post. end of the body.
   O. sinensis. Common form causing the liver fluke disease of Asia.

opisthotic (ŏp″ĭs-thŏt′ĭk). 1. Located behind the ear or in the int. ear. 2. An opisthotic element or bone.
   o. center. Petrous bone's ossification center.

opisthotonos (ŏp″ĭs-thŏt′ō-nŏs). An arched position of the body with feet and head on the floor caused by a tetanic spasm.
   SEE: *emprosthotonos, pleurothotonus, posture.*

opium (ō′pī-ŭm). USP. The dried juice obtained from the unripe capsule of the poppy.
   DOSAGE: Opium: 1 gr. (0.06 Gm.). Tr. opium (laudanum): 10 ℳ (0.6 cc.). Tr. opium camphorated (paregoric): Adult, 1 dram (4 cc.).

opiumism (ō′pī-ŭm-ĭzm). 1. Addiction to use of opium. 2. Physical condition resulting from overuse of opium.

opo-. Prefix meaning *derived from juice.*

opohypophysin (ō″pō-hĭ-pof′ĭ-sĭn). Commercial preparation used in treating acromegaly.

opomam′min. Commercial animal udder extract used in diseases of the uterus.

opoövariin (ō″pō-ō-va′rē-ĭn). Commercial preparation of animal ovaries used in hysteria and diseases of the ovary.

opopros′tatin. Commercial preparation of animal prostate glands used in hypertrophied prostate.

opotherapy (ō-pō-thĕr′ă-pī). 1. Treatment of disease by using animal organs or extracts from them. SYN: *organotherapy.* 2. Use of juice in treatment of disease.

Oppenheim's disease (ŏp′ĕn-hīm). A rare congenital disorder marked by atony of entire bodily musculature. SYN: *amyotonia congenita.*

oppilation (ŏp″pĭ-lā′shŭn). 1. An obstruction. 2. Act or state of being obstructed. 3. Constipation.

oppilative (ŏp′pĭ-lā-tĭv). 1. Closing the pores. 2. Constipating. 3. Obstructive. 4. A constipating agent.

opponens (op-pō′nĕns). Opposing, a term applied to muscles of hand or foot by which 1 of the lateral digits may be opposed to 1 of the other digits.

opposition (ŏp-pō-sĭ′shŭn). Refusal of certain psychopaths to accept suggestions or directions because of retardation,* preoccupation with bizarre concepts, or from fear of the results.

opsialgia (ŏp-sī-al′jĭ-ă). Neuralgic pain of the face.

opsinogen (ŏp-sĭn′ō-jĕn). A substance which stimulates formation of opsonins.

opsinogenous (ŏp-sĭn-oj′ĕn-ŭs). Capable of forming opsonins.

opsiometer (ŏp-sĭ-ŏm′ĕt-ĕr). Apparatus for the measurement of vision. SYN: *optometer.*

opsiuria (ŏp-sī-ū′rĭ-ă). Condition in which excretion of urine is more rapid during fasting than after a meal.

opsogen (ŏp′sō-jĕn). Substance stimulating the formation of opsonins. SYN: *opsinogen.*

opsomania (ŏp-sō-mā′nĭ-ă). Morbid desire for some special article of food.

opsone (ŏp′sōn). Substance in blood serum whose function is to render cell and microörganisms attractive to phagocytes. SYN: *opsonin.*

opsonic (ŏp-sŏn′ik). Pert. to opsonins or their use in therapy.
   o. index. A measure of the resistance of a patient to bacterial invasion.

opsoniferous (op-so-nif′er-us). Carrying or producing opsonin.

opsonification (ŏp-sŏn″ĭ-fĭ-kā′shŭn). Effect of opsonins in rendering cells or bacteria phagocytized more readily.

opsonin (ŏp′sō-nĭn). Substance in blood serum which acts upon microörganisms and other cells, making them more attractive to phagocytes.

opsonization (ŏp-sŏn-ĭ-zā′shŭn). Action of opsonins in making cells or bacteria more attractive to phagocytes. SYN: *opsonification.*

opsonize (ŏp′son-īz). To render more attractive to phagocytes.

opsonocytophagic (op″sŏn-o-sī-tō-fā′jĭk). Pert. to phagocytic action of blood when serum opsonins are present.

opsonogen (ŏp-son′ō-jĕn). A stimulant to opsonin formation.

opsonology (ŏp-sō-nol′ō-jī). Study of opsonins and their function and action.

opsonometry (ŏp-sō-nŏm′ĕt-rī). Estimation of amt. of opsonins in the blood serum. SEE: *opsonic index.*

opsonophilia (ŏp-sŏn-ō-fĭl′ĭ-ă). Attraction for opsonins.

opsonophil′ic. Attractive to opsonins.

opsonotherapy (ŏp-sŏn-ō-thĕr'ă-pĭ). Treatment by stimulation of a specific opsonin with bacterial vaccines. SYN: *vaccine therapy.*

optesthesia (ŏp-tĕs-thē'zĭ-ă). Visual sensibility; perception of visual stimuli.

optic (ŏp'tĭk). Pert. to the eye or the sight.

    o. chiasm, o. commissure. The crossing of the optic nerve fibers in the brain.

    o. disk. Area in retina for entrance of optic nerve; the blind spot.

    o. foramen. Groove for optic nerve and ophthalmic artery at the orbit's apex.

    o. lobes. Upper pair of corpora quadrigemina of the brain.

    o. nerve. Second cranial nerve. FUNCT: Special sense of sight. ORIG: Occipital lobe, cortical center. DIST: Retina.

    o. papilla. SEE: *optic disk.*

    o. thalamus. Mass of gray substance at base of brain which connects with fibers of optic tract. SEE: *thalamic syndrome.*

    o. tract. Fibers running bet. optic chiasm and visual center.

optical (ŏp'tĭ-kăl). Pert. to vision or the eye.

    o. activity. CHEM: The property of rotating the plane of polarized light.

optician (ŏp-tĭsh'ăn). One who makes optical apparatus.

optico-. Combining form meaning *relating to the eye or vision.*

opticociliary (ŏp″tĭ-kō-sĭl'ĭ-ăr-ĭ). Concerning the optic and ciliary nerves.

opticopupillary (ŏp″tĭ-kō-pū'pĭl-ĕr-ĭ). Concerning optic nerve and the pupil.

optics (ŏp'tĭks). The science dealing with light and its relation to vision.

optimum (ŏp'tĭm-ŭm) (pl. *optima*). The condition which is most conducive to favorable activity.

    o. temperature. That temperature which is most suitable for development of bacterial cultures.

opto-. Combining form meaning *vision or eye.*

optogram (ŏp'tō-grăm). Image of ext. object fixed on the retina by photochemical bleaching action of light on the visual purple.

optometer (ŏp-tŏm'ĕt-ĕr). Instrument for measurement of the eye's refractive power.

optometrist (ŏp-tŏm'ĕt-rĭst). Person who measures the eye's refractive powers and fits glasses to correct ocular defects.

optometry (ŏp-tom'ĕt-rĭ). Measurement of the visual refractive power and correction of visual defects with eyeglasses.

optomyometer (ŏp″tō-mĭ-om'ĕt-ĕr). Instrument for determining strength of the muscles of the eye.

optophone (ŏp'tō-fōn). Instrument converting light energy into sound energy. Used by the blind.

optostriate (ŏp-tō-strī'ăt). Concerning the optic thalamus and the corpus striatum.

ora (ō'ra). Plural of os, mouth.

ora (ō'ră). A border or margin.

    o. serrata retinae. BNA. Notched ant. edge of retina.

orad (ō'răd). Toward the mouth or oral region.

oral (ō'răl). Concerning the mouth.

orology (ō-răl'ō-jĭ). 1. The science of oral hygiene. 2. Study of diseases of the mouth.

orbicular (ōr-bĭk'ū-lăr). Circular.

    o. bone. Ossicle frequently becoming attached to the incus. SYN: *os orbiculare.*

    o. ligament. Circular ligament about the neck of the radius. SYN: *ligamentum orbiculare.*

    o. muscle. Muscle about an opening.

    o. process. End of long process of the incus. SYN: *lenticular process.*

orbicularis (ōr″bĭk-ū-la'rĭs). Muscle surrounding an orifice; a sphincter muscle.

    o. oculi. Muscle encircling the opening of orbit of the eye.

    o. oris. Circular muscle surrounding the mouth.

    o. palpebrarum. SEE: *orbicular oculi.*

orbit (or'bĭt). The bony, pyramid-shaped cavity of the skull which holds the eyeball.

orbita (or'bĭ-tă) (pl. *orbitae*). BNA. Latin term for orbit.

orbital (or'bĭ-tăl). Concerning the orbit.

orbitale (or-bĭ-tā'lē). Lowest point on lower orbital margin.

orbitotomy (or-bĭt-ŏt'ō-mĭ). Surgical incision into the orbit.

orchectomy (ŏr-kĕk'tō-mĭ). Surgical removal of a testicle.

orcheoplasty (or'kē-ō-plăs-tĭ). Plastic repair work of the scrotum.

orchialgia (or-kĭ-ăl'jĭ-ă). Pain in the testes. SYN: *orchiodynia.*

orchic (or'kĭk). Concerning the testicle.

orchichorea (or″kĭ-kō-rē'ă). Involuntary jerking movements of the testicles.

orchidalgia (or-kĭ-dal'jĭ-ă). Neuralgia in the testicles. SYN: *orchialgia.*

orchidectomy (or″kĭd-ek'tō-mĭ). Removal of a testicle surgically. SYN: *orchectomy.*

orchidin (or'kĭd-ĭn). Proprietary preparation of testicular extract.

orchido-. Combining form, meaning *testicle.*

orchidocele (or'kĭ-dō-sēl). Scrotal hernia.

orchidocelioplasty (ōr″kĭd-ō-sēl'ĭ-ō-plăs″-tĭ). Surgical transfer of an undescended testicle to the abdominal cavity.

orchidoncus (ŏr-kĭ-dong'kŭs). A neoplasm of the testicle.

orchidopexy (or″kĭd-ō-pĕks″ĭ). Surgical transfer of an imperfectly descended testicle into the scrotum and suturing it there.

orchidoplasty (ŏr′kĭd-ō-plăs″tĭ). Operative transfer of an undescended testicle to the scrotum.

orchidoptosis (ŏr″kĭd-ŏp-tō′sĭs). Dropping of the testicle.

orchidotomy (ŏr-kĭd-ŏt′ō-mĭ). Incision into the testes.

orchiectomy (ŏr-kĭ-ĕk′tō-mĭ). Surgical excision of a testicle. SEE: *castration*.

orchiencephaloma (or″kĭ-ĕn-sef-ă-lō′mă). Tumor of brainlike substance in the testicle. SEE: *orchiomyeloma*.

orchiepididymitis (or″kĭ-ep″ĭ-dĭd-ĭ-mī′tĭs). Inflamed condition of a testicle and epididymis.

orchiocele (or′kĭ-ō-sēl). 1. Scrotal hernia. SYN: *orchidocele*. 2. A tumor of the testicle.

orchiodynia (ŏr-kĭ-ō-din′ĭ-ă). Testicular pain. SYN: *orchialgia, orchidalgia*.

orchiomyeloma (or″kĭ-ō-mĭ-ē-lō′mă). Tumor of the testicle composed of marrowlike cells.

orchioncus (ŏr-kĭ-ong′kŭs). Neoplasm of the testicle. SYN: *orchidoncus*.

orchioneuralgia (or″kĭ-ō-nū-răl′jĭ-ă). Neuralgia of the testicles. SYN: *orchialgia*.

orchiopathy (ŏr-kĭ-op′ăth-ĭ). Any diseased condition of the testes.

orchiopexy (or′kĭ-ō-peks′ĭ). The suturing of an undescended testicle in the scrotum. SYN: *orchidopexy, orchiorrhaphy*.

orchioplasty (or′kĭ-ō-plas′tĭ). Plastic repair of the testicle.

orchiorrhaphy (ŏr-kĭ-or′ră-fĭ). The suturing of an undescended testicle to surrounding tissue in the scrotum. SYN: *orchidopexy, orchiopexy*.

orchiosceocele (or-kĭ-os′kē-ō-sēl). Scrotal hernia with enlargement or tumor of testicle.

orchioscirrhus (or-kĭ-ō-skěr′rŭs). Testicular hardening due to tumor formation.

orchis (ŏr′kĭs). A testicle.

orchitic (or-kit′ik). Concerning or caused by orchitis.

orchitis (ŏr-kī′tĭs). Inflammation of a testis due to trauma, metastasis, mumps, or infection elsewhere in the body.

   o., gonorrheal. Orchitis due to gonococcus.

   o., metastatic. Orchitis due to infection from organisms in blood stream.

   o., syphilitic. SYM: Begins painlessly in body of gland as a rule, apt to be bilateral; causes dense, irregular, knotty induration, but not much increase in size.

   o., tuberculous. Form generally arising in the epididymis. It may be accompanied by formation of chronic sinuses, and destruction of tissues.

orchitolytic (or″kĭt-ō-lĭt′ĭk). Destructive to testicular tissue.

orchotomy (ŏr-kŏt′ō-mĭ). 1. Incision into a testicle. 2. Erroneously, excision of the testes. SYN: *orchectomy*.

orcin, orcinol (or′sĭn, -ol). Antiseptic derived from lichens, used in skin disorders.

orderly (or′dĕr-lĭ). Male attendant in a hospital, other than doctors or interns, responsible for care or preparation of male patients.   [the appetite.

orexigenic (ō-rĕk-sĭ-jĕn′ĭk). Stimulating

oreximania (ō-rĕk-sĭ-mā′nĭ-ă). Abnormal desire for food.

organ (or′găn). A part of the body having a special function.

   o., accessory. One having a subordinate function.

   o., acoustic. SEE: *organ of Corti*.

   o., appendicular. The limbs.

   o., cell. Basic part of a cell, as a nucleus.

   o. of Corti. Terminal acoustic apparatus in the cochlea. SEE: *Claudius' cell, ear*.

   o., end. A termination of a nerve, usually bulbous, and of sensory or motor function.

   o., endocrine. An organ yielding internal secretions. SEE: *endocrine*.

   o., excretory. One secreting waste products of the body.

   o's. of generation. The reproductive organs, external and internal. SEE: *genitalia, male and female*.

   o. of Giraldes. A small body on the spermatic cord, above the epididymis. SYN: *paradidymis*.

   o's, Golgi's. Spindle-shaped structure in muscles.

   o., Jacobson's. Rudimentary canal opening in the nasal septum.

   o., Meyer's. Area on both sides of post. portion of the tongue.

   o. of Rosenmüller. Residual sexual portion of the wolffian body in the broad ligament. SYN: *epoöphoron, parovarium*.

   o. of Ruffini. End organ of the fingertips.

   o., sense. One consisting of a nerve and its terminus, which convert a stimulus into a sensation.

   o., vomeronasal. SEE: *Jacobson's organ*.

   o., Weber's. Residual prostatic pouch in the male, the remains of the müllerian ducts.

organic (or-găn′ĭk). 1. Pert. to an organ or organs. 2. Structural. 3. Pert. to or derived from animal or vegetable forms of life.

   o. acid. Any acid containing or derived from the carboxyl group.

   o. chemistry. Branch dealing with carbon compounds.

   o. disease. One indicating that the structures of an organ are affected.

   o. food nutrients. Those nutrients containing carbon.

   o. reaction types. PSY: A general term applied to those psychoses induced by structural brain changes.

   o. sensation. One which arises from the organs of the body.

organism (or′găn-ĭzm). Any correlated living thing.

organization (or″găn-ĭ-zā′shŭn). 1. Process of correlating. 2. Systematic arrangement. 3. That which is organized; an organism.

organize (or′găn-īz). 1. To correlate or systematize. 2. To furnish with organs.

organogenesis, organogeny (or-găn-ō-jen′-ē-sĭs, -oj′ĕn-ĭ). The formation and development of body organs from embryonic tissues.

organography (or-găn-og'ră-fĭ). The description of the body organs.

organoleptic (or-găn-ō-lep'tĭk). 1. Affecting an organ, esp. the organs of special sense. 2. Susceptible to sensory impressions.

organology (or-găn-ol'ō-jĭ). The science dealing with the body organs.

organoma (or-găn-ō'mă). A tumor composed of definite organs or parts of organs and so arranged as to be a part of the organ or organs concerned.

organon (or'găn-ŏn). An organ.

   o. auditus. BNA. Organ of hearing.

   o. gustus. BNA. Organ of taste.

   o. olfactus. BNA. Organ of smell.

   o. spirale. BNA. Spiral organ in the cochlea. SYN: *organ of Corti.*

   o. visus. BNA. The organ of sight.

   o. vomeronasale. BNA. Canal opening into nasal septum. SYN: *Jacobson's organ.*

organopexia (or"găn-ō-pĕk'sĭ-ă). Surgical fixation of an organ that is detached from its proper position.

organoscopy (or-găn-os'kō-pĭ). Examination of the internal organs of the body.

organotherapy (or"găn-ō-thĕr'ă-pĭ). The treatment of disease by preparations of the endocrine glands of animals, or by extracts made from the same. SEE: *substitution therapy.*

organotrope, organotropic (or-găn'ō-trōp, -trōp'ĭk). Having affinity for tissues, noting substances acting on the organs of the body.

organule (or'gan-ūl). 1. An essential element of a cell or organ. 2. End organ of sensory receptors for the reception of specially complex sensations, such as the *taste bud* of the tongue, the retinal *rods* and *cones* of the eye, and the *organ of Corti* in the internal ear.

orgasm (or'găzm). 1. Paroxysmal emotional excitement. 2. An instance of it, specifically, the climax of sexual passion.

cridine (or'ĭ-dēn). The calcium salt of iodized fatty acids containing 23-25% organic iodine.

   DOSAGE: 1/6 gr. (10 mg.) iodine.

Oriental sore. An ulcerating, chronic, nodular skin lesion prevalent in the Orient and the tropics, due to parasites of the genus Leishmania.

orientation (or"ĭ-ĕn-tā'shŭn). Ability to comprehend and to adjust one's self in an environment with regard to time, location, and identity of persons.

orifice (or'ĭ-fĭs). Mouth, entrance or outlet to any aperture.

   o., anal. The anus.

   o., auriculoventricular. Opening in front and lower part of left and right ventricles of heart, oval in form, connecting with auricle.   [into stomach.

   o., cardiac. Opening of esophagus

   o., pyloric. Opening from stomach into the duodenum. SEE: *pylorus.*

orificial (or-ĭ-fĭsh'ăl). Pert. to or forming an orifice.

orificialist (or-ĭ-fĭsh'ăl-ĭst). One who practices orificial surgery in the treatment of disease.

origin (or'ĭ-jĭn). 1. The source of anything; a starting point. 2. The beginning of a nerve. 3. The more fixed attachment of a muscle. SEE: *cenotype.*

orodiagnosis (or"ō-dī-ăg-nō'sĭs). Diagnosis by using serums or serum reactions.

oroimmunity (or"rō-ĭm-mū-nĭ-tĭ). Immunity acquired by injection of serum from a person or animal who has active immunity against the disease in question. SYN: *passive immunity.*

orolingual (ō"rō-lĭn'gwăl). Concerning the mouth and tongue.

oronasal (ō"rō-nā'zăl). Concerning the mouth and nose.

oropharynx (ō"rō-far'ĭnks). Portion of pharynx between the soft palate and hyoid bone.

orotherapy (ō"rō-thĕr-ă-pĭ). 1. Treatment of disease with serums. SYN: *serotherapy.* 2. Use of whey in treatment.

orrhoimmunity (or"rō-ĭm-mū'nĭ-tĭ). Immunity acquired by serum injections from an animal or individual who is actively immunized against the disease in question. SYN: *passive immunity.*

orrhology (or-rol'ō-jĭ). The study of serums and their reactions. SYN: *serology.*

orrhomeningitis (or"rō-men-ĭn-jĭ'tĭs). Inflamed condition of a serous membrane.

orrhoreaction (or"rō-rē-ăk'shŭn). A reaction from injection of serum. SYN: *seroreaction.*

orrhorrhea (or"rō-rē'ă). 1. A flow of serum. 2. A watery discharge. SYN: *seriflux.*

orrhosis (or-rō'sĭs). Formation of serum.

orrhotherapy (or"rō-thĕr'ă-pĭ). 1. Serum therapy. 2. Whey cure.

or'tal-so'dium. A barbituric acid derivative similar to, but more active than barbital.

   DOSAGE: 3-6 gr. (0.2-0.4 Gm.).

ortho-. Combining form meaning *straight, right.*

orthoarteriotony (or"tho-ăr-tē-rĭ-ot'ō-nĭ). Normal arterial blood pressure.

orthobiosis (or"thō-bī-ō'sĭs). Hygienic living.

orthocephalic (or"thō-sē-făl'ĭk). Noting a head with a height-length index bet. 70 and 75.

orthochorea (or"thō-kō-re'ă). Movements of chorea in erect posture.

orthochromatic (or"thō-krō-mat'ĭk). Having normal color.

orthochromophil (or"thō-krō'mō-fĭl). Staining normally with neutral dyes.

orthocrasia (or"thō-krā'sĭ-ă). Condition in which the body reacts normally to drugs, proteins, and treatment in general.

orthocytosis (or"thō-sī-tō'sĭs). The presence in the blood of mature cells only.

orthodiagraph (or"thō-dī'ă-grăf). An instrument for accurately recording the outlines and positions of organs or foreign bodies as seen by radiographic apparatus.

orthodontia (or″thō-don′shĭ-ă). Division of dentistry dealing with prevention and correction of irregularities of the teeth.

orthoform (or′thō-form). Colorless, crystalline powder used as an anesthetic. DOSAGE: 8-15 gr. (0.5-1.0 Gm.).

orthogenesis (or″thō-jĕn′ē-sĭs). A biological principle that variations in an animal species begin to assume a definite direction, resulting in evolution of a new type, irrespective of ext. factors. SEE: *kinetic system*.

orthogenics (or″thō-jĕn′ĭks). The science dealing with defects, mental and physical, that hinder normal development. SYN: *eugenics*.

orthoglycemic (or″thō-glī-sē′mĭk). Having an average amount of sugar in the blood. [straight jaws.

orthognathous (or-thog′nă-thŭs). Having

orthograde (or′thō-grād). Walking with the body vertical or upright.

ortholiposis (or″thō-lĭ-pō′sĭs). 1. Normal amount of liposin in blood serum. 2. Condition of normal proportion of weight to height.

orthometer (or-thom′ĕt-ĕr). Device for determining the degree of protrusion of the eyes.

orthomorphia (or-tho-mor′fĭ-ă). Correction of a deformity.

orthoneutrophile (or″thō-nū′trō-fĭl, -fīl). Staining normally with neutral dyes.

orthopedia (or″thō-pē′dĭ-ă). Prevention or correction of deformities. SYN: *orthopedics*.

orthopedic (or″thō-pē′dĭk). Concerning orthopedics; prevention or correction of deformities.

   o. surgery. Surgical prevention and correction of deformities. SYN: *orthopedics*.

orthopedics (or″thō-pē′dĭks). The treatment of chronic affections of the spine and joints and the prevention and correction of deformities.

orthopedist (or″thō-pē′dĭst). One who corrects deformities and treats diseases of the joints and spine.

orthopercussion (or″thō-pĕr-kŭsh′ŏn). Percussion with the distal phalanx of the percussing finger held perpendicularly to the surface percussed.

orthophoria (or″thō-fō′rĭ-ă). Parallelism of visual axes, the normal muscle balance.

orthophrenia (or″thō-frē′nĭ-ă). The normal mental state of one who shares his emotional life with the family or a group.

orthopnea (or-thŏp-nē′ă). Respiratory condition in which breathing is possible only when person sits or stands in erect position.

orthopraxy (or′thō-prăk-sĭ). Correction and prevention of deformities by mechanical means. SYN: *orthopedics*.

orthopsychiatry (or″thō-sĭ-kī′ă-trĭ). The study and treatment of conduct disorders, esp. in the young.

orthoptic (or-thŏp′tĭk). Concerning the correction of a deviating eye.

   o. training. Eye muscle exercises for educating the fusion faculty; used in the treatment of squint.

orthoroentgenography (or″thō-rĕnt-gĕn-og′ră-fĭ). Measurement of size and position of internal organs accurately, using radiographic apparatus. SEE: *orthodiagraph*.

orthoscope (or′thō-skōp). Instrument for examining the eyes through a layer of water.

orthoscopic (or″thō-skōp′ĭk). 1. Having correct vision. 2. Seen without distortion. 3. Made to correct optical distortion. [ination with an orthoscope.

orthoscopy (or-thŏs′kō-pĭ). Ocular exam-

orthostatic (or′thō-stăt-ĭk). Concerning an erect position.

orthostatism (or′thō-stăt-ĭzm). An upright standing position of the body.

orthotast (or′thō-tăst). Instrument for straightening bone curvatures.

orthotherapy (or″thō-ther′ă-pĭ). Correction of posture as a means of treatment.

orthotonos, orthotonus (or-thŏt′ō-nos, -nŭs). Tetanic spasm marked by rigidity of the body in a straight line.

orthuria (orth-ū′rĭ-ă). Average frequency of urination.

oryzanin (ō-rī′zăn-ĭn). Concentrated antineuritic vitamin obtained from rice bran. SYN: *Vitamin B₁ or F*.

O. S., o. s. Abbr. for L. *oculus sinister*, left eye.

os (ōs) (pl. *ōra*). Mouth, opening. BNA.

   o. externum. Portion of the cervix uteri opening into the vaginal canal.

   o. internum. Portion of the cervix uteri opening into the uterus.

   o. uteri. Mouth of the uterus.

os (ōs) (pl. *ossa*). Bone.

   o. calcis. Heel bone. SYN: *calcaneum*.

   o. coxae. Hipbone.

   o. hamatum. Hooked bone in second row of carpus. SYN: *unciform bone*.

   o. hyoideum. U-shaped bone at the base of the tongue.

   o. ilium. Haunch bone.

   o. innominatum. SEE: *os coxae*.

   o. interparietale. A bone, occasionally separate, found bet. the frontal, parietal, and sup. occipital bones.

   o. magnum. A carpal bone, the third in the second distal row.

   o. orbiculare. Tiny bone in the ear which usually becomes attached to the incus.

   o. peroneum. Bone occasionally found in tendon of peroneus longus muscle.

   o. planum. 1. Flat bone. 2. Orbital plate of ethmoid bone.

   o. pubis. The pubic bone.

   o. unguis. Lacrimal bone.

osazone (ō′să-zōn, ō″să-zōn′). Any of a series of compounds resulting from heating sugars with acetic acid and phenylhydrazine.

oscedo (os-sē′dō). 1. Yawning. 2. White spots on the mucosa of the mouth. SYN: *aphthae*.

oscheal (os'kē-ăl). Concerning the scrotum.

oscheio-, oscheo-. Combining forms meaning the *scrotum*.

oscheitis (ŏs-kē-ī'tĭs). Inflamed condition of the scrotum.

oscheocele (ŏs'kē-ō-sēl). 1. A scrotal swelling or tumor. 2. Scrotal hernia. SYN: *oscheoma*.

oscheohydrocele (os"kē-ō-hī'drō-sēl). Collection of fluid in the sac of a scrotal hernia.

oscheolith (os'kē-ō-lĭth). A concretion in the scrotal sebaceous glands.

oscheoma (ŏs-kē-ō'mă). Scrotal tumor. SYN: *oscheoncus*.

oscheoncus (ŏs-kē-on'kŭs). A tumor of the scrotum.

oscheoplasty (os'kē-ō-plăs-tĭ). Plastic surgical repair of the scrotum.

oschitis (os-kī'tis). Inflamed condition of the scrotum. SYN: *oscheitis*.

oscillation (ŏs"sĭl-ā'shŭn). A swinging, pendulumlike movement; a vibration.

oscillogram (ŏs'ĭl-ō-grăm). Record made by the oscillograph.

oscillograph (ŏs'ĭl-ō-grăf). Machine for recording electric vibrations, as of the heart or blood pressure.

oscillometer (ŏs-ĭl-om'ĕt-ĕr). Machine to measure oscillations.

oscillometry (os-ĭl-om'ĕ-trĭ). The measurement of oscillations with a machine.

oscilloscope (ŏs-ĭl'ō-skōp). An instrument for making visible the presence or the nature and form of oscillations or irregularities of an electric current.

oscitation (ŏs-ĭ-tā'shŭn). Yawning; gaping.

oscodal (os'kō-dăl). A cod liver oil concentrate containing vitamins A and D.
    DOSAGE: In tablet form, 1-2 tablets t. i. d.

osculum (os'kŭ-lŭm). Any tiny aperture or pore.

-ose. Chemical suffix indicating (a) the presence of carbohydrates, as *glucose*; (b) primary alteration product of a protein, as *proteose*.

-osis. Suffix denoting *caused by, state of, disease, intensive*.

Osler's disease (ōs'lĕr). Rare disease of the blood in which the red cells are increased in number, the spleen becomes enlarged and cyanosis of the mucosa and skin. SYN: *erythremia, polycythemia*.

osmatic (ŏz-măt'ĭk). Having a keen sense of smell.

osmatism (ŏz'mă-tĭzm). A well-developed sense of smell.

osme (ŏz'mē). 1. An odor. 2. The sense of smell.

osmesis (ŏz-mē'sĭs). The sense of smell; act of smelling.

osmesthesia (ŏz-mĕs-thē'zĭ-ă). Olfactory sensibility; power of perceiving and distinguishing odors.

osmic acid (ŏz'mĭk). 1. Volatile, colorless compound formed by heating osmium in air. 2. Compound of osmium trioxide and water (H_2OsO).

osmicate (oz'mĭ-kāt). To impregnate or stain with osmic acid.

osmics (oz'mĭks). The science of odors.

osmidrosis (ŏz-mĭd-rō'sĭs). Condition in which perspiration has a very strong odor. SYN: *bromidrosis*.

osmium (ŏz'mĭ-ŭm). A metallic element; symb. Os.

osmo-. Combining form. 1. (osme) *odor* or *smell*, and 2. (osmos) *threat* or *push*.

osmodysphoria (ŏz-mō-dĭs-fō'rĭ-ă). Abnormal dislike of certain odors.

osmogen (oz'mō-jĕn). Substance from which an enzyme or ferment is derived.

osmolagnia (ŏz-mō-lăg'nĭ-ă). Erotic satisfaction derived from odors, usually of the body.

osmology (ŏz-mŏl'ō-jĭ). 1. The study of odors. SYN: *osphresiology*. 2. Study of osmosis.

osmometer (oz-mŏm'ĕt-ĕr). 1. Device for measuring acuity of sense of smell. 2. Device for measuring velocity of fluids diffused through membranes.

osmonosology (ŏz"mō-nō-sŏl'ō-jĭ). Branch of medicine dealing with diseases of the organs of smell.

os'mophilic. Readily diffused through a membrane.

osmose (ŏz'mōs). 1. To subject to osmosis. 2. To undergo osmosis.

osmosis (ŏz-mō'sĭs). The passage of solvent through a partition separating solutions of different concentrations.

osmotherapy (os-mō-ther'ă-pĭ). Treatment by changing the osmotic pressure of blood and tissues, as by injection of hypertonic solutions into the blood.

osmotic (ŏz-mŏt'ĭk). Pert. to osmosis, the passage of solutions of different concentration through a membrane.
    o. pressure. Unbalanced pressure causing phenomena of osmosis and diffusion.

osphresiolagnia (ŏs-frē"zĭ-ō-lag'nĭ-ă). Excitement of an erotic nature aroused by odors.

osphresiology (ŏs-frē-zĭ-ŏl'ō-jĭ). Science of odors and the sense of smell. SYN: *osmology*.

osphresiometer (ŏs-frē-zĭ-ŏm'ĕt-ĕr). Apparatus for measuring the acuteness of the sense of smell. SYN: *osmometer, 1*.

osphresis (ŏs-frē'sĭs). The sense of smell. SYN: *olfaction*.

osphretic (ŏs-fret'ĭk). Concerning the sense of smell. SYN: *olfactory*.

osphus (os'fŭs). Loin.

osphyalgia (ŏs-fĭ-al'jĭ-ă). Pain of the loins or hips. SEE: *lumbago, sciatica*.

osphyitis (ŏs-fĭ-ī'tĭs). Inflammation in the lumbar region.

osphyomyelitis (ŏs"fĭ-ō-mĭ-ĕl-ī'tĭs). Inflamed condition of the lumbar region of the spinal cord.

os pubis (ŏs pŭ'bĭs). A bone that in adult life unites with the ilium and ischium to form the pelvis. Irregular shape, divided into a horizontal, ascending, and descending ramus. The outer extremity constitutes approximately one-fifth of the acetabulum. The inner unites in middle line with corresponding part of the bone of opp. side, forming the symphysis pubis.

ossa (ŏs'ă) (sing. *os*). Bones.

   o. innominata. The hipbones.

   o. triquetra. Tiny bones in cranial sutures. SYN: *wormian bones.*

ossagen (ŏs'ă-jĕn). Proprietary powder made from red bone marrow, containing calcium salts.

ossein (ŏs'ē-ĭn). The organic substance of bones. SYN: *ostein.*

osseous (ŏs'ē-ŭs). Bonelike; concerning bones. SYN: *bony.*

ossicle (ŏs'ĭ-kl). Any small bone, as 1 of the 3 bones of the ear, the *malleus, incus,* or *stapes.*

ossicula (ŏs-ĭk'ū-lă). Little bones.

ossiculectomy (ŏs″ĭk-ū-lĕk'tō-mĭ). Excision of an ossicle, especially one of the ear.

ossiculotomy (ŏs″ĭk-ū-lŏt'ō-mĭ). Surgical incision of 1 or more of the ossicles of the ear.

ossiculum (ŏs-ĭk'ū-lŭm). Tiny bone, esp. 1 of the 3 in the middle ear.

ossiferous (ŏs-ĭf'ĕr-ŭs). Composed of, or forming bone or bony tissue.

ossific (ŏs-ĭf'ĭk). Producing or becoming bone.

ossification (ŏs″ĭ-fĭ-kā'shŭn). 1. Formation of bone substance. 2. Conversion into bone. SEE: *center, epiotic, centro-sclerosis.*

ossify (ŏs'ĭ-fī). To turn into bone.

ostalgia (ŏs-tăl'jĭ-ă). Pain in a bone. SYN: *osteodynia.*

osteanabrosis (ŏs″tē-ăn-ă-brō'sĭs). Wasting away of bone.

osteanagenesis (ŏs″tē-ăn-ă-jĕn'ē-sĭs). Regeneration or re-formation of bone.

ostearthritis (ŏs″tē-ăr-thrī'tĭs). Inflamed condition of bones and joints.

ostearthrotomy (ŏs″tē-ăr-thrŏt'ō-mĭ). Surgical excision of the articular end of a bone.

ostectomy, osteëctomy (ŏs-tĕk'tō-mĭ, -tē-ĕk'tō-mĭ). Surgical excision of a bone or a portion of one.

osteëctopia (ŏs″tē-ĕk-tō'pĭ-ă). Dislocation of a bone.

ostein (ŏs'tē-ĭn). Organic matter of bone. SYN: *ossein.*

osteitis (ŏs-tē-ī'tĭs). Inflammation of a bone.

   o., condensing. A form in which the marrow changes into bone. SYN: *osteopsathyrosis, q.v.*

   o. deformans. Chronic form with thickening and hypertrophy of the long bones and deformity of the flat bones.

   o. fibrosa. Osteitis in which fibrous tissue replaces bony tissue. SYN: *Recklinghausen's disease.*

   o. f. cystica. Osteitis fibrosa with cyst formation on bones.

   o., gummatous. Chronic osteitis associated with syphilis.

   o., rarefying. Form in which the bone tissue becomes cancellated.

   o., sclerosing. SEE: *condensing osteitis.* [in a bone.

ostemia (ŏs-tē'mĭ-ă). Congestion of blood

ostempyesis (ŏs-tĕm-pī-ē'sĭs). Purulent inflammation within a bone.

osteo-. Combining form meaning *bone.*

osteoaneurysm (ŏs″tē-ō-an'ū-rĭzm). Aneurysm, or dilatation of a blood vessel filled with clotted blood, occurring within a bone.

osteoarthritis (ŏs″tē-ō-ăr-thrī'tĭs). Primarily a disease of the bones with joint involvement and formation of bony excrescences.

osteoarthropathy (ŏs″tē-ō-ar-thrŏp'ăth-ĭ). Any involvement of bones and joints, esp. when associated with disease of the central nervous system, the pleura, and lungs.

   o., hypertrophic pulmonary. An affection characterized by enlargement and curving of the nails of fingers or toes and enlargement of wrist and interphalangeal joints.

osteoarthrotomy (ŏs″tē-ō-ar-throt'ō-mĭ). Excision of joint end of a bone. SYN: *ostearthrotomy.*

osteoblast (ŏs-tē-ō-blăst). Small germinal cell from which bone grows.

osteocampsia (ŏs″tē-ō-kămp'sĭ-ă). Curvature of a bone, as in osteomalacia.

osteocarcinoma (ŏs″tē-ō-kăr-sĭn-ō'mă). 1. Osteoma and carcinoma combined. 2. Carcinoma of a bone.

osteocele (ŏs'tē-ō-sēl). 1. Hardening or bony tumor of testis or scrotum. 2. Bony matter forming in hernial sac.

osteocephaloma (ŏs″tē-ō-sĕf-ă-lō'mă). Encephaloma, a malignant neoplasm of brainlike texture in a bone.

osteochondritis (ŏs″tē-ō-kŏn-drī'tĭs). 1. Inflammation of bone and cartilage. 2. Inflammatory condition in which calcification is defective, with a layer of soft, yellowish-white tissue forming bet. the cartilaginous and calcified parts of a rib.

   o. deformans juvenilis. Chronic inflammation of head of femur in childhood resulting in atrophy and shortening of neck of femur and wide, flat head.

osteochondroma (ŏs″tē-ō-kŏn-drō'mă). Tumor composed of both cartilaginous and bony substance.

osteochondrophyte (ŏs″tē-ō-kŏn'drō-fīt). A tumor composed of cartilage and bone.

osteoclasia, osteoclasis (ŏs″tē-ō-klā'zĭ-ă, -ŏk'lă-sĭs). 1. Fracture of a bone, surgically, to remedy a deformity. 2. Bony tissue destruction.

osteoclast (ŏs'tē-ō-klăst). 1. Device for fracturing bones for therapeutic purposes. 2. Giant, multinuclear cell* found in depressions on the surface of a bone causing entire resorption of bone substance.

osteocope (ŏs'tē-ō-kōp). Severe pain of the bone, esp. at night, usually symptomatic of syphilis.

osteocopic (ŏs″tē-ō-kŏp'ĭk). Concerning pain in the bone.

osteocranium (ŏs″tē-ō-krā'nĭ-ŭm). The bony fetal cranium, as differentiated from the cartilaginous cranium.

osteocystoma (ŏs″tē-ō-sĭs-tō'mă). Cystic tumor of a bone.

osteodermia (ŏs″tē-ō-dĕr′mĭ-ă). Bony portions forming in the skin.

osteodynia (ŏs″tē-ō-din′ĭ-ă). Persistent pain in a bone. SYN: *ostealgia*.

osteodystrophia (ŏs″tē-ō-dĭs-trō′fĭ-ă). Defective bone development.

   o. juvenilis. Defective bone formation in children, in which bone substance is replaced by fibrous tissue. SEE: *osteitis fibrosa*.

osteoencephaloma (ŏs″tē-ō-ĕn″sĕf-ă-lō′mă). Malignant bone tumor, of brainlike texture.

osteoepiphysis (ŏs″tē-ō-ĕp-ĭf′ĭs-ĭs). A small piece of bone which later becomes attached to the larger one.

osteofibroma (ŏs″tē-ō-fĭ-brō′mă). Tumor of bony and fibrous tissues. SYN: *fibroosteoma*.

osteogen (ŏs′tē-ō-jĕn). Substance of the inner periosteal layer from which bone is formed.

osteogenesis, osteogeny (ŏs″tē-ō-jĕn′ĕ-sĭs, -ŏj′ĕ-nĭ). Formation and development of bone taking place in connective tissue or in cartilage.

   o. imperfecta. A congenital bone disease causing the bones to fracture easily.

osteography (ŏs-tē-og′raf-ĭ). Descriptive treatise on the bones.

osteohalisteresis (ŏs″tē-ō-hăl-ĭs-tĕr-ē′sĭs). Deficiency of the mineral constituents in bone causing softening.

osteoid (ŏs′tē-oyd). 1. Resembling bone. 2 A bone tumor.

   o. sarcoma. A rapidly forming sarcoma with bone tissue in it. SYN: *osteosarcoma*.

osteology (ŏs-tē-ol′ō′jĭ). The science of structure and function of bones.

osteolysis (ŏs-tē-ol′ĭs-ĭs). Softening and destruction of bone, as in caries.

osteoma (ŏs-tē-ō′mă) (pl. *osteomata*). A bony tumor; a hard tumor of bonelike structure developing on a bone, and sometimes on other structures.

   o., cancellous. One that is soft and spongy. Its thin and delicate trabeculae enclose large medullary spaces similar to cancellous bone.

   o., cavalryman's. Bony outgrowth of femur at the insertion of the adductor femoris longus.

   o. dentale. A hard, bony outgrowth from the jawbone.

   o. durum. A tumor composed of hard bony tissue.

   o., heteroplastic. An osteoma in an organ or tissue in which bone does not normally occur.

   o. medullare. An osteoma containing medullary spaces.

   o. spongiosum. Soft, spongy tumor in bone.

osteomalacia (ŏs″tē-ō-măl-ā′sĭ-ă). Softening of the bones. SYN: *malacosteon; mollities ossium*.

   o. apsathyros. A form in which bones become flexible like wax.

   o. carcinomatosa. Diffuse cancerous infiltration of medullary tissue of bones with softening.

   o. fracturosa, o. fragilis, o. psathyra. Osteomalacia in which the bones become brittle.

osteomalacic (ŏs″tē-ō-măl-ā′sĭk). Concerning or characterized by softening of the bone.

osteomalacosis (ŏs″tē-ō-măl-ă-kō′sĭs). Softening of the bone. SYN: *osteomalacia*.

osteomatoid (ŏs-tē-ō′mă-toyd). Resembling a tumor of bone tissue.

osteomere (ŏs′tē-ō-mēr). One of a series of similar bone segments, such as any of the vertebrae.

osteometry (ŏs-tē-om′et-rĭ). The study of the measurement of bones.

osteomiosis (ŏs″tē-ō-mĭ-ō′sĭs). Bone disintegration.

osteomyelitis (ŏs″tē-ō-mĭ-ĕl-ī′tĭs). Inflammation of bone marrow, or of the bone and marrow.

   o. fibrosa. Fibroid change in bone in osteitis deformans.

   o., hemorrhagic. Bone marrow inflammation with cyst formation.

   o., hunger. Osteomyelitis in those not properly nourished, displaying early symptoms of osteomalacia.

   o., malignant. Malignant bone marrow tumor.

   o. variolosa. Osteomyelitis as a complication of smallpox.

osteoncus (ŏs-tē-on′kŭs). A bone tumor. SYN: *exostosis, osteoma*.

osteonecrosis (ŏs″tē-ō-nĕ-krō′sĭs). Death of bone.

osteoneuralgia (ŏs″tē-ō-nū-ral′jĭ-ă). Pain of a bone.   [of bone.

osteonosus (ŏs-tē-on′ō-sus). Any disease

osteopath (os′tē-ō-păth). A practitioner of osteopathy, q.v.

osteopathic (ŏs″tē-ō-păth′ĭk). Concerning therapeutic bone manipulation.

osteopathology (os-tē-ō-path-ol′ō-jĭ). Any bone disease.

osteopathy (ŏs-tē-op′ăth-ĭ). 1. Any bone disease.

   2. "A school of medicine based upon the theory that the body is a vital mechanical organism whose structural and functional integrity are coördinate and that the perversion of either is disease, while its therapeutic procedure is chiefly manipulative correction, its name indicating the fact that the bony framework of the body largely determines the structural relation of its tissues." *Committee on Osteopathic Terminology*.

osteopecilia (ŏs″tē-ō-pē-sĭl′ĭ-ă). Disease marked by spontaneous fractures and spotted marble appearance of bones following abnormal skeletal calcification. SYN: *Albers-Schönberg disease*.

osteopedion (ŏs″tē-ō-pe′dĭ-ŏn). A calcified or hardened fetus. SYN: *lithopedion*.

osteoperiosteal (ŏs″tē-ō-per-ĭ-os′tē-ăl). Concerning bone and its periosteum, the protective membrane.

osteoperiostitis (ŏs″tē-ō-per-ĭ-ŏs-tī′tĭs). Combined inflammation of a bone and its protective membrane, the periosteum.

osteopetrosis (ŏs″tē-ō-pĕt-rō′sĭs). Excessive calcification of bones causing spontaneous fractures and marblelike appearance. SYN: *osteosclerosis fragilis generalisata.*

osteophage (ŏs′tē-ō-fāj). Large multinuclear cell which causes absorption of bone. SYN: *osteoclast, 2.*

osteophlebitis (ŏs″tē-ō-flē-bī′tĭs). Inflammation of veins of a bone.

osteophone (ŏs′tē-ō-fōn). Device used by the deaf for conducting sound through facial bones.

osteophyma (ŏs″tē-ō-fī′mă). A swelling or growth of bone.

osteophyte (ŏs′tē-ō-fīt). A bony excrescence or outgrowth, usually branched in shape.

osteoplastic (ŏs″tē-ō-plăs′tĭk). 1. Pert. to bone repair. 2. Concerning bone formation.

osteoplastica (ŏs″tē-ō-plăs′tĭ-kă). An inflammatory disease of the bone with fibrous degeneration and formation of cysts, the femur, humerus, and tibia esp. being affected. SYN: *osteitis fibrosa cystica.*

osteoplasty (ŏs″tē-ō-plăs′tĭ). Plastic repair of the bones.

osteopoikilosis (ŏs″tē-ō-poy-kĭ-lō′sĭs). Disease of bones marked by excessive calcification in spots, causing spontaneous fractures and spotted marble appearance. SYN: *Albers-Schönberg disease.*

osteoporosis (ŏs″tē-ō-por-ō′sĭs). Increased porosity of bone.

   o., parachitic. Osteoporosis with tendency to develop into rickets. Congenital.

osteoporotic (ŏs″tē-ō-pō-rot′ĭk). Concerning enlarged bone spaces.

osteopsathyrosis (ŏs″tē-op-sath″ĭ-rō′sĭs). Fragility or brittleness of·bones. Congenital condition of unknown etiology, in which the long bones seem normal in appearance and chemical composition, but are extremely brittle.

osteorrhagia (ŏs″tē-ō-rā′jĭ-ă). Hemorrhagic flow of blood from a bone.

osteorrhaphy (ŏs-tē-or′ăf-ĭ). Suture of bone or the wiring of bone fragments.

osteosarcoma (ŏs″tē-ō-sar-kō′mă). A malignant sarcoma of the bone. SYN: *myelosarcoma.*

osteosarcomatous (ŏs″tē-ō-sar-kō′măt-ŭs). Concerning or like an osteosarcoma.

osteosarcosis (ŏs″tē-ō-sar-kō′sĭs). Conversion of bone into a fleshy mass.

osteosclerosis (ŏs″tē-ō-sklē-rō′sĭs). Hardening of bone with increased heaviness.

   o. congenita. Defective development of cartilage at epiphyses of long bones resulting in dwarfism. SYN: *achondroplasia.*

   o. fragilis generalisata. Abnormal calcification of the bones, causing spontaneous fractures and spotted marble-like appearance in a roentgenogram. SYN: *Albers-Schönberg disease; marble bones; osteitis, condensing; osteopetrosis; osteopoikilosis.*

osteoscope (ŏs′tē-ō-skōp). Appliance used to test x-ray machines by observing

certain bones of the forearm which are considered as a standard.

osteoseptum (ŏs″tē-ō-sĕp′tŭm). The bony area of the nasal septum.

osteosis (ŏs″tē-ō′sĭs). Formation of bony tissue. SYN: *osteogenesis.*

   o. cutis. Diffuse thickening of skin and subcutaneous tissue. Rare.

osteospongioma (ŏs″tē-ō-spon-jĭ-ō′mă). A spongy neoplasm of bone. SYN: *osteoma spongiosum.*

osteosteatoma (ŏs″tē-ō-stē-ăt-ō′mă). A fatty tumor with bony elements.

osteostixis (ŏs″tē-ō-stiks′ĭs). Therapeutic puncture of a bone.

osteosuture (ŏs″tē-ō-sūt′chūr). Suture or wiring of bone fragments. SYN: *osteorrhaphy.*

osteosynovitis (ŏs″tē-ō-sin-ō-vī′tĭs). Inflammation of a synovial membrane and the surrounding bones.

osteosynthesis (ŏs″tē-ō-sĭn′the-sĭs). Surgical fastening of the ends of a fractured bone mechanically.

osteotabes (ŏs″tē-ō-tā′bēz). Atrophy of the bone in infants, beginning with wasting of the marrow and gradually the rest of the bone.

osteotelangiectasia (ŏs″tē-ō-tĕl-ăn″jĭ-ĕk-tā′zĭ-ă). 1. Dilatation of a bone's small blood vessels. 2. Sarcomatous tumor of the bone containing dilated blood vessels.

osteothrombosis (ŏs″tē-ō-thrŏm-bō′sĭs). Clot formation in the veins of a bone.

osteotome (ŏs′tē-ō-tōm). A chisel beveled on both sides for cutting through bones.

osteotomy (ŏs-tē-ot′ō-mĭ). The surgical section of a bone.

   o., cuneiform. The excision of a wedge of a bone.

   o., linear. Lengthwise division of a bone.

   o., MacEwen's. Supracondylar section of the femur for correction of knock-knee.

   o., subtrochanteric. Gant's operation, division of shaft of femur below lesser trochanter to correct ankylosis of hip joint.

   o., transtrochanteric. Section of the femur through the lesser trochanter for deformity about the hip joint.

osteotrite (ŏs′tē-ō-trīt). Instrument used to scrape away diseased bone.

osthexia (ŏs-thĕks′ĭ-ă). Excessive ossification, esp. in abnormal places.

ostial (os′tĭ-ăl). Concerning an orifice.

ostitis (ŏs-tī′tĭs). Inflammation of a bone. SYN: *osteitis, q.v.*

ostium (ŏs′tĭ-ŭm) (pl. *ostia*). Any small opening.

   o. abdominale. Fimbriated extremity of a fallopian tube.

   o. arteriosum. BNA. Arterial orifice, of ventricle of the heart into the aorta, or pulmonary artery.

   o. internum. Uterine end of a fallopian tube. SYN: *ostium uterinum tubae.*

   o. pharyngeum. Pharyngeal opening of the auditory tube.

o. tympanicum. Tympanic opening of the auditory tube.

o. uterinum tubae. BNA. Uterine opening of an oviduct.

o. vaginae. Ext. opening of the vagina.

ostraco-, ostrac-. Combining form meaning *hard shell.*

ostreotoxismus (ŏs″trē-ō-tŏks-ĭz′mŭs). Poisoning from eating diseased oysters.

Ostrow'ski manumo'bilizer. Apparatus to mobilize finger by stretching contractures and loosening adhesions.

otacoustic (ō″tă-koos′tĭk). 1. Aiding or concerning the hearing. 2. Device to aid hearing.

otalgia (ō-tăl′jĭ-ă). Pain of the ear.

otaphone (ō′tă-fōn). A device used to aid in hearing.

otectomy (ō-tĕk′tō-mĭ). Surgical excision of the contents of the tympanum.

othelcosis (ō-thĕl-kō′sĭs). Ulceration or suppuration of the ear.

othematoma (ō″them-ă-tō′mă). Effusion of blood between perichondrium and cartilage of pinna.

othemorrhea (ō-them-or-rē′ă). Bleeding from the ear.

othygroma (ō-thī-grō′mă). Edema of ear lobe.

otiatrics (ō-tĭ-ăt′rĭks). Treatment of ear diseases.

otic (ō′tĭk). Concerning the ear.

oticodinia (ō″tĭk-ō-dĭn′ĭ-ă). Vertigo due to ear disease.

otitic (ō-tĭt′ĭk). Concerning inflammation of the ear.

otitis (ō-tī′tĭs). Inflamed condition of the ear.

o., furuncular. Furuncle formation in ext. meatus.

o. labyrinthica. Inflammation of the labyrinth.

o. mastoidea. Inflamed condition of the mastoid spaces.

o. mycotica. Fungous inflammation.

o. parasitica. Inflammation caused by a parasitic fungus.

o. sclerotica. Inflammation of inner ear accompanied by hardening of the aural structures.

oto-, ot-. Combining form meaning *ear.*

otoantritis (ō″tō-ăn-trī′tĭs). Inflamed condition of mastoid antrum.

otobiosis (ō″tō-bī-ō′sĭs). Disease of the ear caused by presence of *Otobius.*

Otobius (ō-tō′bĭ-ŭs). Genus of ticks probably transmitting relapsing fever. Certain species bite the ear.

otoblennorrhea (ō″tō-blĕn-or-rē′ă). Mucous discharge from ear.

otocatarrh (ō″tō-kă-tar′). Catarrhal discharge of the ear.

otocerebritis (ō″tō-sĕr-ē-brī′tĭs). Cerebral inflammation resulting from disease of the middle ear.

otocleisis (ō-tō-klī′sĭs). Occlusion of ear.

otoconia, otoconite, otoconium (ō″tō-kō′-nĭ-ă, -tok′ō-nīt, -tō-kō′nĭ-ŭm). Concretion of calcium carbonate on the membranous labyrinth of the ear. SYN: *ear dust, otolith.*

otocrane (ō′tō-krān). The cavity in the petrous bone wherein lodges the internal ear.

otocyst (ō′tō-sĭst). Primordial chamber from which arises the membranous labyrinth. SYN: *auditory vesicle.*

otodynia (ō″tō-din′ĭ-ă). Pain in the ear. SYN: *otalgia.*

otoencephalitis (ō″tō-ĕn-sĕf-ăl-ī′tĭs). Inflammation of brain resulting from disease of the middle ear. SYN: *otocerebritis.*

otoganglion (ō″tō-găng′lĭ-on). Ganglion located below foramen ovale distributing to the tensor tympani and the tensor palati. SYN: *ganglion, otic.*

otography (ō-tog′ră-fĭ). Anatomical description of the ear.

otolith (ō′tō-lith). One of the calcareous deposits resting on sensory nerve fibers within the utricle and saccule; part of the static apparatus. SEE: *otoconia.*

otological (ō″tō-lŏj′ĭ-kl). Rel. to study of diseases of the ear.

otologist (ō-tŏl-ō-jĭst). One versed in diseases of the ear. SYN: *aurist.*

otology (ō-tol′ō-jĭ). The science of the ear, its function, and diseases.

otomassage (ō″tō-mă-săj′). Application of massage to tympanic membrane and auditory ossicles.

otomyasthenia (ō″tō-mī-ăs-thē′nĭ-ă). 1. Weakened condition of the ear muscles. 2. Defective hearing caused by paresis of the tensor tympani and stapedius muscles.

Otomyces (ō″tō-mī′sēz). Fungus infesting the ear.

O. hageni. Form with green conidia, affecting ext. canal.

O. purpureus. A dark red variety.

otomycosis (ō″tō-mī-kō′sĭs). Fungous infection of ext. auditory meatus of the ear. SYN: *otitis mycotica.*

otoncus (ō-tŏng′kŭs). An aural tumor.

otonecrectomy, otonecronectomy (ō″tō-nĕk-rĕk′tō-mĭ, -rō-nĕk′tō-mĭ). Excision of necrosed areas from the ear.

otoneuralgia (ō″tō-nū-răl′jĭ-ă). Pain in the ear. SYN: *otalgia.*

otoneurasthenia (ō″tō-nū-răs-thē′nĭ-ă). Neurasthenia caused by ear disease.

otoneurology (ō″tō-nū-rŏl′ō-jĭ). Study of ear conditions in conjunction with neural complications. SYN: *neurotology.*

otopathy (o-top′ăth-ĭ). Any diseased condition of the ear.

otopharyngeal (ō″tō-far-ĭn′jē-ăl). Concerning the ear and pharynx.

o. tube. Passage bet. tympanic cavity and the pharynx. SYN: *eustachian tube.*

otophone (ō′tō-fōn). Device for assisting deaf to hear.

otopiesis (ō″tō-pī-ē′sĭs). 1. Sinking in or depression of the membrana tympani. 2. Pressure on the labyrinth causing deafness.

otoplasty (ō′tō-plăs-tĭ). Plastic surgery of the ear to correct defects.

otopolypus (ō″tō-pol′ĭp-ŭs). Smooth growth occurring in the ear.

otopyorrhea (ō″tō-pī-ō-re′ă). Purulent ear discharge.

otopyosis (ō″tō-pī-ō′sĭs). Ear disease marked by discharge of pus.

otorhinolaryngology (ō″tō-rī-nō-lăr-ĭn-gŏl′ō-jĭ). The science of ear, nose, and larynx and their functions and diseases.

otorhinology (ō″tō-rī-nŏl′ō-jĭ). Branch of medicine dealing with ear and nose diseases.

otorrhagia (ō-tō-rā′jĭ-ă). Discharge of blood from ear.

otorrhea (ō-tō-rē′ă). Inflammation of ear with purulent discharge.

otosalpinx (ō″tō-săl′pĭnks). Passage connecting pharynx and tympanic cavity. SYN: *eustachian tube.*

otoscleronectomy (ō″tō-sklē-rō-něk′tō-mĭ). Surgical excision of sclerosed and ankylosed ear ossicles.

otosclerosis (ō″tō-sklē-rō′sĭs). Disease of the ear characterized by a patent eustachian tube, normal drum membrane, conversion into sponge of the bony capsule of the labyrinth and fixation of the stapes due to ankylosis in the oval window.

otoscope (ō′tō-skōp). Device for examination of the ear.

otosis (ō-tō′sĭs). Mishearing of spoken sounds.

otosteal (ō-tos′tē-ăl). Concerning the bones or ossicles of the ear.

ototomy (ō-tŏt′ō-mĭ). Incision into or dissection of the ear.

oturia (ō-tū′rĭ-ă). Delusion of urinous discharge from the ear due to metastasis.

O. U. Abbr. for L. *oculus uterque,* for each eye.

ouabain (wăh-băh′ĭn). A glucoside prepared from *Strophanthus gratus,* but more active.

DOSAGE: 1/120 gr. (0.0005 Gm.), intravenously.

Oudin current (oo-dan′). A high frequency oscillating current of higher voltage than the current used ordinarily, employed in therapeutic treatment.

O. resonator. A coil of wire with an adjustable number of turns, designed to be connected to a source of high frequency current, such as a spark gap and induction coil, for the purpose of applying a convective discharge of high voltage current to a patient.

oulitis (oo-lī′tĭs). Inflamed condition of the gums. SYN: *ulitis.*

oulorrhagia (oo-lō-rā′jĭ-ă). Hemorrhage from the gums. SYN: *ulorrhagia.*

ounce (ouns). A measure of weight.

In *apothecaries* or *troy* weight, 1/12 lb. [480 gr. (31.103 Gm.)]. Symb. ℥.

In *avoirdupois* measure, 1/16 lb. [437.5 gr. (28.349 Gm.)]. Abbr. oz.

o., fluid. For liquid medicines, 8 fluid drams [1/16 pint (29.6 cc.)].

out′patient. One receiving treatment at a hospital without being an inmate.

ova (ō′vă) (pl. of *ovum*). 1. Reproductive cells of the female. 2. Eggs. SEE: *ovary; ovum.*

oval (ō′văl). 1. Like or concerning an ovum, the reproductive cell of the female. 2. Shaped like an egg.

o. window. Oval-shaped aperture in the middle ear.

ovalbumin (ō-văl-bū′mĭn). Albumin in egg whites.

ovalocyte (o′văl-ō-sīt). Egg-shaped red blood corpuscle.

ovalocytosis (ō-văl″ō-sī-tō′sĭs). Oval red blood corpuscles in the blood.

ovaraden (ō-văr-ā′děn). A powdered extract from animal ovaries used as a sedative, nerve tonic, and in disorders of the female genitalia.

ovaralgia, ovarialgia (o-var-al′jĭ-ă, -ĭ-al′-jĭ-ă). Ovarian pain. SYN: *oarialgia.*

ovarian (ō-vā′rĭ-ăn). Concerning or resembling the ovary.

o. cyst. A sac containing fluid which develops in the ovary proper.

ovariectomy (ō-vā-rī-ěk′tō-mĭ). Excision of an ovary or a portion of it. SYN: *oöphorectomy.*

ovario-. Combining form meaning *ovary.*

ovariocele (ō-va′rĭ-ō-sēl). Ovarian tumor or hernia.

ovariocentesis (ō-vā-rĭ-ō-sěn-tē′sĭs). Puncture and drainage of an ovarian cyst.

ovariocyesis (ō-vā-rĭ-ō-sī-ē′sĭs). Pregnancy in the ovary, instead of in the uterus.

ovariodysneuria (ō-va″rĭ-ō-dĭs-nū′rĭ-ă). Neuralgia in an ovary.

ovariohysterectomy (ō-vā″rĭ-ō-hĭs-těr-ěk′-tō-mĭ). Excision of the ovaries and uterus. SYN: *oöphorohysterectomy.*

ovariorrhexis (ō-vā″rĭ-ō-rěks′ĭs). Rupture of an ovary.

ovariosalpingectomy (ō-vā″rĭ-ō-săl-pĭn-jěk′tō-mĭ). Removal of an ovary and oviduct. SYN: *oöphorosalpingectomy.*

ovariosteresis (ō-va″rĭ-ō-ster-ē′sĭs). Complete eradication of an ovary.

ovariostomy (ō-vā-rĭ-ŏs′tō-mĭ). Creation of an opening in an ovarian cyst for drainage.

ovariotomist (ō-va″rĭ-ot′ō-mĭst). A surgeon who performs operations on the ovary.

ovariotomy (ō-va″rĭ-ŏt′ō-mĭ). Incision into or removal of an ovary, or of an ovarian tumor.

ovariotubal (ō-va″rĭ-ō-tū′băl). Concerning the ovary and the oviducts.

ovariprival (ō-vā″rĭ-prī′văl). Resulting from loss of the ovaries.

ovaritis (ō-va-rī′tĭs). Inflamed condition of an ovary.

o., acute. Acute, severe inflammation of the ovary.

o., chronic. Inflammation of ovary over a long period of time.

ovarium (ō-va′rĭ-ŭm) (pl. *ovaria*). Ovary.

ovary (ō′va-rĭ). One of 2 glands in the female, producing the reproductive cell, the ovum, and 2 known hormones.

ovate (ō′văt). BACT: Having the outline of an egg.

overdetermination (ō″věr-dē-těr-mĭ-nā-shŭn). PSY: The idea that every symptom and dream may have several meanings, being determined by more than a single association.

overproduction (ō″vĕr-prō-dŭk′shŭn). Destruction of an organic element is followed by overproduction of the element during the reparative process, as excessive callus development after a bone fracture. SYN: *Weigert's law.*

overri′ding. The slipping of 1 end of a fractured bone past the other part.

ov′ertone. A harmonic.

   o., psychic. A dimly perceived associated impression about a mental image.

overwork (ō′vĕr-wŭrk). Excessive work causing exhaustion. SEE: *ergasthenia.*

ovestrin (o-vĕs′trĭn). Hormone from the ovary stimulating the gonads.

ovi-. Combining form meaning *egg.*

ovi albumen (ō′vĭ ăl-bū′mĭn). White of egg.

   o. vitellum. Egg yolk.

ovicapsule (ō″vĭ-kăp′sŭl). The sac enclosing the ovum; outer layer of a graafian follicle. SYN: *ovisac.*

oviduct (ō′vĭ-dŭkt). One of 2 muscular tubes on either side of the uterus, about 4 in. long, forming the path conveying the ovum from the ovary to the uterus.

oviferous (ō-vĭf′ĕr-ŭs). Containing or producing ova.

ovification (ō-vĭ-fĭ-kā′shŭn). The production of ova. SYN: *ovulation.*

oviform (ō′vĭ-form). 1. Having the shape of an egg. 2. Resembling an ovum.

ovigerm (ō′vĭ-jĕrm). The cell which produces or develops into an ovum.

ovigerous (ō-vĭj′ĕr-ŭs). Producing or carrying ova. SYN: *oviferous.*

ovination (ō-vĭn-ā′shŭn). Inoculation with sheep pox virus.

Ovipara (ō-vĭp′ăr-ă). Animals which deposit the ova outside of their bodies. Opp. of *Vivipara.*

oviparous (ō-vĭp′ăr-ŭs). Producing eggs hatched outside the body.

ovisac (ō′vĭ-săk). Outer layer of graafian follicle. SYN: *ovicapsule.*

ovi vitellus (ō′vĭ vĭ-tĕl′ŭs). Egg yolk; pharmaceutical term when used in preparation of emulsions.

ovo-. Combining form meaning *egg.*

ovoferrin (ō″vō-fĕr′rĭn). Commercial name for an albuminate of iron used in anemia.

ovogenesis (ō″vō-jĕn′ĕ-sĭs). Production of ova. SYN: *oögenesis.*

ovoglobulin (ō″vō-glŏb′ŭ-lĭn). The globulin found in egg white. SEE: *albumen, protein.*

ovoid (ō′voyd). Egg shaped. SYN: *oviform.*

   o., fetal. The egg-shaped mass into which the uterine contractions mold the fetus.

ovolemma (ō″vō-lĕm′ă). Membrane enclosing the vitellus of the ovum.

ovomucoid (ō″vō-mŭ′koyd). A glycoprotein principle from egg white.

ovoventer (ō″vō-vĕn′tĕr). The impregnated ovum's centrosome, *q.v.*

ovovitellin (ō″vō-vĭ-tĕl′lĭn). Protein found in an egg yolk.

ovoviviparous (ō″vō-vi-vĭp′ă-rŭs). Reproducing by hatching the eggs within the body.

ovula (ō′vū-lă) (sing. *ovulum*). Little eggs.

   o., Nabothi. Distended mucous follicles in tissues of the cervix uteri.

ovular (ō′vū-lăr). Concerning an ovule or ovum.

ovulation (ō-vū-lā′shŭn). The lunar monthly ripening and rupture of the mature graafian follicle and the discharge of the ovum from the cortex of the ovary, normally occurring 13 times a year.

ovulatory (ō′vū-lă-tō-rĭ). Concerning ovulation.

ovule (ō′vŭl). 1. The unimpregnated ovum before leaving graafian follicle. 2. Any egglike structure.

   o., Naboth's. Distended mucous follicles in the cervix uteri. SYN: *ovula Nabothi.*

   o., primitive. A rudimentary ovum inside the ovary.

ovulin (ō′vū-lĭn). An internal secretion of the ovary, supposed to be 1 of the elements in the hormone oöphorin.

ovulum (ō′vū-lŭm). The ovum contained within the graafian follicle.

ovum (o′vŭm) (pl. *ova*). 1. The fully developed globular cell, about 1/125 of an inch in diameter, which is capable, upon fertilization, of developing into an organism similar to the parent; female sexual cell or egg. 2. An egg.

   o., alecithal. One in which there is little or no food yolk.

   o., apoplectic. One having an extravasation of blood.

   o., blighted. One with arrested development after impregnation.

   o., centrolecithal. One having a large central food yolk.

   o., holoblastic. One having a largely formative yolk.

   o., meroblastic. One having a large yolk.

   o., permanent. One ready for fertilization.

   o., primitive. Cell from which ovule arises.

oxacid (ŏk′să-sĭd). An acid of which oxygen is a constituent.

oxal-, oxalo-. CHEM: Combining forms indicating derivation from *oxalic acid.*

oxalate (ŏk′să-lāt). A salt of oxalic acid. About 5-20 mg. of the oxalates are excreted in urine per day.

oxalemia (ŏk″să-lē′mĭ-ă). An abnormal amount of oxalates in the blood.

oxalic acid (ŏk′săl′ĭk). A white crystalline powder often used about the home as a stain remover or bleach, resembling epsom salts in appearance.

   o. a. diathesis. Chronic state of oxalemia.

oxalism (ŏk′săl-ĭzm). Poisoning from oxalic acid or an oxalate.

oxaluria (ok-sa-lū′rĭ-ă). The abnormal excretion of oxalates in the urine, esp. calcium oxalate.

oxalylurea (ŏk″să-lĭl-ū-rē′ă). An oxidation product of uric acid.

oxidase (ŏk'sĭ-dās). 1. A ferment whose action causes the oxidation process. 2. The inherent substance of the living cell nucleus possessing the power of freeing active oxygen.

oxidation (ŏk″sĭ-dā'shŭn). The process by which a substance combines with oxygen, generally involving a change from a lower to a high positive valence. In the human body the rate of oxidation depends upon cell activity, not the intake of oxygen or food. SEE: *carbonemia*.

oxide (ŏk'sĭd). Any chemical compound in which oxygen is the negative radical.

oxidize (ŏk'sĭ-dīz). 1. To combine with oxygen. 2. To increase the ratio of the negative to the positive radical within a chemical compound, or to form a compound with the principle in question being the positive radical by combining with it any substance that will become the negative radical. SYN: *oxygenize, q.v.*

oxidosis (ŏk″sĭ-dō'sĭs). Decrease in normal alkaline content of blood. SYN: *acidosis*.

oxonemia (ŏk″sō-nē'mĭ-ă). Excess of acetone bodies found in the blood. SYN: *acetonemia*.

oxonuria (ŏk″sō-nū'rĭ-ă). Abnormal number of acetone bodies in urine. SYN: *acetonuria*.

oxos (ŏk'sŏs). Vinegar.

oxy-. Combining form meaning *sharp, keen, acute, acid, pungent.*

oxyacoia, oxyakoia (ŏk″sĭ-ă-koy'ă). Abnormal sensitiveness to noises, as in facial paralysis, esp. if the stapedius muscle is involved.

oxyacusis (ŏk″sĭ-ă-kū'sĭs). Abnormally acute hearing. SYN: *hyperacusis*.

oxyblepsia (ŏk″sĭ-blĕp'sĭ-ă). Extraordinary acuteness of vision.

oxyburserasin (ŏk″sĭ-bŭr-sĕr-ā'zĭn). An extract of resin of myrrh used to aid in healing internal lesions.

oxybutyria (ŏk″sĭ-bū-tĭr'ĭ-ă). Oxybutyric acid in the blood or in the urine.

oxycephalia (ŏk″sĭ-sĕf-ā'lĭ-ă). State of having a high and pointed skull.

oxycephalous (ŏk-sĭ-sĕf'ă-lŭs). Denoting a head that is pointed and conelike.

oxychinolin (ŏk″sĭ-kĭn'ō-lĭn). A quinoline derivative used in disinfecting wounds.

oxychloride (ŏk″sĭ-klō'rĭd). A compound of oxygen and a metal chloride.

oxychlorine (ŏk″sĭ-klō'rēn). Commercial dressing for wounds.

oxychromatic (ŏk″sĭ-krō-măt'ĭk). Staining readily with acid dyes.

oxychromatin (ŏk″sĭ-krō'mă-tĭn). That part of chromatin which stains readily with acid dyes.

oxycinesia (ŏks″ĭ-sĭn-ē'zĭ-ă). Pain experienced on moving.

oxydase (ŏk'sĭ-dās). A ferment causing oxidation. SYN: *oxidase*.

oxydasis (ŏk-sĭ-dā'sĭs). The process of oxidation produced by an oxydase.

oxydesis (ŏk-sĭ-dē'sĭs). Acid fixing capacity, esp. as evidenced in the blood by buffer salts.*

oxydetik (ŏk-sĭ-dē'tĭk). Concerning the acid fixation capacity.

oxyecoia (ŏk″sĭ-ē-koy'ă). Abnormal sensitivity to noises. SYN: *oxyacoia, q.v.*

oxyesthesia (ŏk″sĭ-ĕs-thē'zĭ-ă). Abnormal acuteness of sensation. SYN: *hyperesthesia*.

oxygen (ŏk'sĭ-jĕn). SYMB: O. 1. A nonmetallic element occurring free in the atmosphere as a colorless, odorless, tasteless gas; at. wt., 16. 2. Chlorine used for bleaching purposes.

   o. therapy. Treatment by inhalation of oxygen, as in pneumonia.

oxygenase (ŏk'sĭ-jĕn-ās). A substance in the tissues which takes up oxygen to form an organic peroxide.*

oxygenation (ŏk″sĭ-jĕn-ā'shŭn). Impregnation or combination with oxygen, as the aeration of the blood in the lungs.

oxygenic (ŏk″sĭ-jĕn'ĭk). Concerning, resembling, containing, or consisting of oxygen.

oxygenium (ŏk″sĭ-jĕ'nĭ-ŭm). Oxygen.

oxygenize (ŏk'sĭ-jĕn-īz). To impart oxygen to a substance either by causing chemical union of the substances or by causing absorption or solution of the oxygen by the substance. SYN: *oxidize*.

oxygeusia (ŏk″sĭ-gū'sĭ-ă). Abnormally keen sense of taste.

oxyhemoglobin (ŏk″sĭ-hem-ō-glō'bĭn). The combined form of hemoglobin and oxygen.

   Hemoglobin with oxygen is found in arterial blood and is the oxygen carrier to the body tissues. SYN: *hematoglobulin.* SEE: *respiration.*

oxyhemoglobinometer (ŏk″sĭ-hem-ō-glō″bĭn-ŏm'ĕt-ĕr). Apparatus for measurement of oxygen in the blood.

oxyhydrocephalus (ŏk″sĭ-hī-drō-sĕf'ăl-ŭs). Pointed head shape type of hydrocephalus.

oxyiodide (ŏk″sĭ-ī'ō-dīd). Compound of iodine and oxygen with an element or radical.

oxylalia (ŏk″sĭ-lā'lĭ-ă). Abnormal rapidity of speech.

oxyntic (ŏk-sĭn'tĭk). Producing or secreting acid. SEE: *cell.*

   o. gland. Gland of tubular form found in the body and fundus of the stomach secreting acid of gastric juice.

oxyopia (ŏk″sĭ-ō'pĭ-ă). Unusual acuteness of vision.

oxyopter (ŏk″sĭ-op'tĕr). A unit of visual acuity, being the reciprocal of the visual angle, in degrees.

oxyosis (ŏk″sĭ-ō'sĭs). Decrease in normal alkalinity of the blood. SYN: *acidosis, q.v.*

oxyosmia (ŏk″sĭ-oz'mĭ-ă). Unusual acuity of sense of smell. SYN: *oxyosphresia.*

oxyosphresia (ŏk″sĭ-ŏs-frē'zĭ-ă). Abnormal acuity of the sense of smell.

oxyparaplastin (ŏk″sĭ-păr-ă-plăs'tĭn). Part of paraplastin staining readily with acid dyes.

oxypathia, oxypathy (ŏk″sĭ-păth'ĭ-ă, -sĭp'-ăth-ĭ). 1. Unusual acuity of sensation. 2. An acute condition. 3. Condition of inability to eliminate unoxidizable acids which combine with fixed alkalies of the tissues and harm the organism. SEE: *arthritism, lithemia.*

oxyperitoneum (ŏk″sĭ-pĕr-ĭ-tō-nē′ŭm). Introduction of oxygen into the peritoneal cavity.

oxyphil(e (ok′sĭ-fĭl, -fīl). 1. Staining readily with acid dyes. 2. A cell which stains readily with acid dyes.

oxyphilous (ŏk-sĭf′ĭl-ŭs). Having an affinity for acid dyes. SYN: *oxyphil, 1.*

oxyphonia (ok″sĭ-fō′nĭ-ă). An abnormally sharp or shrill voice.

oxyplasm (ŏk′sĭ-plăzm). The part of the cytoplasm staining readily with acid dyes.

oxyproline (ŏk″sĭ-prō′lēn). An amino acid, a decomposition product of proteins.

oxypurine (ŏk″sĭ-pu′rēn). An oxidation product of purine.

oxyrhine (ŏk′sĭ-rīn). 1. Having a sharp pointed nose. 2. Possessing an acute sense of smell.

oxyrygmia (ŏk″sĭ-rĭg′mĭ-ă). Belching up of acid. SEE: *eructation.*

oxysalt (ŏk′sĭ-sawlt). A salt of an acid of which oxygen is a component.

oxysepsin (ŏk″sĭ-sep′sĭn). An oxidized toxin prepared from cultures of bacilli of tuberculosis in advanced stages.

oxysepsis (ŏk″sĭ-sĕp′sĭs). 1. Decay with development of acidity. 2. Putrefaction developing soon after death.

oxysparteine (ok″sĭ-spär′te-ēn). White crystalline oxidation product of sparteine, used as a cardiac stimulant.

oxytocia (ŏk″sĭ-tō′shĭ-ă). Unusual rapidity of childbirth.

oxytocic (ŏk″sĭ-tō′sĭk). 1. Agent which stimulates uterine contractions. 2. Accelerating childbirth.

oxytocin (ŏk″sĭ-tō′sĭn). Proprietary name for 1 of the 2 hormones from the post. pituitary lobe, which stimulates uterine contractions. SYN: *pitocin.* SEE: *vasopressin.*

oxytoxin (ŏk″sĭ-tŏk′sĭn). An oxidation product of a toxin.

oxytropism (ŏk-sĭt′rō-pĭzm). The tendency of living cells to be attracted by or respond to the stimulus of oxygen.

oxytuberculin (ŏk″sĭ-tū-bĕr′kŭ-lĭn). An oxidized tuberculin.

oxyuriasis (ŏk″sĭ-ū-rī′ās-ĭs). Infestation with pinworms of genus Oxyuris.

oxyuricide (ŏk″sĭ-ū′rĭ-sīd). Destructive to, or an agent that destroys pinworms.

oxyurid (ŏk″sĭ-u′rid). Pinworm.

oxyurifuge (ŏk″sĭ-ū′rĭ-fūj). An agent killing pinworms.

Oxyuris (ŏk″sĭ-ū′rĭs). Genus of nematode worms, the pinworms.

  O. vermicularis. Common pinworm infesting the intestines and causing intense nocturnal itching of the anus.

oxyvaselin (ŏk″sĭ-vas′ē-lēn). Commercial ointment base containing oxygen. SYN: *vasogen.*

Oz., oz. Abbr. for *ounce.*

ozena (ō-zē′nă). Disease of the nose characterized by atrophy of the turbinates and mucous membrane accompanied by considerable crusting and discharge and a very offensive odor.

ozocerite (ō″zō-sē′rīt). Mineral wax used as an ointment base. SEE: *ceresin.*

ozochrotia (ō″zō-krō′shĭ-ă). Strong odor given off by the skin. SYN: *bromidrosis.*

ozokerite (ō″zō-kē′rīt). Mineral wax which is employed as an ointment base. SYN: *ozocerite.*

ozonator (ō′zō-nă-tor). Device for generating ozone.

ozone (ō′zōn). A form of oxygen in which 3 atoms of the element combine to form the molecule, O_3.

ozon′ic e′ther. A mixture of hydrogen peroxide, ether, and alcohol, used in a test for blood in the urine, and in treating diabetes and whooping cough.

ozonization (ō-zō-nĭ-zā′shŭn). The act of converting to, or impregnating with ozone.

ozonize (ō′zō-nīz). 1. To convert oxygen to ozone, i. e., 3 atoms to the molecule of free oxygen. 2. To impregnate the air of a substance with ozone.

ozonometer (ō″zō-nom′ĕt-ĕr). An apparatus for estimating the quantity of ozone in the atmosphere.

ozonophore (ō-zō′nō-fōr). 1. A red blood corpuscle. 2. A protoplasmic granule of a cell.

ozonoscope (ō-zō′nō-skōp). A device for showing the presence or amount of ozone.

ozostomia (ō″zō-stō′mĭ-ă). Fetid breath.

P

P. Symb. of *phosphorus.*

P., p. Abbr. for *para, pupil, pulse, position.*

P₂. Abbr. for *pulmonic second sound.*

pabular (păb'ū-lar). Pert. to nourishment.

pabulin (păb'ū-lĭn). Albuminous and fatty product found in the blood following digestion.

pabulum (păb'ū-lŭm). Food; nourishment.

pacchionian bodies (păk-ē-ō'nĭ-ăn). Enlarged villi, small pedunculated or rounded growths of fibrous tissue along longitudinal fissure of the cerebrum growing on arachnoid membrane.

    p. corpuscle. Small granulation on surface of the dura mater along longitudinal fissure.

    p. depressions. Small pits produced on inner surface of skull by protuberance of pacchionian bodies.

    p. fossae. Depressions upon inner surface of the skull in which are lodged the pacchionian bodies. SYN: *pacchionian depressions.*

    p. glands. SEE: *pacchionian bodies.*

pacemaker (pās'māk-ĕr). The sinuauricular node, so named because cardiac rhythm commences here, taking place near the spot where the large veins empty into the auricle.

pachemia (păk-ē'mĭ-ă). Abnormal thickening of the blood. SYN: *pachyemia.*

pachismus (păk-ĭz'mŭs). Condensation or thickening of an organ or part.

pachometer (păk-ŏm'ĕt-ĕr). Device for determining a body's thickness. SYN: *pachymeter.*

pachy-, pach-. Combining form meaning *thick, large, heavy, massive.*

pachyacria, pachyakria (păk-ĭ-ăk'rĭ-ă). 1. Hypertrophy of soft portions of the extremities. 2. Chronic disease due to overfunction of hypophysis, in which there is enlargement of the face and extremities. SYN: *acromegaly.*

pachyblepharon (păk''ĭ-blĕf'ăr-ŏn). A thickening of border of eyelid.

pachycephalic (păk''ĭ-sĕf-al'ĭk). Possessing a thick skull. SYN: *pachycephalous.*

pachycephalous (păk''ĭ-sĕf'ăl-ŭs). Thick skulled. SYN: *pachycephalic.*

pachycephaly (păk''ĭ-sĕf'ăl-ĭ). Unusual thickness of the skull.

pachychilia (păk''ĭ-kĭ'lĭ-ă). Unusual thickness or swelling of the lips.

pachycholia (păk''ĭ-kō'lĭ-ă). Thickening or inspissation of the bile.

pachychromatic (păk''ĭ-krō-măt'ĭk). Possessing a coarse chromatin network.

pachycolpismus (păk-ĭ-kŏl-pĭz'mŭs). Chronic inflammation of vagina with thickened vaginal walls. SYN: *pachyvaginitis.*

pachydactylia, pachydactyly (păk''ĭ-dăk-til'ĭ-ă, -dak'tĭ-lĭ). Condition marked by unusually large fingers and toes.

pachyderma (păk-ĭ-der'mă). Unusual thickness of the skin.

pachydermatocele (păk''ĭ-dĕr-măt'ō-sēl). A pendulous state of the skin with thickening. SYN: *dermatolysis.*

pachydermatosis (păk''ĭ-dĕr-măt-ō'sĭs). Chronic hypertrophy of the skin. SYN: *pachydermia.*

pachydermatous (păk-ĭ-der'mă-tŭs). Possessing a thick skin.

pachydermia (păk-ĭ-der'mĭ-ă). Progressive hypertrophy of skin and subcutaneous tissues, usually associated with lymphangitis and edema.

    p. laryngis. Irregular thickening and hypertrophy of mucous membrane in the larynx seen in chronic laryngitis.

    p. vesica. Condition in which there is a thickened mucous membrane in the urinary bladder.

pachyemia (păk-ĭ-ē'mĭ-ă). Thickness or coagulation of the blood.

pachyglossia (păk''ĭ-glos'sĭ-ă). Unusual thickness of the tongue.

pachygnathous (păk-ĭg'năth-ŭs). Having a thick or large jaw.

pachygyria (păk-ĭ-jĭ'rĭ-ă). Flat, broad formation of the cerebral convolutions.

pachyhematous (păk-ĭ-hĕm'ăt-ŭs). Having thickened blood.

pachyhemia (păk-ĭ-hē'mĭ-ă). A thickened state of the blood.

pachyleptomeningitis (păk''ĭ-lĕp-tō-mĕn-ĭn-jĭ'tĭs). Inflammation of pia and dura of the brain and spinal cord.

pachylosis (păk-ĭ-lō'sĭs). A rough, dry, thickened, chronic condition of skin. SYN: *xerosis.*

pachymeningitis (păk-ĭ-mĕn-ĭn-jĭ'tĭs). Inflamed condition of the dura mater.

    p. externa. Inflammation of outer layer of dura mater.

    p., hemorrhagic. Circumscribed effusion of blood on inner surface of dura with inflammation.

    p. interna. Inflammation of inner layer of dura mater.

pachymeninx (păk-ĭ-mē'nĭnks). Membrane known as the dura mater.

pachymeter (păk-ĭm'ĕt-ĕr). Instrument for measuring thickness. SYN: *pachometer.*

pachynsis (păk-ĭn'sĭs). Thickening of a substance or part, usually abnormal.

pachyntic (păk-ĭn'tĭk). Thickening, abnormally thickened.

pachyonychia (păk''ĭ-ō-nĭk'ĭ-ă). Thickening of finger or toenails.

pachyostosis (păk''ĭ-ŏs-tō'sĭs). Thickening of the bones.

pachyotia (păk-ĭ-ō'shĭ-ă) Abnormal thickness of the ears.

pachypelviperitonitis (păk″ĭ-pĕl″vĭ-pĕr-ĭt-ō-nī'tĭs). Inflammation of the pelvic and peritoneal membranes with hypertrophy and thickening of their surfaces.

pachyperitonitis (păk-ĭ-pĕr-ĭt-ō-nī'tĭs). Inflammation of the peritoneum with thickening of the membrane.

pachypleuritis (păk-ĭ-plū-rī'tĭs). Inflamed condition of the pleura with thickening of the membrane.

pachypodous (pak-ĭp'ō-dŭs). Having massive feet.

pachysalpingitis (păk-ĭ-săl-pĭn-jī'tĭs). Chronic inflammation of an oviduct with thickening of the muscular coat.

pachysalpingoövaritis (păk″ĭ-săl-pĭn″gō-ō-văr-ī'tĭs). Chronic inflamed condition of an ovary and oviduct with thickening of the membranes.

pachysomia (păk-ĭ-sō'mĭ-ă). Pathological thickening of the soft parts of the body, as in acromegaly.

pachyvaginalitis (păk″ĭ-văj-ĭn-ăl-ī'tĭs). Inflamed condition of the tunica vaginalis with thickening of the membrane.

pachyvaginitis (păk″ĭ-văj-ĭn-ī'tĭs). Chronic inflammation of the vagina with thickening of the membranes. SYN: *pachycolpismus.*

pacinian corpuscles (pă-sĭn'ĭ-ăn). Oval bodies which are end organs of sensory nerve fibers of the skin.

p. fluid. Solution used in making a count of erythrocytes.

pacinitis (pă-sĭn-ī'tĭs). Inflammation of the end organs of the skin, the pacinian corpuscles.

pack (păk). 1. A dry or moist, hot or cold blanket or sheet wrapped around a patient. 2. To fill up a cavity.

p., cold wet sheet. This pack is a physiologic sedative and hypnotic employed for relief of restlessness, insomnia, and used extensively in psychiatric conditions. Effects are similar to those of any cold application except they are more intense, as greater area is covered by the pack.

p., dry. Procedure used in combination with hot bath. When patient leaves hot bath he is placed in dry, warm sheet and wrapped in several warm blankets.

p., full. SEE: *pack, wet sheet.*

p., half. Wet sheet pack but in this type the moist fabric and dry blanket extend from the axilla to below the knees.

p., hot bath. SEE: *pack, dry.*

p., hot blanket. The envelopment of a patient in moist blanket wrung from very hot water (150° to 160° F.). Given to relax contracted muscles, relieve convulsions, or induce profuse perspiration.

p., ice. If icebag is not available, a local cold application may be made by folding a soft towel so it will fit the area and filling it with crushed ice.

p., neutral wet sheet. SEE: *pack, wet sheet.*

p., one sheet. Same as wet sheet pack except only 1 large sheet, 84 x 96 in., is used.

p., partial. SEE: *half and three-quarter packs.*

p., three-quarter. Pack using same temperatures as wet sheet pack but the body is enveloped from below upward as far as the armpits.

p., wet sheet. The envelopment of patient in 1, 2, or 3 linen or soft cotton sheets that have been wrung out of water which is hot, cold, or lukewarm, depending on the purpose. These are held against the body by large woolen blankets.
Temperature of the water used for the sheets varies.

packer (păk'ĕr). Device for packing a cavity, as the uterus or rectum, with gauze, etc.

packing (păk'ĭng). 1. The process of filling a cavity or wound with gauze sponges, etc. 2. Material used to fill a cavity or wound.

pad (păd). Soft cushion or bag to relieve or give pressure, support an organ or part, etc.
Usually cotton, oakum, jute, or wood wool. Surgical cotton is not suitable for open wounds or broken surfaces. Oakum or marine lint is too irritating to place in direct contact with skin.

p., abdominal. Pad for absorbing fluids from surgical wounds, etc., of abdomen. Stock sizes 6 x 7 and 8 x 9 in.

p., dinner. Pad placed on stomach prior to application of a plaster cast.
Pad is then removed, leaving space for abdominal distention after meals.

p., kidney. Air or water pad fixed on abdominal belt for compression over a movable kidney.

p.'s, knuckle. Nodules on dorsal sides of the fingers.

p., Malgaigne's. Mass of fat in knee joint on either side of the patella's upper end.

p., Mikulicz's. One of folded gauze used in surgery.

p., sucking. Mass of fat on inner cheek assumed to aid in sucking.

p., surgical. Soft rubber pad with apron and inflatable rim for drainage of escaping fluids, used in operations and obstetrics.

Pagenstecher's ointment (păhg'ĕn-stĕk-ĕr). Ophthalmic ointment composed of a base of yellow oxide of mercury.

P.'s thread. Suture thread made of linen dipped in celluloid.

Paget's disease (păj'ĕt). 1. Chronic inflammation of bones with thickening and distortion. SYN: *osteitis deformans.*
2. A cancerous dermatosis of nipple area in women, though extramammary cases have been reported.

pain (pān). 1. A protective mechanism of the body; an unpleasant reaction to massive stimulation of the sensory nerve, calling attention to derangement of function, disease, or injury of a part. 2. In the plural refers to contractions of uterus in childbirth.

p., abdominal. Increased with respiration; experienced in broken ribs, intercostal neuralgia, wounds, herpes zoster, pleurisy, pleurodynia, myalgia, periostitis, acute peritonitis, colic; hepatic, gastric, or renal ulcer; gallbladder disorders; carcinoma in late stages, and gummata of this region.

p., absence of. In disorders in which pain should be expected may indicate pressure on the brain. The sudden abatement of pain, when other symptoms continue to be bad, is not a good sign.

p., after-. That following labor, caused by contraction and retraction of uterine muscles during involution.

p., angina pectoris. Paroxysmal, severe pain radiating from the heart to shoulder, thence down the arm, or rarely from the heart to the abdomen. Lasts from a few seconds to several minutes.

p., appendicitis. If acute, abdominal pain, usually severe, generally throughout the abdomen, followed by localization of pain in right lower quadrant of abdomen with tenderness over right rectus muscle with rigidity.

p., bearing-down. Straining and tenesmus with uterine contractions.

p., boring. Pain of a severe, piercing type.

p., cardiac. SEE: *epigastric pain.*

p., cardialgic. SEE: *epigastric pain.*

p., causalgic. A spontaneous pain, esp. burning in character, when associated with anesthesia, or hyperesthesia in a given nerve. SEE: *causalgia.*

p., cephalgic. Head pain, *q.v.*

p., continuous. May indicate persistent obstruction; also a tendency to suppuration.

p., cramplike. Muscular spasm such as epigastric pain. Significance depends upon location of pain.

p., dull. Continuous mild throbbing which attends inflammation of mucous membranes.

p., ear. May indicate inflammation of the ext. auditory canal, except in young children. It also may indicate a furuncle in the meatus, or middle ear disease. SYN: *otodynia.*

p., epigastric. Severe pain occurring in paroxysms in gastric disorders.

p., false. One mistaken for a true labor pain.

p., fixed. Indicates derangement at some special point; the sharper the pain, the deeper seated the trouble.

p., fulgurant. Sudden shooting pain, esp. experienced in locomotor ataxia.

p., gallbladder. In upper right abdominal quadrant, dull pain just below the last rib in infection, or sharp pain in same area radiating to the back and up under right shoulder, esp. if calculi are present. SEE: *epigastric pain.*

p., gastralgic. Severe pain occurring in paroxysms in gastric disorders.

p., girdle. One resembling sensation of a constricting cord around the waist, often associated with syphilis.

p., gnawing. May denote disease of the spinal column, gastric disturbance, and aneurysms.

p., growing. That felt in the joints of growing children.

p., head. It may be due to mental exertion or sympathetic irritation, or intestinal or liver derangements unless it results from catarrh.

p., hunger. Pain due to need for food.

p., ideogenous. Self-induced pain of mental origin.

p., inflammatory. Pain in presence of inflammation which is increased by pressure.

p., lancinating. A short, sharp, cutting pain.

p., lingual. Pain in tongue which may be due to local lesions, glossitis, fissures, pernicious anemia, and malignancies.

p., lung. SEE: *pulmonary pain.*

p., mental. One of psychic origin; mental distress or grief. May, if persistent, cause true physical pathological states.

p., migraine. Headache accompanied by nausea and vomiting. It may arise from a number of causes, esp. those of neurological origin. SEE: *migraine, sick headache.*

p., mind. Pain occurring subsequent to a mental operation or of mental origin. SYN: *psychalgia.*

p., neuralgic. Pain, frequently paroxysmal, occurring along the branches of a nerve. Temporarily relieved by heat or pressure. May be of rheumatic origin, a tic, or inflammation of nerves or nerve trauma.

p., noise. Pain of ear caused by a noise. SEE: *odynacusis.*

p., osteocopic. Pain in bones. SEE: *osteocope.*

p., paresthesic. Stinging or tingling sensation manifested in central and peripheral nerve lesions. SEE: *paresthesia.*

p., pseudomyelic. False sensation of movement in a paralyzed limb, or 1 of no movement in a moving limb. Not a true pain. SEE: *pseudomyelia paresthetica.*

p., pulmonary. Sharp pain in the region of the lungs. Indicates that the pleura are involved. There is no pain when lung substance is involved.

p., referred; p., reflex. Pain seeming to arise in an area or point other than at its origin, as pain from appendicitis which often seems to occur in areas other than that of the appendix. SYN: *synalgia.*

p., regional. Pain in a specific area and its significance.

p., remittent. Pain which subsides temporarily. Characteristic of neuralgia and colic.

p., shifting. Present in rheumatism, hysteria, and locomotor ataxia.

p., shooting. SEE: *fulgurant pain.*

p., soul. SEE: *mind pain.*

p., sympathetic. SEE: *referred pain.*

p., tenesmic. Pain accompanying urination or defecation. SEE: *tenesmus.*

p., thermalgesic. Pain caused by heat. SEE: *thermalgesia.*

p., thoracic. A sharp pain over the sternum, often running down the arm to the elbow.

p., ulcer (*gastric or duodenal*): Sharp, lancinating, or dull and gnawing in precordium, radiating to left of spine posteriorly, on a level with the 10th rib. Burning sensation may be felt in epigastrium. Pain may occur from 10 to 15 minutes after eating, as soon as an excess of hydrochloric acid is secreted. If ulcer is near cardia, pain ensues soon after eating; if near pylorus, pain may not ensue for 2 or 3 hours after eating.

p., urethral. Pain at end of the urethra, without soreness, which may denote presence of gravel or stone in the urinary bladder.

painters' colic (pān'tĕrs). Colic accompanying lead* poisoning.

palatable (păl'ăt-ă-bl). Pleasing to the palate or taste, as food.

palatal (păl'ăt-ăl). Pert. to the roof of the mouth, the palate.

p., paralysis of. May occur in diphtheria, or complications of it, and in severe septic sore throat and quinsy.

p. reflex. Swallowing induced by stimulation of soft palate.

palate (păl'ăt). 1. The horizontal structure separating the mouth and the nasal cavity; the roof of the mouth. 2. Mental taste.

p., artificial. Hard substance molded to fill a cleft in the palate.

p. bones. Bones forming post. part of hard palate and lateral nasal wall bet. the int. pterygoid plate of sphenoid bone and sup. maxilla.

p., cleft. One with congenital opening bet. 2 parts of palate.

p., falling. Abnormally long uvula.

p., hard. Ant. part supported by the maxillary and palatine bones.

p., soft. Post. muscular, membranous fold partly separating the mouth and pharynx. SYN: *velum.*

palatine (păl'ă-tīn). 1. Concerning the palate. 2. The palate bones, *q.v.*

p. arches. Archlike folds or double pillars of mucous membrane formed by descent of the soft palate as it descends toward the pharynx.

p. artery. One of 2 arteries in the face.

p. bone. Palate bones, *q.v.*

palatitis (păl-ăt-ī'tĭs). Inflamed condition of the palate.

palatoglossus (păl"ăt-ō-glŏs'ŭs). Muscle forming undersurface of soft palate, which lifts rear of tongue and narrows the fauces.

palatognathous (păl-ăt-og'nă-thŭs). Having a congenital fissure in the palate.

palatopharyngeus (păl"ăt-ō-făr"ĭn-jē'ŭs).

Muscle arising from soft palate which narrows the fauces.

palatoplasty (păl'ăt-ō-plăs"tĭ). Plastic surgery of the palate, usually to correct a cleft. SYN: *staphylorrhaphy, uranoplasty.*

palatoplegia (păl"ăt-ō-plē'jĭ-ă). Paralysis of muscles of the soft palate. SEE: *palate.*

palatorrhaphy (păl-ă-tor'ă-fĭ). Operation for uniting of a cleft palate. SYN: *staphylorrhaphy.*

palatoschisis (păl-ă-tŏs'kĭs-ĭs). Palate with cleft in it. SYN: *uranoschisis.*

palatostaphylinus (păl"ăt-ō-stă-fĭl-ĭ'nŭs). Group of muscular fibers going from post. nasal spine of palate bone to uvula, helping to raise it.

paleëncephalon, paleoencephalon (pā"lē-ĕn-sĕf'ă-lŏn, -ō-ĕn-sef'ă-lŏn). Phylogenetically older portion of the brain which includes all of it except the cerebral cortex and its allied structures.

paleogenesis (pā"lē-ō-jĕn'ē-sĭs). Reproduction of ancestral characteristics without change, in a later generation, esp. abnormalities.

paleogenetic (pā"lē-ō-jĕn-ĕt'ĭk). Having origin in a previous generation.

paleokinetic (pā"lē-ō-kĭn-ĕt'ĭk). Noting a peripheral motor nervous system controlling automatic associated movements and phylogenetically older than system controlling voluntary movement. SEE: *neokinetic.*

paleontology (pā"lē-ŏn-tŏl'ō-jĭ). Branch of biology dealing with ancient plant and animal life of the earth. SEE: *phylogeny.*

paleopathology (pā"lē-ō-păth-ŏl'ō-jĭ). The study of diseases in remains of bodies and fossils of ancient times.

paleostriatal (pā"lē-ō-strī-a'tăl). Concerning the primitive portion of the corpus striatum.

paleostriatum (pā"lē-ō-strī-ā'tŭm). Primitive portion of corpus striatum, the globus pallidus. SEE: *neostriatum.*

paleothalamus (pā"lē-ō-thăl'ă-mŭs). Medial portion of thalamus, the medullary, or noncortical part which is phylogenetically older. SEE: *thalamus.*

palikinesia (păl"ĭ-kĭn-ē'zĭ-ă). Continued, involuntary, repetitious movements.

palilalia (păl-ĭ-lă'lĭ-ă). Pathologic repetitious use of words and phrases.

palinal (păl'ĭn-ăl). Moved or moving backward.

palindromia (păl-ĭn-drō'mĭ-ă). The recurrence of symptoms of a disease or its turn for the worse. SYN: *relapse.*

palindromic (păl-ĭn-drŏm'ĭk). Recurring, as palindromic rheumatism.

palinesthesia (păl"ĭn-ĕs-thē'zĭ-ă). Return of power of sensation, as after recovery from anesthesia or coma.

palingenesis (păl"ĭn-jĕn'ē-sĭs). 1. Regeneration or restoration of an organism or part of one. 2. Reappearance of ancestral characteristics, esp. abnormal ones. SYN: *atavism, paleogenesis.*

palingraphia (păl"ĭn-grăf'ĭ-ă). Pathologic

repetition of words or phrases in writing.

palinphrasia, paliphrasia (păl-ĭn-frā′zĭ-ă, -ĭ-frā′zĭ-ă). Pathological condition in which there is coherent speech but certain words or phrases are frequently repeated. SYN: *palilalia.*

pallanesthesia (păl″ăn-ĕs-thē′zĭ-ă). Loss of vibration sensation of skin and bones. SYN: *apallesthesia.* SEE: *pallesthesia.*

pallescence (pă-lĕs′ĕns). Diminution of body color; a pale appearance. SYN: *pallor.*

pallesthesia (păl-ĕs-thē′zĭ-ă). The sensation of vibration felt in skin or bones, as that produced by a tuning fork when held against the body.

palliate (păl′ĭ-āt). To ease or reduce in violence, to allay temporarily, as pain, without curing.

palliative (păl′ĭ-a-tĭv). 1. Serving to relieve or alleviate, without curing. 2. An agent which alleviates or eases.

pallid (păl′ĭd). Lacking color, pale, wan.

pallidal (păl′ĭ-dăl). Concerning the pallidum of the brain.

pal′lidin. A preparation made from the lung substance of congenital syphilitics, which is used in the skin test for syphilis.

pallidum (păl′ĭd-ŭm). The globus pallidus of the lenticular nucleus in the corpus striatum.

pallium (păl′ĭ-ŭm). The cerebral cortex with its adjacent white substance, considered as a cover for rest of the brain. SYN: *brain mantle.*

pallor (păl′or). Lack of color; paleness. SEE: *skin.*

palm (pahm). Ant. or flexor surface of the hand from wrist to fingers. SYN: *vola manus.* SEE: *antithenar, thenar.*

palmar (păl′mar). Concerning the palm of the hand.

   p. reflex. Flexion of fingers resulting from irritation of palm of hand.

palmaris (păl-mā′rĭs). One of 2 muscles, *palmaris brevis* and *palmaris longus.*

palm-chin reflex. Contraction of chin muscles resulting when thenar eminence of hand is strongly irritated by a sharp object.

palmicol (pal-mĭ′ăk-ōl). Proprietary creosote derivative used in diseases of the lung.

palmic (pal′mĭk). 1. Concerning palpitation or pulse. 2. Concerning palmus, *q.v.*

palmitic acid (pal-mĭt′ĭk). $CH_3(CH_2)_{14}$-COOH. A fatty acid found in solid fats, animal, and vegetable, palm oil, some waxes and many fatty oils.

palmitin (pal′mĭt-ĭn). An ester of glycerol and palmitic acid, derived from fat of both animal and vegetable origin.

palmomen′tal reflex. Contraction of chin muscles resulting when thenar eminence of hand is strongly irritated by a sharp object.

palmus (păl′mŭs). 1. Palpitation; a throb. 2. Jerking; a disease with convulsive nervous twitching of the leg muscles, similar to jumping. 3. Heartbeat.

palpable (păl′pă-bl). Perceptible, esp. by feeling or touch.

palpate (păl′pāt). To examine by touch; to feel.

palpation (păl-pă′shŭn). Process of examining by application of the hands to the external surface of the body to detect evidence of disease in the various organs.

palpatometer (păl-pă-tom′ĕt-ĕr). Device for determining arterial tension.

palpebra (păl′pe-bră, păl-pē′bră) (pl. *palpebrae*). An eyelid.

   p. inferior. The lower eyelid.

   p. superior. The upper eyelid.

palpebral (păl′pe-brăl). Concerning an eyelid.

   p. cartilages. Thin plates of condensed tissue forming the framework of the eyelid. SYN: *tarsal cartilages.*

   p. fissure. The opening bet. the eyelids.

   p. follicles. Sebaceous follicles in eyelids whose secretion prevents their sticking together. SYN: *meibomian glands.*

   p. muscle. The orbicularis palpebrarum which closes the eyelid.

palpebrate (păl′pē-brāt). 1. To wink. 2. Possessing eyelids.

palpitant (păl′pĭ-tănt). Throbbing; trembling.

palpitate (păl′pĭ-tāt). 1. To cause to throb. 2. To throb or beat intensely or rapidly, usually said of the heart.

palpitation (păl-pĭ-tā′shŭn). Rapid, violent or throbbing pulsation, as an abnormally rapid throbbing, or fluttering of the heart.

   p., arterial. That felt in course of an artery.

palsy (pawl′zĭ). 1. Temporary or permanent loss of sensation, or of ability to move, or to control movement. 2. A person disabled by palsy. SYN: *paralysis.*

   p., Bell's. Palsy of the facial nerve at its periphery.

   p., birth. Palsy arising from an injury received at birth.

   p., crutch. Palsy resulting from pressure on axilla from use of a crutch.

   p., Erb's. A paralysis of the deltoid, biceps, long supinator, and brachialis anticus muscles due to lesion and degenerative changes in spinal cord. Other muscles may sometimes become affected.

   p., lead. Palsy of the forearm as a result of lead poisoning.

   p., night. Form of paresthesia in which numbness is a symptom, esp. at night.

   p., shaking. Progressive muscular weakness and tremor with impaired voluntary motion. SYN: *paralysis agitans, Parkinson's disease.*

   p., wasting. Chronic condition in which there is atrophy and paralysis of muscles which grow progressively worse. SYN: *progressive muscular atrophy.*

paludal (păl′ū-dăl). Concerning, or originating in, marshes. SYN: *malarial.*

paludism (păl′ū-dĭzm). Swamp fever. SYN: *malaria, q.v.*

pampiniform (păm-pĭn'ĭ-form). Convoluted like a tendril.

p. plexus. 1. A mesh of spermatic or ovarian veins. 2. Network of nerves supplying the testicles.

pampinocele (păm-pĭn'ō-sēl). A swollen, painful condition of the veins of the spermatic cord. Syn: *varicocele.*

pan-, pant-. Combining form meaning *all.*

panacea (păn-ă-sē'ă). A remedy for all ills.

panagglutinin (păn-ăg-lū'tĭn-ĭn). Substance capable of agglutinizing corpuscles of every blood group.

Panama fever (păn-ă-mă'). Severe, pernicious, malarial fever peculiar to Panama.

panaris (pă-nă'rĭs, pa'nă-rĭs). Inflammation and infection of part of digit around the nail. Syn: *felon, paronychia, whitlow.*

panarthritis (păn-ar-thrī'tĭs). 1. Inflammation of all parts of a joint. 2. Inflamed condition of all the joints in the body.

panasthenia (păn-ăs-thē'nĭ-ă). Generalized weakness or exhaustion without evidence of organic disease. Syn: *neurasthenia, q.v.*

panatrophy (păn-ăt'rō-fĭ). 1. Wasting away of an entire structure. 2. Generalized wasting away of the body.

pancarditis (păn-kăr-dī'tĭs). Inflamed condition involving all the structures of the heart.

panchreston (păn-krē'stŏn). A remedy for every disease. Syn: *panacea.*

panchromia (păn-krō'mĭ-ă). Power of staining with numerous dyes.

pancreas (păn'krē-ăs). A racemose compound gland, situated behind the stomach in front of the 1st and 2nd lumbar vertebrae, in a horizontal position, its head firmly attached to the duodenum and its tail reaching to the spleen.

p., accessory. Small mass of tissue close to the pancreas, apparently detached from it.

p., little. Semidetached lobular part of post. surface of head of the pancreas, sometimes having a separate duct opening into the principal one.

p., Willis'. See: *little pancreas.*

pancreatalgia (păn"krē-ăt-ăl'jĭ-ă). Painful condition of the pancreas.

pancreatectomy (păn"krē-ăt-ĕk'tō-mĭ). Operation for removal of part or all of the pancreas.

pancreatemphraxis (păn"krē-ăt-ĕm-frăk'-sĭs). Congestion of pancreas due to obstruction of pancreatic duct causing swelling of the gland.

pancreathelcosis (păn"krē-ăth-ĕl-kō'sĭs). Ulcerated condition of the pancreas or its suppurative inflammation.

pancreatic (păn-krē-ăt'ĭk). Concerning the pancreas.

p. juice. An external secretion of the pancreas which acts on food following action of gastric juice in the stomach.

pancreaticocholecystostomy (păn"krē-ăt"-ĭ-kō-kō"le-sĭs-tos'tō-mĭ). Surgical crea-

tion of passage bet. the gallbladder and a fistulous pancreas.

pancreaticoduodenal (păn"krē-ăt"ĭ-kō-dū-ō-dē'năl). Concerning the duodenum and a fistulous pancreas.

pancreaticoduodenostomy (păn"krē-ăt"ĭ-kō-dū"ō-dē-nŏs'tō-mĭ). Surgical creation of a passage bet. a fistulous pancreas and duodenum.

pancreaticogastrostomy (păn"krē-ăt"ĭ-kō-găs-trŏs'tō-mĭ). Surgical creation of a passage bet. a fistulous pancreas and the stomach.

pancreatin (păn'krē-ăt-ĭn). 1. One of the active ferments of the pancreas. 2. USP. A mixture of enzymes obtained from pancreas of ox or hog.

Dosage: 8 gr. (0.5 Gm.).

pancreatism (păn'krē-ăt-ĭzm). Normal activity and functioning of the pancreas.

pancreatitis (păn"krē-ă-tī'tĭs). Inflamed condition of the pancreas.

p., acute. Form characterized by necrosis, suppuration, gangrene, and hemorrhage.

p., centrilobar. Pancreatitis about divisions of the pancreatic duct.

p., chronic. Form marked by formation of scar tissue in pancreas associated with malfunction.

p., hemorrhagic. Form with hemorrhage into pancreatic tissue.

p., perilobar. Fibrosis of the pancreas bet. acinous groups.

p., purulent. Pancreatitis with suppuration.

p., suppurative. Form marked by development of many small abscesses.

pancreatoduodenectomy (păn"krē-ă-tō-dū"ō-dē-nĕk'tō-mĭ). Excision of the head of the pancreas and the adjacent portion of the duodenum.

pancreatogenic, pancreatogenous (păn"krē-ă-tō-jĕn'ĭk, -tŏj'ĕ-nŭs). Produced in or by the pancreas; having origin in the pancreas.

pancreatolith (păn-krē-ăt'ō-lĭth). A calculus of the pancreas.

pancreatolithectomy (păn"krē-ăt-ō-lĭth-ĕk'tō-mĭ). Removal of a concretion from the pancreas. Syn: *pancreatolithotomy.*

pancreatolithotomy (păn"krē-ăt-ō-lĭth-ot'-ō-mĭ). Removal of a concretion from the pancreas. Syn: *pancreatolithectomy.*

pancreatolysis (păn"krē-ăt-ŏl'ĭ-sĭs). Destruction of the pancreatic substance.

pancreatolytic (păn"krē-ăt-ō-lĭt'ĭk). Destructive to the pancreatic tissues. Syn: *pancreolytic.*

pancreatomy (păn-krē-ăt'ō-mĭ). Operation into the pancreas. Syn: *pancreatotomy.*

pancreatoncus (păn-krē-ăt-ong'kŭs). A pancreatic tumor.

pancreatopathy (păn"krē-ăt-op'ă-thĭ). Any pancreatic disease.

pancreatotomy (păn-krē-ă-tŏt'ō-mĭ). Surgical incision into the pancreas. Syn: *pancreatomy.*

pancreëctomy (păn-krē-ek'tō-mĭ). Partial or total excision of the pancreas. See: *preparation for hysteropexy.*

pancreolithotomy (păn"krē-ō-lĭth-ŏt'ō-mĭ).

Surgical removal of a pancreatic concretion.

pancreolytic (păn-krē-ō-lĭt'ĭk). Destructive to the pancreas.

pancreon(e (păn'krē-ōn). A commercial digestive powder obtained from pancreatin.

pancreopathy (păn-krē-ŏp'ăth-ĭ). Any diseased condition of the pancreas. SYN: *pancreatopathy.*

pandemia (păn-dē'mĭ-ă). Epidemic affecting the major portion of the population of a district.

pandemic (păn-dĕm'ĭk). 1. Affecting the majority of the population; said of a disease. 2. A disease affecting the majority of the population of a large region, or which is epidemic at the same time in many different parts of the world.

Pander's layers (păn'dĕr). The mesoblastic layer in which the blood vessels are first formed in the embryo.

pandiculation (păn-dĭk-ŭ-lā'shŭn).Stretching of the limbs and yawning, as on awakening from normal sleep.

pang (păng). 1. A paroxysm of extreme agony. 2. A sudden attack of any emotion.

pangenesis (păn-jĕn'ĕs-ĭs). Darwin's theory of reproduction in which each cell of the parent is represented by a particle in the reproductive cell, and thus each part of the organism reproduces itself in the progeny.

panhidrosis (păn-hĭd-rō'sĭs). Perspiration over the entire surface of the body. SYN: *panidrosis.*

panhydrometer (păn''hĭ-drŏm'ĕt-ĕr). Apparatus for obtaining specific gravity of any fluid.

panhysterectomy (păn-hĭs-tĕr-ĕk'tō-mĭ). Excision of entire uterus including the cervix uteri.

panhysterokolpectomy (păn-hĭs''tĕr-ō-kŏl-pĕk'tō-mĭ). Total excision of the uterus and vagina.

panidrosis (păn-ĭd-rō'sĭs). General perspiration over the body's entire surface.

panighao (păn-ĭ-gä'ō). Eruption due to presence of larva of uncinaria under the skin. SYN: *ground itch.*

panis (păn'ĭs). Bread.

p., mica. Bread crumb.

panmyelophthisis (păn''mī-ĕl-of'thĭ-sĭs). General wasting away of the bone marrow.

panmyelosis (păn''mī-ĕl-ō'sĭs). Increase in all the constituents of the bone marrow.

panneuritis (păn''ū-rī'tĭs). Generalized neuritis.

p. endemica, p. epidemica. Deficiency disease in which there is lack of vitamin B₁. SYN: *beriberi.*

panniculitis (pan-ĭk-ū-lī'tĭs). Inflamed condition of a layer of fatty connective tissue in the abdomen.   [of tissue.

panniculus (păn-ĭk'ū-lŭs). A layer or sheet

p. adiposus. The superficial fascia with fat in its areolar substance.

p. carnosus. Thin layer of muscular tissue in superficial fascia.

pannus (păn'ŭs). Newly formed vascular tissue involving the upper half of the front of the cornea.

panopeptone (păn-ō-pep'tōn). Commercial invalid food composed of bread and peptonized beef.

panophobia (păn-ō-fō'bĭ-ă). Morbid fear of some unknown evil or of everything in general; general apprehension. SYN: *pantophobia.*

panophthalmia, panophthalmitis (păn-ŏf-thăl'mĭ-ă, -mī'tĭs). Inflammation of entire eye.

p. purulenta. Severe form with suppuration.

panoptic (păn-ŏp'tĭk). Making every part visible; completely visible.

p. stain. Stain which causes every part of the tissue to be differentiated.

panoptosis (păn-ŏp-tō'sĭs). General prolapse of the abdominal organs.

panosteitis (păn''ŏs-tē-ī'tĭs). Inflammation of every structure of a bone.

panotitis (păn-ō-tī'tĭs). Inflammation involving all the parts of the ear.

panphobia (păn-fō'bĭ-ă). Groundless fear of everything.

panspermia (păn-spĕr'mĭ-ă). The theory that distribution of disease germs is widespread, accounting for apparent cases of spontaneous generation. SEE: *biogenesis.*

pansphygmograph (păn-sfĭg'mō-grăf). Apparatus for registering cardiac movements, the pulse wave, and chest movements at one time.

pansporoblast (păn-spō'rō-blăst). Reproductive area in the myxosporidia having both germinal and vegetative nuclei.

pant (pănt). 1. To breathe hard; to gasp for breath. 2. A short or labored breath.

pantachromatic (păn''tă-krō-măt'ĭk). Entirely colorless.

pantalgia (păn-tăl'jĭ-ă). Pain felt over the entire body.

pantatrophia, pantatrophy (păn-tăt-rō'-fĭ-ă, -tat'rō-fĭ). Complete lack of nourishment to a part with resultant wasting.

panthodic (păn-thŏd'ĭk). Radiating to all parts of the body, esp. applied to nervous impulses.

panting (pănt'ĭng). 1. Breathing hard; gasping for breath. 2. Labored breathing.

pantophobia (păn-tō-fō'bĭ-ă). Morbid, groundless fear of everything in general. SYN: *panophobia.*

pantopon (păn'tō-pŏn). A mixture of the alkaloids of opium, providing the effects of total opium, but more readily absorbed, and free from nauseating properties.

DOSAGE: From 1/24 to 1/3 gr. (0.0025-0.02 Gm.).

pantoscopic (păn''tō-skŏp'ĭk). Viewing everything; adjusted to both close and far objects.

p. glasses. Glasses with 2 segments of different focal lengths for near and far objects. SYN: *bifocal spectacles.*

pantothenic acid (păn-tō-then'ĭk). Newly

synthesized vitamin found in yeast, molasses, rice hulls, and liver.

pantothermia (păn″tō-thĕr′mĭ-ă). Condition in which there is variation in bodily temperature without apparent reason.

panturbinate (păn-tur′bĭ-nāt). All of the turbinate structure.

pap (păp). 1. Any soft, semiliquid food. 2. The nipple.

papain (pa-pā′ĭn, pa′pā-ĭn). A digestive ferment obtained from the papaw fruit.
Dosage: 2 gr. (0.130 Gm.).

papaverine hydrochloride (pă-păv′ĕr-ēn). The salt of an alkaloid obtained from opium.
Dosage: Average, 1/2 to 1-1/3 gr. (0.03-0.08 Gm.).

paper (pā′pĕr). 1. A substance mechanically woven into thin sheets or strips, with many uses, as for filtering. 2. A piece of paper specially prepared, as by having a medicinal preparation spread out on it.

papilla (pă-pĭl′ă) (pl. *papillae*). 1. The nipple of the breast; any nipplelike protuberance. 2. A small, soft, sensitive eminence in the skin possessing a tactile function.

   p., circumvallate. One of the large papillae near the base on the dorsal aspect of the tongue, arranged in a V-shape.

   p., duodenal. The slight eminence in duodenum indicating opening of ductus choledochus communis.

   p., filiform. One of the very slender papillae at tip of the tongue.

   p., fungiform. One of the broad, flat papillae resembling a fungus, chiefly found on dorsal central area of tongue.

   p., gustatory. Taste papilla of tongue; one of those possessing a taste bud.

   p., hair. A conical process of the corium in which a hair is nourished.

   p., lacrimal. An elevation in edge of eyelid for the lacrimal puncta.

   p., lingual. Tiny eminence covering ant. two-thirds of tongue, including circumvallate, filiform, fungiform, and conical papillae.

   p., nerve. Papilla of skin containing tactile corpuscles. See: *tactile corpuscles.*

   p., optic. Terminus of optic nerve where it enters the eyeball.

   p., primary. A papilla arising directly from the corium.

   p., renal. Apex of a malpighian pyramid in the kidney.

   p., secondary. Papilla arising from a primary papilla.

   p., simple. An undivided papilla arising directly from the corium.

   p., tactile. See: *nerve papilla.*

   p., taste. See: *gustatory papilla.*

   p., vascular. Papilla of skin to the tips of which extend 1 or more capillary loops.

   p. of Vater. See: *duodenal papilla.*

papillary (păp′ĭ-lar-ĭ). 1. Concerning a nipple or papilla. 2. Resembling or composed of papillae.

   p. body. Papillary layer of the corium. Syn: *pars papillaris.*

   p. muscles. Muscular eminences in ventricles of the heart.

   p. tumor. Neoplasm composed of or resembling enlarged papillae. See: *papilloma.*

papillate (păp′ĭl-āt). Bact: Having nipplelike growths on the surface, as a culture.

papillectomy (păp-ĭl-ĕk′tō-mĭ). Excision of any papilla or papillae.

papilledema (păp-ĭl-e-dē′mă). Edema and inflammation of the optic nerve at its point of entrance into the eyeball.

papilliferous (păp-ĭl-ĭf′ĕr-ŭs). Having or containing papillae.

papilliform (pă-pĭl′ĭ-form). 1. Having the characteristics or appearance of papillae. 2. Bact: Denoting a shallow saucer-like form.

papillitis (păp-ĭl-ī′tĭs). Inflammation of optic disk with edema. Syn: *choked disk, optic neuritis.*

papilloadenocystoma (păp″ĭl-ō-ăd″ē-nō-sĭs-tō′mă). A tumor composed of elements of papilloma, adenoma, and cystoma.

papillocarcinoma (păp″ĭl-ō-kăr-sĭn-ō′mă). 1. A malignant tumor of hypertrophied papillae. 2. Carcinoma with papillary growths.

papilloma (păp-ĭ-lō′mă) (pl. *papillomata*). 1. Any benign epithelial tumor. 2. Epithelial tumor of skin or mucous membrane consisting of hypertrophied papillae covered by a layer of epithelium.

   p. durum. A hardened papilloma, as a wart.

   p., hard. Papilloma which develops from squamous epithelium.

   p. molle. A papilloma with only a thin, horny layer covering it.

   p., soft. Papilloma formed from columnar epithelium.

   p., urethral. A painful urethral caruncle or fibrocellular tumor arising from the urethra.

papillomatosis (păp″ĭl-ō-mă-tō′sĭs). 1. Widespread formation of papillomata. 2. Condition of being afflicted with many papillomata.

papilloretinitis (păp″ĭl-ō-rĕt-ĭn-ī′tĭs). Inflamed condition of the papilla and retina extending to the optic disk.

papoid (pa′poyd). Commercial powder given to stimulate digestion.

papula (păp′ū-lă). A pimple. Syn: *papule.*

papular (păp′ū-ler). Of the nature of or concerning pimples.

   p. fever. Mild fever with maculopapular eruptions and rheumatoid pains.

papulation (păp-ū-lā′shŭn). 1. The development of papules. 2. The stage of pimple formation in a disease.

papule (păp′ūl). Red elevated area on the skin, solid and circumscribed, varying from the size of a pinhead to that of a pea.

   p., dry. Hard one that is primary lesion of syphilis.

p., moist; p., mucous. A syphilitic eruption of papules with flat tops. SYN: *condyloma lata.*

papuliferous (păp″ū-lĭf′ĕr-ŭs). Having papules or pimples.

papulo-. Combining form meaning *a pimple, a papule.* [like.

papyraceous (păp-ĭ-rā′shŭs). Parchment-OB: Denoting a fetus retained in the uterus beyond natural term that has assumed a mummified appearance.

Paquelin's cautery (păk-lăn′). A hollow, platinum pointed cautery apparatus kept at a constant temperature by means of benzene vapor.

par. A pair, esp. a pair of cranial nerves.

p. vagum. The vagus or 10th pair of cranial nerves.

para-, par-. Combining forms meaning *alongside of, by, past, beyond, the opposite, abnormal, irregular.*

paraänesthesia (păr″ă-ăn-ĕs-thē′zhĭ-a). Anesthesia of two corresponding sides, esp. of lower half of body.

paraäppendicitis (păr″ă-ăp-ĕnd-ĭ-sī′tĭs). Inflammation involving the connective tissue adjacent to the appendix. SYN: *perityphlitis.*

parabiosis (păr″ă-bī-ō′sĭs). 1. Temporary suppression of excitability and conductivity of a nerve. 2. Anatomical and physiological joining of 2 separate organisms, naturally or artificially formed. SEE: *Siamese twins.*

parabiotik (păr″ă-bī-ŏt′ĭk). Concerning parabiosis.

parablast (păr′ă-blăst). Part of the embryonic mesoblast from which arise the vascular and connective tissue structures.

parablastic (păr″ă-blăst′ĭk). Pert. to the embryonic layer giving rise to the vascular and connective tissue structures.

parablastoma (păr″ă-blăst-ō′mă). A tumor composed of parablastic tissue.

parablepsia, parablepsis (păr″ă-blĕp′sĭ-ă, -sĭs). Abnormality of the visual sensations.

parabulia (păr-ă-bū′lĭ-ă). Perversion or abnormality of will power.

paracentesis (păr-ă-sĕn-tē′sĭs). Puncture of a cavity with evacuation of fluid by tapping, as in dropsy.

p., abdominal. Tapping of the abdomen.

p. capitis. Paracentesis of the cranium.

p. cordis. Surgical puncture of the heart.

p. pericardii. Paracentesis of the pericardial sac.

p. pulmonis. Removal of fluid from a lung.

p. thoracis. Drainage of fluid from the cavity of the chest. SEE: *aspiration.*

p. tunicae vaginalis. Paracentesis of the tunica vaginalis.

p. tympani. Drainage or irrigation through incision of the tympanic membrane.

p. vesicae. Puncture of the wall of the urinary bladder.

paracentetic (păr″ă-sĕn-tet′ĭk). Concerning paracentesis.

paracentral (păr″ă-sĕn′trăl). Located near the center.

p. lobule. Cerebral convolution on mesial surface joining the upper terminations of the ascending parietal and frontal convolutions.

parachlorphenol (păr″ă-klor-fē′nol). Strong antiseptic and disinfectant used in lupus and erysipelas.

paracholia (păr″ă-kō′lĭ-ă). Condition of disturbed bile secretion.

parachordal (păr-ă-kor′dăl). 1. Noting the 2 plates of cartilage, 1 on either side of the ant. portion of the notochord.* 2. A parachordal cartilage.

parachroma (păr-ă-krō′mă). Discoloration, as that of the skin.

parachromatin (păr″ă-krō′mă-tĭn). The portion of the nucleoplasm that forms the spindle threads in karyokinesis.

parachromatopsia (păr″ă-krō-mă-tŏp′sĭ-ă). Color blindness.

parachromatosis (păr″ă-krō-mă-tō′sĭs). Any one of the diseases in which the skin is pigmented.

parachromophoric (păr″ă-krō″mō-for′ĭk). Excreting pigment, but retaining it within the organism.

parachymosin (păr″ă-kī-mō′sĭn). The ferment found in the stomach of both pig and human being.

paracinesia, paracinesis (păr″ă-sĭn-ē′zĭ-ă, -sĭs). Condition in which there is perversion of motor powers; motor abnormality.

paracmastic (păr-ăk-măs′tĭk). Denoting the period of decrease of symptoms.

paracolpitis (păr″ă-kŏl-pī′tĭs). Inflammation of tissues adjoining the vagina.

paracolpium (păr″ă-kol′pĭ-ŭm). The vascular and connective tissue alongside the vagina.

paracrisis (păr-ak′rĭ-sĭs, păr″ă-krī′sĭs). Any abnormality of the secretions.

paracusis (păr-ă-kū′sĭs). Any abnormality or disorder of the sense of hearing.

p. acris. Excessively acute hearing.

p. duplicata. The hearing of 1 sound as 2. SYN: *diplacusis.*

p. loci. Difficulty in estimating the direction of sound.

p. willisiana. An apparent ability to hear better in a noisy place, found in deafness due to stapes fixation and adhesive processes.

paracyesis (păr-ă-sī-ē′sĭs). Extrauterine pregnancy.

paracystitis (păr″ă-sĭs-tī′tĭs). Inflamed condition of connective tissues and other structures around the urinary bladder.

paracystium (păr-ă-sĭs′tĭ-ŭm). The connective tissue surrounding the urinary bladder.

paradenitis (păr″ăd-en-ī′tĭs). Inflammation of areolar tissues close to a gland.

paradidymis (păr-ă-dĭd′ĭ-mĭs). BNA. The atrophic remnants of the tubules of the wolffian body, situated on the spermatic cord above the epididymis. SYN: *massa* *innominata, organ of Giraldès, parepididymis.*

paradoxic, paradoxical (păr″ă-dŏk'sĭk, -sĭ-kal). Seemingly contradictory, but demonstrably true.

   p. contraction. Contraction of a muscle when its origin and insertion are suddenly relaxed or its length shortened, suddenly.

   p. flexor reflex. Extension of great toe when sudden pressure is made on deep flexor muscles of calf of leg.

   p. movement. When diaphragm is paralyzed, it is forced upward during inspiration, and downward during expiration—the reverse of normal.

   p. respiration. A lung is breathing paradoxically when it expands during expiration and contracts during inspiration.

paraffin (păr'ă-fĭn). 1. A waxy, white, tasteless, odorless mixture of solid hydrocarbons obtained from petroleum. 2. A saturated hydrocarbon of the methane series.

   p., hard. Solid paraffin with a melting point bet. 45° C. and 60° C.

   p., liquid. Liquid hydrocarbon. SYN: *liquid petrolatum.*

   p., soft. A semisolid paraffin. SEE: *petrolatum.*

paraffinoma (păr″ă-fĭn-ō'mă). A tumor which arises at site of injection of paraffin.

paraffinum (păr-ă-fe'nŭm). Paraffin, *q.v.*

paraformaldehyde (păr″ă-fŏr-măl'dĕ-hĭd). A white, powdered antiseptic and disinfectant, a polymer of formaldehyde.

paragammacism (păr″ă-găm'mă-sĭzm). Inability to pronounce "g" and "k" sounds, with substitution of other consonants for them.

paraganglin (păr″ă-găng'lĭn). Commercial intestinal tonic prepared from the medulla of the suprarenal glands of oxen.

paraganglioma (păr″ă-găng-lĭ-ō'mă). 1. Tumor composed of cells resembling medullary tissue of the adrenals. 2. Tumor of the adrenal medulla.

paraganglion (păr″ă-găng'lĭ-ŏn) (pl. *paraganglia*). 1. Any structure supplementing, or in the neighborhood of, a ganglion. 2. A mass of cells in the medullary portion of the adrenal bodies. 3. Chromaffin mass found along the branches of the sympathetic nervous system. SEE: *chromaffinoma.*

parageusia, parageusis (păr-ă-gū'sĭ-ă, -sĭs). Disorder or abnormality of the sense of taste.

paraglobulin (păr″ă-glŏb'ū-lĭn). A globulin found in blood plasma, lymph, and other body fluids, associated with coagulation.

paraglobulinuria (păr″ă-glŏb-ū-lĭn-ū'rĭ-ă). Excretion of paraglobulin in the urine.

paraglossa (păr-ă-glŏs'să). 1. Enlargement of the tongue. 2. Congenital hypertrophy of the tongue.

Paragonimus (păr″ă-gŏn'ĭm-ŭs). Genus of trematode worms.

P. westermanii. Lung fluke.

paragraphia (păr-ă-grăf'ĭ-ă). The writing of letters or words other than those intended, due to partial lesion of the visual word center in the brain.

parahepatitis (păr″ă-hĕp-ă-tī'tĭs). Inflamed condition of parts immediately adjacent to the liver.

parainfection (păr″ă-ĭn-fĕk'shŭn). The symptomatology of an infectious disease without evidence of the presence of the microörganism causing the disease.

parakeratosis (păr″ă-kĕr-ă-tō'sĭs). Any disorder affecting the horny layer of the epidermis.

   p. psoriasiformis. Scab formation resembling that of psoriasis.

   p. scutularis. Scalp disease with hairs encircled by epidermic crust formation.

paralalia (păr-ă-lā'lĭ-ă). Any speech defect, characterized by sound distortion.

   p. literalis. Stammering, *q.v.*

paralambdacism (păr″ă-lăm'dă-sĭzm). Inability to sound the letter "l" correctly, substituting some other letter for it.

paralbumin (păr-ăl-bū'mĭn). An albumin found in fluid content in ovarian cysts and in ascites.

paraldehyde (păr-ăl'dĕ-hĭd). USP. $C_6H_{12}O_3$. A liquid polymer of aldehyde which is colorless, with characteristic unpleasant odor and taste.

   DOSAGE: 30 minims (2 cc.) in ice water.

paraldehydism (păr-ăl'dĕ-hĭd-ĭzm). Poisoning from an overdose of paraldehyde, *q.v.*

paralepsy (par'ă-lĕp"sĭ). Temporary attack of mental inertia and hopelessness, or sudden alteration in mood or mental tension. SYN: *psycholepsy.*

paralexia (păr-ă-lĕk'sĭ-ă). Inability to comprehend printed words or sentences with substitution of meaningless combinations of words.

paralysis (pă-ral'ĭ-sĭs). Temporary suspension or permanent loss of function in a living part, esp. loss of sensation or voluntary motion.

   p. of accommodation. Inability of the eye to adjust itself to various distances due to paralysis.

   p., acoustic. Nervous deafness.

   p., acute ascending. Rapidly progressing form of paralysis which begins in the feet and slowly ascends. Fatal. SYN: *Landry's paralysis.*

   p., acute atrophic. SEE: *infantile paralysis.*   [*paralysis.*

   p., acute infectious. SEE: *infantile*

   p. agitans. A basal ganglion disease of late life producing a picture of rigid tremulousness progressive in its course, and marked by weakness, delay of voluntary motion, a peculiar festinating gait, and muscular contraction, causing peculiar and characteristic positions of the limbs and hand.

   p., alcoholic. Paralysis due to habitual drunkenness.

   p., anesthesia. Paralysis which develops following administration of anesthesia.

p., anterior spinal. Inflamed condition of the ant. horns of the spinal cord's gray matter.

p., arsenical. Paralysis following poisoning from arsenic.

p., ascending. Paralysis beginning with the lower limbs and progressing upward.

p., association. SEE: *bulbar paralysis.*

p., Bell's. Facial paralysis.

p., Bernhardt's. Pain and hyperesthesia on the outer femoral surface from lesion or disease of the external cutaneous nerve of the thigh.

p., birth. Paralysis caused by injury received at birth.

p., brachial. Paralysis of 1 or both arms.

p., brachiofacial. Paralysis of the face and an arm.

p., Brown-Sequard's. Paralysis of motion on 1 side and of sensation on the other.

p., bulbar. Paralysis caused by changes in the motor centers of the oblongata.

p., central. Any paralysis from a lesion of the brain or spinal cord.

p., cerebral. Paralysis due to lesion of some portion of the cerebrum.

p., complete. Paralysis in which there is total loss of function.

p., compression. Paralysis due to pressure on a nerve, as by a crutch or during sleep.

p., crossed. Paralysis of the face on 1 side of the body and the limbs on the opposite side.

p., crutch. Paralysis due to pressure in the armpit.

p., decubitus. Paralysis due to pressure on a nerve from lying in 1 position for a long time.

p., diver's. Paralysis due to increase in atmospheric pressure, evidenced on return to normal atmosphere. SYN: *caisson disease.*

p., Erb's. 1. SEE: *birth paralysis.* 2. Partial paralysis of the brachial plexus.

p., exhaustion. Paralysis due to prolonged voluntary movements involving exhaustion of the nerve centers.

p., facial. SEE: *Bell's paralysis.*

p., general. Progressive loss of power and the mental faculties resulting eventually in dementia and death. SYN: *paresis.*

p., ginger. Paralysis of the limbs after drinking Jamaica ginger.

p., glossolabial. SEE: *bulbar paralysis.*

p., histrionic. Paralysis of certain facial muscles, producing a facial expression of some emotion.

p., hysteric. One that may simulate any form of paralysis; it appears to have no adequate causative lesion.

p., incomplete. Partial paralysis of the body or a part.

p., infantile. Motor paralysis with atrophy of a group of muscles following an acute infectious disease in children which is transmitted by a filtrable virus. SYN: *acute anterior poliomyelitis.*

p., Jake. SEE: *ginger paralysis.*

p., Klumpke's. Wasting paralysis of the arms and hands.

p., Kussmaul's; p., Landry's. SEE: *acute ascending paralysis.*   [by lead.

p., lead. Paralysis following poisoning

p., local. Paralysis of a single muscle or 1 group of muscles.

p., nuclear. Paralysis caused by lesion of a nucleus.

p., obstetrical. SEE: *birth paralysis.*

p., periodic. Paralysis which recurs and abates temporarily.

p., progressive bulbar. SEE: *bulbar paralysis.*

p., pseudobulbar. Paralysis caused by cerebral center lesions, which simulates the bulbar types of paralysis.

p., reflex. Paralysis caused by irritation of a periphery. In some cases, secondary changes occur in the spinal cord, and the paralysis ceases to be truly reflex.

p., spastic spinal. Congenital sclerosis of spinal cords' lateral columns with muscular rigidity and exaggerated reflexes. SYN: *Little's disease.*

p., spinal. SEE: *paralysis, anterior spinal.*

p., wasting. Progressive wasting away of the muscles. SEE: *progressive muscular atrophy.*

paralytic (păr-ă-lĭt'ĭk). 1. Concerning paralysis. 2. One afflicted with paralysis.

p. dementia. Progressive paralysis with mental deterioration. SYN: *paresis.*

p. ileus. Paralysis of intestinal wall with distention and symptoms of acute obstruction and prostration.

paralgesia (păr-ăl-jē'zĭ-ă). Any unusual sensation which is painful.

paralgia (păr-al'jĭ-ă). Sensation both abnormal and painful.

parallagma (păr-ăl-ăg'mă). Overlapping or displacement of the fragments of a fractured bone.

parallax (păr'ă-lăks). Apparent displacement of a part due to change in observer's position.

paralogia (păr-ă-lŏ'jĭ-ă). A disorder of the reasoning; a psychosis.

paralysin (păr-ăl'ĭs-ĭn). An antibody causing clumping of cells or bacteria. SYN: *agglutinin.*

paralyzant (păr'ă-lĭz''ănt). 1. Causing paralysis. 2. A drug or other agent that induces paralysis.

paralyze (păr'ă-lĭz). 1. To cause temporary or permanent loss of muscular power or sensation. 2. To render ineffective.

paramastigote (păr''a-măs'tĭ-gŏt). Possessing an accessory flagellum adjacent to a larger one.

paramastitis (păr-ă-măs-tī'tĭs). Inflammation around the mamma.

paramecium (par-ă-mē'cĭ-um). Genus of infusorians, rather long in shape and sometimes large enough to be seen by the naked eye.

paramenia (păr-ă-mē'nĭ-ă). Irregular, abnormal, or difficult menstruation.

parametric (păr-ă-mĕt′rĭk). 1. Concerning the area near the uterus. 2. Rel. to the parametrium, the tissue surrounding the uterus.

parametrismus (păr-ă-mē-trĭz′mŭs). Muscular spasm in the broad ligament accompanied by pain.

parametritis (păr″ă-mē-trī′tĭs). Inflamed condition of parametrium, the cellular tissue adjacent to uterus. SYN: *cellulitis, pelvic.*

parametrium (păr-ă-mē′trĭ-ŭm). Fat and connective tissue around the uterus.

paramimia (păr-ă-mĭm′ĭ-ă). PSY: Disturbance of association tracts bet. motor and sensory centers resulting in misuse of gestures.

paramitome (păr-ă-mī′tōm). Fluid portion of protoplasm of cells. SYN: *hyaloplasm, paraplasm.*

paramnesia (păr-ăm-nē′zĭ-ă). 1. The use of words without meaning. 2. Inability to distinguish imaginary or suggested experiences from those which have actually occurred.   [ity of shape.

paramorphia (păr-ă-mor′fĭ-ă). Abnormal-

paramusia (păr″ă-mū′zĭ-ă). Loss of ability to render music accurately.

paramyoclonus (păr″ă-mĭ-ŏ-klŏ′nŭs). Clonic spasm of symmetrical groups of muscles.

paramyosinogen (păr″ă-mĭ″ō-sĭn′ō-jĕn). Protein derived from muscle plasm.

paramyotonia (păr″ă-mĭ″ō-tō′nĭ-ă). A disorder marked by muscular spasms and abnormal muscular tonicity.

   p. ataxia. Tonic muscular spasm when making any movement, with slight ataxia or paresis.

   p. congenita. Congenital condition of tonic muscular spasms when body is exposed to cold. SYN: *Thomsen's disease.*

   p., symptomatic. Temporary muscular rigidity when first trying to walk, as in paralysis agitans.

paranephrine (păr″ă-nĕf′rĭn). Commercial preparation of extract of the adrenal glands which controls hemorrhage and raises blood pressure.

paranephritis (păr″ă-ne-frī′tĭs). 1. Inflamed condition of the suprarenal capsules. 2. Inflammation of connective tissue about kidney. SYN: *perinephritis.*

paranephros (păr-ă-nĕf′rŏs). A suprarenal or adrenal capsule.

paranesthesia (păr″ăn-ĕs-thē′zĭ-ă). Anesthesia of the lower portion of the body.

paranoia (păr-ă-noy′ă). A chronic, psychotic entity characterized by fixed but ever-expanding systematized delusions of persecution.

   p., alcoholic. This condition simulates true paranoia. Delusions of suspicion, conspiracy, and of superiority are present.

paranoiac (păr-ă-noy′ăk). 1. One suffering from paranoia. 2. Concerning or afflicted with paranoia.

paranoid (păr′ă-noyd). 1. Resembling paranoia. 2. A person afflicted with paranoia.

   p. reaction type. Individual who has fixed, systematized delusions, is suspicious, has a persecution complex and is resentful, bitter, and a megalomaniac.

paranomia (păr-ă-nō′mĭ-ă). Form of aphasia in which there is inability to remember correct name of objects shortly after seeing or using them.

paranuclein (păr″ă-nŭ′klē-ĭn). A protein which does not yield nitrogenous bases when decomposed. SYN: *nucleoalbumin.*

paranucleus (păr″ă-nŭ′klē-ŭs). A small body lying close to a cell nucleus.

paraomphalic (păr″ă-ŏm-făl′ĭk). Adjacent to the navel. SYN: *paraumbilical.*

paraoperative (păr″ă-ŏp′ĕr-ă-tĭv). Concerning all the details and the accessories of operation and preparation of the patient.

paraosteoarthropathy (păr″ă-ŏs″tē-ō-ăr-thrŏp′ăth-ĭ). Paralysis of lower portion of the body in addition to bone and joint disease.

paraparesis (păr″ă-păr-ē′sĭs, -par′ĕ-sĭs). Partial paralysis affecting the lower limbs.

parapathia (păr-ă-păth′ĭ-ă). Emotional aspects of a disorder.

parapedesis (păr″ă-pĕd-ē′sĭs). Secretion through other than normal channels.

parapeptone (păr″ă-pĕp′tōn). Intermediate digestion product of albumin. SEE: *peptone.*

paraphasia (păr-ă-fā′zĭ-ă). The misuse of words or word combinations spoken; a form of aphasia.

paraphemia (păr″ă-fē′mĭ-ă). A disorder marked by consistent use of the wrong words, or mispronunciation of words.

paraphia (păr-ă′fĭ-ă). Irregularity of the sense of touch.

paraphimosis (păr″ă-fī-mō′sĭs). 1. Strangulation of glans penis due to retraction of foreskin. 2. Retraction of eyelid in back of eyeball.

paraphobia (păr-ă-fō′bĭ-ă). A mild form of phobia.

paraphonia (păr″ă-fō′nĭ-ă). Partial loss or weakness or abnormal change of the voice.

paraphora (păr-ăf′ō-ră). 1. A mental disorder of minor degree. 2. The unsteadiness due to drunkenness.

paraphrasia (păr-ă-frā′zĭ-ă). Disorder characterized by incoherent speech. SYN: *paraphasia.*

paraphrenia (păr-ă-fre′nĭ-ă). 1. Dementia precox according to Freud. 2. Paranoid dementia precox according to Kraepelin, behavior disorders and personality defects not being marked.

   p. confabulans. Paraphrenia marked by memory distortions.

   p. expansiva. Paraphrenia with delusions of grandeur, exaltation, and moderate excitement.

   p. phantastica. Paraphrenia with unsystematized delusions.

   p. systematica. Paraphrenia with progressive delusions of persecution, followed by delusions of grandeur, but personality shows no deterioration.

paraphrenitis (păr″ă-frē-nī′tĭs). 1. Inflammation of the tissues around the diaphragm. 2. Mental delirium or derangement.

paraphronia (păr″ă-frō′nĭ-ă). A psychosis with change of the patient's disposition and character.

paraplasm (păr′ă-plăzm). 1. Any abnormal new formation or malformation. 2. The fluid portion of protoplasm. SYN: *hyaloplasm.*

Paraplasma flavigenum (păr-ă-plăz′mă flă-vĭj′ĕn-ŭm).⸱ A parasitic organism in the red blood cells in yellow fever, assumed to be the cause of it. SYN: *Seidelin bodies.*

paraplastic (păr-ă-plăs′tĭk). 1. Pert. to fluid portion of protoplasm. 2. Misshapen; deformed.

paraplastin (păr-ă-plăs′tĭn). A substance found in a cell's nucleus and cytoplasm which resembles parachromatin.

paraplectic (păr-ă-plĕk′tĭk). Afflicted with paralysis of lower extremities. SYN: *paraplegic.*

paraplegia (păr-ă-plē′jĭ-ă). Paralysis of lower portion of the body and of both legs due to injury to spinal cord. SEE: *paralysis.*

  p., alcoholic. Paraplegia of spinal origin due to use of alcohol.

  p., ataxic. Lateral and post. sclerosis of spinal cord, combined, and resulting symptoms.

  p., cerebral. Paraplegia from bilateral cerebral lesion.

  p., cervical. Paraplegia of both arms.

  p. dolorosa. Paraplegia due to pressure of a neoplasm on post. minor roots. Very painful.

  p., ideal. Reflex paraplegia due to [excitement.

  p., peripheral. Paraplegia from neoplastic pressure on nerves with severe pain.

  p., spastic. Paraplegia from primary lateral sclerosis of spinal cord.

  p., s., primary. Paraplegia from degeneration in pyramidal tracts.

paraplegic (păr-ă-plē′jĭk). Concerning, or affected with, paraplegia. SYN: *paraplectic.*

parapleuritis (păr″ă-plū-rī′tĭs). 1. Inflammation in the thoracic wall. 2. Mild inflammation of the pleura. 3. Pain in the pleura. SYN: *pleurodynia.*

paraplexus (păr″ă-plĕk′sŭs). The choroid plexus of the lateral ventricle of the brain.

parapophysis (păr-ă-pŏf′ĭ-sĭs). Elevation on side of a vertebra on which head of a rib fits.

parapoplexy (păr-ăp′ō-plĕk-sĭ). A mild or slight apoplexy with partial stupor; a stupor resembling apoplexy. SYN: *pseudoapoplexy.*

parapraxia, parapraxis (păr-ă-prak′sĭ-ă, -sĭs). Disturbed mental processes producing inaccuracy and forgetfulness and tendency to misplace things and make slips of speech or pen.

paraproctitis (păr″ă-prŏk-tī′tĭs). Inflamed condition of tissues near the rectum.

parapsia, parapsis (păr-ăp′sĭ-ă, -sĭs). Any disorder of touch. SYN: *paraphia.*

parapsoriasis (păr″ă-sō-rī′ă-sĭs). A chronic disorder of the skin marked by scaly red lesions.

parapyknomorphous (păr″ă-pĭk-nō-mor′fŭs). Having cell particles placed so as to stain only moderately well.

paraqueduct (păr-ăk′wē-dŭkt). A lateral protuberance of the aqueduct of the cerebrum.

parareflexia (păr″ă-rē-flĕk′sĭ-ă). Irregularity or disorder of the reflexes.

pararenal (păr-ă-rē′năl). Near the kidneys.

pararhotacism (păr″ă-rō′tă-sĭzm). Constant erroneous use of letter r or the placing of undue emphasis on letter r.

pararrhythmia (păr-ăr-ĭth′mĭ-ă). Disturbed or disordered cardiac rhythm.

pararthria (păr-ärth′rĭ-ă). Disordered articulation of speech.

parasalpingitis (păr″ă-săl-pĭn-jī′tĭs). Inflamed condition of tissues around an oviduct or a eustachian tube.

parasigmatism (păr″ă-sĭg′mă-tĭzm). Imperfect pronunciation of the letter S. SYN: *lisping.*

parasite (păr′ă-sīt). An organism that lives within, upon, or at expense of another organism known as the host.

  p., external. One which lives on the outer surface of its host, bugs, fleas, and lice.

  p., facultative. Parasite capable of living independently of its host at certain times.

  p., internal. One living within its host, as worms and fungi.

  p., obligate. Parasite completely dependent on its host.

parasitic (păr-ă-sĭt′ĭk). Like, caused by, or concerning, a parasite.

parasiticide (păr″ă-sĭt′ĭ-sīd). 1. Killing parasites. 2. An agent that will kill parasites. Ex: *sulfur, iodine, mercurial ointment.*

parasitifer (păr-ă-sĭt′ĭ-fĕr). Organism which acts as the host of a parasite.

parasitism (păr′ă-sĭt-ĭzm). 1. The parasitic condition or state. 2. Disease caused by infestation with parasites.

parasitogenic (păr″ă-sī″tō-jĕn′ĭk). 1. Caused by parasites. 2. Favoring parasite development.

parasitology (păr″ă-sī-tŏl′ō-jĭ). The study of parasites, their effect on the human system, and their elimination.

parasitophobia (păr″ă-sī″tō-fō′bĭ-ă). Unusual fear of parasites.

parasitotropic (păr″ă-sī″tō-trŏp′ĭk). Having attraction for parasites.

paraspadia (păr-ă-spā′dĭ-ă). Condition in which the urethra has an opening into 1 side of the penis.

paraspasm (păr′ă-spazm). 1. Muscular spasm of the lower extremities. 2. Spastic paralysis of the lower extremities.

parasteatosis (păr-ă-stē-ă-tō′sĭs). Any disordered condition of the sebaceous secretions. [side of the sternum.

parasternal (păr-ă-stern′ăl). Along the

p. line. Imaginary vertical line running midway bet. sternal margin and line passing through the nipple.

p. region. Area bet. sternal margin and parasternal line.

parasthenia (păr-ăs-thē'nĭ-ă). Condition characterized by abnormal functioning of organic tissue at odd intervals.

parastruma (păr-ă-strŭ'mă). Goiterlike tumor due to hypertrophy of a parathyroid gland.

parasympathetic (păr"ă-sĭm-pă-thet'ĭk). Term applied to the division of the autonomic* nervous system whose fibers arise from the midbrain, the medulla oblongata and sacral portion of the spinal cord.

p. bodies. Coccygeal gland and the intercoracoid body.

parasynovitis (păr-ă-sin-ō-vī'tis). Inflamed condition of tissues about a synovial sac.

parasyphilitic (păr"ă-sif-ĭl-it'ĭk). Marking diseases assumed to be indirectly due to syphilis, but with none of the usual lesions of that disease.

parasystole (păr-ă-sĭs'tō-lē). Abnormally prolonged interval of rest following the cardiac systole.

paratarsium (păr-ă-tar'sĭ-ŭm). The covering and connective tissues of the tarsus of the feet.

paratenon (păr-ă-těn'ŏn). Fatty tissue surrounding a tendon.

paratereseomania (păr"ă-te-rē"sē-ō-mā'nĭ-ă). Insane desire to investigate new scenes and subjects.

paratherapeutic (păr"ă-thĕr-ă-pū'tĭk). Caused by the treatment used for another disease.

parathesin (păr-ăth'e-sĭn). Proprietary analgesic and local anesthetic.

parathormone (păr-ă-thor'mōn). 1. The substance secreted by the parathyroid glands. 2. Commercial name for this substance.

parathymia (păr"ă-thī'mĭ-ă). Disordered state of the emotions.

parathyrin(e (păr-ă-thī'rĭn, -rēn). The active constituent of the parathyroid glands.

parathyroid (păr-ă-thī'royd). 1. Located close to the thyroid gland. 2. One of 4 small epithelial bodies about the size of a pea on the back of and at lower edge of the thyroid gland.

DOSAGE: Sol. *subcut.* or *intramusc.*, 3-6 gr. (0.2-0.4 Gm.).

parathyroidectomy (păr-ă-thī-royd-ĕk'tō-mĭ). Excision of one or more of the parathyroid glands.

parathyroprivia (păr"ă-thī"rō-prĭv'ĭ-ă). Condition which supervenes when the parathyroids are removed.

parathyroprivic, parathyroprivous (păr-ă-thī-rō-prĭv'ĭk, -us). Resulting from loss of function of, or removal of, parathyroid glands.

paratoloid (păr-ăt'ō-loyd). Substance containing extract from the tubercle bacillus. SYN: *tuberculin.*

paratoxin (păr-ă-tok'sĭn). Product composed of bile, without its pigment, and

cholesterol which is used in treating tuberculosis.

paratrichosis (păr"ă-trĭ-kō'sĭs). Any disorder of hair growth, as growth in abnormal places.

paratrimma (păr-ă-trĭm'mă). Chafing; irritation of the skin. SYN: *intertrigo.*

paratrophic (păr-ă-trō'fĭk). 1. Requiring living substances for food; parasitic. 2. Pert. to abnormal nutrition. 3. Pert. to adiposis dolorosa.

paratrophy (păr-at'rō-fĭ). 1. Localized fatty swellings and nerve lesions in various regions of the body. SYN: *Dercum's disease, adiposis dolorosa.* 2. Defective nutrition. SYN: *dystrophy.*

paratuberculosis (păr"ă-tū-bĕr"kū-lō'sĭs). Disease resembling tuberculosis, but in which the tubercle bacillus cannot be demonstrated.

paratyphlitis (păr"ă-tĭf-lī'tĭs). Inflammation of the connective tissue close to the cecum.

paratyphoid (păr-ă-tī'foyd). Similar to typhoid.

p. fever. An infectious fever resembling typhoid.

paratypic (păr-ă-tĭp'ĭk). Relating to differences due to the influences of environment; diverging from a type.

paraumbilical (păr"ă-ŭm-bĭl'ĭk-ăl). Close to the navel.

paraurethral (păr"ă-ū-rē'thrăl). Located close to the urethra.

parauterine (păr"ă-ū'tĕr-ĭn). Around the uterus. [vagina.

paravaginal (păr"ă-văj'ĭn-ăl). Around the

paravaginitis (păr"ă-văj-ĭn-ī'tĭs). Inflammation of the cellular tissue surrounding the vagina.

paraxanthine (păr-ăk-săn'thĭn). A poisonous leukomaine occurring in healthy urine and in excess in gout.

paraxial (păr-ăk'sĭ-ăl). On either side of the axis of the body, or 1 of its parts.

paraxin (păr-ak'sĭn). Commercial diuretic.

paraxon (păr-ăks'ŏn). A collateral branch of a nerve cell's axis cylinder process.

parched (parchd). Dried to extremity.

paregoric (păr-e-gor'ĭk). 1. Soothing. 2. Camphorated tincture of opium, a narcotic containing drug which in large doses is poisonous.

parencephalia (păr"ĕn-sĕf-a'lĭ-ă). Congenital malformation of the cerebrum.

parencephalitis (păr"ĕn-sĕf-ă-lī'tĭs). Inflamed condition of the cerebellum.

parencephalous (păr-ĕn-sef'ă-lŭs). 1. Having a congenital cerebral deformity. 2. Concerning the cerebellum.

parenchyma (păr-ĕn'kĭ-mă). The essential parts of an organ which are concerned with its function in contradistinction to its framework.

p. disease. Disease affecting the principal tissue of an organ.

parenchymatitis (păr-ĕn-kĭ-mă-tī'tĭs). Inflamed condition of parenchyma, or substance of a gland.

parenchymatous (păr-ĕn-kĭm'ăt-ŭs). Concerning the essential substances of an organ.

p. neuritis. Neuritis of the axis cylinder and its myelin sheath.

p. pain. Pain arising at peripheral end of a nerve.

parent (pār'ent). A father or a mother; one who begets offspring.

p. fixation. Continuation of the childparent affiliation into the adult state, so that the person so afflicted is unable to become interested in a person of the opposite sex.

parenteral (păr-ĕn'tĕr-ăl). Situated or occurring outside of the intestines, as by a subcutaneous method.

p. digestion. Digestion of foreign substances by body cells as opposed to *enteral digestion*, which occurs in the alimentary canal.

p. therapy. Introduction of a substance, esp. nutritive material, into the body by means other than the intestinal tract.

parepididymis (par''ep-ĭ-did'ĭ-mis). A small body to front of the spermatic cord above the epididymis. SYN: *paradidymis*.

parergastic reactions (păr-ĕr-găst'ĭk). A general term used by A. Meyer for the essentials involved in schizoid types but without relation to prognosis.

paresis (pă-rē'sĭs, păr'e-sĭs). 1. Partial or incomplete paralysis. 2. An organic mental disease with somatic, irritative and paralytic focal symptoms and signs running a slow, chronic, progressive course and tending to a fatal termination.

p., juvenile. General paresis due to hereditary syphilis, seen in children.

pareso-analgesia (păr''ĕs-ō-ăn-ăl-jē'zĭ-ă). Painlessness with paralysis of the arms.

paressine (păr'ĕs-ēn). Commercial preparation of paraffin, gum, and wax, used as a covering in burns and frostbites.

paresthesia (păr-ĕs-thē'zĭ-ă). Abnormal sensation without objective cause, such as numbness, pricking, etc.; heightened sensitivity.

Experienced in central and peripheral nerve lesions and in locomotor ataxia.

paretic (pă-rĕt'ĭk, pă-rē'tĭk). Affected with or concerning paresis.

pareunia (păr-ū'nĭ-ă). Sexual intercourse. SYN: *coition, coitus, copulation*.

parhormone (păr-hor'mōn). A waste product having a hormonelike function. SEE: *hormone*.

paridrosis (păr-ĭ-drō'sĭs). Any disordered secretion of perspiration.

paries (pā'rĭ-ēs) (pl. *parietes*). The enveloping wall of any structure; applied especially to hollow organs.

parietal (pă-rī'ĕ-tăl). Pert. to, or forming, the wall of a cavity. SEE: *suture, sagittal*.

p. bone. A bone on each side of the cranium or skull.

p. cells. Large cells on margin of the peptic glands of stomach which supposedly secrete hydrochloric acid. SYN: *border cells*.

p. lobe. A central portion of the cerebrum bet. the parieto-occipital and rolandic fissures above the horizontal branch of the fissure of Sylvius.

parietes (pă-rī'ĕ-tēs). Plural of wall; walls of an organ or hollow part.

Paris green (păr'ĭs grēn). A compound of copper and arsenic, *q.v.*; acetoarsenite of copper.

Parkinson's disease (par'kĭn-sŭn). A chronic nervous disease characterized by a fine, slowly spreading tremor, muscular weakness and rigidity and a peculiar gait.

P.'s mask. Expressionless appearance of the face. Eyebrows are raised, wrinkles are smoothed out, and there is immobility of the facial muscles.

A typical symptom seen in Parkinson's disease and in postencephalitic states.

P.'s syndrome. Symptoms of Parkinson's disease.

paroccipital (păr-ŏk-sĭp'ĭt-ăl). 1. Close to the occipital bone. 2. The paramastoid process.

parodontitis (păr''ō-don-tī'tĭs). Inflamed condition of tissues around a tooth.

parodynia (păr-ō-din'ĭ-ă). 1. Labor pains. 2. Difficult or abnormal labor or birth. SYN: *dystocia*.

p. perversa. Presentation with fetus lying transversely across the uterus. SYN: *cross birth*.

parogen (păr'ō-jĕn). An ointment and liniment base containing liquid petrolatum, oleic acid, and ammoniated alcohol.

paroidin (păr-oy'dĭn). Commercial preparation of parathyroid extract used in treatment of tetany.

parolivary (păr-ŏl'ĭ-va-rĭ). Situated close to the olivary body.

p. bodies. Nuclei in medulla oblongata, lying close to the olivary bodies.

paromphalocele (păr-om'fă-lō-sēl''). Hernia or tumor close to the umbilicus.

paroniria (păr-ō-nī'rĭ-ă). Abnormal dreaming of a terrifying nature.

p. ambulans. Sleepwalking.

p. salax. Restlessness in sleep with lascivious dreams and nocturnal emissions.

paronychia (păr-ō-nĭk'ĭ-ă). Acute or chronic infection of marginal structures about the nail.

p. tendinosa. Inflammation of sheath of a digital tendon.

paroöphoron (păr-ō-ŏf'ō-rŏn). Remnant in the broad ligament of the urinary portion of the wolffian body corresponding to the paradidymis in the male.

parophthalmia (păr-ŏf-thăl'mĭ-ă). Inflamed condition of tissue around the eye.

paropsis (păr-op'sĭs). Any disorder of sense of sight.

parorchidium (păr-ŏr-kĭd'ĭ-ŭm). Abnormal position or nondescent of a testicle. SYN: *ectopia testis*.

parorexia (păr-ō-rĕk'sĭ-ă). An abnormal or perverted craving for special or strange foods. SEE: *appetite, taste*.

parosmia (păr-ŏz′mĭ-ă). Any disorder or perversion of the sense of smell; a false sense of odors or perception of those which do not exist.

parosphresia, parosphresis (păr″ŏs-frē′-zĭ-ă, -sĭs). Disordered sense of smell. SYN: *parosmia, q.v.*

parosteitis, parostitis (păr-ŏs-tē-ī′tĭs, -tī′-tĭs). Inflammation of tissues next to the bone.

parosteosis, parostosis (păr-ŏs-tē-ō′sĭs, -tō′sĭs). Bone formation outside of the periosteum. 2. Bone development in an unusual location.

parotid (pă-rŏt′ĭd). 1. Located near the ear. 2. Parotid gland.

    p. duct. One 2 in. long from ant. border of the parotid gland crossing the masseter and piercing the buccinator, and buccal mucous membrane.

    p. gland. Largest of the salivary glands situated on side of the face below and in front of the ear.

parotidectomy (pă-rŏt-ĭd-ĕk′tō-mĭ). Excision of parotid gland.

parotiditis (pă-rŏt-ĭ-dī′tĭs). Inflamed condition of the parotid gland. SYN: *mumps,* parotitis.*

    p., epidemic. Acute, infectious, contagious inflammation and swelling of parotid gland; mumps.

parotidoscirrhus (pă-rŏt″ĭd-ō-skĭr′ŭs). 1. Hardening of the parotid gland. 2. A scirrhous cancer of the parotid area.

parotitis (pă-rō-tī′tĭs). Inflammation of the parotid gland.

parous (pa′rus). Parturient; fruitful; having borne at least 1 child.

parovarian (par-ō-vār′ĭ-ăn). 1. Situated near or beside the ovary. 2. Pert. to the parovarium, a residual structure in the broad ligament.

parovariotomy (păr-ō-vă-rĭ-ŏt′ō-mĭ). Removal of a parovarian cyst.

parovarium (păr″ō-vār′ĭ-ŭm). Vestigial remnant of the wolffian body found in broad ligament representing the sexual portion. SYN: *epoöphoron.*

paroxyl (păr-ŏk′sĭl). Commercial amebicide. SEE: *acetarsone.*

paroxyntic (păr-ŏk-sĭn′tĭk). Like a convulsion; paroxysmal.

paroxysm (păr′ŏk-sĭzm). 1. A sudden, periodic attack or recurrence of symptoms of a disease; an exacerbation of the symptoms of a disease. 2. A fit or convulsion of any kind. 3. Sudden emotional state, as of fear, grief, or joy.

paroxysmal (păr-ŏk-sĭz′măl). 1. Occurring in or concerning paroxysms. 2. Of the nature of a paroxysm.

parresine (păr′ĕs-ēn). A commercial paraffin mixture used as a protective covering for wounds and burns.

par′rot fever. Contagious disease transmitted by parrots and characterized by high fever and disorder of the lungs. SYN: *psittacosis, q.v.*

Parrot's disease (păr-ō′). The pseudoparalysis of the extremities in infants caused by syphilis.

    P.'s nodes. Bony nodules on skull of infants with syphilis.

    P.'s sign. 1. In meningitis, pupils dilate upon pinching the skin of neck. 2. SEE: *Parrot's nodes.*

    P.'s ulcer. Lesions of thrush or stomatitis.

Parry's disease (păr′ē). Swelling of the thyroid gland with increased rate of basal metabolism in hypersecretion of the thyroid gland. SYN: *goiter, exophthalmic; hyperthyroidism, q.v.*

pars (parz). A part.

    p. basilaris. Basilar process of the occipital bone.

    p. caeca oculi. The blind spot of the eye.

    p. carnea diaphragmatis. Muscular portion of diaphragm.

    p. carnosa urethrae. Membranous portion of urethra.

    p. cartilaginea tubae Eustachii. Cartilaginous portion of eustachian tube.

    p. cavernosa. Cavernous portion of urethra.

    p. cephalica nervi sympathici. Plexuses, ganglia, and nerves derived from sympathetic nerve.

    p. cervicalis nervi sympathici. Ganglia, plexuses, and branches of sympathetic nerve in neck.

    p. ciliaris retinae. Portion of retina situated in front of ora serrata.

    p. flaccida. A portion of membrane of the eardrum which fills the notch of Rivinus. SYN: *Shrapnell's membrane.*

    p. frontalis ossis frontis. Upper, larger portion of frontal bone, excluding orbits and nasal process.

    p. genitales. The genitals.

    p. intestinalis choledochi. Portion of ductus choledochus communis that pierces duodenum.

    p. nervosa. Post. lobe of the pituitary gland.

    p. olfactoria. Part of ant. cerebral commissure of brain the fibers of which, in the shape of a horseshoe, turn toward basal mass of head of corpus striatum.

    p. papillaris. Papillary cutaneous layer.

    p. scleralis corneae. Corneal substance proper.

    p. tendinea diaphragmatis. Tendinous portion of diaphragm.

    p. urethrae cavernosa. Cavernous position of urethra.

    p. urethrae membranacea. Membranous portion of urethra.

parthenogenesis (păr″thĕn-ō-jĕn′ĕ-sĭs). 1. Reproduction without fertilization of egg by a male. 2. Reproduction by fission or division. SYN: *asexual reproduction.*

    p., synthetic. Introduction of chemical stimulus into an egg with its subsequent development, in place of natural fertilization by the male.

parturient (păr-tū′rĭ-ĕnt). 1. Concerning childbirth or parturition.* 2. Bringing forth; giving birth. 3. A woman giving birth.

p. canal. Path from uterine cavity to vulva.

p. woman. One in labor.

parturifacient (păr-tū-rĭ-fā'shĕnt). 1. Inducing or accelerating labor. 2. Drug used to cause delivery of the fetus.

parturiometer (păr-tū-rĭ-ŏm'ĕt-ēr). Instrument for determining the expulsive force of the uterus.

parturition (păr-tū-rĭsh'ŭn). Act of giving birth to young. SYN: *childbirth, delivery.*

partus (păr'tŭs). Labor; parturition.

p. agrippinus. Breech presentation in delivery.

p. caesareus. Delivery by cesarean method.

p. difficilis. Difficult labor. SYN: *dystocia.*

p. immaturus. Premature labor.

p. maturus. Labor at term.

p. serotinus. Prolonged or delayed labor

p. siccus. Dry labor with little amniotic fluid.

parulis (păr-ū'lĭs). Abscess in a gum. SYN: *gumboil.*

parumbilical (păr-ŭm-bĭl'ĭ-kăl). Close to the navel.

paruria (păr-ū'rĭ-ă). Any abnormality in discharge of urine.

parvicellular (păr-vĭ-sĕl'ū-lăr). Concerning, or composed of, tiny cells.

parvule (păr'vŭl). A small pill, pellet, or granule.

Paschen bodies (pä'shĕn). Particles supposed to be the pathogenic virus of vaccinia and variola found in great numbers in skin exanthemas.

passage (păs'āj). 1. A communication bet. cavities and body structures or with the ext. surface of an organ. 2. Act of passing. 3. An evacuation of the bowels. 4. Introduction of a probe or catheter, etc.

p's., alveolar. Sacculated communications into which the bronchioles are transformed and into which infundibula open.

p., lacrimal. Lacrimal and nasal ducts.

passion (păsh'ŭn). 1. Suffering. 2. Great emotion, esp. sexual excitement.

p., ileac. Intestinal colic due to obstruction. SEE: *ileus.*

passional (păsh'ŭn-ăl). Exciting or concerning any passion. SEE: *emotional.*

p. attitudes. The stages of hysteria, as an attitude indicating any great emotion.

passive (păs'ĭv). 1. Submissive. 2. Acted upon. 3. Not active.

p. congestion. Congestion due to obstruction in a part.

p. exercise. Muscular exercise without any effort on part of patient.

p. hyperemia. Blood in a part due to decreased outflow.

p. motion. Same as passive exercise. SEE: *exercise, passive.*

p. movement. SEE: *passive exercise.*

passivism (păs'ĭ-vĭzm). Sexual perversion

with subjugation of the will by that of another, usually of the male by the female.

paste (pāst). 1. To cause to adhere. 2. Any ointment whose base is a nonfatty material. 3. A mixture of flour and water, used as an adhesive. 4. A moist, doughy, plastic substance.

Pasteurella (păs-tēr-ĕl'ă). Genus of family Bacteriaceae, characterized by bipolar staining.

P. pestis. Organism causing bubonic plague. [laremia.

P. tularensis. Organism causing tu-

pasteurellosis (păs-tēr-ĕl-ō'sĭs). Disease caused by infection with bacteria of the *Pasteurella* group inducing hemorrhagic septicemia.

pasteurization (păs-tēr-ĭ-zā'shŭn). Partial sterilization and the arrest of fermentation in a fluid by heating it for 30 minutes at 60°-70° C., without destroying its chemical composition.

Pasteur treatment (păs-tēr'). Inoculation with increasingly virulent doses of dead organism causing rabies prepared from spinal cords of infected rabbits, for prevention of hydrophobia.

pastille (păs-tēl'). 1. A small cone used to fumigate or scent the air of a room. 2. A medicated disk used for local action on the mucosa of the throat and mouth. SYN: *lozenge, troche.* 3. PT: Small disk of paper coated with barium platinocyanide or other substances, used to estimate the amount of x-rays administered, also for testing the intensity of ulraviolet radiations.

p. radiometer. An instrument consisting of a color index by means of which the color changes in the pastilles, before and after exposure to roentgen rays, may be gauged. At one time it was used frequently to estimate the quantity of roentgen rays but is now practically obsolete.

patch (pătsh). A blotch distinct from surrounding surface in character and appearance.

p., herald. Oval patch of efflorescence showing before the general eruption of pityriasis rosea; often several days before.

p., Hutchinson's. Salmon-yellow area seen on cornea in syphilitic keratitis.

p., mucous. A syphilitic eruption having an eroded, moist surface; generally on mucous membrane of mouth or ext. genitals or on surface subject to moisture and heat. SYN: *condyloma latum.*

p., opaline. Whitish patch in mouth, sometimes observed in syphilis.

p's., Peyer's. Masses of lymphoid follicles found on mucous membrane of small intestine. SYN: *noduli lymphatici aggregati.*

p., salmon. Salmon-colored area of cornea in ocular syphilis.

p. test. One to detect hypersensitiveness to food, pollen, or other substances by applying suspected substance to an area on the skin.

patella (pǎ-těl'ǎ). The kneecap, or kneepan; a lens-shaped sesamoid bone situated in front of the knee, in the tendon of the quadriceps extensor.

p., floating. A patella which floats up from the condyles due to a large effusion in the knee.

p., fracture of. TREATMENT: Suture of bone fragments. A plaster is then put on, reaching from the toes to the groin, remaining on for 6-8 weeks. Then gradual exercise and weight upon the leg for a few weeks, after which patient may walk.

p., rider's painful. Tenderness and pain in the patella due to horseback riding.

patellapexy (pǎ-těl'ǎ-pěk"sǐ). Fixation of the patella to the lower end of the femur to stabilize the joint.

patellar (pǎ-těl'ǎr). Concerning the patella.

p. paradoxic reflex. Contraction of ant. muscles when leg is forcibly flexed and immediately released.

p. reflex. Involuntary jerk of leg due to sudden spasm of quadriceps following percussion of patellar ligament. SYN: *knee jerk reflex.*

patelliform (pǎ-těl'ǐ-form). Of the shape of the patella.

patellofemoral (pǎ-těl"ō-fěm'or-ǎl). Concerning the patella and the femur.

patency (pā'těn-sē). The state of being freely open.

patent (pǎt'ěnt, pā'těnt). 1. Wide open; evident; accessible. 2. Protected by a trade mark, as a patent medicine. 3. Secured by law for exclusive manufacture. SYN: *patulous.*

pat'ent med'icine. Packaged remedy for public use which is protected by letters patent and sold without a physician's prescription.

pathema (pǎ-thē'mǎ). Disease.

pathergasia (pǎth-ěr-gā'zǐ-ǎ). Any form of malfunctioning, constitutional or structural, which inhibits self-adjustment.

pathetic (pǎ-thět'ǐk). 1. Arousing the tender emotions, as sorrow. 2. Denoting the sup. oblique muscle or its nerve.

p. muscle. Sup. oblique muscle of the eye.

p. nerve. One of 4th cranial pair of nerves supplying the sup. oblique muscle of the eye.

patheticus (pǎ-thět'ǐk-ŭs). 1. Fourth cranial, or trochlear, nerve which supplies sup. oblique muscle of the eye. 2. Superior oblique muscle of the eye.

pathetism (pǎth'ět-ǐzm). State of overcoming another's will by suggestion. SYN: *hypnotism, mesmerism.*

pathfinder (pǎth'fǐnd-ěr). Instrument for locating stricture of the urethra.

pathic (pǎth'ǐk). 1. Concerning disease. 2. Suffering. 3. One whose sexual perversion causes his submission to unnatural relations.

pathoanatomy (pǎth"ō-ǎn-at'ō-mǐ). Dissection and study of diseased organs.

pathobiology (pǎth"ō-bǐ-ol'ō-jǐ). The study of disease. SYN: *pathology.*

pathobolism (pǎth-ŏb'ō-lǐzm). A condition of abnormal or perverted metabolism; seen in diabetes.

pathocrine (pǎth'ō-krǐn, -krēn, -krǐn). Concerning an endocrine disorder.

pathocrinia (pǎth-ō-krǐn'ǐ-ǎ). Abnormal or disordered endocrine function.

pathodixia (pǎth-ō-dǐk'sǐ-ǎ). Exhibitionism in reference to an injury or to disease.

pathodontia (pǎth'ō-dŏn'shǐ-ǎ). Branch of dentistry dealing with diseases of the teeth.

pathoformic (pǎth-ō-for'mǐk). Concerning the beginning symptoms of a condition, as a mental disease.

pathogen (pǎth'ō-jěn). A microörganism or substance capable of producing a disease.

pathogenesis (pǎth-ō-jěn'ě-sǐs). Origination and development of a disease.

p., drug. 1. Morbid symptoms of disease produced by a drug. 2. Observation of all symptoms which may be produced by a drug.

pathogenetic, pathogenic (pǎth"ō-jěn-ět'ǐk, -jěn'ǐk). Productive of disease. SYN: *morbific.*

p. organism. One that produces disease in the body.

pathogeny (pǎth-ōj'ěn-ǐ). The origin or growth of a disease. SYN: *pathogenesis.*

pathognomonic (pǎth-ŏg-nō-mŏn'ǐk). Indicative of a disease, esp. of 1 or more of its characteristic symptoms.

pathologic, pathological (pǎth-ō-lŏj'ǐk, -ǐ-kǎl). 1. Concerning pathology. 2. Diseased; due to a disease. SYN: *morbid.*

p. histology. Histology of diseased tissues.

p. reflex. One resulting in diseased states.

pathologist (pǎ-thŏl'ō-jǐst). A specialist in diagnosing the morbid changes in tissues removed at operations and postmortem examinations.

pathology (pǎ-thŏl'ō-jǐ). 1. Study of the nature and cause of disease which involves changes in structure and function. 2. Condition produced by disease.

p., cellular. That which is based upon microscopic changes in body cells during disease.

p., comparative. The observation of pathological conditions, spontaneous or artificial, in the lower animals or in vegetable organisms as compared to those of human body.

p., experimental. Study of diseases induced intentionally, esp. in animals.

p., general. The general facts of pathology derived from a comparison of particular diseases with each other.

p., geographical. Pathology in its relations to geographical conditions.

p., medical. The pathology of disorders, the treatment of which does not call for operative interference.

p., special. The pathology of particular diseases.

p., surgical. The pathology of surgical diseases.

patholysis (pă-thŏl'ĭ-sĭs). 1. Dissolution or destruction of disease. 2. Dissolution of diseased tissue.

pathomania (păth-ŏ-mā'nĭ-ă). Moral insanity; irresistible tendency toward forbidden conduct with retention of reasoning power.

pathometabolism (păth"ŏ-me-tăb'ŏ-lĭzm). 1. Metabolism in disease. 2. Disordered metabolism.

pathometry (păth-ŏm'ĕt-rĭ). The estimate of the incidence of a disease.

pathomimesis (păth"ŏ-mĭm-e'sĭs). Intentional or unconscious as well as conscious imitation of a disease.

pathomorphism (păth-ŏ-mor'fĭzm). Study of abnormal form and structure of organisms.

pathonomy (păth-ŏn'ŏ-mĭ). Science of the laws of diseased conditions.

pathophilia (păth-ŏ-fĭl'ĭ-ă). Adjustment of habits to conditions made mandatory by some chronic disease.

pathophobia (păth-ŏ-fō'bĭ-ă). Morbid apprehension of disease.

pathophoresis (păth"ŏ-for-e'sĭs). The transmission of disease-producing organisms.

pathophoric (păth-ŏ-for'ĭk). Carrying or transmitting disease, as certain insects.

pathopleiosis (păth"ŏ-plī-ō'sĭs). The tendency to magnify the gravity of one's disease.

pathopoiesis (păth"ŏ-poy-ē'sĭs). The method of disease production.

pathopsychology (păth"ŏ-sĭ-kŏl'ŏ-jĭ). The branch of psychology dealing with mental processes during disease.

patient (pā'shĕnt). 1. Enduring pain or injury. 2. A person who is receiving treatment for disease.

patulous (păt'ū-lŭs). Open; exposed. SYN: *patent.*

paulocardia (pawl"ŏ-kar'dĭ-ă). 1. Sensation of momentary stoppage of heartbeat. 2. Undue prolongation of the rest period in the cardiac cycle.

pavement (pāv'mĕnt). Any structure resembling a tiled floor, or pavement.

p. epithelium. Flattened, single layer of epithelial cells resembling a tiled floor.

pavilion (păv-ĭl'yŭn). 1. A flaring expansion at the extremity of a canal or tube. 2. A tent-shaped structure.

p. of the pelvis. The flare of the ilia, the expanded part of the pelvis.

pavor (pā'vor). Anxiety, dread.

p. nocturnus. Night terror during sleep in children and the aged.

Pavy's disease (pā'vē). Albuminuria which recurs at periodic intervals.

Pb. SYMB: *plumbum,* lead.

pearl (pĕrl). 1. Small, tough mass in sputum in asthma. 2. Small, hollow glass capsule containing a fluid for inhalation, as amyl nitrite.

p., epithelial. Concentric squamous epithelial cells in carcinoma.

p., gouty. Sodium urate concretion on cartilage of the ear seen in people with gout.

peccant (pek'ant). Corrupt; producing disease. SYN: *pathogenic, unhealthy, morbid.*

peccatiphobia (pĕk-ăt-ĭ-fō'bĭ-ă). Abnormal dread of sinning.

peciloblast (pē-sĭl'ŏ-blăst). Large, malformed, red blood cell. SYN: *poikiloblast, poikilocyte.*

pecilocyte (pē-sĭl'ŏ-sīt). Large red blood cell of irregular shape. SYN: *peciloblast, poikiloblast, poikilocyte.*

pecilocythemia (pē-sĭl"ŏ-sī-thē'mĭ-ă). Pecilocytes in the blood. SYN: *pecilocytosis.*

pecilocytosis (pē-sĭl"ŏ-sī-tō'sĭs). Pecilocytes in the blood stream. SYN: *pecilocythemia.*

pecilothermal (pē-sĭl"ŏ-ther'măl). 1. Not constant in temperature, denoting cold blooded animals. 2. Capable of developing in varying degrees of temperature.

Pecquet's cistern (pē-ka'). A reservoir for chyle at lower end of the thoracic duct. SEE: *chylocyst, receptaculum chyli.*

P.'s duct. Passage from the cisterna chyli to the joining point of the left subclavian and int. jugular veins, acting as a lymph channel.

P.'s reservoir. SEE: *Pecquet's cistern.*

pectase (pĕk'tās). Enzyme facilitating the conversion of pectin into peptic acid.

pecten (pĕk'tĕn). 1. The pubic bone. 2. A comblike organ. 3. Middle portion of anal canal.

p. band. Fiberlike induration of the iliopectineal line.

p. commissurae anterioris. Transverse fibrous bundles of the ant. cerebral commissure.

p. pubis. Ridge on horizontal ramus of the os pubis from its spine, continuous with the *linea arcuata* of the ilium.

p. sclerae. Opening on sclera for passage of the optic nerve.

pectenitis (pĕk-tĕn-ī'tĭs). Inflamed condition of the sphincter ani.

pectenosis (pĕk"tĕn-ō'sĭs). Fibrosis of the pecten which produces the pectenosis band.

pectic acid (pĕk'tĭk). An acid derived from pectin by hydrolyzing the methyl ester group which is found in many fruits.

pectin (pĕk'tĭn). A white, amorphous, plant carbohydrate that forms a gelatinous mass in the cooking of fruits and vegetables, causing them to "jell." SEE: *pectose.*   [a comb.

pectinate (pĕk'tĭn-āt). Having teeth like a comb.

pectineal (pĕk'tĭn'ē-ăl). Relating to the os pubis or the pectineus muscle.

p. line. The line or ridge on the os pubis separating the true from the false pelvis. SYN: *iliopectineal line, linea terminalis.*

p. muscle. Muscle on upper inner portion of thigh aiding in adduction and flexion.

pectineus (pĕk-tĭn'ē-ŭs). A flat, triangular muscle at upper and inner part of thigh arising from iliopectineal line and inserted bet. lesser trochanter and linea aspera of the femur, which flexes and adducts the outward thigh.

pectiniform (pĕk-tĭn'ĭ-form) Toothed like a comb. SYN: *pectinate*.

pectization (pĕk-tĭ-zā'shŭn). In colloidal chemistry, coagulation.

pectoral (pĕk'tō-răl). 1. Concerning the chest. 2. Efficacious in relieving chest conditions, as a cough.

pectoralgia (pĕk-tō-ral'jĭ-ă). Neuralgic pain in the breast.

pectoralis (pĕk-tō-rā'lĭs). One of 4 muscles of the breast.

   p. major. A large triangular muscle extending to the humerus which draws the arm forward and downward and aids in chest expansion.

   p. minor. Muscle beneath pectoralis major, extending to scapula, which lowers the scapula and depresses the shoulder point.

pectoriloquy (pĕk-tō-rĭl'ō-kwĭ). The distinct transmission of vocal sounds to the ear through the chest wall in auscultation.*

   p., aphonic. In auscultation, whispered sound heard over a lung with a cavity or pleural effusion.

   p., whispering. Sound over a lung with a cavity of limited extent when patient whispers, in auscultation of the chest.

pectorophony (pĕk-tō-rof'ō-nĭ). Exaggeration of vocal sounds heard on auscultation of the chest. SYN: *pectoriloquy*.

pectose (pĕk'tōs). A substance found in some fruits and vegetables that yields pectin when it is boiled.

pectunculus (pĕk-tŭn'kū-lŭs). One of the tiny longitudinal ridges on the sylvian aqueduct.

pectus (pĕk'tŭs). The chest; breast; thorax.

   p. carinatum. Abnormal prominence of the sternum. SYN: *chicken* or *pigeon breast*.

pedal (pĕd'ăl, pē'dăl). Concerning the foot.

pederast (pĕd'ĕr-ăst). One who indulges in the unnatural, illegal habit of sexual intercourse with men, esp. young boys, through the anus.

pederasty (pĕd'ĕr-ăs-tĭ). Illicit coitus by the anus with males, esp. with young boys. SYN: *sodomy*.

pedialgia (pĕd-ĭ-al'jĭ-ă, pē-dĭ-al'jĭ-ă). Pain of the foot.

pediatric (pē-dĭ-ăt'rĭk). Concerning the treatment of children.

pediatrician (pē-dĭ-ă-trĭsh'an). A specialist in treatment of children's diseases. SYN: *pediatrist*.

pediatrics (pē-dĭ-ăt'rĭks). Medical science relating to hygienic care of children and treatment of diseases peculiar to them. SYN: *pediatry*.

pediatrist (pē''dĭ-ăt'rĭst). Physician who specializes in treatment of children's diseases.

pediatry (pĕd'ĭ-ăt-rĭ, pē-dĭ'ăt-rĭ). The treatment of children's diseases. SYN: *pediatrics*.

pedicellation (pĕd''ĭ-sĕl-ā'shŭn). Formation and development of a pedicle.

pedicle (pĕd'ĭ-kl). 1. A slender stem, as the attachment of a tumor. 2. The bony process projecting backward which connects the lamina of a vertebra on either side.

pedicular (pē-dĭk'ū-lar). 1. Infested with or concerning lice. 2. Concerning a stalk or stem.

pediculate (pē-dĭk'ū-lāt). Having a pedicle or stem. SYN: *pedunculate*.

pediculation (pē-dĭk-ū-lā'shŭn). 1. Infestation with lice. 2. Development of a pedicle.

pediculicide (pē-dĭk'ū-lĭ-sĭd). Destroying or that which destroys lice.

pediculophobia (pē-dĭk''ū-lō-fō'bĭ-ă). Abnormal dread of lice. SYN: *phthiriophobia*.

pediculosis (pē-dĭk-ū-lō'sĭs). Lousiness; infestation with lice. SEE: *pediculus, 2.*

pediculus (pē-dĭk'ū-lŭs). 1. A pedicle. 2. [C] Genus of parasitic insects; lice.

   P. capitis. A form affecting the scalp.

   P. corporis. The body louse which causes red or purple eruptions on skin as the result of its bite.

   P. pubis. The crab louse affecting the genital, abdominal, and presternal regions, often the result of body contacts. SYN: *morpio*.

   P. vestimenti. SEE: *Pediculus corporis.*

pedicure (ped'ĭ-kūr). 1. Care of the feet. 2. A chiropodist or one who cares for the feet. 3. The care, painting, and polishing of the toenails.

pediluvium (pĕd-ĭ-lū'vĭ-ŭm). A foot bath.

pedionalgia (pĕd-ĭ-ō-nal'jĭ-ă). Neuralgic pain in the sole of the foot. SYN: *metatarsalgia*.

pediophobia (pē-dĭ-ō-fō'bĭ-ă). Unnatural dread of young children or of dolls.

pedobaromacrometer (pē''dō-băr''ō-măk-rŏm'ĕt-ēr). Apparatus for determining measurement and weight of infants.

pedobarometer (pē''dō-băr-om'ĕt-ēr). Apparatus for weighing infants.

pedodontia, pedodontics (pē''dō-don'shĭ-ă, -tĭks). Phase of dentistry dealing with care of children's teeth.

pedodontist (pē''dō-dŏn'tĭst). Dentist who specializes in care of children's teeth.

pedograph (pĕd'ō-grăf). Imprint of the foot on paper.

pedologist (pē-dŏl'ō-jĭst). One who has made a study of children and their development.

pedology (pē-dŏl'ō-jĭ). The study of children and their development.

pedometer (pē-dom'ĕt-ēr). 1. Device for measurement of infants. 2. (pē-dŏm'ĕt-ēr). Watch which indicates number of steps taken in walking.

pedomorphism (pē''dō-mor'fĭzm). Retention of juvenile characteristics in the adult.

pedonosology (pē″dō-nŏs-ŏl′ō-jĭ). The study of children's diseases. SYN: *pediatrics*.

pedophilia (pē″dō-fĭl′ĭ-ă). 1. Fondness for children.
2. PSY: Unnatural desire for sexual relations with children.

peduncle (pē-dung′kl). 1. A stem or stalk. SYN: *pedicle*. 2. A brachium of the brain; a band connecting parts of the brain. SYN: *pedunculus*. SEE: *cimbia, crus, sessile*.

p., callosal. Fibrous band from sylvian fissure to area under the callosum.

p., cerebral. White bundle from upper part of the pons to the cerebrum. SYN: *crus cerebri*.

p., pineal. A band from either side of the pineal gland to the ant. pillars of the fornix.

peduncular (pē-dun′kū-lar). Concerning a peduncle.

pedunculate, pedunculated (pē-dŭn′kū-lāt, -ed). Possessing a stalk or peduncle. SYN: *pediculate*.

pedunculus (pē-dŭn′kū-lŭs). A stalk or peduncle, *q.v.*

p. ant. callosi. Ant. extremity of the *corpus callosum*.

p. flocci. Constricted part of a cerebellar lamina.

p. pulmonum. Root of the lung.

p. trigoni cerebralis ant. Ant. pillar of the fornix.

peinotherapy (pī-nō-thĕr′ă-pĭ). Hunger cure for disease. SYN: *pinotherapy*.

pelada, pelade (pĕ-la′dă, -lăd). 1. Loss of hair on circumscribed areas of the scalp. SYN: *alopecia areata*. 2. Disease resembling pellagra, caused by infected maize.　　　　　　　　[collectively.

pelage (pĕ-lahj′). The hair of the body

pelicology (pĕl-ĭk-ŏl′ō-jĭ). The science of the pelvis and its relation to other structures in the body.

pelidisi (pĕl-ĭd-ē′sē). Pirquet's unit index for the nutritive development of children.

pelioma (pĕl-ĭ-ō′mă). A livid cutaneous patch. SYN: *ecchymosis*.

peliosis (pĕl-ĭ-ō′sĭs). A disease marked by purple patches on the mucous membranes and skin. SYN: *purpura*.

p. rheumatica. An acute affection characterized by inflammation of the joints.

pellagra (pĕl-ā′gră, pĕ-lăg′ră). An endemic deficiency disease affecting chiefly cerebrospinal and digestive systems resulting from improper diet.

p. sine pellagra. Former name for condition due to riboflavin deficiency.

pellagracein (pĕl-ă-gra′sē-ĭn). Poisonous substance in decomposed cornmeal. SYN: *pellagrazein*.

pellagragenic (pĕ-lā-gră-jĕn′ĭk). Producing pellagra.

pellagrazein (pĕl-ă-grā′zē-ĭn). Poisonous substance in cornmeal that has decomposed. SYN: *pellagracein*.

pellagrin (pĕ-lā′grĭn, -lăg′rĭn). A person afflicted with pellagra.

pellagrous (pĕ-lā′grŭs, -lăg′rŭs). Concerning or affected with pellagra.

pellet (pĕl′ĕt). A tiny pill or small ball of medicine or food.

pelletierine tan′nate (pĕl″ĕ-tēr′ĕn). USP. A mixture of the tannates of alkaloids obtained from the pomegranate.

DOSAGE: 4 gr. (0.25 Gm.) in capsule, after adm. of a mild purgative, previous fasting, followed by a purgative. ·

pellicle (pĕl′ĭ-kl). 1. A thin piece of cuticle or skin. 2. Film or surface on a liquid. SYN: *scum*.

pellotine (pĕl′ō-tēn). A white, crystalline alkaloid used as a hypnotic.　　　[parent.

pellucid (pĕ-lū′sĭd). Translucent; transp. zone. Clear layer covering the oöcyte. SYN: *zona pellucida*.

pelveoperitonitis (pĕl″vē-ō-pĕr-ĭ-tō-nī′tĭs). Inflammation of the peritoneum in the pelvic region. SYN: *pelviperitonitis*.

pelvic (pĕl′vĭk). Pert. to the bony basin of trunk formed by innominate bones, sacrum, and coccyx.　　　[nate bones.

p. girdle. Arch made by the innomi-

p. inlet. Upper pelvic entrance, the brim of the pelvis forming its boundary.

p. outlet. Lower pelvic opening.

pelvilithotomy (pĕl″vĭ-lĭ-thŏt′ō-mĭ). Removal of a stone from the renal pelvis. SYN: *nephrolithotomy, pelviolithotomy, pyelolithotomy*.

pelvimeter (pĕl-vĭm′ĕt-ĕr). Device for measuring the pelvis.

pelvimetry (pĕl-vĭm′ĕt-rĭ). Measurement of the pelvic dimensions or proportions.

pelviolithotomy (pĕl″vĭ-ō-lĭ-thŏt′ō-mĭ). Incision of the renal pelvis to remove a calculus.

pelvioperitonitis (pĕl″vĭ-ō-pĕr-ĭ-tō-nī′tĭs). Inflammation of the peritoneum lining the pelvic region.

pelvioplasty (pĕl-vĭ-ō-plăs″tĭ). Enlargement of the outlet of the pelvis. SYN: *hebotomy, symphyseotomy*.

pelvioscopy (pĕl″vĭ-ŏs′kō-pĭ). Inspection of the pelvis.

pelviotomy (pĕl-vĭ-ŏt′ō-mĭ). 1. Incision of pelvic bones, esp. in case of difficult labor. 2. Incision into the renal pelvis.

pelviperitonitis (pĕl″vĭ-pĕr-ĭ-tō-nī′tĭs). Inflammation of the peritoneum in the pelvic region. SYN: *pelveoperitonitis*.

pelvis (pĕl′vĭs) (pl. *pelves*). 1. Any basin-shaped structure or cavity. 2. The bony structure formed by the innominate bones, the sacrum, the coccyx, and the ligaments uniting them, which serves as a support for the post. portion of the limbs. 3. The area included within these bones.

p., aequabiliter justo major. One symmetrically above standard in all its dimensions.

p., aequabiliter justo minor. One with all equally below standard.

p., beaked. One with the pelvic bones laterally compressed and pushed forward so that outlet is narrow and long.

p., brim of. SEE: *inlet of pelvis*.

p., caoutchouc. Same as India rubber pelvis.

p., Capuron's cardinal points of. Four points within the pelvic inlet, the 2 sacroiliac articulations and the 2 iliopectineal eminences.

p., cordate. Pelvis which has a heart shape.

p., coxalgic. One deformed subsequent to hip joint disease.

p., dwarf. An aequabiliter justo minor pelvis.

p., dynamic. The pelvis as related to force, as in labor.

p., elastic. An osteomalacic pelvis.

p., false. Portion above the iliopectineal line.

p., fissured. A rachitic pelvis with ilia pushed forward so as to be almost parallel.

p., fracture of. Bed rest most important. A firm binder is applied round the pelvis and, if the displacement is severe, the legs are placed in Braun's splints with extension. Movements of all joints are allowed. If the fracture is severe the bladder or intestines may be injured; a catheter is usually passed as soon as possible after the accident to see if the urethra or bladder have been injured. The patient must be carefully watched and the urine measured and tested.

p., giant. SEE: *pelvis aequabiliter justo major.*

p., Hauder's. Same as *pelvis spinosa.*

p., inclination of, obliquity of. The angle between the axis of the pelvis and that of the body.

p., India rubber. A pelvis, the bones of which may be stretched out of normal position in osteomalacia. SYN: *caoutchouc pelvis.*

p., inverted. SEE: *split pelvis.*

p., Kilian's. SEE: *osteomalacic pelvis.*

p., kyphotic. Deformed pelvis characterized by increase of the conjugate diameter in the brim with reduction of the transverse diameter at the outlet.

p., lordotic. Deformed pelvis in which the spinal column has an ant. curvature in the lumbar region.

p., malacosteon. SEE: *rachitic pelvis.*

p., masculine. A woman's pelvis that is funnel-shaped like that of a man.

p., Nägele's. Oblique pelvis. Distorted pelvis in which the conjugate diameter takes an oblique direction.

p., osteomalacic. Pelvis distorted as a consequence of osteomalacia.

p., Prague. SEE: *spondylolisthetic pelvis.*

p., pseudoösteomalacic. A rickety pelvis similar to that of a person affected with osteomalacia.

p., rachitic. One deformed from rickets.

p., reduced. SEE: *aequabiliter justo minor.*

p., reniform. Pelvis shaped like a kidney.

p., Robert's. One with an embryonic sacrum and narrowing of the transverse and oblique diameters.

p., Rokitansky's. SEE: *spondylolisthetic pelvis.*

p., rostrate. SEE: *beaked pelvis.*

p., rotunda. A tympanic depression in the inner wall, at the bottom of which is the fenestra rotunda.

p., round. One with a circular inlet.

p., rubber. An osteomalacic pelvis.

p., scoliotic. Deformed pelvis due to spinal curvature.

p., simple flat. One whose deformity is a shortened anteroposterior diameter.

p. spinosa. A rachitic pelvis with a pointed crest of the pubis.

p., split. One with a congenital division at the symphysis pubis.

p., spondylolisthetic. A pelvis in which the last lumbar vertebra is dislocated in front of the sacrum causing occlusion of the brim.

p., triangular. One whose inlet is triangular.

p., triradiate. SEE: *beaked pelvis.*

p., true. The part of the pelvis below the iliopectineal line.

pelvitherm (pĕl'vĭ-thurm). Device for heating the pelvis.

pelvitomy (pĕl-vĭt'ō-mĭ). Incision of the pelvis to aid delivery.

pelvoscopy (pĕl-vŏs'kō-pĭ). Inspection of a pelvis.

pelycalgia (pĕl-ĭ-kăl'jĭ-ă). Pain in the pelvic area.

pelycogram (pĕl'ĭ-kō-grăm). An x-ray of the pelvis.

pelycography (pĕl-ĭ-kŏg'ră-fĭ). Treatise describing the pelvis.

pemphigoid (pĕm'fĭ-goyd). Similar to pemphigus.

pemphigus (pĕm'fĭ-gŭs). An acute or chronic disease of adults characterized by occurrence of successive crops of bullae appearing suddenly on apparently normal skin, and which disappear, leaving pigmented spots.

p. acutus. Butcher's pemphigus. Constitutional symptoms severe and outcome often fatal. Bullae 1-10 cm. in diameter often containing blood and serum. If coalescing, denuded areas are formed.

p. benignus. A mild form of pemphigus.

p. chronicus, p. vulgaris. Uncomplicated form in which replacement of epidermis follows. Lesions round or oval, thin walled, tense, translucent, contents bilateral in distribution, developing suddenly, without scarring resulting.

p. circinatus. Pemphigus with circular eruptions.

p. contagiosa. An infective type of groin and axilla.

p. disseminatus. Pemphigus marked by widely separated bullae.

p. foliaceus. Rare type. Large flaccid bullae developing rapidly, rupture soon, leaving moist, raw surface covered with seropurulent fluid. Bullous contents are purulent from beginning with sickening odor. Chronic course.

p. neonatorum. Pemphigus soon after birth, generally due to septic infection but sometimes luetic.

p. pruriginosus. Pemphigus with severe, continuous itching.

p. syphiliticus. A form due to syphilis.

p. vegetans. Resembles *pemphigus vulgaris* in beginning, but instead of drying up, the lesions persist, resulting in papillary excrescences with no tendency to heal, secreting foul-smelling seropurulent fluid and sodden decomposing masses of epidermis.

pencillin (pĕn-sĭl'ĭn). A substance from the family of molds known as pencillium. A most powerful nontoxic germ killer. Active in dilutions of 1 to 500,000.

pendent (pĕn'dĕnt). Supported from above; hanging.

pendular (pĕn'dū-lĕr). Hanging so as to swing by an attached part; oscillating like a pendulum.

pendulous (pĕn'dū-lŭs). Swinging freely like a pendulum; hanging.

pendulum (pĕn'dū-lŭm). Body suspended from a fixed point and free to swing to and fro.

p. movements. To and fro movement which churns the contents of intestine during digestion, mixing them with ferments without peristaltic action. SEE: *colon, digestion in.*

p. rhythm. Disordered cardiac rhythm in which the diastolic sound resembles the systolic sound so that the completed cardiac cycle sounds like the ticking of a clock.

penetrate (pĕn'e-trāt). To enter into the interior of; to permeate.

penetrating (pĕn'e-trāt-ĭng). Entering beyond the exterior.

p. power. Penetrating capacity of a lens.

p. wound. Wound affecting the interior of an organ or cavity.

penetration (pĕn"e-trā'shŭn). 1. Process of entering within a part. 2. Capacity to enter within a part. 3. Power of a lens to give a clear focus at varying depths.

penetrometer (pĕn-e-trŏm'ĕt-ĕr). PT: An instrument that compares roughly the comparative absorption of roentgen rays in various metals, esp. silver, lead, and aluminum; hence, it gives a rough estimation of hardness of roentgen rays.

penial (pē'nĭ-ăl). Concerning the penis.

penicilliosis (pĕn"ĭ-sĭl'ĭ-ō'sĭs). Infection with the fungi of the genus *Penicillium.*

Penicillium (pĕn"ĭ-sĭl'ĭ-ŭm). A genus of molds seen on fruit, bread, cheese, etc., which affects the skin and mucosa of man.   [SYN: *penile.*

penile (pē'nĭl, -nīl). Pert. to the penis.

p. reflex. 1. Sudden downward movement of penis when the prepuce or gland of a completely relaxed penis is pulled upward. 2. Contraction of bulbocavernous muscle on percussing dorsum of penis. 3. Contraction of bulbocavernous muscle resulting from compression of glans penis.

penis (pē'nĭs) (pl. *penes*). The generative organ of the male.

p. captivus. Forcible retention of the penis in the vagina during copulation due to spasm of the vaginal muscles preventing withdrawal.

p. cerebri. The pineal gland.

p. lunatus. Painful curved erection in gonorrhea. SYN: *chordee, q.v.*

p. muliebris. Clitoris,* the erectile organ of the female.

penitis (pē-nī'tĭs). Inflammation of the penis.

penniform (pĕn'ĭ-form). Feather-shaped.

pennyroyal (pĕn'ĭ-roi'ăl). Name for various plants, esp. Hedeoma and Mentha, which yield commercial oil used as emmenagogue, carminative, and stimulant.

pennyweight (pĕn'ĭ-wāt). Troy weight containing 24 gr. or 1/20 of an ounce.

pension neurosis (pĕn'shŭn nū-rō'sĭs). A condition which develops subsequent to an injury in the belief that compensation can be obtained by being ill. SEE: *neurosis, compensation.*   [*five.*

penta-, pent-. Combining form meaning

pentad (pĕn'tăd). 1. A radical or element with a valence of 5. 2. Group of 5.

pental (pĕn'tăl). C_5H_{10}. Trimethylethylene, a hydrocarbon, used as an anesthetic in minor surgery.

pentamethylendiamine (pĕn"tă-mĕth"ĭl-ĕn-dī'ăm-ēn). A pathogenic ptomaine occurring in tissue decomposition. SYN: *cadaverine, q.v.*

pentane (pĕn'tăn). C_5H_{12}. One of the hydrocarbons of the methane series used as an anesthetic.

pentavalent (pĕn"tă-vā'lĕnt, -tăv'ă-lent). Having a valence of 5. SYN: *quinquivalent.*

pentene (pĕn'tēn). A liquid hydrocarbon used as an anesthetic.

pentnucleotide (pĕnt-nū'klē-ō-tīd). A solution prepared from yeast nucleic acid. DOSAGE: From 10 to 20 cc. intramuscularly.

pentobarbital sodium (pĕn"tō-bar'bĭ-tăl sō'dĭ-ŭm). A barbituric acid derivative used as an analgesic, sedative, and hypnotic, prior to anesthesia.

pentosazon (pĕn"tō-sa'zŏn). Abnormal substance in urine which is incapable of fermentation.

pentose (pĕn'tōs). $C_5H_{10}O_5$. A simple sugar with 5 atoms of oxygen in the molecule.

pentosemia (pĕn"tō-sē'mĭ-ă). Pentose in the blood.

pentoside (pĕn'tō-sĭd). Pentose combined with some other substance.

pentosuria (pĕn"tō-sū'rĭ-ă). A condition in which pentose is found in the urine.

pentothal sodium (pĕn'tō-thăl sō'dĭ-ŭm). Commercial barbituric acid derivative used as an anesthetic and hypnotic.

peonin (pē'ō-nĭn). A dye used as a hydrogen ion concentration test.

peotillomania (pe'ō-tĭl-ō-mā'nĭ-ă). A tic resulting in constant pulling at the penis. SYN: *pseudomasturbation.*

peotomy (pē-ŏt'ō-mĭ). Amputation of the penis.

pepo (pē′pō). USP. Pumpkin seed which is used as an agent to remove tapeworms.

DOSAGE: 1 oz. (30 cc.).

peppermint (pĕp′ĕr-mĭnt). USP. The top and leaves of the plant Mentha piperita from which oil of peppermint is derived.

pepsic (pĕp′sĭk). 1. Concerning digestion. 2. Concerning pepsin. SYN: *peptic*.

pepsin (pĕp′sĭn). The chief enzyme of gastric juice which converts proteins into proteoses and peptones.

DOSAGE: 8 gr. (0.5 Gm.).

p. unit. Standard amount for measurement of ratio of pepsin to gastric juice.

pepsinia (pĕp-sĭn′ĭ-ă). Secretion of pepsin in gastric juice. SEE: *apepsinia, hyperpepsinia, hypopepsinia*.

pepsinogen (pĕp-sĭn′ō-jĕn). A gastric ferment that is converted into pepsin in the stomach during digestion.

pepsinum (pĕp-sī′nŭm). A ferment in the gastric juice which hydrolyzes protein into proteoses and peptones in presence of an acid. SYN: *pepsin, q.v.*

peptarnis (pĕp-tar′nĭs). Preparation of beef peptones.

peptenzyme (pĕpt-ĕn′zīm). Commercial digestive stimulant made of gastric glands.

peptic (pĕp′tĭk). 1. Concerning digestion. 2. Concerning pepsin.

p. cells. Those of the gastric glands secreting pepsin.

p. ulcer. An ulcer of the stomach.

peptide (pĕp′tĭd). Compound formed by hydrolytic cleavage of peptones and which contains 2 or more amino acids.

peptidolytic (pĕp″tĭd-ō-lĭt′ĭk). Causing the splitting up or digestion of peptides.

peptinotoxin (pĕp-tĭn-ō-tŏk′sĭn). Poisonous ptomaine found in the body as a result of disordered or defective digestion.

peptization (pĕp-tĭ-zā′shŭn). In the chemistry of colloids, the process of making a colloidal solution more stable; conversion of a gel to a sol.

peptize (pĕp′tīz). To disperse an insoluble material to a colloidal solution.

peptogenic, peptogenous (pĕp-tō-jĕn′ĭk, -tŏj′ĕn-ŭs). 1. Producing peptones. 2. Promoting digestion.

peptoid (pĕp′toyd). A product of protein digestion which does not give the biuret reaction.

peptolysis (pĕp-tŏl′ĭ-sĭs). The splitting up or hydrolysis of peptones.

peptolytic (pĕp-tō-lĭt′ĭk). Pert. to the splitting up of peptone.

peptone (pĕp′tōn). Secondary protein formed through the action of gastric (pepsin) and pancreatic (trypsin) juices on albumins.

peptonemia (pĕp-tō-nē′mĭ-ă). Peptones in the blood.

peptonization (pĕp″tō-nĭ-zā′shŭn). Process of changing protein substance into peptones by action of proteolytic enzymes.

peptonized milk (pĕp′tō-nīzd). This is milk that has been predigested by the addition of pancreatic extract and sodium bicarbonate, before feeding, to prevent formation of tough curds in stomach.

peptonoid (pĕp′tō-noyd). A substance similar to a peptone.

peptonuria (pĕp-tō-nū′rĭ-ă). Excretion of peptones in the urine.

peptotoxin (pĕp″tō-tŏks′ĭn). A poisonous product found in an early stage of protein decomposition.

per-. Prefix meaning *through, by, by means of.* In chemistry, the *maximum of an element in a combination.*

peracidity (pŭr-ăs-ĭd′ĭt-ĭ). Abnormal acidity.

peracute (pŭr-ăk-ūt′). Very acute or violent.

per anum (pŭr ā′nŭm). Through or by way of the anus.

percaine (pŭr′kā-ĭn). A quinoline derivative used as a local anesthetic, which is powerful and toxic.

perception (pŭr-sĕp′shŭn). 1. Process of being aware of objects; consciousness. 2. The process of receiving sensory impressions. 3. The elaboration of a sensory impression; the ideational association modifying, defining, and usually completing the primary impression or stimulus.

perceptivity (pŭr-sĕp-tĭv′ĭ-tĭ). Power to receive sense impressions.

percolate (pŭr′kō-lāt). 1. To seep through a powdered substance. 2. Any fluid that has been filtered or percolated. 3. To strain a fluid through powdered substances in order to impregnate it with soluble principles of such substances.

percolation (pŭr″kō-lā′shŭn). 1. Filtration. 2. Process of exhausting virtues of a drug of powdered composition by filtering a liquid solvent through it.

percolator (pŭr′kō-lā″tŭr). Apparatus used for extraction of a drug with a liquid solvent.

per contiguum (pŭr kŏn-tĭg′ū-ŭm). Touching, as in the spread of an inflammation from 1 part to a contiguous structure.

per continuum (pŭr kŏn-tĭn′ū-ŭm). Continuous, as the spread of an inflammation from part to part.

percuss (pŭr-kŭs′). To tap parts of the body to aid diagnosis by sound emitted.

percussion (pŭr-kŭsh′ŭn). Tapping the body lightly but sharply to determine position, size and consistency of an underlying structure, the presence of fluid or pus in a cavity and resonance pitch and resistance by the sound emitted.

p., auscultatory. Percussion combined with auscultation.

p., finger. Striking of the finger resting upon the body with a finger of the other hand.

percussor (pŭr-kŭs′or). Device used for diagnosis by percussion, consisting of hammer with rubber or metal head. SEE: *emballometer*.

percutaneous (pŭr″kŭ-tā′nē-ŭs). Effected through the skin, as in inunction and friction.

pereirine (pĕ-rā'rēn). An alkaloid obtained from pereira bark which is used as a tonic, antiperiodic, and antipyretic.

perflation (pŭr-flā'shŭn). The process of blowing air into a cavity to expand its walls or to force out secretions or other matter.

perforans (pŭr'fō'răns). Perforating or penetrating, as a nerve or muscle.

perforate (pŭr'fō-rāt). 1. To puncture or to make holes. 2. Pierced with holes.

perforation (pŭr''fō-rā'shŭn). 1. The act or process of making a hole, such as that caused by ulceration. 2. Hole made through substance or part.

   p. of stomach or intestine. SYM: Abdominal crisis due to escape of contents of the perforated viscus into the peritoneal cavity. Peritonitis certain unless operated upon in time. Onset is accompanied by acute pain over perforated area spreading all over the abdomen which is rigid. Face is anxious with beads of perspiration on it. Nausea and vomiting will occur. Pulse rapid and feeble, respiration rapid and shallow. Temperature drops, but rises as peritonitis sets in, when pulse becomes fuller.

perforator (pŭr'fō-rā-tor). Instrument for piercing the skull and other bones.

   p., tympanum. Instrument for perforating the tympanum.

perfrication (pŭr-frī-kā'shŭn). Thorough rubbing with an ointment or embrocation. SYN: *inunction.*

perfusion (pŭr-fū'zhŭn). Passing of a fluid through spaces.

peri-. Prefix meaning *around, about.*

periacinal, periacinous (pĕr''ī-ăs'ī-năl, -ŭs). Placed around an acinus.

periadenitis (pĕr-ĭ-ă-dē-nī'tĭs). Inflamed condition of tissues surrounding a gland.

perialienitis (pĕr''ī-ă''lī-ĕn-ī'tĭs). Noninfectious inflammation around a foreign body. SYN: *perixenitis.*

periamygdalitis (pĕr''ī-ăm-ĭg''dăl-ī'tĭs). Inflammation of connective tissue around the tonsil. SYN: *peritonsillitis.*

periangiocholitis (pĕr''ī-ăn''jĭ-ō-kō-lī'tĭs). Inflamed condition of tissues around the bile ducts.

periangitis (pĕr''ī-ăn-jī'tĭs). Inflamed condition of tissue around a blood or lymphatic vessel.

periaortitis (pĕr''ī-ă-or-tī'tĭs). Inflamed condition of adventitia and tissues around the aorta.

periapical (pĕr''ī-ăp'ī-kăl). Around the apex of the root of a tooth.

periappendicitis (pĕr''ī-ă-pĕn-dĭ-sī'tĭs). Inflamed condition of appendix with its surrounding tissues. SYN: *perityphlitis.*

   p. decidualis. Decidual cells in the peritoneum of the appendix vermiformis in cases of tubal pregnancy due to adhesions bet. fallopian tubes and the appendix.

periarterial (pĕr''ī-ar-tē'rī-ăl). Placed around an artery.

periarteritis (pĕr''ī-ar-tĕr-ī'tĭs). Inflammation of ext. coat of an artery.

   p. gummosa. Gummas in the blood vessels in syphilis.

   p. nodosa. A multiple, circumscribed inflammation of an outer arterial coat resulting in the formation of nodules along its course.

periarthric (per''ĭ-ar'thrĭk). Surrounding a joint. SYN: *circumarticular.*

periarthritis (pĕr''ī-ar-thrī'tĭs). Inflammation of area around a joint.

periarticular (pĕr''ī-ar-tĭk'ū-lăr). Surrounding a joint. SYN: *circumarticular.*

periaxial (pĕr''ī-ăks'ī-ăl). Located around an axis.   [axilla.

periaxillary (pĕr''ī-ăk'sĭl-ĕ-rī). About the periblast.

periblast (pĕr'ī-blăst). Protoplasm around a cell nucleus. SYN: *periplast.*

peribronchiolitis (pĕr''ī-brŏng''kĭ-ō-lī'tĭs). Inflammation of area around the bronchioles.

peribronchitis (pĕr''ī-brŏng-kī'tĭs). Inflammation of all tissues surrounding the bronchi or bronchial tubes.

pericardiac, pericardial (pĕr-ĭ-kar'dī-ăk, -ăl). Concerning the pericardium.

pericardicentesis (pĕr''ī-kar''dī-sĕn-tē'sĭs). Surgical piercing of the pericardium.

pericardiectomy (pĕr''ī-kar-dī-ĕk'tō-mĭ). Excision of part or all of the pericardium.

pericardiocentesis (pĕr''ī-kar''dī-ō-sĕn-tē'sĭs). Surgical perforation of the pericardium. SYN: *pericardicentesis.*

pericardiolysis (pĕr''ī-kar''dī-ŏl'ī-sĭs). Separation of adhesions bet. the visceral and parietal pericardium.

pericardiomediastinitis (pĕr''ī-kar''dī-ō-mē-dī-ăs''tī-nī'tĭs). Inflamed condition of the pericardium and mediastinum.

pericardiophrenic (pĕr-ĭ-kar''dī-ō-fren'ĭk). Concerning the pericardium and diaphragm.

pericardiopleural (pĕr''ī-kar''dī-ō-plū'răl). Concerning the pericardium and pleura.

pericardiorrhaphy (pĕr''ī-kar''dī-or'ă-fī). Suture of a wound in the pericardium.

pericardiostomy (pĕr''ī-kar''dī-ŏs'tō-mĭ). Formation of an opening into the pericardium for drainage.

pericardiosymphysis (pĕr''ī-kar''dī-ō-sĭm'fi-sĭs). Adhesion bet. the layers of the pericardium.

pericardiotomy (pĕr''ī-kar-dī-ŏt'ō-mĭ). Incision of membranous sac around heart.

pericarditic (pĕr-ĭ-kar-dĭt'ĭk). Concerning the pericardium.

pericarditis (pĕr-ĭ-kar-dī'tĭs). Inflammation of pericardium.

   p. adhesiva. Form in which the layers of pericardium adhere.

   p. callosa. A chronic form with signs of obstructed return flow of venous blood to the heart, but with no other symptoms.

   p. externa. Inflammation of exterior surface of the pericardium.

   p., fibrinous. Membrane is covered with butterlike exudate which organizes and unites the pericardial surfaces.

   p. obliterans. Pericardial inflammation causing adhesions and obliteration of the pericardial cavity.

pericardium (pĕr″ĭ-kar′dĭ-ŭm). The double, membranous, cone-shaped, fibroserous sac enclosing the heart and the roots of the great blood vessels.

   p. externum. The outer fibrous layer of the pericardium.

   p. internum. Serous inner layer of the pericardium.

pericardosis (pĕr″ĭ-kar-dō′sĭs). Bacterial infection of the pericardium.

pericecal (pĕr-ĭ-sē′kăl). Situated around the cecum.

pericecitis (pĕr-ĭ-sē-sī′tĭs). Inflamed condition of area around the cecum. SYN: *perityphlitis.*

pericementitis (pĕr″ĭ-sĕm-ĕn-tī′tĭs). Progressive necrosis of the alveoli of the teeth. SYN: *periodontitis.*

pericementoclasia (pĕr″ĭ-sĕm-ĕn-tō-klā′-zĭ-ă). Dissolution of the pericementum with alveolar absorption. SYN: *pyorrhea alveolaris.*

pericementum (pĕ″rĭ-sĕm-ĕn′tŭm). Fibrous tissue covering the root of a tooth.

pericholangitis (pĕr″ĭ-kō-lăn-jī′tĭs). Inflammation of tissues surrounding a bile duct. SYN: *periangiocholitis.*

pericholecystitis (pĕr″ĭ-kō-lē-sĭs-tī′tĭs). Inflammation of tissues situated around the gallbladder.

perichondral, perichondrial (pĕr-ĭ-kon′drăl, -drĭ-ăl). Concerning the membrane covering cartilage.

perichondritis (pĕr-ĭ-kŏn-drī′tĭs). Inflamed condition of perichondrium.

perichondrium (pĕr-ĭ-kŏn′drĭ-ŭm). Membrane of fibrous connective tissue around surface of cartilage.

perichondroma (pĕr″ĭ-kŏn-drō′mă). A tumor arising from fibrous tissue which covers cartilage.

perichordal (pĕr-ĭ-kor′dăl). Placed around the notochord.

perichorioidal, perichoroidal (pĕr″ĭ-kō-rĭ-oy′dăl, -roy′dăl). Situated around the choroid coat.

perichrome (pĕr′ĭ-krōm). A nerve cell in which the tigroid mass is arranged in rows through the protoplasm.

pericolic (pĕr-ĭ-ko′lĭk). Around or encircling the colon.

pericolitis (pĕr″ĭ-kō-lī′tĭs). Inflammation of area around the colon.

pericolonitis (pĕr″ĭ-kō-lŏn-ī′tĭs). Inflamed condition of region around the colon.

pericolpitis (pĕr″ĭ-kŏl-pī′tĭs). Inflammation of connective tissues surrounding the vagina.

periconchal (pĕr-ĭ-kŏng′kăl). Around the concha of the ear.   [the auricle.

   p. sulcus. Groove on post. surface of

periconchitis (pĕr″ĭ-kŏng-kī′tĭs). Inflamed condition of the lining of the orbit.

pericorneal (pĕr″ĭ-kor′nē-ăl). Placed around the cornea.

pericranitis (pĕr″ĭ-krā-nī′tĭs). Inflamed condition of pericranium.

pericranium (pĕr″ĭ-krā′nĭ-ŭm). Fibrous membrane surrounding the skull bone; periosteum of the skull.

   p. internum. Lining surface of the skull. SYN: *endocranium.*

pericystitis (pĕr″ĭ-sĭs-tī′tĭs). Inflamed condition of tissues about the bladder.

pericytial (pĕr-ĭ-sĭsh′ăl). Placed around a cell.

peridectomy (pĕr-ĭ-dĕk′tō-mĭ). 1. Operation for relief of pannus. 2. Circumcision. SYN: *peritomy.*

peridendric (pĕr-ĭ-dĕn′drĭk). Surrounding a dendrite of a nerve cell.

peridental (pĕr-ĭ-dĕn′tăl). Surrounding a tooth or part of one. SYN: *periodontal.*

peridentoclasia (pĕr″ĭ-dĕn-tō-klā′zĭ-ă). Breaking down of tissues about the teeth.

peridesmitis (pĕr″ĭ-dĕz-mī′tĭs). Inflammation of the areolar tissue around a ligament.

peridesmium (pĕr″ĭ-dĕz′mĭ-ŭm). The connective tissue membrane sheathing a ligament.

peridiastole (pĕr″ĭ-dī-ăs′tō-lē). Interval before onset of the diastole following the systole.

perididymis (pĕr″ĭ-did′ĭ-mĭs). The tunica albuginea of testicles.

perididymitis (pĕr″ĭ-dĭd′ĭ-mī′tĭs). Inflammation of tunica albuginea of the testicles.

peridiverticulitis (pĕr″ĭ-dī-vĕr-tĭk″ū-lī′tĭs). Inflammation of tissues situated around an intestinal diverticulum.

periductal (pĕr-ĭ-duk′tăl). Situated about a duct.

periduodenitis (pĕr″ĭ-dū″o-dē-nī′tĭs). Inflammation around the duodenum due to adhesions attaching it to the peritoneum.

periencephalitis (pĕr″ĭ-ĕn-sĕf-ă-lī′tĭs). Inflamed condition of the surface of the brain.

periencephalomeningitis (pĕr″ĭ-ĕn-sĕf-ă-lō-mĕn-ĭn-jī′tĭs). Inflamed condition of cerebral cortex and the meninges.

periendothelioma (pĕr″ĭ-ĕn″dō-thē-lĭ-ō′mă). A tumor arising from the endothelium of the lymphatics and the perithelium of blood vessels.

perienteritis (pĕr″ĭ-ĕn-tĕr-ī′tĭs). Inflamed condition of peritoneal lining of intestines.

periepithelioma (pĕr″ĭ-ĕp″ĭ-thē″lĭ-ō′mă). A tumor arising in the endothelial lining of blood vessels or lymphatics, as that of the suprarenal body.

periesophagitis (pĕr″ĭ-ē-sŏf-ă-jī′tĭs). Inflamed condition of tissues around the esophagus.

perifistular (pĕr-ĭ-fis′tū-ler). Located around a fistula.

perifolliculitis (pĕr″ĭ-fō-lĭk″ū-lī′tĭs). Inflamed condition of area around the hair follicles.

perigangliitis (pĕr″ĭ-găng-lĭ-ī′tĭs). Inflamed condition of region around a ganglion.

perigastritis (pĕr″ĭ-găs-trī′tĭs). Inflammation of peritoneal lining of stomach.

periglottis (pĕr-ĭ-glŏt′ĭs). The mucosa covering of the tongue.

perihepatitis (pĕr″ĭ-hĕp-ă-tī′tĭs). Inflammation of peritoneal covering of the liver, usually occurring in circumscribed areas.

perijejunitis (pĕr″ĭ-jĕj-ū-nī′tĭs). Inflamed condition of tissues around the jejunum.

perikaryon (pĕr″ĭ-kăr′ĭ-ŏn). Nerve cell exclusive of the nucleus.

perilabyrinthitis (pĕr″ĭ-lab-ĭr-ĭn-thī′tĭs). Inflammation of tissues and parts about the labyrinth.

perilaryngitis (pĕr″ĭ-lăr-ĭn-jī′tĭs). Inflamed condition of tissues around the larynx.

perilymph (pĕr-ĭ-lĭmf). The pale, limpid fluid contained in the space bet. the membranous and bony labyrinth of the internal ear.

perilymphangitis (pĕr″ĭ-lĭmf-ăn-jī′tĭs). Inflammation of tissues around a lymphatic vessel.

perimeningitis (pĕr″ĭ-mĕn-ĭn-jī′tĭs). Inflamed condition of the dura mater. SYN: *pachymeningitis.*

perimeter (pĕr-ĭm′ĕt-ĕr). 1. The outer edge or periphery of a body or measure of the same. 2. Device for determining the extent of the field of vision.

perimetric (pĕr-ĭ-mĕt′rĭk). Concerning the outer surface of a body.

perimetritis (pĕr″ĭ-mē-trī′tĭs). Inflammation of the peritoneal covering of the uterus.
May be associated with parametritis.

perimetrium (pĕr-ĭ-mē′trĭ-ŭm). Peritoneum covering uterus.

perimetry (pĕr-ĭm′ē-trĭ). 1. Circumference, edge, border of a body. 2. Measurement of the scope of the field of vision with a perimeter.

perimyelitis (pĕr″ĭ-mī-ē-lī′tĭs). 1. Inflammation of the pia mater and arachnoid of the brain or spinal cord. SYN: *leptomeningitis.* 2. Inflammation of the endosteum, or membrane around medullary cavity of a bone.

perimyelography (pĕr″ĭ-mī-ē-lŏg′ră-fĭ). X-ray examination of area around the spinal cord.

perimyoendocarditis (pĕr″ĭ-mī″ō-ĕn″dō-kar-dī′tĭs). Inflammation of the muscular wall of the heart, its epithelial lining and the membrane surrounding it.

perimysial (pĕr-ĭ-mĭs′ĭ-ăl). Concerning, or of the nature of, perimysium; sheathing a muscle.

perimysiitis (pĕr-ĭ-mĭs-ĭ-ī′tĭs). Inflamed condition of the perimysium, the sheath surrounding a muscle.

perimysium (pĕr-ĭ-mĭs′ĭ-ŭm). The connective tissue sheath that envelops each primary bundle of muscle fiber.

perineal (pĕr-ĭn-ē′ăl). Concerning or situated on the perineum.
  p. body. Mass of tissue composed of skin, muscle, and fascia bet. vagina and rectum in the female, and the urethra and rectum in the male.
  p. fascia. Three layers bet. muscles of the perineum.
  p. hernia. Hernia perforating the perineum. SYN: *perineocele.*
  p. section. Surgical incision through perineum. SYN: *perineotomy.*

perineo-. Combining form for *region bet. the anus and the scrotum, or the vulva.*

perineocele (pĕr-ĭ-nē′ō-sēl). Hernia in the region of the perineum.

perineocolporectomyomectomy (pĕr-ĭ-nē″-ō-kŏl″pō-rĕk″tō-mī-ō-mĕk′tō-mĭ). Excision of a myoma by incising the perineum, vagina, and rectum.

perineoplasty (pĕr-ĭ-nē′ō-plăs″tĭ). Reparative surgery on the perineum.

perineorrhaphy (pĕr″ĭ-nē-ŏr′ă-fĭ). Suture of the perineum usually following labor.
  p., anterior. Rectifying cystocele.*
  p., colpo-. Removal of part of post. vaginal wall and suturing torn perineal body.
  p., posterior. Removal of rectocele.

perineosynthesis (pĕr-ĭ-nē″ō-sĭn′the-sĭs). Plastic operation for repair of a lacerated perineum; performed by grafting vaginal mucosa over area.

perineotomy (pĕr″ĭ-nē-ŏt′ō-mĭ). Operation of incising the perineum.

perineovaginal (pĕr-ĭ-nē″ō-văj′ĭn-ăl). Concerning the perineum and vagina.

perinephric (pĕr-ĭ-nĕf′rĭk). Located or occurring around the kidney.
  p. abscess. Abscess formation in peritoneal membrane surrounding the kidney.

perinephritis (pĕr″ĭ-ne-frī′tĭs). Inflammation of peritoneal tissues around the kidney. SYN: *paranephritis.*

perinephrium (pĕr-ĭ-nĕf′rĭ-ŭm). The connective and fatty tissue surrounding the kidney.

perineum (pĕr-ĭ-nē′ŭm). The space lying bet. the vulva and the anus in the female; bet. scrotum and anus in male.
  p., tears of the. There are 3 degrees of severity, being caused by overstretching of vagina and perineum in delivery, malposition increasing the tears.
  p., watering-pot. One riddled with fistulas from urethral stricture.

perineurial (pĕr″ĭ-nu′rĭ-ăl). Concerning the perineurium, the sheath around a bundle of nerve fibers.

perineuritis (pĕr″ĭ-nū-rī′tĭs). Inflammation of the sheath enveloping nerve fibers.

perineurium (pĕr-ĭ-nū′rĭ-ŭm). Connective tissue sheath investing a nerve fiber funiculus or bundle.

periocular (pĕr-ĭ-ŏk′ū-ler). Located around the eye. SYN: *circumocular.*

period (pēr′ĭ-ŏd). 1. The time during which anything or at which anything takes place, which is limited by a recurring event. 2. The menses. 3. Time occupied by a disease in running its course, or by a division of the total, as an incubation period.
  p., childbearing. The period in the female during which she is capable of procreation; puberty to the menopause.
  p., incubation. Time from moment of infection until appearance of first symptom.
  p., latent. 1. The time bet. stimulation and the resulting response. 2. Time bet. 4 and 11 years separating infantile sexuality from onset of puberty, the genital sexuality.

p., menstrual. Time for an individual act of menstruation.

p., neonatal. The first 30 days of infant life.

At this time the mortality of all infants under 1 yr. is greatest (67%); usual causes are prematurity, birth injuries, and sepsis.

p., puerperal. The period bet. delivery and first menstruation thereafter; or bet. delivery and normal involution.

periodic (pĕr-ĭ-od'ĭk). Recurring after definite intervals.

p. law. That which states that the chemical and physical properties of the chemical elements are periodic junctions of their atomic weights.

periodicity (pĕr″ĭ-ō-dĭs'ĭ-tĭ). 1. State of being regularly recurrent. 2. PT: The rate of rise and fall or interruption of a unidirectional current. 3. Recurrence of the menses.

periodontal (pĕr″ĭ-ō-don'tăl). Located about a tooth.

periodontitis (pĕr″ĭ-ō-dŏn-tī'tĭs). Inflammation of the tissues sheathing a tooth.

periodontium (pĕr″ĭ-ō-don'shĭ-ŭm). Inflamed condition of membranes enclosing a tooth.

periodontoclasia (pĕr″ĭ-ō-dŏn″tō-klā'zĭ-ă). Dissolution of membrane around a tooth.

periodontology (pĕr″ĭ-ō-dŏn-tŏl'ō-jĭ). Phase of dentistry dealing with treatment of diseases of the tissues around the teeth.

periodoscope (pĕr″ĭ-od'ō-skōp). Table or dial for calculation of expected date of confinement.

periomphalic (pĕr″ĭ-ŏm-făl'ĭk). Located around umbilicus.

perionychium (pĕr″ĭ-ō-nĭk'ĭ-ŭm). The epidermis surrounding a nail.

perionyxis (pĕr″ĭ-ō-nĭk'sĭs). Inflammation of epidermis surrounding a nail.

perioöphoritis (pĕr″ĭ-ō-of″ō-rī'tĭs). Inflammation of the surface membrane of the ovary. Syn: *perioöthecitis.*

perioöphorosalpingitis (pĕr″ĭ-ō-ŏf″ō-rō-sal″pĭn-jī'tĭs). Inflamed condition of tissues around an ovary and oviduct.

perioöthecitis (pĕr″ĭ-ō″ō-the-sī'tĭs). Inflammation of the peritoneal tissues around the ovary. Syn: *perioöphoritis.*

perioöthecosalpingitis (pĕr″ĭ-ō″o-the″kō-săl-pĭn-jī'tĭs). Inflammation of peritoneal membrane around the ovary and oviduct. Syn: *perioöphorosalpingitis, perisalpingoövaritis.*

perioptometry (pĕr″ĭ-op-tŏm'ĕt-rĭ). Measurement of the visual field.

periorbita (pĕr″ĭ-or'bĭ-tă). Periosteum of the socket of the eye.

periorbital (pĕr″ĭ-or'bĭ-tăl). Surrounding the socket of the eye. Syn: *circumorbital.*

periorbititis (pĕr″ĭ-or-bĭ-tī'tĭs). Inflamed condition of the periorbita.

periorchitis (pĕr″ĭ-or-kī'tĭs). Inflamed condition of the tissues investing a testicle.

p. hemorrhagica. Chronic hematocele of the tunica vaginalis coat of the testis.

periosteal (pĕr-ĭ-os'tē-ăl). Concerning the periosteum.

periosteitis (pĕr″ĭ-ŏs-tē-ī'tĭs). Inflammation of membrane investing a bone, the periosteum. Syn: *periostitis.*

periosteoedema (pĕr″ĭ-os″tē-ō-ĕ-dē'mă). Edema of the periosteum, the membrane surrounding a bone.

periosteoma (pĕr″ĭ-ŏs-tē-ō'mă). 1. An abnormal growth surrounding a bone. 2. Tumor of the periosteum, the tissue surrounding a bone.

periosteomedullitis (pĕr″ĭ-os″tē-ō-mĕd-ŭ-lī'tĭs). Inflamed condition of the periosteum and of bone marrow. Syn: *periosteomyelitis.*

periosteomyelitis (pĕr″ĭ-ŏs″tē-ō-mī′ĕ-lī'tĭs). Inflamed condition of the marrow and investing sheath of a bone.

periosteophyte (pĕr″ĭ-ŏs′tē-ō-fīt). Abnormal bony growth on periosteum, or arising from it.

periosteorrhaphy (pĕr″ĭ-ŏs-tē-or′ă-fī). Joining by suture the margins of a severed periosteum.

periosteotome (pĕr″ĭ-ŏs′tē-ō-tōm). Instrument for cutting the periosteum or removing it from the bone.

periosteotomy (pĕr″ĭ-ŏs-tē-ŏt′ō-mĭ). Incision into the periosteum.

periosteous (pĕr″ĭ-ŏs′tē-ŭs). Concerning, or of the nature of, periosteum. Syn: *periosteal.*

periosteum (pĕr-ĭ-ŏs′tē-ŭm). The fibro-vascular membrane that invests and nourishes the bone.

It extends over the whole surface except at the cartilaginous articulations.

p. externum. Periosteum covering ext. surfaces of bones.

p. internum. Int. periosteum lining the medullary canal of a bone.

periostitis (pĕr-ĭ-ŏs-tī'tĭs). Inflamed condition of membrane investing a bone, the periosteum.

p., albuminous. Periostitis with albuminous serous fluid exudate beneath the membrane affected.

p., alveolar. Inflammation of the peridental membrane. Syn: *periodontitis.*

p., dental. Periostitis of a tooth sheath.

p., diffuse. Periostitis of the long bones.

p., hemorrhagic. Periostitis with extravasation of blood under the periosteum.

periostoma (pĕr″ĭ-ŏs-tō'mă). A bony neoplasm around a bone or arising from its membranous sheath.

periostomedullitis (pĕr″ĭ-ŏs″tō-mĕd-ŭ-lī'tĭs). Inflammation of the marrow or sheath of a bone. Syn: *periosteomedullitis, periosteomyelitis.*

periostosis (pĕr″ĭ-ŏs-tō'sĭs). A bony neoplasm around a bone or arising from it.

periostotomy (pĕr″ĭ-ŏs-tŏt′ō-mĭ). Incision of the periosteum, the sheath covering a bone. Syn: *periosteotomy.*

periotic (pĕr-ĭ-ŏt′ĭk). Situated around the internal ear.

p. bone. The mastoid and petrous portions of the temporal bone.

peripachymeningitis (pĕr″ĭ-pak″ĭ-mĕn-ĭn-jī′tĭs). Inflamed condition of connective tissue bet. the dura mater and the bone.

peripancreatitis (pĕr-ĭ-păn-krē-ă-tī′tĭs). Inflammation of the peritoneal tissues covering the pancreas.

peripatetic (pĕr-ĭ-pă-tĕt′ĭk). Moving from place to place, as in walking typhoid.

periphacitis (pĕr-ĭ-fă-sī′tĭs). Inflamed condition of the capsule of the crystalline lens of the eye.

peripherad (pĕr-ĭf′ĕr-ăd). In the direction of the periphery.

peripheral (pĕr-ĭf′ĕr-ăl). Located at or pert. to the periphery.

periphery (pĕr-ĭf′ĕ-rĭ). Outer part or a surface of a body; part away from the center.

periphlebitis (pĕr″ĭ-flē-bī′tĭs). Inflamed condition of external coat of a vein or tissues around it.

periphoria (pĕr-ĭ-fō′rĭ-ă). Tendency for the cornea to deviate from its normal axis. SYN: *cyclophoria.*

periphrastic (pĕr-ĭ-frăs′tĭk). Relating to the use of superfluous words in expressing a thought.

periphrenitis (pĕr″ĭ-frĕn-ī′tĭs). Inflamed condition of the structures around the diaphragm.

periplast (pĕr′ĭ-plăst). 1. Peripheral protoplasm of a cell exclusive of the nucleus. 2. Matrix of a part or organ. 3. A cell wall. SYN: *periblast.*

peripleural (pĕr″ĭ-plū′răl). Encircling the pleura.

peripleuritis (pĕr-ĭ-plū-rī′tĭs). Inflamed condition of the connective tissues bet. the pleura and wall of the chest.

periplocin (pĕr-ĭp′lō-sĭn). $C_{30}H_{48}O_{12}$. Glucoside of *Periploca graeca,* used in treating diseases of the heart.

peripneumonia (pĕr″ĭp-nū-mō′nĭ-ă). Inflammation of the lungs alone or in combination with pleurisy.

p. notha. Congestion of the lungs; term used by older writers.

periproctitis (pĕr″ĭ-prŏk-tī′tĭs). Inflammation of areolar tissues in region of the rectum and anus. SYN: *perirectitis.*

periprostatic (pĕr″ĭ-prŏs-tăt′ĭk). Surrounding or occurring about the prostate.

periprostatitis (pĕr″ĭ-prŏs-tă-tī′tĭs). Inflamed condition of tissues surrounding the prostate.

peripylephlebitis (pĕr″ĭ-pī″le-flē-bī′tĭs). Inflamed condition of tissues about the portal vein.

peripylic (pĕr″ĭ-pī′lĭk). Situated around the portal vein.

peripyloric (pĕr″ĭ-pī-lor′ĭk). Extending around the pylorus.

perirectal (pĕr″ĭ-rĕk′tăl). Extending around the rectum.

perirectitis (pĕr″ĭ-rĕk-tī′tĭs). Inflamed condition of tissues about rectum and anus. SYN: *periproctitis.*

perirenal (pĕr″ĭ-rē′năl). Extending around

the kidney. SYN: *circumrenal, perinephric.*

perirhinal (pĕr″ĭ-rī′năl). Located about the nose or nasal fossae.

perirhizoclasia (pĕr″ĭ-rī″zō-klă′zĭ-ă). Inflammation and destruction of tissues extending around the roots of a tooth.

perisalpingitis (pĕr″ĭ-săl-pĭn-jī′tĭs). Inflamed condition of peritoneal coat about the oviduct.

perisalpingoövaritis (pĕr″ĭ-săl-pĭn″gō-ō-văr-ī′tĭs). Inflammation of peritoneal tissues surrounding the fallopian tubes and ovaries. SYN: *perioöphorosalpingitis, perioöthecosalpingitis.*

perisclerium. Fibrous tissue encircling ossifying cartilage.

periscopic (pĕr″ĭ-skop′ĭk). Viewing on all sides.

perish (pĕr′ĭsh). To disintegrate or die, esp. by other than natural causes.

perisigmoiditis (pĕr″ĭ-sĭg-moi-dī′tĭs). Inflamed condition of peritoneal tissues around sigmoid flexure of the colon.

perisinuitis (pĕr″ĭ-sĭ-nū-ī′tĭs). Inflamed condition of tissue about a sinus, esp. a cerebral one. SYN: *perisinusitis.*

perisinusitis (pĕr″ĭ-sĭ-nū-sī′tĭs). Inflammation of membranes about a sinus, esp. a cerebral sinus. SYN: *perisinuitis.*

perispermatitis (pĕr″ĭ-spĕr-mă-tī′tĭs). Inflamed condition of tissues about spermatic cord.　　　　　　　　　　　[cord.

p. serosa. Hydrocele of spermatic

perisplanchnic (pĕr″ĭ-splănk′nĭk). Extending around a viscus or the viscera.

perisplanchnitis (pĕr″ĭ-splănk-nī′tĭs). Inflamed condition of the tissues around the viscera. SYN: *perivisceritis.*

perisplenitis (pĕr″ĭ-splē-nī′tĭs). Inflammation of peritoneal coat of the spleen, the splenic capsule.

perispondylitis (pĕr″ĭ-spŏn-dĭl-ī′tĭs). Inflamed condition of the parts around a vertebra.

perissad (pĕr-ĭs′ăd, per′ĭs-ad). 1. Radical or element of odd valence. 2. Having odd valence.

perissodactylous (pĕr-ĭs″ō-dăk′tĭ-lŭs). Having an odd number of toes.

peristalsis (pĕr-ĭs-tăl′sĭs). Peculiar, contractile, muscular, vermicular, involuntary movements of any hollow tube of the body, esp. of the alimentary canal.

p., mass. Forced peristaltic movements of short duration moving contents from 1 section of the colon to another, occurring 3 or 4 times daily.

p., reverse. Backward movement of the intestines, a pathological condition often seen in intestinal and pyloric obstruction, and in the presence of diverticula and diverticulitis.

peristaltic (pĕr″ĭ-stăl′tĭk). Concerning, or of the nature of, peristalsis.

p. unrest. Increased peristalsis or abnormal motility of the intestinal tract.

peristaphyline (pĕr″ĭ-stăf′ĭ-lĭn). About the uvula.

peristole (pĕr-ĭs′tō-lē). The tonic power of the stomach to contract around its contents.

peristome (pĕr'ĭs-tōm). Channel leading from the mouth in protozoa.

peristrumitis (pĕr″ĭ-strū-mī'tĭs). Inflamed condition of tissues around a goiter. SYN: *perithyroiditis*.

perisynovial (pĕr″ĭ-sĭn-ō'vĭ-ăl). Extending around a synovial structure.

perisystole (pĕr″ĭ-sĭs'tō-lē). The period preceding the systole in the cardiac rhythm.

peritectomy (pĕr″ĭ-tĕk'tō-mĭ). Surgical removal of a ring of conjunctiva around the cornea.

peritendineum (pĕr″ĭ-tĕn-dĭn'ē-ŭm). The sheath of tissues investing a tendon.

peritendinitis (pĕr″ĭ-tĕn-dĭn-ī'tĭs). Inflamed condition of the sheath of a tendon. SYN: *peritenonitis*.

peritenonitis (pĕr″ĭ-tĕn-on-ī'tĭs). Inflammation of sheath investing a tendon. SYN: *peritendinitis*.

perithelioma (pĕr″ĭ-thē-lĭ-ō'mă). A tumor derived from the perithelial layer of the blood vessels.

perithelium (pĕr-ĭ-thē'lĭ-ŭm). Fibrous outer layer of the blood vessels and capillaries.

perithyroiditis (pĕr″ĭ-thī-roy-dī'tĭs). Inflammation of capsule or tissues sheathing the thyroid gland. SYN: *peristrumitis*.

peritomy (pĕr-ĭt'ō-mĭ). 1. Excision of narrow strip of conjunctiva around the cornea in treatment of pannus. 2. Circumcision. [the peritoneum.

peritoneal (pĕr″ĭ-tō-nē'ăl). Concerning

p. cavity. Region bordered by parietal layer of the peritoneum containing all the abdominal organs exclusive of the kidney. SEE: *cholascos*.

peritonealgia (pĕr″ĭ-tō-nē-al'jĭ-ă). Pain of the peritoneum.

peritoneocentesis (pĕr″ĭ-tō-nē″ō-sĕn-tē'sĭs). Piercing of the peritoneal cavity to obtain fluid. SEE: *paracentesis*.

peritoneoclysis (pĕr″ĭ-tō-nē″ō-klī'sĭs). Introduction of fluid into the peritoneal cavity.

peritoneopathy (pĕr″ĭ-tō-nē-op'ăth-ĭ). Any disordered condition of the peritoneum.

peritoneopexy (pĕr″ĭ-tō-nē'ō-pĕks″ĭ). Fixation of the uterus by way of the vagina.

peritoneoplasty (pĕr″ĭ-tō-nē'ō-plăs″tĭ). Reparative surgery to prevent re-formation of loosened adhesions.

peritoneoscope (pĕr″ĭ-tō-nē'ō-skōp). Long, slender telescope with a tiny electric light on the end as well as a forceps for grasping a small metal fragment or for clamping a bleeding artery in the peritoneum.

peritoneoscopy (pĕr″ĭ-tō-nē-ŏs'kō-pĭ). Examination of peritoneal cavity with the peritoneoscope.

peritoneotomy (pĕr″ĭ-tō-nē-ŏt'ō-mĭ). Process of incising the peritoneum.

peritoneum (pĕr-ĭ-tō-nē'ŭm). The serous membrane reflected over the viscera, and lining the abdominal cavity.

p., abdominal. That part of the peritoneum lining inner surfaces of the abdominal parietes.

p., genitourinary. Retrovesical folds.

p., parietal. Peritoneum lining abdominal and pelvic walls and undersurface of diaphragm.

p., subduodenal. Peritoneal folds and ligaments below the duodenum.

p., supraduodenal. Peritoneal folds and ligaments above the duodenum.

p., visceral. The peritoneum that invests the abdominal organs except the kidneys.

peritonism (pĕr'ĭ-tō-nĭzm). A false peritonitis with symptoms of peritonitis and abdominal rigidity and tenderness, but with no inflammation of the peritoneum.

peritonitic (pĕr-ĭ-tō-nĭt'ĭk). Affected with or concerning peritonitis.

peritonitis (pĕr″ĭ-tō-nī'tĭs). Inflammation of the peritoneum, the membranous coat lining the abdominal cavity and investing the viscera.

p., acute diffuse. Generalized peritonitis of a large area.

p., adhesive. Peritonitis in which the visceral and parietal layers stick together by means of adhesions.

p., chronic. Usually tuberculous, cancerous, or syphilitic; occurs in chronic alcoholism.

p. deformans. Chronic peritonitis with thickened membrane and adhesions contracting and causing retraction of the intestines.

p., diffuse. Peritonitis which is not found in only a circumscribed area.

p., local. Peritonitis confined to 1 limited area of the peritoneum.

p., pelvic. Infection of the peritoneal lining of the pelvic cavity.

p., plastic. A form binding the bowels together with adhesions.

p., puerperal. Peritonitis which develops following childbirth.

p., septic. Peritonitis caused by a pyogenic bacterium.

p., serous. Peritonitis in which there is liquid exudation.

p., traumatic. Peritonitis due to injury or wound infection.

p., tuberculous. Peritonitis caused by numerous tubercle bacilli on the peritoneum. [around a tonsil.

peritonsillar (pĕr″ĭ-ton'sĭl-ăr). Extending

peritonsillitis (pĕr-ĭ-tŏn-sĭl-ī'tĭs). Inflamed condition of tissues around the tonsils. SYN: *periamygdalitis*.

peritrichous (pĕr-ĭt'rĭk-ŭs). BACT: Having cilia or flagella covering the entire surface.

perityphlitis (pĕr″ĭ-tĭf-lī'tĭs). Inflamed condition of tissues around the cecum and appendix. SYN: *appendicitis*.

periureteritis (pĕr″ĭ-ū-rē″tĕr-ī'tĭs). Inflamed condition of parts about the ureter.

periurethral (pĕr″ĭ-ū-rē'thrăl). Located about the urethra.

periuterine (pĕr″ĭ-ū'tĕr-ĭn). Located about the uterus. SYN: *perimetric*.

perivaginitis (pĕr″ĭ-văj-ĭn-ī'tĭs). Inflammation of region around the vagina. SYN: *pericolpitis*.

perivascular (pĕr″ĭ-văs′kū-ler). Located around a vessel, esp. a blood vessel.

perivasculitis (pĕr″ĭ-văs-kū-lī′tĭs). Inflamed condition of tissues surrounding a blood vessel. SYN: *periangitis*.

perivisceritis (pĕr″ĭ-vĭs″ĕr-ī′tĭs). Inflamed condition of the tissues surrounding the viscera.

perixenitis (pĕr″ĭ-zĕn-ī′tĭs). Inflammation of the region around a foreign body.

perlèche (pĕr-lăsh′). Contagious disorder marked by fissures and epithelial desquamation at corners of the mouth, esp. seen in children.

permanent (pŭr′măn-ĕnt). Enduring; without change.

    p. teeth. Teeth developing at the 2nd dentition. SEE: *dens permanens*.

permanganate (pĕr-man′găn-āt). Any one of the salts of permanganic acid.

permeable (pŭr′mē-ă-bl). Capable of or allowing the passage of fluids into or through. SEE: *pervious, porous*.

pernicious (pĕr-nĭsh′ŭs). Destructive; fatal; harmful.

    p. anemia. Severe, often fatal, form of blood disease, marked by progressive decrease in red blood corpuscles, muscular weakness, and gastrointestinal and neural disturbances. SEE: *anemia, pernicious*.

    p. trend. PSY: An abnormal departure from conventional ideas and social interests. Pregenital interests are manifested.

pernio (pŭr′nĭ-ō). Congestion and swelling of the skin, due to cold.

perniosis (pŭr-nĭ-ō′sĭs). A skin disorder due to cold. SEE: *chilblain, pernio*.

pernocton (pŭr-nŏk′tŏn). Barbituric acid derivative used as an anesthetic and hypnotic, as in labor.

pero (pē′rō). The soft outer layer of the olfactory lobe of the brain from which the olfactory nerves arise.

perogen (per′ō-jĕn). A preparation composed of 2 separate mixtures which are united in making an oxygen bath.

peronaeus (pĕr-ō-nē′ŭs). A group of leg muscles controlling motion of the foot.

peroneal (pĕr-ō-nē′ăl). Concerning the fibula.

peroneo-. Combining form, *pert. to the fibula*.

peroneum (pĕr-ō-nē′ŭm). The fibula. SYN: *os peroneum*.

peroneus (pĕr-ō-nē′ŭs). One of several muscles of the leg causing motion in the foot.

peronin (pĕr′ō-nĭn). Proprietary powder, benzylmorphine hydrochloride, used in treating coughs.

    DOSAGE: ⅓ gr. (0.02 Gm.).

Peronospora (pĕr-ō-nŏs′pō-ră). Genus of fungi causing mildew formation.

peroral (pĕr-or′ăl). Via the mouth.

per os. By mouth.

peroxidase (per-ŏks′ĭ-dās). An enzyme which hastens the decomposition of peroxides, esp. of hydrogen peroxide.

peroxide (pŭr-ŏk′sĭd). In chemistry, a compound containing more oxygen than

do the other oxides of the element in question.

perplication (per-plĭ-kā′shŭn). Inserting the cut end of an artery through an incision in its own wall to arrest bleeding.

per primam, per primam intentionem (per prē′măm ĭn-tĕn-tĭ-ō′nĕm). By first intention. SEE: *first intention, healing*.

per rectum (per rĕk′tŭm). By the rectum; through the rectum.

persalt (pursawlt). CHEM: A salt containing largest possible amount of an acid radical.

per secundam (per se-kun′dăm). By second intention. SEE: *healing, second intention*.

perseveration (pŭr-sĕv-ĕr-ā′shŭn). Continued repetition of a meaningless word or phrase, or repetition of answers which are not related to successive questions asked.

personal (pŭr′sō-năl). Characteristic of an individual.

    p. equation. In scientific observation, factors depending on personal qualities of individual observers.

personality (pŭr-sō-năl′ĭ-tĭ). That which constitutes the distinction of person. PSY: Totality of an individual's characteristics; the integrated group of emotional trends, interests and behavior tendencies of an individual. SEE: *idiosyncrasy*.

    p., double. SEE: *dual personality*.

    p., dual. Mental dissociation in which 1 individual shows in alternation 2 very different personalities. SEE: *dual personality*.

    p., multiple. State in which 3 or more personalities alternate in the same individual. SEE: *multiple personality*.

    p., psychopathic. One who, while possessing normal intelligence, by reason of heredity or congenital conditions, becomes constitutionally lacking in moral sensibilities, emotional control and inhibitions of the will.

    p., split. Dissociation of ideas not amenable to conscious control, as in schizophrenia.

perspiration (pŭr-spĭr-ā′shŭn). 1. Sweat. 2. Secretion and exudation of fluid by sweat glands of the skin, about 700 cc. per day.

    p., insensible. Perspiration which evaporates as fast as formed, leaving no moisture on the skin.

    p., sensible. Perspiration which occurs so as to form drops.

perspire (pŭr-spīr′). To excrete fluid through the skin. SYN: *sweat*.

perstriction (pĕr-strĭk′shŭn). Ligation of a bleeding vessel for the arrest of hemorrhage.

persulfate (pŭr-sŭl′fāt). One of a series of sulfates containing more sulfuric acid than the others in same series.

per tertiam intentionem (per tĕr′tĭ-ăm ĭn-tĕn-tĭ-ō′nĕm). By third intention. SEE: *healing, third intention*.

Perthes' disease (păr′tăs). One in which

changes take place in bone at head of femur with deformity resulting.

per tubam (pĕr tū'băm). Through a tube.

pertussin (pĕr-tŭs'ĭn). Proprietary cough remedy.

pertussis (pĕr-tŭs'ĭs). An acute, infectious disease characterized by a catarrhal stage, followed by a peculiar paroxysmal cough, ending in a whooping inspiration.

SYN: *whooping cough.*

pertussoid (pĕr-tŭs'oyd). 1. Of the nature of whooping cough. 2. A cough generally similar to that of whooping cough.

peruol (pĕr'ū-ŏl). Oil derived from balsam of Peru used in scabies.

perversion (pŭr-vŭr'zhŭn). Deviation from the normal path, as in function.

   p., sexual. Maladjustment of sexual life in which satisfaction is sought in ways deviating from the accepted normal.

pervert (pŭr-vŭrt'). 1. v. To turn from the normal. 2. (pŭr'vŭrt). n. One who has turned from the normal or right path, esp. sexually.

   p., sexual. One whose sex conduct is not normal.

pervigilium (pĕr-vĭ-jĭl'ĭ-ŭm). Inability to sleep. SYN: *insomnia, wakefulness.*

pervious (pŭr'vĭ-ŭs). 1. Capable of being penetrated. 2. Penetrating. SYN: *permeable.*

pes (pēz) (pl. *pĕ'dēz*). The foot or a footlike structure.

   p. accessorius. A white projection in the brain at the juncture of descending and post. cornua of lateral ventricle.

   p. anserinus. Three primary branches of the facial nerve after leaving the stylomastoid foramen.

   p. cavus. Abnormal hollowness of the sole of the foot.

   p. corvinus. Wrinkles at outer ocular canthus. SYN: *crow's foot.*

   p. equinus. Deformity marked by walking without touching heel to the ground. SYN: *talipes equinus, q.v.*

   p. hippocampi. Lower portion of the hippocampus major.

   p., infraorbital. Terminal radiating branches of the infraorbital nerve after exit from the infraorbital canal.

   p. planus. Flatfoot.

   p. valgus. Clubfoot in which sole turns outward. SYN: *talipes valgus.*

   p. varus. Clubfoot in which sole turns inward. SYN: *talipes varus.*

pessary (pĕs'ăr-ĭ). 1. A device to insert into the vagina to hold the uterus in position. 2. A vaginal suppository.

   p., cup. One which has a cup-shaped hollow that fits over the os uteri.

   p., diaphragm. Cup-shaped rubber pessary used as a contraceptive device.

   p., Gariel's Inflatable hollow rubber pessary.

   p., Hodge's. Pessary used to correct retrodeviations of the uterus.

   p., lever. Pessary designed according to the principles of a lever.

   p., ring. Round pessary.

   p., stem. Pessary with stem which fits into the uterine canal.

pessima (pĕs'ĭ-mă). A skin affection characterized by pustular lesions, hard and yellowish, surrounded by areola of inflammation appearing over surface of body causing a checkerboard appearance.

pest (pĕst). 1. Fatal epidemic disease, esp. the plague. 2. A destructive insect.

   p.-house. Hospital for those infected with a pestilential or communicable disease.

pestiferous (pĕst-ĭf'ĕr-ŭs). Producing a pestilence; carrying infection. SYN: *pestilential.*

pestilence (pĕst'ĭl-ĕns). 1. An epidemic contagious disease, specifically bubonic plague. 2. An epidemic caused by such a disease.

pestilential (pĕst-ĭ-lĕn'shăl). Concerning or causing a pestilence. SYN: *pestiferous.*

pestis (pĕs'tĭs). The plague.

pestle (pĕs'l). Device for macerating drugs in a mortar.

petechiae (pe-tē'kĭ-ē). 1. Small, purplish, hemorrhagic spots on the skin which appear in certain severe fevers and are indicative of great prostration, as in typhus. 2. Red spots from bite of a flea.

petechial (pe-tē'kĭ-ăl). Marked by presence of petechiae.

petit mal (pĕt'ē măhl). Mild form of epileptic attack.

   Consciousness may be lost, but there is an absence of convulsions. SEE: *epilepsy, pyknolepsy.*

Petit's canal. Canal encircling the lenticular periphery.

   P.'s sinuses. Hollows in aortic and pulmonary arteries behind semilunar valves.

   P.'s triangle. One on lateral abdominal muscular wall.

petrifaction (pĕt-rĭ-făk'shŭn). Process of changing into stone or hard substance.

petrified (pĕt'rĭ-fīd). Changed into stone; rigid. [make rigid.

petrify (pĕt'rĭ-fī). Convert into stone;

pétrissage (pā-trē-sazh'). A kneading movement in massage.

petro-. Combining form meaning *stone.* Pert. to petrous portion of temporal bone.

petrolatoma (pĕt″rō-lă-tō'mă). Tumor or swelling caused by introduction of liquid petrolatum under the skin.

petrolatum (pĕt-rō-lā'tŭm). USP. A purified semi-solid mixture of hydrocarbons obtained from petroleum.

   p. liquid. USP. A mixture of liquid hydrocarbons obtained from petroleum.

   DOSAGE: 4 drams (15 cc.). SEE: *mineral oil, paraffin, liquid.*

petroleum (pĕt-rō'lē-ŭm). An oily inflammable liquid found in the upper strata of the earth, a hydrocarbon mixture.

petrolization (pĕt-rŏl-ĭ-zā'shŭn). The application of kerosene to pools of water for the extermination of mosquito larvae.

petromastoid (pĕt"rō-măs'toyd). Concerning petrous and mastoid portions of the temporal bone.

petrosa (pĕt-rō'să). The petrous part of the temporal bone.

petrosal (pĕt-rō'săl). Of, pert. to, or situated near, the petrous portion of the temporal bone.

petrosalpingostaphylinus (pĕt"rō-săl-pĭn'-gō-stăf-ĭl-ī'nŭs). The levator palati muscle which elevates the soft palate.

petrositis (pĕt"rō-sī'tĭs). Inflamed condition of the petrous region of the temporal bone.

petrous (pĕt'rŭs). 1. Resembling stone. 2. Relating to the petrous portion of the temporal bone. SYN: *petrosal*.

   p. bone. The petrosa, or petrous region of temporal bone.

   p. ganglion. Inf. ganglion of the glossopharyngeal nerve.

pexinogen (pĕks-ĭn'ō-jĕn). The proenzyme which is changed into rennin. SYN: *renninogen*.

Peyer's glands, Peyer's patches (pī'ĕr). Whitish, flat, lymphatic follicles in mucous and submucous layers of the small intestines, chiefly in the ileum ½ to 4 in. long made up of groups of solitary cells. They are the seat of infection in typhoid fever. SEE: *agminated glands*.

Pfeifferella (fī-fĕr-ĕl'ă). A genus of the family Mycobacteriaceae, certain species of which are pathogenic in man.

Pfeiffer's bacillus (fī'fĕr). The microorganism that may be the cause of influenza.

pH. In chemistry, the symbol for hydrogen ion concentration or degree of acidity; more exactly, the logarithm of the reciprocal of the concentration, expressed in terms of normality, of hydrogen ions in a solution.

phacitis (fă-sī'tĭs). Inflamed condition of the crystalline lens. SYN: *phakitis*.

phaco-. Prefix, *pert. to lens of the eye.*

phacoanaphylaxis (făk"ō-ăn-ă-fĭl-ăk'sĭs). Hypersensitivity to protein of the crystalline lens.

phacocele (făk'ō-sēl). Displacement of the crystalline lens into the int. chamber of the eye. [crystalline lens.

phacocyst (făk'ō-sĭst). Capsule of the

phacocystectomy (făk"ō-sĭs-tĕk'tō-mĭ). Surgical excision of part of crystalline lens capsule for cataract.

phacocystitis (făk"ō-sĭs-tī'tĭs). Inflamed condition of capsule of crystalline lens.

phacoeresis (făk"ō-ĕr-ē'sĭs). Removal of crystalline lens by suction method.

phacoglaucoma (făk"ō-glaw-kō'mă). Glaucoma and the changes it induces in the crystalline lens. SEE: *glaucoma*.

phacoid (făk'oyd). Lentil or lens-shaped.

phacoidoscope (făk-oyd'ō-skōp). Instrument for observing accommodative changes of the lens. SYN: *phacoscope*.

phacolysis (făk-ol'ĭ-sĭs). 1. Dissection and removal of the lens of the eye in treatment of cataract. 2. Any dissolution or disintegration of the crystalline lens.

phacomalacia (făk"ō-mal-ā'sĭ-ă). A softening of the lens usually due to a soft cataract.

phacometachoresis (făk"ō-mĕt-ă-kō-rē'sĭs). Dislocation of the crystalline lens. SYN: *phacocele*.

phacometer (făk-ŏm'ĕt-ĕr). Device for ascertaining refractive power of a lens.

phacoplanesis (făk"ō-plăn-ē'sĭs). Abnormal mobility of the crystalline lens.

phacosclerosis (făk"ō-sklēr-ō'sĭs). Hardening of the crystalline lens of eye.

phacoscope (făk'ō-skōp). Instrument for observing change of curvature of crystalline lens during accommodation.

phacotherapy (făk"ō-thĕr'ă-pĭ). Therapeutic use of the sun in treatment of diseases.

phacozymase (făk"ō-zī'măs). Ferment found in the fluid of crystalline lens.

phaeochrome (fē'ō-krōm). Staining readily with chromium salts.

phage (făj). An agent which absorbs bacteria. SYN: *bacteriophage*.

phagedena (făj-ĕd-ē'nă). A sloughing ulcer that spreads.

   p., sloughing. Hospital gangrene.

phagedenic (făj-e-dĕn'ĭk). Concerning, or of the nature of, phagedena.

phagelysis (făj'lĭ-sĭs). 1. Destruction of bacteriophages. 2. Destruction by bacteriophages.

phagocaryosis (făg"ō-kar-ĭ-ō'sĭs). Assumed phagocytic action of a cell nucleus. SYN: *phagokaryosis*.

phagocyte (făg'ō-sīt). An absorbing cell; a white blood corpuscle that destroys microörganisms and foreign particles.

phagocytic (făg"ō-sĭt'ĭk). Concerning phagocytes or phagocytosis.

   p. index. The average number of bacteria absorbed by each leukocyte, after their incubation in a mixture of serum and bacterial culture.

phagocytoblast (făg"ō-sī'tō-blăst). A cell giving origin to a phagocyte.

phagocytolysis (făg"ō-sī-tŏl'ĭ-sĭs). Destruction or disintegration of phagocytes. SYN: *phagolysis*.

phagocytolytic (făg"ō-sī-tō-lĭt'ĭk). Destroying phagocytes.

phagocytosis (făg"ō-sī-tō'sĭs). Ingestion and digestion of bacteria and particles by phagocytes.

   p., induced. Phagocytosis facilitated by action of blood serum.●

   p., spontaneous. Phagocytosis which occurs in any indifferent medium.

phagodynamometer (făg"ō-dī-năm-om'ĕt-ĕr). Device which measures energy expended in chewing.

phagokaryosis (făg"ō-kar-ĭ-ō'sĭs). Phagocytic action which is performed by a cell nucleus.

phagolysis (făg-ol'ĭ-sĭs). Disintegration of phagocytes. SYN: *phagocytolysis*.

phagomania (făg-ō-mā'nĭ-ă). Abnormal craving for food.

phagopyrism (făf"ō-pī'rĭzm). Hypersensitiveness to certain foods which induce symptoms of poisoning upon ingestion.

phagotherapy (făg"ō-thĕr'ă-pĭ). Treatment by feeding or overfeeding.

phakitis (făk-ī'tĭs). Inflamed condition of the crystalline lens. SYN: *phacitis.*

phakolysis (făk-ol'ĭs-ĭs). Disintegration or removal of the crystalline lens. SYN: *phacolysis.*

phalacrosis (făl-ă-krō'sĭs). Baldness. SYN: *alopecia.*

phalacrotic (făl-ăk-rŏt'ĭk). Bald; bald-headed.

phalacrous (făl-ăk'rŭs). Bald. SYN: *phalacrotic.*

phalangeal (fă-lăn'jē-ăl). Concerning a phalanx.

phalangectomy (fă-lăn-jĕk'tō-mĭ). Excision of 1 or more phalanges.

phalanges (fă-lăn'jēz) (sing. *phalanx*). 1. Bones of a finger or toe. SEE: *skeleton.* 2. Any 1 of a set of plates disposed in rows which makes up the lamina reticularis.

    p., Deiter's. Modified plates forming the ends of cells of the reticular membrane of the organ of Corti.

phalangitis (făl-lăn-jī'tĭs). Inflamed condition of 1 or more phalanges.

phalangosis (fă-lăn-gō'sĭs). 1. Arrangement of lashes in rows on the eyelids, a diseased condition. 2. Downward displacement of the eye. SYN: *ptosis.*

phalanx (fă'lănks) (pl. *phalanges*). 1. Any 1 of the bones of fingers or toes. 2. A set of plates in rows composing the lamina reticularis. See: *phalanges.*

    p., distal. The one most remote from the metacarpus or metatarsus.

    p., metacarpal, p., metatarsal. SEE: *proximal phalanx.*

    p., middle. The phalanx (where there are 3) intermediate between distal and proximal phalanges.

    p., proximal. The phalanx articulating with a metacarpal or metatarsal bone.

    p., terminal, p., ungual, p., unguicular. SEE: *distal phalanx.*

phallalgia (făl-ăl'jĭ-ă). Pain in the penis.

phallic (făl'ĭk). Concerning the penis.

phallitis (făl-ī'tĭs). Inflamed condition of the penis.

phallocampsis (făl-ō-kămp'sĭs). Painful downward curvature of penis when erect; seen in gonorrhea. SYN: *chordee.*

phallodynia (făl-ō-dĭn'ĭ-ă). Pain in the penis. SYN: *phallalgia.*

phalloid (făl'oyd). Similar to a penis.

phalloncus (făl-on'kŭs). Tumor or swelling on the penis.

phalloplasty (făl'ō-plăs"tĭ). Reparative or plastic surgery on the penis.

phallorhagia (făl-ō-rā'jĭ-ă). Flow of blood from the penis.

phallus (făl'ŭs). 1. The penis; the male generative organ. 2. An artificial penis, used as a symbol.

phanero-, phaner-. Combining forms meaning *evident, visible.*

phaneromania (făn-ĕr-ō-mā'nĭ-ă). Abnormal tendency to bite the nails, pick or scratch the skin.

phaneroscope (făn-ĕr'ō-skōp). Instrument for securing transparency of skin by illumination.

phaneroscopy (făn-ĕr-ŏs'kō-pĭ). Observation of skin by phaneroscope. Use of a lens to concentrate light in examination of skin lesions.

phanerosis (făn-ĕr-ō'sĭs). The process of becoming visible.

phanic (făn'ĭk). Manifest; apparent.

phanodorn (făn'ō-dorn). A barbital compound, being more rapidly eliminated, its action not so lasting. Use same as barbital.

    DOSAGE: 0.1 Gm. (1½ gr.).

phantasia (făn-tā'zĭ-ă). An appearance that is imaginary.

phantasm (făn'tăzm). An optical illusion; an apparition, or illusion of something that does not exist.

phantasmatomoria (făn-taz"măt-ō-mo'rĭ-ă). Dementia with silly fancies; childishness in the demented.

phantasy (făn'tă-sĭ). A daydream.

phantom (făn'tŭm). 1. An apparition. 2. A model of the body or of 1 of its parts.

    p. corpuscle. A colorless erythrocyte.

    p. tumor. An apparent tumor due to muscular contractions or flatus seen in hysterics. SEE: *pseudocyesis.*

pharmacal (făr'măk-ăl). Concerning pharmacy.

pharmaceutical (făr-mă-sū'tĭk-ăl). Concerning drugs or pharmacy.

pharmaceutics (făr-mă-sū'tĭks). Science of dispensing medicines. SYN: *pharmacy.*

pharmacist (făr'mă-sĭst). A druggist; one licensed to prepare and dispense drugs. SYN: *apothecary.*

pharmaco-. Combining form meaning *drug, medicine, poison.*

pharmacodiagnosis (făr"mă-kō-dī-ăg-nō'sĭs). Use of drugs in making a diagnosis.

pharmacodynamics (făr"mă-kō-dī-năm'ĭks). Study of drugs and their reactions.

pharmacognosy (făr"mă-kog'nō-sĭ). The science of crude drugs, their physical, botanical, and chemical properties.

pharmacography (făr"mă-kog'ră-fĭ). Treatise on the properties of drugs.

pharmacology (făr-mă-kŏl'ō-jĭ). The study of the effects of drugs upon the physical organism. SYN: *pharmacodynamics.*

pharmacomania (făr"mă-kō-mā'nĭ-ă). Abnormal desire for giving or taking medicines.

pharmacopedia (făr"mă-kō-pē'dĭ-ă). Information concernings drugs and their preparation.

pharmacopeia (făr"mă-kō-pē'ă). Authorized treatise on drugs and their preparation, esp. a book containing formulas and information concerning drugs which is a standard for their preparation and dispensation.

pharmacophobia (făr"mă-kō-fō'bĭ-ă). Abnormal fear of taking medicines.

pharmacopsychosis (făr"mă-kō-sī-kō'sĭs). Addiction to drugs.

pharmacotherapy (făr"mă-kō-thĕr'ă-pĭ). Use of medicine in treatment of disease.

pharmacy (făr'mă-sĭ). 1. The practice of compounding and dispensing medicinal preparations. 2. A drugstore. 3. A medicinal preparation.

pharyngalgia (făr-ĭn-găl'jĭ-ă). Pain in the pharynx. SYN: *pharyngodynia*.

pharyngeal (far-ĭn'jē-ăl). Concerning the pharynx.

    p. arches. Cartilaginous embryonic framework forming various structures in neck. SYN: *visceral arches*.

    p. reflex. Attempt to swallow following any application of stimulus to pharynx.

    p. spine. Small elevation on inf. surface of basilar process of occipital bone for attachment of pharynx.

    p. tonsil. Lymphoid tissue on post. sup. wall of the pharynx.

    p. tubercle. SEE: *pharyngeal spine*.

pharyngectomy (făr-ĭn-jĕk'tō-mĭ). Partial excision of the pharynx to remove growths, abscesses, etc.

pharyngemphraxis (făr-ĭn-jĕm-frăks'ĭs). Pharyngeal obstruction.

pharyngismus (făr-ĭn-jĭz'mŭs). Spasm of the muscles in the pharynx. SYN: *pharyngospasm*.

pharyngitis (făr-ĭn-jī'tĭs). Inflammation of pharynx, usually associated with rhinitis.

    p., acute. SYM: Malaise, slight rise in temperature, dysphagia, pain in throat, postnasal secretion.

    p., atrophic. Chronic form with some atrophy of mucous glands and abnormal secretion. SYN: *pharyngitis sicca*.

    p., chronic. Associated with pathology in nose and sinuses, mouth breathing, excessive smoking, and chronic tonsillitis. [false membrane of croup.

    p., croupous. Pharyngitis with the

    p., diphtheritic. Sore throat with general symptoms of diphtheria.

    p., follicular. SEE: *granular pharyngitis*.

    p., gangrenous. Gangrenous inflammation of mucous membrane of pharynx. SYN: *angina maligna, cynanche maligna*.

    p., granular. Pharyngitis with granulations seen on the pharynx. SYN: *clergyman's sore throat*.

    p. hypertrophica. A chronic form with thickened, red mucous membrane on each side with a glazed central portion.

    p. sicca. SEE: *atrophic pharyngitis*.

    p. ulcerosa. Pharyngitis with fever, pain, and the formation of ulcerations.

pharyngo-. Combining form pertaining to the pharynx.

pharyngoamygdalitis (făr-ĭn″gō-ăm-ĭg-dăl-ĭ'tĭs). Inflamed condition of the pharynx and tonsil.

pharyngocele (făr-ĭn'gō-sēl). Hernia through pharyngeal wall.

pharyngodynia (făr-ĭn″gō-dĭn'ĭ-ă). Pain in the pharynx. SYN: *pharyngalgia*.

pharyngolaryngitis (făr-ĭn″gō-lăr-ĭn-jī'tĭs). Inflamed condition of pharynx and larynx.

pharyngolith (făr-ĭn'gō-lĭth). Concretion in pharyngeal walls.

pharyngology (făr-ĭn-gŏl'ō-jĭ). Branch of medicine dealing with the pharynx.

pharyngomycosis (făr-ĭn″gō-mĭ-kō'sĭs). Disease of pharynx due to fungi.

pharyngoparalysis (făr-ĭn″gō-păr-ăl'ĭ-sĭs). Paralysis of the muscles of the pharynx. SYN: *pharyngoplegia*.

pharyngopathy (făr-ĭn-gŏp'ăth-ĭ). Any disorder of the pharynx.

pharyngoperistole (făr-ĭn″gō-pĕr-ĭs'tō-lē). Narrowing or stricture of the lumen of the pharynx.

pharyngoplasty (făr-ĭn'gō-plăs″tĭ). Reparative surgery of the pharynx.

pharyngoplegia (făr-ĭn″gō-plē'jĭ-ă). Paralysis of muscles of pharynx. SYN: *pharyngoparalysis*.

pharyngorhinitis (făr-ĭn″gō-rī-nī'tĭs). Inflamed condition of the nasopharynx.

pharyngorhinoscopy (făr-ĭn″gō-rī-nŏs'kō-pĭ). Inspection of the nasopharynx and posterior nares.

pharyngoscope (făr-ĭn'gō-skōp). Instrument for examination of the pharynx.

pharyngoscopy (făr-ĭn-gos'kō-pĭ). Examination of the pharynx.

pharyngospasm (făr-ĭn'gō-spăzm). Spasmodic contraction of muscles of the pharynx. SYN: *pharyngismus*.

pharyngotherapy (făr-ĭn″gō-thĕr'ă-pĭ). Treatment of pharyngeal disturbances or diseases.

pharyngotome (făr-ĭn'gō-tōm). Instrument for incision of the pharynx.

pharyngotomy (făr-ĭn-gŏt'ō-mĭ). Incision of the pharynx.

pharynx (făr'ĭnks) (pl. *pharynges*). A musculomembranous tube from oral cavity to esophagus.

phase (fāz). 1. A stage of development. 2. A transitory appearance.

phas'ic re'flex. Normal response to stimulation indicated by coördinated movement.

phasin (fā'sĭn). A plant substance which causes erythrocyte agglutination.

phatne (făt'nē). Socket for a tooth.

phatnoma (făt-nō'mă). Tumor of a tooth socket.

phatnorrhagia (făt″nō-rā'jĭ-ă). Hemorrhage from the socket of a tooth.

phatnorrhea (făt-nō-rē'ă). Purulent disintegration of dental periosteum. SYN: *pyorrhea alveolaris*.

phediuretin (fĕd-ū-rē'tĭn). A phenol derivative used as an anodyne and diuretic.

phenacaine (fē'nă-kān, fĕn'ă-kān). A local anesthetic resembling cocaine, but more rapid in effect.

phenacetin (fē-năs'e-tĭn). White crystalline compound commercially prepared as an antipyretic.

    DOSAGE: 5 gr. (0.3 Gm.).

phenalgin (fē-năl'jĭn). A commercial analgesic and antipyretic.

phenate (fē'nāt). A salt of phenic acid.

phenazone (fĕn'ă-zōn). SEE: *antipyrine*.

phenegol (fē'nē-gōl). Antiseptic and emetic formed from mercuric potassium salt of nitroparaphenolsulfonic acid.

phenetidine (fĕn-ĕt'ĭ-dēn). A basic amino derivative used in manufacture of medicine. [etidin in the urine.

phenetidinuria (fĕn-ĕt″ĭd-ĭn-ū'rĭ-ă). Phen-

phenetsal (fĕn-ĕt'săl). A phenetidin derivative, with effects resembling salol.
DOSAGE: 5 to 15 gr. (0.3 to 1 Gm.).

phengophobia (fĕn-gō-fō'bĭ-ă). Abnormal dread of light. SYN: *photophobia*.

phenic acid (fē'nĭk). Carbolic acid, *q.v.*

phenobarbital (fē"nō-bar'bĭ-tăl). A derivative of veronal.
DOSAGE: ¼ to 2 gr. (0.015-0.12 Gm.).

phenobarbital sodium (soluble phenobarbital). More rapidly absorbed than phenobarbital. [Gm.].
DOSAGE: From ½ to 5 gr. (0.03-0.3

phenocoll (fē'nō-kŏl). A white crystalline base from coal tar compounds which are used as analgesics and antipyretics.

phenol (fē'nōl). C₆H₅OH, USP. 1. A crystalline, colorless or light pink, solid melting at 43° C., obtained from the distillation of coal tar, having a characteristic odor, and dangerous because of its rapid corrosive action on tissues. SYN: *carbolic acid.** 2. Any of the aromatic hydroxyl derivatives of benzene of which phenol is the type.
p. coefficient. The germicidal efficiency of phenol as a standard in testing disinfectants in comparison of their potency. SEE: *carbolic acid, phenol.*
p. red. An indicator used in determining hydrogen ion concentration.

phenolin (fĕn'ō-lĭn). Antiseptic prepared from cresol.

phenolization (fē"nō-lĭ-zā'shŭn). Treatment with phenol.

phenology (fē-nōl'ō-jĭ). Branch of biology dealing with the development of animal and plant life as affected by climate.

phenolphthalein (fē"nōl-thăl'ē-ĭn, fē"nōl-thăl'ĕn). USP. A white, yellowish, crystallized powder, produced by the interaction of phenol and phthalic anhydride.
DOSAGE: 1 gr. (0.06 Gm.). SEE: *indicator.*

phenolsulphonphthalein (fē"nōl-sul'fōn-thăl'ĕn). Phenol compound used to test renal function and as an indicator. SYN: *phenol red.*

phenoltetrachlorphthalein (fē"nōl-tĕt"răklōr-thăl'ĕn). A phenol compound used to test function of the liver and as a purgative.

phenoluria (fē"nōl-ū'rĭ-ă). Elimination of phenols in the urine.

phenomenon (fē-nōm'ē-nŏn). A change perceivable by the senses that occurs in an organ or vital function; a symptom.
p., Bell's. Rolling of the eyeballs upward and outward when an attempt is made to close the eye affected in peripheral facial paralysis.

phenopyrine (fē"nō-pī'rēn). Antiseptic composed of equal parts of antipyrine and phenol.

phenoresorcin (fē"nō-rē-sor'sĭn). Compound of resorcin and phenol.

phenosalyl (fē"nō-săl'ĭl). An external antiseptic compound of phenol, salicylic acid, menthol, and lactic acid.

phenyl (fĕn'ĭl). In chemistry, the univalent radical of phenol C₆H₅.

phenyl salicylate (săl-ĭs'ĭl-āt). USP. Compound of salicylic acid and phenol.
DOSAGE: 5 gr. (0.3 Gm.).

phenylhydrazine (fĕn"ĭl-hī'dră-zēn). Oily nitrogenous base used as a test for presence of sugar.

pheochrome (fē'ō-krōm). Staining readily with chromium salts. SYN: *chromaffin.*

pheochromoblast (fē"ō-krō'mō-blăst). A primitive cell which develops into a cell that stains readily with chromium salts, as in adrenal body.

pheochromocyte (fē"ō-krō'mō-sīt). A cell staining readily with chromium salts.

pheochromocytoma (fē"ō-krō-mō-sī-tō'mă). A tumor in the adrenal medulla arising from overgrowth of pheochromocytes.

phesin (fē'sĭn). A commercial antipyretic and antineuralgic.

phial (fī'ăl). A small vessel for medicine; a vial.

phimosis (fī-mō'sĭs). Stenosis or narrowness of preputial orifice so that the foreskin cannot be pushed back over the glans penis.
p. vaginalis. Narrowness or closure of the vaginal orifice.

phlebalgia (flĕb-ăl'jĭ-ă). Pain in varices or venules within or around a nerve.

phlebangioma (flĕb-ăn-jĭ-ō'mă). An aneurysm occurring in a vein.

phlebarteriectasia (flĕb"ăr-tē"rĭ-ĕk-tā'zĭ-ă). Varicose aneurysms; dilatation of blood vessels.

phlebarteriodialysis (flĕb"ăr-tē"rĭ-ō-dī-ăl'ĭs-ĭs). Arteriovenous aneurysm.

phlebectasia, phlebectasis (flĕb-ĕk-tā'zĭ-ă, -ĕk'tă-sĭs). Venous dilatation. SYN: *varicosity.*

phlebectomy (flĕb-ĕk'tō-mĭ). Surgical removal of a vein.

phlebectopia (flĕb-ĕk-tō'pĭ-ă). Abnormal position of a vein.

phlebemphraxis (flĕb-ĕm-frăk'sĭs). Artificial obstruction of a vein.

phlebhepatitis (flĕb-hĕp-ă-tī'tĭs). Inflammation of the hepatic vein.

phlebin (flĕb'ĭn). A pigment assumed to be present in venous blood.

phlebismus (flĕb-ĭz'mŭs). Venous congestion and dilatation. [vein.

phlebitis (flĕ-bī'tĭs). Inflammation of a
p. nodularis necrotisans. Circumscribed inflammation of cutaneous veins resulting in nodules which ulcerate.
p., puerperal. Venous inflammation following childbirth.
p., sinus. Inflammation of a sinus of the cerebrum.

phlebocholosis (flĕb"ō-kō-lō'sĭs). Diseased condition of a vein.

phleboclysis (flĕb-ŏk'lĭ-sĭs). The introduction of an isotonic solution of dextrose or other substances into a vein.
p., drip. Injection, intravenously, drip by drip. SEE: *Murphy drip procedure.*

phlebogram (flĕb'ō-grăm). A tracing of venous movement.

phlebolite, phlebolith (flĕb'ō-lĭt, -lĭth). A venous concretion, caused by calcification of a thrombus.

phlebology (flĕb-ŏl′ō-jĭ). The science of veins and their diseases.

phlebometritis (flĕb″ō-mē-trī′tĭs). Inflammation of uterine veins.

phlebomyomatosis (flĕb″ō-mī″ō-mă-tō′sĭs). Thickening of the tissue of a vein from overgrowth of muscular fibers.

phlebopexy (flĕb′ō-pĕks″ĭ). Extraserous transplantation of the testes for varicocele, with preservation of venous network.

phleboplasty (flĕb′ō-plăs″tĭ). Plastic repair of a wounded vein.

phleborrhaphy (flĕb-or′ăf-ĭ). Suture of a vein.

phleborrhexis (flĕb-or-rĕks′ĭs). Rupture of a vein.

phlebosclerosis (flĕb″ō-sklē-rō′sĭs). Fibrous hardening of a vein's walls.

phlebostasia, phlebostasis (flĕb-ō-stā′zĭ-ă, -ŏs′tă-sĭs). Compression of veins temporarily removing an amount of blood from the general circulation. SYN: *phlebotomy, bloodless.*

phlebothrombosis (flĕb″ō-thrŏm-bō′sĭs). Clotting in a vein; phlebitis with secondary thrombosis.

phlebotome (flĕb′ō-tōm). Lancet used in cutting a vein.

phlebotomist (flĕb-ŏt′ō-mĭst). One who advocates and practices blood letting.

phlebotomy (flĕb-ŏt′ō-mĭ). Opening a vein. SYN: *venesection, q.v.*

p., bloodless. Compression of veins of the extremities, cutting off some of the blood from the general circulation. SYN: *phlebostasia.*

phlegm (flĕm). 1. Thick mucus, esp. that from the respiratory passages. 2. One of the 4 "humors" of early physiology.

phlegmasia (flĕg-mā′zĭ-ă). Inflammation.

p. alba dolens. Acute edema, esp. of leg from venous obstruction, usually thrombosis.

p., cellulitic. Septic inflammation of connective tissue of the leg following childbirth.

p. malabarica. Inflammation with hypertrophy and induration of the skin. SYN: *elephantiasis.*

p., thrombotic. SEE: *phlegmasia alba dolens.*

phlegmatic (flĕg-măt′ĭk). Of sluggish or calm temperament. SYN: *apathetic.*

phlegmon (flĕg′mŏn). Acute suppurative inflammation of subcutaneous connective tissue.

p., bronze. Gaseous phlegmon after a renal operation causing bronze spots near incision.

p., diffuse. Diffuse inflammation of subcutaneous tissues with sepsis.

p., gas. Phlegmon with extensive emphysema.

phlegmonous (flĕg′mŏn-ŭs). Pert. to inflammation of subcutaneous tissues.

phlogistic (flō-jĭs′tĭk). Pert. to or inducing inflammation.

phlogocyte (flō′gō-sīt). A typical cell in tissue during inflammation. SYN: *irritation cell, plasma cell, stimulation cell.*

phlogocytosis (flō″gō-sī-tō′sĭs). Presence of many phlogocytes in the peripheral circulation.

phlogogenic, phlogogenous (flō-gō-jĕn′ĭk, -gŏj′ĕn-ŭs). Producing or exciting inflammation.

phlogosin (flō-gō′sĭn). Substance, isolated from cultures of *Staphylococcus aureus,* producing suppuration.

phlogosis (flō-gō′sĭs). 1. Inflammation. 2. Erysipelas.

phloretin (flor′e-tĭn). Product derived from phlorizin used as a febrifuge.

phlorizin (flor′ĭz-ĭn). A bitter, white, crystalline glucoside used as an antiperiodic and tonic.

phlyctena (flĭk-tē′nă). A thin ichor or lymph containing vesicle, esp. one of many after a first degree burn.

phlyctenoid (flĭk-tē′noyd). Resembling a blister or pustule.

phlyctenosis (flĭk-tē-nō′sĭs). Appearance of blisters or pustules.

phlyctenula (flĭk-tĕn′ū-lă). A tiny vesicle or pustule, esp. that seen on the cornea.

phlyctenular (flĭk-tĕn′ū-lăr). Resembling or pert. to vesicles or pustules.

phlyctenule (flĭk-tĕn′ūl). A small vesicle or blister, as on cornea or conjunctiva.

phlyctenulosis (flĭk-tĕn-ū-lō′sĭs). The formation of many phlyctenules.

phlyzacium (fli-za′sĭ-um). 1. A minute pustule. 2. Inflammatory disease of the skin with large, superficial pustules. SYN: *ecthyma.*   [*fear.*

-phobia. Suffix meaning *dread, horror,*

phobic (fō′bĭk). Concerning a phobia.

phobophobia (fō″bō-fō′bĭ-ă). Morbid fear of acquiring a phobia.

phonacoscope (fō-năk′ō-skōp). A device for increasing the percussion note or voice sounds.

phonacoscopy (fō-năk-ŏs′kō-pĭ). Inspection of the chest with the phonacoscope.

phonal (fō′năl). Concerning the voice.

phonasthenia (fō-năs-thē′nĭ-ă). Abnormal voice sounds due to functional fatigue.

phonation (fō-nā′shŭn). Process of uttering vocal sounds.

phonatory (fō′nă-tō-rĭ). Concerning utterance of vocal sounds.

p. bands. Vocal cords.

phonautograph (fōn-aw′tō-grăf). Device for registering the voice's vibrations.

phoneme (fō′nēm). Auditory hallucination of voices and spoken words.
   May include neologisms. They may repeat a thought or the part of a sentence just read.

phonendoscope (fō-nĕn′dō-skōp). A stethoscope magnifying sounds.

phonendoskiascope (fō-nen″dō-skī′ăs-kōp). Device for observing the cardiac movements and for hearing heart sounds.

phonetics (fō-nĕt′ĭks). Science of speech and pronunciation. SYN: *phonology.*

phonic (fō′nĭk). Concerning the voice or sound.

phonism (fō′nĭzm). An auditory sensation occurring when another sense is stimulated. SEE: *synesthesia.*

phono-. Combining form meaning *sound, voice.*

phonocardiography (fō″nō-kar-dǐ-ǒg-rǎ-fǐ). Mechanical registration of heart sounds.

phonogram (fō′nō-grăm). A graphic curve indicating intensity and duration of a sound.

phonograph (fō′nō-grăf). Appliance used for reproduction of sounds.

phonology (fō-nŏl′ō-jǐ). Science of vocal sounds. SYN: *phonetics.*

phonomassage (fō″nō-măs-sazh′). Exciting movements of the ossicles of the ear by means of noise directed through the ext. auditory meatus.

phonometer (fō-nŏm′ět-ěr). Device for determining intensity of vocal sounds.

phonomyoclonus (fō″nō-mǐ-ok′lō-nŭs). Invisible fibrillary muscular contractions revealed by auscultation.

phonomyogram (fō′nō-mǐ′ō-grăm). A recording of sound produced by action of a muscle.

phonomyography (fō″nō-mǐ-og′rǎ-fǐ). The recording of sounds made by contracting muscular tissue.

phonopathy (fō-nŏp′ăth-ǐ). Any disease of organs affecting speech.

phonophore (fō′nō-fōr). 1. An ossicle of the ear. 2. A form of binaural stethoscope.

phonopneumomassage (fō″nō-nu″mō-măs-sazh′). Massage of the middle ear, and by forcing air into the ext. auditory meatus.

phonopsia (fō-nŏp′sǐ-ă). Perception of certain sounds which cause a subjective color sensation.

phonoscope (fō′nō-skōp). Device for recording photographs of heart sounds.

phoresis (fō-rē′sǐs). PT: The migration of ions through a membrane by the action of an electric current.

phorology (fō-rol′ō-jǐ). Science dealing with disease carriers.

phorometer (fō-rŏm′ět-ěr). Device for examination of the extrinsic ocular muscles.

phorotone (fō′rō-tōn). Device for exercising eye muscles.

phose (fōz). A subjective sensation of light or color.

phosphatase (fŏs′făt-ās). An enzyme which splits phosphoric acid esters.

phosphate (fŏs′făt). A salt of phosphoric acid. [in the blood.

phosphatemia (fŏs-fă-tē′mǐ-ă). Phosphates

phosphatide (fŏs′fă-tīd). One of a group of fatty substances containing phosphoric acid.
　　An example is lecithin. SYN: *phospholipide, phospholipin.*

phosphatine (fŏs′fă-tīn). One of a class of phosphorous compounds found in brain tissue.

phosphatometer (fŏs-fă-tŏm′ět-ěr). Device for measuring the amount of phosphates in the urine.

phosphatoptosis (fŏs-fă-tŏp-tō′sǐs). Spontaneous precipitation of phosphates in urine.

phosphaturia (fŏs-fă-tū′rǐ-ă). Phosphates in the urine.

phosphene (fŏs′fēn). A subjective sensation of light caused by pressure upon the eyeball.

phosphide (fŏs′fīd). Binary compound of phosphorus with an element or radical.

phosphite (fŏs′fīt). A salt of phosphoric acid.

phosphocreatine (fŏs″fō-krē′ă-tēn). A compound found in muscle of equal parts of phosphoric acid and creatine.

phospholipid (fŏs″fō-lĭp′ĭd). A lipoid substance containing phosphorus, fatty acids and nitrogenous base, as lecithin. SYN: *phosphatide.*

phospholipin (fŏs-fō-lĭp′ĭn). A lipoid compound containing phosphorus. SYN: *phosphatide.*

phosphonecrosis (fŏs″fō-nē-krō′sĭs). Necrosis of the alveolar process in those working with phosphorus.

phosphopenia (fŏs″fō-pē′nĭ-ă). Lack of phosphorus in the body.

phosphoprotein (fŏs″fō-prō′tē-ĭn). One of a group of proteins in which the protein is combined with phosphorus other than lecithin or nucleic acid.
　　Formerly called nucleoalbumin.

phosphorated (fŏs″fō-rā-tĕd). Impregnated with phosphorus.

phosphorenesis (fŏs″fō-rĕn′ē-sĭs). Any condition of the body due to excess of calcium phosphate.

phosphorescence (fŏs-fō-rĕs′ĕns). PT: The induced luminescence that persists after cessation of the irradiation that caused it.

phosphoretted (fŏs″fō-rĕt-ĕd). Impregnated with, or charged with phosphorus.

phosphorhidrosis (fŏs″for-hĭd-rō′sĭs). Secretion of phosphorescent perspiration. SYN: *phosphoridrosis.*

phosphoric acid (fŏs-for′ĭk). One of 3 oxygen acids of phosphorus. SEE: *acid.*

phosphoridrosis (fŏs″for-ĭd-rō′sĭs). Secretion of perspiration that is luminous. SYN: *phosphorhidrosis.*

phosphorism (fŏs″for-ĭzm). Chronic poisoning from phosphorus.

phosphorous acid (fŏs-fō′rŭs). Crystalline acid formed when phosphorus is oxidized in moist air. SEE: *acid.*

phosphoruria (fŏs″for-ū′rǐ-ă). Phosphorus in the urine in excess of normal. SYN: *phosphaturia, phosphuria.*

phosphorus (fŏs′fĕr-ŭs). SYMB: P. At. wt. 31.04. A nonmetallic element not found in a free state but in combination with alkalies.

phosphotal (fŏs′fō-tăl). Commercial phosphorus and creosote compound.

phosphuria (fŏs-fū′rǐ-ă). Excess of phosphorus in the urine. SYN: *phosphaturia, phosphoruria.*

photalgia (fō-tăl′jǐ-ă). Pain produced by light. SYN: *photodynia.*

photaugiophobia (fō-tăw-jǐ-ō-fō′bǐ-ă). Intolerance of bright light.

phote (fōt). The unit of photochemical energy, 1 lumen per square centimeter, employed in determination of color solidity in comparison with average noonday solar light.

photesthesis (fō-těs-thē'sĭs). Sensitivity to light.

photic (fō'tĭk). Concerning light.

photism (fō'tĭzm). A subjective sensation of color or light produced by a stimulus of another sense, such as smell, hearing, taste, or touch. SEE: synesthesia.

photo-. Combining form meaning *light*.

photobiotic (fō"to-bī-ŏt'ĭk). Capable of living only in the light.

photocauterization (fō"tō-kaw-tĕr-ĭz-ā'shŭn). Cauterization using radioactive means, as x-rays.

photoceptor (fō"tō-sĕp'tor). A nerve ceptor receiving light ray sensations.

photochemistry (fō"tō-kĕm'ĭs-trĭ). Phase of science dealing with chemical changes produced by light rays.

photodynamic (fō"tō-dī-năm'ĭk). Pert. to the effect of light on organisms.

photodynia (fō"tō-dĭn'ĭ-ă). Pain produced by rays of light. SYN: photalgia.

photodysphoria (fō"tō-dĭs-fō'rĭ-ă). Extreme intolerance of light. SYN: photophobia, phengophobia.

photoelectricity (fō"tō-ē-lĕk-trĭ'sĭ-tĭ). Electricity formed by action of light.

photogene (fō'tō-jēn). Prolonged retinal image. SYN: after-image.

photogenic, photogenous (fō"tō-jĕn'ĭk, -tŏj'ĕn-ŭs). Induced by or inducing light.

photograph'ic radiom'eter. PT: An instrument containing a half-tone color index for strips of photographic paper after exposure to roentgen rays and after development, used to estimate the quantity of roentgen rays.

photohemotachometer (fō"tō-hem"ō-tăk-ŏm'ĕt-ĕr). Device for photographing velocity of blood current.

photoinactivation (fō"tō-ĭn-ăk-tĭ-vā'shŭn). Inactivation of complement by use of light rays.

photokinetic (fō"tō-kĭn-ĕt'ĭk). Reacting with motion to stimulus of light.

photoluminescence (fō"tō-lū-min-ĕs'ĕns). P't: The power of an object to become luminescent when acted on by light.

photolysis (fō-tŏl'ĭs-ĭs). Dissolution or disintegration under stimulus of light rays.

photolytic (fō"tō-lĭt'ĭk). Dissolved by stimulus of light rays.

photomania (fō"tō-mā'nĭ-ă). 1. A psychosis produced by prolonged exposure to intense light. 2. A psychotic desire for light.

photometer (fō-tŏm'ĕt-ĕr). PT: A device for measuring the intensity of light.

photometry (fō-tŏm'ĕt-rĭ). Measurement of light rays.

photomicrograph (fō"tō-mī'krō-grăf). Enlarged photograph of an object under the microscope.

photon (fō'tŏn). A light particle comparable to an electron.

photoncia (fō-tŏn'sĭ-ă). Swelling caused by the action of light.

photonosus (fō-tŏn'ō-sŭs). Disease due to prolonged exposure to intense light.

photoperceptive (fō"tō-pĕr-cĕp'tĭv). Capable of perceiving light.

photophilic (fō-tō-fĭl'ĭk). Seeking or fond of light.

photophobia (fō"tō-fō'bĭ-ă). Unusual intolerance of light.
 Occurs in measles and rubella, meningitis, and inflammations of the eyes. SYN: phengophobia, photodysphoria.

photophone (fō"tō-fōn). Device for production of sound by action of light.

photophore (fō"tō-fōr). Apparatus for examining cavities by electricity.

photopia (fō-tō'pĭ-ă). Adjustment of eye muscles to light.

photopsia, photopsy (fō-tŏp'sĭ-ă, fō"tŏp-sĭ). Subjective sensation of sparks or flashes of light in retinal, optic, or brain diseases.

photoptarmosis (fō"tō-tar-mō'sĭs). Sneezing caused by the action of light.

photoptometer (fō-tō-tŏm'ĕt-ĕr). Device for determining acuteness of vision.

photoreceptive (fō"tō-rē-sĕp'tĭv). Capable of perceiving light rays.

photoreceptor (fō"tō-rē-sep'tor). Nerve ceptor sensitive to light stimuli.

photoscope (fō"tō-skōp). A variety of fluoroscope used to observe light.

photoscopy (fō-tŏs'kō-pĭ). Examination with a fluorescent screen. SYN: fluoroscopy, skiascopy.

photosensitization (fō"tō-sĕn-sĭ-tĭ-zā'shŭn). Process by which phenomena are produced in living system by substances not normally present in these systems which sensitize them to light.

photosensitizer (fō"tō-sĕn-sĭ-tī'zĕr). Sensitizing substance used in light therapy to produce photosensitization, such as fluorescein dyes.

photosynthesis (fō"tō-sĭn'the-sĭs). The process by which plants are able to manufacture carbohydrates from the air in the presence of light.

phototaxis (fō"tō-tăks'ĭs). PT: The reaction and movement of cells and microorganisms under the stimulus of light.

phototherapy (fō"tō-thĕr'ă-pĭ). Light therapy, the use of light in treating disease.

photothermal (fō"tō-thĕr'măl). Concerning heat produced by light.
 p. radiation. Radiation of heat by a source of light, as that from an electric bulb.

phototoxis (fō"tō-toks'ĭs). Disorder produced by effects of overexposure to light or radiation.

photuria (fō-tū'rĭ-ă). Excretion of phosphorescent urine.

phren (frēn). 1. The mind. 2. The diaphragm.

phrenalgia (frē-năl'jĭ-ă). 1. Pain of mental origin or caused by a mental process. SYN: psychalgia. 2. Pain in the diaphragm.

phrenasthenia (fren-ăs-thē'nĭ-ă). Mental deficiency.

phrenetic (fren-ĕt'ĭk). 1. Maniacal; frenzied. 2. A maniac.

phrenic (fren'ĭk). 1. Concerning the diaphragm, as the phrenic nerve. 2. Concerning the mind.

p. avulsion. Elevation of a side of the diaphragm and semicollapse of corresponding lung by means of excision of part of the phrenic nerve.

p. nerve. One arising in the cervical plexus entering the thorax and passing to the diaphragm.

A motor nerve to the diaphragm with sensory fibers to the pericardium. SYN: *nervus phrenicus.*

phrenicectomy (fren-ĭs-ĕk'tō-mĭ). Resection of a part of the phrenic nerve.

phrenicoexairesis (fren"ĭ-kō-ĕks-ĭ-rē'sĭs). Excision of part of the phrenic nerve.

phrenicotomy (fren-ĭk-ŏt'ō-mĭ). Cutting of the phrenic nerve to produce immobilization of a lung by inducing a paralysis of 1 side.

This causes the diaphragm to rise, it compresses the lung, and diminishes respiratory movement, thus resting the viscus.

phrenitis (frē-nī'tĭs). 1. Acute delirium or frenzy. 2. Inflammation of the brain. SYN: *encephalitis.* 3. Inflammation of the diaphragm.

phreno-. Combining form meaning *mind, midriff.*

phrenocardia (frē"nŏ-kar'dĭ-ă). Cardiovascular neurasthenia.

phrenocolopexy (frē"nŏ-kō'lō-pĕks"ĭ). Suture of the transverse colon to the diaphragm.   [diaphragm.

phrenodynia (frē"nŏ-dĭn'ĭ-ă). Pain in the

phrenograph (fren'ō-grăf). Device for registering movements of diaphragm.

phrenology (frē-nol'ō-jĭ). Study of the shape of the skull as indicative of characteristics and mental faculties.

phrenopathy (frē-nŏp'ăth-ĭ). Any mental disorder.

phrenopericarditis (frē"nŏ-pĕr-ĭ-kar-dī'tĭs). Attachment of the heart by adhesions to the diaphragm.

phrenoplegia (frē-nŏ-plē'jĭ-ă). 1. A sudden psychopathic attack. 2. Paralysis of the diaphragm.

phrenosin (fren'ō-sĭn). A nitrogenous principle obtained from brain substance.

phrictopathic (frĭk-tŏ-păth'ĭk). Pert. to or having a shuddering sensation; applied to a shuddering sensation due to irritating a hysterical anesthetic area.

phthiocol (thĭ'ō-kŏl). Oily yellow pigment found in tubercle bacilli.

phthiriasis (thĭr-ĭ'ăs-ĭs). Condition of being infested with lice. SYN: *pediculosis.*

p. palpebrarum. Presence of lice on the eyelashes.

phthiriophobia (thĭr"ĭ-ŏ-fō'bĭ-ă). Abnormal dread of lice.

Phthirius (thĭr'ĭ-ŭs). Genus of crab louse.

phthisic (tĭz'ĭk). 1. Affected with pulmonary consumption. 2. Asthma. 3. One afflicted with phthisis or asthma.

phthisical (tĭz'ĭk-ăl). Concerning, or afflicted with, phthisis.

phthisicky (tĭz'ĭ-kĭ). Suffering from asthma or phthisis.

phthisis (tĭ'sĭs). 1. Pulmonary consumption. SEE: *tuberculosis.* 2. Any wasting or atrophic disease.

p., abdominal. Intestinal tuberculosis.

p., black. Lung disease from inhaled coal dust. SYN: *anthracosis.*

p. bulbi. Atrophy of eyeball following intraocular inflammation.

p., fibroid. 1. Interstitial pneumonia. 2. Pulmonary tuberculosis with dense layers of fibrous tissues surrounding a cavity.

p. mesenterica. Tuberculosis of the mesentery glands.

p., miner's. SEE: *black phthisis.*

p., pulmonary. Tuberculosis of the lungs.

p., stonecutter's. A wasting form of bronchopneumonia due to inhalation of stone dust with consequent irritation. SYN: *chalicosis.*

phygogalactic (fī"gō-găl-ăk'tĭk). Checking or that which checks or arrests milk secretion. SYN: *galactophygous, ischogalactic, lactifuge.*

phylacogen (fī-lăk'ō-jĕn). Commercial bacterial culture filtrate which stimulates defensive protein formation in the body.

phylacogogic (fī-lăk-ō-gŏj'ĭk). Stimulating the formation of protective antibodies.

phylactic (fī-lăk'tĭk). Concerning or producing phylaxis.

p. agent. One with protective power.

p. power. That of an organism to ward off infection.

phylaxin (fī-lăks'ĭn). Substance warding off infection. SEE: *mycophylaxin, toxophylaxin.*

phylaxis (fī-lăks'ĭs). The active defense of the body against infection.

phyllo-. Combining form meaning *leaf.*

phylogenesis (fī-lō-jĕn'ē-sĭs). The growth of a group, race, or species.

phylogenetical (fī"lō-jĕn-ĕt'ĭk-ăl). Concerning the development of a race or group.

phylogeny (fī-lŏj'ē-nĭ). Development and growth of a group or race.

phylum (fī'lŭm). One of the primary divisions of the animal or plant kingdom.

phyma (fī'mă) (pl. *phymata*). A small, rounded skin tumor.

phymatoid (fī'măt-oyd). Like a tumor.

phymatosis (fī-mă-tō'sĭs). A disease marked by the presence of phymata or small nodules in the skin.

phyone (fī'ōn). 1. The growth factor of the ant. pituitary body. 2. Commercial preparation of growth factor of ant. pituitary body.

physaliform, physaliform (fĭs-al'ĭ-form). Resembling a bleb or bubble.

physaliphore (fĭs-al'ĭf-or). A round cavity in a cancer cell.

physalis (fĭs'ăl-ĭs). Huge brood cell from a cancer or sarcoma.

physic (fĭz'ĭk). 1. The art of medicine and healing. 2. A medicine, esp. a cathartic. 3. Drugs in general.

physical (fĭz'ĭk-ăl). Concerning the body.

p. examination. Examination of the body by auscultation, palpation, percussion, and inspection.

p. signs. Disease symptoms revealed by physical examination.

p. therapist. PT: A medical graduate skilled in physical therapy.

p. therapy. The therapeutic use of physical agents other than drugs.

It comprises the use of physical, chemical, and other properties of heat, light, water, electricity, massage, exercise, and radiation. SEE: *breeze, static.*

p. t. technician or aide. A lay assistant or a nurse trained to apply the physical measures of treatment which have been prescribed by a physician. **p. unit.** Coulomb, erg, dyne, etc. SEE: *unit.*

physician (fĭ-zĭsh'ăn). A person authorized by law to treat diseases with medicines.

physicist (fĭz'ĭs-ĭst). One who is versed in the science of physics.

physico-. Combining form meaning *physical, natural.*

physics (fĭz'ĭks). The study of forces and properties of matter, and of natural phenomena.

physinosis (fĭz-ĭn-ō'sĭs). A disease caused by physical agents.

physio-. Combining form meaning *nature.*

physiognomy (fĭz-ĭ-ŏg'nō-mĭ). 1. The countenance. 2. Assumed ability to see the mental or moral character and qualities by the face.

physiognosis (fĭz-ĭ-ŏg-nō'sĭs). Diagnosis determined from one's facial expression and appearance of the eyes.

physiological (fĭz''ĭ-ō-lŏj'ĭk-ăl). 1. Normal; not diseased. 2. Concerning body function.

p. chemistry. Chemistry of living organisms. SEE: *biochemistry.*

p. salt solution. One teaspoonful of salt to a pint of water is a normal salt solution. It may be abbreviated as N. S. Sol.

p. s. s. enema. The distention made by this enema excites peristalsis and evacuation. Often ordered when there is dehydration. SEE: *enema.*

physiology (fĭz-ĭ-ŏl'ō-jĭ). The science of the functions of cells, tissues, and organs of the living organism. SEE: *cerebrophysiology, chemophysiology.*

physiotherapy (fĭz-ĭ-ō-thĕr'ă-pĭ). Treatment with physical and mechanical means, as massage, electricity, etc.

The term "physical therapy" has supplanted it in medical usage.

physo-. Combining form meaning *bladder, bellows, bubble.*

physocele (fĭ'sō-sēl). 1. A tumor filled with gas or circumscribed swelling due to gas. 2. A gas-distended hernial sac.

physohematometra (fĭ''sō-hem-ăt-ō-mē'tră). Gas and blood distending the uterus.

physohydrometra (fĭ''sō-hī-drō-mē'tră). Air or gas and serum in the uterus.

physometra (fĭ-sō-mē'tră). Air or gas in the uterine cavity.

physopyosalpinx (fĭ''sō-pī''ō-săl'pĭnks). Pus and gas in the fallopian tube.

physostigmine salicylate (fĭ-sō-stĭg'mēn

săl-ĭs'ĭl-āt). USP. The salicylate of an alkaloid obtained from the dried Calabar bean.

DOSAGE: In eye, solutions 1%. Internally 1/30 gr. (0.002 Gm.).

phyto-, phyt-. Combining forms meaning a *plant*, or *that which grows.*

phytalbumin (fī-tăl-bū'mĭn). An albumin from plants and vegetables.

phytalbumose (fī-tăl'bū-mōs). An albumose found in plants and vegetables.

phytase (fī'tās). A liver and blood ferment which splits phytin.

phytin (fī'tĭn). Substance derived from plants which is used as a stimulant.

DOSAGE: 4-15 gr. (0.25-1.0 Gm.).

phytobezoar (fī''tō-bē'zōr). A stone composed of vegetable matter found in the stomach. SYN: *food ball.*

phytosis (fī-tō'sĭs). Any disease of vegetable parasitic origin.

pia (pī'ă). Innermost cerebrospinal membrane.

p. arachnoid (ă-răk'noyd). The pia mater and arachnoid membranes, when regarded as 1 structure.

p. cerebral. The pia of the brain, containing in its meshes ramifications of cerebral vessels.

p., external. Pia covering ext. of the brain.

p., internal. Pia within the ventricles of the brain.

p. mater. Innermost vascular membrane covering the spinal cord, nerves, and brain.

p., spinal. SEE: *pia mater.*

pia-arachnitis (pī-ă-ăr-ăk-nī'tĭs). Inflammation of the arachnoid and pia mater. SYN: *leptomeningitis.*

pial (pī'al). Concerning the pia mater.

pialyn (pī'al-in). A fat-splitting enzyme. SYN: *lipase, steapsin.*

pian (pī-ăn'). Contagious skin disease of the tropics. SYN: *frambesia, yaws.*

pianists' cramp (pē'ăn-ĭsts). Spasm or professional neurosis of muscles of fingers and forearms from piano playing.

piarachnitis (pi-ăr-ăk-nī'tĭs). Inflamed condition of the arachnoid and pia mater.

piarachnoid (pĭ-ăr-ăk'noyd). The pia and arachnoid considered as one.

piarrhemia (pī-ar-ē'mĭ-ă). Fat or lipids in the blood. SYN: *lipemia.*

pica (pī'kă). A perversion of appetite, with craving for substance not fit for food.

piceous (pī'sē-ŭs). Like pitch.

Pick's syndrome (pĭk). 1. Effusions in the serous cavities with cardiac decompensation and ascites. 2. Progressive dementia.

picrate (pĭk'rāt). A salt of picric acid.

picric ac'id (pĭk'rĭk). Bitter yellow crystalline substance formed by action of nitric acid on phenol or allied compounds.

Used as a dye, an antiseptic, and in treating burns.

picro-, picr-. Combining forms meaning *bitter.*

picrocarmine (pĭk-rō-kar'mĭn). A stain used in microscopy.

picroformal (pĭk-rō-for'mal). Solution of picric acid, formaldehyde and water used as a fixing agent.

picrol (pĭk'rōl). Antiseptic powder used as a dressing.

piebald skin (pī'bawld). Skin with spots or pigmentation or patches with loss of pigment. SEE: *leukoderma, vitiligo.*

piedra (pī-ā'drä). Disease in which hard nodules form on the hair shafts.

    p. nostras. Piedra affecting the beard.

piesesthesia (pī-es-ĕs-thē'zĭ-ä). Sensibility to pressure. SYN: *pressure sense.*

piesimeter, piesometer (pī-ē-sĭm'ĕt-ĕr, -sŏm'ĕt-ĕr). Device for measurement of skin's sensitiveness to pressure.

pigment (pĭg'mĕnt). Any coloring matter. SEE: *albino, "chrom-" words.*

    p., biliary. Bilirubin, biliverdin, q.v.

    p., blood. Hematin, hemoglobin, oxyhemoglobin, q.v.

    p., endogenous. A pigment produced within the body, as melanin.

    p., exogenous. A pigment produced outside the human body.

    p., hematogenous. Pigment from hemoglobin of erythrocytes.

    p., hepatogenous. Pigment from hemoglobin destruction in the liver. SYN: *bile pigment.*

    p., urinary. Urobilin, q.v.

    p., uveal. That in cells on inner or post. surface of the iris, choroid, and ciliary processes.

pigmentary (pĭg'mĕn-tĕr-ĭ). Concerning, or like, a pigment.

pigmentation (pĭg-mĕn-tā'shŭn). Localized coloration due to deposition of pigments.

    p., lymphatic. Arrest of granules of pigment by lymph nodules in tattooing.

pigmentolysin (pĭg"mĕn-tŏl'ĭ-sĭn). An antibody that destroys pigment.

pigmentolysis (pĭg"mĕn-tŏl'ĭ-sĭs). Disintegration of pigment.

pigmentophage (pĭg-mĕn'tŏ-fāj). Cell which absorbs pigment.

pigritis (pī-grī'tĭs). Stuporous condition due to alcoholism.

piitis (pī-ī'tĭs). Inflamed condition of the pia mater.

Pil. Abbr. of L. *pilula*, pill, or pl. *pilulae*, pills.

pilar, pilary (pī'lar, pĭl'ă-rĭ). Concerning, or covered with, hair.

pilaster (pĭ-lăs'ter). A prominent line on the femur.

pile (pīl). 1. A single hemorrhoid. SEE: *piles.* 2. The hair. 3. A battery for production of electricity.

pileous (pī'lē-ŭs). Hairy; hirsute.

piles (pīls). Dilated blood vessels in the rectal mucosa forming a vascular tumor. SYN: *hemorrhoids, q.v.*

pileus (pī'lē-ŭs). A nipple shield.

    p. ventriculi. The upper part of the duodenum. SYN: *duodenal bulb.*

piliation (pĭl-ĭ-ā'shŭn). Formation and development of hair.

piliform (pĭl'ĭ-form). Hairlike.

pill (pĭl). Medicine in the form of a tiny rounded mass to be taken whole.

pillar (pĭl'ĕr). An upright support; column, or structure resembling a column.

    p. of the abdominal ring. One of the columns on either side of abdominal ring.

    p., ext., of abdominal ring. Outer aponeurotic margin of ext. abdominal ring, formed by portion of Poupart's ligament.

    p., int., of abdominal ring. Inner aponeurotic margin of ext. abdominal ring.

    p's. of Corti. Two layers resting on membrana basilaris in the ear. SYN: *rods of Corti.*

    p's. of diaphragm. Bundles of tendinous fibers arising on right side from ant. surfaces of 1st, 2nd, and 3rd lumbar vertebrae and the intervertebral fibrocartilages, and on the left side from the ant. surfaces of 2nd and 3rd lumbar vertebrae, passing upward and outward, to form an arch over the aorta.

    p's. of the fauces. Folds of mucous membrane on each side of the fauces, bet. which is situated the tonsil. SEE: *fauces.*

    p's., ant., of fornix. Two diverging columns extending downward from ant. extremity of body of the fornix.

    p's., posterior, of fornix. Two bands forming prolongation of fornix posteriorly.

pilleus, pilleum (pĭl'ē-ŭs, -ŭm). A membrane sometimes covering a baby's head at birth. SYN: *caul.*

    p. ventriculi. The 1st portion of the duodenum. SYN: *pyloric cap.*

pillion (pĭl'yŭn). Artificial leg, esp. in form of a stump.

pilo-. Combining form meaning *hair.*

pilocarpine hydrochlor'ide (pī"lō-kar'pēn). Hydrochloride of an alkaloid obtained from leaves of the plant.

    DOSAGE: 1/12 gr. (0.005 Gm.).

    p. ni'trate. USP. Nitrate of the alkaloid obtained from pilocarpus.

    DOSAGE: Same as pilocarpine hydrochloride.

pilocystic (pī-lō-sĭs'tĭk). Encysted and containing hair, said of a dermoid cyst.

pilomotor (pī-lō-mō'tor). Causing the movements of hairs, as the *arrectores pilarum.*

    p. reflex. Gooseflesh formation when skin is stroked.

pilonidal (pī-lō-nī'dăl). Containing hairs in a cyst in nest formation.

    p. fistula. Fistula near the rectum resulting from a growth of subcutaneous hair.

    p. sinus. A pilonidal fistula.

pilose (pī'lōs). Hairy, downy.

pilosebaceous (pī"lō-sē-bā'shŭs). Concerning the hair ánd sebaceous glands.

pilosis (pī-lō'sĭs). Excessive formation of hair.

pilosity (pī-lŏs'ĭ-tĭ). Hairiness.

pilous (pī'lŭs). Covered with hair; hirsute.

Piltz's reflex (pĭltz). Change in size of pupil on sudden fixation of attention.

pilula (pĭl′u-lă) (pl. *pilulae*). A small, solid body of medicine of a globular, ovoid or lenticular shape, intended to be swallowed whole and produce medicinal action.

pilular (pĭl′ū-lar). Pert. to, or of the nature of, pills.

pilus (pī′lŭs) (pl. *pili*). A hair.

pimel-. Combining form or prefix meaning *fat* or *associated with fat*.

pimelitis (pĭm-ĕl-ī′tĭs). Inflammation of adipose and of connective tissue in general.

pimeloma (pĭm-ĕl-ō′mă). A fatty tumor. SYN: *lipoma*.

pimelorrhea (pĭm-ĕl-or-ē′ă). Discharge of fat in loose stools.

pimelosis (pĭm-ĕl-ō′sĭs). 1. A conversion into fat. 2. Fatty degeneration of any tissue. 3. Corpulence; obesity.

pimeluria (pĭm-ĕl-ŭ′rĭ-ă). Excretion of fat or oil in urine. SYN: *lipuria*.

pimple (pĭm′pl). A tiny, sharp-pointed protuberance of the skin, sometimes going on to suppuration. SYN: *papule*, *pustule*.

pincement (pans-mong′). Pinching or nipping of the flesh in massage.

pineal (pĭ′nē-ăl) (pĭn′ē-ăl). 1. Shaped like a pine cone. 2. The small red gland attached to post. part of 3rd ventricle of brain.

pinealectomy (pĭ″nē-ăl-ĕk′tō-mĭ). Removal of the pineal body.

pinealism (pĭ′nē-ăl-ĭzm). Disorder caused by abnormality of the secretion of the pineal body.

pinealoma (pĭ-nē-ăl-ō′mă). A tumor of the pineal body.

pinealopathy (pĭ″nē-ăl-op′ăth-ĭ). Any disorder of the pineal gland.

pine tar (pīn). USP. A product obtained from the distillation of pine wood.

DOSAGE: 8 gr. (0.5 Gm.). Externally, 50% ointment in petrolatum. SYN: *pix liquida*.

pinguecula (pĭn-gwĕk′ū-lă). BNA. Yellowish thickening of bulbar conjunctiva, triangular in shape, on inner and outer margins of the cornea.

pinhole (pĭn′hōl). Small perforation made by, or size of that made by, a pin.

p. os. A very small os uteri in young women.

p. pupil. Extreme contraction of the iris.   [cone.

piniform (pĭn′ĭ-form). Shaped like a pine

pink disease (pĭnk). Rare disease of children marked by swelling and redness of feet and hands, sweating, itching and polyarthritis. SYN: *acodynia,** *erythredema*.

p. eye. Epidemic form of acute conjunctivitis* from Koch-Weeks bacillus.

pinna (pĭn′ă) (pl. *pinnae*). The auricle or projecting part of the ext. ear.

p. nasi. Protruding cartilaginous extension on each nostril. SYN: *ala nasi*.

pinocytosis (pī″nō-sī-tō′sĭs). Term for the absorption of liquids by phagocytic cells.

pinotherapy (pī-nō-thĕr′ă-pĭ). Hunger cure. SYN: *nestotherapy, peinotherapy*.

pint (pĭnt). Measure of capacity equal to one-half a quart; 16 fluid ounces; 28.875 cu. in.

pinworm (pĭn′wurm). Parasitic worm found in the intestines and rectum. SYN: *ascaris, oxyuris*.

pioepithelium (pī″ō-ĕp-ĭ-thē′lĭ-ŭm). Epithelium that has undergone fatty degeneration, or which contains fat globules.

pionemia (pī-ō-nē′mĭ-ă). Fat in the blood SYN: *lipemia*.

pioscope (pī′ō-skōp). Device for estimating the fat content of milk.

piper (pī′pĕr). Pepper.

pipet, pipette (pĭ-pĕt′). Narrow glass tube with both ends open for transferring and measuring liquids, using suction principle.

Pirogoff's amputation (pĭr′ō-gŏf). Foot amputation, removing part of the os calcis.

Piroplas (pĭ″ăl-ăz′mă). A genus of Sporo parasitic to ma

p.
cause

piroplas fectio

Pirquet culosi

pisiform pealli Pea-

pit (pĭt). 1. A tiny hollow or pocket. SYN: *depression, fossa*. 2. To be or become marked with a shallow depression; to cause a depression on pressure in edema.

p's. nasal; p's., olfactory. Two small depressions on ant. cerebral vesicle, from which the nasal fossae develop.

p. of the stomach. 1. Depression at end of the ensiform process. 2. The center of the abdominal region above the navel.

p's., stomach. Openings of gastric tubules in the mucous surface of the stomach. SYN: *stomach cells, stomach ducts*.

p., tear. The lacrimal sinus.

pithecoid (pĭth′ē-koyd). Apelike; resembling an ape.

pithiatism (pĭth-ī′ăt-ĭzm). 1. Hysteria induced by suggestion. 2. Mental disorder cured by suggestion.

pithiatric (pĭth-ī-at′rĭk). Capable of being soothed or relieved by persuasion or by suggestion.

pithing (pĭth′ing). Destruction of the central nervous system by the piercing of brain or spinal cord, as in vivisection, etc. SYN: *decerebration*.

pitocin (pĭt-ō′sĭn). An aqueous solution containing the oxytocic principle of the post. lobe of pituitary gland.

DOSAGE: From 5 to 15 ℔ (0.3-1 cc.) intramuscularly.

Pitres's sections (pē-trē′). Series of 6 coronal vertical brain sections for study of this organ.

pitressin (pĭt-rĕs′ĭn). A product obtained

from the post. lobe of the pituitary gland.

DOSAGE: From 5 to 15 ♏ (0.3-1 cc.) intramuscularly. SEE: *vasopressin*.

pitting (pĭt′ĭng). The formation of pits or depressions or scars, as in smallpox.

pituglandol (pĭt-ū-glăn′dŏl). Commercial extract of infundibular area of pituitary body.

pituita (pĭt-ū′ĭ-tă). A glairy or viscid mucus, as a thick nasal secretion.

pituitarism (pĭt-ū′ĭ-tă-rĭzm). Any disorder of the pituitary gland.

pituitary (pĭt-ū′ĭ-tăr-ĭ). 1. Concerning phlegm. 2. The pituitary body.

  p. body, p. gland. Small, reddish body; weight 5 to 10 grains; situated in sella turcica or pituitary fossa of sphenoid bone, just back of root of nose.

  p. extract. Extract of the internal secretions of the pituitary gland.

  p. membrane. Schneiderian membrane of nose.

[text obscured by damage]

...zoa, some of which are parasitic...

...n and beast.

...**hominis.** A parasite assumed to...

...Rocky Mountain spotted fever.

...**mosis** (pī′rō-plăz-mō′sĭs). An in-...

...n caused by Piroplasma.

...**test** (pĕr-kā′). Test for tuber-...

...s by means of a skin reaction.

...(pī′sĭ-form). 1. Name of small,...

...e sesamoid bone of the wrist. 2.

...shaped.

pituitrism (pĭt-u′ĭ-rĭzm). Any disorder of the pituitary gland.

pityriasis (pĭt-ĭr-ī′ăs-ĭs). A skin disease characterized by branny scales.

  p. alba atrophicans. Cutaneous disorder with scaling and atrophy. SYN: *atrophoderma albidum*.

  p. capitis. Dandruff. SYN: *dermatitis seborrhoica*.

  p. lichenodes seborrhoica chronica. Maculopapular erythrodermia.

  p. linguae. Transitory benign plaques of the tongue.

  p. maculata et circinata. SEE: *pityriasis rosea*.

  p. nigra. The dark brown or black patches in pityriasis versicolor in warm climates.

  p. pilaris. SEE: *pityriasis rubra*.

  p. rosea. A skin disease characterized by development of distributed patches which are circinate in outline, slightly scaly, a faint red color. SYN: *pityriasis maculata et circinata*.

  p. rubra. Persistent general exfoliative dermatitis.

  p. rubra pilaris. A chronic disease with formation of subacute inflammatory papules around the hair follicles. These coalesce and form infiltrated plaques of scaling dermatitis.

  p. versicolor. Contagious skin disease marked by yellow patches, scales and itching. [bran.

pityroid (pĭt′ĭr-oyd). Branny; resembling pix (pĭks). Pitch.

  p. liquida. Tar.

placebo (plă-sē′bō). Inactive substance given to satisfy patient's demand for medicine, such as a bread pill.

placenta (plă-sĕn′ta) (pl. *placentae*). The oval or discoid spongy structure in the uterus through which the fetus derives its nourishment.

  p. accreta. A placenta in which the cotyledons have invaded the uterine musculature and, as a result of this, separation of the placenta is very difficult or even impossible.

  p., adherent. One that remains adherent to the uterine wall after normal period following childbirth.

  p., annular. A placenta that extends like a belt around the interior of the uterus.

  p., basal; p., basilar. A free central placenta, 1 in which the ovules are borne on a column rising free from the bottom of the ovary.

  ...insertion... ...argin of... ...ds out to...

  ...acenta. ...ided into...

  ...-shaped. ...appear-...

  ...placenta having a heart shape.

  p., deciduate. A placenta of which the maternal part escapes with delivery.

  p., diffused. A villous* placenta.

  p., discoid. Placenta which constitutes practically 1 mass, circumscribed and circular in form.

  p., disseminated. SEE: *villous placenta*.

  p., domelike. One in which the chorionic villi persist at the upper pole of chorion, disappearing from lower pole.

  p., double. A placental mass of the 2 placentae of a twin gestation.

  p., duplex. Same as *placenta bipartita*.

  p. fenestrata. One so formed that at some point not involving the periphery, its substance is lacking, the chorion being free from villi at that point and transparent like a window.

  p., fetal. That part of the placenta formed by aggregation of chorionic villi in which the umbilical vein and arteries ramify. [centa.

  p., free central. Same as *basal placenta*.

  p., fundal. One attached to the uterine wall within the fundal zone.

  p., horseshoe. A formation in which the 2 placentae of a twin gestation are united.

  p., incarcerated. One retained in the uterus by irregular uterine contractions after delivery.

  p., lateral. One attached to lateral wall of uterus.

  p., marginate. One with a large amount of tissue elevated on the edge.

p., maternal. That part of the placenta originally consisting of the superficial part of the decidua serotina, and forming a thin, translucent, whitish gray layer attached to uterine surface of the fetal placenta so as to be separable only in small pieces.

p., membranous. A thinning of the placenta from atrophy.

p., nondeciduate. One that does not shed the maternal portion.

p. previa. Placenta which is implanted in the lower uterine segment. There are 3 types: *Centralis, lateralis,* and *marginalis. Placenta previa centralis* is the condition where the placenta has been implanted in the lower uterine segment and has grown to completely cover the cervical os. *Placenta previa lateralis* is the condition when the placenta lies just within the lower uterine segment. *Placenta previa marginalis* is the condition where the placenta partially covers internal cervical os.

p. reniformis. A kidney-shaped half of a *placenta dimidiata.*

p., retained. One not expelled for 2 hours after 2nd stage of labor.

p. sanguinis. A blood clot.

p. spuria. An outlying portion of placenta which has not maintained its vascular connection with the decidua vera.

p. succenturiata. An accesory placenta.

p. tripartita. A 3-lobed placenta.

p., triple. A placental mass of 3 placentae of a triple gestation.

p., uterine. Same as *maternal placenta.*

p., velamentous. A placenta having the umbilical cord attached at 1 end.

p., villous. A placental formation with cotyledons scattered and having the form of chorionic villi.

p., zonary. Same as *annular placenta.*

placental (plă-sĕn'tăl). Relating to the placenta.

p. bruit, p. souffle. Sound heard in auscultation over the placenta in pregnancy due to circulation of the blood.

placentation (plă-sĕn-tā'shŭn). The process of formation and attachment of the placenta.

placentin (plă-sĕn'tĭn). Extract of placenta used for cutaneous reaction in testing for pregnancy.

placentitis (plă-sĕn-tī'tĭs). Inflamed condition of placenta.

placentography (plă-sĕn-tŏg'ră-fĭ). Examination of the placenta by x-ray.

placentoid (plăs-ĕn'toyd). Like the placenta.

placentolysin (plă-sĕn-tŏl'ĭs-ĭn). A lysin obtained by injecting placental tissue into an animal, the serum thus obtained being destructive to placental cells of the species of animal from which the placenta was taken.

placentoma (plă-sĕn-tō'mă). A new growth derived from retained placental tissue.

placentotherapy (plă-sĕn″tō-thĕr'ă-pĭ). Therapeutic use of placental extract.

Placido's disk (pla-sē'dō). A disk marked with black and white circles used in determining amt. and character of corneal astigmatism.

placuntitis (plă-kŭn-tī'tĭs). Inflamed condition of the placenta. SYN: *placentitis.*

pladarosis (plad-ar-ō'sĭs). A soft growth like a wart on the eyelid.

plagiocephalic (plă-jĭ-ō-sĕf-ăl'ĭk). Marked by or relating to plagiocephaly.*

plagiocephalism, plagiocephaly (plă″jĭ-ō-sĕf'ăl-izm, plă″jĭ-ō-sĕf'ă-lĭ). Condition of malformation of the skull, it being developed more ant. than post.

plague (plăg). 1. Any widespread contagious disease of great mortality. 2. A deadly acute infection caused by *Pasteurella pestis.* SYN: *black death, bubonic plague.*

p., ambulatory. Mild but often fatal form.

Patient does not take to his bed.

p., bubonic. SEE: *plague,* 2.

plane (plān). 1. A level surface. 2. An ideal plane as a standard of reference by which positions of parts of a body are indicated.

p's., Addison's. Planes used as landmarks in thoracoabdominal topography.

p., Aeby's. One perpendicular to the median plane of the cranium through the *basion* and *nasion.*

p., alveolocondylar. One tangent to the alveolar point and most prominent points on lower aspects of condyles of the occipital bone.

p., Baer's. One through upper border of the zygomatic arches.

p., coccygeal. The 4th parallel one of the pelvis.

p., coronal. Vertical plane at right angles to a sagittal plane dividing the body into ant. and post. portions.

p., datum. An assumed horizontal plane from which craniometric measurements are taken.

p., Daubenton's. One passing through the opisthion and inferior borders of the orbits.

p's., focal. Two planes through ant. and post. principal foci of a dioptric system and perpendicular to the line connecting the two.

p., glabello-occipital. The vertical plane of maximum anteroposterior diameter of the skull.

p., Hodge's. One parallel to the plane of the pelvic inlet and passing through the 2nd sacral vertebra and upper border of the os pubis.

p's., inclined, of the pelvis. According to Lusk, "The sciatic spines divide the pelvic cavity into 2 unequal sections. In the larger, anterior section, the lateral walls slope toward the symphysis and arch of the pubes, while posteriorly the walls slope in the direction of the sacrum and coccyx. The declivities in front of the spines are termed the anterior inclined planes of the plevis, over which rotation of the occiput takes place in the mechanism of normal labor. Behind the spines the lateral slopes are known as the posterior inclined planes."

p., Listing's. A transverse vertical plane perpendicular to anteroposterior axis of eye, containing center of motion of the eyes; in it also lie the transverse and vertical axes of voluntary ocular rotation.

p., Meckel's. One through the auricular and alveolar points.

p., medial; p., median; p., mesial. One usually anteroposterior dividing a body or organ into 2 equal and symmetrical parts. The median plane of the body is known as the *meson.*

p., Morton's. One passing through the most projecting points of the parietal and occipital protuberances.

p., nuchal. Outer surface of occipital bone between the foramen magnum and the sup. curved line.

p., occipital. Outer surface of occipital bone above the sup. curved line.

p., orbital. 1. Orbital surface of the maxilla. 2. One passing through the visual axis of the eye.

p's., parallel, of the pelvis. Those intersecting at right angles the axis of the pelvic canal. The 1st is the plane of the superior strait; the 2nd the plane extending from middle of the sacral vertebra to level of the subpubic ligament; the 3rd the plane at level of spines of the ischia; the 4th at the outlet.

p's. of the pelvis. Imaginary ones touching the same parts of the pelvic canal on both sides.

p., popliteal. The popliteal space.

p. of refraction. One passing through a refracted ray of light and drawn perpendicular to the surface at which refraction takes place.

p. of regard. One through the fovea of the eye and fixation point.

p., sagittal. The median anteroposterior plane of the body.

p., sternal. Ant. surface of sternum.

p., temporal. Depressed area on side of skull below the inf. temporal line.

p., visual. One passing the visual axis of the eye.

planocellular (plā″nō-sĕl'ū-lăr). Composed of or concerning flat cells.

planoconcave (plā″nō-kon'kāv). Flat on 1 side and concave on the other.

planoconvex (plā″nō-kŏn'vĕks). Flat on 1 side and on the other convex.

planocyte (plā'nō-sīt). A meandering cell. SYN: *ameboid cell.*

plant (plănt). Organized being of vegetable life that is nonsentient and lacks voluntary motor power. SEE: *chloroplast.*

p. acids. Acids containing carbon; organic acids found in many fruits.

planta (plan'tă). BNA. The sole of the foot.

plantar (plăn'tăr). Concerning the sole of foot.

p. arch. Vascular arch in sole of foot. The union of the plantar and dorsalis pedis arteries in the sole. SYN: *arcus plantaris.*

p. reflex. Contraction of toes upon irritation of the sole.

plantaris (plăn-tăr'ĭs). An extensor muscle found in the calf of the leg.

planuria (plăn-ū'rĭ-ă). The voiding of urine from an abnormal passage of the body.

plaque (plăk). 1. A patch on the skin or on a mucous surface. 2. A *blood platelet.**

plasma (plăz'mă). 1. The liquid part of the lymph and of the blood. 2. Protoplasm, cell substance outside the nucleus. 3. An ointment base of glycerol and starch.

p., blood. Fluid in which float the corpuscles. [cell.

p., germ. Protoplasm of the germinal

p., histogenetic. Protoplasm controlling tissue development.

p., lymph. Lymph without its corpuscles.

p., muscle. Muscle juice that forms myosin on coagulation.

p., somatic. That of body cells other than the germ cells.

plasmacule (plăz'mă-kūl). One of the minute particles said to be found in the blood plasma giving it its vital power. SYN: *hemokonia.*

plasmacyte (plăz'mă-sīt). A plasma cell, 1 of those found in connective tissue with an eccentrically placed round nucleus and filled with a chromatin mass that stains deeply.

plasmacytosis (plăz-mă-sī-tō'sĭs). Plasma cells in the blood.

plasmameba (plăz-mă-mē'bă). An amebic parasitic organism in blood during dengue, possibly causing that disease.

plasmapheresis (plăz-mă-fĕr'ē-sĭs). The removal of fluid portion of blood from the body by venesection, centrifugalization, and replacement of the corpuscles into the blood stream.

plasmase (plăz'măs). Substance in serum which combines with fibrinogen to form fibrin. SYN: *fibrin ferment.*

plasmasome (plăz'măs-ōm). A leukocyte granule; nucleolar substance (nonchromatin staining) in the cytoplasm.

plasmatic (plăz-măt'ĭk). 1. Relating to plasma. 2. Formative or plastic.

p. layer. Blood plasma adjacent to the capillary walls. SYN: *plasmic.*

plasmatorrhexis (plăz'măt-ō-rĕks'ĭs). Rupture of a cell with loss of its plasma from internal pressure due to swelling.

plasmic (plăz'mĭk). Concerning plasma. SYN: *plasmatic.*

plasmochin (plăz'mō-kĭn). An oxyquinoline derivative, in the form of a tasteless salt.

DOSAGE: Adult, 1/6 gr. (0.01 Gm.).

plasmocyte (plăz'mō-sīt). 1. Any cell except blood corpuscles free in blood plasma. 2. A parasite in the blood plasma.

plasmodium (plăz-mō'dĭ-ŭm) (pl. *plasmodia*). Protoplasm formed by 2 or more amebiform bodies fusing with each other.

Plasmodium (plăz-mō'dĭ-ŭm). Genus of malarial parasites.

P. falciparum. The parasite of pernicious anemia.

P. malariae. A protozoan parasite found in the blood of those with malaria.

plasmogen (plăz'mō-jĕn). Essential part of protoplasm. SYN: *bioplasm*.

plasmology (plăz-mŏl'ō-jĭ). The study of the cells and plasma. SYN: *histology*.

plasmolysis (plăz-mŏl'ĭs-ĭs). Shrinking of cytoplasm in a living cell due to loss of water by osmosis.

plasmorrhexis (plăz-mor-ĕks'ĭs). Rupture of a cell with loss of plasma. SYN: *erythrocytorrhexis, erythrorrhexis, plasmatorrhexis*.

plasmoschisis (plăz-mos'kĭs-ĭs). The splitting of a cell.

plasmosome (plăz'mō-sōm). 1. The nucleolus of a cell. 2. A granular structural element of a cell.

plasmotomy (plăz-mŏt'ō-mĭ). Mitosis in which the cytoplasm divides into 2 or more masses.

plasmotropism (plăz-mŏt'rō-pĭzm). The action of spleen, liver, and bone marrow, causing the destruction of red blood cells.

plasmozyme (plăz'mo-zīm). A substance in blood plasma which probably becomes thrombin when activated by thrombokinase. SYN: *thrombogen*.

plasome (plăz'ōm). Smallest hypothetical unit of protoplasm capable of life.

plasson (plăs'ŏn). Primitive protoplasm in the cytode or non-nucleated stage.

plastein (plăs'tē-ĭn). One of several proteinlike substances produced by the action of proteolytic enzymes, as pepsin, on digestion products of protein.

plaster (plăs'tŭr). Medicinal preparation, to be used externally, in which the constituents are formed into a tenacious mass of substance harder than an ointment and spread upon muslin, linen, skin, or paper.

p., adhesive. Plaster made of resin, wax, and olive oil used to immobilize a part, to relieve pressure upon sutures, to protect wounds, to secure traction in fractures, to exert pressure, to hold dressings in place, etc.

p. bandage. Bandage stiffened with plaster of Paris.

p., blistering. Plaster made of cantharides.

p., court-. Plaster made of isinglass on silk, used for superficial wounds.

p. jacket. Plaster for the trunk made of plaster of Paris.

p., mustard. Plaster made of powdered mustard paste spread on cloth, used as a rubefacient.

p. of Paris. Calcined gypsum mixed with water to form a paste which sets rapidly, used to make casts and stiff bandages.

p., porous. Perforated plaster.

p., resin; p., rosin. Plaster containing resin, wax, and lead plaster, used as a soothing agent, esp. for children.

p., rubber. SEE: *adhesive plaster*.

p., warming. Plaster of cantharides and pitch employed as a counterirritant.

plas'ter cast. Rigid dressing made of gauze impregnated with plaster of Paris, used to immobilize an injured part, esp. in bone fractures.

plastic (plăs'tĭk). 1. Capable of being molded. 2. Contributing to building tissues.

p. bronchitis. Bronchitis with fibrin exudate adhering in the form of a cast to the bronchial tubes.

p. force. The impetus that builds tissues; generative force.

p. linitis. Cirrhosis of the stomach.

p. lymph. The exudate covering inflamed serous surfaces, as in wounds.

p. surgery. The restoration and repair of external physical defects by use of grafts of bone or tissues. SEE: *chalinoplasty*.

plasticity (plăs-tĭs'ĭ-tĭ). The ability to be molded.

plastid (plăs'tĭd). Area having special chemical activity in the cells for the production of special substances, such as the starch grains in plant cells; a cytode or elementary organism.

plastidule (plăs'tĭd-ūl). Smallest unit of protoplasm capable of life.

plastin (plăs'tĭn). 1. The principal proteid of protoplasm. 2. Chromatin granules in a cell nucleus. SYN: *linin*.

plastocyte (plăs'tō-sīt). A blood platelet.

plastocytopenia (plăs"tō-sī"tō-pē'nĭ-ă). Lack of the normal number of blood platelets.

plastocytosis (plăs"tō-sī-tō'sĭs). Abnormal increase in the quantity of blood platelets.

plate (plāt). A flattened process, chiefly of bone. SYN: *lamina, lamella*.

p., approximation. A disk of decalcified bone used in intestinal surgery.

p., auditory. Bony roof of the ext. auditory meatus.

p., axial. The primitive streak of the embryo.

p., blood. Platelet.

p., bone. Flat, round, or oval decalcified bone metal or hard rubber disk, employed in pairs, used in approximation.

p. culture. Bacterial culture in agar or gelatin on a plate.

p., dorsal. One of 2 prominences of the notochord in the embryo.

p., end-. Termination expanded of a nerve fibril in muscular tissue.

p., foot. Flat portion of stapes. BNA. *basis stapedis*.

p., medullary or **neural.** Central portion of the ectoderm developing into neural canal.

p., palate. Part of the palate bone forming a lateral half of roof of mouth.

p., tympanic. Bony plate between ant. wall of the ext. auditory meatus and the tympanum.

platelet (plăt'lĕt). A round or oval disk, 1/3 to 1/2 the size of an erythrocyte found in the blood.

platiculture (plă'tĭ-kŭl'chur). Cultivation of bacterial plates. SYN: *plate culture.*

platinum (plăt'ĭn-ŭm). Heavy silver-white metal. SYMB: Pt. At. wt. 195.2. Sp. gr. 21.5.

platy-. Combining form meaning *broad.*

platycelous (plăt-ĭ-sē'lŭs). Concave ventrally and convex dorsally, said of vertebrae.

platycephalic, platycephalous (plăt'ĭ-sē-făl'ĭk, -sĕf'ă-lŭs). Having a wide skull with vertical index less than 70.

platycnemia, platycnemism (plat-ĭk-nē'mĭ-ă, -mĭzm). 1. Having an unusually broad tibia. 2. Broadlegged.

platycnemic (plăt-ĭk-nē'mĭk). Having unusually broad tibiae.

platycyte (plăt'ĭs-ĭt). A form of cell found in tubercle nodules.
   It is bet. a leukocyte and a giant cell in size.

Platyhelminthes (plăt'ĭ-hĕl-mĭn'thēz). A phylum of flatworms. SEE: *Cestoda, Trematoda.*

platyhieric (plat-e-hi-er'ĭk). Having a broad sacrum with a sacral index over 100.   [usually broad femur.

platymeric (plăt-ĭ-mē'rĭk). Having an un-

platyopia (plăt-ĭ-ō'pĭ-ă). Having a very broad face.

platypellic, platypelvic (plăt'ĭ-pĕl'ĭk, -vĭk). Having a broad pelvis.

platypodia (plăt-ĭ-pō'dĭ-ă). Condition of being flat-footed.

platyrrhine (plăt'ĭr-ĭn). 1. Having a very wide nose in proportion to length. 2. Pert. to a skull with a nasal index bet. 51.1 and 58.

platysma myoides (plăt-ĭz'mă mĭ-oy'dēz). Broad, thin muscular layer on either side of the neck under the superficial fascia.

platysmal reflex. Dilation of pupil resulting from sharp pinching of platysma myoides.

platyspondylisis (plăt'ĭ-spŏn-dĭl'ĭs-ĭs). Flatness of the vertebral bodies.

platytrope (plăt'ĭ-trōp). One of a pair of bilateral symmetrical parts of the body on either side.

Plaut's angina (plawt's ăn-jī'nă). Ulceromembranous form of contagious disease of the oral mucosa, with inflammation of the tonsil. SYN: *trench mouth, Vincent's angina.*

pleas'ure prin'ciple. PSY: The avoidance of pain and the seeking of pleasure, indicative of the early stages of man's development. SYN: *hedonism.*

pledget (plĕj'ĕt). Small, flat, lint compress, used to apply or absorb fluid, as a protector, to exclude air, etc.

plegaphonia (pleg-af-ō'nĭ-ă). A sound produced in percussion of the larynx when the glottis is open during auscultation of the chest.

pleio-, pleo-, plio-. Combining forms meaning *more.*

pleochroic, pleochromatic (plē-ō-krō'ĭk, -măt'ĭk). Pert. to property of crystals and some other bodies of showing various colors when seen from different axes.

pleocytosis (plē"ō-sī-tō'sĭs). Increased number of lymphocytes in the cerebrospinal fluid.

pleomastia, pleomazia (plē"ō-măs'tĭ-ă, -mā'zĭ-ă). The state of having more than 2 mammae. SYN: *polymastia.*

pleomorphic (plē-ō-mor'fĭk). Having many shapes.

pleomorphism (plē-ō-mor'fĭzm). 1. Property of crystallizing into 2 or more different forms. 2. Occurrence of more than 1 form in a life cycle.

pleomorphous (plē-ō-mor'fŭs). Having many shapes or crystallizing into several forms.

pleonasm (plē'ō-năzm). State of having more than normal number of organs or parts.

pleonectic (plē-ō-nĕk'tĭk). 1. Being saturated with more than the normal amount of oxygen; said of blood. 2. Relating to excessive urge to possess; greedy. SEE: *mesectic, mionectic.*

pleonexia (plē"ō-nĕk'sĭ-ă). Having morbid desire for possession.

plesiomorphous (plē-sĭ-ō-mor'fŭs). Of like or nearly the same in form.

plessesthesia (plĕs-ĕs-thē'zĭ-ă). Palpatory percussion with left middle finger pressed against body and the index finger of right hand percussing in contact with left finger.

plessimeter (plĕs-im'et-er). A disk held over the body which is struck in mediate percussion. SYN: *pleximeter.*

plessor (plĕs'sor). A hammer for performing percussion. SYN: *plexor.*

plethora (plĕth'ō-ră). 1. Overfullness of blood vessels or of the total quantity of blood or other fluid in the body. 2. Congestion causing distention of blood vessels. SEE: *sanguine.*

plethoric (plĕth-or'ĭk). Pert. to or characterized by plethora; overfull.

plethysmograph (plē-thĭz'mō-grăf). Device for finding variations in size of a part, due to vascular changes.

pleura (plū'ră) (pl. *pleurae*). Serous membrane that enfolds lungs and is reflected upon the walls of the thorax and diaphragm. SEE: *mediastinum, thorax.*

   p., costal or **parietal layer.** Extends from roots of the lungs covering the sides of the pericardium to chest wall and backward to the spine. The visceral and costal pleural layers are separated only by a lubricating secretion. These layers may become adherent or separated by fluid or air in diseased conditions.

   p. diaphragmatica. That covering upper surface of diaphragm.

   p. pericardiaca. That covering the pericardium.   [*matica.*

   p. phrenica. SEE: *pleura diaphrag-*

p. pulmonalis. BNA. The pleura investing the lungs and fissures bet. the lobes.

p., visceral. Invests the lungs and enters into and lines the interlobar fissures. It is loose at the base and at sternal and vertebral borders to allow for lung expansion.

pleural (plū'răl). Concerning the pleura.

p. cavity. Space bet. the parietal and visceral layers of the pleura. SEE: *chylothorax.*

pleuralgia (plū-răl'jĭ-ă). Pain in the pleura, or in the side. SYN: *neuralgia, intercostal.*

pleurapophysis (plū-ră-pop'ĭs-ĭs). A rib or a vertebral lateral process.

pleurectomy (plū-rĕk'tō-mĭ). Excision of part of the pleura.

pleurisy (plū'rĭs-ĭ). Inflammation of pleura—may be primary or secondary; unilateral, bilateral, or local; acute or chronic; fibrinous, serofibrinous, or purulent. SEE: *Andral's decubitus.*

p., acute. Chilliness, stabbing pain or stitch in affected side, intensified by coughing or deep breathing. Fever, 101°-103°; cough short, dry, partially suppressed; face pale, anxious; patient usually lies on affected side. An effusion of any kind remaining unabsorbed constitutes a chronic pleurisy.

p., diaphragmatic. Inflammation of diaphragmatic pleura.

p., dry. Condition in which the pleural membrane is covered with a fibrinous exudate.

p., embolic. Pleurisy resulting from a pulmonary embolus.

p., encysted. Pleurisy with effusion limited by adhesions.

p., fibrinous. Pain severe and continuous. Aspiration gives negative results, later much retraction of affected side.

p., hemorrhagic. Pleurisy with hemorrhage.

p., interlobar. Pleurisy in interlobar spaces.

p., purulent. High, irregular fever; sweats; chills; anemia; sometimes pitting from edema of surface; purulent effusion found on aspiration.

p., secondary. Infectious pleurisy resulting from some specific inflammation.

p., serofibrinous. Pleurisy with fibrinous exudate and serous effusion.

p., suppurative. SEE: *purulent pleurisy.*

p., tuberculous. Most common cause of pleurisy that is apparently primary is tuberculosis. May be secondary to pulmonary phthisis. Effusion apt to be bloody, but presents same symptoms as ordinary serofibrinous pleurisy.

pleuritic (plū-rĭt'ĭk). Relating to, or like, pleurisy.

pleuritis (plū-rī'tĭs). Inflammation of the pleura. SYN: *pleurisy.*

pleurocele (plū'rō-sēl). 1. Hernia of lungs or of pleura. 2. A serous pleural effusion.

pleurocentesis (plū″rō-sĕn-tē'sĭs). Surgi-

cal puncture of the pleural cavity. SYN: *thoracentesis.*

pleurocentrum (plū-rō-sĕn'trŭm) (pl. *pleurocentra*). The lateral element of the centrum or vertebral column.

pleurocholecystitis (plū″rō-kō-lē-sĭst-ī'tĭs). Inflamed condition of the pleura and gallbladder.

pleuroclysis (plū-rŏk'lĭs-ĭs). Injection of fluid into the pleural cavity.

pleurodynia (plū″rō-dĭn'ĭ-ă). Pain in intercostal muscles of sharp intensity, due to chronic inflammatory changes in chest fasciae; pain of the pleural nerves.

p., epidemic diaphragmatic. Epidemic disease with sudden attack of pain in the chest, fever, and a tendency to recrudescence on the 3rd day. SYN: *devil's grip.*

pleurogenic (plū-rō-jĕn'ĭk). Arising in the pleura. SYN: *pleurogenous.*

pleurogenous (plū-rŏj'ĕn-ŭs). Having origin in the pleura. SYN: *pleurogenic.*

pleurography (plū-rŏg'ră-fĭ). X-ray examination of the lungs and pleura.

pleurohepatitis (plū″rō-hĕp-ă-tī'tĭs). Inflammation of pleura and the liver.

pleurolith (plū'rō-lĭth). A calculus in the pleura.

pleurolysis (plū-rŏl'ĭ-sĭs). Loosening of pleura that has become thickened from intrathoracic fascia, to relieve contraction of the lungs. SYN: *pneumolysis.*

pleuroparietopexy (plū″rō-păr-ī'ĕt-ō-pĕk″-sĭ). Fastening the lung to the wall of the chest by binding the visceral pleura to the wall of its cavity.

pleuropericarditis (plū″rō-pĕr″ĭ-kar-dī'tĭs). Pleuritis accompanied by pericarditis.

pleuroperitoneal (plū″rō-pĕr-ĭ-tō-nē'ăl). Relating to the pleura and peritoneum.

p. cavity. The body cavity. SYN: *celom.*

pleuropneumonia (plū″rō-nū-mō'nĭ-ă). Pleurisy accompanied by pneumonia.

pleuropneumonolysis (plū″rō-nū-mōn-ŏl'ĭ-sĭs). Resection of 1 or more ribs from 1 side to collapse the lung in unilateral pulmonary tuberculosis.

pleurorrhea (plū″rō-rē'ă). Effusion of fluid into the pleura.

pleuroscopy (plū-rŏs'kō-pĭ). Inspection of the pleural cavity through an incision into the thorax.

pleurothotonos (plū-rō-thŏt'ō-nos). Tetanic spasm in which the body position is arched to 1 side.

pleurotomy (plū-rŏt'ō-mĭ). Incision of the pleura.

pleurotyphoid (plū-rō-tī'foyd). Typhoid fever with pleural involvement.

pleurovisceral (plū″rō-vĭs'ĕr-ăl). Concerning the pleura and the viscera.

plexal (plĕks'ăl). Pertaining to, or of the nature of, a plexus.

plexalgia (plĕks-ăl'jĭ-ă). General fatigue, multiple pains, excitability, paresthesia, and insomnia seen in soldiers after long exposure to cold and wet; a symptom complex.

plexiform (plĕk'sĭ-form). Resembling a network or plexus.

pleximeter (plĕks-ĭm′ĕt-ĕr). Device made of many kinds of material, for receiving the blow of the percussion hammer.

plexor (plĕks′or). Hammer or other device for striking upon the pleximeter in percussion.

plexus (plĕk′sus) (pl. *plexūs* or *plexuses*). A network of nerves or blood vessels.

pliability (plī-ă-bĭl′ĭ-tĭ). Capacity of being bent or twisted easily.

plica (plī′kă) (pl. *plicae*). A fold.

   p. circularis. One of the transverse folds in the intestinal mucosa.

   p. epiglottica. One of 3 folds of mucosa bet. the tongue and the epiglottis.

   p. lacrimalis. Mucosal fold at the lower orifice of the nasolacrimal duct.

   p. neuropathica. Curly hair due to a nervous disorder.

   p. palmatae. Radiating fold in the uterine mucosa.

   p. polonica. Tangled matted hair in which crusts and vermin are embedded.

   p. semilunaris. Mucosal fold at the inner canthus of the eye.

   p. transversalis recti. One of the mucosal folds in the rectum.

plicate (plī′kāt). Braided or folded.

plication (plī-kā′shŭn). Stitching folds in an organ's walls to reduce its size.

plicotomy (plī-kŏt′ō-mĭ). Section of the post. fold of the tympanic membrane.

plombage (plŭm-bazh′). A method of collapsing the apex of lung by stripping the parietal pleura from the chest wall at the site of desired collapse and packing the space bet. the lung and chest wall with a foreign substance, such as adipose tissue, muslin, gauze, or paraffin wax.

plough (plow) (*nasal*). Triangular gouge used with Woake's forceps for excision of nasal tissue.

plug (plŭg). A mass obstructing or for closing a hole.

   p., cervical. One forming in cervix after conception for duration of pregnancy.

   p., laryngeal. Bulb-shaped laryngeal dilator.

   p., suprapubic urethral. A stem mounted upon a disk used to maintain the patency of an artificial suprapubic urethra and to prevent dribbling of urine.

   p., vaginal. Closed tube for maintaining patency of vagina following operation for fistula.

plumbago (plŭm-bā′gō). Graphite; a native carbon.

plumbic (plŭm′bĭk). Pertaining to, or containing, lead.

plumbism (plŭm′bĭzm). Poisoning from lead, *q.v.*

plumbotherapy (plŭm″bō-ther′ă-pĭ). Treatment of disease with lead.

plumbum (plŭm′bŭm). Lead; a bluish-white metal. Symb: Pb. At. wt. 207.10. Sp. gr. 11.38. Syn: *lead.*

plumose (plū′mōs). Having a delicate, feathery growth.

plumper (plŭm′pĕr). Pad for filling out sunken cheeks, sometimes in form of extended artificial dentures.

pluri-. Combining form meaning *several.*

pluriceptor (plū-rĭ-sĕp′tor). A receptor which has more than 2 groups uniting with the complement.

pluridyscrinia (plū″rĭ-dĭs-krĭn′ĭ-ă). Disorder of several endocrine organs at the same time.

pluriglandular (plū″rĭ-glăn′dū-ler). Concerning more than 2 glands.

   p. syndrome. Term concerned with any group of endocrinologic symptoms.

plurigravida (plū-rĭ-grăv′ĭd-ă). A woman who has had 2 or more children.

plurilocular (plū-rĭl-ŏk′ū-lar). Composed of many cells. Syn: *multilocular.*

plurimenorrhea (plū-rĭ-mĕn-ō-rē′ă). Abnormal frequency of menstrual periods.

pluripara (plū-rĭp′ă-ră). A woman who has given birth to 3 or more children.

pluripar′ity. Condition of having borne 3 or more children.

plutomania (plū″tō-mā′nĭ-ă). Delusion that one is very rich.

pnein (nē′ĭn). A substance assumed to be present in the tissues which hastens their oxidizing activities.

pneocardiac reflex (nē-ō-kar′dĭ-ăk). Change in rate and rhythm of heart and circulatory changes as blanching, flushing, or sweating, when an irritant vapor enters air passages.

pneodynamics (nē″ō-dī-năm′ĭks). Branch of science which treats of respiration. Syn: *pneumodynamics.*

pneograph (nē′ō-grăf). Apparatus for registering respiratory movements.

pneometer (nē-ŏm′ĕt-ĕr). Instrument for measuring lung respiration. Syn: *spirometer, q.v.*

pneophore (nē′ō-for). Device to aid artificial respiration.

pneopneic reflex (nē-ŏp-nē′ĭk). Change in respiratory depth and rate, coughing, suffocation, and pulmonary edema, when an irritant vapor enters air passages.

pneoscope (nē′ō-skōp). Device for measuring movements of respiration.

pneumarthrosis (nū-mar-thrō′sĭs). Accumulation of gas or air in a joint.

pneumascope (nū″mă-skōp). 1. Device for estimating gas in expired air. 2. Instrument for internal auscultation of the thorax. 3. Device for discovering foreign bodies in mastoid sinuses. 4. Apparatus for measurement of the movements of respiration. Syn: *pneumatoscope.*

pneumathemia (nū-mă-thē′mĭ-ă). Accumulation of air or gas in blood vessels.

pneumatic (nū-măt′ĭk). 1. Concerning gas or air. 2. Relating to respiration. 3. Relating to rarefied or compressed air.

   p. cabinet. Cabinet for treatment of a part with rarefied or compressed air.

pneumatinuria (nū″măt-ĭn-ū′rĭ-ă). Excretion of urine containing free gas. Syn: *pneumaturia.*

pneumatocardia (nū″măt-ō-kar′dĭ-ă). Air or gas in the heart chambers.

pneumatocele (nū-măt′ō-sēl). 1. Hernial protuberance of lung tissue. 2. A swelling containing a gas or air, esp. of the scrotum. SYN: *pneumonocele.*

pneumatodyspnea (nū″măt-ō-dĭsp-nē′ă). Dyspnea caused by pulmonary emphysema.

pneumatogram (nū-măt′ō-grăm). A tracing or record made by a pneumatograph.

pneumatograph (nū-măt′ō-grăf). Device for registering respiratory movements. SYN: *pneograph.*

pneumatology (nū-mă-tŏl′ō-jĭ). Science of gases and air, their chemical properties and use in treatment.

pneumatometer (nū-măt-ŏm′ĕt-ĕr). Device for measuring quantity of air involved in inspiration and expiration. SYN: *spirometer.*

pneumatometry (nū-măt-ŏm′ĕt-rĭ). Measurement of respiratory force as a means of diagnosis.

pneumatorachis (nū-măt-or′ă-kĭs). Air in the spinal canal.

pneumatoscope (nū-măt′ō-skōp). 1. Device for ascertaining presence of foreign bodies in mastoid sinuses. 2. Apparatus used to measure the gas in expired air. 3. Apparatus for internal thoracic auscultation. 4. Instrument used to measure the respiratory movements. SYN: *pneumascope.*

pneumatosis (nū-mă-tō′sĭs). Accumulation in any part of the body of gas, esp. in the intestinal tract.

pneumatotherapy (nū″măt-ō-thĕr′ă-pĭ). Treatment by means of rarefied or compressed air.

pneumatothorax (nū″măt-ō-thō′răks). Air or gas accumulation in the pleural cavities. SYN: *pneumothorax.**

pneumaturia (nū-măt-u′rĭ-ă). Excretion of urine containing free gas.

pneumatype (nū′mă-tĭp). Deposit of moisture on glass from the breath exhaled through the nostrils with the mouth closed for purpose of diagnosis.

pneumectomy (nū-měk′tō-mĭ). Excision of all or part of a lung.

pneumo-, pneumono-. Combining forms meaning *air; lung.*

pneumobacillus (nū″mō-bă-sĭl-ŭs). The bacillus causing pneumonia. SYN: *B. pneumoniae.*

pneumocele (nū′mō-sēl). 1. A swelling containing air or gas, esp. of the scrotum. 2. Hernia of lung tissue through chest wall. SYN: *pneumatocele.*

pneumocentesis (nū″mō-sĕn-tē′sĭs). Paracentesis* or surgical puncture of a lung to evacuate a cavity.

pneumocephalus (nū″mō-sĕf′ă-lŭs). Gas or air in the cavity of the cranium.

pneumocholin (nū″mō-kō′lĭn). Commercial preparation of pneumococci in sodium taurocholate used as prophylactic agent in Type I.

pneumochysis (nū-mŏk′ĭs-ĭs). Edema of the lung.

pneumococcal (nū-mō-kŏk′ăl). Concerning or caused by pneumococci.

pneumococcemia (nū″mō-kŏk-sē′mĭ-ă). Presence of pneumococci circulating in the blood.

pneumococcolysis (nū″mō-kŏk-ŏl′ĭ-sĭs). Destruction or lysis of pneumococci.

pneumococcus (nū-mō-kŏk′ŭs). The pathogenic microörganism causing pneumonia of which there are 33 known strains or types.

   p. antibody solution. A colorless, clear, aqueous solution containing antibodies from antipneumococcic serum in normal saline, combining Types I-II-III. It is free from serum proteins, is miscible with body fluids and quickly absorbed.

   p., how to recognize in sputum. Detected by paired arrangements and slightly curved, long, thin, appearance. Commonly seen in clumps, in short chains of 4 to 6. It takes a gram-positive stain.

pneumoconiosis (nū″mō-kō-nĭ-ō′sĭs). A condition of the respiratory tract due to inhalation of dust particles.

pneumoderma (nū-mō-dĕr′mă). Emphysema under the skin.

pneumodynamics (nū″mō-dī-năm′ĭks). Branch of science treating with force employed in respiration.

pneumoempyema (nū″mō-ĕm-pī-ē′mă). Empyema accompanied by an accumulation of gas.

pneumoenteritis (nū″mō-ĕn-tĕr-ī′tĭs). Pneumonia and enteritis combined.

pneumogalactocele (nū″mō-găl-ăk′tō-sēl). A breast tumor containing milk and gas.

pneumogastric (nū″mō-găs′trĭk). Concerning the lungs and stomach.

   p. nerve. The 10th cranial nerve.

pneumogram (nū′mō-grăm). Device for recording respiratory movements. SYN: *pneumatogram.*

pneumograph (nū′mō-grăf). Device for measuring and recording movements of respiration.

pneumography (nū-mŏg′ră-fĭ). 1. A descriptive treatise on the lungs. 2. A tracing of the respiratory movements.

pneumohemopericardium (nū″mō-hem″ō-pĕr-ĭ-kar′dĭ-ŭm). The accumulation of air and blood in the pericardium.

pneumohemorrhagia (nū″mō-hem-or-hā′-jĭ-ă). Hemorrhage into pulmonary air cells; apoplexy of the lungs.

pneumohemothorax (nū″mō-hem″ō-thō′-răks). Gas or air and blood collected in the pleural cavity.

pneumohydropericardium (nū″mō-hī″drō-pĕr-ĭ-kar′dĭ-ŭm). Air and fluid accumulated in the pericardium.

pneumohydrothorax (nū″mō-hī-drō-thō′-răks). Gas or air and fluid in the pleural cavity.

pneumohypoderma (nū″mō-hī-pō-dĕr′mă). Air in the tissues under the skin.

pneumokidney (nū″mō-kĭd′nĭ). X-ray of the kidney following introduction of oxygen into renal pelvis. SYN: *pneumopyelography.*

pneumolith (nū′mō-lĭth). A pulmonary calculus.

pneumolithiasis (nū″mō-lĭth-ĭ′ăs-ĭs). Formation of concretions in the lungs.

pneumology (nū-mŏl′ō-jĭ). The scientific

study of diseases of the lungs and air passages.

pneumolysis (nū-mŏl'ĭs-ĭs). Separation of an adherent lung from costal pleura.

pneumomalacia (nū″mō-mă-lā'sĭ-ă). Abnormal softening of the lung.

pneumomassage (nū″mō-măs-sazh′). Massage of the tympanum with air to cause movement of the ossicles.

pneumomelanosis (nū″mō-mĕl-ăn-ō'sĭs). Pigmentation of lung seen in pneumoconiosis.

pneumometer (nū-mŏm'ĕt-ĕr). Instrument for measuring amt. of air inspired and expired in respiration. SYN: *spirometer, q.v.*

pneumomycosis (nū″mō-mĭ-kō'sĭs). A fungous pulmonary disease. SYN: *pneumonomycosis.*

pneumomyelography (nū″mō-mĭ-ĕl-ŏg'ră-fĭ). X-ray inspection of the spinal canal.

pneumonectasia, pneumonectasis (nū-mŏn-ĕk-tā'zĭ-ă, -ĕk'tă-sĭs). Distention of lungs with air.

pneumonectomy (nū-mŏn-ĕk'tō-mĭ). Removal of a lung. SYN: *pulmonectomy, pneumectomy.*

pneumonemia (nū-mō-nē'mĭ-ă). Congestion of the lungs.

pneumonia (nū-mō'nĭ-ă). Inflammation of the lungs with exudation into the lung tissue and high temperature.

  p., acute lobar. Pneumonia of one or more lobes of the lungs.

  p., broncho-. SEE: *catarrhal pneumonia.*

  p., catarrhal. Inflammation of terminal bronchioles and air vesicles, with scattered areas of consolidation, usually secondary to bronchitis.

  p., chronic interstitial. Chronic disease of lung with overgrowth of fibrous tissue.

  p., croupous. SEE: *lobar pneumonia.*

  p., double. That affecting both lungs or both lobes of 1 lung.

  p., hypostatic. Pneumonia caused by constantly remaining in same position.

  p., lobar. An acute specific disease characterized by inflammation of lungs, followed by a rapid infiltration of their alveoli.

  p., typhoid. Pneumonia associated with typhoid symptoms; headache; muttering delirium; stupor; dry, brown tongue, etc.

pneumonic (nū-mon'ĭk). Concerning the lungs or pneumonia.

  p. phthisis. Tuberculosis of an entire pulmonary lobe.

pneumonitis (nū-mō-nī'tĭs). Inflammation of the lung. SYN: *pneumonia.*

pneumono- (nū-mon-ō). Prefix: *pert. to the lungs.*

pneumonocele (nū-mō'nō-sēl). A pulmonary hernia. SYN: *pneumocele.*

pneumonocirrhosis (nū″mō-nō-sĭr-ō'sĭs). Interstitial pneumonia; cirrhosis of the lung.

pneumonoconiosis (nū″mō-nō-kō-nĭ-ō'sĭs). Fibrous inflammation or chronic induration of the lungs resulting from inhala-

tion of dust. SEE: *anthracosis, chalicosis, siderosis.*

pneumonograph (nū-mō'nō-grăf). Roentgen ray picture of the lungs.

pneumonography (nū-mō-nŏg'ră-fĭ). The taking and developing of x-ray pictures of the lungs.

pneumonolysis (nū-mō-nŏl'ĭs-ĭs). Loosening of an adherent lung from the pleura. SYN: *pneumolysis.*

pneumonomelanosis (nū″mō-nō-mĕl-ăn-ō'sĭs). Pigmentation and disease of the lung due to inhalation of dust.

pneumonometer (nū-mō-nŏm'ĕt-ĕr). Device to measure amt. of inspired and expired air during respiration. SYN: *spirometer.*

pneumonomoniliasis (nū″mō-no-mō″nĭl-ī'-ăs-ĭs). Infestation of lungs and bronchi by Monilia.

pneumonomycosis (nū-mō-nō-mĭ-kō'sĭs). Disease of the lungs caused by schizomycetes. SYN: *pneumomycosis.*

pneumonopathy (nū-mō-nŏp'ăth-ĭ). Any diseased condition of the lung.

pneumonoperitonitis (nū″mō-nō-pĕr″ĭ-tō-nī'tĭs). Peritonitis with gas in the peritoneal cavity.

pneumonopexy (nū″mō-nō-pĕk'sĭ). Surgical attachment of the lung to the chest wall. SYN: *pneumopexy.*

pneumonophthisis (nū″mō-nŏf'thĭs-ĭs). Tuberculosis of the lungs.

pneumonorrhaphy (nū-mō-nor'ă-fĭ). Suture of a lung.   [nary disease.

pneumonosis (nū-mō-nō'sĭs). Any pulmo-

pneumonotomy (nū-mō-nŏt'ō-mĭ). Incision into the lung. SYN: *pneumotomy.*

pneumopaludism (nū″mō-păl'ū-dĭzm). Malarial symptom complex of the lungs.

pneumoparesis (nū″mō-păr-ē'sĭs). Progressive congestion of the lungs.

pneumopericardium (nū″mō-pĕr-ĭ-kar'dĭ-ŭm). Air or gas in the pericardial sac.

pneumoperitoneum (nū″mō-pĕr-ĭ-tō-nē'-ŭm). Condition in which air or gas is collected in the peritoneal cavity.

pneumoperitonitis (nū″mō-pĕr-ĭ-tō-nī'tĭs). Peritonitis with gas accumulation.

pneumopexy (nū′mō-pĕks′ĭ). Surgical attachment of a lung to the thoracic wall.

pneumopleuritis (nū″mō-plū-rī'tĭs). Inflamed condition of lungs and pleura.

pneumopleuroparietopexy (nū″mō-plū″rō-pă-rī′ĕt-ō-pĕk″sĭ). The operation of attaching the lung with its parietal pleura to the border of a thoracic wound.

pneumopyelography (nū″mō-pī-ĕ-lŏg'ră-fĭ). Making of a skiagram of the renal pelvis and ureters after they are injected with oxygen.

pneumopyopericardium (nū″mō-pī″ō-pĕr-ĭ-kar'dĭ-ŭm). Air, gas, and pus collected in the pericardial sac.

pneumopyothorax (nū″mō-pī″ō-thō'răks). Air and pus collected in the pleural cavity.

pneumorrhachis (nū-mor-ră'kĭs). Gas accumulation in the spinal canal.

pneumoradiography (nū″mō-rā-dĭ-ŏg'ră-fĭ). Injection of air into a part for taking an x-ray picture.

pneumorrhagia (nŭ-mor-ā'jĭ-ă). Pulmonary hemorrhage. SYN: *hemoptysis*.

pneumosan (nŭ'mō-san). Commercial remedy for pulmonary tuberculosis.

pneumoscope (nŭ'mō-skōp). Device for estimating the respiratory force.

pneumoserosa (nŭ''mō-sē-rō'să). Introduction of air into a joint cavity.

pneumoserothorax (nŭ''mō-sē-rō-thō'rāks). Air or gas and serum collected in the pleural cavity.

pneumosillicosis (nŭ''mō-sĭl-ĭ-kō'sĭs). Silica particles in the lungs.

pneumotachograph (nŭ''mō-tăk'ō-grăf). Device for registering velocity of inspiration and expiration of air.

pneumotherapy (nŭ-mō-ther'ă-pĭ). 1. Treatment of diseases of the lungs. 2. Use of compressed air in treatment. SYN: *pneumatotherapy*.

pneumothermomassage (nŭ''mō-ther''mō-măs-sazh'). Application to the body of air of varying temperature and pressure.

pneumothorax (nŭ-mō-thō'rāks). A collection of air or gas in the pleural cavity.

   p., artificial. Pneumothorax induced intentionally by artificial means employed in the treatment of pulmonary tuberculosis or pneumonia.

   p., spontaneous. Spontaneous entrance of air into the pleural cavity.

   p., valvular. That which is characterized by an opening through the pleura which has a slit with a valvelike action allowing the air to pass in but not out.

pneumotomy (nŭ-mŏt'ō-mĭ). Incision of the lung.

pneumotoxin (nŭ''mō-tŏks'ĭn). A toxin produced by the pneumococcus.

pneumotyphus (nŭ''mō-tī'fŭs). 1. Typhoid fever with pneumonia at onset. 2. Development of pneumonia during typhoid fever.

pneumouria (nŭ''mō-ū'rĭ-ă). Excretion of urine with free gas. SYN: *pneumaturia*.

pneumoventricle (nŭ''mō-vĕn'trĭ-kl). Air accumulation in the cerebral ventricles.

pneumoventriculography (nŭ''mō-vĕn-trĭk''ū-lŏg'ră-fĭ). Radiography of the lateral ventricles of the brain, after removal of fluid content and injection with air. SYN: *ventriculography*.

pneusimeter, pneusometer (nŭ-sĭm'ĕt-ĕr, -sŏm'ĕt-ĕr). Device used as a spirometer to measure vital capacity of the chest in respiration.

pnigophobia (ni-gō-fō'bĭ-ă). Morbid fear of choking; sometimes experienced in angina pectoris.

pock (pŏk). A pustule of an eruptive fever, esp. of smallpox.

   p.-marked. Pitted or marked with cicatrices of smallpox pustules.

pocket (pŏk'ĕt). A saclike cavity.

pocketing (pŏk'ĕt-ĭng). Method of treating the pedicle in ovariotomy by enclosing it within the edges of the wound.

podagra (pŏd-ăg'ră). Gout, esp. of the foot's joints or of the great toe.

podalgia (pod-ăl'jĭ-ă). Pain in the feet.

podalic (pŏd-ăl'ĭk). Pert. to the feet.

   p. version. Shifting position of a fetus to bring the feet to the outlet in labor.

podarthritis (pŏd-ar-thrī'tĭs). Inflammation of joints of the feet. SYN: *podagra*.

podo-, pod-. Combining forms meaning *foot*.

podiatrist (pŏd-ī'ăt-rĭst). Specialist in foot diseases. SYN: *chiropodist*.

podiatry (pŏd-ī'ăt-rĭ). Treatment of foot disorders. SYN: *chiropody*.

podobromidrosis (pŏd''ō-brō-mĭ-drō'sĭs). Offensive perspiration of the feet.

pododynamometer (pŏd''ō-dī-năm-ŏm'ĕt-ĕr). A device for testing strength of the leg and foot muscles.

pododynia (pŏd-ō-dĭn'ĭ-ă). Pain in the feet, esp. a neuralgic pain in the heel with swelling and redness.

podogram (pŏd'ō-grăm). An imprint of the sole of the foot.

podology (pŏd-ŏl'ō-jĭ). The study of the anatomy and physiology of the foot.

podophyllum (pŏd-ō-fĭl'ŭm). USP. Mandrake; May apple. An herb grown extensively in eastern U. S. and parts of the South.

   p., resin of.
   DOSAGE: 1/6 gr. (0.01 Gm.).

pogoniasis (pō-gō-nī'ăs-ĭs). 1. Excessive growth of the beard. 2. Growth of a beard in a woman.

pogonion (pō-go'nĭ-ŏn). The most anterior projecting midpoint of the chin.

-poietic (poy-ĕt'ĭk). Suffix meaning making or producing.

poikilocyte (poy'kĭl-ō-sīt). A large, irregular, malformed blood corpuscle.

poikilocytosis (poy''kĭl-ō-sī-tō'sĭs). Variation in shape of red blood corpuscles; a condition characterized by poikilocytes in the blood.

poikiloplastocyte (poy''kĭl-ō-plăs'tō-sīt). A blood platelet of irregular form.

poikilothermal (poy''kĭl-ō-thĕr'măl). Varying in temperature according to environment.

point (poynt). 1. The sharp end of any object. 2. Point at which an abscess is about to rupture on a surface. SEE: *fixation*. 3. A minute spot. 4. Position in space, time, or degree.

   p., absolute near. The nearest point at which normal vision is retained.

   p., anterior focal. Same as focal point.

   p., anterior nodal. SEE: *nodal points*.

   p., apophysial. Tender spot over a vertebral spinous process, beneath which neuralgic nerves exit.

   p., auricular. Center of external orifice of auditory canal.

   p., Boas'. Tender spot in gastric ulcer left of 12th thoracic vertebra.

   p., boiling. The temperature at which a liquid vaporizes.

   p., Brewer's. Costovertebral triangle which in kidney infection is tender to pressure.

   p., Broca's. Center of the ext. auditory meatus; the *auricular point*.

p's., Capuron's. Four fixed points in pelvic inlet, the iliopectineal eminences and the sacroiliac joints.

p's., cardinal. Six points determining direction of light rays emerging from and entering the eye and of 4 points of the pelvic inlet toward 1 of which the head of the fetus is presented. SEE: *principal points, focal points, nodal points.*

p., craniometric. One of the fixed points of the skull used in craniometry.

p., critical, of gases. Temperature at or above which a gas can no longer be liquefied by pressure.

p., critical, of liquids. Temperature above which no pressure may retain a body in a liquid form.

p's., deaf, of the ear. Point at lower end of tragus and 1 where helix intersects line of motion when vibrating tuning fork held in front of ear cannot be heard when started from the lower edge of the zygoma and moved backward toward the occiput.

p., dew. The temperature at which moisture begins to be deposited as dew.

p., disparate. Points on the retinae unequally paired.

p., external orbital. The prominent 1 at outer edge of orbit above the fronto-malar suture.

p., far. The point (20 ft. or more) at which distinct vision is possible without aid of the muscles of accommodation. It is nearer than 20 ft. according to degree of myopia. There is no far point in the hypermetropic eye.

p., fixation. That at which the 2 visual axes converge.

p., freezing. Temperature at which liquids become solid.

p's., hysterogenic. Circumscribed areas of the body which produce symptoms of a hysterical aura, and eventually a hysterical attack when rubbed or pressed.

p's., identical retinal. Points in the 2 retinae upon which the images are seen as one.

p., jugal. Posterior border of frontal process of the malar bone where cut by a line tangent to upper border of zygoma.

p., lacrimal. Outlet of lacrimal canaliculus. SYN: *puncta lacrimalia.*

p., Lanz's. One on line bet. 2 ant. sup. iliac spines, 1/3 distant from right spine, indicating origin of the vermiform appendix.

p., Lian's. One at junction of outer and middle thirds of a line from the umbilicus to ant. sup. spine of ilium where trocar may be introduced safely for paracentesis.

p., malar. The most prominent point on ext. tubercle of the malar bone.

p., Mayo-Robson's. 1. One just above and right of the umbilicus, pressure over which causes tenderness in the pancreas. 2. One on 1/3 of distance from umbilicus to right nipple showing great-est tenderness in gallbladder inflammation.

p., McBurney's. One bet. 1½ and 2 in. above ant. sup. spine of ilium, on line bet. the ilium and umbilicus, where pressure shows tenderness in acute appendicitis.

p., Morris'. Point of tenderness on pressure on line bet. umbilicus (1½ in. from it) and right ant. sup. spine of ilium. Present in irritation near the vermiform appendix.

p., motor. The point at which a motor nerve enters a muscle, where an electrode may produce the maximum electrical contraction of that muscle.

p., Munro's. One halfway bet. left ant. iliac spine and the umbilicus.

p's., nasal genital. Point at ant. end of lower turbinated bone, and 1 at the tuberculum septi, irritation of which, when in a hyperesthetic state, produces pain in the hypogastrium and in sacral region.

p., near. Nearest one at which the eye can accommodate itself for distinct vision.

p's., nodal. An ant. and post. cardinal point on the surface of lens of the eye so related that every ray directed toward the ant. point is represented after refraction by a ray emanating from the post. point.

p's., painful. Points over which a neuralgic nerve is tender on pressure.

p's., pressure. The points of emergence of the infraorbital and supra-orbital, and sometimes branches of facial nerve, in vicinity of margins of the orbit, pressure upon which may arrest blepharospasm.

p's., principal. Two points so situated that the optical axis is cut by the 2 principal planes.

p., Robson's. SEE: *Mayo-Robson's point.*

p's., Valleix's. Tender spots upon pressure over the course of a nerve in neuralgia.

pointillage (pwähn-tĭ-yahzh'). Massage with the finger tips.

points douloureux (pwähnt doo-loo-rōō'). Painful points in peripheral neuralgia when the nerves pass through bony canals or openings in fascia. SYN: *Valleix's points.*

Poiseuille's law (pwä-sŭ-ēz'). The rapidity of the capillary currents is in proportion to the square of the diameter of their capillary tubes.

P.'s layer or **space.** The inert capillary current in which leukocytes move slowly, the erythrocytes moving more rapidly in the middle current.

poison (poy'zn). Any substance which, taken into the system, will produce an injurious or deadly effect.

p., acid. SEE: *acid poisoning.*

p., alkali. SEE: *alkali poisoning.*

p., atropine. SEE: *atropine poisoning.*

p., belladonna. SEE: *belladonna poisoning.*

Some Common Poisons and Treatment

Poison	Lavage or Emetic	Antidote	Other Treatment
Aconite.	Lavage or emetic.	Tr. digitalis or liq. atropinae, ♏ ii.	Keep flat with head low. Stimulants. Treat for shock. Unceasing artificial respiration.
Alcohol.	Lavage or emetic.		Strychnine, gr. 1/20. Cold douche, etc. Leave coffee in stomach after lavage.
Ammonia.	None.	Weak acetic acid or vinegar.	Olive oil and demulcents. Treat shock. Morphine. (Tracheotomy may be necessary.)
Antimony (tartar emetic).	Not usually required.	Tannin.	Alcohol. Strong tea or coffee. Warmth. Treat shock. Keep prone. Give demulcents.
Arsenic.	Lavage or emetic.	Dialyzed iron, ℥ i every 2 hours for some hours.	Large dose of castor oil to clear out intestines. Demulcent drinks.
Belladonna and atropine.	Lavage or emetic.	Tannin or tea, morphine, gr. 1/2.	Free stimulation. Artificial respiration.
Camphor.	Lavage or emetic.		Stimulants. Alternate hot and cold douches. Oils.
Carbolic, Lysol, etc.	Lavage with very soft tube.	Mag. sulph.	Albumen water, oil, milk. Treat shock.
Caustic potash. Caustic soda.	Neither.	Dilute vinegar or lemon juice.	Treat shock. Oils and butter. Demulcents.
Chloral hydrate.	Lavage or emetic.	Strychnine, gr. 1/20, or atropine, gr. 1/25.	Stimulants. Artificial respiration. External warmth. Rouse patient.
Cocaine.	Lavage or emetic.	Strychnine, gr. 1/20.	Stimulants. Artificial respiration. External warmth. Rouse patient.
Corrosive sublimate. Digitalis.	SEE: Mercury. Emetic and lavage (zinc sulphate, gr. 1/2).	Opium and tannin.	Keep in horizontal position. Free stimulation. Alcohol.
Fungi.	Emetic or lavage.	Atropine or morphine.	Free stimulation and friction.
Hydrochloric acid (spirits of salt).	Same as for sulphuric acid.		
Hydrocyanic acid (prussic acid).	Lavage or rapid emetic.	Ammonia inhalation. Ferri-sulph.	Alternate hot and cold douches. Artificial respiration. Treat for shock.

Some Common Poisons and Treatment (*Continued*)

Poison	Lavage or Emetic	Antidote	Other Treatment
Iodine.	Emetic or lavage (*used continuously*).	Starch in water.	Demulcent drinks. Bread, arrowroot, flour.
Laudanum (*opium*).	SEE: Morphine.		
Lead salts.	Lavage or emetic.	Sulphate of zinc.	Demulcents. Epsom salts. White of egg.
Mercury.	Emetic or lavage.		Demulcents. Treat for shock. White of egg.
Morphine.	Lavage with pot. permanganate or emetic (*apomorphine, gr. 1/10*).	Pot. permanganate. Atropine.	Stimulation. Prevent sleep. Artificial respiration if necessary.
Nitric acid.	Neither.	Alkalis.	Demulcents. Magnesia, lime water, or albumen water.
Nux vomica.	SEE: Strychnine.		
Opium.	SEE: Morphine.		
Oxalic acid.	Lavage or emetics.	Lime water and chalk.	Castor oil. Free stimulation. Demulcents. Treat shock.
Phosphorus.	Lavage or emetics. ($CuSO_4$.)	Permanganate of potash, gr. 5, in 1 oz. of water. Also $CuSO_4$, gr. 5.	Avoid oils but give French oil of turpentine. Purgatives. Demulcents.
Ptomaines.	Lavage with **Condy's** fluid.		Purgation and colonic lavage. Salines. Strychnine. Treat for shock.
Silver nitrate (*lunar caustic*).	Lavage and emetics.	Large doses of common salt.	White of egg, milk, and water.
Soda, caustic.	SEE: Caustic soda.		
Strychnine.	Lavage before spasms appear. Emetic (*apomorphine, gr. 1/10*).	Tannin or charcoal. Chloral, pot. bromide.	Chloroform inhalation. Morphine. Artificial respiration.
Sulphuric acid (*oil of vitriol*).	Neither.	Dilute alkalis, *e. g.*, lime, soap, chalk, magnesia, etc.	Wall plaster in warm water. Oils. Demulcents.
Tobacco.	Emetics.	Tannin.	Free stimulation. Strychnine. Recumbent position.
Turpentine.	Emetics.	Mag. sulph.	Albumen water or milk.
Veronal.	Lavage.	Strychnine.	Artificial respiration. Keep warm.
Zinc chloride.	Cautious lavage, emetic (*apomorphine, gr. 1/10*).		Tannin. Egg albumen. Oils. Give demulcents freely.

p., blood. SEE: *bacteremia, pyemia, septicemia, toxemia.*

p., convulsive. SEE: *convulsive poisoning.*

p., corrosive. SEE: *corrosive poisoning.*

p., fish. Treat as for *black widow spider.*

p., ivy. SEE: *ivy poisoning.*

p., mushroom. SEE: *mushroom poisoning.*

p., narcotic. SEE: *name of.*

p., sedative. SEE: *sedative poisoning.*

p., toadstool. SEE: *toadstool poisoning.*

p., unknown. In case no information is available about the character of the poison taken, and the symptoms and signs are not characteristic, it is evident that the exact antidote cannot be administered.

poitrinaire (pwah-trē-när′). One with chronic disease of the chest or with pulmonary tuberculosis.

polar. Concerning a pole.

p. compounds. Those formed by an exchange of electrons.

polarimeter (pō-lar-ĭm′ĕt-ĕr). Instrument for measuring amount of polarization of light, or rotation of polarized light.

polarimetry (pō-lar-ĭm′ĕt-rĭ). Measurement of the amount and rotation of polarized light.

polariscope (pō-lar′ĭ-skōp). Apparatus used in measurement of polarized light.

polarity (pō-lar′ĭt-ĭ). P.T. 1. The quality of having poles. 2. The exhibition of opposite effects at the 2 extremities.

polarization (pō-lăr-ĭ-zā′shŭn). 1. Condition in a ray of light in which vibrations occur in only 1 plane or in curves. 2. In a galvanic battery, collection of hydrogen bubbles on negative plate and oxygen on the positive plate, whereby generation of current is impeded.

pole (pōl). 1. The extremity of any axis about which forces acting on it are symmetrically disposed. 2. One of 2 points in a magnet, cell, or battery having opposite physical qualities.

p., animal. One opposite the yolk in an ovum near which is the protoplasm of the germinal vesicle.

p., antigerminal. That of an ovum opp. the germinal pole where is situated the food yolk.

p., cephalic. End of the ovoid formed by the fetus at which the head is formed.

p's. of the chorion. The upper and lower extremities of the chorion, analogous to the fundus and os uteri.

p's. of the eye. The ant. and post. extremities of the optic axis.

p., frontal. Most projecting part of the ant. extremity of both cerebral hemispheres.

p., germinal. The pole of an ovum at which the development begins.

p's. of the kidney. The kidney's upper and lower extremities.

p., negative. That electrode or cathode portion of a battery connected with its electropositive element.

p., nutritive. Antigerminal* pole.

p., occipital. The post. extremity of the occipital lobe.

p., pelvic. Breech of a fetus.

p., placental, of the chorion. Spot at which the domelike placenta is situated.

p., positive. That electrode (anode) or other portion of the apparatus of a battery connected with its electronegative element.

p's. of the testicle. The upper and lower extremities of a testicle.

p., vegetative. Part of the egg containing the food yolk.

p., Vitelline. Antigerminal* pole.

policlinic (pŏl-ĭ-klĭn′ĭk). A city hospital or clinic for outpatients. SYN: *polyclinic.*

polioencephalitis (pŏl″ĭ-ō-ĕn-sĕf-ăl-ĭ′tĭs). An infectious inflammatory disease of the gray matter of the brain.

p. acuta. Acute inflammation of the cerebral cortex giving rise to infantile cerebral palsy in children.

p., anterior superior. Polioencephalitis of the 3rd ventricle and ant. portion of the 4th of the brain.

p., infective. Encephalitis lethargica.

p., inferior. Bulbar paralysis.

polioclastic (pŏl″ĭ-ō-klăs′tĭk). Destructive of the gray matter of the nervous system.

polioencephalomeningomyelitis (pŏl″ĭ-ō-ĕn-sĕf″ăl-ō-men-ĭng-ō-mĭ-ĕl-ĭ′tĭs). Inflammation of the gray matter of the brain and spinal cord and their meninges.

polioencephalomyelitis (pŏl″ĭ-ō-ĕn-sĕf″ăl-ō-mĭ-ĕl-ĭ′tĭs). Inflamed condition of the gray matter of the brain and spinal cord. SYN: *Heine-Medin disease.*

polioencephalopathy (pŏl″ĭ-ō-ĕn-sĕf-ăl-ŏp′ăth-ĭ). Diseased condition of the gray matter of the brain.

poliomyelencephalitis (pŏl″ĭ-ō-mĭ-ĕl-ĕn″-sĕf-ăl-ĭ′tĭs). Poliomyelitis with polioencephalitis.

poliomyeliticidal (pŏl″ĭ-ō-mĭ-ĕl-ĭt-ĭs-ĭ′dăl). Having power to destroy or neutralize poliomyelitis virus.

poliomyelitis (pŏl″ĭ-ō-mĭ-ĕl-ĭ′tĭs). Inflammation of the gray matter of the spinal cord.

p., acute anterior. An acute infectious inflammation of ant. horns of the spinal cord.

p., anterior. Inflamed state of spinal cord's ant. horns.

p., chronic, anterior. Progressive wasting of the muscles.

poliomyelopathy (pŏl″ĭ-ō-mĭ-ĕl-ŏp′ăth-ĭ). Any diseased condition of the gray matter of the spinal cord.

polioplasm (pŏl′ĭ-ō-plăzm). Granular protoplasm.

poliosis (pŏl-ĭ-ō′sĭs). Absence of pigment in the hair. SYN: *calvities; grayness.*

Po′lish plait. Matted hair due to disease of the scalp and want of cleanliness. SYN: *plica polonica.*

politzerization (pŏ-lĭt-zĕr-ĭ-zā'shŭn). The inflation of the middle ear using a Politzer bag.

Politzer's bag (pŏl'ĭts-ĕr). Soft rubber bag with rubber tip for inflating the middle ear.

pollaccine (pŏl-ăk'sĭn). A pollen preparation used in testing for sensitivity and in treatment of asthma and hay fever.

pollakiuria (pŏl-ăk-ĭ-ū'rĭ-ă). Abnormally frequent passage of urine.

pollen (pŏl'ĕn). The male element in flowering plants.

pollenogenic (pŏl''ĕn-ō-jen'ĭk). Due to the pollen of plants or producing plant pollen.

pollenosis (pŏl-ĕn-ō'sĭs). Hay fever; disease due to pollen.

pollex (pŏl'ĕks). The thumb.

p. flexus. Permanent flexion of the thumb.

p. pedis. The great toe. SYN: *hallux.*

pollinosis (pŏl-ĭn-ō'sĭs). Nasal congestion of mucous membranes due to contact with pollen. SYN: *hay fever.*

pollution (pol-ū'shun). 1. State of making impure or defiling. 2. Emission of semen at other times than in coition.

polonium (pō-lo'nĭ-ŭm). Radioactive metal isolated from pitchblende. SYN: *radium F.*

polus (pō'lŭs). Pole.

poly-. Prefix meaning *many* or *much.*

poly. (pŏl'ĭ). Abbr. for *polymorphonuclear leukocyte.*

polyadenia (pŏl''ĭ-ăd-ē'nĭ-ă). Enlargement of the lymph glands. SYN: *pseudoleukemia.*

polyadenomatosis (pŏl''ĭ-ăd-ē-nō-mă-tō'sĭs). Adenomas in many glands.

polyadenous (pŏl-ĭ-ad'ē-nŭs). Involving or relating to many glands.

polyalgesia (pŏl''ĭ-ăl-je'zĭ-ă). A single stimulus of a part, producing sensation in many parts.

polyandry (pŏl''ĭ-an'drĭ). The practice of having more than 1 husband at the same time. SEE: *polygamy.*

polyarteritis (pŏl''ĭ-ar-ter-ī'tĭs). Inflammation of more than 1 or 2 arteries at the same time.

p. nodosa. Polyarteritis with nodules on smaller arterial branches.

polyarthric (pŏl''ĭ-ar'thrĭk). Affecting or pert. to several joints.

polyarthritis (pŏl-ĭ-ar-thrī'tĭs). Inflammation of a number of joints.

p. rheumatica acuta. Acute articular rheumatism.

p., vertebra. Intervertebral inflammation of the disks without vertebral caries.

polyarticular (pŏl''ĭ-ar-tĭk'ū-lar). Affecting many joints. SYN: *multiarticular.*

polyatomic (pŏl''ĭ-ă-tom'ĭk). Having several atoms or more than 2 replaceable hydrogen atoms.

polyaxon (pol-ĭ-ak'son). Neuron with more than 2 axons.

polyblast (pŏl'ĭ-blăst). Large mononuclear phagocyte present in inflammation derived from an embryonic wandering cell.

polyblenia (pŏl-ĭ-blĕn'nĭ-ă). Secretion of more mucus than normal.

polyceptor (pŏl-ĭ-sep'tor). An amboceptor having several complementophile groups.

polycholia (pŏl-ĭ-kō'lĭ-ă). Abnormal secretion of bile.

polychrest (pol'ĭ-krĕst). A medicine useful in many diseases.

polychromasia (pŏl''ĭ-krō-mā'zĭ-ă). Quality of having many colors.

polychromatic (pŏl''ĭ-krō-măt'ĭk). Multicolored.

polychromatophile (pŏl''ĭ-krō-măt'ō-fĭl). Stainable with more than 1 kind of stain.

polychromatophilia (pol''ĭ-krō-măt-ō-fĭl'ĭ-ă). 1. The quality of being stainable with more than 1 stain. 2. Polychromatophil cells in the blood to excess.

polychromemia (pŏl-ĭ-krō-mē'mĭ-ă). Increase in the blood's coloring matter.

polychromia (pŏl''ĭ-krō'mĭ-ă). Increased or excessive pigmentation.

polychylia (pŏl''ĭ-kī'lĭ-ă). Excessive secretion of chyle.

polyclinic (pŏl-ĭ-klĭn'ĭk). Hospital or clinic treating many diseases; a general hospital.

polyclonia (pŏl''ĭ-klō'nĭ-ă). A disease characterized by many clonic spasms but distinct from chorea or tic.

polycoria (pŏl-ĭ-kō'rĭ-ă). The state of having more than 1 pupil in 1 eye.

polycrotic (pŏl-ĭ-krŏt'ĭk). Having several pulse waves for each cardiac systole.

polycrotism (pŏl-ĭk'rŏt-ĭzm). Condition of having several pulse waves for each cardiac systole.

polycyesia, polycyesis (pŏl-ĭ-sĭ-ē'zĭ-ă, -sĭs). 1. Pregnancy with more than 1 fetus in the uterus. 2. Frequent pregnancy.

polycystic (pŏl-ĭ-sĭs'tĭk). Composed of many cysts.

polycythemia (pŏl''ĭ-sĭ-thē'mĭ-ă). An excess of red blood cells. SEE: *erythrocytosis.*

p. megalosplenica; p., myelopathic; p. rubra; p., splenomegalic; p. vera. A slowly progressive disease characterized by an increased number of red blood cells and increase in total blood volume.

polycytosis (pŏl''ĭ-sī-tō'sĭs). Increased number of red and white blood corpuscles in the blood.

polydactylism (pŏl''ĭ-dăk'tĭl-ĭzm). State of having supernumerary fingers or toes.

polydipsia (pŏl-ĭ-dĭp'sĭ-ă). Excessive thirst.

polyemia (pol-ĭ-ē'mĭ-ă). Abnormal amount of blood in the system. SYN: *polycythemia.*

p. aquosa. Physiological excess of water in the blood after drinking much fluid.

p. hyperalbuminosa. Excessive amt. of albumin in the blood plasma.

p. polycythaemica. An increase of red corpuscles.

p. serosa. Increase of blood serum.

polyesthesia (pŏl''ĭ-ĕs-thē'zĭ-ă). Disturbed sensation of touch in which an external stimulus or touch is felt as several.

polyesthetic (pŏl''ĭ-ĕs-thĕt'ĭk). Exciting

sensation in several different points when only 1 is stimulated.

polygalactia (pŏl″ĭ-găl-ăk′shĭ-ă). Excessive secretion or flow of milk.

polygamy (pō-lĭg′ă-mĭ). Practice of having several wives or husbands at the same time, esp. wives.

polygen (pŏl′ĭ-jĕn). 1. Serum derived from more than 1 antigen. 2. Element capable of combining in several proportions.

polygenesis (pŏl″ĭ-jĕn′ĕ-sĭs). Theory that 2 or more branches of the human race evolved independent of each other.

polyglandular (pŏl″ĭ-glăn′dū-lar). Pert. to or affecting many glands. SYN: *pluriglandular*.

polyglobulia, polyglobulism (pŏl″ĭ-glŏ-bū′lĭ-ă, -glŏb′ū-lĭzm). Increase in number of red corpuscles in the blood. SYN: *polycythemia*.

polygram (pŏl′ĭ-grăm). Sphygmographic record made by polygraph of pulse beats simultaneously.

polygraph (pŏl′ĭ-grăf). A device which records simultaneously tracings of several different pulsations, as arterial and venous pulse waves, apex beat of heart, and other pulsations. SYN: *sphygmograph*.

polygroma (pŏl-ĭ-grō′mă). A large sac distended with fluid. SYN: *hygroma*.

polygyria (pŏl-ĭ-jĭ′rĭ-ă). Excess of the number of convolutions in the brain.

polyhedral (pŏl-ĭ-hē′drăl). Having many surfaces.

polyhemia (pŏl″ĭ-hē′mĭ-ă). Abnormal increase in amount of the blood. SYN: *polyemia*.   [perspiration.*

polyhidrosis (pŏl-ĭ-hĭ-drō′sĭs). Excessive

polyhydramnios (pŏl-ĭ-hĭ-drăm′nĭ-ŏs). An excess of amniotic fluid in the bag-of-waters in pregnancy. SEE: *amnion*.

polyhydruria (pŏl″ĭ-hĭ-drū′rĭ-ă). Excessive amt. of water in urine.

polyhypermenorrhea (pŏl″ĭ-hī-pĕr-mĕn-ō-rē′ă). Frequent menstruation with excessive discharge.

polyhypomenorrhea (pŏl-ĭ-hī-pō-mĕn-ō-rē′ă). Frequent menstruation with scanty discharge.

polyinfection (pŏl″ĭ-ĭn-fĕk′shŭn). Infection with 2 or more microörganisms. SYN: *multiinfection*.

polykaryocyte (pŏl-ĭ-kar′ĭ-ō-sīt). A cell possessing several nuclei.

polyleptic (pŏl″ĭ-lĕp′tĭk). Characterized by numerous remissions and exacerbations, as malaria.

polymastia, polymazia (pŏl-ĭ-măs′tĭ-ă, -mă′zĭ-ă). Condition of having more than 2 mammae.

polymastigate (pŏl-ĭ-măs′tĭg-āt). Possessing several flagella.

polymenia (pŏl-ĭ-mē′nĭ-ă). Excessive and frequent menstrual flow. SYN: *menorrhagia, polymenorrhea*.

polymenorrhea (pŏl″ĭ-mĕn-or-rē′ă). Excessive menstrual flow occurring too frequently. SYN: *menorrhagia, polymenia*.

polymer (pŏl′ĭ-mer). One of 2 or more

compounds of same elements in same proportion by weight, but differing in molecular weight, formed by polymerization, as paraformaldehyde from formaldehyde.

polymeria (pŏl-ĭ-mē′rĭ-ă). 1. Condition of having supernumerary parts of the body. 2. A chain of atoms.

polymeric (pŏl-ĭ-mĕr′ĭk). 1. Consisting of the same elements in same proportions by weight, but differing in molecular weight. 2. Said of muscles derived from more than 1 myotome.

polymerism (pŏl″ĭ-mĕr-ĭzm, pō-lĭm′ĕr-ĭzm). 1. Condition of having more than normal number of parts. 2. Isomerism in which the molecular weights of the polymers are multiples of each other.

polymerization (pŏl″ĭ-mĕr-ĭ-zā′shŭn). Process of changing into another compound having same elements in same proportions, but a higher molecular weight.

polymitus (po-lĭm′ĭ-tŭs). Stage in reproduction of microörganisms with threads of protoplasm which, being detached, constitute the microgamete.

polymorphic (pŏl-ĭ-mor′fĭk). Occurring in more than 1 form.

polymorphism (pŏl-ĭ-mor′fĭzm). 1. Capacity for appearing in many forms. 2. Existence of several types in the same group or species. SYN: *pleomorphism*.

polymorphocellular (pŏl″ĭ-mor-fō-sĕl′ū-lar). Composed of cells of many forms.

polymorphonuclear (pŏl″ĭ-mor-fō-nū′klē-ar). Having nuclei of varied forms, esp. a common variety of leukocytes.

p. leukocyte, p. neutrophil leukocyte. Finely granular cell with an affinity for acid and neutral dyes with an irregularly formed nucleus. SEE: *leukocyte*.

polymorphous (pŏl-ĭ-mor′fŭs). Appearing in many forms. SYN: *polymorphic*.

p. perverse. PSY: Term for pregenital expressions of sex activities natural in babies, but which become abnormal when expressed in adult life. EX: *cruelty, exhibitionism*.

polymyoclonus (pŏl-ĭ-mī-ŏk′lō-nŭs). A shocklike muscular contraction, occurring in various parts at the same time. SYN: *myoclonus multiplex, paramyoclonus*.

polymyositis (pŏl-ĭ-mī-ō-sī′tĭs). Simultaneous inflammation of many muscles.

polynesic (pŏl-ĭ-nē′sĭk). Appearing in many separate locations or foci.

polyneural (pŏl-ĭ-nū′răl). Pert. to, innervated, or supplied by, many nerves.

polyneuralgia (pŏl″ĭ-nū-ral′jĭ-ă). Neuralgia in several nerves.

polyneuritic (pŏl″ĭ-nū-rĭt′ĭk). Suffering from inflammation of several nerves at once.

p. psychosis. Psychosis seen in chronic alcoholism with disturbed orientation, polyneuritis, hallucinations, falsification of memory, etc.

polyneuritis (pŏl-ĭ-nū-rī′tĭs). A neuritis involving 2 or more nerves; usually a large number.

polynuclear (pŏl″ĭ-nū′klē-ar). Possessing more than 1 nucleus.

polynucleosis (pŏl″ĭ-nū-klē-ō′sĭs). Many polynuclear cells in the blood or in a pathologic exudate. SYN: *leukocytosis, polymorphonuclear.*

polyodontia (pŏl″ĭ-ō-dŏn′shĭ-ă). State of having supernumerary teeth.

polyopia, polyopsia (pŏl-ĭ-ō′pĭ-ă, -ŏp′sĭ-ă). Multiple vision; perception of more than 1 image of the same object.

polyorchidism (pŏl″ĭ-or′kĭd-ĭzm). Condition marked by having more than 2 testicles.   [than 2 testicles.

polyorchis (pŏl-ĭ-or′kĭs). One with more

polyorrhomenitis (pŏl-ĭ-or″ro-mĕn-ĭ′tĭs). Malignant inflammation and wasting of serous membranes. SYN: *Concato's disease.*

polyotia (pŏl-ĭ-ō′shĭ-ă). State of having more than 2 ears.

polyp (pŏl′ĭp). A tumor with a pedicle, esp. on mucous membranes of *nose, bladder, rectum, uterus.* SYN: *polypus.*

polyparesis (pŏl″ĭ-par′ĕs-ĭs). General progressive paralysis of paralytic dementia.

polypathia (pŏl-ĭ-păth′ĭ-ă). The presence of several diseases at 1 time, or their frequent recurrence.

polypeptide (pŏl-ĭ-pĕp′tĭd). A union of 3 or more amino acids. SEE: *peptide.*

polypeptidemia (pŏl″ĭ-pĕp-tĭd-ē′mĭ-ă). Polypeptides present in the blood.

polypeptidorrhachia (pŏl″ĭ-pĕp-tĭd-ō-ră′-kĭ-ă). Polypeptides in the cerebrospinal fluid.

polyphagia (pŏl-ĭ-fā′jĭ-ă). Eating abnormally large amounts of food at a meal.

polyphalangism (pŏl″ĭ-făl-ăn′jĭzm). An extra number of phalanges on a finger or toe.

polypharmacy (pŏl-ĭ-far′mă-sĭ). 1. Excessive use of drugs or overdose of a drug. 2. Prescription of many drugs given at 1 time.

polyphobia (pŏl-ĭ-fō′bĭ-ă). Excessive or abnormal fear of a number of things.

polyphrasia (pŏl-ĭ-frā′zĭ-ă). Excessive talkativeness, a manifestation of insanity. SYN: *verbigeration.*

polyplast (pŏl′ĭ-plăst). 1. Composed of many different substances. 2. Experiencing many structural modifications during development.

polyplastic (pŏl-ĭ-plăs′tĭk). 1. Having had many evolutionary modifications. 2. Having many substances in cellular composition.

polyplastocytosis (pŏl″ĭ-plăs-tō-sĭ-tō′sĭs). Increase of blood platelets formation.

polyplegia (pŏl-ĭ-plē′jĭ-ă). Paralysis affecting several muscles.

polypnea (pŏl-ĭp-nĭ′ă). Very rapid breathing. SYN: *panting.*

polypodia (pŏl″ĭ-pō′dĭ-ă). Possession of more than normal number of feet.

polypoid (pŏl′ĭ-poyd). Like a polyp.

polyposis (pŏl-ĭ-pō′sĭs). The presence of numerous polypi.

   p. ventriculi. Warty condition of the gastric mucosa accompanied by catarrh and hypertrophy.

polypotome (pol-ĭp′o-tōm). Instrument for excision of a polypus.

polypus (pŏl′ĭ-pŭs) (pl. *polypi*). A pedunculate tumor growing from a mucous membrane.

   p., bleeding. Angioma of nasal mucous membrane.

   p., cellular. Mucous polypus.

   p., cervical. A polyp, either fibrous or mucous, on the cervical mucosa.

   p., fibrous. A pedunculated fibroid tumor within the uterine or cervical cavities.

   p., fleshy. A submucous myoma in the uterus.

   p., placental. A polyp composed of retained placental tissue.

polyrrhea, polyrrhoea (pol-ĭr-rē′ă). Excessive secretion of fluid.

polysaccharid (pŏl″ĭ-săk′kă-rĭd) $(C_6H_{10}O_5)$ n. One of a carbohydrate group which on hydrolysis yields 2 or more molecules of simple sugars. Ex: Starch, which on hydrolysis yields maltose.

polysaccharose (pŏl″ĭ-săk′ă-rōs). The name for 1 of a *group* of carbohydrates which yields simple sugar.

polysarcia (pŏl″ĭ-sar′shĭ-ă). Fleshiness; obesity.   [fat.

polysarcous (pŏl″ĭ-sar′kŭs). Very fleshy;

polyscelia (pŏl″ĭ-sē′lĭ-ă). Condition of having more than the normal number of legs.

polyscope (pŏl′ĭ-skōp). Instrument for illumination and examination of cavities.

polyserositis (pŏl″ĭ-sē-rō-sī′tĭs). General progressive inflammation of all the serous membranes.

polysinuitis, polysinusitis (pŏl″ĭ-sīn-ū-ī′tĭs, -sī″nŭs-ī′tĭs). Inflammation of several sinuses simultaneously.

polyspermia, polyspermism (pŏl″ĭ-sper′-mĭ-ă, -mĭzm). 1. Excessive secretion of seminal fluid. 2. Entrance of several spermatozoa into 1 ovum.

polystichia (pŏl-ĭ-stĭk′ĭ-ă). Condition in which there are more than 2 rows of eyelashes.

polysyphilide (pŏl″ĭ-sĭf′ĭl-īd). Having numerous syphilitic lesions.

polythelia, polythelism (pŏl″ĭ-thē′lĭ-ă, -lĭzm). Presence of more than 1 nipple on a mamma.

polytocous (pŏl-ĭt′ō-kŭs). Producing several offspring at 1 time.

polytrichia, polytrichosis (pŏl-ĭ-trĭk′ĭ-ă, -ō′sĭs). Excessive growth of hair. SYN: *hypertrichiasis.*

polytrophia, polytrophy (pŏl-ĭ-trō′fĭ-ă, -ĭt′rō-fĭ). Excessive or abundant nutrition.

polyuria (pŏl-ĭ-ū′rĭ-ă). Excessive secretion and discharge of urine.

polyvalent (pŏl-ĭ-vā′lĕnt, pŏ-lĭv′ă-lent). 1. Multivalent; having a combining power of more than 2 atoms of hydrogen.

   p. serum. One with antibodies produced by injecting several strains of microörganisms of the same species or by injecting different species.

   p. vaccine. One produced from cultures of a number of strains of the same species.

pomade (po'mād). A perfumed ointment, esp. 1 for the hair. SYN: *pomatum*.

pomatum (pō-mā'tŭm). A perfumed unguent, esp. 1 used on the hair. SYN: *pomade*.

pompholyx (pŏm'fō-lĭks). Acute inflammatory affection characterized by bullae limited to hands and feet.

pomphus (pŏm'fŭs) (pl. *pomphi*). A blister or a circumscribed elevation on the skin; a wheal.

pomum (pō'mŭm). An apple.

p. Adami. Prominence in middle line of throat, caused by junction of 2 lateral wings of the thyroid cartilage.

p. oculi. The eyeball.

ponogen (pŏn'ō-jĕn). Any waste matter of tissues derived from the nervous system. SYN: *fatigue poison*.

ponograph (pŏn'ō-grăf). Device for measuring and registering sensitiveness to pain or fatigue.

ponopalmosis (pŏn''ō-păl-mō'sĭs). Palpitation of the heart produced by slight exertion. SYN: *neurocirculatory asthenia*.

ponophobia (pŏn-ō-fō'bĭ-ă). 1. Abnormal distaste for exerting one's self. 2. Dread of pain.

pons (pl. *pontes*). 1. A process of tissue connecting 2 or more parts. 2. Pons Varolii, *q.v.*

p. hepatis. Part of liver extending sometimes from quadrate lobe to left lobe across the umbilical fissure.

p. Varolii. The eminence caused by a convex mass of white nerve tissue connecting cerebrum, medulla oblongata and cerebellum.

pontic (pŏn'tĭk). 1. An artificial tooth set in a bridge. 2. Concerning the pons.

ponticular (pŏn-tĭk'ū-lar). Relating to the ponticulus or ridge bet. the pyramids of the pons and oblongata.

ponticulus (pŏn-tĭk'ū-lŭs). The transverse ridge bet. the pyramids of the pons and oblongata. SYN: *propons*.

pontile, pontine (pŏn'tĭl, -tēn). Pert. to the pons Varolii.

p. hemiplegia. One due to lesion of the pons. The arm and leg on 1 side and face on the other are affected.   [pons.

p. nuclei. The gray matter in the

pontocaine hydrochloride (pŏn'tō-kān). A white crystalline powder, the base of which belongs to the procaine type.

DOSAGE: ½% strength recommended for the eye, 2% for nose and throat.

popliteal (pŏp-lĭt'ē-ăl, -lĭt-ē'ăl). Concerning the post. surface of the knee.

popliteus (pŏp-lĭt'ē-ŭs, -lĭt-ē'ŭs). Muscle located in hind part of the knee joint which flexes the leg and aids it in rotating.

poradenitis (pŏr-ăd-ĕ-nī'tĭs). Formation of small abscesses in the iliac glands.

porcellaneous, porcellanous (pŏr-sĕ-lā'nē-ŭs, -sel'ăn-ŭs). Translucent or white like porcelain, as the skin.

porcupine disease (por'kū-pīn). A chronic skin disease with scaly epidermal plates. SYN: *ichthyosis*.

pore (pōr). A small orifice in membrane or tissue, the mouth of a duct, for absorption or excretion; as orifices of sweat glands of skin.

porencephalia, porencephalus (pōr-ĕn-sĕf-ā'lĭ-ă, -sĕf'ā-lŭs). Depressions on surface of the brain, congenital or acquired.

porencephalitis (pōr-ĕn-sĕf-ăl-ī'tĭs). Inflammation of the brain with development of depressions on its surface.

porencephalous (por-ĕn-sĕf'ăl-ŭs). Affected with depressions on the brain surface.

pornography (pŏr-nŏg'rā-fĭ). 1. Obscene writing or painting. 2. Description of prostitutes or prostitution.

porocele (pō'rō-sēl). Scrotal hernia with indurated and thickened coverings.

porocephaliasis, porocephalosis (pō''rō-sĕf-ăl-ī'ă-sĭs, -ō'sĭs). Infection with a species of Porocephalus.

Porocephalus (pō''rō-sĕf'ă-lŭs). A genus of parasites or their larvae which infest animals and man.

porokeratosis (pō''rō-kĕr-ăt-ō'sĭs). Skin disease marked by thickening of stratum corneum in linear arrangement, followed by its atrophy.

poroma (pō-rō'mă). Inflammatory hardening or callosity.

porosis (pō-rō'sĭs). 1. A callus formed about the ends of a fractured bone. 2. A thickened induration. 3. A condition marked by pore formation.

porosity (pō-rŏs'ĭ-tĭ). 1. The state of being porous. 2. Pore.

porotomy (pō-rŏt'ō-mĭ). Incision of urethral meatus to enlarge it.

porous (pō'rŭs). Full of pores; able to admit passage of a liquid.

porphyria (por-fĭ'rĭ-ă). Porphyrin in the blood.

porphyrin (por'fĭ-rĭn). One of a group forming basis of animal and plant respiratory pigments, obtained from hemoglobin and chlorophyll.

porphyrinuria (por''fĭ-rĭn-ū'rĭ-ă). The excretion of porphyrin in the urine.

porphyrization (por''fĭr-ĭ-zā'shŭn). Process of pulverizing.

porphyruria (por-fĭr-ū'rĭ-ă). Excretion of porphyrin in urine.

porrigo (pō-rī'gō). Any disease of scalp involving scaling or loss of hair.

p. decalvans. Baldness in patches. SYN: *alopecia areata*.

p. favosa. Tiny, contiguous ulcer and crust formation. SYN: *favus.**

p. furfurans. Ringworm of the scalp. SYN: *tinea* tonsurans*.

p. larvalis. Eczema of the scalp with impetigo.

Porro's operation (por'ōz). Removal of a pregnant uterus, the ovaries and tubes through an incision in the abdominal wall.

porta (por'tă). 1. The point of entry of nerves and vessels into an organ or part. 2. Passage bet. the 3rd and lateral ventricles of the brain. SEE: *hilum*.

p. hepatis. The fissure of the liver where the portal vein enters.

p. lienis. Hilus of the spleen where vessels enter.

p. pulmonis. Pulmonary hilus for entry and exit of the bronchi, nerves, and vessels.

p. renis. Hilus of the kidney for entry of the vessels.

portal (por'tăl). Concerning a porta or entrance to an organ, esp. that through which the blood is carried to liver.

p. circulation. That of blood brought by the portal vein into the liver and out by the hepatic vein.

p. system. Branches of portal vein by which blood is taken up from abdominal viscera and carried through portal capillaries of liver, finally entering inf. vena cava.

p. vein. One formed by the veins of the splanchnic area conveying its blood into the liver.

It is made of the combined sup. and inf. mesenteric, splenic, gastric, and cystic veins.

port-caustic (pōrt'kaws'tĭk). Contrivance for handling a caustic.

porte-, port- (pōrt). To carry.

porte-caustic (pōrt''kŏs-tēk'). Device for handling a caustic.

porte-fillet (pōrt''fĭl'ĕt). Appliance for passing a cord around a fetus, employed in breech presentation.

portenoeud (pōrt-ned'). Instrument for applying a ligature around an artery or the pedicle of a tumor.

portio (pōr'shĭ-ō). A part.

p. dura. The 7th cranial or facial nerve.

p. intermedia. A small nerve bet. the facial and acoustic nerves, the sensory root of the facial nerve. SYN: *pars intermedia of Wrisberg*.

p. major. BNA. The larger sensory part of the trigeminal nerve.

p. minor. BNA. The smaller motor part of the trigeminal nerve.

p. mollis. The 8th cranial or acoustic nerve.

p. vaginalis. The part of the cervix within the vagina.

port-wine mark or **stain.** A purplish-red, superficial birthmark. SYN: *nevus.**

porus (pō'rŭs). A meatus or foramen; a tiny aperture in a structure; a pore.

p. acusticus externus. Ext. acoustic or auditory meatus.

p. acusticus internus. Int. acoustic or auditory foramen.

p. opticus. Aperture containing the optic disk, the point where the optic nerve pierces the sclera.

posiomania (pos''ĭ-ō-mā'nĭ-ă). Addiction to alcoholic drinks. SYN: *dipsomania.*

position (pō-zĭsh'ŭn). 1. Place in which a thing is put. 2. Manner in which a body is arranged, as by the nurse or physician for examination. 3. OB: The relation of some arbitrarily chosen portion of the child in the pelvis to the right or left side of the mother, the occiput, chin, and sacrum being the points used. SEE: *posture.*

p., dorsal. Position in which patient is on his back.

p., d. elevated. On back, head and shoulders elevated at angle of 30° or more. Employed in digital examination of genitalia and in bimanual examination.

p., d. recumbent. On back, extremities moderately flexed and rotated outward. Employed in application of obstetrical forceps, repair of lesions following parturition, vaginal examination, bimanual palpation.

p., dorsosacral. Same as *lithotomy position.*

p., Edebohl's. Same as *Simon's position.*

p., Elliott's. Position in which supports are placed under small of back so that patient resembles a double inclined plane.

p., English. SEE: *left lateral recumbent position.*

p., erect. Occiput and heels on line, also nose, groins, and great toes in same vertical plane. Employed in practice of ballottement, differentiation of tumors, cystic and solid hernia.

p., Fowler's. Position when the head of the patient's bed is raised above the level about 1½ ft.

p., genucubital. Patient on knees, thighs upright, body resting on elbows, head down on hands. Employed when not possible to use the classic knee-chest position.

p., genupectoral. Patient on knees, thighs upright, head and upper part of chest resting on table, arms crossed above head. Employed in displacement of prolapsed fundus, dislodgement of impacted head, management of transverse presentation, replacement of retroverted uterus or displaced ovary, flushing of intestinal canal.

p., horizontal. Lying supine, feet extended. Employed in palpation, in auscultation of fetal heart and in operative procedures.

p., h. abdominal. Patient flat on abdomen, feet extended. Employed in examination of back and spinal column.

p., jackknife. Patient on back, shoulders elevated, legs flexed on thighs, thighs at right angles to abdomen. Employed when passing urethral sound.

p., knee-chest. SYN: *genupectoral position.*

p., knee-elbow. SEE: *genucubital position.*

p., kneeling-squatting. Patient stooping, knees pressed on abdomen trunk erect. Employed in childbirth in difficult cases and in uncivilized nations.

p., lateroprone. Same as *Sims' position.*

p., laterosemiprone. Same as *Sims' position.*

p., left lateral recumbent. Patient on left side, right knee and thigh drawn up. Employed in childbirth.

p., lithotomy. Patient on back, thighs flexed on abdomen, legs on thighs, thighs abducted. Employed in operation on genital tract, in vaginal hysterectomy, diagnosis and treatment of diseases of urethra and bladder.

p., obstetrical. SEE: *left lateral recumbent position.*

p., prone. Position in which patient is lying face downward.

p., reclining. SEE: *jackknife position.* [*position.*

p., side, semiprone. Same as *Sims'*

p., Simon's. Exaggerated lithotomy position. Patient flat on back, legs flexed on thighs, thighs on abdomen, hips somewhat elevated, thighs strongly abducted. Employed in operations on vagina.

p., Sims'. Patient on left side, right knee and thigh drawn well up above left, left arm back of patient and hanging over edge of table, chest inclined forward so that patient rests upon it. Employed in curettement of uterus, intrauterine irrigation after labor, tamponade of vagina, rectal exploration, operations on cervix.

p., Trendelenburg. Dorsal position, body elevated at angle of about 45°, feet and legs hanging over end of table, head down. Employed in abdominal surgery to favor gravitation upward of abdominal viscera.

p., Walcher. The patient with hips on the edge of the table and the lower extremities hanging down.

positive (pŏz'ĭt-ĭv). 1. Definite affirmative; opposed to negative. 2. Indicating the reaction in laboratory work. 3. Indicating an abnormal condition in examination and diagnosis. 4. Indicates pathological change in post-mortem examination. 5. Noting a quantity greater than zero.

Indicated by the plus (+) sign.

p. pole. The electrode of a battery which is connected with the negative plate. SEE: *anode.*

posological (pŏs″ō-loj'ĭ-kăl). Concerning dosage.

posology (pō-sŏl'ō-jĭ). Branch of scientific study dealing with dosage.

possession (pŏ-zĕsh'ŭn). State of being dominated by an idea, a passion or a mental obsession.

p., demoniacal. Belief of being under the influence of an evil spirit or demon.

post-. A prefix meaning *behind* or *after.*

postabortal (pōst″ăb-or'tăl). Happening subsequent to abortion.

postaxial (pōst-ăks'ĭ-ăl). Situated or happening behind an axis.

postcava (pōst-kā'vă). The ascending or inf. vena cava.

postcaval (pōst-kā'văl). Concerning the postcava.

postcentral (pōst-sĕn'trăl). 1. Situated or happening behind a center. 2. Located behind the fissure of Rolando.

postcibal (pōst-sī'băl). Occurring after meals.

postclavicular (pōst″klă-vĭk'ū-lăr). Located or occurring behind the clavicle.

postclimacteric (pōst-klī-măk-tĕr'ĭk). Occurring after the menopause.

postcoital (pōst-kō'ĭt-ăl). Subsequent to sexual intercourse.

postcommissure (pōst-kŏm'ĭs-ūr). The post. commissure of the brain.

postconnubial (pōst-kŏn-ū'bĭ-ăl). Occurring after marriage.

postconvulsive (pōst-kŏn-vŭl'sĭv). Occurring after a convulsion.

postcornu (pōst-kor'nū). The post. horn of the lateral ventricle of the brain.

postdiastolic (pōst-dĭ-ăs-tŏl'ĭk). Occurring after the cardiac diastole.

postdicrotic (pōst-dĭ-krŏt'ĭk). Occurring after the dicrotic pulse wave.

p. wave. A recoil or second wave (not always present) in a sphygmographic tracing.

postencephalitis (pōst″ĕn-sĕf-ăl-ī'tĭs). The condition sometimes remaining after convalescence from epidemic encephalitis.

postepileptic (pōst″ĕp-ĭ-lĕp'tĭk). Following an epileptic seizure.

posterior (pŏs-tē'rĭ-or). 1. Toward the dorsal or back aspect; opposed to anterior. 2. Situated behind; coming after.

postero-. Prefix meaning *hinder, situated back.*

posteroexternal (pŏs″tĕr-ō-ĕks-tŭr'năl). On the outer side of a back aspect, as the posteroexternal column of the spinal cord.

posterointernal (pŏs″tĕr-ō-ĭn-tŭr'năl). On the inner side of a back part.

posterolateral (pŏs″tĕr-ō-lăt'ĕr-ăl Located behind and at the side of a part.

posteromedian (pŏs-tĕr-ō-mē'dĭ-ăn). Located at the middle of a posterior aspect.

posterosuperior (pŏs-tĕr-ō-sū-pē'rĭ-or). Located behind and above a part.

posterula (pŏs-ter'oo-lă). Portion of nasopharynx bet. the salpingopalatal fold and the post. nares, a small space between the turbinal bones and the posterior nares.

postesophageal (pōst″ē-sō-făj'ē-ăl). Located behind the esophagus.

postethmoid (pōst-ĕth'moyd). Located behind the ethmoid bone.

postfebrile (pōst-fē'brĭl). Occurring after a fever.

postgeminum (pōst-jĕm'ĭn-ŭm). The post. pair of corpora quadrigemina.

postgeniculatum, postgeniculum (pōst″jē-nĭk-ū-lă'tŭm, -nĭk'ū-lŭm). The inner elevation on optic thalamus, the internal geniculate body of the brain.

posthetomy (pŏs-thĕt'ō-mĭ). Surgical removal of all or part of the foreskin. SYN: *circumcision.*

posthioplasty (pŏs'thĭ-ō-plas″tĭ). Plastic surgery of the prepuce or foreskin.

posthitis (pŏs-thī'tĭs). Inflamed condition of the foreskin.

posthumous (pŏs'tū-mŭs). Born after the father's death.

Sometimes refers to a child taken from dead body of mother.

posthypnotic (pŏst″hĭp-nŏt′ĭk). Occurring or performed subsequent to the hypnotic state.

p. suggestion. One offered during the hypnotic state influencing a later action when individual returns to normal state.

posticus (pŏs-tī′kŭs). Posterior.

postmedian (pŏst″mē′dĭ-ăn) Behind the middle transverse line of the body.

post-mortem (pŏst-mor′tĕm). After death.

p. examination. Dissection of a dead body to ascertain cause of death and the changes wrought by disease. SYN: *autopsy*.

postnatal (pŏst-nā′tăl). Happening after birth.

postoblongata (pŏst-ŏb-long-gah′tă). Caudal portion of the oblongata below the pons.

postocular (pŏst-ŏk′ū-lar). Behind the eye.

p. neuritis. Inflammation of the optic nerve behind the eyeball.

postolivary (pŏst-ŏl′ĭv-a-rĭ). Behind the olivary body; back of the ant. pyramid of the medulla.

postoperative (pŏst-ŏp′ĕr-ā-tĭv). After or following a surgical operation.

postoperculum (pŏst-ō-per′kū-lŭm). The fold covering the insula that is formed of part of the supertemporal gyrus. SYN: *operculum temporal*.

postoral (pŏst-ō′răl). Behind or in the posterior part of the mouth.

postpallium (pŏst-păl′ĭ-ŭm). That part of the cerebral cortex behind the fissure of Rolando.

postpaludal (post-pal′ū-dăl). After a malarial attack.

postparalytic (pŏst-par-ă-lĭt′ĭk). Subsequent to an attack of paralysis.

postpartum (pŏst-par′tŭm). After parturition.

p. hemorrhage. Hemorrhage which occurs after childbirth.

postpontile (pŏst-pŏn′tĭl). Situated behind the pons Varolii.

p. recess. The foramen caecum.

postpyramidal (pŏst″pĭr-ăm′ĭd-ăl). Behind the pyramidal tract.

p. nucleus. Mass of gray matter in post. column of the medulla. SYN: *nucleus funiculi gracilis*.

postural (pos′tū-răl). Pert. to or effected by posture.

p. drainage. Drainage of secretions from the bronchi or a cavity in the lung by placing the patient's head lower than the area to be drained.

posture (pŏs′tūr). 1. Posture is the adaptation of the body to the laws of gravity. SYN: *body mechanics, position*. 2. Attitude or position of the body, esp. in relation to disease.

p., coiled. Body on 1 side with legs drawn up to meet the trunk. Noted in cerebral diseases, hepatic, intestinal or renal colic.

p., dorsal inertia. Patient on back, with tendency to slip down in bed or to either side. Seen in great weakness,

in acute infectious diseases such as typhoid in mental apathy or muscular weakness.

p., dorsal, rigid. Posture on back with both legs drawn up. Seen in peritonitis, meningitis, ascites, tympanites. In appendicitis the right leg is drawn up. Also occurs in pelvic inflammation or peritonitis of right side, renal calculus in right ureter, and in psoas abscess.

p., emprosthotonos. The body is incurved and rests upon the forehead and feet with face downward. It is rarely seen in tetanus and strychnia poisoning.

p., opisthotonos. An uncommon dorsal position in which the body rests upon the head and heels, with the trunk arched upward. It is seen in strychnia poisoning, tetanus, hysteria, epilepsy, the convulsions of rabies, and to a slight extent in meningitis. In the latter case, the neck is rigid and the head retracted, seeming to press into the pillow. SEE: *opisthotonos*.

p., orthopnea. Patient sitting upright, hands or elbows resting upon some support. Seen in spasmodic asthma, emphysema, dyspnea, abdominal dropsy, effusions into the pleural and pericardial cavities, and in late stages of diseases of the heart.

p., orthotkos. Neck and trunk extended rigidly in straight line, in tetanus, strychnine poisoning, rabies or meningitis.

p., pleurothotonos. Lateral position with body arched in acute pleural involvement or spinal affection.

p., prone. Posture assumed after abdominal colic or because of tuberculosis of spine, eroded vertebrae, abdominal pain or gastric ulcer.

p., semireclining. Used in diseases of heart and interference with respiration in asthma and pleural effusions.

p., unilateral. Patient on right side in acute pleurisy, lobar pneumonia of right side and in a greatly enlarged liver, or left side in lobar pneumonia, or pleurisy on that side, and in large pericardial effusions.

postuterine (pŏst-ū′tĕr-ĭn). Situated behind the uterus.

postvaccinal (pŏst-văk′sĭn-ăl). Following vaccination.

postvermis (pŏst-vĕr′mĭs). The inferior vermiform process of the cerebellum.

potable (pō′tă-bl). Suitable for drinking.

potamophobia (pŏt″ăm-ō-fō′bĭ-ă). A morbid fear of large bodies of water.

potash (pŏt′ăsh). SEE: *potassium carbonate or potassium hydroxide, q.v.*

potassa sulfurata (pō-tăs′a sŭl-fū-rā′ta) USP. (Liver of sulfur.) Greenish yellow pieces containing 12.8% sulfur in the combination as a sulfide.

DOSAGE: For application in 5% solution.

potassemia (pō-tăs-sē′mĭ-ă). The presence of an excessive quantity of potassium in the blood.

potassic (pō-tas′ĭk). Composed of or containing potash.

potassium (pō-tas′ĭ-ŭm). Symb: K. At. wt. 39.10. Sp. gr. 0.865. An alkaline mineral element found in combination with other elements in the body.

   p. acetate. USP. A white powder or crystalline flakes.
     Dosage: 15 gr. (1 Gm.).

   p. bicarbonate. USP. White crystals or powder.
     Dosage: 15 gr. (1 Gm.). See: *potassium chromate.*

   p. bitartrate. USP. Cream of tartar. A white powder or crystalline salt.
     Dosage: 30 gr. (2 Gm.).

   p. bromide. USP. White cubical crystals of powder.
     Dosage: 15 gr. (1 Gm.).

   p. chlorate. USP. An explosive, white crystalline salt, used in diseases of mouth and throat.

   p. citrate. USP. Transparent prismatic crystals.
     Dosage: 15 gr. (1 Gm.).

   p. cromate. Used as dye, furniture stain, in manufacture of batteries, in photography and in medicine for cauterization.

   p. cyanide. See: *cyanide.*

   p. hydroxide. Grayish-white compound used in various shops, and in preparation of soap.

   p. iodide. USP. Colorless or white crystals having a faint odor of iodine.
     Dosage: 5 gr. (0.3 Gm.).

   p. permanganate. USP. Dark purple prisms, odorless, with sweet taste.
     Dosage: 1 gr. (0.06 Gm.).

   p. sulfate. USP. A laxative and a purgative, but because of its irritant qualities not to be recommended.
     Dosage: 20 gr. to 2 drams (1.3-8 Gm.).

potency (pō′těn-sĭ). 1. Strength of a medicine. 2. Ability of male to perform coitus. 3. Strength; force; power.

potent (pō′těnt). 1. Powerful. 2. Highly effective medicinally. 3. Having power of procreation.

potentia coeundi (pō-těn′shĭ-ă kō-ĕ-ŭn′dē). Complete ability to perform sexual intercourse in a normal manner.

potential (pō-těn′shăl). 1. Latent; existing in possibility. 2. PT: The condition of electrical tension in a body, manifested by the production of electrical effects in other bodies of different potential, or in a different state of electrical tension.

potion (pō′shŭn). A drink or draught; a dose of poison or liquid medicine.

potomania (pō-tō-mā′nĭ-ă). Delirium tremens, *q.v.*

Pott's disease (pŏts). Caries or osteitis of the vertebrae, usually of tuberculous origin; tubercular inflammation of bodies of the vertebrae.

   A disease usually found in children between ages of 3 and 10 years, of poor parents, and esp. those of tubercular families. No age or class exempt, however. Syn: *spondylitis.*

   P.'s fracture. Fracture of lower end of fibula with dislocation of foot outwards and backwards.

pouch (powch). Any pocket or sac. Syn: *sacculation.*

   p., Broca's. A sac in tissues of the labia majora.

   p., laryngeal. Blind pouch of mucosa entering the ventral portion of the ventricle of the larynx.

   p., pressure. An esophageal bulge due to weakness of the wall.

   p., rectouterine. Pouch bet. ant. rectal wall and post. uterine wall. Syn: *Douglas' cul-de-sac.*

poultice (pōl′tĭs). A hot, moist mass of linseed, bread, mustard, or soap and oil bet. 2 pieces of muslin applied to the skin to relieve congestion or pain, to stimulate absorption of inflammatory products, and to hasten suppuration. Syn: *cataplasm.* See: *plaster, sinapism.*

   p., bread. The crumb of bread is moistened by pouring boiling water over it; the water is then pressed out, and the bread mash spread between old linen and applied.

   p., charcoal. Used for foul septic wounds. It can either be made in the same way as a mustard poultice in the proportion of 1 to 3, or an ordinary linseed poultice can be made and the charcoal powdered over the top; the former method is the more usual.

   p., flaxseed. Aim: To apply moist heat for the relief of congestion and the promotion of suppuration.

   p., jacket. One made both for the chest and back; used in acute lobar pneumonia.

   p., linseed. Have everything heated before commencing. Pour 1 teacupful of boiling water into hot bowl and add heated linseed (about 3 cupfuls) handful by handful, stirring all the time. Should be a stiff paste which does not stick to the sides of the bowl.
   On the flannel spread the paste ¼ to ½ in. thick with the hot moist spatula, fold over the edges of the flannel. The poultice is then rolled on itself, carried bet. 2 hot plates to the bedside. Apply to the part, cover with wool, and bandage. The fresh poultice is rolled on as the old one is removed. The skin must not be exposed.

   p., mustard. Dry mustard is added to the dry linseed in proportions of 1 to 8 for adults, but 1 to 12 to 1 to 16 for children; the poultice is then made as for an ordinary linseed poultice.

   p., starch. Used in eczema and other skin affections.

pound (pownd). Symb: lb. A measure of weight, commonly 12 or 16 ounces.

   p., avoirdupois. Sixteen ounces, 7000 grains.

   p., foot-. Power necessary to raise 1 pound 1 foot high.

   p., troy. Twelve ounces, 5760 grains.

Poupart's ligament (pŏō-parz′). The ligament which is the lower border of aponeurosis of external oblique muscle bet. ant. sup. spine of the ilium and spine of the pubis. SYN: *inguinal ligament*.

powder (pow'dĕr). 1. Aggregation of particles. 2. Fine particles of 1 or more substances that may be passed through fine meshes. 3. A dose of such a powder, contained in a paper.

power (pow'er). 1. PT: Rate at which work is done. 2. Capacity for action. The electrical unit of power is the watt, *q.v.*

pox (pŏx). 1. An eruptive, contagious disease. 2. A papular eruption that becomes pustular.
SEE: *chickenpox, smallpox, etc.*

P. P. D. Abbr. *purified protein derivative,* substance used in intradermal test for tuberculosis.

P. P. F. Abbr. meaning the *pellagra preventive factor* in Vitamin B.

Ppt. Abbr. for *precipitate.*

Pr. Abbr. for *presbyopia.*

P. r. Abbr. of *punctum remotum* meaning *far point.*

practice (prăk'tĭs). Phase of medicine dealing with professional diagnosis and treatment of disease.

practitioner (prăk-tĭsh'ŭn-ĕr). One who practices the profession of medicine.

prae-. For words beginning thus, see *pre-.*

pragmatagnosia (prăg"măt-ăg-nō'zĭ-ă). Inability to recognize objects once familiar.

pragmatamnesia (prăg"măt-ăm-nē'zĭ-ă). Inability to recall the appearance of an object.
p., visual. Name for the mental condition making possible pragmatamnesia.

pragmatic (prăg-măt'ĭk). Pert. to, or concerned with, the practical side of anything.

pragmatism (prăg'mă-tĭzm). A belief that the practical application of a principle should be the determining factor.

pragmatist (prăg'mă-tĭst). One who believes that practical application should be the determining factor of a principle.

prasoid (prā'soyd). 1. Leek green. 2. Commercial mixture of globularin and globularetin used in treatment of rheumatism and gout.

praxinoscope (prăk-sĭn'ō-skōp). Contrivance for studying the larynx.

pre-. Prefix meaning *before,* or in *front of.*

preagonal (prē-ăg'ō-năl). Pert. to condition immediately before death agony.

prealbuminuric (prē"ăl-bū"mĭn-ū'rĭk). Before the appearance of albuminuria.

preanal (prē-ā'năl). In front of the anus.

preanesthetic (prē"ăn-ĕs-thĕt'ĭk). Preliminary drug given to facilitate induction of general anesthesia.

preantiseptic (prē"ăn-tĭ-sĕp'tĭk). Before the adoption of antisepsis in surgery.

preaortic (prē-ā-or'tĭk). Located in front of the aorta.

preataxic (prē-ăt-ăk'sĭk). Occurring before the onset of ataxia.

preaxial (prē-ăk'sĭ-ăl). In front of the axis of a limb or of the body.

precancerous (prē-kan'sĕr-ŭs). Taking

place before the development of a carcinoma.

precava (prē-kā'vă). The descending or superior vena cava.

precentral (prē-sĕn'trăl). In front of a center, as the central fissure of the brain.
p. convolution. The ascending frontal convolution.

prechordal (prē-kor'dăl). In front of the primitive backbone or notochord.

precipitant (prē-sĭp'ĭt-ănt). A substance bringing about precipitation.

precipitate (prē-sĭp'ĭt-āt). 1. A deposit separated from a suspension or solution by precipitation, the reaction of a reagent, which causes the deposit to fall to the bottom or float near the top. 2. To separate as a precipitate. 3. Hasty.

precipitation (prē-sĭp"ĭ-tā'shŭn). Process of a substance being separated from a solution by action of a reagent.
p. test. One in which positive reaction is indicated by formation of a precipitate in the solution being tested.

precipitin (prē-sĭp'ĭt-ĭn). Substance, formed in blood serum, producing precipitation of solubles utilized for biological identification of unknown proteins, for determining types of pneumococcus, for diagnosis of echinococcus, etc., and to discriminate bet. human and animal blood.

precipitinogen (prē-sĭp"ĭt-ĭn'ō-jĕn). Any protein which, acting as an antigen, stimulates the production of a specific precipitin.

precipitoid (prē-sĭp'ĭt-oyd). Precipitin which can no longer cause precipitation due to subjection to heat.

precipitophore (prē-sĭp'ĭt-ō-fōr). Group in a precipitin which produces precipitation. OPP: *haptophore precipitum.*

preclinical (prē-klĭn'ĭ-kăl). Before the development or onset of disease.
p. medicine. Practice of health examinations at stated intervals in order to detect presence of disease.

preclival (prē-klī'văl). In front of the cerebellar clivus.

precoital (prē-kō'ĭt-ăl). Prior to sexual intercourse.

precommissure (prē-kŏm'ĭs-ūr). The ant. commissure of the brain.

preconscious (prē-kŏn'shŭs). Not present in consciousness but able to be recalled as desired.

preconvulsive (prē-kŏn-vŭl'sĭv). Before a convulsion.

precordia (prē-kor'dĭ-ă). The epigastric region including ant. part of lower thorax. SYN: *epigastrium, precordium.*

precordial (prē-kor'dĭ-ăl). Pert. to the precordia or epigastrium.

precordialgia (prē"-kor-dĭ-ăl'jĭ-ă). Pain in the chest or precordial area.

precordium (prē-kor'dĭ-ŭm). A rectangular space over the heart, its blood vessels and the pericardium.

precornu (prē-kor'nū). Anterior horn of lateral ventricle of the brain.

precuneus (prē-kū'nē-ŭs). The quadrate

lobule of the parietal lobe of the cerebrum.

prediastolic (prē-dī-ăs-tŏl'ĭk). Before the diastole, or interval in the cardiac cycle that precedes it.

predicrotic (prē-dī-krŏt'ĭk). Preceding the dicrotic wave of the sphygmographic tracing.

predigestion (prē-dī-jĕs'chŭn). Artificial proteolysis or digestion of proteins and amylolysis of starches before ingestion for use in illness.

predisposing (prē-dĭs-pōz'ĭng). Conferring a tendency to or susceptibility to disease.

predisposition (prē''dĭs-pō-zĭ'shŭn). A tendency to develop a certain disease, either acquired or hereditary, such as nervous disorders, malformations, etc.

    p., acquired. Principally subject to diseases made possible by lowered resistance. This class includes such factors as age, sex, climate, racial differences, environment, and occupation.

preëclampsia (prē''ĕk-lămp'sĭ-ă). A toxemia of pregnancy characterized by hypertension which increases, headaches, albuminuria, and edema of the lower extremities.

preflagellate (prē-flăj'ĕl-āt). Before the flagellate stage; noted in protozoa.

prefrontal (prē-frŏn'tăl). 1. The middle portion of the ethmoid bone. 2. In ant. part of the frontal lobe of the brain.

pregeniculatum, pregeniculum (prē''jē-nĭk''ū-lā'tŭm, -nĭk'ū-lŭm). The external geniculate body; 1 of 2 flattened bodies on the post. inf. part of the optic thalamus.

pregenital (prē-jĕn'ĭt-ăl). Psy: Relating to that period when erotic interest is not yet organized about the reproductive organs and functions.

preglobulin (prē-glŏb'ū-lĭn). A proteid in cell protoplasm derived from cytoglobulin.   [being with child.

pregnancy (prĕg'năn-sĭ). The condition of

    p., abdominal. Implantation of the ovum in the abdominal cavity.

    p., bigeminal. Pregnancy with twins *in utero.*

    p., cervical. Implantation of the ovum in the cervical canal.

    p., cornual. Pregnancy in 1 of the horns of a bicornuate uterus.

    p., ectopic. SEE: *extrauterine pregnancy.*

    p., extrauterine. Pregnancy outside the uterine cavity.

    p., heterotropic. Combined intrauterine and extrauterine pregnancies.

    p., interstitial. Pregnancy occurring in the uterine wall which forms part of the oviduct.

    p., mask of. Area of brown pigmentation sometimes appearing on the face during pregnancy.

    p., multiple. State of having more than 1 fetus in the uterus at the same time.

    p., ovarian. Implantation of the fertilized ovum in the substance of the ovary.

    p., phantom. Enlargement of the abdomen simulating pregnancy. SEE: *pseudocyesis.*

    p. table. SEE: Table for calculation of expected date of delivery from the first day of the last menstrual period.

pregnant (prĕg'nănt). Having conceived; with child. SYN: *gravid.*

pregniotin (prĕg-nī'ŏt-ĭn). Preparation, no longer available commercially, of antigen from human placenta which was supposed to determine pregnancy when injected intradermally.

pregravidic (prē-grăv-ĭd'ĭk). Before pregnancy.

prehallux (prē-hăl'ŭks). A supernumerary bone or accessory *naviculare pedis* or sometimes a prolongation inward of it on the foot.

prehemiplegic (prē-hĕm-ĭ-plē'jĭk). Occurring before an attack of hemiplegia.

prehensile (prē-hĕn'sĭl). Capable of grasping.

prehension (prē-hĕn'shŭn). The act of grasping or seizing.

prehyoid (prē-hī'oyd). Before the hyoid bone.

prehypophysis (prē''hī-pof'ĭs-ĭs). The anterior and larger part of the hypophysis or pituitary gland.

preimmunization (prē-ĭm''ū-nĭ-zā'shŭn). Immunization produced artificially in very young infants.

preinsula (prē-ĭn'sū-lă). The cephalic area of the island of Reil, the insula, a group of several small convolutions at bottom of the fissure of Sylvius.

Preiser's disease (prī'zĕr). A porous condition of bone, osteoporosis, caused by trauma and affecting the carpal scaphoid bone of the wrist.

prelimbic (prē-lĭm'bĭk). Situated before a margin.

    p. fissure. Ant. part of the fissure of the corpus callosum and marginal gyri of the brain.

prelipoid (prē-lĭp'oyd). Before conversion into the lipoid state.

    p. substance. Nerve tissue broken down, but not yet converted into fat.

prelum (prē'lŭm). A press.

    p. abdominale. Squeezing of abdominal viscera in defecation, urination, and parturition, bet. the diaphragm and abdominal wall.

premature (prē-mă-tūr'). Not mature; before term or full development.

    p. beat. A cardiac contraction occurring before the normal one. SYN: *extrasystole.*

    p. infant. One born before term.

    p. labor. Onset of labor before full term.

premaxilla (prē''măks-ĭl'ă). The intermaxillary bone forming median ant. part of sup. maxillary bones.

premaxillary (prē-măk'sĭ-lĕr-ĭ). Located before the maxilla.

    p. bone. The intermaxillary bone. SYN: *incisive bone.*

premedication (prē-mĕd-ĭ-kā'shŭn). Induction of unconsciousness by internal

PREGNANCY TABLE

Find the date of the first day of the last menstrual period in the top line and the date below this will be the expected day of delivery.

	1	2	3	4	5	6	7	8	9	10	11	12	13	14	15	16	17	18	19	20	21	22	23	24	25	26	27	28	29	30	31	→
Jan.	1	2	3	4	5	6	7	8	9	10	11	12	13	14	15	16	17	18	19	20	21	22	23	24	25	26	27	28	29	30	31	
Oct.	8	9	10	11	12	13	14	15	16	17	18	19	20	21	22	23	24	25	26	27	28	29	30	31	(1	2	3	4	5	6	7	**Nov.**
Feb.	1	2	3	4	5	6	7	8	9	10	11	12	13	14	15	16	17	18	19	20	21	22	23	24	25	26	27	28				
Nov.	8	9	10	11	12	13	14	15	16	17	18	19	20	21	22	23	24	25	26	27	28	29	30	(1	2	3	4	5				**Dec.**
Mar.	1	2	3	4	5	6	7	8	9	10	11	12	13	14	15	16	17	18	19	20	21	22	23	24	25	26	27	28	29	30	31	
Dec.	8	9	10	11	12	13	14	15	16	17	18	19	20	21	22	23	24	25	26	27	28	29	30	31	(1	2	3	4	5	6	7	**Jan.**
Apr.	1	2	3	4	5	6	7	8	9	10	11	12	13	14	15	16	17	18	19	20	21	22	23	24	25	26	27	28	29	30		
Jan.	8	9	10	11	12	13	14	15	16	17	18	19	20	21	22	23	24	25	26	27	28	29	30	31	(1	2	3	4	5	6		**Feb.**
May	1	2	3	4	5	6	7	8	9	10	11	12	13	14	15	16	17	18	19	20	21	22	23	24	25	26	27	28	29	30	31	
Feb.	8	9	10	11	12	13	14	15	16	17	18	19	20	21	22	23	24	25	26	27	28	(1	2	3	4	5	6	7	8	9	10	**Mar.**
June	1	2	3	4	5	6	7	8	9	10	11	12	13	14	15	16	17	18	19	20	21	22	23	24	25	26	27	28	29	30		
Mar.	8	9	10	11	12	13	14	15	16	17	18	19	20	21	22	23	24	25	26	27	28	29	30	31	(1	2	3	4	5	6		**April**
July	1	2	3	4	5	6	7	8	9	10	11	12	13	14	15	16	17	18	19	20	21	22	23	24	25	26	27	28	29	30	31	
Apr.	8	9	10	11	12	13	14	15	16	17	18	19	20	21	22	23	24	25	26	27	28	29	30	(1	2	3	4	5	6	7	8	**May**
Aug.	1	2	3	4	5	6	7	8	9	10	11	12	13	14	15	16	17	18	19	20	21	22	23	24	25	26	27	28	29	30	31	
May	8	9	10	11	12	13	14	15	16	17	18	19	20	21	22	23	24	25	26	27	28	29	30	31	(1	2	3	4	5	6	7	**June**
Sept.	1	2	3	4	5	6	7	8	9	10	11	12	13	14	15	16	17	18	19	20	21	22	23	24	25	26	27	28	29	30		
June	8	9	10	11	12	13	14	15	16	17	18	19	20	21	22	23	24	25	26	27	28	29	30	(1	2	3	4	5	6	7		**July**
Oct.	1	2	3	4	5	6	7	8	9	10	11	12	13	14	15	16	17	18	19	20	21	22	23	24	25	26	27	28	29	30	31	
July	8	9	10	11	12	13	14	15	16	17	18	19	20	21	22	23	24	25	26	27	28	29	30	31	(1	2	3	4	5	6	7	**Aug.**
Nov.	1	2	3	4	5	6	7	8	9	10	11	12	13	14	15	16	17	18	19	20	21	22	23	24	25	26	27	28	29	30		
Aug.	8	9	10	11	12	13	14	15	16	17	18	19	20	21	22	23	24	25	26	27	28	29	30	31	(1	2	3	4	5	6		**Sept.**
Dec.	1	2	3	4	5	6	7	8	9	10	11	12	13	14	15	16	17	18	19	20	21	22	23	24	25	26	27	28	29	30	31	
Sept.	8	9	10	11	12	13	14	15	16	17	18	19	20	21	22	23	24	25	26	27	28	29	30	(1	2	3	4	5	6	7	8	**Oct.**

drugs prior to administration of inhalation anesthesia.

premenstrual (prē-měn'strū-ăl). Before menstruation.

premenstruum (prē-měn'strŭ-ŭm). The period prior to menstruation.

premolar (prē-mō'ler). 1. A bicuspid tooth. 2. Before a molar tooth.

premonition (prē-mō-nĭsh'ŭn). A feeling of an impending event.

premonitory (prē-mon'ĭ-tō-rĭ). Giving a warning; foreboding or forewarning.

premonocyte (prē-mon'ō-sīt). An embryonic cell transitional in development prior to a monocyte.

premunition (prē-mū-nĭsh'ŭn). Immunity conferred by preventive vaccination.

premunitive (prē-mū'nĭ-tĭv). Pert. to, or resulting from, preventive vaccination.

premyelocyte (prē-mī'ěl-ō-sīt). An embryonic myeloblast.

prenarcosis (prē-nar-kō'sĭs). Induction of unconsciousness by int. drugs before general inhalation anesthesia. SYN: *premedication.*

prenatal (prē-nā'tl). Before birth.

preoperculum (prē''ō-pěr'kū-lŭm). The frontal part of the convolutions covering the island of Reil, the operculum.

preoptic (prē-ŏp'tĭk). In front of the optic lobes. [mouth.

preoral (prē-ō'răl). In front part of the

prepallium (prē-păl'ĭ-ŭm). The part of the brain cortex ant. to the fissure of Rolando.

preparalytic (prē''păr-ă-lĭt'ĭk). Before the appearance of paralysis.

prepatellar (prē-pă-těl'ar). In front of the patella.

   p. bursitis. Inflammation of the bursa in front of patella. SYN: *housemaid's knee.* SEE: *bursitis.*

prephthisis (prē-tĭ'sĭs). 1. The pretuberculous stages of pulmonary phthisis. 2. Predisposition to tuberculosis.

prephyson (prē-fi'son). Hormone elaborated by the ant. pituitary lobe which aids in metabolic regulation.

prepuce (prē'pūs). The foreskin or fold of skin over the glans penis in the male.

   p. of the clitoris. Fold of the labia minora which covers the clitoris. SEE: *clitoris.*

preputial (prē-pū'shăl). Concerning the prepuce.

   p. glands. Small sebaceous glands of the corona of the penis which secrete an odoriferous discharge. SYN: *Tyson's glands.*

preputium (prē-pū'shĭ-ŭm) (pl. *preputia*). The fold of skin which covers the glans penis. SYN: *prepuce, q.v.*

   p. clitoridis. Prepuce of the clitoris, the 2 layers of the labia pudendi minora which split at their junction anteriorly.

presbyacusia, presbyacousia (prěz''bĭ-ă-kū'sĭ-ă). Hearing less acutely, due to old age. SYN: *presbycusis.*

presbyatrics, presbyatry (prěz-bĭ-ăt'rĭks, prěz'bĭ-ăt-rĭ). That branch of medicine dealing with the diseases of old age.

presbycusis, presbykousis (prěz-bĭ-kū'sĭs). Impairment of acute hearing in old age. SYN: *presbyacusia.*

presbyophrenia (prěz-bĭ-ō-frē'nĭ-ă). Senile psychotic syndrome involving confabulation and disorientation with preservation of mobility, loquacity, and good spirits. SYN: *Wernicke's syndrome.*

presbyopia (prěz-bĭ-ō'pĭ-ă). Defect of vision in ad''ancing age involving loss of accommodation or recession of near point.

   Usually occurs between 40 and 45 years of age. SEE: *farsightedness.*

presbytiatrics (prěz-bĭt-ĭ-ăt'rĭks). Science of old age and its treatment. SYN: *geriatrics, presbyatrics, presbyatry.*

prescription (prē-skrĭp'shŭn). A written order for dispensing drugs signed by a physician.

   p. carbons. PT: Carbons impregnated with various substances for use in treatment of specific conditions.

presentation (prē-zěn-tā'shŭn). OB: Term applied to the manner of the fetus presenting itself to the examining finger at the mouth of the uterus.

   p., breech. When pelvic extremity presents.

   p., brow. When the brow presents.

   p., cephalic. Presentation of the head in any position.

   p., face. When the head is sharply extended so that the face presents.

   p., footling. Presenting feet first.

   p., placental. Presentation of the placenta first. SYN: *placenta previa.*

   p., sinciput. When the large fontanel presents.

   p., transverse. With fetus lying crosswise.

   p. vertex. Presentation of the upper and back part of the head.

presphenoid (prē-sfē'noyd). Ant. region of the body of the sphenoid bone.

presphygmic (prē-sfĭg'mĭk). Pert. to period preceding the pulse wave.

prespinal (prē-spī'năl). Before the spine, or ventral to it.

prespondylolisthesis (prē-spŏn''dĭl-ō-lĭs-thē'sĭs). A congenital defect of a lumbar vertebra without displacement, which predisposes to spondylolisthesis.

pressinervoscopy (prěs''ĭ-něr-vŏs'kō-pĭ). Diagnosis by pressing upon the pneumogastric and sympathetic nerves.

pressor (prěs'ŏr). 1. Stimulating, increasing the activity of a function, especially of vasomotor activity, as a nerve. 2. A substance in the pituitary body capable of raising blood pressure.

   p. base or *substance.* One of several products of intestinal putrefaction found in normal urine which, when injected, raises blood pressure in animals.

   p. nerves. Those nerves which under stimulation cause reaction of the vasomotor centers.

   p. reflex. Any reflex in which the response to stimulation is increased activity of a motor center.

Terms Used in Prescription Writing

Abbreviation	Word or Phrase	English Equivalent
āā or a	ana	of each
ads. feb.	absente febre	fever being absent
ad	ad	to, up to
add.	adde	add
ad. feb.	adstante febre	fever being present
adhib.	adhibendus	to be administered
ad. lib.	ad libitum	at pleasure
admov.	admove	apply
ante cib. or A. C.	ante cibum	before food
aq. bull.	aqua bulliens	boiling water
aq. dest.	aqua destillata	distilled water
aq. font.	aqua fontis	spring water
aq. pur.	aqua pura	pure water
bene	bene	well
b. i. d.	bis in die	twice daily
bull.	bulliat	let (it) boil
c̄	cum	with
cap.	capsula	a capsule
chart. or cht.	chartula	a small medicated paper
coch. mag.	cochleare magnum	a tablespoonful
coch. med.	cochleare medium	a dessertspoonful
coch. parv.	cochleare parvum	a teaspoonful
collyr.	collyrium	an eyewash
comp.	compositus	compounded of
cong.	congius	a gallon
cont. rem.	continuantur remedia	continue the medicine
cras mane sum.	cras mane sumendus	take tomorrow morning
cuj. lib.	cujus libet	of any you please
d., det.	da, detur	give, let be given
d. d. in d.	de die in diem	from day to day
dent. tal. dos.	dentur tales doses	give of such doses
dieb. alt.	diebus alternis	every other day
dieb. tert.	diebus tertiis	every 3rd day
dil.	dilue, dilutus	dilute, diluted
dim.	dimidius	one-half
div.	divide	divide
div. in p. aeq.	dividatur in partes aequales	let it be divided into equal parts
donec alv. sol. ft.	donec alvus soluta fuerit	until bowels are open
dos.	dosis	dose
dur. dolor.	durante dolore	while pain lasts
emp.	emplastrum	plaster
emuls.	emulsio	an emulsion
ft.	fiat	let be made
garg.	gargarisma	a gargle
grad.	gradatim	by degrees
gr.	granum	a grain
gtt.	gutta, guttae	a drop, drops
guttat.	guttatim	by drops
haust.	haustus	a draught
hor. decub.	hora decubitus	bed hour
hor. som. or h. s.	hora somni	bed time
hor. 1 spat.	horae unius spatio	one hour's time
ind.	indies	daily
inf.	infusum	let it infuse
int.	intime	thoroughly
lin.	linimentum	a liniment
lot.	lotio	a lotion
M.	misce	mix
mac.	macera	macerate
man. prim.	mane primo	first thing in the morning
mas.	massa	mass
med.	medicamentum	a medicine

Abbreviation	Word or Phrase	English Equivalent
m. et n.	mane et nocte	morning and night
mitt.	mitte	send
mitt. x tal.	mitte decem tales	send 10 like this
mod.	modicus	moderate sized
mod. praesc.	modo praescripto	in the manner written
moll.	mollis	soft
mor. dict.	more dicto	in the manner directed
mor. sol.	more solito	as accustomed
ne tr. s. num.	ne tradas sine nummo	deliver not without the money
no.	numerus	number
noct. maneq.	nocte maneque	night and morning
non. rep., n. r.	non repetatur	let it not be repeated
o.	octarius	a pint
omn. bih.	omni bihoris	every 2nd hour
omn. hor.	omni hora	every hour
om. ¼ h.	omni quadrantae horae	every 15 minutes
om. mane vel. noc.	omni mane vel nocte .?	every morning or night
p. c.	post cibum	after meals
pil.	pilula	a pill
p. p. a.	phiala prius agitata	the bottle being first shaken
p. r. n.	pro re nata	as occasion arises
pro. rat. aet.	pro ratione aetatis	according to patient's age
pulv.	pulvis	powder
q. h.	quaque hora	every hour
q. l.	quantum libet	as much as pleases
q. s.	quantum sufficiat	as much as suffices
quotid.	quotidie	daily
red. in pulv.	redactus in pulverem	reduced to powder
repetat., rep.	repetatur	to be repeated
sec. a., or s. a.	secundem artem	according to art
semih.	semihora	half an hour
sig.	signa	write
sing.	singulorum	of each
sol.	solutio	solution
s. o. s.	si opus sit	if need exists
solv.	solve	dissolve
ss.	semi or semisse	a half
stat.	statim	immediately
st.	stet or stent	let it (or them) stand
subind.	subinde	frequently
sum.	sume	take
sum. tal.	sumat talem	take 1 such
suppos.	suppositoria	a suppository
tab.	tabella	a tablet
tere	tere	rub
tere bene	tere bene	rub well
t. i. d.	ter in die	thrice daily
trit.	tritura	triturate or grind
ult. praes.	ultimus praescriptus	the last ordered
ut dict.	ut dictum	as directed
vitel.	vitellus	yolk of an egg

Weights and Measures.

℔   Minimum, -i, n., minim, of a fluidram.
Gtt.   Gutta, -ae, f., a drop.
gr.   Granum, -i, n., a grain.
Ɔ   Scrupulus, -i, m., a scruple, 20 grains.
ʒ   Drachma, -ae, f., a dram, 60 grains.
f ʒ   Fluidrachma, -ae, f., a fluidram, 60 minims.
ℨ   Uncia, -ae, f., a troy ounce, 480 grains.
f ℨ   Fluiduncia, -ae, f., a fluidounce, 8 fluidrams.
lb.   Libra, -ae, f., a pound (troy), 5760 grains.
O.   Octarius, -i, m., a pint, 16 fluidounces.
C.   Congius, -i, m., a gallon, 8 pints.
ss.   Semis, indecl., a half.

Quantities are designated by Roman numerals following the symbol for denomination
SEE: *charting.*

p. X. An animal extract which raises blood pressure and decreases kidney function.

pressure (prĕsh'ŭr). 1. A compression. 2. Stress or force exerted on a body, as by tension, weight, pulling, etc. 3. PSY: Quality of sensation aroused by moderate compression of the skin. 4. In physics, the quotient obtained by dividing a force by the area of the surface on which it acts.

p., after. A feeling of pressure which remains for a few seconds after removal of a weight or other pressure.

p., arterial. Pressure of blood in the arteries.

p., atmospheric. Pressure of weight of atmosphere; at sea level it averages about 760 mm. of mercury.

p., blood. Pressure exerted by blood against the walls of blood vessels.

p., diastolic. Arterial pressure during dilatation of the heart cavities; diastole.

p., intracranial. Pressure of the cerebrospinal fluid, which in a recumbent position is from 60 to 120 mm.

p., intraocular. Normal tension within the eyeball, equal to 25 mm. of mercury.

p., intrathoracic. Pressure within the thorax but outside of the lungs. In quiet expiration it is about — 4.5 mm., and in forced inspiration, as high as — 30 mm., but in quiet inspiration, — 7.5 mm.

p., intraventricular. Pressure within the ventricles of the heart during different phases of diastole and systole.

p., osmotic. The force with which the solvent passes through a semipermeable septum bet. solutions, which is measured by determining the hydrostatic (mechanical) pressure which must be opposed to the osmotic force to bring the passage to a standstill. The osmotic pressure of blood serum and of solutions isotonic* with it is 6.7 atmospheres.

p. palsy. Temporary paralysis due to pressure on a nerve trunk.

p. paralysis. Paralysis due to pressure on the spinal cord.

p. points. Areas for exerting pressure to control bleeding.

p., pulse. The difference between systolic and diastolic pressures; normally about 120, —70 equalling 50 mm.

p. sore. A bed* sore, one caused by pressure on a certain area or by a splint. SYN: decubitus.

p., systolic. Arterial pressure at time of the contraction of the ventricles; the cardiac systole.

presternum (prē-ster'nŭm). Upper part of sternum. SYN: manubrium, sterni.

presuppurative (prē-sŭp'ū-rā-tĭv). Relating to period of inflammation before suppuration.

presylvian fissure (pre-sil'vĭ-ăn). The anterior division of the sylvian fissure.

presystole (prē-sĭs'tō-lē). The period in the heart's cycle just before the systole.

presystolic (prē-sĭs-tol'ĭk). Before the systole of the heart.

pretarsal (prē-tar'săl). In front of the tarsus.

pretibial (prē-tĭb'ĭ-ăl). In front of the tibia.

preurethritis (prē"ū-re-thrī'tĭs). Inflammation around the urethral orifice of the vaginal vestibule.

preventive (prē-vĕn'tĭv). Warding off. SYN: prophylactic.

p. medicine. That branch of medicine concerned with the prevention of disease.

preventorium (prē-vĕn-to'rĭ-ŭm). An institution for those threatened with tuberculosis.

prevertebral (prē-ver'te-brăl). In front of a vertebra.

prevertiginous (prē-ver-tĭj'ĭn-ŭs). Having a tendency to fall forward. SYN: dizzy.

prezymogen (prē-zī'mō-jĕn). A granular substance in the cell nucleus which changes into zymogen when discharged into the cytoplasm. SYN: prozymogen.

priapism (prī'ăp-ĭzm). Abnormal, painful, and continued erection of the penis due to disease, usually without sexual desire.

priapitis (prī-ăp-ī'tĭs). Inflammation of the penis.

prickle cell (prĭk'l). A cell with rod-shaped processes connecting with similar adjoining cells.

p. layer. Outer layer of the epidermal stratum mucosum. SYN: stratum spinosum.

prickly heat (prĭk'lĭ hēt). Noncontagious, cutaneous eruption of red pimples, with itching and tingling of the affected parts, seen usually in hot weather.

Priessnitz compress (prēs'nĭtz). A wet cold compress. SEE: Neptune girdle.

primae viae (prī'mē vī'ē). The alimentary canal; the secondary ones consisting of the lacteals.

primary (prī'mă-rĭ). First in time or order. SYN: principal.

p. amputation. One before inflammation has set in.

p. bubo. An adenitis, of simple character, of an inguinal gland. SYN: bubon d'emblée.

p. cell. PT: A device consisting of a container, 2 solid conducting elements and an electrolyte, for the production of electric current by chemical energy.

p. dementia. A psychosis of youth.

p. hemorrhage. Bleeding at time of an injury.

p. lesion. 1. An original one from which a 2nd one originates. 2. Lesion of syphilis, a chancre.*

p. sore. The initial sore or hard chancre of syphilis.

primate (prī'māt). Highest order of Primates, mammals, including man and the apes, monkeys, lemurs, and marmosets.

prime (prīm). Period of greatest health and strength.

primigravida (prī-mĭ-grăv'ĭ-dă). A woman during her 1st pregnancy.

primipara (prī-mĭp'ă-ră). A woman who has had or who is giving birth to her 1st child.

primiparity (prĭ-mĭp-ăr'ĭt-ĭ). Condition of having given birth to only 1 child.

primiparous (prī-mĭp'ă-rŭs). Pert. to a primipara, a woman giving birth to, or having had, 1st child.

primitiae (prī-mĭsh'ĭ-ē). Liquor amnii appearing before the fetus at birth. SEE: *amnion, bag-of-waters, liquor amnii, labor.*

primitive (prĭm'ĭ-tĭv). Original; early in point of time; embryonic.

   p. groove. Deepening of the primitive streak.

   p. streak, p. trace. One indicating 1st appearance of the embryo which develops at margin of the germinal disk.

primordial (prī-mor'dĭ-ăl). Existing first. SYN: *original, primitive, rudimentary.*

princeps (prĭn'sĕps). 1. Original; first. 2. A principal artery.

principal (prĭn'sĭ-păl). 1. Chief. 2. Outstanding, main.

principle (prĭn'sĭ-pl). A constituent of a compound representing its essential properties.

   p., proximate. A substance that may be extracted from its complex form without destroying or altering its chemical properties.

   p., ultimate. Any element within a compound body.

prism (prĭzm). A solid with sides which are parallelograms whose bases are similar plane figures.

prismoptometer (prĭz-mŏp-tŏm'ĕt-ēr). Device for estimating abnormal refraction of the eye by using prisms.

privates (prī'vĕts). The ext. genitalia of the male or female.

p. r. n. As circumstance may require.

pro-. Prefix meaning *for, in front of, before, from, in behalf of, on account of*, etc.

proamnion (prō-ăm'nĭ-ŏn). The primitive amnion, at the cephalic extremity which at first is without the mesoderm.

probang (prō'băng). Rod and sponge used in treatment of larynx.

   p., foreign body. Web catheterlike tube with circle of bristles or sponge tip for removal of foreign bodies from the esophagus.

probationary (prō-bā'shŭn-ar-ĭ). One who is on trial. Waiting, as for admission or for a test.

   p. ward. One for the temporary detention of patients suspected of having a communicable disease.

probationer (prō-bā'shŭn-ēr). A person on trial for a period of time, as a newly admitted student nurse.

probe (prōb). Slender, flexible rod for exploring suppurative tracts, cavities, or for locating foreign bodies.

procaine hydrochlor'ide (prō'kăn). USP. White, colorless, crystalline compound.

   DOSAGE: Subcutaneously (having no effect when applied on the surface), from ½ to 1%. SYN: *novocain, q.v.*

procatarctic (prō''kăt-ark'tĭk). Predisposing or 'nciting, a.. the cause of a disease.

procatarxis (prō''kăt-ark'sĭs). Inception

of a disease through a predisposing cause.

procelous (prō-sē'lŭs). Concave anteriorly.

procephalic (prō-sē-făl'ĭk). Of or relating to the ant. part of the head.

process (prŏs'ĕs). 1. A method of action. 2. State of progress of a disease. 3. A projection, as of the extremity of a bone.

   p., acromion. Summit of the acromion.

   p., alveolar. Thick curved border of either maxilla containing the alveoli.

   p., basilar. Narrow part of the base of occipital bone, in front of foramen magnum, articulating with the sphenoid bone. SYN: *pars basilaris.*

   p., ensiform. The xiphoid cartilage of the sternum.

   p., ethmoidal. A small projection on the upper surface of the inferior turbinated bone which articulates with the uncinate process of the ethmoid bone.

   p., lenticular. A knob on the malleus in the ear which articulates with the stapes.

   p., mastoid. Projection of mastoid process of the temporal bone.

   p., orbicular. SEE: *process, lenticular.*

processus (prō-sĕs'ŭs) (pl. *processūs*). Process or processes.

   p. brevis. Short process of the malleus; also, short process of the incus.

   p. clavatus. A thickening on posterior pyramid of medulla, near apex of 4th ventricle.

   p. cochleariformis. Bony plate bet. the canal for eustachian tube from that of tensor tympani.

   p. e cerebello ad medullam. Inf. peduncle of the cerebellum.

   p. e cerebello ad pontem. The center peduncles of cerebellum.

   p. e cerebello ad testes. Superior cerebellar peduncles.

   p. gracilis. The long process below neck of the malleus.

   p. hamatus. SEE: *processus, uncinatus processus.*

   p. lenticularis. Knob at tip of incus articulating with the stapes.

   p. longus. 1. Long process of incus. 2. Long process of malleus.

   p. uncinatus. Sickle-shaped 1 on inner surface of the ethmoidal labyrinth.

Prochownick's diet (prō-kŏv'nĭk). A restricted 1 for women with a narrow pelvis who are pregnant.

   Carbohydrates and liquids are reduced.

procidentia (prō-sĭ-dĕn'shĭ-ă). A complete prolapse, esp. of the uterus which lies outside of the vulva, with inverted vaginal walls.

procreate (prō'krē-āt). To beget; to bring forth young.

procreation (prō''krē-ā'shŭn). The act or state of bringing forth young. SYN: *reproduction.*

proctagra (prŏk-tag'ră). Sudden rectal pain.

proctalgia (prŏk-tăl'jĭ-ă). Pain in or about the anus and rectum.

proctatresia (prŏk-tăt-rē'zĭ-ă). Imperforate condition of the anus.

proctectomy (prŏk-tĕk'tō-mĭ). Excision of the rectum or anus.

proctenclisis (prŏk-tĕn-klĭ'sĭs). Stricture of the anus or rectum.

procteurynter (prŏk-tū-rĭn'tĕr). Instrument for dilation of the anus or rectum.

proctitis (prŏk-tī'tĭs). Inflammation of rectum and anus. SEE: *bicho, rectitis*.

 p., catarrhal, acute and chronic. SYM: Mucus in each stool and some blood, finally dysenteric stool.

 p., diphtheritic. Diphtheritic membrane forms over surface of mucous membrane, forms sort of albuminous membrane. Headache, roaring in ears. Constipation, gas, neurasthenia, bloating.

 p., dysenteric. May result from ordinary diarrhea, affects upper part the most. May have ulcers, afterwards cicatricial scars.

 p., gonorrheal. Gonorrheal infection.

 p., traumatic. SYM: Pain, pressure as if bowels were going to move; irritable; mucous membrane red, eroded. Surface tissues sensitive to touch. Chronic constipation.

procto-, proct-. Combining forms meaning the *anus* and *rectum*.

proctocele (prŏk'tō-sēl). A protrusion of the rectal mucosa. [mucosa.

 p., vaginal. Prolapsus of the vaginal

proctoclysis (prŏk-tŏk'lĭ-sĭs). A continuous injection into the rectum and colon in which the solution is introduced drop by drop.

proctococcypexia, proctococcypexy (prŏk''tō-kŏk-sĭ-pĕk'sĭ-ă, -kŏk'sĭ-pĕk''sĭ). Suture of rectum to the coccyx.

proctocolitis (prŏk''tō-kō-lī'tĭs). Inflamed condition of colon and rectum.

proctocolonoscopy (prŏk''tō-kō''lŏn-ŏs'kō-pĭ). Examination of interior of rectum and lower colon.

proctocystotomy (prŏk''tō-sĭs-tŏt'ō-mĭ). Incision into the bladder through the rectum.

proctodeum (prŏk-tō-dē'ŭm). The primitive fold which becomes the anus.

proctodynia (prŏk-tō-dĭn'ĭ-ă). Pain in the rectum or about the anus.

proctologist (prŏk-tŏl'ō-jĭst). One who specializes in diseases of the rectum and anus.

proctology (prŏk-tol'ō-jĭ). Phase of medicine dealing with treatment of diseases of rectum and anus.

proctoparalysis (prŏk-tō-păr-ăl'ĭs-ĭs). Paralysis of the anal sphincter muscle.

proctopexia, proctopexy (prŏk-tō-pĕks'ĭ-ă, prŏk'tō-pĕks''ĭ). Suture of the rectum to some other part.

proctophobia (prŏk''tō-fō'bĭ-ă). Abnormal apprehension in those suffering from rectal disease.

proctoplasty (prŏk'tō-plăs-tĭ). Plastic surgery of the anus or rectum.

proctoplegia (prŏk''tō-plē'jĭ-ă). Paralysis of the anal sphincter. SYN: *proctoparalysis*.

proctoptosis (prŏk-tŏp-tō'sĭs). Prolapse of the rectum. SEE: *procidentia*.

proctorrhaphy (prŏk-tŏr'ă-fĭ). Suturing of rectum or anus.

proctorrhea (prŏk-tŏr-ē'ă). Mucous dis◀ charge from the rectum.

proctoscope (prŏk'tō-skōp). Instrumen◀ for inspection of the rectum.

proctoscopy (prŏk-tŏs'kō-pĭ). Instrumen◀ tal inspection of the rectum.

proctosigmoiditis (prŏk''tō-sĭg-moyd-ī'tĭs) Inflamed condition of the rectum an◀ sigmoid.

proctospasm (prŏk'tō-spăzm). Recta◀ spasm.

proctostenosis (prŏk''tō-stĕn-ō'sĭs). Stric◀ ture of the anus or rectum.

proctostomy (prŏk-tŏs'tō-mĭ). Creatio◀ of a permanent opening into the rec◀ tum.

proctotome (prŏk'tō-tōm). Knife for in◀ cision into rectum.

proctotomy (prŏk-tŏt'ō-mĭ). Incision o◀ the rectum or anus.

proctotoreusis (prŏk-tō-tō-rū'sĭs). Th◀ making of an opening in an imperforat◀ anus.

proctovalvotomy (prŏk-tō-văl-vŏt'ō-mĭ)◀ Incision of the rectal valves.

procumbent (prō-kŭm'bĕnt). Lying fac◀ down.

procursive (prō-kūr'sĭv). Having an in◀ voluntary tendency to run forward, a◀ in procursive epilepsy.

prodromal (prŏd'rō-măl). Pert. to the inf◀ tial stage of a disease; the interval bet◀ the earliest symptoms and the appear◀ ance of the rash or fever.

 p. rash. One that precedes the tru◀ rash of an infectious disease.

prodrome (prō'drŏm). A symptom indica◀ tive of an approaching disease.

product (prŏd'ŭkt). Anything which ▮ made naturally or artificially. SEE◀ *catabolin, catabolite*.

production (prō-dŭk'shŭn). Developmen◀ or formation of a substance. SEE: *chro◀ moparic*.

productive (prō-dŭk'tĭv). Forming, as ne◀ tissue.

 p. inflammation. Inflammation pro◀ ducing new tissue with or without a◀ exudate.

proenzyme (prō-ĕn'zīm). 1. Substanc◀ from which an enzyme is derived. 2◀ Microörganism causing fermentation◀ SYN: *zymogen*.

proferment (prō-fer'mĕnt). 1. Substanc◀ which develops into an enzyme. 2. Mi◀ croörganism causing fermentation.

professional (prō-fĕsh'ŭn-ăl). 1. Pert. t◀ a profession. 2. Caused by the practic◀ of a profession, as *writer's cramp*.

profondometer (prō-fŏn-dŏm'ĕt-ĕr). De◀ vice for locating a foreign body wit◀ the fluoroscope.

progeny (prŏj'ĕn-ĭ). Offspring.

progeria (prō-jē'rĭ-ă). Premature senilit◀ supervening upon infantilism. Rare.

progesterone (prō-jĕs'tĕr-ōn). The hor◀ mone found in corpora lutea which pre◀ pares the endometrium for nidation o◀ the embryo.

progestin (prō-jĕs'tĭn). A corpus luteu◀

hormone which prepares the endometrium for the fertilized ovum. SYN: *progesterone.*

proglossis (prō-glŏs'ĭs). The tip of the tongue.

prognathism (prŏg'nă-thĭzm). Projection of jaws beyond upper face.

prognathous (prŏg'năth-ŭs). Having jaws projecting forward beyond rest of the face.

prognosis (prŏg-nō'sĭs). Prediction of course and end of disease, and outlook based on it.

   p. anceps. Doubtful prognosis.
   p. fausta. Favorable prognosis.
   p. infausta. Unfavorable prognosis.

prognostic (prŏg-nŏs'tĭk). Affording an indication as to outcome of a disease.

prognosticate (prŏg-nŏs'tĭ-kāt). To make a statement on the probable outcome of an illness.

progonasyl (prō-gō-nă'zĭl). A medicinal vegetable and mineral oil containing an emulsifier and iodine, used to spread over vaginal tissues as a preventive against venereal disease for both sexes.

progressive (prō-grĕs'ĭv). Advancing.

   p. muscular atrophy. Gradual advancing atrophy of groups of muscles due to spinal cord degeneration. SEE: *atrophy.*
   p. ossifying myositis. Tendency to bony deposits in the muscles with chronic inflammation.

progynon (prō'jĭn-ōn). Commercial preparation of female sex hormone extracted from the placenta.

proiosystole (prō-ĭ-ō-sĭs'tō-lē). A cardiac contraction occurring before its normal time.

proiosystolia (prō-ĭ-ō-sĭs-tō'lĭ-ă). A condition marked by occurrence of systoles before the normal time.

proiotia (prō-ĭ-ō'shĭ-ă). Genital precocity.

projec'tile vomiting. Vomiting not preceded by nausea in which the stomach contents ɼ are forcibly ejected.

   Seen in some cerebral diseases and in pyloric obstruction.

projection (prō-jĕk'shŭn). 1. The act of throwing forward. 2. A part extending beyond the level of its surroundings. 3. PSY: Distortion of a perception as a result of its repression, resulting in such a phenomenon as hating without cause one who has been dearly loved, seen in paranoiac delusions of persecution.

   p. erroneous. Inability to correctly judge the position of an object due to weak ocular muscles.

prolabium (prō-lā'bĭ-ŭm). The exposed ext. ɽd border of the lip.

prolactin (prō-lăk'tĭn). Hormone, derived from the ant. pituitary lobe, which stimulates lactation. SYN: *galactin, mammotropin.*

prolamin(e (prō-lăm'ĭn, prō'lă-mĭn). Any one of a class of proteins found in seeds, soluble in alcohol, and insoluble in water and absolute alcohol. SYN: *gliadin.*

prolan (prō'lan). A hormone from the ant. pituitary body. It consists of:

   p. A. Which stimulates the ovary to formation of ripe graafian follicles and the secretion of estrin, and
   p. B. Which acts on the ovary to stimulate the formation of progestin by the corpora lutea. SEE: *hormone, prolactin.*

prolapse (prō-lăps'). 1. A dropping of an int. part of the body, as of the uterus or rectum. 2. To drop down, noted of an organ. SYN: *ptosis.*

   p. of the cord. Expulsion of umbilical cord prematurely. SEE: *labor.*
   p. of rectum. Seen in children under 3 years of age. Sometimes in old people.

prolapsus (prō-lăp'sŭs). A falling or downward displacement of some part of the body, as the uterus.

   p. ani. Dropping down of the anus.
   p. uteri. Dropping down of the uterus. SYN: *descensus uteri.*

prolepsis (prō-lĕp'sĭs). Return of paroxysmal attacks at successively shorter intervals.

proleptic (prō-lĕp'tĭk). Recurring before the time expected, said of paroxysms.

proleukemia (prō-lū-kē'mĭ-ă). A condition marked by both leukemia and pernicious anemia. SYN: *leukanemia.*

proleukocyte (prō-lū'kō-sīt). An undeveloped leukocyte. SYN: *leukoblast.*

proliferate (prō-lĭf'ĕr-āt). To increase by reproduction of similar forms.

proliferation (prō-lĭf'ĕr-ā'shŭn). 1. Reproduction rapidly and repeatedly of new parts, as by cell division. 2. Process or result of rapid reproduction. SEE: *auxesis.*

proliferous (prō-lĭf'ĕr-ŭs). 1. Multiplying, as by formation of new tissue cells. 2. Bearing offspring.

   p. cyst. One with epithelial lining, proliferating and projecting from inner surface of the cyst.

prolific (prō-lĭf'ĭk). Fruitful; reproductive. SYN: *fertile.*

proligerous (prō-lĭj'ĕr-ŭs). Producing offspring. SYN: *germinating.*

   p. disk. Collection of cells of the graafian vesicle surrounding the ovum. SYN: *discus proligerous.*

prolin(e (prō'lēn, -lĭn). An important amino acid, formed by protein decomposition, having the formula: C_4H_9N-COOH.

promegaloblast (prō''mĕg'ăl-ō-blăst). A cell intervening bet. a megaloblast and a lymphoidocyte.

promin (prō'mĭn). Commercial preparation of follicular sex hormone.

prominentia (prŏm-ĭn-ĕn'shĭ-ă). A projection.

   p. laryngea. BNA. The laryngeal prominence; Adam's apple. SYN: *pomum adami.*

promontory (prŏm'un-tō-rĭ). A projecting process or part.

   p. of the sacrum. Promontory between upper extremity of the sacrum and 5th lumbar vertebra.

promyelocyte (prō''mī'ĕl-ō-sīt). 1. A large mononuclear myeloid cell seen in the blood in leukemia. 2. Cell development bet. myeloblast and a myelocyte, resembling a myeloblast.

pronation (prō-nā'shŭn). The act of lying with face downward, or having the palms face downward. The opp. of *supine.* [vagina.

pronaus (prō'nā-ŭs). The vestibule of the

prone (prōn). Lying horizontal. with face downward; of the hand, with the palms turned downward. OPP: *supine.*

pronephron, pronephros (prō-nĕf'ron, -ros). The primitive kidney. SEE: *wolffian duct.*

pronograde (prō'nō-grād). Walking on hands and feet or resting with the body in a horizontal position. OPP: *orthograde.*

pronometer (prō-nŏm'ĕt-ĕr). Device for showing amount of pronation or supination of forearm.

prontosil (pron'tō-sĭl). A less toxic sulfanilamide derivative.

prontylin (prŏn'tĭl-ĭn). A commercial brand of sulfanilamide, *q.v.*

pronucleus (prō-nū'klē-ŭs). Nucleus of the ovum, the female pronucleus, or of the spermatozoon, the male pronucleus, after the fertilization of the ovum.

proötic (prō-ōt'ĭk, -ō'tĭk). In front of the ear.

propagation (prŏp'ă-gā'shŭn). Act of reproducing or giving birth. SYN: *generation, reproduction.*

propagative (prŏp'ă-gā-tĭv). Pert. to or taking part in reproduction.

propalinal (prō-păl'ĭn-ăl). Applied to a backward and forward movement, as of the jaws.

prop cells (prŏp). 1. Nerve cells bet. the granular and molecular layers of the cerebellar cortex. SYN: *Purkinje's cells.* 2. Columnar or fusiform cells bet. rods and hair cells of the organ of Corti. SYN: *Deiter's cells.*

propeptone (prō-pĕp'tōn). An intermediate product in the digestive conversion of protein into peptone. SYN: *hemialbumose.*

propeptonuria (prō'pĕp-tō-nū'rĭ-ă). Excretion of propeptone in the urine. SYN: *hemialbumosuria.*

prophase (prō'fāz). First stage of indirect cell division.
    SEE: *centriole, "meta-" words, mitosis, "tele-" words.*

prophylactic (prō-fĭl-ăk'tĭk). 1. Warding off disease. 2. Agent which wards off disease.

prophylaxis (prō-fĭl-ăks'ĭs). 1. Observance of rules necessary to prevent disease. 2. In dentistry, cleansing of the teeth's surface.

proplex, proplexus (prō'plĕks, prō-plĕk'sŭs). The choroid plexus of the lateral ventricles of the cerebrum.

propons (prō'pŏnz). White fibers passing transversely across the ant. margin of the pyramid and just below the pons Varolii. SYN: *ponticulus.*

proposote (prō'pō-sōt). A condensation product containing 50% creosote.
    DOSAGE: 10 minims (0.6 cc.).

proprietary medicine (prō-prī'ĕ-tar"ĭ). "Any chemical, drug, or similar preparation used in the treatment of diseases. if such article is protected against free competition, as to name, product, composition, or process of manufacture, by secrecy, patent, or copyright, or by another means." *American Medical Association.* SEE: *patent medicine.*

proprioceptive (prō"prī-ō-sĕp'tĭv). Noting impulses from afferent nerves in an organism stimulated by its own tissues.

proprioceptor (prō"prī-ō-sep'tor). A receptor stimulated by action of the organism itself. SEE: *receptor.*

proptometer (prŏp-tŏm'ĕt-ĕr). An instrument for measuring extent of exophthalmos.

proptosis (prŏp-tō'sĭs). A downward displacement, as of the uterus or of the eyeball in exophthalmic goiter, or in inflammatory conditions of the orbit.

propulsion (prō-pŭl'shŭn). 1. A tendency to push or fall forward in walking. 2. A condition seen in paralysis agitans. SEE: *festination.*

pro re nata (prō rā nah'tă). According to the circumstances.

prorennin (prō-rĕn'ĭn). The preliminary material which is converted into rennin. SYN: *mother substance, renninogen, zymogen.* [or front.

prorsad (pror'săd). Toward the anterior

prosecretin (prō"sē-kre'tĭn). Preliminary substance which develops into secretin.

prosector (prō-sĕk'tor). One who prepares cadavers for dissection or dissects for demonstration.

prosencephalon (prŏs-ĕn-sef'ăl-ŏn). Part of embryonic brain from which arise the cerebral hemispheres, corpora striata. corpus callosum, olfactory lobes, and the fornix. SYN: *forebrain.*

prosodemic (prŏs-ō-dĕm'ĭk). Spread by individual contact; said of a disease.

prosogaster (prŏs-ō-găs'tĕr). Embryonic forerunner of the digestive tract. SYN: *foregut.*

prosopalgia (prŏs-ō-păl'jĭ-ă). Neuralgic pain in the trigeminal nerve and its branches. SYN: *prosopodynia.*

prosopantritis (prŏs-ō-păn-trī'tĭs). Inflamed condition of the frontal sinuses.

prosopectasia (prŏs"ō-pĕk-tā'zĭ-ă). Abnormal size of the face.

prosoplasia (prŏs"ō-plā'zĭ-ă). 1. Progressive cellular changes toward a more complex state. 2. Unusual cell differentiation beyond the normal.

prosopodiplegia (prŏs"ō-pō-dĭ-plē'jĭ-ă). Paralysis of 1 lower extremity and the face.

prosopodynia (prŏs"ō-pō-dĭn'ĭ-ă). Pain in the face. SYN: *tic douloureux.*

prosoponeuralgia (prŏs"ō-pō-nū-răl'jĭ-ă). Facial neuralgia. SYN: *prosopalgia.*

prosopoplegia (prŏs"ō-pō-plē'jĭ-ă). Paralysis of the face.

prosopoplegic (prŏs"ō-pō-plē'jĭk). Relating to, or afflicted with, facial paralysis.

prosoposchisis (prŏs-ō-pōs'kĭ-sĭs). Congenital cleft of the face.

prosopospasm (prŏs'ō-pō-spazm). Facial spasm.

prosopotocia (prŏs"ō-pō-tō'shĭ-ă). Presentation of the face in parturition.

prostatalgia (prŏs-tă-tal'jĭ-ă). Pain of the prostate gland.

prostatauxe (pros-tat-awks'e). Enlargement of the prostate gland.

prostate (prŏs'tăt). A male body, partly glandular, partly muscular, surrounding proximal portion of the male urethra and the neck of the bladder, consisting of a median lobe and 2 lateral lobes, the glandular matter emptying through ducts into the post. urethra, and the muscular fibers encircling the urethra.

prostatectomy (prŏs-tă-tĕk'tō-mĭ). Excision of part or all of the prostate gland.

prostatic (prŏs-tăt'ĭk). Concerning the prostate gland.

   p. calculus. A stone in the prostate.

   p. plexus. 1. Veins around the base and neck of the bladder and prostate gland. 2. Nerves from the pelvic plexus to the prostate gland, erectile tissue of the penis, and to the seminal vesicles.

   p. urethra. Part of the urethra surrounded by the prostate gland.

prostatism (prŏs'tă-tĭzm). Condition induced by chronic prostatic disease.

prostatitis (prŏs-tă-tī'tĭs). Inflamed condition of the prostate gland.

   May be a complication of gonorrheal infection.

   p., acute. Discomfort and pain in perineal area. Frequent urination; later, retention of urine. If severe, marked malaise, rise of temperature, constipation, thirst, furred tongue, rigors, and vomiting.

   p., chronic. Dull, aching pain in perineal region. Discharge from the penis.

prostatocystitis (prŏs"tăt-ō-sĭs-tī'tĭs). Inflammation of the prostatic urethra involving the bladder.

prostatocystotomy (prŏs"tăt-ō-sĭs-tŏt'ō-mĭ). Surgical incision of the prostate and the bladder.

prostatodynia (prŏs"tăt-ō-dĭn'ĭ-ă). Pain in the prostate gland. SYN: *prostatalgia.*

prostatomegaly (prŏs"tăt-ō-mĕg'ăl-ĭ). Enlargement of the prostate gland.

prostatometer (prŏs-tăt-ŏm'ĕt-ĕr). Device for measuring enlargement of the prostate.

prostatomyomectomy (prŏs"tăt-ō-mī-ō-mĕk'tō-mĭ). Surgical excision of a prostatic myoma.   [the prostate.

prostatomy (prŏs-tăt'ō-mĭ). Incision into

prostatorrhea (prŏs-tăt-or-rē'ă). Abnormal discharge from the prostate gland.

prostatotomy (prŏs-tă-tŏt'ō-mĭ). Incision into prostate gland.

prostatovesiculectomy (prŏs"tăt-ō-vĕs-ĭk"ū-lĕk'tō-mĭ). Removal of the prostate gland and seminal vesicles.

prostatovesiculitis (prŏs"tăt-ō-vĕs-ĭk-ū-lī'tĭs). Inflammation of the seminal vesicles and prostate gland.

prosternation (prō-stĕr-nā'shŭn). Habitual flexion of the trunk forward. SYN: *camptocormia.*

prostheon (prŏs'thē-ŏn). The alveolar point; midpoint of lower border of upper alveolar arch.

prosthesis (prŏs'thē-sĭs). 1. Replacement of a missing part by an artificial substitute. 2. An artificial organ or part.

   p., dental. Mechanical dentistry.

   p., maxillofacial. Repair and artificial replacements of face and jaw.

   p., paraffin. Subcutaneous injection of paraffin to restore the natural contour of a part or to replace cartilaginous part of the nasal septum.

prosthetics (prŏs-thĕt'ĭks). The making and application of an artificial part to remedy a want or defect of the body, as a wooden leg.

prosthetist (prŏs'thē-tĭst). 1. Specialist in artificial dentures. 2. Maker of artificial limbs.

prosthodontist (prŏs-thō-dŏn'tĭst). A dentist who specializes in the mechanics of making and fitting artificial teeth.

prostigmine (prō-stĭg'mēn). A synthetic intestinal stimulant resembling in some effects physostigmine.

   p. bromide. USES: Orally, for the treatment of myasthenia gravis.

   DOSAGE: 0.015 Gm.

   p. methylsulfate. USES: For prevention and treatment of postoperative distention.

   DOSAGE: For prophylactic, 1 cc. 1-4000; for treatment, 1 cc. 1-2000 solution.

prostitution (prŏs-tĭ-tū'shŭn). Profession practiced, esp. by women, in which sexual gratification is exchanged for hire.

prostration (prŏs-trā'shŭn). Absolute exhaustion.

   p., nervous. General physical and nervous exhaustion. SYN: *neurasthenia.*

protagon (prō'tăg-ŏn). White, crystalline mixture of lipids obtained from the brain.

protamine (prō'tă-mēn). One of a class of simple proteins which are strongly basic, noncoagulable in heat and yield diamino acids when hydrolyzed.

   p. insulin, p. zinc insulin. Preparations of insulin which are more slowly dissolved and absorbed by body tissues than ordinary insulin. Act longer and keep the blood sugar normal for 20 to 24 hr. One injection is sufficient for this period.

protan (prō'tăn). A chemical combination of casein and tannic acid, containing 50% tannic acid.   [0.6 Gm.].

   DOSAGE: For children, 5 to 10 gr. (0.3-

protanopia (prō-tăn-ō'pĭ-ă). Defect in color vision in which there is condition of red blindness.

protargol (prō-tar'gŏl). A compound of silver albumose containing approximately 8% silver.

   DOSAGE: For application to mucous membrane from 0.5% to 2%.

protean (prō'tē-ăn). Having the ability to change form, as the ameba. 2. One of the primary derivatives of protein resulting from action of water, enzymes, or dilute acids.

protease (prō′tē-as). A protein-splitting enzyme.*

protectin (prō-těk′tĭn). A substance in blood serum protecting corpuscles against a hemolytic action.

protective (prō-těk′tĭv). 1. Covering or guarding. 2. An agent that will mechanically protect the part to which applied. Ex: *collodion, plaster*. SYN: *dressing*.

proteid (prō′tē-ĭd). One of a class of constituents essential to all living organisms. SYN: *protein, q.v.*

proteidin (prō′tē-ĭd-ĭn). A bacteriolytic substance formed in the body.

proteidogenous (prō″tē-ĭd-ŏj′ĕn-ŭs). Producing proteins.

protein (prō′tē-ĭn, prō′tēn). One of a class of nitrogenous compounds which occur naturally, give amino acids when hydrolyzed, and are essential to all living organisms.

p., conjugated. Those containing the protein molecule with some other molecule or molecules.

p., derived. The product of hydrolytic changes of the protein molecule with only slight alteration.

p. high diet. 1.5-2 Gm. protein per kg. ideal body weight.

p. low diet. 0.65 Gm. protein per kg. ideal body weight. Supplied by means of protein of good biological value.

p. sensitization. Condition in which patient is hypersensitive to foreign proteins, so that severe reaction occurs upon their administration.

p. shock therapy. Introduction into the body of a nonspecific protein substance, such as milk, egg albumin, or whole blood in treatment of disease. Sometimes used in rheumatoid arthritis, disseminated sclerosis, gonorrhea, and syphilis.

p., simple. Those which produce alpha amino acids on hydrolysis.

proteinase (prō′tē-ĭn-ās). A colloid enzyme which splits protein.

proteinemia (prō-tē-ĭn-ē′mĭ-ă). Excessive amount of protein in the blood.

proteinic (prō-tē-ĭn′ĭk). Relating to protein.

proteinivorus (prō-tē-ĭn-ĭv′ō-rŭs). Living on protein.

proteinogenous (prō-tē-ĭn-ŏj′ĕn-ŭs). Developing from a protein.

proteinophobia (prō″tē-ĭn-ō-fō′bĭ-ă). Aversion to foods containing protein.

proteinotherapy (prō″tē-ĭn-ō-thěr′ă-pĭ). Treatment by the injection of proteins not normally present in the body.

proteinuria (prō-tē-ĭn-ŭ′rĭ-ă). Protein or albumin in the urine.

proteoclastic (prō″tē-ō-klăs′tĭk). Having the ability to split up proteins.

proteogens (prō′tē-ō-jěns). Preparations of plant proteins for injection hypodermically.

proteolysin (prō-tē-ŏl′ĭs-ĭn). A specific substance causing decomposition of proteins.

proteolysis (prō-tē-ŏl′ĭs-ĭs). 1. The conversion of proteins by ferments into peptones. 2. The process of disintegrating dissolved antigens by immune sera, lysin being the antibody.

proteolytic (prō-tē-ō-lĭt′ĭk). In the chemistry of enzymes, hastening the hydrolysis of proteins.

proteometabolism (prō″tē-ō-mē-tăb′ō-lĭzm). Digestion, absorption, and assimilation of proteins.

proteopeptic (prō″tē-ō-pěp′tĭk). Pert. to the digestion of protein.

proteopexic (prō-tē-ō-pěks′ĭk). Pert. to fixation of proteins within the organism.

proteopexy (prō″tē-ō-pěks′ĭ). The fixation of proteins within the body.

proteose (prō′tē-ōs). One of the class of intermediate products of proteolysis bet. protein and peptone.

p., primary. First formed products during proteolysis of proteins.

p., secondary. Proteose resulting from further hydrolysis of primary proteoses.

proteosotherapy (prō″tē-ōs-ō-thěr′ă-pĭ). Treatment by introduction of foreign proteose intravenously, or subcutaneously. SYN: *protein therapy*.

proteosuria (prō″tē-ōs-ū′rĭ-ă). Proteose in urine. SYN: *albumosuria*.

proteotherapy (prō″tē-ō-thěr′ă-pĭ). Introduction of proteins parenterally in treating disease. SYN: *proteinotherapy*.

proteotoxin (prō″tē-ō-tŏk′sĭn). Product from reaction bet. serum of a host and a foreign protein. SYN: *anaphylatoxin, endotoxin*.

proteuria (prō-tē-ū′rĭ-ă). Proteins in the urine. SYN: *proteinuria*.

Proteus (prō′tē-ŭs). A genus of family Bacteriaceae found in intestines and decaying material, which cause protein decomposition.

prosthesis (prŏth′ĕs-ĭs). Replacement by an artificial part. SYN: *prosthesis*.

prothrombase (prō-thrŏm′bās). A substance which becomes a fibrin ferment when activated by thrombokinase. SYN: *prothrombin, thrombogen*.

prothrombin (prō-thrŏm′bĭn). A chemical substance existing in circulating blood, and which, through the medium of *thrombokinase*, interacts with calcium salts to produce thrombin. SYN: *thrombogen*.

protistologist (prō-tĭs-tŏl′ō-jĭst). One who studies the Protista, the unicellular organisms.

protistology (prō-tĭs-tŏl′ō-jĭ). The science of Protista or animal unicellular plant and microörganisms. SYN: *microbiology*.

proto-. 1. A prefix signifying *first*. 2. The lowest of a series of compounds having the same elements.

protobe (prō′tōb). d'Herelle's term for the bacteriophage. SYN: *protobios*.

protobiology (prō″tō-bī-ŏl′ō-jĭ). The phase of science dealing with the forms more minute than bacteria, as the ultraviruses and bacteriophages.

protobios (prō-tō-bī′ŏs). A term suggested by d'Herelle for the minute forms parasitic to other organisms. SYN: *bacteriophage*.

protoblast (pro″to-blăst). 1. A naked cell with no cell wall yet formed. 2. Blastomere of segmenting ovum which is parent cell of a part or organ.

protoblastic (pro″to-blăs′tĭk). Pert. to a protoblast.

protocol (pro′to-kŏl). 1. A clinical report from first notes taken. 2. Minutes of a meeting. 3. Description of steps taken in an experiment.

protoerythrocyte (pro″to-ĕr-ĭth′ro-sīt). An embryonic erythroblast with deeply staining nucleus.

protogala (pro-tŏg′ăl-ă). A mother's first milk after birth of a child. SYN: *colostrum.*

protogaster (pro″to-găs′ter). Embryonic part from which stomach arises. SYN: *foregut.*

protogen (pro′to-jĕn). 1. Any albuminoid substance which, when heated, does not coagulate. 2. Dietary preparation formed by action of formaldehyde on egg albumin.

protoglobulose (pro″to-glŏb′u-lōs). A primary product in the digestion of protein.

protoleukocyte (pro″to-lu′ko-sīt). A minute lymphoid cell in red bone marrow and in the spleen.

protomyosinose (pro″to-mī-o′sĭn-ōs). An albumose formed in the primary digestion of protein.

proton (pro′tŏn). 1. Embryonic trace which is forerunner of a part. PT: The nucleus of the hydrogen atom.

protone (pro′tŏn). Any 1 of the peptonelike substances formed as primary decomposition products of the protamines.

protonephron, protonephros (pro″to-nĕf′ron, -pro-to-nĕf′rōs). The primitive kidney of the embryo. SYN: *pronephros, wolffian body.*

protoneuron (pro″to-nu′rŏn). A bipolar neuron connecting a sense organ with the central nervous system.

protoplasm (pro′to-plăzm). 1. A vaguely used word for the essential, living material in an organism. 2. The primitive organic cell matter.

protoplasmic (pro″to-plăz′mĭk). Pert. to protoplasm or composer of it.

  p. process. A dendrite. SEE: *nerve.*

protoplast (pro′to-plăst). 1. First hypothetical specimen of a race. 2. A primitive cell. 3. A unicellular organism. 4. Vital substance of an organism. SYN: *protoplasm.*

protospasm (pro′to-spăzm). One which begins in 1 area and which extends to other parts.

prototoxin (pro″to-tŏks′ĭn). Dissociation product of a toxin, having greatest affinity for the antitoxin.

prototrophic (pro″to-trō′fĭk). Requiring simple inorganic elements as food.

prototvertebra (pro″to-vĕr′te-bră). Primitive vertebra in the notochord. SYN: *metamere, somite.*

prototoxoid (pro-tŏks′oyd). Hypothetical nonpoisonous substance from prototoxin

which has stronger affinity for the antitoxin than the toxin has. SEE: *toxoid.*

protozoa (pro-to-zo′ă) (sing. *protozoon*). The division of animal kingdom characterized by being unicellular and reproducing by fission.

protozoacide (pro-to-zo′ă-sīd). Destructive to, or that which kills, protozoa.

protozoal (pro″to-zo′ăl). Pert. to protozoa, unicellular organisms.

  p. diseases. Those produced by single-celled organisms, such as amebic dysentery, malaria, and syphilis.

protozoan (pro-to-zo′ăn). 1. One organism of the protozoa. 2. Pert. to protozoa. SEE: *Cercomonas intestinalis.*

protozoölogy (pro″to-zo-ŏl′o-jĭ). Phase of science dealing with study of protozoa.

protozoon (pro″to-zo′ŏn) (pl. *protozoa*). Unicellular organism. SEE: *protozoa.*

protozoöphage (pro″to-zo′o-făg, -făj). A phagocyte which ingests protozoa.

protozoötherapy (pro″to-zo-o-thĕr′ă-pĭ). Treatment of conditions due to protozoa.

protractor (pro-trăk′tŏr). 1. Instrument for removing foreign bodies from wounds. 2. A muscle that draws a part forward. OPP: *retractor.*

protuberance (pro-tu′bĕr-ăns). 1. A part that is prominent beyond a surface, like a knob. 2. Quality of projecting.

proud flesh (prowd). A mass of excessive granulation, formed when a wound shows no other sign of healing or tendency to cicatrization.

provertebra (pro-ver′te-bră). A mesoblastic segment on the notochord of the embryo from which vertebra arises. SYN: *protovertebra, somite.*

proviron (pro-vī′rŏn). A hormone producing secondary male characteristics.

provisional (pro-vĭzh′ŭn-ăl). Serving a temporary use.

provitamin (pro-vī′tăm-ĭn). The forerunner of a vitamin.

Prowazekia (pro-wă-zē′kĭ-ă). A genus of flagellate protozoans.

prowazekiasis (pro-wă-zē-kī′ăs-ĭs). Infestation with Prowazekia.

proximad (prŏk′sĭm-ăd). Toward the proximal or central point.

proximal (prŏks′ĭm-ăl). Nearest the point of attachment.

proximate (prŏks′ĭm-ăt). 1. Next to; immediate.

  2. In chemistry, elemental, the opposite of ultimate.

proximoataxia (prŏk-sĭ-mo-ă-tăk′sĭ-ă). Lack of coördination in muscles of the proximal area of an extremity, as the arm, forearm, thigh, or leg.

prozymogen (pro-zī′mo-jĕn). An intranuclear substance that becomes zymogen. SYN: *prezymogen.*

pruriginous (pru-rĭj′ĭn-ŭs). Pert. to, or of the nature of, prurigo.

prurigo (pru-rī′go). A chronic skin disease marked by constantly recurring, discrete, pale, deep-seated, intensely itchy papules on extensor surfaces of limbs.

p. aestivalis. Prurigo recurring every summer and continuing during hot weather.

p. agria. Very severe prurigo with great itching.

p. infantilis. Prurigo in children during eruption of milk teeth.

p. nodularis. Eruption in skin of hard nodules with great itching.

p. simplex. Simple form of prurigo with recurring tendency.

pruritus (prū-rī'tŭs). Severe itching. May be symptomatic, or occur idiopathically as a neurosis without structural change.

p. aestivalis. Pruritus with prickly heat occurring in hot weather. SYN: *summer itch.*

p. ani. Itching about the anus. May be due to threadworms, fistula in ani, hemorrhoids, or irritation.

p., essential. Pruritus without apparent skin lesion.

p. hiemalis. Winter itch, occurring in cold weather.

p. senilis. Pruritus in aged with degenerative skin changes.

p., symptomatic. Pruritus as a symptom of some other disorder.

p. vulvae. Disorder marked by severe itching of ext. female genitalia. Often an early sign of diabetes mellitus.

Prussak's space (prŏŏs'ăk). Tiny space in middle ear bet. Shrapnell's membrane laterally and neck of malleus medially.

prussic acid (prŭs'ĭk, prŏŏ'sĭk). A violent and rapid poison. SYN: *acid, hydrocyanic, q.v.*

psalis (sā'lĭs). The cerebral fornix, a fibrous arch connecting cerebral hemispheres.

psalterium (săhl-tē'rĭ-ŭm). Longitudinal fibers on floor of the aqueduct of Sylvius, the post. portion of cerebral fornix. SYN: *lyra.*

psammoma (săm-ō'mă). A small tumor of the brain, the choroid plexus and other areas, containing calcareous particles.

psammosarcoma (săm″ō-sar-kō'mă). A sarcoma composed of spots of calcareous degeneration.

psammotherapy (săm″ō-thĕr'ă-pĭ). The application of sand baths in treatment.

pselaphesia, pselaphesis (sĕl-ă-fē'zhĭ-ă, -sĭs). 1. Active sense of touch, including muscle sense. 2. Plucking at bedclothes with the fingers, a sign observed in low delirium. SYN: *carphology.*

psellism, psellismus (sĕl'ĭzm, sĕl-ĭz'mŭs). Defective pronunciation, stuttering or stammering.

p. mercurialis. Jerking, hurried, unintelligible speech in mercurial tremor.

pseudacousma (sū″dă-kŭz'mă). Condition in which all sounds are heard falsely, seeming to be altered in quality of pitch, or imaginary sounds are heard.

pseudacusis (sū″dă-kū'sĭs). State in which sounds are heard falsely or imagined. SYN: *pseudacousma.*

pseudaphia (sū-dăf'ĭ-ă). A false or defective perception of touch. SEE: *paraphia, pseudesthesia.*

pseudarthritis (sū″dar-thrī'tĭs). Hysterical disease of the joints.

pseudarthrosis (sū-dar-thrō'sĭs). A false joint developing after a fracture that has not united.

pseudesthesia (sū-dĕs-thē'zĭ-ă). 1. An imaginary or false sensation, as that after amputation felt in the lost part. 2. Sense of feeling not caused by ext. stimulation. SEE: *paraphia, pseudaphia.*

pseudo- (sū'dō). A prefix meaning *false.*

pseudoanemia (sū″dō-ăn-ē'mĭ-ă). Pallor of mucous membranes and skin without other signs of true anemia.

pseudoangina (sū″dō-ăn'jĭ-nă). False symptoms resembling angina pectoris of nervous origin.

pseudoapoplexy (sū″dō-ăp'ō-plĕk-sĭ). Condition simulating apoplexy but not accompanied by cerebral hemorrhage.

pseudoataxia (sū″dō-ă-tăks'ĭ-ă). Condition resembling ataxia not due to *tabes dorsalis.*

pseudobacterium (sū″dō-băk-tē'rĭ-ŭm). Any microscopic cell similar to a bacterium.

pseudoblepsia, pseudoblepsis (sū″dō-blĕp'sĭ-ă, -sĭs). False or imaginary vision. SYN: *parablepsia, pseudopsia.*

pseudobulbar paralysis (sū″dō-bŭl'ber). Paralysis resembling bulbar paralysis, but due to lesion of cortical centers.

pseudocartilaginous (sū″dō-kar-tĭ-lăj'ĭn-ŭs). Pert. to, or formed of, a substance resembling cartilage.

pseudocast (sū'dō-kăst). A sediment in urine resembling a true cast.

pseudocele (sū'dō-sēl). The 5th ventricle of the brain. SYN: *cavum septi pellucidi.*

pseudochorea (sū″dō-kō-rē'ă). Hysterical state resembling chorea. SYN: *spurious chorea.*

pseudochromesthesia (sū″dō-krō-mĕs-thē'zĭ-ă). A condition in which sounds, esp. of the vowels, seem to induce a sensation of a distinct visual color. SEE: *phonism, photism.*

pseudocirrhosis (sū″dō-sĭr-ō'sĭs). A condition with symptoms of cirrhosis of liver, due usually to pericarditis.

pseudocoele (sū'dō-sēl). The 5th ventricle of brain. SYN: *pseudocele.*

pseudocoloboma (sū″dō-kŏl-ō-bō'mă). A scarcely noticeable scar on the iris from an embryonic fissure.

pseudocrisis (sū-dō-krī'sĭs). A temporary fall of body temperature which may be followed by a rise.

pseudocroup (sū'dō-kroop). False croup. SYN: *laryngismus stridulus.*

pseudocyesis (sū″dō-sī-ē'sĭs). A condition in which the abdomen enlarges and the menses cease when the patient thinks that she is pregnant but is not.

pseudocyst (sū'dō-sĭst). A dilatation resembling a cyst.

pseudodementia (sū″dō-dĕ-mĕn'shĭ-ă). Exaggerated indifference to environment without impairment of mind.

pseudodiphtheria (sū″dō-dĭf-thē′rĭ-ă). A condition resembling diphtheria but not due to Klebs-Löffler bacillus.

p. bacillus. A nonpathogenic one resembling the true diphtheria bacillus.

pseudoedema (sū″dō-ē-dē′mă). A puffy condition of the skin simulating edema.

pseudoemphysema (sū″dō-ĕm-fĭz-ē′mă). A bronchial condition with blocking simulating emphysema.

pseudoencephalitis (sū″dō-ĕn-sĕf-ă-lī′tĭs). A false encephalitis, due to profuse diarrhea.

pseudoerysipelas (sū″dō-ĕr-ĭ-sĭp′ĕl-ăs). An inflammation of subcutaneous cellular tissue simulating erysipelas.

pseudoesthesia (sū″dō-ĕs-thē′zĭ-ă). An imaginary sensation or a false one. SYN: *pseudesthesia.*

pseudoganglion (sū″dō-găn′glĭ-ŏn). A slight thickening of a nerve resembling a ganglion.

pseudogeusesthesia (sū″dō-gū-sĕs-thē′zĭ-ă). A sense of color accompanying sensations of taste.

pseudogeusia (sū″dō-gū′sĭ-ă). A subjective sensation of taste not produced by external stimulus.

pseudoglioma (sū″dō-glī′ō-mă). Exudate in the vitreous giving a yellowish reflex as seen in glioma of retina.

pseudoglobulin (sū″dō-glŏb′ū-lĭn). One of 2 globulins comprising paraglobulin, *q.v.*

pseudoglottis (sū″dō-glŏt′ĭs). Area bet. false vocal cords.

pseudohemoptysis (sū″dō-he-mŏp′tĭs-ĭs). Spitting of blood which does not arise from the bronchi or the lungs.

pseudohermaphroditism (sū″dō-hĕr-măf′rō-dīt″ĭzm). A congenital abnormality of the ext. genitalia and of the body in which one resembles the other sex; not a true hermaphroditism. SEE: *hermaphroditism.*

p. femininus. One with a large clitoris resembling the penis and with hypertrophied labia majora resembling the scrotum, thus resembling a male.

p. masculinus. A male with a small penis and perineal hypospadias; and scrotum without testes, the condition resembling the vulva.

pseudohernia (sū-dō-hĕr′nĭ-ă). An empty hernial sac simulating a strangulated, inflamed hernia.

pseudohydrophobia (sū″dō-hī-drō-fō′bĭ-ă). Disorder simulating hydrophobia in its symptoms. SYN: *lyssophobia.*

pseudohypertrophic (sū″dō-hī-pĕr-trō′fĭk). Pert. to a false hypertrophy.

p. paralysis. Paralysis with enlargement and loss of motion of muscles.

pseudohypertrophy (sū″dō-hī-per′trō-fĭ). Increase of size of an organ or part with diminution of function.

pseudoleukemia (sū″dō-lū-kē′mĭ-ă). Progressive anemia with lymphomata, generally fatal. SYN: *Hodgkin's disease.*

p., infantile. Anemia in children caused by rachitic tendencies.

pseudoleukocythemia (sū″dō-lū″kō-sī-thē′mĭ-ă). Progressive anemia with lymphomata, characteristic of several conditions. SYN: *pseudoleukemia.*

pseudologia (sū-dō-lo′jĭ-ă). Falsification in writing or in speech, a form of pathological lying.

p. fantastica. Pathological lying; one of the forms of the psychopathic state.

A moral deficiency exists and punishment therefore is useless.

pseudomania (sū″dō-mā′nĭ-ă). 1. A psychosis in which the patient falsely accuses himself of crimes which he thinks he has committed. 2. Pathological lying.

pseudomasturbation (sū″dō-măs-tur-bā′-shŭn). A nervous habit of pulling at the penis. SYN: *peotillomania.*

pseudomelanosis (sū″dō-mĕl-ăn-ō′sĭs). Discoloration of tissues after death.

pseudomembrane (sū″dō-mĕm′brăn). A false membrane, as in diphtheria.

pseudomembranous (sū″dō-mĕm′bră-nŭs). Pert. to or marked by false membranes.

pseudomeningitis (sū″dō-mĕn-ĭn-jī′tĭs). A condition resembling symptoms of meningitis without lesions of meningeal inflammation.

pseudomnesia (sū″dŏm-nē′zĭ-ă). A memory perversion in which patient remembers that which never occurred.

Pseudomonas (sū-dō-mō′năs). A genus of saprophytic bacteria found in soil and water which produces blue-green pigment.

pseudomucin (sū-dō-mū′sĭn). A variety of mucin found in proliferative ovarian cysts.

pseudomyelia paresthetica (sū″dō-mī-ē′lĭ-ă păr-ĕs-thĕt′ĭk-ă). False sense of motion in paralyzed limb or of no motion in a moving limb. SEE: *pain.*

pseudoneuroma (sū″dō-nū-rō′mă). A growth of connective tissue of a nerve including medullary layer of nerve fiber. SYN: *neurofibroma.*

pseudonuclein (sū″dō-nū′klē-ĭn). A combination of albumin with metaphosphoric acid. SYN: *paranuclein.*

pseudoparalysis (sū″dō-pă-răl′ĭ-sĭs). A loss of muscular power not due to lesion of the nervous system.

pseudoparaplegia (sū″dō-păr-ă-plē′jĭ-ă). Seemingly paralysis of the lower extremities without impairment of the reflexes.

pseudoparasite (sū″dō-păr′ă-sīt). 1. Anything resembling a parasite. 2. Organism which can live as a parasite, although it is normally not one. SYN: *commensal.* SEE: *facultative parasite.*

pseudoparesis (sū″dō-par-e′sĭs, -par′e-sĭs). A condition simulating paresis but unlike the ordinary forms and due to hysteria.

pseudopepsin (sū″dō-pĕp′sĭn). A proteolytic ferment secreted by some of the gastric glands.

pseudopeptone (sū″dō-pĕp′tōn). A mucoid substance derived from egg white.

pseudophthisis (sū-dŏf-thī′sĭs, -dō-tī′sĭs). Progressive emaciation not due to pulmonary tuberculosis.

pseudoplegia (sū″dō-plē′jĭ-ă). Paralysis

of hysterical origin. SYN: *pseudoparalysis*.

pseudopod (sū'dŏ-pŏd). Protruding protoplasmic process of a temporary nature in protozoa for taking up food and aiding in locomotion. SYN: *pseudopodium*.

pseudopodium (sū"dŏ-pō'dĭ-ŭm) (pl. *pseudopodia*). A temporary protruding process of a protozoan aiding in locomotion and prehension of food. SYN: *pseudopod*.

pseudopsia (sū-dŏp'sĭ-ă). Visual hallucinations or false perceptions. SYN: *pseudoblepsis*.

pseudorabies (sū"dŏ-rā'bēz, -rā'bĭ-ēz). Condition simulating rabies due to fear of the disease. SYN: *lyssophobia, pseudohydrophobia*.

pseudoscarlatina (sū"dŏ-skar-lă-tē'nă). A septic febrile condition with rash resembling scarlatina.

pseudosclerosis (sū"dŏ-sklē-rō'sĭs). A condition with the symptoms, but without the lesions, of multiple sclerosis of the nervous system.

pseudosmia (sū-dŏz'mĭ-ă). An olfactory hallucination or perversion of the sense of smell.

pseudostoma (sū-dŏs'tŏ'mă). An apparent aperture bet. endothelial cells that have been stained.

pseudosyphilis (sū"dŏ-sĭf'ĭ-lĭs). A nonspecific condition resembling syphilis.

pseudotabes (sū"dŏ-tā'bēz). A neural disease simulating tabes dorsalis.

pseudotetanus (sū"dŏ-tĕt'ăn-ŭs). Persistent muscular contractions resembling tetanus.

pseudotuberculosis (sū"dŏ-tū-ber"kŭ-lō'sĭs). Disease like tuberculosis not caused by the tubercle bacillus.

pseudotympany (sū"dŏ-tĭm'pă-nĭ). Flattening of arch of diaphragm, swelling of abdomen with increased respiration.

It disappears under anesthesia and is of purely nervous origin. SYN: *accordion abdomen*.

pseudotyphoid (sū"dŏ-tī'foyd). Condition resembling typhoid fever, not caused by the typhoid bacillus.

pseudoxanthoma (sū"dŏ-zăn-thō'mă). Chronic degenerative cutaneous disease marked by yellow patches and stretching of the skin; resembles xanthoma.

psilosis (sī-lō'sĭs). 1. Falling out or removal of hair.

2. Tropical diarrhea of severe, often fatal form. SYN: *sprue*.

psittacosis (sĭt-ă-kō'sĭs). A fatal, infectious disease of parrots and other birds that may be transmitted to man.

psoas (sō'ăs). One of 2 muscles of the loins.

p. abscess. A cold abscess in sheath of the psoas major muscle.

psoitis (sō-ī'tĭs). Inflammation of the psoas msucles or of the area of the loins.

psora (sō'ră). 1. An itching disease of the skin; scabies. 2. Psoriasis, an erythematous, scaling, cutaneous eruption. 3. Hahnemann's name for the theory that

chronic diseases are a manifestation of a suppressed itch or an itch dyscrasia.

psorelcosis (sō-rĕl-kō'sĭs). Ulceration occurring as a result of scabies.

psoriasis (sō-rī'ăs-ĭs). Chronic inflammatory skin disease of many varieties characterized by formation of scaly red patches on extensor surfaces of body.

p. buccalis. Variety with white patches on tongue and cheek. SYN: *leukoplakia buccalis*.

p. circinata. Form with ring-shaped lesions with healing beginning in the center.

p. diffusa. Psoriasis with more or less coalescence of lesions.

p. punctata. Psoriasis with papular red eruptions tipped with white scales.

psorocomium (sō-rō-kō'mĭ-ŭm). Hospital for patients with the itch.

psorophthalmia (sō-rŏf-thăl'mĭ-ă). Marginal inflammation of the eyelids with ulceration.

psorosperm (sō'rŏ-sperm). A unicellular, protozoan, parasitic organism. SYN: *coccidium, sporozoon*.

psorospermosis (sō"rō-sperm-ō'sĭs). Morbid condition caused by presence of psorosperms.

psorous (sō'rŭs). Related to or affected with itch.

psychalgia (sī-kăl'jĭ-ă). 1. dental distress or pain, esp. in melancholia. 2. Pain of hysterical origin. SYN: *mind* or *soul pain, phrenalgia*.

psychanalysis (sī-kăn-ăl'ĭ-sĭs). Discovery of the pathogenic links bet. the objective and subjective consciousness by a system of recall. SYN: *psychoanalysis, q.v.*

psychanopsia (sī-kăn-ŏp'sĭ-ă). Sight with failure to recognize anything seen, due to brain lesion. SYN: *psychic blindness*.

psychasthenia (sī-kăs-thē'nĭ-ă). A neurotic condition marked by sense of inadequacy, unreality, anxiety, and doubt.

psychataxia (sī"kă-tăk'sĭ-ă). Disordered power of concentration.

psyche (sī'kē). All that constitutes the mind and its processes. SYN: *soul*.

psycheclampsia (sī-kĕk-lămp'sĭ-ă). Acute mania or mental convulsions.

psychiatric (sī-kĭ-ăt'rĭk). 1. Pert. to psychiatry, the science dealing with mental ailments. 2. One who has a psychosis or tendency toward one.

p. habits. *The Confused*: May not realize the incongruity of an act as related to the environment.

The Deluded: May have phobias or specific fears which control some of their habits.

The Depressed: May ignore everything because of their misery, which engages all of their attention.

The Excited: May be unable to concentrate.

The Feeble: May be unable to control themselves because of weakness.

The Hallucinated: Habits may be affected by "voices," etc.

psychiatrist (sī-kī'ă-trĭst). A physician

who specializes in study and treatment of mental disorders.

psychiatry (sĭ-kī'ă-trĭ). That branch of medicine which treats of mental and neurotic disorders and the pathologic, or psychopathologic changes associated with them.

psychic (sī'kĭk). 1. Concerning the mind, or soul. 2. One said to be endowed with semisupernatural powers, such as the ability to read the mind of others, or to foresee coming events; one apparently sensitive to nonphysical forces.

  p. blindness. Sight without recognition of that which is seen.

  p. contagion. Communication of another's nervous disorder by imitation, as a tic.   [sounds heard.

  p. deafness. Inability to recognize

  p. determinism. The theory that mental processes are determined by conscious or unconscious motives, and are never irrelevant.

  p. force. One generated apart from physical energy.

  p. infection. Mental condition due to an influence upon the mind.

psychical (sī'kĭ-kăl). Pert. to mind or soul. Syn: *psychic.*

psychinosis (sī-kĭn-ō'sĭs). Any functional disease affecting the mind.

psychoanalysis (sī''kō-ăn-ăl'ĭ-sĭs). Method of obtaining a detailed account of past and present mental and emotional experiences and repressions, in order to determine the source and eliminate the pathologic mental or physical state produced by these mechanisms.

psychobiological formula (sī''kō-bī-ō-lŏj'ĭ-kăl). A series of questions, used in studying a psychobiological problem, as to what constitutes the facts of mental phenomena, the factors and their grouping, and the conditions and results involving such facts and how they may be tested or modified.

psychobiology (sī''kō-bī-ŏl'ō-jĭ). Study of mental life and behavior in its interrelationship with other biological processes.

psychocardiac reflex (sī''kō-kar'dĭ-ăk). Change in circulatory rate and consciousness of heart thumping resulting from memory of, or subconscious dream state recollection of, an emotional impression or experience.

psychochrome (sī'kō-krōm). Color impression resulting from sensory stimulation of a part other than the visual organ. See: *psychochromesthesia.*

psychochromesthesia (sī''kō-krōm-ĕs-thē'-zĭ-ă). Color sensation produced by the stimulus of sense organ other than that of vision.

psychocoma (sī-kō-kō'mă). Condition of mental stupor.

psychocortical (sī''kō-kor'tĭ-kăl). Pert. to the cerebral cortex as the seat of sensory, motor, and psychic functions.

  p. center. The cerebral center supposed to be the seat of motor, sensory, and psychic activity.

psychodometry (sī''kō-dŏm'ĕ-trĭ). Measurement of rate of mental activity.

psychodynamics (sī''kō-dī-năm'ĭks). The scientific study of mental action or force.

psychogenia (sī''kō-jē'nĭ-ă). Disease resulting from disturbed psychic activity.

psychogenesis (sī''kō-jĕn'ĕs-ĭs). The origin and development of mind; the formation of mental traits.

psychogenetic (sī''kō-jĕn-ĕt'ĭk). 1. Originating in the mind, as a disease. 2. Concerning formation of mental traits.

psychogenic (sī-kō-jĕn'ĭk). 1. Of mental origin. 2. Concerning the development of the mind. Syn: *psychogenetic.*

psychogram (sī'kō-grăm). A subjective visualization of a mental concept.

psychokinesia (sī''kō-kĭn-ē'zĭ-ă). Explosive or impulsive maniacal action due to defective inhibition. Syn: *psycheclampsia.*

psycholepsy (sī''kō-lĕp'sĭ). Sudden alteration of moods in which mental inertia and hopelessness are manifested.

psycholeptic (sī''kō-lĕp'tĭk). Concerning sudden shifting of moods, particularly to 1 marked by hopelessness and mental inertia.

psychological (sī''kō-lŏj'ĭ-kal). Pert. to study of the mind in all of its relationships, normal and abnormal.

psychologist (sī-kŏl'ō-jĭst). One who specializes in the mental phenomena of consciousness and behavior or mental activity.

psychology (sī-kŏl'ō-jĭ). The science which deals with the mental processes, both normal and abnormal, and their effects upon behavior.

  p., abnormal. The study of irregular or pathological mental phenomena.

  p., experimental. Study of mental acts by tests and experiments.

  p., genetic. Study of the evolution of mind in the individual and the race.

psychometry (sī-kŏm'ĕt-rĭ). Measurement of work accomplished, time consumed, and precision of mental operations; intelligence testing.

psychomotor (sī-kō-mō'tor). Concerning, or causing, voluntary movement.

psychoneurosis (sī''kō-nū-rō'sĭs). A functional disease or disorder of mental origin without demonstrable lesion. Value of reality remains unchanged, but the individual uses reality to excess or to a minimum.

  p., defense. Condition due to attempt to dismiss from the mind ideas and sensations that are painful. This results in buried subconscious memories producing psychoneurosis.

psychoneurotic (sī''kō-nū-rŏt'ĭk). Pert. to a functional disorder of mental origin.

psychonomy (sī-kŏn'ō-mĭ). The science of the laws of the mind and its functions.

psychonosis (sī''kō-nō'sĭs). Any mental disorder.

psychoparesis (sī''kō-păr-ē'sĭs). Weakness or enfeeblement of the mind.

psychopath (sī'kō-păth). One with a constitutional lack of moral sensibility, although possessing normal intelligence. SYN: *psychopathic personality.*

psychopathic (sī″kō-păth′ĭk). 1. Concerning or characterized by a mental disorder. 2. Concerning treatment of mental disorders.

   p. personality. "One who, though possessing normal intelligence, is or becomes, by reason of heredity or congenital conditions, constitutionally lacking in moral sensibility, emotional control, and the inhibition of will."—Dr. C. H. Patten.

   p., transportation of. 1. Be sure you have necessary legal papers.

   2. Learn all you can about patient before starting.

   3. Ascertain, if suicidal, epileptic, destructive, or dangerous.

   4. If so (No. 3), do not travel with patient without assistance.

   5. See that patient has nothing that may be used for violence or self-destruction.

   6. If on train or boat, use a compartment.

   7. If patient is dangerous, notify the transportation company in advance.

   8. Do not hesitate to call upon local police or trainmen if necessary.

   9. Be sure you have enough money for the journey and your own return.

   10. Ascertain names of physicians who may be called en route if needed.

   11. Secure copy of inventory of patient's effects from hospital, with statement as to any bruises or injuries suffered by patient.

psychopathology (sī″kō-păth-ŏl′ō-jĭ) Cause and nature of diseased mental processes.

psychopathosis (sī″kō-păth-ō′sĭs). Any disease of the mind in the psychopathic group.

psychopathy (sī-kŏp′ăth-ĭ). Any mental disease, esp. 1 characterized by defective character or personality.

   p., bisexual. Disorder including those who find sexual gratification from either sex.

   p., sexual. A term for the group of disorders in which exist perversions of sex.

psychophysical (sī″kō-fĭz′ĭ-kăl). Concerning the relation of the physical and the mental.

   p. law. Intensity of sensation increases as the logarithms of the stimuli.

psychophysics (sī″kō-fĭz′ĭks). 1. The study of mental processes in relation to physical processes. 2. The study of stimuli in relation to the effects they produce.

psychophysiology (sī″kō-fĭz-ĭ-ŏl′ō-jĭ). Physiology of the mind; science of the correlation of body and mind.

psychoplegic (sī-kō-plē′jĭk). An agent reducing excitability of the cerebrum.

psychoreaction (sī″kō-rē-ăk′shŭn). Ability of serum from one having dementia precox or manic-depressive psychosis to inhibit hemolysis caused by cobra venom. SYN: *Much-Holzmann reaction.*

psychorhythmia (sī″kō-rĭth′mĭ-ă). Involuntary repetition by the mind of its former actions.

psychorrhea (sī-kor-ē′ă). A disorder manifested by an incoherent stream of thought.

psychosensory (sī″kō-sĕn′sor-ĭ). 1. Understanding and interpreting sensory stimuli. 2. Concerning perceptions not arising in sensory organs, as hallucinations.

psychosexual (sī″kō-sĕks′ū-ăl). Concerning the emotional components of sexual instinct.

   p. development. Evolution of personality through infantile and pregenital periods to sexual maturity.

psychosin (sī-kō′sĭn). A cerebroside occurring in brain tissue.

psychosis (sī-kō′sĭs) (pl. *psychoses*). Any mental derangement. SEE: *neurosis, psychoneurosis, psychotherapy.*

   p., affective. Psychosis marked by moods of exaltation and depression, with flight or retardation of ideas, and nervous manifestations, hallucinations, and delusions. SYN: *manic-depressive psychosis.*

   p., anxiety. Functional disturbance of mind marked by anxiety, depression, and restlessness.

   p., barbed wire. A psychosis involving irritability and loss of memory; seen in prisoners of war.

   p., exhaustion. Confusional psychosis following an operation, tragic event, infection, or shock.

   p., involutional. Psychosis following the menopause, or in senility.

   p., manic-depressive. One manifesting excitement and overactivity, or depression and psychomotor retardation, or a mixed condition.

   p., organic. The result of a pathological condition of the central nervous system, such as paresis.

   p., polyneuritic. Korsakoff's psychosis, seen in chronic alcoholism, with hallucinations, falsification of memory, wrist drop, and disturbed orientation as symptoms.

   p., situation. Transitory psychosis caused by an unpleasant situation.

   p., toxic. One resulting from toxic agents, as drugs.

   p., traumatic. One resulting from head injuries and belonging to the organic group.

psychotechnics (sī″kō-tĕk′nĭks). Application of psychological methods in the study of economic and social problems.

psychotherapy (sī-kō-thĕr′ă-pĭ). Any mental method of treating diseases, esp. nervous disorders, by means such as suggestion, hypnotism, psychoanalytic therapy, persuasion, etc.

psychroalgia (sī-krō-ăl′jĭ-ă). Painful sensation of cold.

psychroesthesia (sī″krō-ĕs-thē′zĭ-ă). 1. A sensation of cold in a part of the body, although it is warm. 2. The sensation that perceives cold.

psychrometer (sĭ-krŏm′ĕ-tĕr). Device for measuring relative humidity of the atmosphere.

psychrophilic (sĭ-krō-fĭl′ĭk). Preferring cold, as bacteria which thrive best at low temperature.

psychrophobia (sĭ-krō-fō′bĭ-ă). Abnormal aversion or sensitiveness to cold.

psychrophore (sĭ′krō-fōr). Apparatus for applying cold to the urethra, or other canal.

psychrotherapy (sī″krō-thĕr′ă-pĭ). Treatment of disease by administration of cold.

psyllium seed (sĭl′ĭ-ŭm). The dried, ripe seed of a plant grown in France, Spain, and India.

DOSAGE: From 1 to 4 drams (4-15 Gm.) in orange or prune juice.

ptarmic (tar′mĭk). 1. Causing sneezing. SYN: *sternutatory*. 2. That which causes sneezing.

pterion (tē′rĭ-ŏn). Point of suture of frontal, parietal, temporal, and sphenoid bones.

pterygium (tĕr-ĭj′ĭ-ŭm). OPHTH: Triangular thickening of bulbar conjunctiva on the cornea with apex toward pupil.

p., progressive. Stage in which the growth extends toward center of cornea.

p., stationary. Stage in which the head of pterygium remains permanently attached to the same point upon the cornea.

pterygoid (tĕr′ĭ-goyd). Wing-shaped. SYN: *alate*.

p. fossa. Notch bet. the ext. and int. plates of the sphenoidal pterygoid process.

p. processes. Two big processes which are part of the sphenoid bone.

pterygomaxillary (tĕr″ĭ-gō-măks′ĭl-ă-rĭ). Concerning the pterygoid process and the upper jaw.

pterygopalatine (tĕr″ĭ-gō-păl′ă-tĭn). Relating to the pterygoid process and the palate bone.

ptilosis (tĭl-ō′sĭs). Loss of eyelashes.

ptomaine (tō′mān). One of a class of nitrogenous organic bases formed in the action of putrefactive bacteria on proteins and amino acids.

p. poisoning. An unsatisfactory term for food poisoning which has been dropped from good medical usage.

ptomainemia (tō″măn-ē′mĭ-ă). Conditions caused by ptomaines in the circulating blood.

ptosis (tō′sĭs). Dropping or drooping of an organ or part, as the upper eyelid from paralysis, or the visceral organs from weakness of the abdominal muscles.

p., abdominal. Sagging of transverse colon; sometimes almost to the pelvic floor.

ptyalagogue (tĭ-ăl′ă-gŏg). Causing or that which causes a flow of saliva. SYN: *sialogogue*.

ptyalin (tĭ′ă-lĭn). A salivary amylolytic enzyme converting starch into maltose and dextrin. SEE: *enzyme, ptyalinogen, ptyalism, saliva*.

ptyalinogen (tĭ-ăl-ĭn′ō-jĕn). A hypothetical substance in the salivary glands from which ptyalin is formed.

ptyalism (tĭ′ăl-ĭzm). Excessive secretion of saliva.

ptyalith (tĭ′ă-lĭth). A calculus in a salivary gland.

ptyalocele (tĭ-ăl′ō-sēl). A salivary cystic tumor or cystic dilatation of a salivary duct.   [origin.

ptyalogenic (tĭ″ăl-ō-jĕn′ĭk). Of salivary

ptyalogogue (tĭ-ăl′ō-gŏg). That which produces saliva. SYN: *sialogogue*.

ptyalogram (tĭ-ăl′ō-grăm). An x-ray film of the salivary glands.

ptyalography (tĭ-ăl-ōg′ră-fĭ). X-ray inspection of the salivary glands and ducts. SYN: *sialography*.

ptyalolith (tĭ′ă-lō-lĭth). A salivary concretion.

ptyalolithotomy (tĭ″ăl-ō-lĭth-ŏt′ō-mĭ). Surgical removal of a concretion from a salivary duct or gland.

ptyalorrhea (tĭ″ă-lō-rē′ă). An excessive flow of saliva.

ptyocrine, ptyocrinous (tĭ′ō-krĕn, tĭ-ŏk′rĭn-ŭs). Secreting part of the protoplasm, said of a gland cell. OPP: *diacrinous, exocrine*.

puber (pū′bŭr). One at onset of puberty.

puberal (pū′bĕr-ăl). Concerning puberty.

puberty (pū′bĕr-tĭ). Period in life at which 1 of either sex becomes functionally capable of reproduction.

pubes (pū′bēz) (sing. *pubis*). 1. Ant. part of innominate bone; *os pubis*. 2. The pubic region. 3. Hair of the pubic region.

pubescence (pū-bĕs′sĕns). 1. Puberty or its approach. 2. Covering of fine, soft hairs on the body. SYN: *lanugo*.

pubescent (pū-bĕs′ĕnt). 1. Reaching puberty. 2. Covered with downy hair.

pubetrotomy (pū′bē-trŏt′ō-mĭ). Section through the pubes.

pubic (pū′bĭk). Concerning the pubes.

p. bone. The lower ant. part of the innominate bone. SYN: *os pubis*.

p. hair. Hair over the pubes which appears at onset of sexual maturity.

pubio-, pubo-. Combining forms meaning the *pubic hair, pubic bone* or *region*.

pubiotomy (pū-bĭ-ŏt′ō-mĭ). Incision across the pubis in order to enlarge the pelvic passage, facilitating the delivery of the fetus when pelvis is malformed.

pubis (pū′bĭs). 1. Pubic bone. 2. BNA. Hair over pubic bone.

pubofemoral (pū″bō-fĕm′or-ăl). Pert. to the os pubis and the femur.

puboprostatic (pū″bō-prŏs-tăt′ĭk). Relating to the os pubis and prostate gland.

pubovesical (pū″bō-vĕs′ĭ-kl). Pert. to the os pubis and bladder.

pudenda (pū-dĕn′dă) (sing. *pudendum**). The ext. genitalia, esp. of the female. SYN: *vulva*.

pudendagra (pū′den-dăg′ră). Pain in the ext. genitals.

p. pruriens. Intense itching of ext. female genitals. SYN: *pruritus vulvae*.

pudendal (pū-dĕn′dăl). Relating to the ext. genitals of female.

pudendum (pū-dĕn′dŭm) (pl. *pudenda*). The ext. genitals, esp. those of the female; the vulva.

  p. muliebre. BNA. Ext. genitals of the female.

pudic (pū′dĭk). Concerning ext. female genitalia. SYN: *pudendal.*

puericulture (pū-er′ĭ-kŭl″chūr). Science concerned with prenatal care of unborn children and the art of raising and training children.

puerile (pū′ĕ-rĭl). Concerning a child; childlike.

  p. respiration. That heard in auscultation of healthy children.

puerilism (pū′ĕr-ĭl-ĭzm). Childishness.

puerpera (pū-er′pĕr-ă). Woman during the period following the 3rd stage of labor, lasting until there is complete involution of the pelvic viscera.

puerperal (pū-er′pur-ăl). Concerning childbirth.

  p. eclampsia. Convulsions during parturition.

  p. fever. Septicemia following childbirth. SYN: *childbed fever.*

  p. insanity. A psychosis resulting during the puerperium.

  p. period. Period immediately following after childbirth.

  p. sepsis. A toxemia of puerperium accompanied by a rise in temperature during the first 21 days.

puerperalism (pū-er′pŭr-ăl-ĭzm). Pathological conditions of the puerperal state.

  p., infantile. Any pathogenic condition of the newly born.

  p., infectious. Puerperal disease caused by infection.

puerperant (pū-er′pŭr-ănt). A woman in labor or one who recently has been delivered.

puerperium (pū-er-pē′rĭ-ŭm). Period following the 3rd stage of labor, lasting until involution of pelvic organs takes place; usually 3 to 6 weeks.

puerperous (pū-ūr′pŭr-ŭs). In the period following childbirth. SYN: *puerperal.*

pulmo-. Combining form meaning *lung.*

pulmoaortic (pŭl″mō-ā-or′tĭk). 1. Concerning the lungs and the aorta. 2. Relating to the pulmonary artery and aorta.

pulmometer (pŭl-mŏm′ĕt-ĕr). Device for measuring the lung capacity. SYN: *spirometer.*

pulmometry (pŭl-mŏm′ĕt-rĭ). Determination of capacity of the lungs.

pulmonary (pŭl′mō-na-rĭ). Concerning or affected by the lungs. SEE: *caverniloquy.*

  p. circulation. Passage of blood from heart to lungs and back again for purification.

  p. incompetence, p. insufficiency. Failure of the pulmonary valve to close properly.

  p. reflex. Contraction of lung induced by sudden stimulation of thoracic wall.

  p. stenosis. Narrowing of opening into the pulmonary artery from right cardiac ventricle.

pulmonectomy (pŭl-mō-nĕk′tō-mĭ). Removal of part or all of a lung's tissue. SYN: *pneumonectomy.*

pulmonic (pŭl-mŏn′ĭk). 1. Relating to or affecting the lungs. SYN: *pulmonary.* 2. Relating to the pulmonary artery. 3. Having origin at or by the pulmonic valve, as a *murmur.*

  p. circulation. Flow of blood from right cardiac ventricle to the lungs, returning to the left ventricle.

  p. fever. Lobar pneumonia.

pulmonitis (pŭl-mō-nī′tĭs). Inflamed condition of the lung. SYN: *pneumonia.*

pulmotor (pŭl-mō′tor). Apparatus for inducing artificial respiration by forcing oxygen into the lungs, or for expelling gas in case of asphyxiation.

pulp (pŭlp). 1. The soft part of fruit. 2. The soft part of an organ. 3. Chyme.

  p. cavity. Hollow space within a tooth containing dental pulp.

  p. cells. Those in the pulp cavity of any organ.   [cavity of a tooth.

  p., dental. The soft tissue filling the

  p., digital. Elastic, soft prominence on the palmar or plantar surface of the last phalanx of a finger or toe.

pulpal (pŭl′păl). Relating to pulp.

pulpefaction (pŭl-pē-făk′shŭn). Conversion into pulpy substance.

pulpy (pŭl′pĭ). Resembling pulp; flabby. SYN: *pultaceous.*

pulsate (pŭl′săt). To throb or beat in rhythm.

pulsatile (pŭl′să-tĭl). Pulsating; characterized by a rhythmic beat. SYN: *throbbing.*

pulsation (pŭl-sā′shŭn). The rhythmic beat, as of the heart and blood vessels; a throbbing. SEE: *pulse.*

pulse (pŭls). 1. Edible leguminous seeds, as peas, beans. 2. Rhythmical throbbing. 3. Throbbing caused by the regular contraction and alternate expansion of an artery; the periodic thrust felt over arteries in time with the heartbeat.

  Normal pulse rate of adult is 70 to 75 and is usually observed in radial artery of the wrist.

  p., accelerated. A common symptom in all fevers. The pulse of the adult rarely exceeds 150 beats per minute even in acute inflammatory infections; when it runs above 170 it *may* portend a fatal issue.

  p., anacrotic. One showing a secondary wave on ascending limb of the main wave.

  p., ardent. One that seems to strike the finger at a single point.

  p., asymmetrical radial. May result from anomalies of distribution, size, and division of 1 of the vessels; aortic aneurysm; embolism; an atheromatous plate within a vessel; fractures; luxations causing compression of a vessel, or compression of a vessel by tumors within or without the thorax.

  p., bigeminal. Two regular beats followed by a longer pause. It has the same significance as an irregular pulse.

p., capillary. Alternating redness and pallor of capillary region, as in the matrices beneath the nails, occurring chiefly where an excessive cardiac impulse coincides with general arterial narrowing.

p., caprizant. An irregular, peculiar, weak pulsation succeeded by a stronger one.

p., catacrotic. One showing 1 or more secondary waves on descending limb of the main wave.

p., changeable. Denotes nervous derangement and sometimes organic heart disease.

p., collapsing. One feebly striking the finger, then subsiding abruptly and completely.

p., Corrigan's. One of aortic insufficiency. SEE: *water-hammer pulse.*

p., dicrotic. A double beat, 1 heartbeat for 2 arterial pulsations, or a seeming weak wave bet. the usual heartbeats. This weak wave should not be counted as a regular beat. It is indicative of low arterial tension, and is noted in fevers, in low states of the nervous system, and sometimes in typhoid fever.

p., febrile. A full, bounding pulse at onset of fever, becoming feeble and weak when fever subsides or on prostration.

p., female. More frequent than male pulse by 10 or 15 beats. There is an important correlation bet. the pulse, respiration and temperature which must be considered in most disease states.

p., fine, scarcely perceptible. Denotes great exhaustion and approaching death. May be caused by wasting disease or by hemorrhage.

p. frequency. Depends upon sex, age, exertion, position of body and health. It is higher in children and increases with very old age. It is slower in tall persons than it is in short ones. It is 10 to 12 beats more frequent in standing than sitting. Muscular exertion, as dancing, will raise it from 75 to 125 or higher. Eating and drinking likewise increase heart action. It is less frequent when sleeping or lying down.

p., full. A distended one giving a tense feeling; observed in sthenic inflammation.

p., gaseous. SEE: *hemorrhagic pulse.*

p., goat-leap. SEE: *caprizant pulse.*

p., hard. One with sensation of hardness due to changes in the arterial wall or to vascular distention.

p., hemorrhagic. A soft, full, and readily compressible 1 marking a distended artery that has lost its tone.

p., hepatic. One due to expansion of veins of the liver at each ventricular contraction.

p., high-tension. One in which force of beat is relatively increased and which may be roughly estimated by noting the amount of pressure of the fingers that is required to arrest the beat. It is observed in many conditions, notably: cardiac diseases, such as hypertrophy; chronic nephritis; cerebral affections; irritation of the vasomotor center, as in apoplexy, tumors, and beginning meningitis; also after the use of certain drugs, such as digitalis, ergot, and alcoholic stimulants; and in chills, angina pectoris, epileptic and hysterical seizures, lithemia, gout, and uremia.

p., incident. One with 2nd beat weaker than 1st, the 3rd weaker than the 4th, followed by a stroke as strong as the 1st.

p., infrequent. Observed in organic heart disease, especially fatty degeneration, and fibroid induration; jaundice; pressure at base of brain sufficient to irritate the vagus, as in beginning meningitis; and at the close of febrile diseases, as in typhoid fever, and pneumonia. May follow the use of certain drugs, such as digitalis, aconite, and opium. Physiological slowness is noted in repose, during fasting, in the puerperium, and old age; it is habitual in certain people (40 to 60 beats per minute).

p., intermittent. One in which occasional beats are skipped.
   Caused by an apparent drop of a heartbeat. It is not inconsistent with health; yet it is commonly an indication of disease, frequently from gastric, hepatic, uterine, and renal causes. It is common in lithemia and fatty degeneration of the heart and is habitual in certain people after exercise, eating, excitement, or after the use of tobacco, tea, coffee, or other stimulants.

p., irregular. One when there is a variation in "force" and "frequency." Has same significance as intermittent pulse. Common in myocarditis and valvular diseases, esp. in mitral regurgitation. Heart trouble may be noted by long continued irregular pulse. Excess of tea, coffee, tobacco, or exercise may cause an irregular pulse.

p., jerking. That of aortic regurgitation, because from a state of emptiness the artery is suddenly filled with blood.

p., jugular. Venous pulse, q.v.

p., long. One in which duration of the systolic wave is comparatively long.

p., low-tension. One with sudden onset, short duration and rapid decline; esp. noted in degeneration of the heart, collapse, in debility, fevers, and low states of the nervous system.

p., male. From 70-75 beats per minute, but not as invariable rule, as some are healthy with a pulse rate of 50 or even 90.

p., monocrotous. One with a sphygmogram showing a simple ascending and descending, uninterrupted line and no dicrotism, indicative of a grave condition of the circulation and of impending death.

p., myurous. One with gradually weaker beats of diminishing amplitude.

p., paradoxical. One which is more or less suppressed at close of each full inspiration. Thought to be due to compression of the great vessels by inflammatory adhesion; the latter being stretched during act of inspiration. Frequently noted in adherent pericardium.

p., plateau. One slowly rising but which is maintained.

p. pressure. The difference bet. the systolic and the diastolic pressure.

This is really expressive of the tone of the arterial walls. Ex:

120 is systolic pressure.
100 is diastolic pressure.

20 is the pulse pressure.
130 is the systolic pressure.
90 is the diastolic pressure.

40 is the pulse pressure.

Normal pulse pressure: The systolic pressure must be about 40 points over the diastolic pressure in comparison. *Abnormal pulse pressure:* A pulse pressure over 50 points and under 30 points is considered abnormal.

p., quick, full, bounding. Indicates inflammation or fever of acute inflammatory character.

p., quick, hard. Characteristic of diphtheria and scarlatina. It also indicates inflammation or fever of acute inflammatory nature.

p., rapid. SEE: *accelerated pulse.*

p. rate.

Average Normal Expansile

Pulse of embryo, average per minute	150
At birth	140-130
During 1st year	130-115
During 2nd year	115-100
During 3rd year	100- 90
About 7th year	90- 85
About 14th year	85- 80
In middle life	75- 70
Old age	65- 50

p., regular. When the "force" and "frequency" are the same, that is, when the length of beat and number of beats per minute and the strength are the same.   [from kidney disease.

p., renal. A hard and full one in coma

p., respiratory. Alternate dilatation and contraction of the large veins of the neck occurring simultaneously with inspiration and expiration following rapid exercise.

p., senile. That of the aged. The sphygmogram shows a high position of the secondary waves in descent with great size of the 1st secondary wave as compared with the 2nd.

p., short. One with a short, quick systolic wave.

p., shuttle. One that feels as though it is floating something solid as well as fluid.

p., slow. A very slow pulse, fully accentuated often found among the aged, and it is a habitual rate among those inclined to be slow and easy in their actions. Such a pulse rate ranges bet. 40 and 60 beats per minute.

p., sluggish, full. Evinces want of nervous energy. Usual slowness, chiefly met with in chronic softening and tuberculous affections of brain. Also common in diseases attended with coma resulting from concussion or compression of brain.

p., small and rapid. Seen in great prostration from wasting diseases or hemorrhage.

p., soft. One which may be stopped by digital compression.

p., steel hammer. It is abrupt and energetic, as the rebound of a smith's hammer. One observed in arteries near a joint in rheumatism.

p., systolic. The period of the contraction of the heart causing the greatest arterial pressure, which normally is 100. Two or 3 beats followed by a longer pause. It has the same significance as the irregular pulse.

p., thready. A scarcely appreciable one observed in syncope.

p., tremulous. One in which a series of oscillations is felt with each beat.

p., trigeminal. Three regular beats followed by a pause. SEE: *irregular pulse.*

p., undulating. One that seems to have several successive waves.

p., unequal. One that varies in strength of its beats.

p., vaginal. Arterial pulse perceptible in the vagina in inflammatory disease or in pregnancy.

p., venous. Pulsation noted in jugular vein, often noted in tricuspid regurgitation. A venous pulse on dorsum of hand may be due to forcible propulsion of blood through the capillaries, as in aortic regurgitation, with great hypertrophy of left ventricle, or to extreme relaxation of arterioles and capillaries, permitting the transmission of the pulse wave, as in grave cachexia and anemia.

p., vermicular. A small, frequent one with a wormlike feeling.

p., vibrating. A jerking pulse, *q.v.*

p., water-hammer. Characterized by a short, powerful, jerky beat which suddenly collapses. The peculiar pulsation may be distinctly visible, not only in the carotids, but throughout the brachial artery.   [wire or firm cord.

p., wiry. A tense one that feels like a

pulsimeter (pŭl-sĭm'ĕt-ĕr). Contrivance for measuring frequency and force of the pulse. SYN: *sphygmometer.*

pul'sion. A veering of the individual from one side to another.

pulsus (pŭl'sŭs). Pulse.

p. alternans. A succession of strong and weak beats alternating.

p. bigeminus. Paired beats.

p. celer. Fast pulse, particularly that associated with high pulse pressure in aortic regurgitation.

p. paradoxus. One in which pulse becomes weaker during inspiration.

p. tardus. Slow pulse, particularly seen in aortic stenosis.

pultaceous (pŭl-tā'shŭs). Resembling a poultice. Syn: *pulpy.*

pulv. Abbr. *pulvis,* powder.

pulverization (pŭl-vĕr-ĭ-zā'shŭn). The crushing of any substance to powder or tiny particles.

pulverulent (pŭl-vĕr'ŭ-lĕnt). Of the nature of, or resembling, powder. Syn: *powdery.*

pulvinar (pŭl-vī'nĕr). The post. prominence of the optic thalamus.

pulvinate (pŭl'vĭn-āt). Very convex; shaped like a cushion.

pulvis (pŭl'vĭs). Powder.
The 6 official powders are mixtures of powdered medicinal substances.

pump (pŭmp). 1. Apparatus that transfers fluids or gases by pressure or suction. 2. To force air or fluid into a cavity, as heart pumps blood.

  p., air. Device for forcing air in or out of a chamber.

  p., breast. Apparatus for removing milk from the breasts.

  p., dental. Apparatus for removing saliva during operation on teeth or jaws.

  p., stomach. Apparatus for removing contents of stomach.

puncta (pŭnk'tă). (sing. *puʾu tum*). Points.

  p. dolorosa. Painful points in course of or at exit of nerves affected by neuralgia.

  p. lacrimalia. Orifices of lacrimal canaliculi about 6 mm. from inner canthus in the eyelids.

  p. vasculosa. Minute red areas which mark the cut surface of white central substance of the brain, from blood escaping from divided blood vessels.

punctate (pŭnk'tāt). Having pinpoint punctures or depressions on the surface; marked with dots.

  p. rash. One with minute red points.

punctiform (pŭnk'tĭ-form). 1. Formed like a point. 2. Bact: Referring to pinpoint colonies of less than 1 mm. in diameter.

punctograph (pŭnk'tō-grăf). Device employing radiography for localization of foreign bodies in the tissues.

punctum (pŭnk'tŭm) (pl. *puncta*). Point.

  p. caecum. Spot in fundus of the eyeball where the optic nerve enters. Syn: *blind spot.*

  p. lacrimale. Outlet of lacrimal canaliculus.

  p. nasale inferius. Lower portion of suture joining the nasal bones. Syn: *rhinion.*

  p. proximum. Point nearest the eye at which an object may be seen clearly. Syn: *near point.*

  p. remotum. Farthest spot at which there is clear vision. Syn: *far point.*

  p. saliens. First trace of the embryonic heart.

puncture (pŭnk'chūr). 1. A hole or wound made by a sharp pointed instrument. 2. To make a hole with such an instrument.

  p., exploratory. Removal of fluid or pus from a cavity or cyst for examination by piercing it.

  p., lumbar. Puncture of the lumbar spinal membranes to relieve dropsy or for examination of spinal fluid. See: *cisternal puncture, lumbar puncture, spinal fluid, spinal puncture.*

  p., spinal. See: *lumbar puncture.*

  p. wound. A wound made by piercing with a sharp instrument.

pungency (pŭn'jĕn-sĭ). Quality of being sharp, strong or bitter, as an odor or taste.

pungent (pŭn'jĕnt). Acrid, sharp, as applied to an odor or to taste.

P. U. O. Abbr. for *pyrexia of unknown origin,* or for *trench fever.*

pupil (pū'pĭl). The contractile opening at the center of the iris for the transmission of light.

  p., Argyll*-Robertson. Symptom of locomotor ataxia in which there is accommodation but light reflex is lost.

  p., bounding. Rapid dilatation of pupil alternating with contraction.

  p., occlusion of. One with opaque membrane shutting off the pupillary area.

pupillary (pū'pĭ-lĕr'ĭ). Concerning the pupil.

  p. contraction reflex. Pupillary contraction resulting from endeavoring forcibly to close eyelids which are held apart.

  p. reflexes. Those concerning passage of light through or dilation or contraction of pupil.

pupillometer (pū-pĭl-ŏm'ĕt-ĕr). Device for measurement of pupil's diameter.

pupilloscopy (pū-pĭl-os'kŏ-pĭ). 1. Measurement of eye refraction by effect of light and shadow on the retina. Syn: *skiascopy.* 2. Examination of the pupil.

pupillostatometer (pū'pĭl-ō-stăt-ŏm'ĕt-ĕr). Device for measuring distance between centers of the pupils.

purgation (pŭr-gā'shŭn). 1. Evacuation of the bowels caused by action of a purgative medicine. Syn: *catharsis.* 2. Cleansing.

purgative (pŭr'gă-tĭv). 1. Cleansing. 2. An agent that will cause watery evacuation of the intestinal contents.

  p. enema. A strong, high one that produces evacuation when other enemas fail. See: *enema.*

purge (pŭrj). 1. To evacuate the bowels by means of a cathartic. 2. A drug that causes evacuation of the bowels.

puriform (pū'rĭ-form). Resembling pus.

purin(e (pū'rēn, -rĭn). Parent of a group of heterocyclic nitrogen compounds including purine itself, $C_5H_4N_4$, and caffeine, theobromine, theophylline, xanthine, prepared from uric acid.

  p. body, base. Purine or any base derived from it.
Those mentioned in the foregoing plus paraxanthine and heteroxanthine.

  p. free diet. Any fruit excepting cranberries and prunes. Milk, butter, cream, cheese, rice, flour, tapioca, cabbage, cauliflower, sugar, macaroni, white bread.

p. low diet. Excludes meat, fish, fowl, spinach, lentils, mushrooms, peas, asparagus, coffee, tea, cocoa, spices, etc.

purinemia (pū-rĭn-ē′mĭ-ă). Purine bodies in the blood.

Purkinje's cells (poor-kĭn′yĕ). Large ganglionated cells of middle layer of the cerebellar cortex.

P's. corpuscles. SEE: *Purkinje's cells.*

P's. figures. Dark lines produced by the vessels of the retina.

P's. network. Fibrous network of large muscle cells found in cardiac muscle beneath the endocardium.

P. vesicle. The nuclear portion of an ovum. SYN: *germinal vesicle.*

Purkinje-Sanson's images (poor-kĭn′yĕ-sähn-son′). Three images of 1 object seen in the pupil of the eye.

purohepatitis (pū″rō-hep-ă-tī′tĭs). Purulent inflammation of the liver.

puromucous (pū″rō-mū′kŭs). Both purulent and mucus.

purpura (pûr′pū-ră). Purplish blotches beneath skin due to hemorrhage, serious symptom in many diseases.

p. annularis telangiectodes. Eruption of ring-shaped spots on lower limbs with pronounced telangiectasia.

p. haemorrhagica. Severe systemic disease with eruption progressing from legs over entire body. SYN: *land scurvy.*

p., malignant. Cerebrospinal fever.

p. rheumatica. Purpura with fever, swelling and severe rheumatic pains.

p. senilis. In debilitated and aged persons, ecchymoses and petechiae on legs.   [or suffering from, purpura.

purpuric (pûr-pū′rĭk). Pert. to, resembling,

purpurin (pûr′pū-rĭn). An acid dye used to stain nuclei.

purpurinuria (pûr″pū-rĭn-ū′rĭ-ă). Purpurin in urine. SYN: *porphyrinuria.*

purring thrill (pûr′ĭng). Thrill or vibration like a cat's purring, due to mitral stenosis, aneurysm, or valvular erosion of the heart felt by palpation over the precordium.

purulence, purulency (pûr′ū-lĕns, pûr′ū-lĕn-sĭ). The state of containing pus. SYN: *suppuration.*

purulent (pûr′ū-lĕnt). Suppurative; forming or containing pus, *q.v.* SEE: *sputum.*

puruloid (pûr′ū-loyd). Like pus. SYN: *puriform.*

pus (pŭs). Liquid product of inflammation composed of albuminous substances, a thin fluid, and leukocytes or their remains, generally yellow in color.
   If *red* it suggests rupture of small vessels. If *blue* or *green* it indicates presence of *B. pyocyaneus.*

p., cheesy. Very thick pus.

p., concrete. Fibropurulent coagula seen in infective endocarditis.

p., healthy. Same as laudable pus.

p., ichorous. Pus that is thin with shreds of sloughing tissue. It may have a fetid odor.

p., laudable. Obsolete term referring to typical pus considered as essential in healing wounds.

p., sanious. Pus colored by blood.

p., serous. Pus mostly of thin serum containing flakes.

p. in urine. Condition when there are more than the normal number of pus or white blood cells in the urine. It may be due to cystitis, pyelitis, urethritis, tuberculosis of the kidney, or any infection of the genitourinary tract. May also be caused by trauma. SYN: *pyuria.*

pustulant (pŭs′tū-lănt). 1. Causing pustules. 2. Agent which produces the formation of pustules, such as Croton oil and antimony; seldom used any more.

pustular (pŭs′tū-lĕr). Pert. to, or characterized by, pustules.

pustulation (pŭs-tū-lā′shŭn). The development of pustules.

pustule (pŭs′tūl). Small elevation of skin filled with lymph or pus.

p., malignant. Severe infectious disease with formation of hard pustule and symptoms of collapse. SYN: *anthrax.*

pustulocrustaceous (pŭs″tū-lō-krŭs-tā′-shŭs). Characterized by formation of pustules and crusts.

pustulosis (pŭs-tū-lō′sĭs). A generalized eruption of pustules.

putamen (pū-tā′mĕn). BNA. The darker, outer layer of the lenticular nucleus.

putrefaction (pū″trē-făk′shŭn). Decomposition of animal matter, esp. protein, associated with malodorous and poisonous products, such as the ptomaines, mercaptans, and hydrogen sulfide, caused by certain kinds of bacteria and fungi.

putrefactive (pū-trē-făk′tĭv). 1. Causing, or pert. to, putrefaction. 2. Agent promoting putrefaction.

p. alkaloid. A ptomaine, a base formed by action of bacteria on an amino acid.

putrefy (pū′trē-fī). To cause to decompose offensively.

putrescence (pū-trĕs′ĕns). Decay; rottenness.

putrid (pū′trĭd). Decayed; rotten; foul.

putrilage (pū′trĭl-ăj). Product of putrefaction.

pyarthrosis (pī-ar-thrō′sĭs). Pus in the cavity of a joint.

pycnemia (pĭk-nē′mĭ-ă). Thickening of the blood. SYN: *pyknemia.*

pycno- (pĭk′no). Combining form meaning *dense, thick.*

pycnosis (pĭk-nō′sĭs). 1. Thickening. SYN: *inspissation.* 2. A degenerative cellular change with shrinking of the cell. SYN: *pyknosis.*

pyecchysis (pī-ĕk′ĭs-ĭs). An effusion of pus.

pyelectasia, pyelectasis (pī-ĕl-ĕk-tā′zĭ-ă, -ek′tăs-ĭs). Dilatation of the renal pelvis.

pyelitic (pī-ĕ-lĭt′ĭk). Relating to or affected with pyelitis.

pyelitis (pī-ĕl-ī′tĭs). Inflammation of the kidney pelvis and its calices.

pyelo-. Combining form meaning the *pelvis.*

pyelocystitis (pī″ĕl-ō-sĭs-tī′tĭs). Inflamed

condition of the kidney, pelvis, and bladder.

pyelocystostomosis (pī″ĕl-ō-sĭs″tō-sto-mō′-sĭs). Establishment of surgical communication bet. the kidney and the bladder.

pyelogram, pyelograph (pī′ĕl-ō-grăm, -grăf). A roentgen picture of the ureter and renal pelvis.

pyelography (pī-ĕ-lŏg′rȧ-fĭ). Radiography of a renal pelvis and ureter.

pyelolithotomy (pī″ĕl-ō-lĭth-ŏt′ō-mĭ). Removal of calculus from the pelvis of a kidney through an incision.

pyelometer (pī-ĕl-ŏm′ĕt-ĕr). Device to measure the pelvic diameters. SYN: *pelvimeter.*

pyelometry (pī-ĕl-ŏm′ĕ-trĭ). 1. Measurement of the kidney's pelvis. 2. Measurement of the diameters of the pelvis. SYN: *pelvimetry.*

pyelonephritis (pī″ĕl-ō-nef-rī′tĭs). Inflammation of kidney substance and pelvis.

pyelonephrosis (pī″ĕl-ō-nef-rō′sĭs). Disease of the pelvis of the kidney.

pyelopathy (pī-ĕl-ŏp′ȧth-ĭ). Any disease of the pelvis of the kidney. SYN: *pyelonephrosis.*

pyeloplasty (pī′ĕl-ō-plăs″tĭ). Reparative operation on the kidney pelvis.

pyeloplication (pī″ĕl-ō-plĭ-kā′shŭn). Shortening of the wall of a dilated renal pelvis by taking tucks in it.

pyeloscopy (pī-ĕl-ŏs′kō-pĭ). Examination of the pelvis of the kidney using an x-ray.   [opening into renal pelvis.

pyelostomy (pī-ĕl-ŏs′tō-mĭ). Creation of

pyelotomy (pī-ĕl-ŏt′ō-mĭ). Incision of renal pelvis.

pyelovenous backflow (pī-ĕl-ō-vē′nŭs). Drainage from the renal pelvis into the venous system because of back pressure.

pyemesis (pī-ĕm′ĭs-ĭs). The vomiting of pus.

pyemia (pī-ē′mĭ-ȧ). Blood poisoning caused by pus absorption; a form of septicemia.

    p., cryptogenic. Pyemia, the focus of which is hidden in the deeper tissues.

    p., metastatic. Multiple abscess resulting from infected pyemic thrombi.

    p., portal. Suppurative inflammation of portal vein.

pyemic (pī-ē′mĭk). Relating to or affected with blood poisoning.

pyemid (pī-ē′mĭd). A cutaneous eruption in pyemia from metastasis.

pyencephalus (pī-en-sef′al-us). A brain abscess with suppuration within the cranium. SYN: *pyocephalus.*

pyesis (pī-ē′sĭs). The formation of pus. SYN: *suppuration.*

pygal (pī′găl). Concerning the buttocks.

pygalgia (pī-găl′jĭ-ȧ). Pain in the rump or buttocks.

pygo-. Combining form meaning the *rump.*

pyin (pī′ĭn). A substance of albuminous nature sometimes present in pus.

pyknemia (pĭk-nē′mĭ-ȧ). Thickening of the blood.

pyknic type (pĭk′nĭk). One with broad head, thick shoulders, large chest, short neck, and stocky body.

pyknocardia (pĭk-nō-kar′dĭ-ȧ). Rapid pulse. SYN: *tachycardia.*

pyknohemia (pĭk-nō-hē′mĭ-ȧ). Thickening of the blood. SYN: *pyknemia.*

pyknolepsy (pĭk-nō-lĕp′sĭ). Attacks similar to petit mal or minor epileptic seizures, usually occurring in childhood.

pyknometer (pĭk-nŏm′ĕt-ĕr). 1. Device for determining specific gravity of anything. 2. Device for measurement of the thickness of a substance.

pyknomorphous (pĭk″nō-morf′ŭs). Characterized by compact arrangement of the stainable portions, said esp. of certain nerve cells.

pyknophrasia (pĭk″-nō-frā′zĭ-ȧ). Thickness of words uttered in speech.

pyknosis (pĭk-nō′sĭs). Inspissation; thickness, esp. shrinking of cells through degeneration.

pyla (pī′lȧ). Opening connecting the 3rd ventricle to the sylvian aqueduct.

pyle-. Combining form meaning *orifice,* esp. that of the portal vein.

pylemphraxis (pī-lĕm-frăk′sĭs). Occlusion of the portal vein.

pylephlebectasia, pylephlebectasis (pī-le-flē-bĕk-tā′zĭ-ȧ, -bĕk′tȧ-sĭs). Distention of the portal vein.

pylephlebitis (pī-le-flē-bī′tĭs). Inflamed condition of the portal vein, generally suppurative.

    p., adhesive. Thrombosis of the portal vein.

    p. obturans. Pylephlebitis with obstructed flow in the portal vein.

pylethrombosis (pī-le-thrŏm-bō′sĭs). Occlusion of portal vein by a thrombus.

pylometer (pī-lŏm′ĕt-ĕr). Device for measuring obstructions at vesical opening.

pyloralgia (pī″lō-răl′jĭ-ȧ). Pain around the pylorus.

pylorectomy (pī-lō-rĕk′tō-mĭ). Surgical removal of the pylorus.

pyloric (pī-lor′ĭk). Pert. to the opening bet. the stomach and duodenum.

    p. cap. Portion of duodenum next to pylorus.

    p. gland. A gland of the stomach near the pylorus secreting pepsin.

    p. orifice. Opening or passage bet. the stomach and duodenum.

    p. stenosis. Narrowing of the pyloric orifice.

    Often due to contraction following healing of a peptic ulcer.

pyloristenosis (pī″lō-rĭ-stĕn-ō′sĭs). Constriction of the pylorus.

pyloritis (pī-lō-rī′tĭs). Inflamed condition of the pylorus.

pyloro-. Combining form meaning *gatekeeper;* applied to the *pylorus.*

pyloroduodenitis (pī″lor-ō-dū″ō-dē-nī′tĭs). Inflammation of the mucosa of the pylorus and duodenum.

pylorogastrectomy (pī-lō″rō-găs-trĕk′tō-mĭ). Excision of pyloric portion of the stomach.

pyloromyotomy (pī-lō″rō-mī-ŏt′ō-mĭ). Incision and suture of the pyloric sphincter.

pyloroplasty (pī-lor'ō-plǎs"tǐ). Operation to repair the pylorus, esp. 1 to increase the caliber of the pyloric opening by stretching.

pyloroptosia, pyloroptosis (pī-lo"rŏp-tō'sǐ-ǎ, -rŏp'tō-sǐs). Displacement downward of the pyloric end of the stomach.

pyloroscopy (pī-lō-rŏs'kō-pǐ). Fluoroscopic examination of the pylorus.

pylorospasm (pī-lō'rō-spǎzm). Spasmodic contraction of the pyloric orifice.

pylorostenosis (pī-lō"rō-stěn-ō'sǐs). Contraction of the pylorus.

pylorostomy (pī-lor-ŏs'tō-mǐ). Formation of an opening through the abdominal wall into the pylorus.

pylorotomy (pī-lor-ŏt'ō-mǐ). Incision of the pyloric submucosa to relieve hypertrophic stenosis.

pylorus (pī-lōr'ŭs). The lower orifice of the stomach opening into the duodenum.

    p., glands of. Those in the stomach near the pylorus secreting pepsin.

    p., spasm of. Usually secondary to hyperperistalsis, hyperacidity, or the ingestion of irritating foods.

pyo-, py-. Combining forms meaning *pus*.

pyocele (pī'ō-sēl). A hernia or distended cavity containing pus.

pyocelia (pī-ō-sē'lǐ-ǎ). Pus formation in the abdominal cavity.

pyocephalus (pī"ō-sěf'ā-lŭs). Effusion of purulent nature within the cranium.

    p., circumscribed. Abscess of the brain.

    p., external. Suppuration of the meninges.

    p., interval. Pus in the cerebrospinal fluid.

pyochezia (pī"ō-kē'zǐ-ǎ). Pus in the feces.

pyococcus (pī"ō-kŏk'ŭs). A micrococcus which causes suppuration, as the *Streptococcus pyogenes*.

pyocolpocele (pī-ō-kŏl'pō-sēl). A vaginal tumor containing pus. SEE: *pyocolpos*.

pyocol'pos. Accumulation of pus in the vagina.

pyoculture (pī'ō-kŭl-chūr). Comparative tests for cultivation of pus from a wound, a portion being left in the collecting tube and a portion being cultivated on bouillon.

pyocyst (pī'ō-sĭst). A cyst holding pus.

pyocyte (pī'ō-sīt). A pus corpuscle, considered a leukocyte. SYN: *pus cell.*

pyodermatitis (pī"ō-dŭr-mǎ-tī'tǐs). Pyogenic infection of the skin causing a dermatitis.

pyodermatosis (pī"ō-děr-mǎ-tō'sǐs). Any skin condition of pyogenic origin. SYN: *pyodermia.*

pyodermia (pī"ō-děr'mǐ-ǎ). Any suppurative skin disease.

pyofecia (pī"ō-fē'sǐ-ǎ). Pus in the stools.

pyogenesis (pī"ō-jěn'ěs-ĭs). The development of pus.

pyogenic (pī-ō-jěn'ĭk). Producing pus.

    p. microörganisms. Microörganisms forming pus.

pyohemia (pī"ō-hē'mǐ-ǎ). Blood poisoning with multiple abscess formation. SYN: *pyemia.*

pyohemothorax (pī"ō-hěm-ō-thō'rǎks). Pus and blood in the pleural cavity.

pyoid (pī'oyd). Resembling pus.

pyoktanin (pī-ŏk'tǎn-ĭn). Commercial preparation of methyl violet; a germicide used in cystitis, gonorrhea, and infections of the eyes, ears, nose, and throat.

pyolabyrinthitis (pī"ō-lǎb-ĭ-rĭn-thī'tǐs). Inflammation with suppuration of the labyrinth of the ear.

pyometra (pī-ō-mē'trǎ). Retained pus accumulation in the uterine cavity.

pyometritis (pī"ō-mē-trī'tǐs). Purulent inflammation of the uterus.

pyonephritis (pī"ō-nef-rī'tǐs). Inflammation of the kidney, suppurative in character.

pyonephrolithiasis (pī"ō-nef-rō-lĭth-ī'ǎs-ĭs). Pus and calculi formation in the kidney.

pyonephrosis (pī"ō-nef-rō'sǐs). Pus accumulation in the pelvis of kidney.

pyoövarium (pī"ō-ō-vā'rǐ-ŭm). Abscess formation in an ovary.

pyopericarditis (pī"ō-pěr-ĭ-kar-dī'tǐs). Pericarditis with suppuration.

pyopericardium (pī"ō-pěr-ĭ-kar'dǐ-ŭm). Pus formation in the pericardium.

pyoperitoneum (pī"ō-pěr-ĭ-tō-nē'ŭm). Pus formation in the peritoneal cavity.

pyoperitonitis (pī"ō-pěr-ĭ-tō-nī'tǐs). Purulent inflammation of the lining of peritoneum.

pyophagia (pī"ō-fā'jǐ-ǎ). Swallowing of purulent substance.

pyophthalmia, pyophthalmitis (pī"ŏf-thǎl'-mǐ-ǎ, -thǎl-mī'tǐs). Suppurative inflamed condition of the eye.

pyophylactic (pī"ō-fī-lǎk'tǐk). Guarding against formation of pus.

    p. membrane. Lining membrane of an abscess cavity separating it from healthy tissue.

pyophysometra (pī"ō-fī-sō-mē'trǎ). Pus and gas accumulation in the uterus.

pyoplania (pī"ō-plā'nǐ-ǎ). Spreading of pus by infiltration into tissue.

pyopneumocholecystitis (pī"ō-nū"mō-kō-lē-sĭs-tī'tǐs). Dilatation of the gallbladder with air and pus.

pyopneumocyst (pī"ō-nū'mō-sĭst). A cyst enclosing pus and gas.

pyopneumopericardium (pī"ō-nū"mō-pěr-ĭ-kar'dǐ-ŭm). Pus and air or gas in pericardium.

pyopneumoperitonitis (pī"ō-nū"mō-pěr-ĭ-tō-nī'tǐs). Pus and air in the peritoneal cavity complicating peritonitis.

pyopneumothorax (pī"ō-nū"mō-thō'rǎks). Pus and gas or air accumulated in the pleural cavity.

    p., subphrenic. Pus and air accumulated beneath the diaphragm.

pyopoiesis (pī"ō-poy-ē'sǐs). Development of pus. SYN: *pyogenesis, suppuration.*

pyopoietic (pī"ō-poy-ět'ĭk). Secreting or forming pus. SYN: *suppurative.*

pyoptysis (pī-ŏp'tǐs-ĭs). Spitting of pus.

pyorrhagia (pī-or-ā'jǐ-ǎ). Profuse flow of pus, as when an abscess ruptures.

pyorrhea (pī-ō-rē′ă). A discharge of purulent matter.

p. alveolaris. Inflammation of periosteum of the tooth socket.

p. salivaris. Flow of pus from a salivary duct.

pyosalpingitis (pī″ō-săl-pĭn-jī′tĭs). Retained pus in the oviduct with inflammation.

pyosalpingoöophoritis (pī″ō-săl-pĭn″gō-ō-ŏf-ō-rī′tĭs). Inflammation of ovary and oviduct with suppuration.

pyosalpinx (pī″ō-săl′pĭnks). Pus in the fallopian tube. SEE: *pyosalpingitis.*

pyosapremia (pī″ō-săp-rē′mĭ-ă). Purulent infection of the blood; blood poisoning. SYN: *pyemia.*

pyoscheocele (pī-ŏs′kē-ō-sēl). Swelling and suppuration of the scrotum.

pyosepticemia (pī″ō-sĕp-tĭ-sē′mĭ-ă). Condition in which pyogenic and pathogenic bacteria are in the blood; blood poisoning with suppuration. SYN: *septicopyemia.*

pyosin (pī′ō-sĭn). A substance found in plasma of pus cells.

pyosis (pī-ō′sĭs). Formation of pus. SYN: *suppuration.*

pyospermia (pī″ō-spĕr′mĭ-ă). Pus in the semen.

pyostatic (pī-ō-stăt′ĭk). 1. Agent checking the development of pus. 2. Preventing pus formation.

pyotherapy (pī″ō-thĕr′ă-pĭ). Treatment of disease with pus.

pyothorax (pī″ō-thō′răks). Pus in the pleural cavity. SYN: *empyema.*

p. subphrenic. An abscess below the diaphragm.

pyotorrhea (pī″ō-tor-ē′ă). Purulent discharge from the ear.

pyotoxinemia (pī″ō-tŏk-sĭ-nē′mĭ-ă). Infection from toxic products of pus organisms in the blood.

pyoturia (pī″ō-tū′rĭ-ă). Pus cells in the urine. SYN: *pyuria.*

pyourachus (pī″ō-ū′ră-kŭs). Accumulation of pus in the urachus.

pyoureter (pī″ō-ūr′ĕt-ĕr, -ū-rē′tĕr). Pus collection in a ureter.

pyovesiculosis (pī″ō-vĕs-ĭk-ū-lō′sĭs). Pus collection in the seminal vesicles.

pyramid (pĭr′ăm-ĭd). 1. A solid on a base with 3 or more sides, the triangular planes of which meet at an apex. 2. Any part of the body resembling a pyramid. 3. A compact bundle of nerve fibers in the medulla oblongata. 4. Petrous portion of temporal bone.

p. of cerebellum. A conical projection near the center of the inf. vermiform process.

p., Ferrein's. Any one of the renal medullary rays.

p., Lalouette's. Pyramid of the thyroid.

p., malpighian. Any 1 of the pyramidal masses of the renal cortex made up of glomeruli, blood vessels, and convoluted tubules. SYN: *cones of Malpighi.*

p. of the medulla. (Ant.) A pair of oblong bodies on ant. surface of the medulla. (Post.) The 2 expanded portions of the funiculus gracilis at lower angle of the 4th ventricle.

p., renal. Same as *malpighian pyramid.*

p. of the thyroid. A conical process sometimes arising from the thyroid gland up to the hyoid bone, the median lobe.

p. of the tympanum. A hollow projection on inner wall of the tympanum through which passes the stapedius muscle.

pyramidal (pĭ-răm′ĭd-ăl). In the shape of a pyramid.

p. bone. The cuneiform bone of the carpus.

p. cell. Pyramid-shaped cell of cerebral cortex.

p. tract. A large bundle of medullated nerve fibers in the medulla oblongata carrying motor nerves downward to the spinal cord.

pyramidalis (pī-răm″ĭ-dā′lĭs). Abdominal muscle sometimes present in front of the rectus aiding inspiration.

pyramidon (pĭ-răm′ĭd-ŏn). Proprietary preparation of amidopyrine; a yellowish-white powder.

DOSAGE: 5-8 gr. (0.32-0.51 Gm.) every 2 hours.

pyrazine -2, 3- dicarboxylic acid (pĭr′ă-zēn dī″kar-bŏk-sĭl′ĭk). Compound used successfully in treating pellagra, *q.v.*

p. monocarboxylic acid. Compound used successfully in treatment of pellagra.

pyrectic (pī-rĕk′tĭk). Feverish. SYN: *pyretic.*

pyrenemia (pī-rē-nē′mĭ-ă). Condition in which there are nucleated red cells in the blood.

pyrenin (pī-rē′nĭn). The oxyphilic substance found in a nucleolus.

pyrenoid (pī′rē-noyd). A colorless, highly refractive body in certain protozoan chromatophores.

pyretherapy (pī-rē-thĕr′ă-pĭ). 1. Artificial fever treatment. 2. Treatment of febrile conditions. SYN: *pyretotherapy.*

pyretic (pī-rĕt′ĭk). 1. Concerning fever. 2. Remedy for fever.

p. therapy. Treatment of disease by artificial induction of fever, either by physical agents or the inoculation of malarial organisms.

pyreticosis (pī-rĕt-ĭ-kō′sĭs). Feverishness.

pyreto-. Prefix meaning *fever.*

pyretogen (pī-rĕt′ō-jĕn). A substance producing fever.

pyretogenesia, pyretogenesis (pī″rĕt-ō-jĕn-ē′zĭ-ă, -jĕn′ĕs-ĭs). Origin and production of fever.

pyretogenic, pyretogenous (pī″ret-ō-jĕn′-ĭk, -ŏj′ĕn-ŭs). Producing or causing fever.

p. bacteria. Pathogenic bacteria causing fever.

p. stage. Period in a fever when it is rising slowly.

pyretography (pī-rĕt-ŏg′ră-fĭ). A treatise on fever,

pyretology (pī-rĕt-ŏl'ō-jĭ). Science of fevers and their characteristics.

pyretolysis (pī-rĕt-ŏl'ĭs-ĭs). 1. Reduction of fever. 2. Hastening of lysis by elevation of temperature.

pyretotherapy (pī''rē-tō-thĕr'ă-pĭ). 1. Treatment by artificially raising the patient's temperature. 2. Treatment of fever.

pyretotyphosis (pī-rĕt-ō-tĭ-fō'sĭs). The delirious or stuporous symptom of fever.

pyrexia (pī-rĕk'sĭ-ă). Condition in which the temperature is above normal. SYN: *fever.*

Some classify it as:

Low .... 99°—101° F.
Moderate .... 101°—103° F.
High .... 103°—105° F.

p., local. Acute inflammation of a part.

pyrexial (pī-rĕks'ĭ-ăl). Concerning fever.

3-pyridinecarboxylic acid (pĭr''ĭd-ēn-kar''bŏk-sĭl'ĭk). Organic substance obtained by oxidizing nicotine. SYN: *nicotinic acid.* SEE: *pellagra.*

pyridium (pī-rĭd'ĭ-ŭm). A commercial brick red powder, belonging to the group of azo dyes.

DOSAGE: 1½ gr. (0.1 Gm.) application, 0.125%-0.5% solution as irrigation.

pyriform (pĭ'rĭ-form). Shaped like a pear.

pyrimidine (pī-rĭm'ĭd-ēn). The parent of a group of heterocyclic nitrogen compounds. $C_4H_4N_2$, including uracil, cytosine, and thymine, some of which are components of nucleic acid.

pyro-. Prefix meaning *heat* or *fire.*

pyrocatechinuria (pī''rō-kăt-ĕ-kĭn-ū'rĭ-ă). Pyrocatechin in the urine.

pyrodox'in. Vitamin* B_6, of the B complex group.

pyrogallol, pyrogallic acid (pī''rō-găl'ŏl, -ĭk). USP. A substance obtained by the decomposition of gallic acid.

DOSAGE: Externally, 2 to 10% ointment, with caution.   [to fever.

pyrogenic (pī''rō-jĕn'ĭk). Producing or due

pyrolagnia (pī''rō-lăg'nĭ-ă). Insane desire to see or produce fires accompanied by sexual gratification.

pyrolysis (pī-rŏl'ĭs-ĭs). Disintegration of organic matter when there is a rise in temperature.

pyromania (pī''rō-mā'nĭ-ă). Fire madness; mania for setting fires or seeing them.

pyrometer (pī-rŏm'ĕt-ĕr). Device for measuring extreme degrees of heat.

pyronyxis (pī-rō-nĭks'ĭs). Treatment or cauterization by puncturing a part with hot needles. SYN: *ignipuncture.*

pyrophobia (pī-rō-fō'bĭ-ă). Abnormal fear of fire.

pyroptothymia (pī-rŏp-tō-thī'mĭ-ă). A psychosis in which one imagines himself surrounded by flames.

pyropuncture (pī''rō-pŭnk'chŭr). Treatment by puncture of a part with hot needles. SYN: *pyronyxis.*

pyrosis (pī-rō'sĭs). A burning sensation in the epigastric and sternal region, with raising of acid liquid from stomach. SYN: *heartburn, waterbrash.*

pyrotic (pī-rŏt'ĭk). 1. Caustic. 2. Pert. to pyrosis.

pyrotoxin (pī-rō-tŏks'ĭn). A toxin generated by a febrile process.

pyroxylin (pī-rŏk'sĭl-ĭn). A product obtained by the action of a mixture of nitric and sulfuric acids on cellulose.

Pyst'yan pack. A mud pack.

pythogenesis (pī-thō-jĕn'ĕs-ĭs). 1. Generation from decayed matter or decomposition. 2. The cause of decay.

pythogenic, pythogenous (pī-thō-jĕn'ĭk, -thŏj'ĕn-ŭs). Arising from putrefaction or decomposition.

p. fever. Typhoid fever, *q.v.*

pyuria (pī-ū'rĭ-ă). Pus in the urine; evidence of renal disease.

Q

Q. 1. Abbr. for *electric quantity, quart.* 2. Symb. for *coulomb.*

Q. d., q. d. Abbr. for L. *quater in die,* four times a day.

Q. h., q. h. Abbr. for L. *quaque hora,* every hour.

Q. i. d., q. i. d. Abbr. for *quater in die,* four times a day.

Q. L., q. l. Abbr. for *quantum libet,* as much as one pleases.

Q. S., q. s. Abbr. for *quantum sufficit,* as much as necessary.

quack (kwăk). One who pretends to have knowledge or skill in medicine. SYN: *charlatan.*

quackery (kwăk′ĕr-ĭ). The practice or pretensions of a quack. SYN: *charlatanry.*

quadrangular (kwŏd-răng′ū-lĕr). Having 4 angles and 4 sides.

quadrant (kwŏd′rănt). 1. The 4th of a circle. 2. One of 4 corresponding regions, as of the abdomen, divided for diagnostic purposes.

quadrantanopsia (kwŏd-rănt-ăn-ŏp′sĭă). Loss of sight in approximately ¼ of the visual field.

quadrate (kwŏd′rāt). Square or having 4 equal sides.

  q. lobe. One of the smaller hepatic lobes.

  q. lobule. The precuneus; a part of the cerebral parietal lobe.

quadri-, quadr-. Combining forms meaning *having four; consisting of four.*

quadriceps (kwŏd′rĭ-sĕps). Four-headed, noting a large muscle, the *quadriceps extensor femoris;* the extensor of the leg, having 4 heads, rectus femoris, vastus internus, vastus externus, and crureus.

quadrigemina (kwŏd-rĭ-jĕm′ĭn-ă). The corpora quadrigemina.

quadrigeminal (kwŏd-rĭ-jĕm′ĭn-ăl). Fourfold; having 4 symmetrical parts.

quadrilateral (kwŏd-rĭ-lăt′ĕr-ăl). Having 4 sides.

quadripara (kwŏd-rĭp′ă-ră). A woman in her 4th confinement or who has had 4 children.

quadripartite (kwŏd-rĭ-par′tīt). Divided into 4 parts.

quadripedal reflex (kwŏd-rĭp′ĕd-ăl). Extension of flexed arm on assuming quadripedal posture.

quadriplegia (kwŏd-rĭ-plē′jĭ-ă). Paralysis affecting all 4 limbs.

quadrisect (kwŏd′rĭ-sĕkt). To divide into 4 parts.

quadritubercular (kwŏd″rĭ-tū-bur′kŭ-lĕr). Having 4 tubercles or cusps.

quadrivalent (kwŏd-rĭ-vā′lĕnt, -rĭv′ăl-ĕnt). Having ability to replace 4 atoms of hydrogen in a compound.

quadroon (kwŏd-rōōn′). The offspring of a white person and a mulatto, thus having one-quarter Negro blood.

quadruplet (kwŏd′rū-plĕt). One of 4 children born of the same mother at same labor. SEE: *Hellin's law.*

quale (kwā′lē). The quality of anything, as of a sensation.

qualimeter (kwŏl-ĭm′ĕt-ĕr). Device to determine hardness of the x-rays. SEE: *penetrometer.*

qualitative (kwŏl′ĭ-tā-tĭv). Referring to the quality of anything.

  q. analysis. CHEM: One that determines the nature of the elements of a compound. SEE: *quantitative.*

quality (kwŏl′ĭ-tĭ). That which constitutes or characterizes a thing; nature.

quanta (kwŏn′tă). Plural of quantum, *q.v.*

quantimeter (kwŏn-tĭm′ĕt-ĕr). Colorimetric standard for measuring quantity of x-rays to which a subject is exposed.

quanti-Pirquet (kwŏn-tĭ-pēr′kă). Quantitative cutaneous test of amt. of sensitiveness to tuberculin by use of graduated dilutions. [quantity.]

quantitative (kwŏn-tĭ-tā′tĭv). Concerning

  q. analysis. One that determines the proportionate parts of elements in a compound. SEE: *qualitative.*

quantity (kwŏn′tĭ-tĭ). Amount; portion.

  q., unit of. Coulomb, the measure of amt. of electric current passing a given point in a conductor in a given time.

quantum (kwŏn′tŭm). 1. A unit of radiant energy. 2. A definite amount.

  q. libet. As much as desired.

  q. limit. Shortest wave length in x-ray spectrum. SYN: *minimum wave length.*

  q. sufficit. As much as needed.

  q. theory. Radiation is an intermittent emission of energy in varying multiples of quanta action; not continuous.

quarantine (kwor′ăn-tēn). 1. The period of debarring from entrance to a country, or the isolation of persons exposed to infectious diseases; formerly 40 days. 2. Period of isolation from public communication following onset of a contagious disease. 3. To so restrict from public communication. SEE: *contagious diseases, isolation.*

  q., chickenpox. Until skin is free of all crusts. From 2 to 3 weeks.

  q., diphtheria. Until patient is free of the Klebs-Loeffler bacillus as demonstrated by 1 or more laboratory examinations of cultures that have been obtained for this purpose. Average time for uncomplicated cases about 3 weeks.

  q., measles. Until eruption has disappeared and temperature has remained normal for 48 hours. Average time, 10 days for uncomplicated cases.

q., mumps. Minimum period, 10 days. Preferably, 2 weeks.

q., poliomyelitis. From 3 to 4 weeks.

q., scarlet fever. Time depends chiefly on severity and presence or absence of complications. Under any circumstances, the patient should be found free of hemolytic streptococci by laboratory examination. Average time, 3 to 4 weeks for uncomplicated cases.

q., smallpox. Until patient is clinically well and skin is free of all crusts. About 3 weeks for discrete cases.

q., typhoid fever. To the 2nd week of convalescence, and preferably until examination of feces demonstrates the absence of the *Bacillus typhosus.*

q., typhus fever. From 3 to 4 weeks.

q., whooping cough. Average period, 3 weeks from the beginning of the catarrhal stage appears to be sufficient.

quart (kwort). A fluid measure; two pints.

quartan (kwor'tăn). 1. Occurring every 4th day. 2. Malarial fever with a paroxysm every 4th day, figuring from and including the 1st day of paroxysm. See: *fever, malaria.*

quartile (kwor'tĭl). One of the 2 middle values of each half of a series of variables.

quartipara (kwor-tĭp'ä-ră). A woman who has borne her fourth child.

quartiparous (kwor-tĭp'är-ŭs). Having given birth to 4 children or having been in labor 4th time.

quartz (kwortz). Silicon dioxide, the principal ingredient of sandstone (crystallized silica; rock crystal).

q. applicator. Quartz rod of various shapes and angles to conduct (by total internal reflection) ultraviolet radiation from a water-cooled mercury arc quartz lamp.

q. glass. Crystalline quartz is used for prisms and lenses, fused quartz for windows, etc., through which ultraviolet radiations are freely transmitted.

quassation (kwă-să'shŭn). A beating, a shaking; breaking up of crude materials into small pieces.

quassia (kwŏsh'ă). The wood of a tree grown chiefly in Jamaica.

Dosage: From 5 to 10 gr. (0.3-0.6 Gm.). For injections, an infusion of 2 oz. to a pint of water.

quaternary (kwă-tĕr'nă-rĭ). 1. The 4th in order. 2. Composed of 4 elements.

Queckenstadt's sign. Upon compression of the veins of the neck, unilaterally or bilaterally, cerebrospinal fluid pressure rises rapidly in healthy persons; this disappears when pressure is released. In vertebral canal block, the pressure is scarcely affected by this procedure.

querulent (kwĕr'ū-lĕnt). 1. Complaining; fretful. 2. One who is dissatisfied, complaining, and suspicious.

quickening (kwĭk'ĕn-ĭng). First movements of the fetus felt in *utero.* [cury.

quicksilver (kwĭk'sĭl-vĕr). The metal mercury.

quillaja (kwĭl-ā'yă) (soap bark). The inner bark of a tree grown in Chile.

Quincke's disease (kvĭng'kĕh). Angioneurotic edema of skin; reddening and blanching of fingernails.

Q.'s pulse. Capillary pulse; by pressure with each systole; a sign of aortic insufficiency.

Q.'s puncture. Lumbar puncture to determine tension of, or to remove some of, the spinal fluid.

quinidine sulfate (kwĭn'ĭd-ēn). USP. The sulfate of an alkaloid obtained from cinchona, being a white, crystalline substance with a bitter taste.

Dosage: 3 gr. (0.2 Gm.) with caution.

quinine (kwī'nĭn, kwī'nēn). Bitter, crystalline, white alkaloid derived from cinchona bark.

Dosage: As *tonic,* 1½ gr. (0.1 Gm.); as *antimalarial,* 15 gr. (1.0 Gm.).

q. bisulfate. USP. The acid sulfate of quinine.

Dosage: Same as quinine sulfate.

q. hydrochloride. USP. The hydrochloride of quinine.

Dosage: Same as quinine sulfate.

q. sulfate. USP. The sulfate of an alkaloid obtained from cinchona.

Dosage: 15 gr. (1 Gm.) for malaria; as a tonic, 1½ gr. (0.1 Gm.).

q. tannate. USP. A nearly tasteless and odorless compound of quinine and tannic acid.

Dosage: 3 gr. (0.2 Gm.).

q. and urea hydrochloride. USP. The compound of quinine hydrochloride and urea hydrochloride.

Dosage: Antimalarial, 15 gr. (1 Gm.) daily. Local anesthetic, 0.25 to 1% solution.

quininism (kwī'nĭn-ĭzm, kwī-nēn'ĭzm). Poisoning by cinchona or its alkaloids. Syn: *cinchonism.*

quiniobine (kwĭn-ĭ'ō-bēn). A commercial solution of quinine bismuth iodide in olive oil.

Dosage: For adults, 1 to 2 cc. twice a week, usually for 12 injections.

quinisal (kwĭn'ĭs-ăl). A commercial compound of quinine and salicylic acid.

Dosage: From 5 to 8 gr. (0.3-0.5 Gm.).

quinone (kwĭn-ōn'). 1. Yellow, crystalline oxidation product of quinic acid. 2. Class of organic compounds in which 2 atoms of hydrogen are replaced by oxygen.

quinoxyl (kwĭn-ŏk'sĭl). See: *chiniofon.*

Quinquad's disease (kăn-kōz'). Purulent inflammation of scalp's hair follicles with bald patches as a result.

quinqu-. Combining form meaning *five.*

quinquina (kwĭn-kwī'nă, -kĭn-kē'nă). Cinchona, *q.v.*

quinsy (kwĭn'zē). Acute inflammation of the tonsil and of the peritonsillar tissue usually forming an abscess. Peritonsillar abscess.

q., lingual. Phlegmonous inflammation of the lingual tonsil.

quintan (kwĭn'tăn). 1. Occurring every 5th day. 2. Intermittent fever, the paroxysms occurring every 5th day with intermission of three days.

quinti-. Combining form meaning *fifth*.

Quintin treatment (kăn-tăn'). The therapeutic injection of sea water.

quintipara (kwĭn-tĭp'ă-ră). A woman in her 5th confinement or who has had 5 children.

quintuplet (kwĭn'tū-plĕt). One of 5 children born of 1 mother during the same confinement. See: *Hellin's law, twins.*

quiz (kwĭz). 1. A series of questions to be given a student. 2. The administering of such questions.   [instructor.

    q. class. A class questioned by an

quotidian (kwō-tĭd'ĭ-ăn). Occurring daily.

    q. fever. A malarial fever characterized by daily paroxysms.

quotient (kwō'shĕnt). Number of times 1 number is contained in another.

    q., blood. A color index obtained by finding the number of erythrocytes in the percentage of hemoglobin shown by a percentage of the normal number in the same specimen.

    q., caloric. Result obtained by dividing heat (in calories) by the oxygen consumed (in milligrams) in metabolism.

    q., D. The ratio of glucose to nitrogen in the urine.

    q., growth. Percentage of the food energy utilized for growth; estimated at 5%.

    q., intelligence. Division of the patient's mental age by his actual age.

    q., protein. The number obtained by dividing the amount of globulin by the albumin in a specimen of blood plasma.

    q., respiratory. The result of dividing amt. of carbon dioxide in expired air by the oxygen inhaled, normally 0.9.

q.v. 1. Abbr. for L. *quantum vis*, as much as you like. 2. Abbr. for L. *quod vide*, meaning *which see.*

R

R. Abbr. for *Réaumur, roentgen, respiration, right.* ℞. Symb. for L. *recipe,* to take.

Ra. Chemical symb. for *radium.*

rabbetting (răb'ĕt-ĭng). Interlocking of the jagged edges of a fractured bone.

rabiate (rā'bĭ-āt). Suffering from rabies. SYN: *rabid.*

rabiator (rā'bĭ-ā-tor). One affected with rabies.

rabic (răb'ĭk). Concerning rabies.

rabicidal (răb-ĭ-sī'dăl). Destructive to causative agent of rabies (*Bacillus lyssae*).

rabid (răb'ĭd). Pert. to or affected with rabies. SYN: *rabiate.*

rabies (rā'bēz). An extremely fatal infectious disease communicated to man by bite of a rabid animal, usually a dog. SYN: *hydrophobia, lyssa.* SEE: *dog bite.*

race (rās). 1. A class of individuals with common interests, characteristics, appearance, habits, etc., as if derived from a common ancestor. 2. State of being 1 of a special group. 3. Division of mankind with traits sufficient to mark it as a distinct human type.

racemose (răs'ē-mōs). Resembling a clustered bunch of grapes, as a gland, divided and subdivided, ending in a bunch of follicles.

rachi-, rachio-. Combining forms meaning *rib of a leaf, ridge, spine.*

rachialbuminimeter (rā″kĭ-ăl-bū-mĭn-ĭm'ĕt-ĕr). Device for estimating amt. of albumin in the cerebrospinal fluid.

rachialbuminimetry (rā″kĭ-ăl-bū-mĭn-ĭm'ĕt-rĭ). The estimation of amt. of albumin in the cerebrospinal fluid.

rachianalgesia (rā″kĭ-ăn-ăl-jē'zĭ-ă). Spinal anesthesia. SYN: *rachianesthesia.*

rachialgia (rā-kĭ-ăl'jĭ-ă). Pain in the spine.

rachianesthesia (rā″kĭ-ăn-ĕs-thē'zĭ-ă). Spinal anesthesia.

rachicentesis (rā″kĭ-sĕn-tē'sĭs). Puncture into the spinal canal.

rachidian (ra-kĭd'ĭ-ăn). Relating to the spinal column.

rachigraph (rā'kĭ-grăf). Device for outlining the curves of the spine.

rachilysis (rā-kĭl'ĭs-ĭs). Mechanical treatment of lateral curvature of the spine.

rachiocampsis (rā-kĭ-ō-kamp'sĭs). Curvature of spine.

rachiochysis (rā-kĭ-ok'ĭs-ĭs). Accumulation of fluid within the spinal canal.

rachiodynia (rā-kĭ-ō-dĭn'ĭ-ă). Painful condition of spinal column. SYN: *rachialgia.*

rachiometer (rā-kĭ-ŏm'ĕt-ĕr). Instrument for measuring a curvature of the spine.

rachiomyelitis (rā″kĭ-ō-mī-ĕ-lī'tĭs). Inflamed condition of spinal cord. SYN: *myelitis.*

rachioplegia (rā″kĭ-ō-plē'jĭ-ă). Paralysis of spine.

rachiotome (rā'kĭ-ō-tōm). Instrument for dividing the vertebrae.

rachiotomy (rā-kĭ-ŏt'ō-mĭ). Surgical cutting of the vertebral column.

rachis (rā'kĭs) (pl. *rachises*). The spinal column. [fissure; congenital.

rachischisis (rā-kĭs'kĭs-ĭs). Spinal column

rachistovainization (rā″kĭs-tō-vā-nĭ-zā'-shŭn). Spinal injection of stovaine to produce anesthesia.

rachitic (rā-kĭt'ĭk). Pert. to or affected with rickets.

   r. flat pelvis. Pelvic deformity due to having had rickets in childhood.

   r. rosary. Beadlike prominences at junction of the ribs with their cartilages.

rachitis (ra-kī'tĭs). Inflammation of the spine, commonly rickets, *q.v.* SEE: *rachitic beads.*

   r. fetalis annularis. Enlargement of epiphyses of long bones; congenital.

   r. fetalis micromelica. Congenital shortness of the bones.

rachitome (rā'kĭ-tōm). Instrument employed for opening spinal canal.

radiability (rā-dĭ-ă-bĭl'ĭ-tĭ). Capability of being penetrated readily by the x-ray.

radiad (rā'dĭ-ăd). In direction of the radial side.

radial (rā'dĭ-ăl). 1. Radiating out from a given center. 2. Pert. to the radius.

   r. reflex. Flexion of forearm resulting when lower end of radius is percussed.

radiant (rā'dĭ-ant). 1. Emitting beams of light. 2. Transmitted by radiation. 3. Emanating from a common center.

radiate (rā'dĭ-āt). 1. Spreading from a common center. 2. To spread from a common center.

radiation (rā-dĭ-ā'shŭn). 1. Process by which energy is propagated through space or matter not affected by it. 2. Emission of rays in all directions from a common center. 3. Treatment with a radioactive substance.

   r., far ultraviolet. Ultraviolet radiation of short wave length; farthest away from the visible spectrum.

   r., infrared. Near or short infrared extends from 7200 A. U. to 14,000 A. U. Far or long infrared from 15,000 to 150,-000 A. U.

   r., photochemical. From a therapeutic standpoint the electromagnetic spectrum divided into photothermal and photochemical radiations. Photochemical radiations penetrate only to fractions of millimeters, are absorbed by protoplasm, and cause physical and biological changes which manifest themselves after several hours from exposure.

r., photothermal. Photothermal radiations penetrate subcutaneous tissues, heat the blood, accelerate vital reactions and act instantaneously. SEE: *photochemical radiation.*

r., solar. Radiations of the sun, 60% in infrared region and 40% visible and ultraviolet, shortest wave length is 2900 A. U.

r., ultraviolet. Radiant energy extending from 3900 to 1800 A. U. Divided into "near ultraviolet," extending from 3900 to 2900 A. U., and "far ultraviolet," from 2900 to 1800 A. U.

r. unit. SEE: *Angström unit, Maché unit.*

r., visible. Visible spectrum may be broken up into different wave lengths representing different colors:

Violet	4000-4500 A. U.
Blue	4500-4900 " "
Green	4900-5500 " "
Yellow	5500-5900 " "
Orange	5900-6300 " "
Red	6300-7800 " "

SEE: *spectrum.*

radiator (rā'dĭ-ā-tor). Device for radiating heat or light.

r., infrared. Device for transmitting infrared rays. SEE: *heater, radiant.*

radical (răd'ĭ-kal). 1. A group of elements acting as a single element, passing without change from 1 compound to another one, but not able to exist in a free state. 2. Anything that reaches the root or origin; original. 3. A foundation or principle.

r. treatment. A treatment that seeks an absolute cure, as radical surgery; not palliative.

radicle (răd'ĭ-kl). 1. A structure resembling a rootlet, as a radicle of a nerve or vein. 2. Group of elements unaffected by chemical change, unable to exist in the free state.

radicotomy (răd-ĭ-kŏt'ō-mĭ). Section of a nerve, esp. post. spinal nerve roots. SYN: *rhizotomy.* SEE: *radiculectomy.*

radiculalgia (răd-ĭ-kū-lăl'jĭ-ă). Neuralgia of roots of nerves.

radicular (răd-ĭk'ū-lar). Concerning a root or radicle.

r. arteries. Those accessory to spinal nerve roots.

r. fibers. Those associated with spinal nerve roots.

r. syndrome. Symptoms due to interference with intradural part of spinal nerve roots.

r. vessels. Those supplying spinal nerves and their roots.

radiculectomy (răd-ĭk-ū-lĕk'tō-mĭ). 1. Excision of a spinal nerve root. 2. Resection of post. spinal nerve root. SEE: *radicotomy.*

radiculitis (răd-ĭk-ū-lī'tĭs). Inflammation of spinal nerve roots, accompanied by pain and hyperesthesia.

radiculomeningomyelitis (răd-ĭk″ū-lō-mē-nĭn″gō-mī-ĕl-ī'tĭs). Inflamed condition of nerve roots, meninges, and spinal cord. SYN: *rhizomeningomyelitis.*

radioactive (rā″dĭ-ō-ăk'tĭv). Exhibiting radioactivity.

r. constant. That part of the whole amt. of radioactive substance which, in a given unit of time, will disintegrate. SYMB: λ

radioactivity (rā″dĭ-ō-ăk-tĭv'ĭ-tĭ). The ability to emit rays or particles of matter, which can penetrate various substances, as radium.

r., induced. Temporary radioactivity of a substance which has been within the sphere of influence of a radioactive element.

radioanaphylaxis (rā″dĭ-ō-ăn-ă-fĭ-lăks'ĭs). Sensitization to radioactive energy.

radiocarpal (rā″dĭ-ō-kar'păl). Concerning the radius and carpus.

radiochemistry (rā″dĭ-ō-kĕm'ĭs-trĭ). The phase of chemistry dealing with radioactive phenomena.

radiochroism (rā″dĭ-ō-krō'ĭzm). The ability of a substance to absorb radioactive rays.

radiochrometer (rā″dĭ-ō-krŏm'ĕt-ĕr). Device for testing penetrating powers of x-rays and the character of roentgen tubes. SEE: *penetrometer.*

radiode (rā'dĭ-ōd). Metal container for radium, used in therapeutic application.

radiodermatitis (rā″dĭ-ō-dĕr″mă-tī'tĭs). Inflammation of the skin caused by roentgen rays or radiation from radioactive elements. SYN: *actinodermatitis, q.v.*

radiodiagnosis (rā″dĭ-ō-dī-ăg-nō'sĭs). Diagnosis by means of x-ray.

radioelement (rā″dĭ-ō-ĕl'e-mĕnt). An element possessing power of radioactivity.

radioepidermitis (rā″dĭ-ō-ĕp-ĭ-der-mī'tĭs). Irritation of the skin due to radioactive rays.

radioepithelitis (rā″dĭ-ō-ĕp-ĭ-thē-lī'tĭs). Disintegration of epithelium due to exposure to irradiation.

radiogen (rā'dĭ-ō-jĕn). Any substance containing radioactive elements. SYN: *actinogen.*

radiogenic (rā″dĭ-ō-jĕn'ĭk). 1. Due to irradiation. 2. Producing rays. SYN: *actinogenic.*

radiogenol (rā″dĭ-ō-jĕn'ŏl). A commercial emulsion of radioactive substances for injection into tumors.

radiogram (rā'dĭ-ō-grăm). X-ray picture, esp. of internal organs. SYN: *actinogram.*

radiograph (rā'dĭ-ō-grăf). A record produced on a photographic plate, film, or paper by the action of roentgen rays or radium; specifically an x-ray photograph.

radiographer (rā″dĭ-ŏg'ră-fer). A person skilled in making roentgenograms, or radiographs.

radiography (rā-dĭ-ŏg'ră-fĭ). The making of x-ray pictures. SYN: *roentgenography, skiagraphy.*

radiohumeral (rā″dĭ-ō-hū'mĕr-ăl). Concerning the radius and humerus.

radiologist (rā-dĭ-ŏl'ō-jĭst). One who practices diagnosis and treatment by radiant energy.

radiology (rā-dǐ-ol'ō-jǐ). The branch of science which deals with roentgen rays, radium rays, and other radiations, and their curative properties.

radiolucency (rā″dǐ-ō-lū'sĕn-sǐ). Property of being partly or wholly permeable to radiant energy.

radiolus (rā-dǐ'ō-lǔs). A sound; a probe.

radiometallography (rā″dǐ-ō-mĕt″ăl-ŏg'rä-fǐ). The study of metals by means of x-rays.

radiometer (rā-dǐ-ŏm'ĕt-ĕr). 1. An instrument used to estimate the quantity of roentgen rays, usually with pastilles or pieces of photographic paper.

2. An instrument in which radiant heat and light may be directly converted into mechanical energy as devised by Sir William Crookes.

3. An instrument for measuring intensity of radiant energy.

radion (rā'dǐ-ōn). One of the particles of the alpha, beta rays, or cathode rays, given off by radioactive matter.

radionecrosis (rā″dǐ-ō-nĕ-krō'sǐs). Disintegration of tissue by exposure to radiant energy.

radioneuritis (rā″dǐ-ō-nū-rī'tǐs). Neuritis caused by exposure to radioactive substance.

radiopaque (rā-dǐ-ō-pāk'). Impenetrable to the x-ray or other forms of radiation.

radioparent (rā″dǐ-ō-par'ĕnt). Penetrable by the x-ray or other rays.

radiopelvimetry (rā″dǐ-ō-pĕl-vǐm'ĕt-rǐ). Measurement of the pelvis by the x-ray.

radiopraxis (rā″dǐ-ō-prăks'ǐs). Diagnosis or use in treatment of some radioactive substance, as x-ray or ultraviolet ray. Syn: *actinopraxis*.

radioreceptor (rā″dǐ-ō-rē-sĕp'tor). Receptor responding to stimuli of radioactive elements, as to light and temperature. See: *receptor*.

radiosclerometer (rā″dǐ-ō-sklē-rŏm'ĕt-ĕr). An instrument that records penetration and intensity of the x-ray. Syn: *penetrometer, q.v.*

radioscopy (rā-dǐ-ōs'kō-pǐ). Inspection and examination of the inner structures of the body by means of roentgen ray. Syn: *actinoscopy*.

radiosensibility (rā″dǐ-ō-sĕn″sǐ-bǐl'ǐ-tǐ). Quality of sensitivity to radioactive substances.

radiosensitive (rā″dǐ-ō-sĕn'sǐ-tǐv). Capable of being destroyed by radiation, as a tumor by x-rays.

radiosurgery (rā″dǐ-ō-sur'jer-ǐ). The use of radium in surgery.

radiotherapist (rā″dǐ-ō-ther'ä-pǐst). One trained in use of radiant energy for therapeutic purposes.

radiotherapy (rā″dǐ-ō-ther'ä-pǐ). The treatment of disease by application of roentgen rays, radium, ultraviolet, and other radiations.

radiothermitis (rā″dǐ-ō-ther-mī'tǐs). Dermatitis caused by exposure to x-rays or other radiant substances.

radiothermy (rā″dǐ-ō-ther'mǐ). Use of heat, in treatment, obtained from radio-active substances by specially built short wave apparatus.

radiotoxemia (rā″dǐ-ō-tŏks-ē'mǐ-ă). Toxemia produced by exposure to radioactive substance. Syn: *actinotoxemia*.

radiotransparent (rā″dǐ-ō-trăns-par'ĕnt). Penetrable by x-ray or other forms of radiation.

radiotropic (rā″dǐ-ō-trŏp'ǐk). Affected by radiation.

radioulnar (rā″dǐ-ō-ǔl'nar). Concerning the radius and ulna.

radio wave (rā'dǐ-ō wāv). Electric wave produced by or employing radiant energy.* See: *radiothermy*.

radium (rā'dǐ-ŭm). Symb: Ra. A metallic element found in very small quantities in pitchblende. At. wt. 226.4. See: *"actin-" words*.

r. emanation. Heavy, colorless, gaseous element given off in disintegration of radium. Syn: *radon*.

Its concentration is measured in terms of the Maché unit, abbr. *m. u.*

r. intratumoral application. Implanting radium into tumors for therapeutic purposes.

r. needles. Radium needles contain from 2 to 12½ milligrams of radium element. The usual material employed for needle containers is a steel alloy. The wall thickness is from 0.2 to 0.4 millimeters.

radiumization (rā″dǐ-ŭm-ǐ-za'shŭn). Exposure to action of radium rays.

radiumologist (rā″dǐ-ŭm-ŏl'ō-jǐst). One who specializes in radium therapy.

radiumology (rā″dǐ-ŭm-ŏl'ō-jǐ). The science of radium therapy.

radium therapy (rā'dǐ-ŭm ther'ă-pǐ). The treatment of disease by means of radium, radon, its emanation, or its active deposit.

radius (rā'dǐ-ŭs). 1. The outer and shorter bone of the arm which revolves partially about the ulna. 2. A line extending from a circle's center point to its circumference.

r., fracture of. Colles' Fracture: A fracture and dislocation of lower end of radius, generally caused by falling on the outstretched hand.

radix (ra'dǐks) (pl. *radices*). 1. The root portion of a cranial or spinal nerve. 2. The root of a plant.

radon (rā'dŏn). A heavy radioactive gas given off in the disintegration of radium. Syn: *niton, radium emanation*.

ragsorters' disease (răg'sort'ers). A febrile pulmonary disease arising in persons who sort paper and rags due to inhalation of bacillus causing anthrax, *q.v.*

railway spine (rāl'wǎ). A traumatic neurasthenia due to injuries in railway accidents.

raised (rāzd). Bact: Having a thick, elevated growth with terraced edges.

râle (rahl). Bubbling sound heard in bronchi in inspiration and expiration in disease.

r., bronchiectatic. Heard over bronchiectatic cavities filled with accumulated secretion. Disappears with expectoration.

r., bubbling medium. Heard in inspiration and expiration; produced by passage of air through mucus in the larger tubes; character, larger than the small bubbling moist râle; heard in capillary bronchitis, esp. in children.

r., cavernous. Heard in inspiration and expiration; produced by passage of air through a small cavity with flaccid walls that collapse with expiration; character, hollow and metallic; heard in the 3rd stage of pulmonary tuberculosis.

r., clicking. Heard in inspiration only; produced by passage of air through softening material in smaller bronchi; character, small, sticky; heard in pulmonary tuberculosis, early stage.

r., coarse. Originates in the larger bronchi.

r., crackling, medium. Heard chiefly in inspiration; produced by fluid in the finer bronchi; character, larger than the small, crackling, dry; heard in softening of the tubercular deposit, or pneumonic exudation.

r., crepitant. Heard at end of inspiration; produced by passage of air into collapsed vesicles containing fibrinous exudation, usually at base of lungs; character, small, like rubbing hair bet. the fingers; heard in pneumonia, in early stage edema of lungs, hypostatic pneumonia. It is localized in pulmonary tuberculosis.

r., dry. Heard in inspiration and expiration; produced by narrowing of the bronchial tubes from thickening of their mucous lining, from spasmodic contraction of the muscular coat, viscid mucus within or pressure from without; character, large and sonorous, small, hissing or whistling; heard in bronchitis, asthma, and localized in beginning pulmonary tuberculosis.

r., friction. Heard in inspiration and expiration, most distinct at end of respiration, produced by the rubbing together of serous surfaces roughened by inflammation or deprived of their natural secretions; character, grazing, rubbing, grating, creaking, or crackling; heard in pleurisy and pericarditis.

r., gurgling. Heard in inspiration and expiration; produced by passage of air through fluid in cavities of large bubbles; heard in pulmonary tuberculosis after formation of cavities.

r., moist. Produced by passage of air through bronchi containing fluid.

r., mucous (of Laennec). Heard in inspiration and expiration; produced by viscid bubbles bursting in the bronchial tubes; character, modification of the subcrepitant; heard in pulmonary emphysema.

r. redux, r. de retour. Heard in inspiration and expiration; produced by passage of air through fluid in bronchial tubes; character, crackling, unequal; heard in pneumonia, in the stage of resolution.

r., sibilant. High pitched, whistling, and frequent at end of inspiration.

r., sonorous. Low snoring, greater in volume, continuing during inspiration.

r., subcrepitant. Heard in inspiration and expiration; produced by passage of air through mucus in the capillary bronchial tubes; character, small, moist; heard in capillary bronchitis.

r., submucous. Higher pitched and more numerous than large mucous râle. Heard in interscapular and supramammary regions and indicating involvement of many tubes of small caliber.

rami (rā′mī). Plural of *ramus,* a branch.

ramification (răm-ĭ-fĭ-kā′shŭn). 1. Process of branching. 2. A branch. 3. Arrangement in branches.

ramify (răm′ĭ-fī). To branch; to spread out in different directions.

ramisection (răm′ĭ-sĕk″shŭn, răm″ĭ-sĕk′shŭn). Section of nerve fibrils bet. the spinal and sympathetic systems.

ramisectomy (răm-ĭs-ĕk′tō-mĭ). Excision of a ramus, specifically ramus communicans. SEE: *ramisection.*   [mation.

ramitis (răm-ī′tĭs). A nerve root inflam-

ramollissement (rah″mo-lēs-mon′). Morbid softening of some organ or tissue, esp. of brain.

ramus (rā′mŭs) (pl. *rami*). 1. A branch of 1 of the divisions of a forked structure. 2. Post. portion of lower jawbone. 3. BNA. Primary division of a blood vessel or nerve.

r. communicans. Small nerve fiber passing bet. fibers from ant. roots of the spinal cord and a sympathetic ganglion. SEE: *sympathetic nervous system.*

rancid (răn′sĭd). Offensive; having a sour smell or taste from partial decomposition, as a *fat.*

range of accommodation. Difference bet. least and greatest distance of distinct vision. SEE: *accommodation.*

ranine (rā′nīn). 1. Pert. to a ranula or to the region beneath the tip of the tongue. 2. Branch of the lingual artery supplying that area.

Ranvier's nodes (ron-vē-ās′). Constrictions in the medullary substance of a nerve fiber at more or less regular intervals. SEE: *nerve.*

ranula (răn′ū-lă). A large cystic tumor seen on underside of tongue on either side of the frenum.

r. pancreatica. Cystic disease of pancreas due to obstruction of its ducts.

rape (rāp). 1. Coitus with a woman without her consent and accomplished by force or intimidation. 2. To commit rape upon. SYN: *stupration.*

raphania (răf-ā′nĭ-ă). A spasmodic disease caused by eating seeds of the wild radish; allied to ergotism, *q.v.* SYN: *rhaphania.*

raphe (rā′fē). 1. A crease or ridge or seam noting union of the halves of a part, as the division of the 2 lateral halves of the scrotum. 2. A suture.

rapport'. PSY: A relationship of sympathy and confidence.

rarefaction (rar″ē-făk'shŭn). Process of decreasing density and weight, as of *air*.

r. of bone. The process of making bone more porous because of absorption of lime salts.

rar'efy″ing os″tei'tis. Chronic bone inflammation marked by development of granulation tissue in marrow spaces with absorption of surrounding hard bone. SEE: *osteitis.*

rash (răsh). Temporary eruption on skin, with little or no elevation. SYN: *exanthema.* SEE: *lesion, roseola.*

r., drug. One caused by use of certain drugs, such as *bromide* or *iodine.* SEE: *idiosyncrasy.*

r., enema. One caused by too much soap in an enema; resembles measles.

r., gum. A red, papular eruption of the mouth, a form of miliaria, seen esp. in infants, due to intestinal disturbances. SYN: *strophulus.*

r., mulberry. Rash seen in typhus fever; dusky in color.

r., nettle. Smooth, elevated, itchy, white patches. SYN: *hives, urticaria.*

r., red. SEE: *gum rash.*   [*roseola.*

r., rose. Any rose-colored rash. SYN:

r., tooth. SEE: *gum rash.*

raspatory (răs'pă-tō″rĭ). File used in surgery, esp. for trimming surfaces of bone.

rasura, rasure (ră-sū'ră, ră'zhur). 1. Process of scraping, or shaving. 2. Scrapings or filings.

rat (răt). A rodent found in and around human habitations.

r. unit. Greatest dilution of an estrus-producing hormone which will cause desquamation and cornification of vaginal epithelium during 1st day, if given to a mature spayed rat in 3 injections, 1 every 4 hours.

ratbite fever. An infectious disease transmitted by bite of a rat, caused by infection with *Spirillum minus.*

rate (răt). 1. Valuation based on comparison with a standard. 2. Measure of a thing.

Rathke's columns (raht'keh). Two cartilages elongated at ant. extremity of chorda dorsalis.

R.'s diverticulum, R.'s pouch. A pouch in bucco-pharyngeal embryonic membrane from which is developed the ant. lobe of the hypophysis cerebri.

ratio (rā'shĭ-ō). Proportion.

ration (rā'shŭn). Fixed allowance of food and drink for a certain period.

rational (răsh'ŭn-ăl). 1. Of sound mind. SYN: *sane.* 2. Reasonable or logical. 3. Employing treatments based on reasoning or general principles, opposed to empiric.

r. formula. A chemical one, written in symbols showing the constituents of a molecule and the atomic arrangement and relationship in it.

r. symptom. One discovered by questioning instead of by physical examination.

rationalization (răsh-ŭn-ăl-ĭ-zā'shŭn). PSY: Rational or plausible explanation of behavior or belief activated by unknown motives.

rattle (răt'l). A sound or râle heard on auscultation.

r., death. A gurgling sound or subcrepitant râle heard in the trachea of the dying.

Rau's process (rowz). Slender, long process of the malleus. SYN: *processus gracilis mallei.*

Rauber's layer (row'ber). The external layer of cells partially composing the ectoderm of the primitive embryo.

raucous (raw'kŭs). Hoarse, strident, as the sound of a voice.

rave (rāv). To talk irrationally, as in delirium.

raving (rāv'ĭng). 1. Irrational utterance. 2. Talking irrationally.

ravish (răv'ĭsh). 1. To commit rape upon a girl or woman. 2. To remove or carry away by force.

ray (rā). 1. One of a number of lines diverging from a common center. 2. Line of propagation of any form of radiant energy, esp. light or heat; loosely, any narrow beam of light.

r., actinic. A solar ray of the spectrum capable of producing chemical changes.

r., alpha. Ray composed of positively charged particles of helium derived from atomic disintegration of radioactive elements.   [2700 to 3020 A. U.

r., antirachitic. Ultraviolet ray from

r., bactericidal. Ray bet. 1850 and 2600 A. U. which is strongly bactericidal

r's., Becquerel's. Those from radium uranium, and other radioactive substances.

r's., beta. Negatively charged electrons expelled from atoms of disintegrating radioactive elements.

r's., Blondlot's. SEE: *n-rays.*

r's., border; r's., borderline; r's. Bucky. SEE: *Grenz rays.*

r's., canal. Positive rays in a vacuum tube going from anode toward cathode Old name for positive ray.

r's., cathode. Negatively charged electrons discharged by the cathode through a vacuum, moving in a straight line and upon hitting solid matter produce roentgen rays.

r., characteristic. Secondary roentgen rays, the wave lengths of which are determined by the chemical constitution of the object that emits, transmits or scatters them.

r., chemical. SEE: *actinic ray.*

r., cosmic. SEE: *Millikan's rays.*

r's., delta. Highly penetrative ether waves given off by radioactive substances.

r's., dynamic. Rays which are physically or therapeutically active.

r., erythema-producing. Ray bet. 1800 and 4000 A. U., which produces erythema; those around 2540 and bet. 2050 and 3100 A. U. being most effective.

r., Finsen (or light). Ultraviolet radiation from the Finsen lamp.

r's., fluorescent roentgen. Secondary rays whose wave lengths are characteristic of the substance which emits them.

r. fungus. Genus of parasitic fungi with radiating formation.

r., gamma. Heterogeneous vibrations caused by electronic disturbance in atoms of radioactive elements during their disintegration and appear identical with roentgen rays except that the wave lengths range from about 1.4 to 0.01 angströms. They have high velocity and penetrative power. They lie bet. ultraviolet and roentgen rays.

r., Grenz. Soft roentgen ray with an average wave length of 2 angströms (range from 1 to 3 angströms); obtained with peak voltage of less than 10 kilovolts.

r's., hard. X-rays of short wave length and great penetration.

r's., heat. Visible rays from 4000 to 7000 A. U. and infrared rays from 6000 to 14,000 A. U. The heating effect of visible rays on deeper tissue is proportionately stronger than that of infrared rays, on account of greater penetrating power. See: heat.

r's., Hertzian. Electromagnetic waves of great wave length. Used in radio communication.

r's., infrared. Radiations just beyond the red end of the spectrum. Their wave lengths range bet. 7700 and 500,000 angströms. The therapeutic range extends from about 7700 to about 14,000 angströms.

r's., Lenard's. Cathode rays that have passed outside the discharge tube. See: cathode ray.

r., luminous. Visible ray.

r., medullary. Cortical protuberance from a bundle of tubules in a renal pyramid.

r's., Millikan. Electromagnetic waves coming from unknown sources, resembling the gamma rays, but their penetration is greater and their wave length shorter.

r's., monochromatic. Rays characterized by a definite wave length, as secondary rays.

r's., n. Radiant energy emitted by active nerves and muscles, affecting a fluorescent screen similar to x-rays; discovered by Blondlot.

r's., pigment-producing. Rays at 2500 and 3000 A. U. are most effective in causing pigmentation, a local response to irritation of cutaneous prickle cells.

r., positive. Ray of positively charged ions which, in a discharge tube, go from the anode toward the cathode.

r., primary. Ray discharged directly from a radioactive substance, as the alpha, beta, and gamma rays.

r., roentgen. X-rays discovered by Wilhelm Konrad Roentgen. They have a penetrative power through opaque substances.

r's., scattered. Roentgen rays or gamma rays which, in their passage through a substance, have deviated in direction and also may have been changed by an increase in wave length.

r's., Schumann. Rays in the region bounded bet. 1220 and 1850 angströms.

r's., secondary. Roentgen rays emitted in all directions by any matter irradiated with roentgen rays.

r's., ultraviolet. Invisible rays of the spectrum which are beyond the violet rays, and of varying wave lengths.

r's., x-. See: roentgen rays.

Raynaud's disease (rä-nōz'). Severe, paroxysmal, nervous disorder causing disturbances of the circulation in the extremities.

Rb. Symb. for rubidium.

R. C. P. Royal College of Physicians.

R. C. S. Royal College of Surgeons.

R. D. A. Right dorsoanterior presentation position of the fetus.

R. D. P. Right dorsoposterior presentation position of the fetus.

R. E. Abbr. for radium emanation and for right eye.

re-. Prefix meaning back or again.

reaction (rē-ăk'shŭn). 1. Mutual action of chemical agents upon each other. 2. Response of a muscle or nerve to stimulation, including its rebound or opp. movement. 3. Emotional and mental state created by a situation.

r., cutaneous deep. Psy: Diminution or abolition of pressure, musculoarticular, or osseous sensibility occurs with conservation of thermic, tactile and pain sensibility.

r. of degeneration. The change in muscle reactivity to electricity, seen in lower motor neuron paralysis.

r. formation. The checking of infantile impulses and tendencies which might become those of an antisocial nature later, or which might hold the individual upon an infantile level and the attributes developed from such partial repressions, such as modesty, shame, or disgust.

r., miostagmin. Diagnostic test for syphilis, malignant tumors, and typhoid involving determination of surface tension of blood serum.

r., ophthalmic. Ocular reaction to introduction of toxins of tuberculosis and typhoid fever; more severe in those having the diseases.

r. period. See: reaction time.

r's. of sensibility. Tests to determine forms of sensibility by pressure, tactile means, heat, pain, etc.

r. time. Time elapsing bet. giving a stimulus word and the response to it.

reactive depression (rē-ăk'tĭv dē-prĕsh'-ŭn). Psy: A psychosis resulting from bereavement, sadness, or a situation causing such emotions, lasting longer and more marked than the normal reaction.

reagent (rē-ā'jĕnt). 1. A substance which may be added to a solution to detect the presence or absence of a certain substance, or to produce a chemical reaction. 2. PSY: Subject of a psychological experiment, esp. one reacting to a stimulus.

reality principle (rē-ăl'ĭ-tĭ). The effect of necessity or external consideration, acting to control self-gratification, or of the ego's self-protective influences.

reapers' keratitis (rēp'ĕrs kĕr-ă-tī'tĭs). Keratitis caused by dust from grain.

Réaumur's thermometer (rā'o-mur). A thermometric scale having 0° for the freezing point, and 80° for the boiling point of water.

rebreathing (rē-brēth'ĭng). Administration of oxygen to a patient under a general anesthetic for speedy elimination of the anesthetic.

recall (rē-kawl'). PSY: Act of bringing back to mind that which has been previously learned or experienced; reproduction.

recapitulation theory (rē″kă-pĭt-ū-lā'shŭn). The idea that man's development from the ovum to maturity repeats and represents all the stages of evolution through which he is supposed to have developed.

receiver (rē-sēv'er). Container for holding a gas or a distillate.

receptaculum (rē-sĕp-tăk'ū-lŭm). A vessel or cavity in which a fluid is contained.
  r. chyli. Inferior, pear-shaped, expanded portion of the lower end of the thoracic duct, near 1st and 2nd lumbar vertebrae, into which certain lymphatics discharge.
  r. seminis. Post. *cul-de-sac* of the vagina, so named because it was once assumed to be a receptacle for the semen during sexual intercourse.

receptor (rē-sĕp'tor). 1. Molecular group in cells which have a special affinity for toxins, amboceptors, etc. SEE: *Ehrlich's side chain theory.* 2. Group of cells functioning in reception of stimuli; a sense organ; endings of afferent (sensory) nerves.
  r. neuron (sensory). One carrying impulses from the periphery to the center.

recessus (rē-sĕs'ŭs). A small hollow or recess.
  r. cochlearis. Hollow or inner wall of the labyrinthine vestibule, perforated for passing of nerves supplying the ductus cochlearis.
  r. opticus. BNA. Optic recess above the optic chiasm.
  r. parotideus. Deep recess in front of the mastoid in which is lodged the parotid gland.
  r. pharyngeus. Fossa in nasopharynx on either side of the eustachian tubes.

recipe (rĕs'ĭ-pē). 1. Take, indicated by the sign ℞. 2. A prescription or formula for a medicine.

recipient (rē-sĭp'ĭ-ĕnt). One who receives anything, esp. the blood in transfusion. SEE: *donor.*

reciprocal (rē-sĭp'rō-kăl). Interchangeable in character.
  r. reception. Articulation with convex surface in 1 direction and concave surface in another.

Recklinghausen's canals (rek'lĭng-how-zĕn). Tiny channels conveying lymph in connective tissue which are continuations of the lymphatics, being their roots.
  R.'s disease. 1. A condition characterized by pigmentation of the skin and multiple neurofibromata of trunk and scalp. SYN: *Von Recklinghausen's disease.* 2. Generalized fibrocystic bone disease. 3. Arthritis with deformity and neoplastic formations.

reclination (rĕk-lĭ-nā'shŭn). The turning of the eye lens covered with a cataract over into the vitreous to remove it from line of vision.

recline (rē-klīn'). To be in recumbent position; to lie down.

Reclus' disease (rē-klū'). Multiple, benign, cystic growths in the mammary gland.
  R.'s method. The use of cocaine to produce local anesthesia.
  R.'s operation. Creation of an artificial anus in cancer of the rectum.

reconstituent (rē″kŏn-stĭt'ū-ĕnt). An agent that improves or strengthens 1 or more parts or functions of the body by replacing lost material. Ex: *calcium, iron, phosphorus.* SYN: *tonic.*

recrement (rĕk're-mĕnt). Secretion which, after having performed its function as the saliva or part of the bile, is reabsorbed into the blood.

recrementitious (rĕk″rē-mĕn-tĭsh'ŭs). Of the nature of a secretion which, having performed its function, is reabsorbed into the blood.

recrudescence (rē-krū-dĕs'ĕns). Return of symptoms. SYN: *relapse.*

recrudescent (rē-krū-dĕs'ĕnt). Assuming renewed activity.

rectal (rĕkt'ăl). Pert. to the rectum.
  r. alimentation. Rectal feeding, *q.v.*
  r. anesthesia. Introduction of anesthetic into rectum for local desensitization, used esp. in labor. SEE: *anesthesia, labor.*
  r. crisis. Tenesmus and rectal pain in locomotor ataxia.
  r. feeding. The introduction of nutrients in fluid form into the colon through the rectum. SYN: *nutrient enema, q.v.*
  r. reflex. The normal desire to evacuate feces present in rectum.

rectalgia (rĕk-tăl'jĭ-ă). Pain in rectum.

rectectomy (rĕk-tĕk'tō-mĭ). Excision of the rectum or anus. SYN: *proctectomy.*

rectification (rĕk″tĭ-fĭ-kā'shŭn). 1. The process of refining or purifying a substance. 2. Act of straightening or correcting.

rectified (rĕk'tĭ-fīd). Made pure or straight. Set right.
  r. spirit. One resulting from fractional or repeated distillation of alcohol, as whisky.

rectifier (rĕk'tĭ-fī"ĕr). A device for obtaining a unidirectional current from an alternating current.

rectitis (rĕk-tī'tĭs). Inflamed condition of the rectum. SYN: *proctitis.*

recto-. Combining form meaning *straight, the rectum.*

rectocele (rĕk'tō-sēl). Protrusion of post. vaginal wall with ant. wall of rectum through the vagina.

rectoclysis (rĕk-tŏk'lĭs-ĭs). Slow introduction of fluid into rectum. SYN: *Murphy drip, proctoclysis.*

rectococcypexia (rĕk"tō-kŏk-sĭ-pĕks'sĭ-ă). Fixation of rectum by suturing it to coccyx.

rectocolitis (rĕk"tō-kō-lī'tĭs). Inflamed condition of rectum and colon. SYN: *proctocolitis.*

rectocystotomy (rĕk"tō-sĭs-tŏt'ō-mĭ). Incision of the bladder through rectum, usually to remove a calculus.

rectopexy (rĕk'tō-pĕks-ĭ). Fixation of rectum by suturing to another part. SYN: *proctopexy.*

rectophobia (rĕk"tō-fō'bĭ-ă). Morbid fear in those patients with rectal disease.

rectoplasty (rĕk'tō-plăs"tĭ). Plastic operation on the anus and rectum. SYN: *proctoplasty.*

rectorrhaphy (rĕk-tor'ră-fĭ). Suture of rectum and anus. SYN: *proctorrhaphy.*

rectoscope (rĕk'tō-skōp). A speculum to examine the rectum.

rectosigmoid (rĕk"tō-sĭg'moyd). Upper part of rectum and adjoining portion of sigmoid colon.   [ture of rectum.

rectostenosis (rĕk"tō-stĕn-ō'sĭs). Stric-

rectostomy (rĕk-tŏs'tō-mĭ). Creation of an artificial opening into the rectum to relieve stricture. SYN: *proctostomy, q.v.*

rectotomy (rĕk-tŏt'ō-mĭ). Incision for stricture of the rectum or other purposes. SYN: *proctotomy, q.v.*

rectourethral (rĕk"tō-ū-rē'thrăl). Concerning the rectum and urethra.

rectouterine (rĕk"tō-ū'tĕr-ĭn). Concerning the rectum and uterus.

rectovaginal (rĕk"tō-văj'ĭn-ăl). Concerning the rectum and vagina.

rectovesical (rĕk"tō-vĕs'ĭk-ăl). Concerning the rectum and bladder.

rectum (rĕk'tŭm). Lower part of large intestine, about 5 in. (12 cm.) long, bet. sigmoid flexure and the anus.

rectus (rĕk'tŭs). 1. Straight; not crooked. 2. Any straight muscle.
    r. muscles. 1. Two ext. abdominal muscles, 1 on each side, from pubic bone to the ensiform cartilage and 5th, 6th, and 7th ribs. 2. Four short muscles of the eye, *ext., int., sup.,* and *inf.*

recumbent (rē-kŭm'bĕnt). 1. Lying down. SEE: *left lateral recumbent position, prone.* 2. One who is lying down.

recuperation (rē-kū"per-ā'shŭn). Restoration to normal health.

recurrence (rē-kŭr'ĕns). Return of symptoms after a period of quiescence, as in recurrent fever and in yellow fever. SYN: *relapse.*

recurrent (rē-kur'ĕnt). Returning at intervals, as a fever.

recurrentotherapy (rē-kur"rĕnt-ō-ther'ă-pĭ). Therapeutic inoculation with organisms of a recurrent fever.

recurve (rē-kurv'). Bend backward.

red (rĕd). A primary color of the spectrum.
    r. blindness. Inability to see red hues. The most frequent color blindness.
    r. blood cell. Blood corpuscle containing hemoglobin. SYN: *erythrocyte, q.v.*   [minium.
    r. lead. Lead tetroxide, Pb_3O_4;
    r. nucleus. Gray matter in the tegmentum. SYN: *nucleus ruber.*
    r. precipitate. Red mercuric oxide.
    r. softening. Hemorrhagic softening of the brain and cord.
    r. streak. One lasting more than 14 seconds when the skin is stroked with a pressure of about 10 oz. by a hard object followed by a white line in a few seconds which lasts a minute or 2; a reflex vasodilatation.

redintegration (rĕd-ĭn-tĕ-grā'shŭn). 1. Restitution of a part. 2. Restoration to health. 3. Recall by mental association.

redressment (rē-drĕs'mĕnt). 1. Correction of a deformity. 2. Dressing of a wound more than once.

reduce (rē-dūs'). 1. To restore to usual relationship, as the ends of a fractured bone. 2. To weaken, as a solution. 3. To diminish, as in bulk or weight.

reducible (rē-dūs'ĭ-bl). Capable of being replaced in a normal position, as a dislocated bone, a hernia, etc.

reductase (rē-dŭk'tās). An enzyme accelerating process of reduction of chemical compounds.

reduction (rē-dŭk'shŭn). 1. Restoration to normal position, as a hernia. 2. CHEM: A type of reaction in which hydrogen is taken up by the given compound, or oxygen is removed, or the valence of the metallic element is lowered. *Cf. oxidation.*
    r. diet. One that eliminates fat-producing foods.
    Normal metabolism must be preserved. Bulk, mineral, protein, vitamin, and water requirements must be maintained. Energy value should be 600 to 1500 calories below maintenance requirements. Not over 10 to 20 Gm. of fat per day. Carbo., 52 Gm.; Pro., 60 Gm.; Fat, 45 Gm.; Cal., 850.
    r. d., modified, Evans-Strang. 970 Cal. diet: Carbo., 50 Gm.; Pro., 80 Gm.; Fat, 50 Gm. 1500 Cal. diet: Carbo., 115 Gm.; Pro., 80 Gm.; Fat, 80 Gm. 1800 Cal. diet: Carbo., 180 Gm.; Pro., 85 Gm. Emphasis placed on avoidance of food poor in vitamins and minerals and high in calories. SEE: *obesity diet.*

reduplicated (rē-dū'plĭ-kā"tĕd). 1. Doubled. 2. Bent backward upon itself, as a fold.

reduplication (rē-dū"plĭ-kā'shŭn). 1. A doubling, as of the heart sounds in some morbid conditions. 2. A fold.

reëducation (rē″ĕd-ū-kā'shŭn). 1. Training of a disabled or mentally disordered individual to restore to him at least partial competence. 2. Physical means for restoring muscular tone and activity.

referred pain (rē-ferd' pān). Pain felt in a part removed from its point of origin. SYN: *synalgia*.

refine (rē-fīn'). To purify or render free from foreign material.

reflection (rē-flĕk'shŭn). 1. Process or condition of bending back. 2. The throwing back of a ray of radiant energy from a surface not penetrated. 3. Mental consideration of some subject matter.

reflector (rē-flĕk'tor). Device or surface which reflects waves of radiant energy or sound.

reflex (rē'flĕks). 1. Turned backward. 2. Pert. to a reflex action. 3. An involuntary act in response to a nervous impulse transmitted inward by afferent fibers to a nerve center and outward by efferent fibers to an effector, as a muscle or gland; the process culminating in such an act, called reflex action.

  r. action. The transmission of an impulse from a sensory to a motor nerve. SEE: *reflex, 3.*

  r. arc. The structures which are concerned with reflex action, *i. e.*, receptor and effector nerves and a nerve center.

  r. center. Spot in spinal cord or brain where a sensory impression is converted into a motor impulse.

  r., conditioned. A reflex which arises as a response to some particular situation, the reflex being aroused and modified by association with some past experience. The majority of the bodily acts are reflex in type, *e. g.*, sneezing, blinking, coughing, etc.

  r., deep. One caused by stimulation of parts beneath skin, like tendons or bones, as the jaw, elbow, wrist, triceps, knee, and ankle jerk reflexes.

  r., delayed. One not taking place until some seconds after application of stimulus.

  r., elbow jerk; r., biceps. Normal reflex caused by tapping of tendon on the biceps.

  r., excitomotor. Organic, as in defecation, urination, respiration.

  r., knee jerk. This is illustrative of a series of so-called deep muscular reflexes. If one strikes the patellar tendon, the quadriceps femoris contracts, extending the leg.

  r., myenteric. Contraction above the stimulation point of intestines and relaxation below it.

  r., organic. One of natural phenomena as those of defecation and urination.

  r., patellar. SEE: *knee jerk.*

  r., pathologic. Abnormal reflex due to disease and seen as one of its symptoms.

  r., pupillary. A beam of light striking the retina normally causes the pupil to contract (protective against excessive stimulation). The same effect results with accommodation to near objects.

  r., superficial (cutaneous). Reflex caused by irritation of the skin or areas depending upon the spinal cord as a motor center, such as the *scapular, epigastric, abdominal, cremasteric, gluteal,* and *plantar reflexes,* or upon *centers in the medulla,* as *conjunctival, pupillary,* and *palatal reflexes.*

  r., tendon. Deep reflex obtained by tapping skin over tendon of a muscle sharply.

  It is exaggerated in disease of an upper motor neuron, and diminished or lost in disease of lower neuron.

reflexogenic (rē-flĕks″ō-jĕn'ĭk). Causing a reflex action.

reflexograph (rē-flĕks'ō-grăf). Device for charting a reflex.

reflexometer (rē-flĕks-ŏm'ĕt-ĕr). Instrument for measuring force of the tap required to excite a reflex.

reflexophil (rē-flĕks'ō-fĭl). Characterized by activity of, or exaggerated, reflexes.

reflexotherapy (rē-flĕks-ō-ther'ă-pĭ). Treatment by manipulation, anesthetizing, or cauterizing an area distant from seat of the disorder. SEE: *spondylotherapy, zone therapy.*

reflux (rē'flŭks). A return or backward flow. SYN: *regurgitation, 2.*

refract (rē-frăkt'). 1. To turn back. 2. To deflect a light ray. 3. To detect errors of refraction in the eyes and to correct them.

refracta dosi (rē-frak'tă dō'sĭ). In divided doses, denoting a definite amt. of a drug taken within a given time in a number of fractional equal parts.

refraction (rē-frăk'shŭn). 1. Deflection from a straight path, as of light rays as they pass through media of different densities; the change of direction of a ray when it passes from one medium to another of a different density. 2. Determination of amount of ocular refractive errors and their correction. SEE: *catadioptric.*

refractionist (rē-frăk'shŭn-ĭst). One skilled in determining and correcting ocular refractive errors by means of glasses.

refractive (rē-frăkt'ĭv). Concerning refraction.

refractometer (rē-frăk-tŏm'ĕt-ĕr). Device for measuring the refractive power, as of the eye.

refractory (rē-frăk'tō-rĭ). Not responsive to ordinary treatment.

  r. period. A short period in muscle and nerve functioning after activity when stimuli will not excite tissue.

refractoscope (rē-frăk'tō-skōp). Device for auscultation of heart sounds.

refracture (rē-frăk'chŭr). 1. To break again, as a bone set wrongly. 2. Rebreaking of a fracture previously united in the wrong position.

refrangible (rē-frăn'jĭ-bl). Capable of refraction.

refresh (rē-frĕsh'). 1. To restore strength; to relieve from fatigue; to renew; to revive. 2. To scrape epithelial covering from 2 opposing surfaces of a wound to cause them to unite.

refrigerant (rē-frĭj'ĕr-ănt). 1. Allaying heat or fever; cooling. 2. Medicine or agent which relieves thirst and is cooling or reduces a fever. SEE: *algefacient*.

r. gases. A number of these gases are used in ordinary household mechanical refrigerators; poisoning due to leaks, faulty connections or breakage, and gas dissipated into atmosphere may occur.

refrigeration (rē-frĭj″ĕr-ā'shŭn). In physical therapy the therapeutic application of low temperatures, as with solid carbon dioxide.

refusion (rē-fū'zhŭn). 1. Process of melting again. 2. The return of blood to the circulation after being temporarily cut off by a ligature.

regeneration (rē-jĕn″ĕr-ā'shŭn). Repair, regrowth, or restoration of a part, as tissues. Opp. of *degeneration, q.v.*

r., pathological. Renewal of injured tissues by pathological rather than by physiological processes.

regimen (rĕj'ĭ-mĕn). 1. Regulation of diet, sleep, exercise, and manner of living to improve or maintain health. 2. Hygiene.

region (rē'jŭn). A portion of the body with natural or arbitrary boundaries. SEE: *abdomen*.

regional (rē'jŭn-ăl). Concerning a region.

registrant (rĕj'ĭs-trănt). A nurse who is named on the books of a registry as being "on call" for duty.

registrar (rĕj'ĭs-trar). The official manager of a registry.

registry (rĕj'ĭs-trĭ). An office or book where a list of nurses ready for duty is kept; a placement bureau for nurses.

regression (rē-grĕsh'ŭn). 1. Abatement or return of symptoms. 2. Degeneration. 3. PSY: The turning back of the libido, upon encountering difficulties, to an early fixation, from a higher to a lower level. 4. BIOL: Reversion of offspring from the mean of parental traits to normal type.

regressive (rē-grĕs'sĭv). Concerning or marked by regression.

regular (rĕg'ū-lar). 1. Conforming to rule or custom. 2. Methodical, steady in course, as pulse. SYN: *normal, typical.*

r. practitioner. A physician of the regular school of medicine.

r. school. That system of medicine to which the greatest number of physicians belong; erroneously called the *allopathic school*; founded on scientific facts and the knowledge gained by experience.

regurgitant (rē-gŭr'jĭt-ănt). Throwing or flowing back.

regurgitation (rē-gŭr-jĭ-tā'shŭn). 1. Return of solids or fluids to the mouth from the stomach. 2. Reflux of blood from the ventricles into the auricles when the heart valves are defective.

r., cardiac. Backward flow of blood through the *aortic mitral*, and *tricuspid* valves due to incomplete closure.

rehabilitation (rē″hă-bĭl″ĭ-tā'shŭn). Process of restoring, or of undergoing restoration, to health or efficiency, as a person physically handicapped.

rehalation (rē-ha-lā'shŭn). Rebreathing process occasionally employed in anesthesia.

Reichart's cartilage (rī'kerts). The hyoid cartilaginous arch of the embryo which becomes the styloid process, stylohyoid ligaments, and lesser cornua of the hyoid bone.

Reichmann's disease (rīk'mahnz). Excessive gastric secretion, without intermission. SYN: *gastrochronorrhea, gastrorrhea, gastrosuccorrhea.*

Reid's base line (rēds). One extending from lower edge of the orbit to center of aperture of ext. auditory canal backward to center of occipital bone.

Reil's island (rīlz). Three or more small convolutions at bottom of fissure of Sylvius. SYN: *the insula, island of Reil, q.v.*

reimplantation (rē″ĭm-plăn-tā'shŭn). Replacement of a part from where it has been taken out, as a tooth.

reinfection (rē″ĭn-fĕk'shŭn). Infection after recovery or during convalescence from the original disease.

reinforcement (rē″ĭn-fors'mĕnt). Strengthening of the response to one stimulus by concurrent action of another; the exaggeration of a reflex by nervous activity elsewhere.

reinnervation (rē″ĭn-ner-vā'shŭn). Anastomosis of a paralyzed part with a living nerve.

reinoculation (rē″ĭn-nŏk-ū-lā'shŭn). A second inoculation with the same virus following a previous one. SEE: *reinfection.*

Reinsch's test (rīnsh'ez). One for presence of arsenic.

reinversion (rē″ĭn-ver'shŭn). Correction of an inverted organ, as of an inverted uterus, by pressure on the fundus.

Reissner's canal (rīs'nerz). A canal in the cochlea following convolutions of the lamina spiralis. SYN: *cochlear canal.*

R's. corpuscles. Epithelial cells covering Reissner's membrane.

R.'s membrane. Delicate membrane separating the cochlear canal from scala vestibuli. SYN: *membrana vestibularis.*

rejuvenation (rē-jū-ve-nā'shŭn). A return to youthful conditions or to the normal.

r. operation. One to restore virility or for renewing youth by ligating the vas deferens of the male. SYN: *Steinach's operation.*

rejuvenescence (rē-jū-ve-nĕs'ĕns). The renewal of youth or return to earlier stage of existence.

relapse (re-lăps'). Recurrence of grave symptoms during convalescence.

relapsing (rē-lăps'ĭng). Recurring after beginning of convalescence.

r. fever. A contagious disease marked by intermittent attacks of high fever.

relative (rĕl'ă-tĭv). Existing in connection with another object or person.

r. field. That area in the cerebral cortex in which a lesion may or may not cause a spasm or paralysis.

r. humid'ity. Ratio of amt. of moisture in the atmosphere to amt. present if air is saturated at the same temperature. SEE: *humidity.*

r. near point. Nearest point at which clear vision is possible. SEE: *near point.*

relaxant (rē-lăks'ănt). 1. Loosening; laxative. 2. An agent diminishing tension, or loosening the bowels.

relaxation (rē-lăks-ā'shŭn). A lessening of tension or activity in a part.

r., complete. Relaxation, whether general or local, is complete if it proceeds to the zero point of contraction for the part or parts involved.

r., differential. Absence of an undue degree of contraction in the muscles employed during an act, while other muscles not so needed remain flaccid.

r., general. Relaxation which includes practically the entire body lying down.

r., local. Relaxation limited to a particular muscle group or to a part.

relaxed move'ment (rē-lăksd'). Form of bodily movement which the operator carries through without the assistance or resistance of the patient. SYN: *passive exercise.*

relaxin (rē-lăks'ĭn). Extract of corpora lutea which relaxes the pelvic ligaments, as in pregnancy.

relief (rē-lēf'). Alleviation or removal of a distressing or painful symptom.

r. incision. One made to relieve tension.

Remak's axis cylinder (ra'mahk). The conducting part of a nerve.

R.'s fibers. The nonmedullated nerve fibers.

R.'s ganglion. A ganglion of nerve cells near the sup. vena cava.

R.'s sign. A double sensation after pricking with a needle, the 2nd one being painful. Seen in *tabes dorsalis.*

R.'s symptom. Delayed appearance of pain.

R.'s type of palsy. Paralysis of muscles of the arm.

remedial (rē-mē'dĭ-ăl). 1. Curative; intended for a remedy. 2. Something used as a remedy.

remedy (rĕm'ĕd-ĭ). 1. Anything that relieves or cures a disease. 2. To cure or relieve a disease. SEE: *catholicon.*

r., local. Agent to relieve a local condition, as a sore.

r., systemic. Agent to relieve or cure a disease affecting the entire organism.

remission (rē-mĭsh'ŭn). Lessening of severity, or abatement of symptoms.

remittent (rē-mĭt'ĕnt). Alternately abating and returning at certain intervals.

r. fever. A malarial* fever with alternate periods of high and low temperature, but not below normal.

r. temperature. One that varies 2 or more degrees but which does not reach the normal.

ren (pl. *renes*). The kidney.

r. amyloidens. Amyloid degeneration of the kidneys.

r. mobilis. Movable kidney.

r. unguiformis. Horseshoe kidney.

renal (rē'năl). 1. Pert. to the kidney. 2. Shaped like a kidney.

renicapsule (ren-ĭ-kap'sŭl). The suprarenal capsule of the kidneys.

renifleur (rā-nĭ-flur'). One stimulated sexually by certain odors, esp. by the urine of others.

reniform (ren'ĭ-form). Shaped like a kidney.

reniportal (rĕn-ĭ-por'tăl). 1. Concerning the portal system of the kidney. 2. Pert. to the kidney's venous capillary circulation.

renipuncture (rĕn"ĭ-pŭnk'chŭr). Surgical puncture of capsule of kidney to relieve albuminuria.

rennet (rĕn'nĕt). 1. An infusion of inner coat of calf's stomach. 2. A fluid containing rennin,* a coagulating enzyme, used for making junket.

rennin (rĕn'ĭn). A proteolytic, coagulating enzyme found in the stomach which is afterwards converted into an active enzyme of milk, causing its curdling.

renninogen, rennogen (rĕn-ĭn'ō-jĕn, rĕn'ō-jĕn). Antecedent or zymogen in the gastric glands from which rennin is formed.

renogastric (rĕn-ō-găs'trĭk). Concerning the kidney and stomach.

renopathy (rĕn-ŏp'ăth-ĭ). Any pathological condition of the kidneys.

repair (rē-pār'). To remedy, replace, or heal, as a wound or a lost part.

repellent (rē-pĕl'ĕnt). 1. Reducing a swelling. 2. That which lessens a swelling.

repercolation (rē"per-kō-lā'shŭn). Repeated percolation using same materials.

repercussion (rē-per-kŭsh'ŭn). 1. Reciprocal action. 2. Action involved in causing subsidence of a swelling, tumor, or eruption. 3. OB: Diagnosis of pregnancy by insertion of a finger into the vagina to push the uterus, causing embryo to rise and fall. SYN: *ballottement.*

repletion (rē-plē'shŭn). 1. Condition of being full or satisfied. 2. Fullness of blood. SYN: *plethora.*

report'able diseases. Diseases which must be reported by the physician to the health authorities.

List of Reportable Diseases

1. Actinomycosis.
2. Acute infectious conjunctivitis (ophthalmia neonatorum).
3. Ankylostomiasis (hookworm).
4. Anthrax.
5. Botulism and other forms of food poisoning.
6. Chancroid.
7. Chickenpox.
8. Cholera (Asiatic).
9. Dengue.
10. Diphtheria.
11. Dog bites.
12. Dysentery (amebic).
13. Dysentery (bacillary and other infectious types).

14. Epidemic (lethargic) encephalitis.
15. Erysipelas.
16. Favus.
17. German measles.
18. Glanders.
19. Gonorrhea.
20. Granuloma inguinale.
21. Impetigo contagiosa (in institutions).
22. Influenza, epidemic.
23. Leprosy.
24. Malaria.
25. Measles.
26. Meningitis, epidemic (cerebrospinal fever, meningococcus meningitis).
27. Mumps.
28. Pellagra.
29. Paratyphoid fever.
30. Plague.
31. Pneumonias, the primary and the pneumonias complicating influenza, measles, and whooping cough.
32. Poisonings, heavy metals, drugs, occupational, and other poisonings.
33. Poliomyelitis, acute anterior (infantile paralysis).
34. Psittacosis.
35. Puerperal septicemia.
36. Rabies.
37. Rocky Mountain spotted or tick fever.
38. Scarlet fever.
39. Septic sore throat.
40. Smallpox.
41. Syphilis.
42. Tetanus.
43. Trachoma.
44. Trichinosis.
45. Tuberculosis (pulmonary).
46. Tuberculosis (other than pulmonary).
47. Tularemia.
48. Typhoid fever.
49. Typhus.
50. Undulant fever and Malta fever (brucellosis).
51. Vincent's angina and other anginas.
52. Whooping cough.
53. Yellow fever.

reposition (rē-pō-sĭsh'ŭn). Act of replacing a part.

repositor (rē-pŏz'ĭt-or). Instrument for replacing a part.

   r., inversion. Instrument for replacement of an inverted uterus.

   r., uterine. A lever to replace the uterus when out of normal position.

repression (rē-prĕsh'ŭn). PSY: Refusal to entertain distressing or painful ideas, thus submerging them in the unconscious where they continue to exert their influence upon the individual.

reproduction (rē-prō-dŭk'shŭn). 1. Conscious repetition of recognized sensations. SYN: *recall.* 2. Process by which plants and animals give rise to offspring. 3. Process of regeneration, as of tissue.

   r., asexual. Reproduction without sexual contact, intercourse, or seminal implantation.

reproductive (rē-prō-dŭk'tĭv). Concerning, or employed in, reproduction.

renography (rē-nŏg'ră-fĭ). Study of the kidney by means of an x-ray picture.

renointestinal (rĕn″ō-ĭn-tĕs'tĭn-ăl). Concerning the kidney and the intestine.

repulsion (rē-pŭl'shŭn). 1. Act of driving back. 2. The force exerted by one body on another to cause separation.

   r., capillary. Repulsion from forces causing movements of liquid in small vessels.

   r., electric. Like charges of electricity repel each other.

resection (rē-sĕk'shŭn). Partial excision of a bone or other structure.

resectoscope (rē-sĕk'tō-skōp). An instrument for resection of prostate gland through the urethra.

resectoscopy (rē-sĕk-tŏs'kō-pĭ). Resection of the prostate through the urethra.

reserve (rē-zerv'). 1. That which is held back for future use. 2. Self control of one's feelings and thoughts.

   r. air. Additional amount of air that can be expelled from the lungs over the normal quantity, 1200-1600 cc.

   r., alkali. Alkali content of body available for neutralization of acid. SEE: *alkaline reserve.*

reservoir of Pecquet (rĕz'ĕr-vwor pĕ-kā'). Expansion beginning at the thoracic duct opp. 12th dorsal vertebra. SYN: *receptaculum chyli.*

residual (rē-zĭd'ū-ăl). 1. Relating to that which is left as a residue. 2. PSY: Any internal aftereffect of experience influencing later behavior.

   r. air. That remaining in the lungs after normal expiration.

   r. urine. That left in bladder after urination; occurring in cases of enlarged prostate.

residue (rĕz'ĭd-ū). That which remains after a part is removed.

   r. free diet. One without cellulose or roughage.

   Purées and semisolids and bland foods are included.

   r., high, diet. A diet with increased amounts of cellulose (fiber), water, mineral salts, and vitamins (esp. vitamin B).

   r., low, diet (solid). An inadequate diet including solid food in which residue is reduced to a minimum. SEE: *nonlaxative diet.*

residuum (rē-zĭd'ū-ŭm). Residue; the remainder.

resilience (rē-zil'ĭ-ĕns). The quality of coming back to normal after straining, as a stretched rubber band when released. SYN: *elasticity.*

resilient (rē-zil'ĭ-ĕnt). Elastic.

resin (rĕz'ĭn). An amorphous, nonvolatile solid or soft solid substance, a natural exudation from plants; it is practically insoluble in water, but soluble in alcohol. EX: *Guaiac, rosin.*

resinous (rĕz'ĭn-ŭs). Of the nature of or pert. to resin.

resistance (rē-zĭs'tăns). 1. BIOL: Opposition to disease offered by plants and animals. 2. PSY: Force accounting for repression which opposes attempts to penetrate the unconscious. 3. ELECT: The opposing influence of a body (solid, liquid, or gaseous) to the passage of an electric current.

r., unit of. Expressed in ohms; 1 ohm of resistance will permit the flow of a current of 1 ampere as the result of a pressure of 1 volt.

resolution (rĕz-ō-lū'shŭn). 1. Decomposition; absorption or breaking down of the products of inflammation. 2. Cessation of inflammation without suppuration. The return to normal.

resolvent (rē-zŏl'vĕnt). 1. Promoting disappearance of inflammation. 2. That which causes dispersion of inflammation.

resonance (rĕz'ō-năns). 1. A sound heard on percussing or on auscultating a part, esp. the lungs. 2. PT: Resonance of an electric circuit is similar to the resonance of a mechanically vibrating body, such as a tuning fork.

r., amphoric. Sound, as that when blowing across the mouth of an empty bottle.

r., bell-metal. Sound heard in pneumothorax in auscultation when chest is percussed with 2 coins.

r., skodaic. Increased percussion sound over upper lung when there is pleural effusion in lower part.

r., tympanic. Hollow percussion sound over large air-filled cavities. [nance.

r., vesicular. Normal pulmonary reso-

r., vocal. The vibrations of the voice transmitted to the ear, normally more marked over the right apex.

r., whispering. Auscultation sound heard when patient whispers.

resonator (rĕz'ō-nā"tor). Apparatus for exhibiting effects of resonance on an electrical circuit in which oscillations of a certain frequency are set up by oscillations of the same frequency in another circuit. When this occurs, the circuits are said to be in syntony.

resorbent (rē-sor'bĕnt). An agent that promotes the absorption of abnormal matter, as exudates or blood clots. Ex: *Potassium iodide, ammonium chloride.*

resorcin, resorcinol (re-zor'sĭn, -ŏl). USP. Nearly colorless, needle-shaped crystals with a sweetish taste.

DOSAGE: 2 gr. (0.12 Gm.). Externally, 1 to 4% solution or ointment.

resorption (rē-sorp'shŭn). 1. Act of removing by absorption of an exudate or pus. 2. Loss by lysis. 3. Absorption not dependent upon mechanical laws of diffusion, as *intestinal absorption.*

respirable (rē-spīr'ă-bl, rĕs'pĭr-ă-bl). Fit or adapted for respiration.

respiration (rĕs-pĭr-ā'shŭn). The act of breathing.

r., abdominal. Respiration where the diaphragm chiefly exerts itself, while walls of chest are nearly at rest, as in acute pleurisy, pericarditis, fracture of rib.

r., accelerated. Considered accelerated when more than 25 per minute, after 15 years of age.

r., artificial. Artificial methods to restore respiration in cases of suspended breathing. SEE: *artificial respiration.*

r., Cheyne-Stokes. The respirations gradually increase in rapidity and volume until they reach climax, then gradually subside and finally cease entirely for from 5 to 50 seconds, when they begin again.

r., decreased. It obtains in uremia, diabetic coma, affections of the brain, in shock, hysteria, stenosis of the larynx, in chronic fibroid phthisis, on approaching death, and in poisoning with opium or its derivatives.

r., edematous. Breathing moist, rattling sounds, due to air passing through fluid from the blood infiltrated into air cells.

r., external. The mechanical process, involving contractions of muscles and movements of ribs and sternum, whereby air is aspirated (inspiration) into the lungs and then released (expiration), liberating carbon dioxide.

r., forms of. Jerking, spasmodic, stertorous, stridulous, whistling, wavy, lack of evenness, abdominal, or thoracic.

r., frequent. Common in all febrile and inflammatory diseases, esp. in children. As a rule, rapid breathing is a sign of thoracic disease. In hysteria patient often breathes 60 to 70 times per minute. It may occur in acute respiratory affections, lesions of medulla, or it may be induced by atropine, carbon dioxide, cocaine.

r., internal. The carriage of oxygen and carbon dioxide by the blood, the passage of oxygen into the cells, its utilization there and the reverse processes with carbon dioxide.

r., method of counting. With the hand in the same position as when taking the pulse, watch the patient's chest, without his knowledge if possible, as breathing is controlled by both the voluntary and involuntary muscles. Count each inspiration and expiration as 1 breath for 1 full minute by watching rise and fall of chest or upper abdomen. When the movements are scarcely perceptible, place the hand gently but firmly on the chest or back and count in this manner. *Note* hour, frequency, any abnormal condition such as pain associated with breathing.

Respiration, Pulse, and Temperature Ratio

Respiration	Pulsations	Temperature
18	80	99° F.
19 (plus)	88	100
21	96	101
23	104	102
25 (minus)	112	103
27	120	104
28	128	105
30	136	106

r., slow. Generally result of some structural or functional derangement of the nervous system.

r., thoracic. Respiration when abdomen does not move, being performed entirely by expansion of the chest. Observed when peritoneum, diaphragm, or its pleural cavity is inflamed.

respirator (rĕs'pĭ-rā″tor). 1. A device by which inspired air is purified, warmed, or medicated when passing through it. 2. A machine for prolonged artificial respiration. SEE: *Drinker's respirator.*

respiratory (rē-spīr'ă-tō-rĭ, rĕs'pĭ-ră-tō-rĭ). Pertaining to respiration.

r. center. A region in the medulla oblongata which regulates movements of respiration.

r. system. The lungs, pleura, bronchi, pharynx, larynx, tonsils, and the nose.

respirometer (rĕs″pĭr-ŏm'ĕt-ĕr). Instrument to ascertain character of respirations.

rest (rĕst). 1. Repose of body due to sleep. 2. Freedom from activity, as of mind or body. 3. To lie down; to cease from motion.

r. cure. Method of treatment of nervous diseases described by S. Weir Mitchell, consisting of isolation, rest in bed, forced feeding, massage, and hydrotherapy.

restibrachium (rĕs″tĭ-brā'kĭ-ŭm). Bundle of nerve fibers on both sides of the medulla, inferior peduncles of cerebellum. SYN: *corpus restiforme, myelobrachium.*

restiform (rĕs'tĭ-form). Ropelike; rope-shaped.

r. body. Inferior peduncle of the cerebellum. SYN: *corpus restiforme, restibrachium.*

restis (rĕs'tĭs). The restiform body, the inf. cerebellar peduncle.

restitution (rĕs-tĭt-ū'shŭn). 1. A return to a former status. 2. The act of making amends. 3. The turning of the fetal head to the right or left after it has completely emerged through the vulva.

restorative (rē-stōr'ă-tĭv). An agent that restores lost tone or function. Ex: *Preparations of iron, arsenic, mercury, etc.*

restraint (rē-strănt'). 1. Process of hindering from any action, mental or physical. 2. State of being hindered. 3. That which hinders or restricts; device or method used to keep a patient from injuring himself. SEE: *knot.*

r. in bed. Move bed against wall, place straight backed chairs along open side of bed. Tie them into place by interlacing with rope and then tying to foot and head of bed, or place a wide board the length of bed on either side and fasten through 3 or 4 holes bored near ends of the boards. Place a folded sheet across chest under each armpit with ends of sheet tied to end of bed. Bring patient's arms along sides and place them in a wide pillow slip under back with the open end of the slip pulled to armpits and closed end tucked under buttocks. The weight of body holds pillow slip in place.

r. of the lower extremities. Tie a sheet across knees and tie feet together with a figure-of-eight bandage. (Start loop under ankles, cross between feet and bring ends around feet and tie on top.)

resuscitation (rē-sŭs-ĭ-tā'shŭn). Act of bringing one back to full consciousness.

retardation (rē-tar-dā'shŭn). 1. A holding back or slowing down; delay. 2. Delayed mental or physical response due to pathological conditions, and seen in manic-depressive psychosis.

retard'ed depres'sion. The depressed state of manic-depressive psychosis.

retch (rĕtch). To make an involuntary attempt to vomit, *q.v.*

retching (rĕtch'ĭng). An involuntary attempt to vomit.

rete (rē'tē) (pl. *retia*). A network. A plexus of nerves or blood vessels.

r. Malpighii. Same as *rete mucosum.*

r. mirabile. BNA. A plexus formed by sudden division of a vessel into small twigs, which unite again to form 1 vessel, as in the vessel tufts of the kidneys.

r. mucosum. Three lower layers of the epidermis.

retention (rē-tĕn'shŭn). Retaining in the body that which does not belong there, or which should be excreted, as urine, feces, or perspiration. SEE: *chloruremia.*

r. cyst. One caused by retention of a secretion in a gland.

r. defect. Inability to recall a name, number, or fact shortly after the subject was requested to remember it.

r. enema. Enema to be retained to provide nourishment, medicate the mucosa or for anesthesia. SEE: *enema, retention.*

r. memory. It is affected in senile psychoses, paresis, arteriosclerosis, alcoholic hallucinosis, and in Altheimer's disease. Memory of long-past events is affected in senile dementia, dementia precox, paresis, epilepsy, and arteriosclerosis.

r. of urine. This is failure to expel the urine in the bladder.

r. with overflow. Spasm of sphincter, causing failure to empty the bladder at one voiding, only overflow dribbling away, due to above causes.

reticular (rē-tĭk'ū-lăr). Meshed, as a network, or distributed as the fibers of a leaf.

r. tissue. Connective tissue formed of a fibrous network containing lymphoid cells. SEE: *tissue.*

reticulated (rē-tĭk'ū-lă-tĕd). Netlike; pert. to a reticulum. SYN: *reticular.*

reticulation (rē-tĭk-ū-lā'shŭn). The formation of a network mass.

reticulin (rē-tĭk'ū-lĭn). An albuminoid or scleroprotein substance in the connective tissue framework of lymphatic tissues.

reticulocyte (re-tĭk'ū-lō-sīt). A reticulated red blood cell in process of active blood regeneration.

reticulocytopenia (re-tĭk″ū-lō-sī″tō-pē'-

nĭ-ă). Lowering of the number of the reticulocytes of the blood.

reticulocytosis (re-tĭk″ū-lō-sĭ-tō′sĭs). Presence of numerous reticulocytes during active blood regeneration. SYN: *reticulosis*.

reticuloendothelial system (re-tĭk′ū-lō-ĕn″dō-thē′lĭ-ăl). A cell group having the same behavior toward dyes, and with endothelial and reticular qualities. They are found in the bone marrow, liver, spleen, and hemolymph nodes. They are assumed to aid in making new blood cells and in disintegrating old ones.

reticuloendothelioma (re-tĭk″ū-lō-ĕn″dō-thē-lĭ-ō′mă). Reticuloendothelial tissue tumor.

reticuloendotheliosis (re-tĭk″ū-lō-ĕn″dō-thē-lĭ-ō′sĭs). Hyperplasia of reticuloendothelium.

reticuloendothelium (re-tĭk″ū-lō-ĕn″dō-thē′lĭ-ŭm). Tissue of the reticuloendothelial system.

reticuloma (re-tĭk-ū-lō′mă). Reticuloendothelial cell tumor.

reticulosis (re-tĭk-ū-lō′sĭs). Presence of more than the normal percentage of reticulocytes in the peripheral blood during active blood regeneration.

reticulum (re-tĭk′ū-lŭm). A network in cells.

  r. cell. A parent stem cell which in fetal life is responsible for the formation of the blood elements, the erythrocytes,* leukocytes,* monocytes,* lymphocytes,* and the thrombocytes.*

retiform (rĕt′ĭ-form). Resembling a network. SYN: *reticular*.

retina (rĕt′ĭ-nă) (pl. *retinae*). Innermost or 3rd tunic of the eye which receives image formed by the lens and is immediate instrument of vision.

retinaculum (rĕt-ĭn-ăk′ū-lŭm). A band or membrane holding any organ or part in its place.

  r. costae ultimatae. Lumbocostal ligament.

  r. ligamenti arcuati. Short, external, lateral ligament of the knee joint.

  r. morgagni of the ileocecal valve. Ridge formed by the coming together of valve segments at each end of opening bet. the ileum and cecum.

  r. peroneorum inferius. Fibrous band over peroneal tendons on outer side of calcaneum.

  r. peroneorum superius. External annular ligament of ankle joint.

  r. tendinum. Annular ligament of the ankle or wrist.

retinal (rĕt′ĭn-ăl). Concerning the retina.

retinitis (rĕt-ĭn-ī′tĭs). Inflamed condition of the retina.

  r., actinic. Retinitis due to exposure to intense light or other forms of radiant energy.

  r. albuminurica. Retinitis associated with chronic kidney disease.

Shows not only general signs of retinitis but is distinguished by white patches in the fundus, esp. surrounding the papilla and in the macular region.

  r., diabetic. Retinitis seen in diabetes. Picture may resemble albuminuric retinitis.

  r. pigmentosa. Chronic progressive degeneration consisting of atrophy of retina with characteristic deposit of pigment.

  r., proliferating. Vascularized masses of connective tissue which project from retina into the vitreous. End result of recurrent hemorrhage from retina into the vitreous. Found in tuberculosis.

  r., syphilitic. Retinitis generally associated with choroiditis.

retinochoroiditis (rĕt″ĭn-ō-kō-royd-ī′tĭs). Inflamed condition of retina and choroid.

retinocystoma (rĕt″ĭn-ō-sĭs-tō′mă). Glioma of the retina

retinoid (rĕt′ĭn-oyd). Like the retina.

retinopapillitis (rĕt″ĭ-nō-pă-pĭl-ī′tĭs). Inflamed condition of retina and optic papilla. SYN: *papilloretinitis*.

retinoscope (rĕt′ĭn-ō-skōp). An instrument used in performing retinoscopy.

retinoscopy (rĕt-ĭn-ŏs-kō′pĭ). Shadow test or refraction of eyes by effect of lights and shadows. SYN: *skiascopy*.

retinosis (rĕt-ĭn-ō′sĭs). A degeneration of the retina.

retisolution (rĕt-ĭ-sō-lū′shŭn). Dissolution of the Golgi structures.

retispersion (rĕt″ĭ-sper′zhŭn). Transference of Golgi structures to periphery of the cell.

retort (rē-tort′). A flasklike, long-necked vessel used for distilling.

retothelioma (rē″tō-thē-lĭ-ō′mă). A tumor of the retothelium.

retothelium (rē″tō-thē′lĭ-ŭm). Cellular layers covering reticular tissue. SYN: *reticuloendothelium, reticulothelium*.

retractile (rē-trăkt′ĭl). Capable of being drawn back or in.

retraction (rē-trăk′shŭn). A shortening. The act of drawing backward or state of being drawn back.

  r. ring. A ridge sometimes felt on uterus above the pubes, marking line of separation bet. upper contractile and lower dilatable segments of the uterus. Seen in prolonged or obstructed labor. SYN: *Bandl's ring*.

  r., uterine. The process by which muscular fibers of the uterus remain permanently shortened to a small degree following each contraction or labor pain.

retractor (rē-trăk′tor). 1. Instrument for holding back the margins of a wound. 2. Muscle which draws in any organ or part.

retro-. Prefix meaning *backward*.

retroauricular (rē″trō-aw-rĭk′ū-lar). Behind the auricle or ear.

retrobuccal (rē″trō-bŭk′ăl). Concerning the back part of the mouth or area behind the mouth.

retrobulbar (rē″trō-bŭl′bar). 1. Behind the eyeball. 2. Post. to the medulla oblongata.

retrocedent (rē″trō-sē′dĕnt). Going backward.

r. gout. Gout in which inflammation of the joint disappears with appearance of an internal affection.

retrocervical (rē″trō-sẽr′vĭ-kăl). Back of the cervix uteri.

retrocession (rē″trō-sĕsh′ŭn). 1. A going back; a relapse. 2. Metastasis of a condition from the surface to an internal organ. 3. Indication of an abnormal (further back) position of the uterus.

retroclusion (rē″trō-klū′zhŭn). Passing a pin over and under a vessel in compression of a bleeding artery.

retrocolic (rē″trō-kol′ĭk). Back of the colon. [back of the neck.

retrocollic (rē″trō-kŏl′ĭk). Concerning the **r. spasm.** Wryneck with spasms affecting post. muscles of neck.

retrocollis (rē″trō-kŏl′ĭs). Spasm of post. muscles of the neck with torsion. SYN: *torticollis.*

retrocursive (rē″trō-kẽr′sĭv). Stepping or turning backward.

retrodeviation (rē″trō-dē″vĭ-ā′shŭn). Backward displacement, as of an organ.

retrodisplacement (rē″trō-dĭs-plās′mĕnt). Displacement backwards of a part.

retroesophageal (rē″trō-ē-sŏf-ā′jē-ăl). Located behind the esophagus.

retroflexed (rē″trō-flĕkst). Bent backward.

retroflexion (rē″trō-flĕk′shŭn). A bending or flexing backward.
r. of uterus. A condition of the womb in which its body is bent backward at an angle with the cervix whose position usually remains unchanged.

retrogasserian (rē″trō-găs-sē′rĭ-ăn). Referring to the post. root of the gasserian ganglion.

retrograde (rĕt′rō-grād, rē′trō-grād). Moving backward; degenerating from better to worse state.
r. amnesia.* Loss of memory for events and situations just preceding time of patient's illness.

retrography (rē-trŏg′ră-fĭ). Mirror writing, a symptom of certain brain diseases.

retrogression (rĕt′rō-grĕsh′ŭn, rē″trō-grĕsh′ŭn). 1. Atrophy or degeneration, esp. of tissue. 2. Transition of tissue from a higher to a lower type of structure. SEE: *catagenesis.*

retrogressive changes (rē″trō-grĕs′ĭv). Changes to lower type of organization, such as in atrophy, degeneration, necrosis, hypertrophy, etc.

retroinfection (rē″trō-ĭn-fĕk′shŭn). Infection communicated by the fetus *in utero* to the mother.

retroinsular (rē″trō-ĭn′sū-lar). Situated behind the island of Reil.

retrolabyrinthine (rē″trō-lăb-ĭ-rĭn′thĭn). Situated behind the labyrinth of the ear.

retrolingual (rē″trō-lĭng′gwal). Situated behind the tongue.

retromammary (rē″trō-măm′mă-rĭ). Located behind the mammary gland.

retromandibular (rē″trō-măn-dĭb′ū-lar). Located behind the lower jaw.

retromastoid (rē″trō-măs′toyd). Situated behind the mastoid process.

retromorphosis (rē″trō-mor′fō-sĭs). Change in shape accompanying a transition from a higher to a lower type of structure. SEE: *catabolism.*

retronasal (rē″trō-nā′zăl). Relating to or situated at the back part of the nose.

retroöcular (rē″trō-ŏk′ū-lar). Located behind the eye.

retroperitoneal (rē″trō-pĕr-ĭ-tō-nē′ăl). Located behind the peritoneum.

retroperitoneum (rē″trō-pĕr-ĭ-tō-nē′ŭm). The space behind the peritoneum.

retroperitonitis (rē″trō-pĕr-ĭ-tō-nī′tĭs). Inflammation behind the peritoneum.

retropharyngeal (rē″trō-făr-ĭn′jē-ăl). Behind the pharynx.
r. abscess. Acute or chronic abscess behind the pharynx.

retropharyngitis (rē″trō-făr-ĭn-jī′tĭs). Inflammation of the retropharyngeal tissue.

retroplacental (rē″trō-plă-sĕn′tăl). Behind the placenta.

retroplasia (rē″trō-plā′zĭ-ă). Degenerative change of a cell or tissue into a more primary form.

retroposed (rē-trō-pōsd′). Displaced backward.

retropulsion (rē″trō-pŭl′shŭn). 1. Pushing back of any part, as of the fetal head in labor. 2. A walking or running backward, involuntarily, seen in some nervous disorders.

retrosternal (rē″trō-stẽr′năl). Behind the sternum.
r. pulse. Venous pulse felt over suprasternal notch.

retrotarsal (rē-trō-tar′săl). Located behind the tarsus of the eye.

retrouterine (rē″trō-ū′tẽr-ĭn). Located behind the uterus.

retroversion (rĕt″rō-vẽr′shŭn, rē″trō-vẽr′shŭn). A turning or state of being turned back.
r. of uterus. Displacement of the uterus backward with cervix pointing forward toward symphysis pubis.

Retzius, lines of (ret′zē-ŭs). Brownish, concentric lines in the enamel of a tooth.
R., s ace of. Triangular space bet. peritoneum and ant. abdominal wall filled with connective tissue.
R., veins of. Veins forming communications bet. the mesenteric veins and inf. vena cava.

Reuss' test (rois′ez). Test for atropine employing sulfuric acid and an oxidizing agent.

revellent (rē-vel′ent). 1. Producing revulsion, the diversion of disease or blood from one part of the body to another. 2. Agent producing revulsion.

revivification (rē-vĭv″ĭ-fĭ-kā′shŭn). 1. Attempt to restore life to those apparently dead; restoration to life or consciousness. Also restoring life in local parts, as a limb after freezing. SEE: *resuscitation, artificial respiration.* 2. Paring of surfaces to facilitate healing, as in a wound.

revulsant (rē-vŭl′sănt). 1. Causing transfer of disease or blood from one part of the body to another. 2. Drug which draws blood to an inflamed part.

revulsion (rē-vŭl'shŭn). 1. Act of driving backward, as diverting disease from one part to another by a quick withdrawal of the blood from that part. 2. PT: Circulatory changes obtained by sudden and intense reactions to applications of heat and cold.

revulsive (rē-vŭl'sĭv). 1. Causing revulsion. 2. A counterirritant.

Rhabditis (răb-dī'tĭs). A genus of small nematode worms, some of which are parasitic.

rhabdo-. Combining form meaning *rod.*

rhabdomyoma (răb″dō-mī-ō'mă). A striated muscular tissue tumor.

Rhabdonema (răb″dō-nē'mă). A genus of minute nematode worms, some of which are parasitic.

rhabdophobia (răb-dō-fō'bĭ-ă). Abnormal fear of being chastised, or of anything that might be used for such a purpose, as a *rod.* [spine.

rhachialgia (rā″kĭ-ăl'jĭ-ă). Pain in the

rhachiocampsis (rā″kĭ-ō-kămp'sĭs). Curvature of spine.

rhachioplegia (rā″kĭ-ō-plē'jĭ-ă). Spinal paralysis.

rhachioscoliosis (rā″kĭ-ō-skō-lĭ-ō'sĭs). Curvature of the spine laterally.

rhachis (rā'kĭs). Spinal column.

rhachischisis (rā-kĭs'kĭs-ĭs). A congenital cleft in the spinal column.

rhachitis (rā-kī'tĭs). Constitutional disease of infancy marked by faulty nutrition and bone deformity. SYN: *rachitis, rickets, q.v.*

rhacoma (rā-kō'mă). 1. Ragged, irregular abrasion, usually of the skin. 2. Relaxation of integument of scrotum.

rhagades (răg'ăd-ēz). Linear fissures appearing in skin, esp. at the corner of the mouth or anus, causing pain.
    If due to syphilis, they form a radiating scar on healing.

rhagadiform (răg-ăd'ĭ-form). Fissured; having cracks.

-rhagia. Suffix meaning *bleeding.*

rhaphania (răf-ă'nĭ-ă). Spasmodic disease caused by eating the wild radish. SYN: *raphania.*

rhaphe (rā'fē). A seam or ridge. SYN: *raphe.*

rhegma (rĕg'mă). Rupture, fracture, or rent, as of vessel walls, a bone, or of an abscess.

rheo-. Combining form meaning *current, stream.*

rheobase (rē-ō-bās). In unipolar testing with the galvanic current using negative as active pole, the minimal voltage required for a response when the make of the current is determined.

rheochord (rē-ō-kord). Type of rheostat used for measuring resistance of an electric current. SEE: *rheostat.*

rheometer (rē-ŏm'ĕt-ĕr). 1. Instrument for qualitative determination of presence of an electric current. SYN: *galvanometer.* 2. Device for measuring rapidity of the blood current.

rheonome (rē'ō-nōm). Device for ascertaining the effect of irritation on a nerve.

rheophore (rē'ō-fōr). A cord conducting an electrical current, as one bet. patient and electrical apparatus. SYN: *electrode.*

rheoscope (rē'ō-skōp). Device indicating the existence of an electric current. SYN: *galvanoscope.*

rheostat (rē'ō-stăt). A device maintaining fixed or variable resistance for controlling the amount of current entering a circuit.

rheostosis (rē-ŏs-tō'sĭs). A hypertrophying and condensing osteitis in streaks, involving long bones.

rheotachygraphy (rē-ō-tă-kĭg'ră-fĭ). Graphic recording of variation of electromotive force in a muscle.

rheotaxis (rē′ō-tăks'ĭs). Reaction to a current of fluid causing the part acted upon to move against the current.

rheotome (rē′ō-tōm). An interrupter with an adjustable speed control.

rheotrope (rē′ō-trōp). An instrument for automatically reversing a current of electricity.

rhestocythemia (rĕs″tō-sī-thē'mĭ-ă). Condition of degenerated red blood cells in the peripheral circulation.

rheum, rheuma (rūm, rūm'ă). Any catarrhal or watery discharge.
    r., salt. Moist tetter and similar skin eruptions; chronic eczema.

rheumarthrosis (rū-mar-thrō'sĭs). Chronic rheumatic pain in the joints; articular rheumatism.

rheumatalgia (rū″mă-tăl'jĭ-ă). Rheumatic pain.

rheumatic (rū-măt'ĭk). Pert. to rheumatism.
    r. fever. Acute articular rheumatism.

rheumaticosis (rū″măt-ĭ-kō'sĭs). General condition caused by rheumatism in children.

rheumatid (rū'mă-tĭd). A skin lesion sometimes seen in rheumatic conditions.

rheumatism (rū'măt-ĭzm). A disease with fever, pain, inflammation, and swelling of the joints. SEE: *arthritis.*
    r., acute articular; r., inflammatory. Acute general disease, characterized by irregular fever, acid sweat, inflammation of joints and marked tendency to involve the heart.
    r., chronic. Usually begins as chronic infection.
    r., gonorrheal. Joint affections associated with gonorrhea.
    r., muscular. An affection of the voluntary muscles characterized by pain, tenderness, and rigidity.
    r., palindromic. Recurring attacks of acute arthritis and periarthritis at irregularly spaced intervals.

rheumatismal (rū-mă-tĭz'măl). Of the nature of rheumatism.
    r. edema. Rheumatism accompanied by painful subcutaneous swellings.

rheumatoid (rū'mă-toyd). Of the nature of rheumatism.

r. arthritis. Form with inflammation of the joints, stiffness, swelling, cartilaginous hypertrophy, and pain. SEE: *arthritis.*

rheumatopyra (rū″măt-ō-pī′ră, rū-mă-top′-ĭ-ră). Febrile infectious disease with pain and swelling of the joints and cardiac involvement. SYN: *rheumatic fever.*

rheumatosis (rū-mă-tō′sĭs). Any disorder believed to be of rheumatic origin, as *erythema nodosum.*

rheumic (rū′mĭk). Concerning a rheum or flux.

r. diathesis. Predisposition to rheumatismal conditions.

rhexis (rĕks′ĭs). The rupture of any organ, blood vessel, or tissue.

rhinal (rī′năl). Concerning the nose. SYN: *nasal.*   [sal neuralgia.

rhinalgia (rī-năl′jĭ-ă). Pain in nose; na-

rhinencephalon (rī-nĕn-sĕf′ăl-ŏn). BNA. The olfactory portion of the brain; consisting of the olfactory lobe, the ant. perforated substance, the subcallosal gyrus, and the parolfactory area.

rhinesthesia (rī-nĕs-thē′zĭ-ă). The sense of smell.

rhineurynter (rī-nū-rĭn′tĕr). Elastic bag used for dilating the nostrils.

rhinion (rĭn′ĭ-on). Lower end of the suture bet. nasal bones. A craniometric point. SYN: *punctum nasale inferius.*

rhinitis (rī-nī′tĭs). Inflammation of the nasal mucosa. SEE: *endorrhinitis, ozena.*

r., acute catarrhal. Acute congested condition of nose with increased secretion of mucus. SYN: *common head cold, coryza.*

r., atrophic. Chronic inflammation with marked atrophy of mucous membrane with considerable dry crusting and disturbance in the sense of smell.

r., chronic hyperplastic. Chronic inflammation of mucous membrane accompanied by polypoid formation and underlying sinus pathology. SEE: *sinus.*

r., chronic hypertrophic. Inflammation of the mucous membrane of the nose characterized by hypertrophy of the mucous membrane of the turbinates and the septum.

r., hyperesthetic. Nonseasonal symptom complex depending on a conditioning predisposition of eyes and respiratory tract.

r., intumescent. Chronic rhinitis with unilateral, bilateral, or alternating swelling of the inf. turbinates.

r., specific. Tuberculosis or syphilis with ulceration or gumma in respiratory tract.

r., suppurative. Seen in suppurative sinus disease such as complication of severe rhinitis.

r., vasomotor. SEE: *hyperesthetic rhinitis.*

rhino-. Combining form meaning *the nose.*

rhinoantritis (rī″nō-ăn-trī′tĭs). Inflamed condition of the nasal cavities and one or both maxillary antra.

rhinobyon (rī-nō-bī′ŏn). A tampon or plug for the nose.

rhinocanthectomy (rī″nō-kăn-thĕk′tō-mĭ). Excision of inner canthus of the eye. SYN: *rhinommectomy.*

rhinocele (rī′nō-sēl). The ventricle or hollow of the olfactory lobe or *rhinoencephalon.*

rhinochiloplasty (rī″nō-kī′lō-plăs-tĭ). Plastic surgery of the nose and upper lip.

rhinocleisis (rī-nō-klī′sĭs). Nasal obstruction.

rhinodacryolith (rī-nō-dăk′rĭ-ō-lĭth). A nasal calculus.

rhinodynia (rī-nō-dĭn′ĭ-ă). Nasal pain. SYN: *rhinalgia.*

rhinogenous (rī-nŏj′ĕn-ŭs). Originating in the nose.

rhinolalia (rī-nō-lā′lĭ-ă). Nasal quality of voice.

r. aperta. Rhinolalia caused by undue patency of posterior nares.

r. clausa. Rhinolalia caused by closure of nasal passages.

rhinolaryngitis (rī″nō-lăr-ĭn-jī′tĭs). Inflammation of mucosa of nose and larynx at the same time.

rhinolite (rī′nō-līt). A nasal calculus; stone in the nose.

rhinolith (rī′nō-lĭth). Nasal concretion.

rhinolithiasis (rī″nō-lĭth-ī′ă-sĭs). The formation of nasal calculi.

rhinologist (rī-nŏl′ō-jĭst). A specialist in diseases of the nose.

rhinology (rī-nŏl′ō-jĭ). Science of the nose and its diseases.

rhinomanometer (rī″nō-măn-ŏm′ĕt-ĕr). A device for measuring the amount of nasal obstruction.

rhinometer (rī-nŏm′ĕt-ĕr). Device for measurement of the nose.

rhinomiosis (rī-nō-mī-ō′sĭs). Surgical reduction in size of the nose.

rhinommectomy (rī-nŏm-mĕk′tō-mĭ). Surgical excision of the inner canthus.

rhinomycosis (rī″nō-mī-kō′sĭs). Fungi in mucous membranes and secretions of the nose.

rhinonecrosis (rī″nō-nē-krō′sĭs). Necrosis of the nasal bones.

rhinopathy (rī-nŏp′ă-thĭ). Any nasal diseases.

rhinopharyngitis (rī″nō-făr-ĭn-jī′tĭs). Inflamed condition of the nasopharynx.

rhinopharyngocele (rī″nō-făr-ĭn′gō-sēl). A nasopharyngeal tumor.

rhinopharyngolith (rī″nō-făr-ĭn′gō-lĭth). Concretion in the nasal pharynx.

rhinopharynx (rī″nō-făr′ĭnks). Upper portion of pharynx continuous with the nasal passages.

rhinophonia (rī″nō-fō′nĭ-ă). A nasal tone in speaking.

rhinophyma (rī-nō-fī′mă). Lobular hypertrophy of nose, with red coloration, congestion, and retention of sebum. SYN: *acne rosacea.*

rhinoplasty (rī′nō-plăs-tĭ). Plastic surgery of the nose.

rhinopolypus (rī-nō-pŏl′ĭp-ŭs). Polypus of the nose.

rhinoreaction (rī″nō-rē-ăk′shŭn). Moeller's test for tuberculosis, a nasal tuberculin reaction.

rhinorrhagia (rī-nō-rā'jī-ă). Profuse hemorrhage from nose. SYN: *epistaxis, nosebleed.*

rhinorrhea (rī-nō-rē'ă). Thin, watery discharge from nose.
Progesterone reduces discharge and congestion.

r., cerebrospinal. Discharge of spinal fluid from nose due to defect in cribriform plate.

rhinosalpingitis (rī"nō-săl"pĭn-jī'tĭs). Inflammation of the mucosa of the nose and eustachian tube.

rhinoscleroma (rī-nō-skle-rō'mă). Nodular enlargement of nose and other portions of upper air passages.

rhinoscope (rī'nō-skōp). Instrument for examination of the nose.

rhinoscopy (rī-nŏs'kō-pĭ). Examination of nasal passages.

r., anterior. Examination through anterior nares.

r., posterior. Examination through posterior nares usually with small mirror in nasopharynx.

rhinostenosis (rī"nō-sten-ō'sĭs). Obstruction of the nasal passages. SYN: *rhinocleisis.*

rhinotomy (rī-nŏt'ō-mĭ). Incision of the nose.

rhinovaccination (rī"nō-văk-sĭn-ā'shŭn). Vaccine applied to the mucosa of the nose.

rhitidectomy (rī-tĭ-děk'tō-mĭ). Removal of wrinkles by operation. SYN: *rhytidectomy.*

rhitidosis (rī-tĭ-dō'sĭs). 1. Wrinkling of face without corresponding signs of age. 2. Wrinkling of the cornea, indicating its disintegration. SYN: *rhytidosis.*

rhizo-. Combining form meaning *root.*

rhizodontropy (rī-zō-dŏn'trō-pĭ). Process of pivoting an artificial crown upon the root of a tooth.

rhizodontrypy (rī-zō-dŏn'trī-pĭ). Puncture of root of a tooth.

rhizoid (rī'zoyd). BACT: 1. Having branched growth as *B. mycoides;* rootlike. 2. A rootlike plant filament.

rhizome (rī'zōm). A more or less underground and horizontal root stem of a plant. Ex: *hydrastis, valerian, ginger.*

rhizomelic (rī-zō-měl'ĭk). Concerning the hips and shoulders, in man the roots of the extremities.

rhizomeningomyelitis (rī"zō-me-nĭng"gō-mĭ-ĕl-ī'tĭs). Inflammation of roots of a nerve, the meninges, and spinal cord. SYN: *radiculomeningomyelitis.*

rhizoneure (rī'zō-nūr). A nerve cell having a fiber contributing to formation of a nerve root.

Rhizopoda (rī-zop'ō-dă). A class of Sarcodina without axial filaments, as the amebas.

rhizotomy (rī-zŏt'ō-mĭ). Section of post. roots of the spinal nerves for pain or spastic paralysis. SYN: *Dana's operation.*

rhodocyte (rō'dō-sīt). A red blood cell.

rhodogenesis (rō'dō-jĕn'ĕs-ĭs). Regeneration of visual purple bleached by light.

rhodophane (rō'dō-fān). A red pigment found in retinal cones.

rhodophylaxis (rō-dō-fī-lăks'ĭs). Ability of the retinal epithelium to regenerate visual purple which has been bleached by light.

rhodopsin (rō-dŏp'sĭn). Visual purple, a pigment in outer segment of retinal rods.

rhombencephalon (rŏm-bĕn-sĕf'ă-lon). The hind brain (metencephalon) with the after brain (myelencephalon).

rhombocele (rŏm'bō-sēl). Dilatation in the sacral region of the cavity of the spinal cord.

rhomboid (rŏm'boyd). Shaped like a rhomb.

r., fossa, r., sinus. The 4th ventricle of the brain.

rhomboideus (rŏm-boi'dē-ŭs). One of 2 muscles beneath the trapezius muscle.

rhoncal, rhonchial (rong'kal, rŏng'kĭ-ăl). Pert. to or produced by a rhonchus, or rattle in the throat.

rhonchus (rŏn'kŭs). A râle or rattling in the throat, esp. when it resembles snoring.

rhotacism (rō'tăs'ĭzm). Overuse or improper utterance of *r* sounds, with too much emphasis upon this letter.

rhyostomaturia (rī"ō-sto-mă-tū'rī-ă). The elimination of urinary elements by the salivary glands.

rhyparia (rī-pa'rī-ă). 1. Foul substance in mouth in low fevers. SYN: *sordes.* 2. Filth.

rhypophagy (rī-pŏf'ă-jī). The eating of filth. SYN: *scatophagy.*

rhypophobia (rī-pō-fō'bĭ-ă). Abnormal disgust at the act of defecation, feces, or filth.

rhythm (rĭth'ŭm). 1. A measured time or movement; regularity of occurrence. 2. Marking the intermenstrual periods of fertility and sterility in the female. SEE: *cacorhythmic.*

r., cantering. Abnormal heart rhythm comparable to the cantering of a horse.

r., coupled. One in which every other heartbeat produces no pulse at the wrist.

r., gallop. Same as *cantering rhythm.*

r., idioventricular. An automatic rhythm in complete heart block.

r., nodal. Rhythm caused by contraction starting from the atrioventricular instead of sinoauricular node.

r., pendulum. Rhythm with the 2 heart sounds alike, with the sound of a ticking clock.

r., respiratory. Successive and measured movements in breathing.

r., sinus. The normal cardiac rhythm proceeding from the sinoauricular node.

r., ventricular. Very slow ventricular contractions in heart block.

rhythmotherapy (rĭth"mō-ther'ă-pĭ). Application of different forms of rhythm in treatment of disease.

rhytidectomy (rĭt-ĭd-ĕk'tō-mĭ). Excision of wrinkles by plastic surgery.

rhytidosis (rĭt-ĭd-ō'sĭs). 1. Wrinkling of the skin. 2. Wrinkling of cornea.

Occurs in cases of great diminution in tension of eyeball, particularly after the escape of aqueous or vitreous, usually near death. SYN: *rhitidosis*.

rib (rĭb). One of the 24 bones enclosing the chest.

r's., false. Five ribs on each side not directly attached to the sternum.

r's., floating. Two lower ribs not attached to the sternum.

r's., true. The upper 7 ribs on each side which join the sternum by separate cartilages.

Ribes' ganglion (rēbz). Small ganglion of the sympathetic nervous system situated on the ant. communicating artery of brain.

riboflavin (rĭb″ō-flāv-ĭn). This is vitamin B_2 complex and was formerly called bactoflavin.

DOSAGE: Experimentally, 2 to 3 mg., higher in lactation and pregnancy.

rice water stools. Those of cholera which resemble water in which rice has been boiled.

Richter's hernia (rĭk′terz). Strangulated hernia with only a part of the gut constricted.

rickets (rĭk′ĕts). A disease of metabolism affecting children, characterized by defective nutrition and often resulting in deformities.

r., fetal. Defective cartilage formation at epiphyses of long bones in fetus producing a dwarfed body.

r., renal. A disturbance in epiphyseal growth during childhood due to severe chronic renal insufficiency.

Dwarfism and failure of gonadal development result.

Rickettsia (rĭk-ĕt′sĭ-ă). Minute organisms found in typhus fever, trench fever, and Rocky Mountain spotted fever. SEE: *spotted fever, tick fever*.

rickety (rĭk′ĕt-ĭ). Affected with or resembling rickets. SYN: *rachitic*.

Riddock's mass reflex. Flexion of 1 or both lower extremities with involuntary emptying of bladder and sweating in lower regions when stimulation is applied below level of a spinal cord injury.

riders' bone (rī′derz). Bony formation in adductor muscle of leg from pressure on the saddle. SYN: *cavalry bone*.

r. leg, r. sprain. Sprain of adductor muscles of the thigh. [border.

ridge (rĭj). Narrow, elongated or elevated

r., epicondylic. One of 2 ridges for muscular attachments on the humerus.

r., gastrocnemial. A ridge on post. femoral surface for attachment of gastrocnemius muscles.

r., gluteal. A ridge extending obliquely downward from great trochanter of femur for the attachment of the gluteus maximus muscle.

r., interosseous. A ridge on the fibula for attachment of the interosseous membrane.

r., pronator. Oblique ridge on the ant. surface of ulna, giving attachment to the pronator quadratus.

r., pterygoid. One at angle of junction of temporal and infratemporal surface of great wing of the sphenoid bone.

r., superciliary; r., supraorbital. Curved ridge of the frontal bone over supraorbital arch.

r., supracondylar. Epicondylic ridge.

r., tentorial. One on upper inner surface of the cranium to which is attached the tentorium.

r., trapezoid. An oblique ridge on the upper surface of the clavicle giving attachment to the trapezoid ligament.

r., wolffian. Ridge in the embryo from which the wolffian body develops.

ridgel, ridgil, ridgling (rĭj′ĕl, -ĭl, -lĭng). One with 1 testicle removed.

Riedel's lobe (rē′dĕl). A tongue-shaped process of liver, frequently found protruding over gallbladder in cases of chronic cholecystitis.

Riegel's test meal (rē′gĕl). Mutton broth, 200 cc.; beefsteak, 200 Gm.; mashed potato, 50 Gm.; bread or rolls, 50 Gm.; water, 200 cc. The stomach contents are expressed in 6 hours.

Riga's disease (rē′gä). Ulceration of frenum of the tongue with membrane formation.

Rigg's disease (rĭg). Formation of pus in teeth sockets with inflammation of the gums. SYN: *pyorrhea alveolaris, q.v.*

rigidity (rĭj-ĭd′ĭ-tĭ). Tenseness; immovability; stiffness; inability to bend or be bent.

rigor (rī′gŏr, rĭg′or). 1. A sudden, paroxysmal chill with high temperature, called the *cold stage*, followed by a sense of heat and profuse perspiration, called the *hot stage*. 2. A state of hardness and stiffness, as in a muscle. Rigor chills may be coarse, fine, diffuse, trembling.

r. mortis. The stiffness seen in corpses.

The rigidity of death which begins after 8, 10, or 20 hr. and may last 9 days. SEE: *dead, care of the; Nysten's law*. [or crack.

rima (rī′ma) (pl. *rimae*). A slit, fissure.

r. cornea'lis. Groove in the sclera holding edge of the cornea. SYN: *corneal cleft*.

r. glottidis. Interval bet. the true vocal cords. SYN: *glottis vera*.

r. oris. Aperture of the mouth.

r. palpebrarum. Slit bet. the eyelids.

r. pudendi. Space bet. the labia majora. SYN: *pudendal slit, vulvar slit, urogenital cleft*.

r. respiratoria. Space behind the arytenoid cartilages.

r. vestibuli. BNA. Space bet. the false vocal cords. SYN: *glottis spuria*.

r. vocalis. SEE: *rima glottidis*.

rimmose, rimose (rĭm′ōs, rī′mōs). Fissured or marked by cracks.

rimous (rī′mŭs). Filled with cracks or fissures. SYN: *rimmose*.

rimula (rĭm′ū-lă). A minute fissure or slit, esp. of the spinal cord or brain.

rind (rĭnd). The skin or cortex of an organ or person.

r. tumor. Neoplasm arising from lining membrane tissue of the embryo. SYN: *lepidoma*.

ring (rĭng). 1. Any round organ or band around a circular opening. 2. ANAT: A circular structure. SYN: *annulus*. 3. BACT: A growth like a ring around upper margin of a liquid culture, adhering to the glass more or less closely.

Ringer's solution (rĭng'er). An aqueous solution containing 0.7% sodium chloride, 0.03% potassium chloride, and 0.025% calcium chloride.

DOSAGE: From 500 to 1000 cc., all parenteral routes, chiefly subcutaneously.

ringworm (rĭng'wûrm). Contagious skin disease due to a species of *Trichophyton*, a fungous parasite.

r., crusted. Contagious skin affection caused by parasitic fungus with formation of honeycomblike crusts over hair follicles, itching, and moldy odor. SYN: *favus*.

r., honeycomb. SEE: *crusted ringworm*.

Rinne test (rĭn'nĕh). A test to ascertain condition of various parts of the ear with a vibrating tuning fork held over the mastoid process. SEE: *test*.

Riolan's arch (rē-ō-lahn'). Arch of transverse mesocolon.

R.'s bouquet. Two ligaments and 3 muscles attached to styloid process of temporal bone.

R.'s muscle. Ciliary portion of orbicularis palpebrarum. SYN: *musculus ciliaris*.

ripa (rī'pă). Any line of reflection of the endyma of the brain from a ventricular surface.

Ripault's sign (rē-pōz'). Change in shape of pupil produced by unilateral pressure upon eyeball, transitory phase during life, but permanent after death.

risorius (rī-sō'rĭ-ŭs). Muscular fibrous band arising over masseter muscle and inserted into tissues at the corner of the mouth.

risus (rī'sŭs). Laughter; a laugh.

r. sardonicus. A peculiar grin, as seen in tetanus, caused by acute spasm of facial muscles.

Ritter's disease (rĭt'ĕr). 1. Severe inflammation of skin with scaling, seen in infants. SYN: *dermatitis exfoliativa infantum*. 2. Fatal disease of infants, marked by hemorrhage, jaundice, and cyanosis.

Ritter-Valli law (rĭt"ĕr-văl'ĭ). Increased irritability from center outward if a nerve is cut off from its center or if the latter is destroyed.

Irritability is soon lost.

ri'valry strife. Alternate sensations of color and shape when the fields of vision of the 2 eyes cannot combine in 1 visual image.

Rivalta's disease (rē-val'tă). Chronic inflammation with lumpy formations and suppuration about the jaws. SYN: *actinomycosis, lumpy jaw*.

Rivinus' canals or ducts (re-ve'nŭs). Ducts of sublingual gland.

R.'s glands. Sublingual glands.

R.'s ligament. Small portion of the drum membrane in notch of Rivinus. SYN: *Shrapnell's membrane*.

R.'s notch. Cleft in upper part of long tympanic ring, filled by Shrapnell's membrane. [grains.

riziform (rĭz'ĭ-form). Resembling rice

RLS person. One who stammers and usually mispronounces these letters.

R. M. A. Abbr. of *right mentoanterior presentation of the fetal face*.

R. M. P. Abbr. of *right mentoposterior presentation of the fetal face*.

R. N. Abbr. for *Registered Nurse*.

Robertson's pupil. Pupil in which there is no light reflex, but power of contraction during accommodation remains unchanged. Same as *Argyll-Robertson pupil*.

roborant (rŏb'ō-rănt). 1. A tonic. 2. Strengthening.

Rochelle salt (rō-shĕll'). USP. Potassium and sodium tartrate, a colorless, transparent powder, having a cooling and saline taste.

DOSAGE: From 1 to 4 drams (4-15 Gm.).

Rocky Mountain spotted fever. An infectious disease caused by a parasite and transmitted by a wood tick; marked by fever, pains in bones and muscles, and profuse reddish eruption.

rod (rŏd). 1. Slender, straight bar. 2. One of the slender, long sensory bodies in retina responding to faint light. 3. Bacterium shaped like a rod.

r's. and cones. Sensory ending of the retina composing the 2nd layer.

rodent ulcer (rō'dĕnt). A slow growing, gnawing cancer which steadily eats into tissues, causing great destruction.

The most usual sites are on outer angle of the eye, near side, and on tip of nose, and edges of the scalp. SEE: *ulcer, rodent*.

rodonalgia (rō-dŏn-ăl'jĭ-ă). Vasomotor condition marked by redness and neuralgic pain of the extremities and swelling, and fever. SYN: *erythromelalgia*.

roentgen (rĕnt'gĕn). The international unit of quantity of roentgen rays adopted by the Second International Congress of Radiology at Stockholm in 1928.

roentgen rays. X-rays.

r. r. crystallography. The study of the arrangement of the atoms in a crystal by the deflection of roentgen rays by the atoms of the crystal.

r. r. photograph. A photograph taken with roentgen rays. SYN: *roentgenogram*.

r. r., quality of. Hardness, that quality of roentgen rays which determines their penetrating power, the hardness increasing as wave length shortens.

r. r., quantity of. The product of intensity and time. Quantity is used here in a sense different from that customary in other fields, such as radiant energy in general. It is not proportional to energy, but rather to the product of energy density and a coefficient expressing the ability to cause ionization.

r. r. spectrometer. An instrument used for determining the wave length of roentgen rays.

r. r. spectrum. The spectrum of a heterogeneous beam of roentgen rays produced by a suitable grating, generally a crystal.

r. r. tube. A glass vacuum bulb containing 2 electrodes. Electrons are obtained either from gas in the tube or from a heated cathode. When suitable potential is applied, electrons travel at high velocity from cathode to anode, where they are suddenly arrested, giving rise to roentgen rays.

roentgenism (rĕnt′gĕn-ĭzm). Disease produced by the use of roentgen rays.

roentgenization (rĕnt-gĕn-ĭ-zā′shŭn). The act of subjecting a patient, animal, or other object to the action of roentgen rays.

roentgenocinematography (rĕnt″gĕn-ō-sĭ″ne-măt-ŏg′rȧ-fĭ). Photography with roentgen rays of the internal organs' movements.

roentgenogram (rĕnt′gĕn-ō-grăm). A photographic record made with roentgen rays of the relative transparency of the various parts of an object to roentgen rays.

roentgenographer (rĕnt-gĕn-ŏg′rȧ-fer). A physician skilled in roentgen diagnosis.
Applies specifically to the making of photographic records as distinguished from roentgenoscopy.

roentgenography (rĕnt-gĕn-ŏg′rȧ-fĭ). The art of producing roentgenograms or photography with roentgen rays.

roentgenologist (rĕnt-gĕn-ŏl′ō-jĭst). A physician skilled in roentgen diagnosis, roentgen therapy, or both.

roentgenology (rĕnt-gĕn-ŏl′ō-jĭ). The science of applying roentgen rays for diagnostic and therapeutic purposes.

roentgenometer (rĕnt-gĕn-ŏm′ĕ-tĕr). An instrument for measuring the quantity, dosage, or intensity of roentgen rays.

roentgenometry (rĕnt-gĕn-ŏm′ĕ-trĭ). Measurement of penetrating capacity of the x-ray and of its therapeutic doses.

roentgenoscope (rĕnt′gĕn-ō-skōp). Device for holding the fluorescent screen in roentgen ray examinations. SYN: *fluoroscope.*

roentgenoscopy (rĕnt-gĕn-ŏs′kō-pĭ). The examination of a patient or object by direct visualization of shadows cast on a roentgenoscope, fluoroscope, or fluorescent screen by a beam of roentgen rays.

roentgenotherapy, roentgentherapy (rĕnt-gĕn-ō-ther′ȧp-ĭ, rĕnt-gĕn-ther′ȧ-pĭ). The treatment of disease by exposure of the patient to roentgen rays.

r., radicular. The application of roentgen rays to the roots of nerves where they emerge from the spinal cord.

roentgography (rĕn-tŏg′rȧ-fĭ). The making of x-ray pictures. SYN: *roentgenography, skiagraphy.*

roeteln, roetheln (ret′ĕln). German measles, *q.v.* SYN: *rubella.*

Rokitansky's disease (rō-kĭt-ăn′skĭ). Acute yellow atrophy of the liver.

Rolan′do's area. Motor area in the cerebral cortex.

R. fissure. Fissure bet. parietal and frontal lobes. SYN: *sulcus centralis.*

roller (rōl′er). 1. Strip of muslin or other cloth rolled up in cylinder form for surgeon's use. 2. A roller bandage. SEE: *bandage.*

Rollier technic (rōl′ē-ā). Method of using heliotherapy in which the body is gradually exposed to the sun's rays.

Roman numerals. Those used by the Romans in contradistinction to the Arabic numerals which we now use.

In Roman notations values are increased either by adding 1 or more symbols to the initial symbol, as III for 3, or by subtracting a symbol from 1 or more to the right of it, as IV for 4, IX for 9, etc., as shown in the following table:

Arabic	Roman	Arabic	Roman
1	I	18	XVIII
2	II	19	XIX
3	III	20	XX
4	IV	30	XXX
5	V	40	XL
6	VI	50	L
7	VII	60	LX
8	VIII	70	LXX
9	IX	80	LXXX
10	X	90	XC
11	XI	100	C
12	XII	500	D
13	XIII	900	CM
14	XIV	1,000	M
15	XV	1,900	MCM
16	XVI	1,000,000	M̄
17	XVII		

A line placed over a letter increases its value 1000 times, as M̄ is equal to 1000 times 1000 for which the M stands.

romanopexy (rō-man′ō-pĕks″ĭ). Fixation of the sigmoid flexure for prolapse of the rectum. SYN: *sigmoidopexy.*

romanoscope (rō-măn′ō-skōp). Instrument for examining the sigmoid flexure.

Romberg's sign (rŏm′bĕrg). Inability to maintain the body balance when the eyes are shut and the feet close together; a characteristic sign of locomotor ataxia.

rongeur (ron-zhŭr′). A gouge forceps, an instrument for removing tiny fragments of bone.

roof nucleus (rŭf nū′klē-ŭs). Small mass of gray matter in white substance of vermis of the cerebellum. SYN: *nucleus fastigii.*

root (rūt). 1. The underground part of a plant. Ex: *Stillingia, Glycyrrhiza, Belladonna.* 2. Proximal end of a nerve. 3. Portion of an organ implanted in tissues.

r. arteries. Artery accompanying nerve roots into the spinal cord. SYN: *radicular vessels.*

r. canal. Pulp cavity of root of a tooth.

r. sheath. Epithelium covering the hair follicle.

r. zone. Burdach's column of the spinal cord. Outer tract of post. funiculus or white column of the cord. SYN: *fasciculus cuneatus.*

R. O. P. Abbr. for *right occipitoposterior presentation, i. e.,* the occiput of fetus being in relation to the right sacroiliac joint of the mother.

rosa (rō′zä). Rose.

r. asturica. Deficiency disease due to lack of vitamin B₂. SYN: *pellagra.*

rosacea (rō-zā′sē-ä). Chronic hyperemic disease of the skin, esp. of the nose. SYN: *acne* rosacea.*

rose cold or **rose fever.** Summer or June cold; hay fever of early summer attributed to inhaling rose pollen. SEE: *hay fever.*

Rosenbach's sign (rō′zĕn-bähk). One of 4 signs; absence of abdominal reflex in intestinal inflammation.

Rosenheim's enema (rō′zĕn-hīm). A nutrient enema containing cod liver oil, sugar, and peptone in a 3% soda solution. SEE: *enema.*

Rosenmüller's body (rō′zĕn-mŭ-ler). Rudimentary tubule in the mesosalpinx bet. the fallopian tube and ovary. SYN: *epoöphoron, parovarium.*

R.'s cavity, R.'s fossa. Slitlike depression in the pharyngeal wall behind opening of the eustachian tube.

roseo-. 1. Combining form meaning *rose-colored.* 2. A prefix in chemical terms.

roseola (rō-zē′ō-lä). 1. Skin condition marked by maculae or red spots of varying sizes on the skin; a rose-colored rash. 2. Measles or German measles. SEE: *roseolous, rose rash.*

r. idiopathica. Macular eruptions not associated with any well-defined symptoms.

r. symptomatica. Macular eruption occurring in well-defined diseases.

roseolous (rō-zē′ō-lŭs). Resembling or pert. to roseola.

rose rash (rōz răsh). Any red colored eruption. SYN: *roseola.*

Roser's position (rō′zer). Head downward for operations on the air passages.

R.'s sign. No pulsation of dura mater after trephining, indicative of a subjacent lesion.

rose water (rōz wau′ter). Saturated aqueous solution of the oil of rose.

rosin (rŏz′ĭn). Substance distilled from oil of turpentine and used as adhesive and stimulant on plasters.

Rossbach's disease (rŏs′bähks). Excessive secretion of gastric juice. SYN: *gastroxynsis, hyperchlorhydria.*

Rossolimo's reflex (rŏs-ō-lē′mō). Extension or abduction of great toe resulting from light percussion or stroking of its plantar surface.

Ross' bodies (rŏs). Bodies sometimes found in tissue fluids in syphilis.

rostellum (rŏs-tĕl′lŭm). The ant. part of the head of worms equipped with a row of hooks.

rostral (rŏs′trăl). 1. Beaklike. 2 Toward the front or cephalic end of the body.

rostrate (rŏs′trāt). Having a beak or hook formation.

rostrum (rŏs′trŭm). Any hooked or beaked structure.

rosulate (rŏs′ū-lāt). Shaped like a rosette.

rotate (rō′tāt). To twist or revolve.

rotation (rō-tā′shŭn). Process of turning on an axis.

r., fetal. Twisting of the fetal head as it follows the curves of the birth canal, downward.

rotator (rō-tā′tor) (pl. *rotatores*). A muscle revolving a part on its axis.

r., uterine. An elevator or replacer used to push or rotate the uterus when it is out of its natural position.

röteln, rötheln (re′teln). German measles. SYN: *rubella.*

Rothera's test (rŏth′ē-rä). Method for finding acetone bodies in urine. SEE: *acetone.*

rotula (rŏt′ū-lä). 1. The kneecap. SYN: *patella.* 2. A medicated disk. SYN: *lozenge, troche.*

rotular (rŏt′ū-lar). Concerning the patella or kneecap.

rouge (rŭzh). A powder prepared by calcining ferrous sulfate used in polishing metal and glass instruments.

roughage (rŭf′ij). Indigestible fiber of fruits, vegetables, and cereals which acts as a stimulant to aid intestinal peristalsis.

r. diet. Diet with large amounts of cellulose, water, mineral salts, and vitamins. SYN: *high residue diet.*

rough on rats. A proprietary rat poison.

rouleau (roo-lō) (pl. *rouleaux*). A group of red blood corpuscles arranged like a roll of coins.

round (rownd). Circular in shape.

r. ligament. 1. Curved fibrous cord attached to center of articular surface of head of femur. 2. Two round cordlike structures passing from front of the body of the uterus in ant. wall of broad ligament, below the fallopian tubes, outward through the inguinal canals to soft tissues of the labia majora. 3. Fibrous cord which is the remnant of umbilical vein.

r.-worm. Common intestinal parasite, esp. in children. SYN: *Ascaris lumbricoides.*

roust (rowst). Delivery room nurse who carries out unsterile tasks.

R. Q. Abbr. for *respiratory quotient.*

-rrhagia (rä′jĭ-ä). Combining form indicating *abnormal discharge, hemorrhage.*

rubber dam. Thin rubber tissue used by dentists, and as covering for dry dressings.

r. tissue. Gutta percha sheets used for protecting dry dressings.

rubedo (rū-bē′dō). Temporary redness of the skin. SYN: *blushing.*

rubefacient (rū″be-fā′shĕnt). 1. Causing redness, as of the skin. 2. Agent which reddens the skin, producing a local congestion, the vessels becoming dilated and the supply of blood increased.

rubella (rū-bĕl′lä). Acute infectious disease, resembling both scarlet fever and measles, but differing from these in its short course, slight fever, and freedom from sequelae. Syn: *German measles, röteln.*

r. scarlatinosa. A mild, exanthematous, contagious disease similar to scarlatina, measles, and rubella.

rubeola (rū-bē′ō-lă). 1. Acute, contagious disease, marked by fever, catarrhal symptoms, and a typical cutaneous eruption. Syn: *measles.* 2. Term occasionally applied to acute infectious disease with mild symptoms and rose-colored macular eruption. Syn: *German measles, rubella.* [flushing.

rubescent (rū-bĕs′ĕnt). Growing red;

rubidium (rū-bĭd′ĭ-um). A metallic, silvery white metal used for same purpose as sodium salts or potassium. Symb: Rb. At. wt. 85.44.

rubiginous (rū-bĭj′ĭn-ŭs). Rusty or rust-colored.

rubigo (rū-bī′gō). Rust; mildew.

Rubin's test (rū′bĭn). Transuterine insufflation with carbon dioxide to test the patency of the fallopian tubes. See: *sterility.*

rubor (rōō′bor). Discoloration or redness due to inflammation.

One of the classical symptoms of inflammation.

rubrospinal (rū″brō-spī′năl). Concerning the red nucleus and the spinal cord.

rubrum (rū′brum). Reddish nucleus of gray matter in crus cerebri near optic thalamus.

r. scarlatinum. N.F.: Scarlet red, a substance used as a healing agent and stain.

ructus (rŭk′tŭs). Belching of wind from stomach.

rude respira′tion (rūd). Respiration having both bronchial and normal vesicular qualities.

rudiment (rū′dĭm-ĕnt). 1. That which is undeveloped. 2. Biol: A part just beginning to develop. 3. An organ arrested in an early stage of development. 4. Remains of a part functional only at an earlier stage of an individual or in his ancestors.

rudimentary (rū-dĭm-ĕn′tă-rĭ). 1. Elementary. 2. Undeveloped; not fully formed; remaining from an earlier stage. Syn: *vestigial.*

rufous (rū′fŭs). Ruddy; having a ruddy complexion and reddish hair.

ruga (rū′gă) (pl. *rugae*). A fold or crease.

r. vaginae. Transverse ridges of ant. and post. walls of the vagina.

Ruggeri's reflex. Increase in pulse rate when eyes are strongly converged on a near object.

rugose, rugous (rū′gōs, -gŭs). Wrinkled and rough in short, irregular folds. Syn: *corrugated.*

rugosity (rū-gos′ĭ-tĭ). 1. Condition of being folded or wrinkled. 2. A ridge or wrinkle.

Ruhmkorff coil (rōōm′korf). An induction coil with an immovable secondary coil

fixed at point of maximum intensity.

rumination (rū-mĭn-ā′shŭn). Regurgitation, esp. with rechewing, of previously swallowed food. [buttocks.

rump (rŭmp). Post. end of the back; the

Rumpf's symptom (rŭmpf). 1. In neurasthenia, the pulse is quickened to 20 beats per minute if pressure is exerted over a painful spot. 2. Twitching, after strong faradization, in traumatic neuroses.

run (rŭn). To exude pus or mucus.

run-around, runround (rŭn′ă-rownd, -rownd). Superficial infection fingernail. Syn: *felon, paronychia, whitlow.*

rupia (rū′pĭ-ă). A cutaneous eruption, usually of tertiary syphilis, with large elevations of the epidermis, filled with a clear or bloodstained serum, soon becoming turbid and purulent.

rupophobia (rū″pō-fō′bĭ-ă). Abnormal dislike for dirt or filth. Syn: *rhypophobia.*

rupture (rŭp′tūr). A breaking apart, as of an organ. Syn: *hernia, q.v.*

r. of membranes. Rupture of amniotic sac as normal result of dilatation of the cervix uteri in labor.

r. of perineum. Rupture of perineum, a condition the obstetrician seeks to avoid; more frequent in *primiparae.*

r. of tubes. Rupture of a fallopian tube; a serious event in extrauterine pregnancy which may occur without the woman's knowledge of her pregnancy.

r. of uterus. Rare and due to unrelieved obstructed labor.

Russell's bodies (rŭs′ĕl). Hyaline, small, spherical bodies in cancerous and simple inflammatory growths.

Russian bath. Hot vapor bath followed by friction and plunge in cold water.

Rust's disease (rŭst). Tuberculosis of 2 upper cervical vertebrae and their articulations.

rusty (rŭst′ĭ). Reddish in color; containing rust. Syn: *rubiginous.*

r. sputum. Reddish sputum expectorated in pneumonia.

rut-formation. Loss of interest in environment, fixation upon a single object, and concentration of emotional or other interests in a groove or rut.

ruthenium (rū-thē′nĭ-ŭm). A hard, brittle, metallic element of platinum group. Symb: Ru. At. wt. 101.7.

rutidosus (rūt-ĭ-dō′sŭs). Contraction or puckering of cornea just before death.

rutilism (rū′tĭl-ĭzm). Red-headedness.

ruyschian membrane, r. tunic (rĭsh′ĭ-an). Middle layer of the choroid. Syn: *lamina choriocapillaris, entochoroidea.*

r. muscle. Muscular tissue of the fundus uteri.

rytidosis (rĭt-ĭ-dō′sĭs). Wrinkling or contraction of cornea preceding death. Syn: *rutidosis.*

ryzamin-B (rī′ză-mĭn). A proprietary preparation of concentrated vitamin B_1 obtained from rice polishings, and having a potency of 50 I. U. per cake.

Dosage: As indicated, ½ Gm. being equivalent in B_1 potency to 3 cakes of yeast.

S

S. Abbr. for *signa*, mark, term used in prescription writing; *sinister*, left; *semis*, half; *spherical* or *spherical lens*.

S. Symb. of *sulfur*.

Sabatier's suture (sab-ă-tē-āz′). Method using oiled cardboard inserted into the intestine for closing of wounds.

saber shin. Ant. border of the tibia marked with sharp convexity found in hereditary syphilis.

sabulous (săb′ū-lŭs). Gritty; sandy.

saburra (să-bŭr′ră). Foulness of stomach or mouth; vitiated matter accumulated in stomach from indigestion. Syn: *sordes*.

saburral (să-bŭr′ăl). 1. Pert. to foulness of mouth or stomach due to accumulation of undigested material. 2. Pert. to sand, as in application of a hot sand bath for relief from pain, as in muscular rheumatism.

sac (săk). A baglike part of an organ; a cavity or pouch, sometimes containing fluid. See: *cyst*.

   s., air. An air cell in the lung.

   s., allantoid. Embryonic organ forming part of the umbilical cord, its expanded extremity uniting with the chorion to form the placenta.

   s., amniotic. A thin membrane, containing a serous fluid, enclosing the embryo. Syn: *amnion*.

   s., aneurysmal. Dilatation of a blood vessel forming wall of an aneurysm.

   s., embryonic. The embryo at an early period when it resembles a sac.

   s., fetal. Sac containing the fetus in extrauterine pregnancy.

   s., hernial. Covering of a hernia from a pouch of peritoneum.

   s., lacrimal. Upper dilated portion of the lacrimal duct.

   s., vitelline. Umbilical vessel surrounding the yolk in the embryo.

   s., yolk. Part of vitelline sac which is outside the embryonic body connected to it by umbilical duct. Syn: *umbilical vesicle*.

saccate (săk′āt). 1. Pert. to, like, or enclosed in a sac. Syn: *encysted*. 2. Bact: Marking a sac-shaped form, as in a type of liquefaction.

saccharephidrosis (săk″ă-rĕf-ĭ-drō′sĭs). Sugar in the perspiration, giving it a sweet odor.

saccharide (săk′ă-rĭd). One of the carbohydrate group containing sugar, made up of monosaccharoses, disaccharoses, and polysaccharoses, *q.v.*

sacchariferous (săk-ă-rĭf′ĕr-ŭs). Producing or containing sugar.

saccharification (săk″ă-rĭ-fĭ-kā′shŭn). Process of changing into sugar.

saccharimeter (săk-ă-rĭm′ĕ-tĕr). Device for determining amount of sugar in a solution. Syn: *saccharometer*. See: *hydrometer, polarimeter*.

saccharin (săk′ă-rĭn). USP. ($C_6H_4SO_2$-NHCO.) A sweet, white, powdered, synthetic product derived from coal tar, 300 to 500 times as sweet as sugar.

   Dosage: ¼ gr. (0.015 Gm.) in place of 1 lump of sugar; 2 ½ gr. tablets will sweeten 4 oz. of fluid. Syn: *gluside, 2*.

saccharine (săk′ă-rĭn, -rīn). Of the nature of, or having the quality of, sugar. Syn: *sweet*.

saccharo-. Combining form meaning sugar.

saccharogalactorrhea (săk″ă-rō-găl-ăk-tō-rē′ă). Excessive lactose secreted in milk.

saccharolytic (săk″ă-rō-lĭt′ĭk). Able to split up sugar.

saccharometabolic (săk″ă-rō-mĕt-ă-bŏl′ĭk). Concerning the metabolism of sugar.

saccharometabolism (săk″ă-rō-mĕ-tăb′ō-lĭzm). The chemical changes involved in utilization of sugar by the body. Syn: *glycometabolism*.

saccharometer (săk-ă-rŏm′ĕt-ĕr). Device for determining amount of sugar in a solution.

   Used in testing urine. Syn: *saccharimeter*.

Saccharomyces (săk″ă-rō-mī′sēz) (pl. *saccharomycetes*). A genus of fungi, reproducing by budding. Syn: *yeasts*.

saccharomycetolysis (săk″ă-rō-mī-sĕt-ŏl′ĭ-sĭs). Splitting up of sugar by a yeast fungus.

saccharomycosis (săk″ă-rō-mī-kō′sĭs). Disease due to yeast fungi. Syn: *blastomycosis*.

   s. hominis. Pyemia induced by a pathogenic yeast.

saccharorrhea (săk-ă-rō-rē′ă). Secretion of sugar in the body fluids, as in urine or perspiration. See: *diabetes mellitus, glycosuria*.

saccharose (săk′ăr-ōs). 1. Sucrose; cane, beet, or maple sugar. 2. One of the group of carbohydrates having the same chemical formula, $C_{12}H_{22}O_{11}$.

saccharosuria (săk″ă-rō-sū′rĭ-ă). Saccharose in the urine.

saccharum (săk′ăr-ŭm). Sugar, the term being used in the pharmacopeia.

   s. album. Pure or white crystallized sugar.

   s. canadense. Maple sugar.

   s. candidum. Rock candy.

   s. lactis. Sugar of milk. Syn: *lactose*.

   s. purificatum. Pure white sugar.

saccharuria (săk-ă-rū′rĭ-ă). Sugar in the urine.

sacciform (săk′sĭ-form). Bag-shaped or like a sac. Syn: *saccate*.

sacculated (săk′ū-lāt-ĕd). Consisting of small sacs or saccules.

sacculation (săk″ū-lā′shŭn). 1. Formation into a sac or sacs. 2. Group of sacs, collectively.

saccule (săk′ūl). 1. A small sac. 2. One of the sacs of the vestibular membrane of the ear, the other being the utricle.

  s., vestibular. SEE: *saccule, 2.*

sacculocochlear (săk″ū-lō-kŏk′lē-ar). Concerning the saccule of the vestibule, and the cochlea.

sacculus (săk′ū-lŭs) (pl. *sacculi*). A saccule or little sac.

  s. alveolaris. An air cell of the lung.

  s. chylifer. The receptaculum* chyli.

  s. cordis. Sac surrounding the heart. SYN: *pericardium.*

  s., Horner's. Saccular fold of the rectal mucosa forming anal pocket.

  s. lacrimalis. Expanded portion of nasolacrimal duct.

  s. laryngis. Pouch bet. sup. vocal bands and inner surface of the thyroid cartilage.

saccus (săk′ŭs). A sac or pouch.

  s. endolymphaticus. BNA. Dilated, blind end of the *ductus endolymphaticus.*

  s. lacrimalis. BNA. The lacrimal sac, into which empty the 2 lacrimal ducts.

sacrad (sā′krăd). In the direction of the sacrum.

sacral (sā′krăl). Relating to the sacrum.

  s. bone. A triangular bone made up of 5 vertebrae just above the coccyx.

  s. canal. Continuation of the vertebral canal in the sacrum.

  s. flexure. Rectal curve in front of the sacrum.

  s. index. Sacral breadth multiplied by 100 and divided by sacral length.

  s. nerves. Two spinal nerves of motion and sensation which emerge from the sacral foramina.

  s. vertebra. Fused segments forming the sacrum.

sacralgia (sā-krăl′jĭ-ă). Pain in the sacrum. SYN: *hieralgia.*

sacralization (sā-krăl-ĭ-zā′shŭn). Union of the sacrum and the 5th lumbar vertebra.

sacra media (sā′kră mē′dĭ-ă). Middle sacral artery.

sacrectomy (sā-krĕk′tō-mĭ). Excision of part of sacrum.

sacrificial operation. One in which some organ is removed for the patient's good.

sacro- (sā′krō). Prefix denoting the *sacrum.*

sacroanterior (sā″krō-ăn-tē′rĭ-or). Denoting a fetus having the sacrum directed forward.

sacrococainization (sā″krō-kō-kān-ĭ-zā′shŭn). Injection of cocaine through the sacrolumbar space into the spinal cord.

sacrococcygeal (sā″krō-kŏk-sĭj′ē-ăl). Concerning the sacrum and coccyx.

sacrocoxalgia (sā″krō-kŏks-ăl′jĭ-ă). Pain in sacroiliac joint, usually due to inflammation. SEE: *sacrocoxitis.*

sacrocoxitis (sā″krō-kŏks-ī′tĭs). Inflammation of the sacroiliac joint, frequently tuberculous.

sacrodynia (sā-krō-dĭn′ĭ-ă). Pain in the region of the sacrum.
  Sometimes referred in neurasthenia or hysteria.

sacroiliac (sā″krō-ĭl′ĭ-ăk). Of, or pert. to the sacrum and ilium.

  s. disease. Tuberculous disease of the sacroiliac joint.

  s. joint. The articulation bet. the hipbone and sacrum.
  There is no movement normally in this joint in men, but in the pregnant woman it becomes movable, allowing the pelvis to tip slightly during labor.

  s. synchondrosis. Meeting point of the sacrum and ilium.

sacrolumbar (sā″krō-lŭm′bar). Of, or concerning the sacrum and loins.

  s. angle. Angle formed by articulation of the last lumbar vertebra and the sacrum.

sacroposterior (sā″krō-pŏs-tē′rĭ-or). Having the fetal sacrum directed backward.

sacrosciatic (sā″krō-sī-ăt′ĭk). Concerning the sacrum and ischium.

sacrospinal (sā″krō-spī′năl). Relating to the sacrum and spine.

sacrotomy (sā-krŏt′ō-mĭ). Surgical excision of the lower part of the sacrum.

sacrouterine (sā″krō-ū′tĕr-ĭn). Concerning the sacrum and uterus.

sacrovertebral (sā″krō-ver′tē-brăl). Concerning the sacrum and the vertebrae.

  s. angle. Promontory of the sacrum.

sacrum (sā′krŭm). The triangular bone situated dorsal and caudal from the 2 ilia bet. the 5th lumbar vertebra and the coccyx.

  s., assimilation. A sacrum with a lumbar vertebra fused to the sacrum, or 1 with the 1st sacral vertebra free, resembling a lumbar vertebra. SEE: *pelvic, sacroiliac.*

sacto-. Combining form meaning *stuffed,* as sactosalpinx, an overfilled tube.

sactosalpinx (săk″tō-săl′pĭnks). Dilated fallopian tube due to retention of secretions, as in pyosalpinx or hydrosalpinx.

saddle joint (săd′l). Joint with articulating surfaces convex in 1 direction and concave in the other.

  s. nose. A nose with a depressed bridge.

sadism (sā′dĭzm, săd′ĭzm). A morbid phenomenon named after the Marquis de Sade, a French pervert of the 18th century, in which gratification is obtained by hurting a loved person.

Saemisch's ulcer (sā′mĭsh). Serpiginous, infectious ulcer of the cornea.

safety symbolism. Engagements to marry, the engagement ring, the wedding, the wedding ring, marriage, itself, the public announcement of wedding anniversaries, the advent of children, are all symbols which announce to the world that a man or a woman is the possession of one or the other; a warning, as it were, to protect the other partner from the attentions of one of the opposite sex.

sagittal (săj′ĭ-tăl). Arrowlike; in an anteroposterior direction.

s. line. An anteroposterior line.

s. plane. A bilateral symmetrical plane representing an imaginary line from the tip of the nose, tip of chin, and the occipital protuberance, dividing the head and the rest of the body medially.

s. sinus. The sup. longitudinal sinus.

s. sulcus. Groove on int. surface of skull.   [bones.

s. suture. Suture bet. the 2 parietal

sago (sā'gō). COMP: A substance prepared from the vegetable cells of various palms. A carbohydrate food made up entirely of starch.

s. spleen. The spleen in state of amyloid degeneration resembling sago.

Sahli's motor and secretory test meal (sah'lǐ). Test for both motor and secretory functions.

Saint Anthony's fire. Any of certain inflammations or gangrenous skin conditions, esp. erysipelas, hospital gangrene, and ergotism, *q.v.*

Saint Gotthard's disease. Condition due to presence of hookworms in intestinal tract. SYN: *ankylostomiasis.*

Saint Vitus' dance. Nervous disease with involuntary, jerking motions. SYN: *chorea.*

sajodin (săj'ō-dǐn). A brand of calcium iodobehenate. USP. A preparation from calcium and iodine, containing 17% iodine.

    DOSAGE: 8 gr. (0.5 Gm.).

sal (săl). Salt.

s. ammoniac. Chloride of ammonia.

salaam convulsion (sa-lahm'). Clonic muscular spasm of the trunk resulting in a bowing movement. SYN: *nodding spasm.*

salacious (sa-lā'shŭs). Lustful or inciting to lust.

salethyl carbonate. A proprietary salicylic acid derivative.

    DOSAGE: 5-15 gr. (0.3-1 Gm.).

salicylate (săl'ǐ-sǐl''āt, săl-ǐs'ǐl-āt). Any salt of salicylic acid.

s., methyl. The principal constituent of oil of wintergreen. It is applied externally for acute rheumatism.

s., sodium. White crystalline substance with disagreeable taste, in some cases even nauseating.

    DOSAGE: 15-30 gr. (1.2 Gm.).

salicylated (săl-ǐs'ǐl-āt-ēd). Impregnated with salicylic acid.

salicylism (săl'ǐs-ǐl-ǐzm). Toxic condition caused by salicylic acid or its derivatives.

salicyl-sulfonic acid test. Test for albumen in urine. SEE: *albumen.*

salicyluric acid (săl-ǐs-ǐl-ū'rǐk). Acid in urine after taking salicylic acid or its derivatives.

salifiable (săl-ǐf-ǐ'ā-bl). Capable of forming a salt by combining with an acid.

salihexin (săl-ǐ-hĕks'ǐn). A proprietary salicylic acid derivative combining the effects of the salicylates and methenamine.

    DOSAGE: 5-10 gr. (0.3-0.6 Gm.).

salimiter (săl-ǐm'ǐt-er). Device for testing strength of saline solutions.

saline (sā'lǐn). 1. Containing or pert. to salt; salty. 2. A mineral salt that produces evacuation of the intestinal contents. EX: *magnesium sulfate, sodium sulfate, potassium citrate,* and *potassium tartrate.*

s. enema. Enema used to excite peristalsis and evacuation.

    Magnesium sulfate, 1 oz. in 2 oz. of very warm water (115° F.), given with a small bore tube. SEE: *normal salt solution enema.*

s. purgative. Any salt producing evacuation, as Epsom salts.

s. solution. A solution of sodium chloride and distilled water; in biological laboratory parlance, a 0.9% solution of sodium chloride.

Salisbury treatment (sawlz'bĕr-ǐ). Treatment of obesity with meat and hot water diet.

saliva (să-lī'vă). The 1st digestive secretion emitted from the salivary glands into the mouth. SYN: *spittle.*

s., chorda. Saliva from the submaxillary gland obtained by irritation of the chorda tympani.

s., sympathetic. Saliva produced by stimulus to sympathetic nerve fibers supplying the glands; more scanty, but thicker than that of the chorda saliva.

salivant (săl'ǐv-ănt). Stimulating or that which stimulates the secretion of saliva.

salivary (săl'ǐv-ĕr-ǐ). Pert. to, producing, or formed from, saliva.

s. calculus. Concretion in a salivary duct.   [bodies in saliva.

s. corpuscles. Nucleated, spherical

s. diastase. Enzyme in saliva acting on starch. SYN: *ptyalin.*

s. digestion. The 1st digestive process taking place in the mouth.

s. glands. Three pairs of glands including the: (1) *Parotid* glands, 1 on each side of the face below the ear; secrete *ptyalin;* (2) *submaxillary* glands, principally in the floor of mouth; secrete *ptyalin* and *mucin;* (3) *sublingual* glands, principally in floor of mouth; secrete *mucin* and *mucinogen;* (4) *buccal* glands, scattered beneath the mucous membrane of lips and cheeks. They form a secretion that is mixed with the saliva.

salivation (săl-ǐ-vā'shŭn). 1. The secretion of saliva. 2. Excessive secretion of saliva. SYN: *ptyalism.*

salivatory (săl'ǐ-vā'tō-rǐ). Producing secretion of saliva. SYN: *salivant.*

salivin (săl'ǐv-ǐn). Enzyme in saliva acting on starch. SYN: *ptyalin.*

sallow (săl'ō). Of a pale, yellowish color, usually said of complexion or skin.

sallowness (săl'ō-nĕs). Brownish-yellow tint combined with pallor of skin; normal to brunettes. SEE: *skin, face, facies.*

salmine (săl'mēn, -mǐn). $C_{30}H_{57}N_{14}O_6$. A protamine obtained from spermatozoa of salmon. SEE: *protamine, protein.*

sal mirabile (săl mǐ-răb'ǐ-lē). A purgative salt. SYN: *Glauber's salt, sodium sulfate, q.v.*

salmon patch (săm'ŭn). Salmon-colored area of the cornea in syphilitic keratitis. SYN: *Hutchinson's patch.*

Salmonella (săl-mō-nĕl'ă). A genus of Gram-negative bacteria, some of them being intestinal pathogens.

    S. aertrycke (ā-ĕr'trĭk-ē). A medium-sized, motile, Gram-negative rod present in meat poisoning and in paratyphoid fevers.

    S. enteritidis. Gärtner's bacillus, a species causing meat poisoning.

    S. hirschfeldii. A species found in paratyphoid fever, Type C.

    S. paratyphi. A species causing paratyphoid fever, Type A.

    S. psittacosis. A species found on parrots.

    S. schottmülleri. Species causing paratyphoid fever, Type B.

salmonellosis (săl-mō-nĕ-lō'sĭs). Infestation with bacteria of genus *Salmonella.*

Salmon's operation (să'mŭn). Incision along an anal fistula; back-cut of Salmon.

salpingectomy (săl-pĭn-jĕk'tō-mĭ). Excision of an oviduct.

salpingemphraxis (săl"pĭn-jĕm-frăks'ĭs). Obstruction of the eustachian tube causing deafness, or of a fallopian tube.

salpingian (săl-pĭn'jĭ-ăn). Concerning an oviduct, or the eustachian tube.

salpingion (săl-pĭn'jĭ-ŏn). A point at inf. surface of the apex of the petrous portion of temporal bone.

salpingitis (săl-pĭn-jī'tĭs). Inflammation of the fallopian tube, or, less commonly, of the eustachian tube.

    s. profluens. Salpingitis with sudden discharge of secretions gathered in the fallopian tube.

salpingo-. Combining form meaning *trumpet* or *tube.*

salpingocatheterism (săl-pĭng"gō-kăth'ĕt-ĕr-ĭzm). Application of a catheter to the eustachian tube.

salpingocele (săl-pĭn'gō-sēl). Hernial protrusion of an oviduct.

salpingocyesis (săl-pĭng"ō-sī-ē'sĭs). Pregnancy where fetus begins to develop in an oviduct; tubal pregnancy.

salpingo-oöphorectomy (săl-pĭng"gō-ō"ō-for-ĕk'tō-mĭ). Excision of an oviduct and ovary.

salpingo-oöphoritis (săl-pĭng"ō-o"ō-for-ī'-tĭs). Inflammation of the tube and ovary. SYN: *salpingo-oöthecitis.*

salpingo-oöphorocele (săl-pĭng"gō-ō-of'or-ō-sēl). Hernia enclosing the ovary and fallopian tube.

salpingo-oöthecitis (săl-pĭng"gō-ō"ō-thē-sī'tĭs). Inflammation of a fallopian tube and ovary. SYN: *salpingo-oöphoritis.*

salpingo-oöthecocele (săl-pĭng"gō-ō"ō-thē'kō-sēl). Hernia of both ovary and fallopian tube.

salpingo-ovariectomy (săl-pĭng"gō-o"var-ĭ-ĕk'tō-mĭ). Surgical removal of an oviduct and ovary. SYN: *salpingo-oöphorectomy.*

salpingopexy (săl-pĭng"o-pĕks'ĭ). Fixation of a fallopian tube.

salpingopharyngeus (săl-pĭng"ō-făr-ĭn'jē-ŭs). The muscle arising in cartilage of the eustachian tube which raises soft palate.

salpingorrhaphy (săl-pĭng-or'ă-fĭ). Suture of an oviduct.

salpingosalpingostomy (săl-pĭng"gō-săl-pĭng-gŏs'tō-mĭ). The operation of attaching 1 fallopian tube to the other.

salpingoscope (săl-pĭng'gō-skōp). Device for examining the nasopharynx and eustachian tube.

salpingostaphylinus (săl-pĭng"gō-stăf-ĭl-ī'-nŭs). The muscle which tightens soft palate.

salpingostomatomy (săl-pĭng"gō-stō-măt'ō-mĭ). Creation of an artificial opening in a fallopian tube after it has been occluded by inflammation.

salpingostomy (săl-pĭng-gŏs'tō-mĭ). Surgical opening of a fallopian tube which has been occluded, or for drainage.

salpingotomy (săl-pĭng-ŏt'ō-mĭ). Section of a fallopian tube.

salpingo-ureterostomy (săl-pĭng"ō-ūr-ĕt"-ĕr-ŏs'tō-mĭ). Surgical connection of the ureter and the fallopian tube.

salpingysterocyesis (săl-pĭn-jĭs"ter-ō-sī-ē'-sĭs). Pregnancy partly in a fallopian tube and partly in the uterus.

salpinx (săl'pĭnks) (pl. *salpinges*). The fallopian or eustachian tube.

salt (sawlt). SYMB: NaCl. 1. White crystalline compound occurring in nature, known chemically as sodium chloride. 2. Containing, tasting of, or treated with salt. 3. To treat with salt. 4. *plural.* Any mineral salt or saline mixture used as an aperient or cathartic, esp. Epsom salts or Glauber's salt. 5. CHEM: A compound consisting of a positive ion other than hydrogen, and a negative ion other than hydroxyl. 6. A chemical compound, usually crystalline, resulting from the interaction of an acid and a base.

    s., buffer. A salt found in the blood which fixes excess amounts of acid or alkali, without a change in hydrogen-ion concentration.

    s., Epsom. Magnesium sulfate.

    s., Glauber's. Sodium sulfate.

    s., iodized. Salt containing 1 part sodium or potassium iodide to 5000 parts of sodium chloride.

    s., Rochelle. Sodium and potassium tartrate.

    s., rock. Native sodium chloride.

    s. solution, normal. SEE: *physiological salt solution.*

    s. s., physiological. Solution containing 0.9% of salt, which resembles in density the proportion in the blood. SYN: *saline solution.*

saltation (săl-tā'shŭn). 1. Act of leaping dancing, as in chorea. 2. Abrupt variation in character of a species. SYN: *mutation.* 3. A spurting forth of arterial blood.

saltatory (săl'ta-tō-rĭ). Marked by dancing or leaping.

s. spasm. Tic of muscles of lower extremity, causing convulsive leaping upon attempt to stand. SEE: *palmus*.

salt-free diet. One with no more than 2 Gm. of salt allowed, as in *edema*.

salt glow. Name given to a rub of the entire body with moist salt for stimulation.

salt, low diet. No salt allowed on patient's tray. No salty food served.

s. poor diet. All food prepared and served without the addition of salt, including salt-free bread and butter. Milk intake is limited. Protein caloric fluid level governed by orders of physician.

saltpeter (sawlt″pē′ter). A common name for potassium nitrate.

s., chile. A common name for sodium nitrate. NaNO₃. Crystalline powder, saline in taste and soluble in water.

    DOSAGE: 1-2 drams (4-8 Gm.).

salt rheum (sawlt room). Any one of a variety of skin affections of the eczematous type. SEE: *eczema*.

salts. Plural of salt. SEE: *salt, 4.*

salubrious (săl-ū′brĭ-ŭs). Promoting or favorable to health. SYN: *wholesome*.

salutary (săl′ū-ta-rĭ). Healthful; promoting health; curative.

salvarsan (săl′var-săn). An arsenical, yellowish powder preparation (606) given intramuscularly or intravenously for syphilis.

salvatella (săl-văt-ĕl′ă). A small vein on the dorsum of the little finger and hand. SYN: *vena salvatella*.

salve (săv). 1. An ointment applied to wounds. 2. PHARM: Any ointment or cerate made with a base of a fat, oil, petrolatum, resin, etc.

salyrgan (săl-ĭr′găn). A synthetic mercurial compound containing about 40% mercury.

    DOSAGE: 10% solution intravenously or intramuscularly, 0.5 cc. increased to 1 cc. or a maximum of 2 cc. if required. Injections are made at intervals of 3-5 days. SYN: *mersalyl*.

s. suppositories. Each suppository contains 0.4 Gm. salyrgan.

    DOSAGE: 1 suppository.

Salzer's double test meal (sahlz′er). Beef, 40 Gm., scraped and broiled; milk, 250 cc.; boiled rice, 50 Gm.; 1 soft cooked egg. Four hours later give Ewald-Boas test meal and express 1 hour later.

sanative (săn′ă-tĭv). Of a healing nature. SYN: *curative*.

sanatorium (săn-ă-tō′rĭ-ŭm) (pl. *sanatoriums* or *-ria*). An establishment for preservation of health or the treatment of the chronically sick; esp. a private one. SYN: *sanitarium*.

sanatory (săn′ă-tō-rĭ). Curative; conducive to health.

sand (sănd). Fine grains of disintegrated rock.

s. auditory. Calcareous concretion in labyrinth of the ear. SYN: *otolith*.

s. bath. Therapeutic covering of the body with hot sand.

s., brain. Concretion of matter near base of the pineal gland. SYN: *acervulus cerebri*.

s. tumor. One in membrane of the brain, choroid plexus, and other areas made up of calcareous particles. SYN: *psammoma*.

Sand'with's bald tongue. Abnormally clean tongue seen in late stages of pellagra.

sane (sān). Sound of mind; mentally normal.

Sänger's operation (seng′er). A form of cesarean section by which the uterus is taken out before the fetus.

sanguicolous (săng-gwĭk′ō-lŭs). Inhabiting the blood, as a parasite.

sanguifacient (săng-gwĭf-ă′shĕnt). Making blood.

sanguiferous (săng-gwĭf′ĕr-ŭs). Conducting blood, as the circulatory organs.

sanguification (săng-gwĭf-ĭk-ā′shŭn). Conversion into, or formation of, blood. SYN: *hematopoiesis*.

sanguimotor, sanguimotory (săng″gwĭ-mō′tor, -tō-rĭ). Pert. to the blood circulation.

sanguinal (săng′gwĭn-ăl). A blood preparation used in chlorosis and anemia.

sanguine (săng′gwĭn). 1. Hopeful. 2. Plethoric, bloody; marked by abundance and active blood circulation. 3. Pert. to or consisting of blood.

sanguineous (săng-gwĭn′ē-ŭs). 1. Bloody; relating to blood. 2. Having an abundance of blood. SYN: *plethoric*.

sanguinolent (săng-gwĭn′ō-lĕnt). Containing, or tinged with, blood.

sanguinopoietic (săng″gwĭn-ō-poy-ĕt′ĭk). Generating blood. SYN: *hematopoietic, sanguifacient*.

sanguirenal (săng″gwĭ-rē′năl). Pert. to the blood supply of the kidneys.

sanguis (săng′gwĭs). Blood.

sanguisuga (săng-gwĭs-ū′gă). A leech or bloodsucker. SEE: *Hirudo*.

sanies (să′nĭ-ēz). A thin, fetid, greenish discharge from a wound or ulcer, presenting appearance of pus tinged with blood.

saniopurulent (să″nĭ-ō-pū′rŭ-lĕnt). Having characteristics of sanies and pus; pert. to a fetid, serous, blood-tinged discharge containing pus.

sanioserous (să″nĭ-ō-sē′rŭs). Composed of sanies* and serum.

sanious (să′nĭ-ŭs). Of the nature of fetid, purulent fluid from an ulcer; sanies.

sanitarium (săn-ĭ-tā′rĭ-ŭm) (pl. *sanitariums* or *-ria*). Institution for treatment and recuperation of persons having physical or mental disorders; occasionally limited to place where conditions are prophylactic rather than therapeutic. SYN: *sanatorium*.

sanitary (săn′ĭ-tar-ĭ). Promoting, or pert. to conditions improving health.

sanitation (săn″ĭ-tā′shŭn). The use of measure to promote and establish conditions favorable to health, esp. public health. SEE: *assanation, hygiene*.

sanity (săn′ĭt-ĭ). Soundness of health or mind; normal mentality. SEE: *sane*,

santal oil (săn'tăl). USP. Sandalwood oil. A volatile oil distilled from the wood of the plant.

DOSAGE: 8 ɱ (0.5 cc.) in capsules.

santonin (săn'tō-nĭn). USP. A colorless crystalline substance obtained from the dried flower heads of the plant *santonica*.

DOSAGE: 1 gr. (0.06 Gm.).

Santorini's canal (săn-tō-rē'nē). Same as *Santorini's duct*.

S.'s cartilage. Nodules of cartilage on tips of the arytenoid cartilages.

S.'s duct. An accessory duct of the pancreas.

S.'s fissures. A fissure in cartilage of the ext. auditory meatus and one in the tragus.

S.'s muscle. The risorius muscle, which compresses the cheek and draws angle of mouth out.

S.'s veins. Veins from scalp passing to the cerebral sinus.

sap (săp). 1. Any fluid essential to life and vitality of a living structure. 2. To cause gradual exhaustion of, as the strength.

s., nuclear. Liquid portion of a cell nucleus. SYN: *karyolymph*.

saphena (să-fē'nă) (pl. *saphenae*). Name given to two large veins of the leg.

saphenous (saf-ē'nŭs). Pert. to or associated with a saphenous vein or nerve in the leg.

s. nerves. Two nerves accompanying each saphenous vein.

s. opening. An aperture in the fascia, oval in shape, in inner and upper part of thigh transmitting the saphenous vein below Poupart's ligament. SYN: *fossa ovalis*.

s. veins. Two veins, long and short, passing up the leg, the long from the foot to the saphenous opening, the short one behind outer malleolus up back of leg joining the popliteal. SEE: *vein, saphenous*.

sapid (săp'ĭd). Savory; tasty; opp. of insipid.

sapo (sā'pō). USP. Soap prepared from pure olive oil and sodium hydroxide.

sapocrinin (săp'ō-krĭn'ĭn). The secretion of the intestinal mucous membrane after a soap enema or rub.

saponaceous (săp-ō-nā'shŭs). Soapy; resembling soap in feel or quality.

saponification (sa-pŏn''ĭ-fĭ-kā'shŭn). 1. Conversion into soap; chemically, the hydrolysis or the splitting of fat by an alkali yielding glycerol and 3 molecules of alkali salt of the fatty acid, the soap. 2. CHEM: Hydrolysis of an ester into corresponding alcohol and acid (free or in form of a salt).

s. number. In analysis of fats, the number of milligrams of potassium hydroxide needed to neutralize the fatty acids in 1 Gm. of oil or fat.

saponify (sa-pŏn'ĭ-fī). To convert into a soap, as when fats are treated with an alkali to produce a free alcohol plus the salt of the fatty acid.

saponin(e (săp'ō-nĭn, -nēn). Unabsorbable glucoside contained in the roots of some plants forming a lather in an aqueous solution.

saporific (săp''ō-rĭf'ĭk). Imparting a taste or flavor.

sapphism (săf'ĭzm). Sexual desire of women for their own sex.

sapremia (săp-rē'mĭ-ă). A toxic condition caused by the absorption into the blood of toxins or poisons produced by saprophytes or putrefactive bacteria. SEE: *septicemia*.

sapro-. Combining form meaning *putrid*.

saprodontia (săp-rō-dŏn'shĭ-ă). Caries of the teeth; tooth decay.

saprogen (săp'rō-jĕn). Any microörganism causing or produced by putrefaction.

saprogenic (săp''rō-jĕn'ĭk). Causing decay or resulting from it.

saprophilous (săp-rof'ĭl-ŭs). Living on decaying or dead substances, as a microörganism. SYN: *saprophytic*.

saprophyte (săp'rō-fīt). Any organism living on decaying or dead organic matter. Most of the higher fungi are saprophytes. SEE: *parasite*.

saprophytic (săp-rō-fĭt'ĭk). Living or growing in decaying or dead matter; characteristic of a saprophyte.

sapropyra (săp-rō-pī'rä). 1. Typhus fever. 2. Any fever caused by putrid infection. SYN: *saprotyphus*.

saprotyphus (săp''rō-tī'fŭs). 1. Putrid or typhus fever. 2. Fever due to putrid infection.

saprozoic (săp-rō-zō'ĭk). Living on decaying or dead organic matter.

sarcin (sar'sĭn). A leukomaine found during decomposition of proteins in muscles and other tissues. SYN: *hypozanthine*.

Sarcina (sar'sĭ-nă). A genus of nonflagellated bacteria of the family *Coccaceae* which has cells dividing in 3 directions. Majority are harmless and produce pigments.

S. ventriculi. Sarcina found in the stomach of man.

sarcitis (sar-sī'tĭs). Inflammation of muscle tissue. SYN: *myositis*.

sarco-. Combining form meaning *flesh*.

sarcoadenoma (sar''kō-ăd''en-ō'mä). A fleshy tumor of a gland. SYN: *adenosarcoma*.

sarcoblast (sar'kō-blăst). 1. A protoplasmic germinal mass. 2. Embryonic cell which develops into a muscle cell.

sarcocarcinoma (sar''kō-kar-sĭn-ō'mä). A tumor of malignant growth of sarcomatous and carcinomatous types.

sarcocele (sar'kō-sēl). A fleshy tumor of the testicle.

Sarcocystis (sar''kō-sĭs'tĭs). A genus of parasitic microörganisms found in the muscles of swine and other animals.

S. miescheriana. A parasite found in pork and beef.

sarcode (sar'kōd). Protoplasm of body of a unicellular animal.

Sarcodina (sar-kō-dī'nă). The lowest class of protozoa including the Amoebae.

sarcoenchondroma (sar"kō-ĕn-kŏn-drō'mă). Tumor composed of cartilaginous and fleshy elements. SEE: *enchondroma, sarcoma.*

sarcogenic (sar"kō-jĕn'ĭk). Producing flesh.

sarcoglia (sar-kŏg'lĭ-ă). Protoplasmic matter containing granules and nuclei composing the eminences of Doyen or point of entrance of a motor nerve into a muscular fiber.

sarcoid (sar'koyd). 1. A sarcomalike tumor. 2. Resembling flesh. 3. A nodule or plaque of the skin which leaves atrophic scars.

sarcolemma (sar"kō-lĕm'ă). A delicate membrane surrounding each striated muscle fiber. SEE: *muscle.*

sarcology (sar-kŏl'ō-jĭ). Branch of medicine dealing with study of the soft tissues of the body.

sarcolysis (sar-kŏl'ĭ-sĭs). Decomposition of the soft tissues or flesh.

sarcolyte (sar'kō-līt). A multinucleated cell concerned in the decomposition of the soft tissues.

sarcolytic (sar"kō-lĭt'ĭk). Decomposing flesh.

sarcoma (sar-kō'mă) (pl. *sarcomas, -mata*). A tumor of nonepithelial, modified, embryonic, connective tissue, esp. a malignant one.

s., alveolar. Sarcoma principally in bone, skin, and muscle with largely developed stroma and alveoli.

s., angiolithic. Small tumor containing granular calcareous concretions in the cerebral meninges.

s., chondro-. One composed of masses of cartilage.

s., fibro-. A malignant tumor with fibrous tissue and many spindle cells and dilated vessels.

s., giant-celled. Sarcoma from cancellous bone tissue with large cells with many nuclei.

s., lymphangio-. Sarcoma arising from endothelium of lymph vessels in a lymph gland.

s., melanotic. Sarcoma containing melanin.

s., myeloid. Same as giant-celled sarcoma.

s., myxo-. A tumor of loose connective tissue containing a viscid fluid, mucin.

s., osteo-. One composed of osseous tissue or bone containing variously shaped cells.

s., round-cell. One containing small and large closely packed round cells resembling leukocytes.

s., spindle-cell. One consisting of small and large spindle-shaped cells.

sarcomatoid (sar-kō'mă-toyd). Resembling a sarcoma.

sarcomatosis (sar"kō-mă-tō'sĭs). Condition marked by presence and spread of a sarcoma; sarcomatous degeneration.

sarcomatous (sar-kō'măt-ŭs). Of the nature of, or like, a sarcoma.

sarcomere (sar'kō-mēr). A segment into which a muscle fibril is divided by transverse septa.

sarcomphalocele (sar-kŏm-făl'ō-sēl). Fleshy tumor at the umbilicus.

sarcophagy (sar-kŏf'ă-jĭ). Practice of eating flesh.

sarcoplasm (sar'kō-plăzm). Hyaline, semifluid, interfibrillary substance of striated muscle fibers.

sarcoplast (sar'kō-plăst). A cell bet. muscular fibrils developing into muscular fiber.

sarcopoietic (sar"kō-poy-ĕt'ĭk). Forming muscle or flesh.

Sarcoptes (sar-kŏp'tēz). A genus of mites.

S. scabiei. A species that produces the itch or scabies, *q.v.*

sarcosis (sar-kō'sĭs). 1. The development of multiple fleshy tumors. 2. Abnormal formation of flesh.

sarcosome (sar'kō-sōm). Contractile part of a muscle fibril.

Sarcosporidia (sar"kō-spō-rĭd'ĭ-ă). An order of protozoans parasitic in muscle fiber.

sarcosporidiosis (sar"kō-spō-rĭd-ĭ-ō'sĭs). Infestation with Sarcosporidia or condition produced by them.

sarcostosis (sar-kŏs-tō'sĭs). Ossification of fleshy or muscular tissue.

sarcostyle (sar'kō-stīl). Any one of the fine longitudinal fibrillae of a striated muscle fiber.

sarcotherapeutics (sar"kō-ther-ă-pū'tĭks). Treatment of disease with animal extracts or glands. SYN: *organotherapy.*

sarcotherapy (sar"kō-ther'ă-pĭ). Use of animal extracts and glands in treatment. SYN: *organotherapy, sarcotherapeutics.*

sarcotic (sar-kŏt'ĭk). 1. Producing or pert. to flesh formation. 2. Agent producing growth of flesh.

sarcous (sar'kŭs). Concerning flesh or muscle.

s. element. One of the dark prisms of ultimate fibrils of striated muscle fibers.

s. substance. Substance of a sarcous element.

sardon'ic laugh. Old term for a spasmodic affection of facial muscles, giving an appearance of laughter. SYN: *risus sardonicus.*

sartorius (sar-tō'rĭ-ŭs). A long, ribbon-shaped muscle of the thigh.

satellite (săt'ĕl-īt). 1. ANAT: Structure associated with another, esp. vein accompanying an artery. 2. A tiny lesion near a big one.

satellitosis (săt-ĕl-ĭ-tō'sĭs). Accumulation of free cell nuclei around the ganglion cells of the cortex of the brain, seen in paralysis and other affections.

satiety (sa-tī'ĕt-ĭ). Fullness or gratification beyond desire.

saturated (sat'ū-rā-tĕd). Holding all of a substance that can be combined.

s. compounds. Those incapable of additional products, as any in the methane series. SEE: *unsaturated compounds.*

s. solution. One containing as much of the solid drug as it can dissolve.

saturation (săt″ū-rā′shŭn). 1. The holding in solution of all of a solid that can be dissolved therein. 2. Administration of an erythema dose of radiant energy, followed by smaller doses for a period of time.

s., high frequency. Rarely employed modification of a monoterminal high frequency treatment.

saturnine (săt′ŭr-nĭn). Concerning or produced by lead.

s. breath. Sweet breath produced by lead* poisoning.

saturnism (săt′ŭrn-ĭzm). Lead poisoning, *q.v.*

satyriasis (sat-ĭ-rī′ă-sĭs). Great mental excitement with abnormal sex desire in the male.

satyromania (săt″ĭr-ō-mā′nĭ-ă). Excessive sexual desire in the male. SYN: *satyriasis.*

Sauerbruch's cabinet (sow′ĕr-brook). An airtight cabinet for operation on the chest under negative pressure.

The patient's head is outside the cabinet and his body and the surgeon's are within it.

sauriasis (saw-rī′ăs-ĭs). Ichthyosis* with marked thickness of the skin.

sauriderma (saw-rĭ-der′mă). Skin disease with thick, elevated scale formation. SYN: *ichthyosis hystrix.*

sauriosis (saw-rĭ-ō′sĭs). Cutaneous disorder in which there is cornification of epithelial layers. SYN: *ichthyosis.*

Savill's disease (să′vĭl). An epidemic skin disease with papular rash, followed by branny desquamation. May be fatal. SYN: *dermatitis exfoliativa epidemica, epidemic eczema.*

Saviotti's canals (sah-vē-ŏt′ĭ). Artificially formed passages bet. secreting cells of pancreas.

savory (sā′vō-rĭ). Having a pleasant or appetizing taste or odor.

saw (saw). Instrument for cutting, esp. bone, its cutting edge being toothed.

saxifragant (săks-ĭf′răg-ănt). Dissolving or breaking calculi, esp. in the bladder.

Sayre's jacket (sārz). A jacket of plaster-of-Paris worn to support the spine in vertebral diseases.

Sb. Symb. for *antimony.*

SbCl₃. Antimony trichloride.

Sb₂O₅. Antimonic oxide; antimony pentoxide.

Sb₂O₃. Antimonious oxide.

scab (skăb). 1. Crust of a cutaneous sore, wound, ulcer, or pustule formed by drying up of the discharge. 2. To become covered with a crust.

scabies (skā′bĭ-ēs). 1. A skin disease caused by an animal parasite, the Acarus scabei. SYN: *itch.* 2. A form of vesicles associated with pustules.

scabrities (skă-brĭsh′ĭ-ēz). 1. Scaly, roughened condition of the skin. 2. A morbid roughness of inner surface of eyelids, causing sensation as if sand were in eyes.

s. unguium. Morbid degeneration of the nails, making them rough, thick, distorted, and separated from the flesh at the root. Symptomatic of syphilis and leprosy.

scala (skā′lă). Any one of the 3 spiral passages of the cochlea. SEE: *ear.*

s. media. It contains the organ of Corti.

s. tympani. BNA. The part of the spiral canal of the cochlea which is situated below the lamina spiralis.

s. vestibuli. BNA. The part of the spiral canal above the lamina spiralis.

scald (skawld). 1. Burn to skin or flesh caused by moist heat and hot vapors, as steam. 2. To cause a burn with hot liquid or steam. 3. Cutaneous disease marked by scab formation on the head. It is deeper than dry heat, and should be treated as a burn, *q.v.* Healing is slower and scar formation greater. SEE: *burn.*

scald head (skawld′ hĕd). Any one of several contagious affections of the scalp excited by Achorion Schönleinii.

scale (skāl). 1. A small, thin, dry exfoliation shed from upper layers of skin. 2. Film of tartar incrusting the teeth. 3. To form a scale on. 4. To shed scales. 5. An instrument for weighing. 6. A graduated or proportioned measure, series of tests, or instrument for measuring quantities or for rating, as individual intelligence. SEE: *Binet.*

s., absolute. A scale used for indicating low temperatures based on absolute zero. SEE: *absolute temperature, absolute zero.*

s., centigrade. Thermometric scale running from 0°, the melting point of ice, and 100°, the boiling point of water. SEE: *centigrade, thermometer.*

s., Fahrenheit. One in which the freezing point of water is 32° and the boiling point is 212°. SEE: *Fahrenheit, thermometer.*

s., Réamur. Scale which runs bet. freezing point of water at 0° and the boiling point at 80°. SEE: *Réamur, thermometer.*

scalene (skā-lēn′). 1. Having unequal sides and angles, said of a triangle. 2. Designating a scalenus muscle.

s. tubercle. One on upper surface of 1st rib, the insertion of the scalenus anticus muscle. SYN: *Lisfranc's tubercle.*

scaleniotomy (skā-lēn″ĭ-ŏt′ō-mĭ). Incision of scalenus muscles near their insertion to check expansive movements in tuberculosis of the apex of the lung.

scalenus (skā-lē′nŭs). One of 3 deeply situated muscles on each side of the neck, extending from the transverse processes of 2 or more cervical vertebrae to the 1st or 2nd rib; known as scalenus anterior, medius, posterior.

s. anticus syndrome, s. syndrome. A symptom complex characterized by brachial neuritis with or without vascular or vasomotor disturbance in the upper extremities.

scall (skawl). A crusty eruption of the skin or scalp. SYN: *favus, impetigo, eczema, psoriasis.*

scalp (skălp). The hairy integument of the head.

In anat. includes skin, dense subcutaneous tissue, occipitofrontalis muscle with the galea aponeurotica, loose subaponeurotic tissue, and the cranial periosteum.

scalpel (skăl'pĕl). A straight, small surgical knife with a convex edge and thin, keen blade. [of a chisel.

scalpriform (skăl'prĭ-form). In the shape

scalprum (skăl'prŭm) (pl. *scalpra*). 1. A toothed instrument for removal of carious bone or for trephining. 2. A large scalpel. 3. Cutting edge of an incisor tooth.

scaly (skā'lĭ). Resembling or characterized by scales.

scan'ning speech. Pronunciation of words in syllables, or slowly and hesitatingly; a symptom of disseminated sclerosis.* SEE: *speech.*

scanty (skăn'tĭ). Not abundant; insufficient, as a secretion.

scapha (skā'fā). BNA. Elongated depression of the ear bet. the helix and anthelix.

scapho-. Combining form meaning *boat.*

scaphocephalic, scaphocephalous (skăf″ō-sĕf-ăl'ĭk, -sĕf'ăl-ŭs). Having a deformed head, projecting like a boat's keel.

scaphocephalism (skăf″ō-sĕf'ăl-ĭzm). Condition of having a deformed head, projecting like the keel of a boat.

scaphoid (skăf'oyd). 1. A proximal, boat-shaped bone of the carpus on radial side. SYN: *os scaphoides.* 2. A boat-shaped bone on inner side of the tarsus between the astragalus and 3 cuneiform bones. 3. Boat-shaped, navicular, hollowed.

s. abdomen. One with hollowed anterior wall.

s. bone. SEE: *scaphoid, 1 and 2.*

scaphoiditis (skăf-oyd-ī'tĭs). Inflamed condition of the scaphoid bone.

scapula (skăp'ū-lă) (pl. *scapulae, -as*). The large, flat, triangular bone of the shoulder.

s. alata. Winglike appearance of the scapula in thin and weak muscled persons.

scapulalgia (skăp-ū-lăl'jĭ-ă). Pain in the region of the shoulder blade.

scapular (skăp'ū-lar). Of or pert. to the shoulder blade.

s. reflex. Scapular muscular contraction following percussion or stimulus bet. the scapulas.

scapulary (skăp'ū-la-rĭ). A shoulder bandage bifurcated with the 2 ends over the shoulders, the single end passing down the back, the 3 fastened to a body bandage.

scapulectomy (skăp-ū-lĕk'tō-mĭ). Surgical excision of the scapula.

scapulo-. Combining form meaning *shoulder.*

scapuloclavicular (skăp″ū-lō-klă-vĭk'ū-lar). Concerning the scapula and the clavicle.

scapulodynia (skăp″ū-lō-dĭn'ĭ-ă). Inflammation and pain in the shoulder muscles.

scapulohumeral (skăp″ū-lō-hū'mer-ăl). Concerning the scapula and the humerus.

s. reflex. When inner margin of scapula is percussed upper arm is adducted and rotated outwards.

scapulopexy (skăp″ū-lō-pĕks'ĭ). Fixation of the scapula to the ribs.

scapulothoracic (skăp″ū-lō-thō-răs'ĭk). Concerning the scapula and the thorax.

scapus (skā'pŭs). The stem or shaft of the hair which includes the *cuticle, cortex,* and *medulla.*

scar (skar). Mark left in skin or internal organ by healing of a wound, sore or injury because of replacement by connective tissue of the injured tissue.

s., cicatricial. A scar or cicatrix with considerable contraction.

It may be necessary to divide the scar and graft on new skin, as in burns.

s., keloid. A red, raised, smooth scar containing blood vessels, often irritable.

Seen in the tuberculous, after superficial septic wounds, as from infected vaccination scars.

s., painful. One due to involvement of a nerve during healing.

The end of the nerve may become bulbous.

scarfskin (skarf'skĭn). Epidermis* or outermost layer of the skin.

scarification (skăr-ĭ-fĭ-kā'shŭn). Making of numerous slight incisions in the skin, over a part.

scarificator (skăr'ĭf-ĭk-ā-tor). Instrument for making small incisions in the skin.

scarifier (skăr'ĭ-fī-er). Instrument used for withdrawal of blood by incision with circular cutting edge and blades operated by springs.

scarlatina (skar-lă-tē'nă). An acute, contagious disease characterized by sore throat, fever, punctiform scarlet rash, and rapid pulse. SYN: *scarlet fever.*

s. anginosa. Scarlatina with throat symptoms. SEE: *scarlatina.*

s. haemorrhagica. Scarlatina with blood extravasated into mucous membranes and the skin.

s. latens. Scarlatina without rash. but complicated by nephritis.

s. maligna. Scarlatina with great prostration and severe symptoms. SEE: *scarlatina.*

s. rheumatica. Scarlatina with severe pain. SYN: *dengue.*

scarlatinal (skar-lă-tē'năl). Concerning or due to scarlatina.

scarlatinella (skar-lă-tĭn-el'lă), A mild disease resembling measles and scarlet fever. SYN: *fourth disease, rubella scarlatinosa.*

scarlatiniform, scarlatinoid (skar-lă-tĭn'ĭ-form, -lăt'ĭ-noyd). Resembling scarlatina or its rash.

scarlet (skar'lĕt). A bright red color, as that of a rash.

s. fever. Acute, contagious, febrile disease marked by sore throat, and a scarlet rash. SYN: *scarlatina, q.v.*

s. rash. A rose-colored rash, specifically that of German* measles.

scar'let red. An azo dye, of the color its name suggests.

DOSAGE: 4 to 8% ointment. SYN: *rubrum scarlatinum.*

Scarpa's fascia (skar'pa). Deep layer of superficial abdominal fascia around edge of the subcutaneous inguinal ring.

S's. fluid. Fluid in membranous labyrinth of the ear. SYN: *endolymph.*

S's. foramina. Bony passages opening into the incisor canal for passage of the nasopalatine nerves.

S's. liquor. SEE: *Scarpa's fluid.*

S's. membrane. Membrane that closes the fenestra rotunda of the tympanic cavity.

S's. triangle. Triangular space bounded laterally by inner edge of sartorius, above by Poupart's ligament, and medially by the adductor longus.

scatacratia (skăt-ă-krā'shĭ-ă). Fecal incontinence.

scatemia (skăt-ē'mĭ-ă). Intestinal toxemia from retained fecal matter.

scatology (skăt-ŏl'ō-jĭ). 1. Scientific study and analysis of the feces. SYN: *coprology.* * 2. Interest in obscene things, esp. literature.

scatoma (skă-tō'mă). Mass of inspissated feces in colon or rectum resembling an abdominal tumor. SYN: *coproma, fecaloma, stercoroma.*

scatophagy (skă-tŏf'ăj-ĭ). The eating of excrement. SYN: *coprophagy.*

scatoscopy (skă-tŏs'kō-pĭ). Examination of excreta for diagnostic purposes.

scavenger cells (skăv'ĕn-jer). Wandering phagocytic cells, common in the nervous system, that aid in removing disintegrated tissue.

scelalgia (skē-lăl'jĭ-ă, sē-lăl'jĭ-ă). Pain in a leg.

s. puerperarum. Painful swelling of the leg due to septic infection in the puerperium. SYN: *phlegmasia alba dolens.*

Schacher's ganglion (shah'ker). The ophthalmic ganglion.

Schachowa's spiral tube (shah-ko'vah). Part of a uriniferous tubule between a looped tubule and a convoluted one.

Schafer's method of artificial respiration (shā'fer). Patient placed face down and intermittent pressure is applied to area over the lower thorax. SEE: *artificial* respiration.*

Schäffer's reflex (shā'fer). Dorsal flexion of toes and flexion of foot resulting when middle portion of tendo Achillis is pinched.

Schede's method (shā'dē). Treatment of caries of bone by scraping away dead tissue and allowing cavity to fill with a blood clot.

S's. operation. A radical thoracoplasty.   [arsenite.

Scheel's green (shā'lēz, shēlz). Copper

schematic (skē-măt'ĭk). Pert. to a diagram or model; showing part for part in a diagram.

s. eye. A diagram or model showing proportions of a typical eye.

Scheurlen's bacillus (shor'lĕnz). A bacillus once thought to cause carcinoma.

Schick's method (shĭk). Injection of a mixture or toxin and antitoxin to cause immunity to diphtheria.

Schiller's test (shĭl'er). One for superficial cancer, esp. of the cervix uteri.

Paint with solution of iodine. Cancer cells not containing glycogen fail to stain, thus revealing their presence.

Schilling's hem'ogram (shĭl'ĭng). Method of taking a differential blood count by separating the polymorphonuclear neutrophils into 4 categories according to number and arrangement of the nuclei in the cells.

schindylesis (skĭn-dĭ-lē'sĭs). A form of synarthrosis* in which the receptor of a plate of one bone fits into a fissure of another one. SEE: *gomphosis, synchondrosis.*

schistasis (skĭs'tăs-ĭs). A splitting; specifically, a congenital fissure of the body.

schistocelia (skĭs-tō-sē'lĭ-ă). Congenital abdominal fissure.

schistocyte (skĭs'tō-sīt). 1. A blood cell in process of segmentation. 2. A very tiny red blood corpuscle.

schistocytosis (skĭs"tō-sī-tō'sĭs). 1. Schistocytes in the blood. 2. Segmentation process of blood corpuscles.

schistoglossia (skĭs"tō-glos'ĭ-ă). A cleft tongue.

schistoprosopia (skĭs"tō-prō-sō'pĭ-ă). Congenital fissure of the face.

schistorrhachis (skĭs"tor'ă-kĭs) Protrusion of membranes through a congenital cleft in lower vertebral column. SYN: *spina bifida.*

Schistosoma (skĭs"tō-sō'mă). A genus of trematode parasitic worms. SYN: *flukes.*

schistosomiasis (skĭs"tō-sō-mī'ăs-ĭs). Infestation with Schistosoma.

schistothorax (skĭs"tō-thō'răks). Fissure of the thorax.

schizaxon (skĭs-ăks'ŏn). A neuraxon that divides in 2 equal or nearly equal branches.

schizo-. Combining form meaning to *split.*

schizocyte (skĭs'ō-sīt). 1. A blood cell in process of segmentation. 2. A tiny red blood cell. SYN: *schistocyte.*

schizocytosis (skĭs"ō-sī-tō'sĭs). Schistocytes in the blood. SYN: *schistocytosis.*

schizogenesis (skĭz"ō-jĕn'ĕs-ĭs). BIOL: Reproduction by fission.*

schizogyria (skĭz-ō-jĭ'rĭ-ă). A break or cleft in the cerebral convolutions.

schizoid (skĭz'oyd). Similar to schizophrenia, name applied to one unduly given to introspection and the inner rather than the outer life.

Schizomycetes (skĭz"ō-mī-sē'tēz). Class of plant microorganisms or fungi which multipy by fission.

schizomycosis (skĭz"ō-mī-kō'sĭs). Disease caused by Schizomycetes.

schizont (skǐz'ont). A form of protozoa showing alternation* of generation.

schizonychia (skǐz″ō-nǐk′ǐ-ǎ). Split condition of the nails.

schizophasia (skǐz-ō-fā′zǐ-ǎ). Muttered and incomprehensible speech of the schizophrenic.

schizophrenia (skǐz-ō-frē′nǐ-ǎ). The most important of the psychoses, characterized by loss of contact, with the environment and by disintegration of personality.

schizophrenic (skǐz″ō-frěn′ǐk). Afflicted with or person afflicted with schizophrenia.

schizophrenosis (skǐz″ō-frē-nō′sǐs). Any of the types of schizophrenia.

schizothemia (skǐz-ō-thē′mǐ-ǎ). Psy: Hysterical resort to reminiscences during a conversation.   [the hair.

schizotrichia (skǐz″ō-trǐk′ǐ-ǎ). Splitting of

Schlemm's canal (shlěm). Irregular space or spaces in the sclerocorneal region of the eye.

    S.'s ligament. One of 2 ligaments of the shoulder joint. Syn: *glenoideobrachial ligament.*

Schmidt's intestinal test (shmǐt). Test diet given for indigestion.

Schmidt-Strassburger motor test meal. An intestinal motility test meal.

schneiderian membrane (shnī-dē′rǐ-ǎn). The nasal mucosa. Syn: *pituitary membrane.*

    s. reflex. Contraction of facial muscles due to irritation of nasal mucosa.

Schönlein's disease (shen′līn). An acute disease characterized by purpuric spots, urticaria, sore throat, and inflammation of the joints resembling rheumatism. Syn: *peliosis, purpura rheumatica.*

Schott method (shŏt). Resisting exercises and special baths in the treatment of heart disease.

Schüller's ducts (shil′er). Those of Skene's glands.

    S.'s glands. The glands of the urethra.

    S.'s phenomenon. Turning to the sound side in walking, in functional hemiplegia, but to the affected side in cases of organic lesion.

Schultze's bundle. Longitudinal mass of descending fibers shaped like a comma, in the fasciculus cuneatus of spinal cord.

    S.'s cells. Olfactory cells.

    S.'s granule masses. Fine, granular masses formed by breaking up of plaques in the blood.

    S.'s method. A method of resuscitating an asphyxiated infant at birth.

    The 1st and 2nd fingers are placed in child's axillae, with thumbs over shoulders. The child is held firmly, and swung at arm's length above head of nurse, which brings the legs of the infant on to the abdomen, thereby compressing the chest. On swinging child down again, the chest becomes expanded, and so inspiration takes place.

Schwabach test (shvah′bahkh). A test for hearing by use of 5 tuning forks, each of a different tone. See: *test.*

Schwann's primitive bundle (shvan). A muscular fiber.

    S.'s sheath. The neurilemma of a nerve fiber. Syn: *neurilemma.*

    S.'s white substance. Myelin of a medullated nerve fiber.

schwannoma (shvan-nō′mǎ). A tumor having its origin in Schwann's sheath.

sciage (se-ahzh′). A movement in massage resembling that in sawing.

sciatic (sī-ǎt′ǐk). 1. Pert. to the hip or ischium. 2. Pert. to, due to, or afflicted with, sciatica.

    s. nerve. Largest nerve in the body arising from sacral plexus on either side, passing from pelvis to greater sciatic foramen, down back of thigh, where it divides into tibial and peroneal nerves.

    s. n., great. Has 2 divisions—external and internal popliteal.

    s. n., small. Ischiatic nerve; a cutaneous nerve supplying skin of buttocks, perineum, popliteal region, and back of thigh. Lesions of: Result in flaccidity of affected buttock, difficult extension of thigh.

sciatica (sī-ǎt′ǐ-kǎ). Inflammation and pain along the sciatic nerve felt at back of thigh running down the inside of the leg. See: *meralgia; sciatic, lesions of.*

science (sī′ĕns). 1. Any branch of systematized knowledge considered as a distinct field of investigation or object of study. 2. Knowledge accumulated and classified and made available for work.

scieropia (sī-ĕr-ō′pǐ-ǎ). Abnormal vision in which things appear to be in shadow.

scillaren (sǐl′ǎ-rēn). A mixture of glucosides obtained from squill.

    Dosage: 1/40 gr. (1.6 mg.).

scintillascope (sǐn-tǐl′ǎ-skōp). Device for estimating physical properties of radium. Syn: *spinthariscope.*

scintillation (sǐn-tǐl-lā′shŭn). Sparkling; a subjective sensation, as of seeing sparks.

scirrho-. Combining form meaning *hard,* as *scirrhus,* a hard tumor.

scirrhoid (skǐr′oyd). Pert. to or like a hard carcinoma or scirrhus.

scirrhoma (skǐr-ō′mǎ). A hard carcinoma or scirrhus.

scirrhosarca (skǐr-ō-sar′kǎ). Hardening of the flesh, esp. of the newly born. Syn: *sclerema neonatorum, scleroderma.*

scirrhous (skǐr′rŭs). Hard, like a scirrhus.

scirrhus (skǐr′ŭs). A hard, cancerous tumor due to overgrowth of fibrous tissue. A hard form of cancer.

    s., atrophic. Tumor resulting from the fatty degeneration and absorption of the epithelial cells. Perhaps induced by unusually abundant development of the fibrous stroma, contracting so as to diminish the blood supply to the cells. Leaves little more than a mass of fibrous tissue, with here and there a few cells surrounded by débris. Although tumor is slower in its growth and rather diminishes than increases in size, its malignancy is not lost, the ultimate result being same. Syn: *witherings.*

s. of breast. SYM: Scirrhus forms an irregular, nodulated, somewhat rounded, stony, hard, heavy mass, inseparable from the glandular tissue, possessing no defined outline, but gradually merging into the healthy mammary tissue, with which it freely moves. Soon it adheres to the skin which becomes dimpled, and later to the pectoral muscle, thus at first being partially, then immovably, fixed to chest wall; grows slowly, nipple gradually becomes retracted, but growth never attains large size.

s. of testicle. Presents no features peculiar to the locality; is very rare.

s. ventriculi. 1. Induration and diffuse thickening of wall of stomach, esp. of the pylorus. 2. A form of chronic gastritis.

scissor leg (sĭz'or lĕg). Abnormal crossing of both legs, the result of adduction at both hips. SYN: *x-leg.*

s. l. gait. Crossing the legs in walking. SEE: *gait.*

scissors (sĭz'ors). A cutting instrument composed of 2 opposed cutting blades with handles, held together by a central pin.

sclera (sklē'rä) (pl. *sclerae*). BNA. The white or sclerotic outer coat of the eye. It extends from optic nerve to cornea. SYN: *sclerotica.*

scleradenitis (sklē-rad-ĕn-ī'tĭs). Inflammation and induration of a gland.

scleral (sklē'răl). Concerning the sclera.

sclerectasia (sklĕr-ĕk-tā'zĭ-ä). Protrusion of the sclera.

sclerectoiridectomy (sklĕr-ĕk″tō-ĭr-ĭ-dĕk'tō-mĭ). Formation of a filtering cicatrix in glaucoma by combined sclerectomy and iridectomy.

sclerectoiridodialysis (sklĕr-ĕk″tō-ĭr-ĭd-ō-dī-ăl'ĭ-sĭs). Sclerectomy and iridodialysis for relief of glaucoma.

sclerectomy (sklē-rĕk'tō-mĭ). 1. Excision of a portion of the sclera. 2. Removal of adhesions in chronic otitis media.

sclerema (sklē-rē'mä). Hardening of the skin. SYN: *scleroderma.*

s. neonatorum. Progressive hardening of the skin in the newly born; usually fatal.

scleriasis (sklē-rī'ăs-ĭs). Progressive hardening of the skin. SYN: *scleroderma.*

scleriritomy (sklēr-ĭ-rĭt'ō-mĭ). Incision of iris and sclera.

scleritis (sklē-rī'tĭs). Inflammation of the sclera; superficial and deep. SEE: *episcleritis.*

scleroblastema (sklē″rō-blăs-tē'mä). The embryonic tissue from which formation of bone takes place.

scleroblastemic (sklē″rō-blăs-tĕm'ĭk). Relating to or derived from scleroblastema.

sclerocataracta (sklē″rō-kăt-ä-răkt-ä). A hard cataract.

sclerochoroiditis (sklē″rō-kō-roy-dī'tĭs). Inflammation of the sclera and choroid coat of the eye.

sclerocornea (sklē″rō-kor'nē-ä). The sclera and cornea together considered as one coat.

sclerodactylia (sklē″rō-dăk-tĭl'ĭ-ä). Induration of the skin of the fingers and toes.

scleroderma (sklē-rō-der'mä). Hard, thickened, rigid disease of the skin resulting in a hidebound condition.

s., circumscribed. Skin disease with pink, firm patches which atrophy, leaving scars. SYN: *morphea.*

s. neonatorum. Hardness and tightness of the skin in early infancy. SYN: *sclerema.*

sclerodermitis (sklē″rō-der-mä-tī'tĭs). Induration and inflammation of the skin.

sclerogenous (sklē-rŏj'ĕn-ŭs). Causing sclerosis or hardening of tissue.

scleroiritis (sklē″rō-ĭ-rī'tĭs). Inflammation of both sclera and iris.

sclerokeratitis (sklē″rō-ker-ă-tī'tĭs). Cellular infiltration with inflammation of the sclera and cornea.

sclerokeratoiritis (sklē″rō-ker″ă-tō-ĭ-rī'tĭs). Inflamed condition of the sclera, cornea, and iris.

scleroma (sklē-rō'mä). Indurated, circumscribed area of granulation tissue in mucous membrane or skin. SEE: *sclerosis.*

scleromere (sklē'rō-mēr). Any homologous segment of the skeleton.

scleronyxis (sklē-rō-nĭks'ĭs). Puncture of the sclera.

sclero-oöphoritis (sklē″rō-ō″ŏf-or-ī'tĭs). Induration and inflammation of the ovary.

sclerophthalmia (sklēr-ŏf-thăl'mĭ-ä). Congenital condition in which opacity of the sclera advances over the cornea.

scleroprotein (sklē″rō-prō'tē-ĭn). One of group of simple proteins* forming the skeletal structure of animals marked by their insolubility.

sclerosarcoma (sklē″rō-sar-kō'mä). A fleshy, fibrous tumor of the gums. SEE: *epulis.*

sclerosed (sklē-rōsd', sklē'rōsd). Having sclerosis; hardened. SYN: *indurated.*

sclerosing (sklē-rō'sĭng). Causing or suffering from sclerosis.

sclerosis (sklē-rō'sĭs). An induration of inflammatory nature, esp. of the nervous system; also a chronic thickening of the arteries' coats due to inflammation.

s., Alzheimer's. Hyaline degeneration affecting the small blood vessels of brain.

s., amyotrophic lateral. Progressive muscular atrophy affecting lateral columns of the spinal cord and ending in bulbar paralysis.

s., arterial. Hardening of the coats of the arteries. SYN: *arteriosclerosis.*

s., diffuse. Sclerosis affecting large areas of the brain and spinal cord.

s., disseminated. Condition characterized by inflammatory patches which become sclerosed, freely scattered through the brain and spinal cord.

s., insular. Multiple sclerosis, q.v.

s., lateral. Sclerosis of a lateral column of the spinal cord.

s., multiple. Chronic induration in patches scattered over the nervous system

s., neural. Sclerosis with chronic inflammation of a nerve trunk with branches.

s., vascular. Same as arterial sclerosis, *q.v.*

scleroskeleton (sklē″rō-skěl′ě-tŏn). Skeletal parts resulting from ossification of fibrous structures, such as ligaments, fasciae, and tendons.

sclerostenosis (sklē″rō-sten-ō′sĭs). Contraction and induration of tissues.

s. cutanea. Induration of the skin. SYN: *scleroderma.*

sclerostomy (sklē-rŏs′tō-mĭ). Formation of an opening in the sclera.

sclerothrix (sklē′rō-thrĭks). Brittleness of the hair.

sclerotic (sklē-rŏt′ĭk). 1. Pert. to or affected with sclerosis. 2. Hard.

s. acid. An amorphous, brown powder from ergot. A hemostatic and oxytocic.

s. coat. The membrane forming the ext. coat of the eye. SYN: *sclera, sclerotica.*

s. teeth. Hard, yellowish ones almost immune to caries.

sclerotica (sklē-rŏt′ĭ-kă). The ext. white coat of the eye. SYN: *sclera, sclerotic coat.*

scleroticectomy (sklē-rŏt-ĭ-sěk′tō-mĭ). Excision of a part of the sclera. SYN: *sclerectomy.*

scleroticochoroiditis (sklē-rŏt″ĭ-kō-kō″roy-dī′tĭs). Inflammation of sclerotic and choroid coats of the eye. SYN: *sclerochoroiditis.*

scleroticonyxis (sklē-rŏt-ĭk-ō-nĭks′ĭs). Puncture of the sclera. SYN: *scleronyxis.*

scleroticopuncture (sklē-rŏt″ĭk-ō-pŭnk′tūr). Surgical puncture of the sclera. SYN: *scleronyxis, scleroticonyxis.*

scleroticotomy (sklē-rŏt-ĭk-ŏt′ō-mĭ). Incision of the sclerotic coat of the eye. SYN: *sclerotomy.*

sclerotitis (sklē-rō-tī′tĭs). Inflammation of the sclera. SYN: *scleritis.*

sclerotium (sklē-rō′shĭ-ŭm). Hardened mass formed of mycelium and food débris, the resting stage of certain fungi.

sclerotome (sklē′rō-tōm). 1. Knife used in incision of the sclera. 2. Embryonic mass of tissue from which part of the skeleton arises.

sclerotomy (sklē-rŏt′ō-mĭ). Simple division of sclera.

s., anterior. Incision at angle of anterior chamber in glaucoma.

s., posterior. Opening through sclera into the vitreous for detached retina, removal of foreign body, etc.

scolecology (skō″lē-kŏl′ō-jĭ). The study of parasitic worms. SYN: *helminthology.*

scolectomy (skō-lěk′tō-mĭ). Operation for removal of the vermiform appendix. SYN: *appendectomy.*

scoledocostomy (skō-lěd-ō-kŏs′tō-mĭ). Creation of an opening into the vermiform appendix. SYN: *appendicostomy.*

scoliometer (skō-lĭ-ŏm′ět-ěr). Device for measuring curves, esp. lateral ones of the spine.

scoliorachitic (skō″lĭ-ō-ra-kĭt′ĭk). Pert. to or afflicted with spinal curvature from rickets.

scoliosiometry (skō″lĭ-ō-sĭ-ŏm′ě-trĭ). Measurement of degree of spinal curvature.

scoliosis (skō-lĭ-ō′sĭs). Lateral curvature of the spine.

Usually consists of 2 curves, the original one and a compensatory curve in the opp. direction.

s., cicatricial. Scoliosis due to cicatricial contraction resulting from necrosis.

s., coxitic. Scoliosis in the lumbar spine due to tilting of the pelvis in hip disease.

s., empyematic. Scoliosis following empyema and retraction of one side of the chest.

s., habit. Scoliosis due to habitually assumed improper position.

s., inflammatory. Scoliosis due to disease of the vertebrae.

s., ischiatic. Scoliosis due to hip disease.

s., myopathic. Weakening of spinal muscles causing a lateral curvature.

s., ocular; s., ophthalmic. Scoliosis from tilting of the head in astigmatism.

s., osteopathic. Same as scoliosis myopathic, *q.v.*

s., paralytic. Lateral curvature of the spine due to paralysis of the muscles.

s., rachitic. Scoliosis due to rickets.

s., rheumatic. Scoliosis due to rheumatism of dorsal muscles.

s., sciatic. Lateral curvature in sciatica.

s., static. That due to difference in length of legs.

scoliosometry (skō″lĭ-ō-sŏm′ět-rĭ). Determination of degree of spinal curvature SYN: *scoliosiometry.*

scoliotic (skō-lĭ-ŏt′ĭk). Suffering from or related to scoliosis.

scoliotone (skō′lĭ-ō-tōn). An apparatus for correcting the curve in scoliosis by stretching the spine.

scolopsia (skō-lŏp′sĭ-ă). A suture bet. 2 bones which permits reciprocal motion

scoop (skōōp). Surgical spoon-shaped instrument.

s., bone. Instrument for scraping or removing necrosed bone or contents of suppurative tracts. Volkmann's Schede's, Von Bruns, Hebras, Treves.

s., bullet. Instrument for dislodging bullets.

s., cataract. Instrument for removing fluids, foreign growths, for exerting pressure or center pressure.

s., ear. Instrument for removing middle ear granulations.

s., lithotomy. Instrument for dislodging encysted calculi, removing stones débris, etc.

s., mastoid. Instrument used in mastoid operations.

s., renal. Instrument to dislodge or remove small stones from pelvis or kidney.

scopograph (skŏp′ō-grăf). A fluoroscope

and radiographic unit combined in one device.

scopolamine hydrobromide (sko-pol'ă-mēn hī"drŏ-brŏ'mĭd). USP. The hydrobromide of alkaloids obtained from plants of the nightshade family.
DOSAGE: 1/120 gr. (0.5 mg.).

scopophobia (skō"pō-fō'bĭ-ă). Abnormal fear of being seen.

scopophobiac (skō"pō-fō'bĭ-ăk). One who is afraid of being seen.

scoptolagniac (skŏp-tō-lăg'nĭ-ăk). One who derives sexual gratification from observing objects or situations. SYN: *voyeur, q.v.* SEE: *scoptophilia.*

scoptophilia (skŏp-tō-fĭl'ĭ-ă). Sexual pleasure derived from visual sources, such as nudity, obscene pictures, etc.

scoptophobia (skŏp-tō-fō'bĭ-ă). Aversion to being seen.

scoptophobiac (skŏp"tō-fō'bĭ-ăk). One who dreads being seen.

-scopy. Combining form meaning *examination.*

scoracratia (skōr-ăk-rā'shĭ-ă). Inability to retain the feces. SYN: *scatacratia.*

scorbutic (skor-bū'tĭk). Concerning or affected with scurvy.

scorbutus (skor-bū'tŭs). A deficiency disease due to lack of vitamin C in fresh vegetables and fruits. SYN: *scurvy, q.v.* SEE: *deficiency diseases, vitamin.*

scordinema (skor-dĭn-ē'mă). Yawning and stretching with heaviness of the head, a prodrome of an infectious disease.

scoretemia (skor-ĕ-tē'mĭ-ă). Autointoxication resulting from absorption of feces in the intestine. SYN: *scatemia.*

scorpion bite (skor'pĭ-ŏn). The symptoms are similar to those from a spider bite.

scotodinia (skō-tō-dĭn'ĭ-ă). Vertigo with black spots before the eyes and faintness.

scotogram, scotograph (skŏt'ō-grăm, -grăf). A print from an x-ray plate. SYN: *skiagram.*

scotography (skō-tŏg'ră-fĭ). Making of x-ray photographs. SYN: *skiagraphy.*

scotoma (skō-tō'mă) (pl. *scotomata*). Islandlike blind gap in the visual field.
s., absolute. An area in the visual field in which there is absolute blindness.
s., annular. A scotomatous zone which encircles the point of fixation like a ring, not always completely closed, but leaves the fixation point intact.
s., central. One which involves the point of fixation, seen in lesions of the macula.
s., color. Color blindness in the involved area.
s., flittering. Same as scintillating scotoma.
s., negative. One not perceptible by the patient.
s., physiological. Blind spot where optic nerve enters the retina.
s., positive. One which patient perceives in his visual field as a dark spot.
s., relative. One in which perception of the object is impaired but not completely lost.

s., scintillating. An irregular outline around a luminous patch in the visual field following mental or physical labor or eyestrain or in migraine.

scotomagraph (skō-tō'mă-grăf). Instrument for automatically recording the shape and size of a scotoma.

scotomameter (skō"tō-măm'ĕ-ter). Instrument for measuring the size of a scotoma. [*toma.*

scotomata (skō-tō'mă-tă). Plural of *sco-*

scotomatous (skō-tom'ă-tŭs). Relating to, of the nature of, or afflicted with, scotoma.

scotometer (skō-tŏm'ĕt-ĕr). Device for detecting and measuring a dark spot in visual field.

scotometry (skō-tom'ĕ-trĭ). The locating and measurement of scotomata.

scotomization (skō-tō-mĭz-ā'shŭn). PSY: A sadistic expression seen in compulsion neuroses and schizophrenia by which the victim indulges in self-punishment as an expression of hatred for another.

scotophilia (skō-tō-fĭl'ĭ-ă). Preference for darkness or for the night. SYN: *nyctophilia.*

scotophobia (skō-tō-fō'bĭ-ă). Abnormal dread of darkness.

scotopia (skō-tō'pĭ-ă). The adjustment of vision for darkness.

scotoscopy (skō-tŏs'kō-pĭ). Examination of internal organs by use of the fluoroscope. SYN: *skiascopy.*

scototherapy (skō"tō-ther'ă-pĭ). Treatment of disease by keeping patient in a dark room and by exclusion of light, as in malaria.

scratch (skrătsh). A mark or superficial injury produced by scraping with the nails or a rough surface.

screatus (skre-ā'tŭs). A neurosis characterized by paroxysmal fits of hawking.

scriveners' palsy (skrĭv'ner). Occupational neurosis caused by excessive use of the hand in writing. SYN: *writers' cramp.*

scrobiculate (skrō-bĭk'ū-lāt). Having shallow depressions; pitted.

scrobiculus (skrō-bĭk'ū-lŭs). A small groove or pit.
s., cordis. Pit of the stomach; precordial or epigastric depression.

scrofula (skrŏf'ū-lă). A constitutional, tuberculous condition characterized by glandular swelling in the neck and inflammations of joints and mucous membranes followed by cheesy degeneration; tuberculosis of the glands, joints, bones.
s., erethistic. Less tendency to glandular enlargement. Individuals are dark colored, nervous temperament subject to catarrhal affections.
s., torpid. Most characteristic. Such children have light or reddish hair, a sallow or pasty complexion, puffy cheeks, protruding lips. Eyelids and conjunctivae often seat of a chronic inflammation. Catarrhal affections of nose and ear often exist; skin is eczematous and cervical glands enlarged.

scrofulide (skrof'ū-līd). Any scrofulous skin disease. SYN: *scrofuloderm, scrofuloderma*.

scrofuloderm, scrofuloderma (skrŏf'ū-lō-derm, -der'mă). Any tuberculous skin disease. SYN: *scrofulide*.

scrofulosis (skrŏf-ū-lō'sĭs). Predisposition to scrofula.

scrofulous (skrŏf'ū-lŭs). Of the nature of, or afflicted with, scrofula.

scrotal (skrō'tăl). Concerning the scrotum.

   s. reflex. Slow vermicular contraction of scrotal muscle when perineum is stroked or cold applied.

   s. tongue. A furrowed tongue.

scrotectomy (skrō-těk'tō-mĭ). Excision of part of the scrotum.

scrotitis (skrō-tī'tĭs). Inflamed condition of the scrotum.

scrotocele (skrō'tō-sēl). Hernia in the scrotum.

scrotum (skrō'tŭm) (pl. *scrota*). The double pouch containing the testicles and part of the spermatic cord.

   s., lymph. Dilatation of scrotal lymphatics. SYN: *elephantiasis of scrotum.*

scrub'bing. Term applied to sterilization of the hands for surgical operations.

scrub nurse. Term applied to operating room nurse who hands instruments to the surgeon, and who has previously sterilized her hands and wears sterile rubber gloves.

scruple (skrū'pl). Twenty grains apothecaries' weight; 1/3 dram. SYMB: ℈.

Scultetus bandage (skŭl-tē'tŭs). A many-tailed bandage used in compound fractures.

   S. position. One with head low and the body on an inclined plane.

scum (skŭm). BACT: Slimy floating islands of bacteria or impurities on the surface of a culture; an interrupted pellicle of bacterial growth.

scurf (skurf). A branny desquamation of the epidermis, esp. on the scalp. SEE: *dandruff.*

scurvy (skur'vĭ). A disease due to lack of fresh fruits and vegetables, and of vitamin C in diet.

   s., infantile. A form of scurvy which sometimes follows the prolonged use of condensed milk, sterilized milk or proprietary foods. SYN: *Barlow's disease.*

   s., land. Disease characterized by hemorrhage of the mucosa, ecchymoses and prostration. SYN: *purpura haemorrhagica.*

scute (skūt). A plate or thin lamina forming outer wall of the attic separating it from the tympanum.

   s., tympanic. A crescentic plate.

scutiform (skū'tĭ-form). Shield-shaped.

scutulum (skū'tū-lŭm) (pl. *scutula*). 1. Any of the thin crusts of favus. 2. The shoulder blade. SYN: *scapula.*

scutum (skū'tŭm). 1. Plate of bone resembling a shield. 2. The thyroid cartilage. 3. The kneecap. SYN: *patella.*

   s. cordis. The sternum.

   s. genu. The patella.

   s. pectoris. The thorax.

   s. thoracis. The sternum.

scybalous (sĭb'ăl-ŭs). Of the nature of hard fecal matter.

scybalum (sĭb'ăl-ŭm) (pl. *scybala*). A hard, rounded mass of fecal matter.

scypho-. Combining form meaning *cup.*

scyphoid (si'foyd). Cup-shaped.

scythian disease (sĭth'ĭ-ăn). Atrophy of male ext. genitalia with corresponding tendency to perversion and feminine manners.

scytitis (sī-tī'tĭs). Inflammation of the skin. SYN: *dermatitis.*

scytoblastema (sī'tō-blăs-tē'mă). Skin in embryonic stage of its development.

scytoblastesis (sī'tō-blăs-tē'sĭs). The condition and progressive development of the embryonic skin.

séance (sāns). A treatment, as by electricity or massage.

searcher (serch'er). Instrument for locating opening of ureter previous to inserting catheter, exploring sinuses, and esp. for detecting stones in the bladder. SYN: *sound.*

seasickness (sē'sĭk-něs). Disorder due to motion of a vessel at sea, or riding in cars, trains, and elevators. A similar condition affects some air travelers.

seat worm (sēt' worm). A genus of nematode worms, *Oxyuris vermicularis*, found in the sigmoid colon and the rectum.

sebaceous (sē-bā'shŭs). Containing or pert. to sebum, an oily, fatty matter secreted by the sebaceous glands.

   s. cyst. A cyst filled with sebaceous material from a distended sebaceous gland.

   s. gland. Oil-secreting gland of the skin.

   SEE: *seborrhea, sebum, steatoma, steatorrhea.*

sebastomania (sē-băs-tō-mā'nĭ-ă). Religious insanity.

sebiagogic (seb-ĭ-ă-goj'ĭk). Forming fat or sebaceous matter. SYN: *sebiferous, sebiparous.*

sebiferous (sē-bĭf'ĕr-ŭs). Producing fatty or sebaceous matter. SYN: *sebiagogic, sebiparous.*

sebip'arous. Producing sebum or sebaceous matter. SYN: *sebiagogic, sebiferous.*

sebolite, sebolith (sĕb'ō-līt, -lĭth). Concretion in a sebaceous gland.

seborrhagia (sĕb-ō-rā'jĭ-ă). Excessive secretion of sebaceous glands. SYN: *seborrhea.*

seborrhea (sĕb-or-ē'ă). Functional disease of the sebaceous glands marked by increase in the amount and often alteration of the quality of the sebaceous secretion.

   s. capillitii. Scalp seborrhea.

   s. congestiva. Facial form with elevated patches with red borders and covered with crusts and scars. SYN: *lupus erythematosus.*

   s. corporis. Seborrhea of the trunk.

   s. faciei. Seborrhea of the face.

   s. nigra, s. nigricans. Dark-colored crusts in seborrhea.

s. oleosa. Seborrhea in which fat elements predominate. Shows shiny skin with widely dilated follicular orifices, many of which contain comedones.

s. sicca. Seborrhea with grayish-brown or yellow scale and crust formation in addition to abnormal oiliness.

seborrheic (sĕb-or-rē'ĭk). Afflicted with or like seborrhea.

seborrheid (sĕb-ō-rē'ĭd). A seborrheic eruption.

seborrhoea (sĕb-or-ē'ä). Disease of the sebaceous glands marked by increased discharge and altered quality of the secretion. SYN: *seborrhea, q.v.*

seborrhoic (sĕb-or-ō'ĭk). Suffering from or like seborrhea.* SYN: *seborrheic.*

sebum (sē'bŭm). A fatty secretion of the sebaceous glands of the skin.

secernent (sē-ser'nĕnt). 1. Secreting. 2. A secreting organ.

seclusio pupillae. Shutting off of the pupil due to adherence of iris to the lenticular capsule. SYN: *synechia, annular posterior.*

s. p. siderosis bulbi. Deposit of iron pigment within the eyeball.

Seen in cases of retained iron foreign body in the eye.

seconal (sē'kŏn-ăl). A barbituric acid derivative.

DOSAGE: 1.5 gr. (0.1 Gm.).

second cranial nerve (sĕk'und). The optic nerve which controls sight.

s. intention. Healing by granulation or indirect union.

s. sight. Alteration in refractive powers of the lens so that reading again is possible without glasses in incipient cataract. SYN: *gerontopia.**

s. stage of labor. Period bet. complete dilatation of cervix and delivery of the child.

During this stage pains become severe. It lasts normally 2-4 hr. in primiparae and up to 1 hr. in multiparae.

secondary (sek'ŭn-dar-ĭ). 1. Next to or following; second in order. 2. Produced by a primary cause. SYN: *subordinate.*

s. areola. Pigmentation around the nipples during pregnancy. SEE: *areola.*

s. disease. One following a previous disease.

s. hemorrhage. 1. One after an injury or operation coming on more than 24 hr. afterward and which is due to sepsis and septic ulceration into a blood vessel. 2. Uterine bleeding due to septic infection or from infant's umbilicus due to same cause. SEE: *hemorrhage.*

secreta (sē-krē'tä). The products of secretion.

secretagogue (sē-krē'tă-gog). 1. Causing secretion. 2. That which stimulates secreting organs, as "substances present in food or produced by the digestion or decomposition of food which excite the secretion of digestive juice either by acting locally or by being absorbed into the blood or lymph or by causing a hormone to be formed." (A. C. Ivy.)

secrete (sē-krēt'). To separate a constituent from the blood, elaborate and discharge it; said of a gland.

secretin (sē-krē'tĭn). 1. A hormone formed in the mucous membrane of the duodenum through the influence of acid contents from the stomach whose function is to stimulate the flow of pancreatic juice. 2. A substance of unknown chemical composition, prepared by extraction from the mucous membrane of the duodenum and causing, when injected intravenously, an increased secretion of pancreatic juice.

SEE: *duodenal and intestinal digestion, gastrin.*

secretion (sē-krē'shŭn). 1. A process in physiology whereby certain materials are separated, by the activity of a gland, from the blood, and made into something useful to the body. 2. Substance secreted. Fluids of the body.

s., antilytic. Watery saliva excreted continuously by submaxillary gland with intact nerves after division of the chorda tympani of the other side.

s., external. Secretion discharged from the body.

s., internal. Secretion imparted to the blood instead of being eliminated by a duct.

s., nervous. Secretion that depends upon activity of secretory nerves.

s., paralytic. Abundant watery secretion continuously from a gland after section of its secretory nerves.

secretodermatosis (sē-krē"tō-der-mă-tō'sĭs). Condition resulting from disorder of the secretory function of the skin.

secretogogue (sē-krē'tō-gŏg). 1. Causing secretion. 2. That which stimulates secretion.

secretoinhibitory (sē-krē"tō-ĭn-hĭb'ĭ-tō-rĭ). Checking secretion.

secretomotor, secretomotory (sē-krē"tō-mō"tor, -ĭ). Stimulating or promoting secretion.

secretory (sē-krē'tō-rĭ, sē'krē-tō-rĭ). Pert. to or promoting secretion; secreting.

s. capillaries. Very small canaliculi receiving secretion discharged from gland cells.

s. fibers. Centrifugal nerve fibers which excite secretion.

sectarian (sĕk-tār'ĭ-ăn). A medical man who "follows a dogma, tenet, or principle based on the authority of its promulgator to the exclusion of demonstration and practice" (Judicial Council A. M. A.).

sectile (sĕk'tĭl). Capable of being cut.

section (sĕk'shŭn). 1. Process of cutting. 2. A division or segment of a part. 3. A surface made by cutting.

s., abdominal. Any abdominal operation. SYN: *laparotomy, q.v.*

s., cesarean. Incision of uterus for delivery of a fetus through abdominal wall or through the vagina. SEE: *cesarean section.*

s., frontal. One dividing the body into 2 parts, *dorsal* and *ventral.*

s., occipital. Transverse section through middle of the occipital lobe.

s., parietal. Transverse vertical section through ascending parietal convolution.

s., perineal. External incision into urethra to relieve stricture.

s., sagittal. One parallel with the sagittal suture.

s., serial. Microscopic sections made and arranged in consecutive order.

s., sigaultian. Resection of the symphysis pubis. SYN: *symphysiotomy*.

s., vaginal. Incision into the abdominal cavity through the vagina.

sectioning (sĕk-shŭn'ĭng). The slicing of thin sections of tissue for examination under the microscope.

sector (sĕk'tor). The area of a circle included bet. 2 radii and an arc.

sectorial (sĕk-tō'rĭ-ăl). Cutting, as teeth.

secundae viae (sē-kŭn'dē vi'ē). Secondary passage in the body for nutrients, the lacteals, and blood vessels. SEE: *via*.

secundigravida (sē-kŭn″dĭ-grăv'ĭd-ă). A woman in her 2nd pregnancy.

secundinae (sĕk″ŭn-dē'nē). The membranes discharged after birth of the child. SYN: *afterbirth*.

secundines (sĕk'ŭn-dīns). The placenta and fetal membranes expelled during the 3rd stage of labor. SYN: *afterbirth*.

secundipara (sĕk″ŭn-dĭp'ă-ră). A woman who has borne 2 children at separate labors.

secundum artem (sē-kun'dŭm ar'tĕm). In an approved manner; according to rule or science.

S. E. D. Abbr. for *skin erythema dose*.

Sed. Abbr. of *sedes*, stool.

sedation (sē-dā'shŭn). 1. Process of allaying nervous excitement. 2. State of being calmed.

Usually effected by means of a drug.

sedative (sĕd'a-tĭv). 1. An agent allaying irritability or nerve action. 2. Quieting.

s., cardiac. One that decreases the heart's force.

s. enema. Retention enema given for its soothing action and to allay irritability. SEE: *enema, sedative*.

s., nervous. Sedative affecting nervous system.

s. poisons. TREATMENT: Administer large amounts of fluids and induce vomiting.

sedentary (sĕd'ĕn-ta-rĭ). 1. Sitting. 2. Pert. to an indoor occupation in which physical exercise is impossible.

sediment (sĕd'ĭ-mĕnt). The substance settling at bottom of a liquid. SYN: *hypostasis*. SEE: *precipitate*.

sedimentation (sĕd″ĭ-mĕn-tā'shŭn). Formation or depositing of sediment.

s. rate. Speed at which erythrocytes settle when an anticoagulant is added to blood. SYN: *suspension stability*.

sedimentator (sĕd-ĭ-mĕn-tā'tor). A centrifuge for separating urinary sediment.

seed (sēd). 1. The part of the fruit containing the germ. Ex: *nux vomica, mustard, colchicum seed*. 2. Sperm; semen.

3. Capsule containing radon, radium etc., for use in treatment of cancer. 4. Offspring. 5. To introduce microörganisms into a culture medium.

segment (sĕg'mĕnt). 1. A part or section esp. a natural one, of an organ or body 2. One of the serial divisions of an ani mal. SYN: *metamere*.

segmental (sĕg-mĕn'tăl). Relating to o forming a segment.

segmentation (sĕg″mĕn-tā'shŭn). 1. Divi sion into similar parts. SEE: *merogene sis*. 2. Formation of many cells from single cell. SYN: *cleavage*.

s. cavity. Central space in blastula stage of segmentation of an ovum.

s. nucleus. Nucleus developing fron union of the male and female pronucleï

s., rhythmic. Division of chyme inte segments by intestinal contractions SEE: *intestinal digestion*.

s. sphere. Cells of an ovum during early stages of segmentation when nu cleus is dividing.

segregator (sĕg're-gă-tor). Instrumen composed of 2 catheters for securing urine from each kidney separately.

Séguin's signal symptom (sa-ganz'). Contraction of muscles constituting a fore-runner of an epileptic attack.

Seidelin bodies (sī'de-lĭn). Parasitic organisms in the erythrocytes in yellow fever, the probable cause of the disease

Seidlitz powder (sĕd'lĭts, sīd'lĭtz). Effervescent cathartic composed of tartaric acid, sodium bicarbonate, and sodium and potassium tartrate.

seisesthesia (sī-zĕs-thē'zĭ-ă). The perception of a concussion.

seismesthesia (sīz-mĕs-thē'zĭ-ă). Perception of vibrations.

seismotherapy (sīz-mō-thĕr'ă-pĭ). Treatment of disease by vibratory massage. SYN: *sismotherapy*.

seizure (sē'zhŭr). A sudden attack of pain or of a disease, or of certain symptoms.

s., psychic. Appearance of morbid sensations, such as palpitation, with temporary disturbance of consciousness.

self-abuse'. Unnatural method of bringing about the venereal orgasm by mechanical friction, in either sex. SYN: *masturbation*.

self-diges'tion. Destruction or disintegration of a cell or tissue by its own juice, as that of the walls of the stomach by the gastric juice occurring in certain diseases of that organ. SYN: *autodigestion*.

self-induc'tance. Tendency in a conductor to oppose changes in current by formation of a counter electromotive force. SEE: *inductance*.

self-lim'ited disease. Disease that, without treatment, runs a definite course within a limited time.

self-pollu'tion. Sexual self-abuse. SYN: *masturbation*.

self-suspen'sion. Suspension of the body for extension by stretching of the vertebral column.

sella turcica (sĕl'ä tŭr'sĭ-ka). Pituitary fossa of middle of the sphenoid bone enclosing the pituitary body.

sellar (sĕl'ar). Pert. to the sella turcica, depression for pituitary body in sphenoid bone.

Selters water, Seltzer water (sĕl'ters, sĕlt'-ser). Effervescent mineral water containing carbonates of sodium, calcium, chloride of sodium, and magnesium.

semeiology (sē″mĭ-ŏl'ō-jĭ). The branch of medicine dealing with the study of symptoms. SYN: *symptomatology.*

semeiosis (sē-mĭ-ō'sĭs). Study of diseases by symptoms.

semeiotic (sē″mĭ-ot'ĭk). Of or pert. to symptoms. SYN: *symptomatic.*

semeiotics (sē″mĭ-ŏt'ĭks). 1. Phase of medical science treating of symptoms. 2. Symptoms of a disease in a particular case considered as a whole. SYN: *semiotics. symptomatology.*

semel (sĕm'ĕl). Once. SEE: *charting, prescription writing.*

semelincident (sĕm-ĕl-ĭn'sĭd-ĕnt). Occurring only once in the same person.

semen (sē'mĕn) (pl. *semina*). A thick, opalescent, viscid secretion discharged from the urethra of the male at the climax of sexual excitement (orgasm) which fertilizes the female ovum.

semenuria (sē″mĕn-ū'rĭ-ä). Excretion of semen in the urine. SYN: *seminuria, spermaturia.*

semi-. Prefix meaning *half.*

semicanal (sĕm″ĭ-kăn-ăl'). A duct open on one side.

semicircular (sĕm″ĭ-sĭr'kŭ-lar). In the form of a half circle.

  s. canals. Sup., post., and inf. passages forming back part of ear, *q.v.*

semicoma (sĕm″ĭ-kō'mä). Mild degree of coma from which it is possible to arouse the patient.

semicomatose (sĕm″ĭ-kō'măt-ōs). In a condition of unconsciousness from which patient may be aroused.

semiflexion (sĕm″ĭ-flē'shŭn). Position of a segment of a limb midway bet. flexion and extension.

semilunar (sĕm″ĭ-lū'nar). Crescentic in shape.

  s. bone. Halfmoon-shaped bone of carpus.

  s. cartilages. Two crescentic cartilages (int. and ext.) in the knee joint bet. the femur and tibia.

  s. ganglions. Two small nervous ganglions of the abdominal cavity, supplying solar plexus.

  s. lobe. One on upper surface of the cerebellum.

  s. notch. Notch in scapula for passage of the suprascapular nerve.

  s. valves. Valves of aorta and pulmonary artery. SEE: *Arantius' body.*

semimembranosus (sĕm″ĭ-mĕm-brăn-ō'sŭs). Large muscle of inner and back part of thigh.

seminal (sĕm'ĭn-ăl). Concerning the semen.

  s. emission. Involuntary loss of seminal fluid, usually during sleep, esp. in the adolescent male.

  s. filament. Male seed. SYN: *spermatozoon.*

  s. fluid. Semen, male fertilizing fluid.

  s. vesicle. Sac, on either side, in male connected with seminal duct and serving to store semen temporarily. SYN: *vesicula seminalis.*

semination (sĕm-ĭn-ā'shŭn). Introduction of semen into the uterus during sexual intercourse or artificially. SYN: *insemination.*

  s., artificial. Introduction of prepared semen into the uterus. SYN: *artificial insemination.*

seminiferous (sĕm-ĭn-ĭf'ĕr-ŭs). Producing or conducting semen, as the tubules of the testes.

seminoma (sĕm-ĭ-nō'mä). A tumor of the testis.

seminormal (sĕm″ĭ-nor'măl). One-half the normal standard.

  s. solution. One having half the quantity of the substance in the normal solution.

seminuria (sē″mĭn-ū'rĭ-ä). Seminal discharge present in the urine. SYN: *semenuria, spermaturia.*

semiology (sē″mĭ-ŏl'ō-jĭ). Phase of medicine dealing with study of symptoms. SYN: *semeiology, symptomatology.*

semiotic (sē-mĭ-ŏt'ĭk). Like or pert. to symptoms of disease. SYN: *semeiotic, symptomatic.*

semiotics (sē″mĭ-ŏt'ĭks). Scientific study of symptoms as a whole or in one particular case. SYN: *semiology, symptomatology.*

semiparasite (sĕm″ĭ-par'ä-sīt). 1. Organism usually a parasite, but capable of living as a saprophyte. 2. An organism with mild infectiousness for living tissue.

semipermeable (sĕm″ĭ-per'mē-ă-bl). Half permeable; said of a membrane which will allow fluids but not the dissolved substance to pass through it. SEE: *membrane, osmosis.*

semiprone (sĕm-ĭ-prōn'). In a position on left side and chest, with both thighs flexed on abdomen, the right higher than the left, and left arm back. SYN: *Sims' position, q.v.*

semirecumbent (sĕm″ĭ-rē-kŭm'bĕnt). Reclining, but not fully recumbent.

semis (sē'mĭs). Half.

  Abbreviated to *ss* after sign indicating the measure in prescriptions.

semisideratio, semisideration (sĕm″ĭ-sĭd-ĕr-ä'shĭ-ō, -ä'shŭn). Paralysis on one side of the body. SYN: *hemiplegia.*

semisopor (sĕm-ĭ-sō'por). Light coma from which patient can be roused. SYN: *semicoma.*

semispinalis (sĕm″ĭ-spĭ-na'lĭs). Deep layer of muscle of back on either side of spinal column, divided into 3 parts.

semisulcus (sĕm″ĭ-sŭl'kŭs). A slight depression or groove which forms a sulcus by uniting with a similar groove on the adjoining structure.

semisupination (sĕm″ĭ-sū-pĭn-ā′shŭn). A position halfway bet. supination and pronation.

semitendinosus (sĕm″ĭ-tĕn-dĭn-ō′sŭs). Fusiform muscle of post. and inner part of thigh.

semper-. Combining form meaning *always*.

senescence (sĕn-es′ĕns). The process of growing old, or the period of old age.

senile (sē′nīl, -nĭl). Pert. to growing old or to the aged.

senilism (sē′nĭl-ĭzm, -nĭl-ĭzm). Old age, particularly when premature. SEE: *progeria*.

senility (sē-nĭl′ĭ-tĭ). 1. The state of being old. 2. Weakness of old age, mental or physical.

   s., premature. Onset of characteristics before the normal time.
   May be due to dissipation, privation, or congenital structural defects.

   s., psychosis, of. Mental disorder in old age.

senium (sē′nĭ-ŭm). Old age, esp. its debility.

   s. precox. PSY: Mental disorder resembling senile dementia occurring before 60, usually showing incoherent delusions.

senna (sĕn′a). USP. The dried leaves of the plant *Cassia acutifolia* and *C. angustifolia*.

   DOSAGE: 30 gr. (2 Gm.).

Senn's bone plates (sĕn). Plates of decalcified bone used for intestinal anastomoses.

senopia (sĕn-ō′pĭ-ă). Improvement in visual power of old people usually due to incipient cataract. SYN: *gerontopia*.

sensation (sĕn-sā′shŭn). 1. State resulting when a stimulus is conveyed to the brain by the action of an afferent nerve and projected *externally* in the form of sight, smell, taste, hearing, heat, cold, or pressure, or *internally* as in hunger, pain, thirst, fatigue, sexual desire, etc. SEE: *receptor*. 2. Power or act of responding to stimulation.

   s., articular. Sensation caused by moving of joint surfaces.

   s., common. The sum total of all bodily sensations.

   s., cutaneous. Sensation through medium of the skin.

   s., delayed. Sensation not experienced immediately following a stimulus.

   s., epigastric. A sinking feeling in the stomach.

   s., external. Effect upon the mind of any stimuli from peripheral nerves.

   s., general. One of the body as a whole and not referred to any particular external object. SEE: *subjective sensation*.

   s., girdle. A painful sensation, as a bandage tightened about a limb or the trunk as in spinal disease. SYN: *zonesthesia*.

   s., gnostic. Nerve sensations, as those of touch and vibration.

   s., internal. A subjective one.

   s., palmesthetic. Sensation felt in the skin from vibration.

   s., referred. Same as reflex sensation.

   s., reflex. Sensation felt elsewhere than at point of stimulus.

   s., subjective. Sensation not resulting from any external stimulus and perceptible only by the subject.

   s., tactile. Sensation produced through the sense of touch.

   s., transferred. Same as a reflex sensation.

sense (sĕns). 1. To perceive through a sense organ. 2. The general faculty by which conditions outside or inside the body are perceived. 3. Any special faculty of sensation connected with a particular organ. 4. Normal power of understanding.

   s., acid. Ability of the stomach to regulate as needed the secretion of hydrochloric acid.

   s. body. The peripheral termination of nerve of special sensation.

   s. capsule. Hollow, cuplike receptacle of a peripheral sense organ.

   s., color. The perception of various colors.

   s., concomitant. A secondary sensation along with a primary one.

   s., cutaneous. Sensation felt through the skin.

   s., dermal. A sensation felt through the skin.

   s. epithelium. A tract of epithelium having a specialized function of sensation.

   s., genesic. The sexual instinct.

   s., kinesthetic. SEE: *muscular sense*.

   s., light. Perception of degree of light.

   s., muscle, muscular. Consciousness of muscular movement required in a given act.   [taste.

   s's., nutritive. Senses of smell and

   s. organ. The organ which receives a stimulus and converts it into a sensation.

   s., posture. Ability through muscle sense to differentiate positions of the body or its structures.

   s., pressure. Faculty of feeling various degrees of pressure on the body surface.

   s., seventh. Subjective sensations of internal organs.

   s. shock. Condition in hysterics at moment of awakening, the sensation rising from feet or hands and disappearing in the sense of having been struck a blow in the head.

   s., sixth. General feeling of normal functioning of the bodily organs. SYN: *cenesthesia*.

   s., space. That sense by which we recognize objects in space, their relationship and dimensions.

   s's., special. Sight, hearing, smell, touch, and taste.

   s., stereognostic. Ability to judge consistency and shape of objects held in the fingers.

   s., temperature. Ability to detect differences of temperature.

   s., time. Ability to detect differences in time intervals, as in sound.

s., tone. Ability to distinguish bet. different tones.

s., visceral. Perception of the sensations of the internal organs. SYN: *seventh sense.*

sensibilin (sĕn'sĭ-bĭl-ĭn). A specific antibody formed at first injection of a foreign protein, derived from sensibilisinogen.

sensibilisatrice (sĭn-se-be-le-să-trēs). An immune body. SYN: *amboceptor, q.v.*

sensibilisin (sĕn-sĭ-bĭl'ĭ-sĭn). A specific antibody produced by introduction of a foreign protein and arising from a substance in it. SYN: *anaphylactin.*

sensibilisinogen (sĕn-sĭ-bĭl-ĭs-ĭn'ō-jĕn). A substance in an antigen that, when injected, produces a specific antibody, *sensibilisin.* SEE: *allergen.*

sensibility (sĕn-sĭ-bĭl'ĭ-tĭ). Capacity to receive and respond to stimuli.

s., bone. Sensation like that received from the vibration of a tuning fork. SYN: *pallesthesia.*

s., deep. 1. The sensibility existing after an area is made anesthetic. 2. Sensation by which the position of a limb and estimation of difference in weight and tension is apparent.

s., epicritic. The sensibility which makes fine discriminations of touch and temperature.

s., mesoblastic. SEE: *deep sensibility.*

s., palmesthetic. SEE: *bone sensibility.*

s., protopathic. The sensibility to strong stimulations of pain and temperature, which exists in the skin and in the viscera.

s., recurrent. Sensibility in the ant. root of a spinal nerve when distal portion is stimulated after section.

s., somesthetic. Sensory consciousness of bodily movements.

s., splanchnesthetic. Consciousness or sensibility from splanchnic receptors.

sensibilization (sĕn-sĭ-bĭl-ĭz-ā'shŭn). 1. The process of making sensitive. 2. Production of hypersusceptibility to a foreign substance by injecting it into the body. SYN: *anaphylaxis, sensitization.*

sensibilizer (sĕn'sĭ-bĭl-ī-zer). Substance in blood serum normally or after inoculation which is active in cytolysis. SYN: *amboceptor, immune body, sensitizer.*

sensible (sĕn'sĭ-bl). 1. Capable of being perceived by the senses; perceptible. 2. Capable of receiving sensations. SYN: *sensitive.* 3. Having reason. SYN: *intelligent.* 4. Conscious, as opposed to insensible.

sensiferous (sĕn-sĭf'ĕr-ŭs). Conducting or transmitting sensations. [sensation.

sensigenous (sĕn-sĭj'ĕn-ŭs). Producing

sensimeter (sĕn-sĭm'ē-ter). Machine for recording the degree of sensitiveness of various areas of the body.

sensitinogen (sĕn-sĭ-tĭn'ō-jen). The antigens collectively which sensitize the body.

sensitive (sĕn'sĭ-tĭv). 1. Capable of transmitting a sensation. 2. Able to respond

to a stimulus. 3. Subject to destructive action of a complement. 4. Susceptible to suggestions, as a hypnotic. 5. Abnormally susceptible to a substance, as a drug or foreign protein.

sensitization (sĕn'sĭ-tĭ-zā'shŭn). 1. A condition of being made sensitive to specific stimulus. 2. Rendering of a cell sensitive to the action of a complement by uniting it with a specific amboceptor. 3. Process of making a person susceptible to a substance by repeated injections of it, as a serum. SYN: *anaphylaxis.*

sensitized (sĕn'sĭ-tĭzd). Made susceptible to a specific substance.

s. vaccine. A live culture which has been mixed with its antiserum before introduction.

sensitizer (sĕn'sĭ-tī'zer). An antibody producing susceptibility to cytolysis. SYN: *amboceptor.*

sensitometer (sĕn-sĭ-tŏm'ĕt-ĕr). Device for determining the penetrating power of light.

sensomobile (sĕn-sō-mō'bĭl). Capable of responding to a stimulus.

sensomotor (sĕn"sō-mō'tor). Both sensory and motor, esp. a nerve with both afferent and efferent fibers. SYN: *sensorimotor.*

sensoparalysis (sĕn"sō-păr-ăl'ĭ-sĭs). Paralysis of a sensory nerve.

sensorial (sĕn-sō'rĭ-ăl). Pert. to the sensorium, the seat of sensation.

sensorimotor (sĕn-sō-rĭ-mō'tor). Both sensory and motor. SYN: *sensomotor.*

sensorium (sĕn-sō'rĭ-ŭm) (pl. *sensoriums, -ria*). 1. Brain center of a nerve and its special sense organ. 2. The sensory apparatus of the body taken as a whole.

s., clear. Normal correct memory and orientation.

sensory (sĕn'sō-rĭ). 1. Conveying impulses from sense organs to the reflex or higher centers. SYN: *afferent.** 2. Pert. to sensation.

s. amusia. Inability to produce or understand musical sounds.

s. aphasia. Loss of memory for words. SEE: *aphasia.*

s. crossway. Part of the internal capsule behind lenticular nucleus at place where afferent fibers send forth sensory impulses to the opposite side.

s. decussation. The sup. pyramidal decussation.

s. epilepsy. Disturbances of sensation that replace epileptic convulsions.

s. nerve. An afferent nerve conveying sensory impressions to the sensorium, or one composed of sensory fibers.

sensual (sĕn'shū-ăl). Concerning or consisting in the gratification of the senses.

sensuous (sĕn'shū-ŭs). Pert. to or affecting the senses; susceptible to influence through the senses.

sentient (sĕn'shĭ-ĕnt). Capable of sensation. SYN: *sensitive.*

separator (sĕp'ar-ā-tor). 1. Anything which prevents 2 substances from mingling. 2. Device to prevent mingling in the bladder of urine from the 2 ureters.

separatorium (sĕp-ar-ă-tō'rĭ-ŭm). Instrument for separating pericranium from skull.

separatory (sĕp'ar-ă-tō"rĭ). Device for keeping objects or substances apart. SYN: *separator.*

sepedogenesis (sē"pĕd-ō-jĕn'ĕ-sĭs). Development of putrefaction.

sepsis (sĕp'sĭs). Poisoned state due to absorption of pathogenic bacteria and their products into the blood stream. SYN: *putrefaction, septicemia, q.v.*

 s., gas. Sepsis due to the gas bacillus, *Bacillus aerogenes capsulatus.*

 s., intestinal. Poisoning due to ingestion of decaying food.

 s. lenta. A more or less localized and slowly developing infection from *Streptococcus viridans.*

 s., puerperal. Infection of the genital tract following childbirth.

sepsometer (sĕp-sŏm'ĕ-ter). Device for detecting organic impurities in the air. SYN: *septometer,* ɠ.

septal (sĕp'tăl). Concerning a septum.

septan (sĕp'tăn). Recurring every 7th day, as the paroxysms of malarial fever.

septate (sĕp'tāt). Having a dividing wall.

septectomy (sĕp-tĕk'tō-mĭ). Excision of a septum, esp. the nasal septum or a part of it.

septemia (sĕp-tē'mĭ-ă). Invasion of the blood by pathogenic bacteria or their toxins. SYN: *septicemia.*

septic (sĕp'tĭk). Caused by or relating to putrefaction.

 s. fever, s. infection. Fever or infection due to presence of pathogenic organisms or their products in the blood. SYN: *septicemia.*

 s. sore throat. Streptococcic inflammation of throat with fever and marked prostration.

septicemia (sĕp-tĭ-sē'mĭ-ă). Morbid condition from absorption of septic products into blood and tissues or of pathogenic bacteria which may rapidly multiply there.

 s., bronchopulmonary. Septicemia following operation on the larynx resulting in infected secretions from the wound entering the bronchial tubes.

 s., Bruce's. Same as melitensis septicemia.

 s., cryptogenic. Septicemia in which cannot be found any primary focus of infection.

 s., melitensis. Infectious disease marked by remittent fever, weakness, perspiration, neuralgia, and swelling in the joints. SYN: *Malta fever, undulant fever.*

 s., puerperal. Septicemia occurring following childbirth due to a lesion in the genital tract. SEE: *puerperal sepsis.*

septicemic (sĕp-tĭ-sē'mĭk). Relating to, resulting from, or of the nature of, septicemia.

septicophlebitis (sĕp"tĭ-kō-flē-bī'tĭs). Septic inflammation of a vein.

septicopyemia (sĕp"tĭ-kō-pī-ē'mĭ-ă). Septicemia and pyemia together.

septiferous (sĕp-tĭf'ĕr-ŭs). Carrying or transmitting septic poisoning.

septile (sĕp'tĭl). Relating to a septum. SYN: *septal.*

septimetritis (sĕp"tĭ-mē-trī'tĭs). Inflammation of uterus due to sepsis.

septipara (sĕp-tĭp'ă-ră). A woman who has borne 7 children separately or is pregnant for the 7th time.

septivalent (sĕp-tĭ-vā'lĕnt, -tĭv'ă-lĕnt). Having a valency of 7 or combining with or replacing 7 hydrogen atoms.

septometer (sĕp-tŏm'ĕt-ĕr). 1. Calipers for measuring nasal septum. 2. Device for determining atmospheric impurity.

septopyemia (sĕp"tō-pī'ē-mĭ-ă). Pyemia and septicemia together. SYN: *septicopyemia.*

septotome (sĕp'tō-tōm). An instrument for cutting or removing a section of the nasal septum.

septotomy (sĕp-tŏt'ō-mĭ). Incision of a septum, esp. the nasal septum.

septum (sĕp'tŭm) (pl. *septa*). A membranous wall dividing two cavities.

 s. atriorum, BNA, **s. auricularum.** A wall bet. the atria of the heart.

 s., crural. A mass of fat obstructing the femoral ring.

 s. lucidum. 1. A translucent septum, the int. boundary of lateral ventricles of the brain. 2. The stratum corneum layer of the epidermis.

 s., nasal. The partition which divides the 2 nasal cavities.

 s. pectiniforme. Comblike partition that separates the corpora cavernosa.

 s., rectovaginal. Partition bet. the rectum and the vagina.

 s. scroti. BNA. Partition dividing the 2 chambers of the scrotum.

 s. ventriculorum. BNA. Partition bet. the ventricles of the heart.

septuplet (sĕp'tŭp-lĕt). One of 7 children born from the same gestation.

séquardin (sā-kwar'dĭn). Commercial sterilized testicular extract.

sequela (sē-kwē'lă) (pl. *sequelae*). A condition following and resulting from a disease.

sequester (sē-kwĕs'tĕr). 1. To isolate. 2 A piece of necrosed bone separated from surrounding tissue. SYN: *sequestrum.*

sequestration (sē-kwĕs-tra'shŭn). 1. The formation of sequestrum. 2. Isolation of a patient for treatment or quarantine 3. Reduction of hemorrhage of head or trunk by temporarily stopping circulation with bands on the thighs and arms

sequestrectomy (sē-kwĕs-trĕk'tō-mĭ). Excision of a necrosed piece of bone.

sequestrotomy (sē-kwĕs-trŏt'ō-mĭ). Operation for removal of a sequestrum, a fragment of necrosed bone. SYN: *sequestrectomy.*

sequestrum (sē-kwĕs'trŭm). Fragment o a necrosed bone that has become sep arated from surrounding tissue.

sera (sē'ră). Pleural of *serum.* [blood

seralbumin (sĕr-ăl-bū'mĭn). Albumin of th

serial (sē'rĭ-ăl). In numerical order, in continuity or sequence, as in a series.

sericeps (sĕr'ĭ-sĕps). Silk sac used in making traction on fetal head.

series (sēr'ēz). 1. Arrangement of objects in succession or in order. 2. ELECT: A mode of arranging the parts of a circuit by connecting them successively end to end to form a single path for the current. The parts so arranged are said to be "in series."

seriflux (sē'rĭf-lŭks). A profuse, serous, or watery discharge. SYN: orrhorrhea.

seriscission (sĕr-ĭ-sĭsh'ŭn). Division of soft tissues, as a pedicle, by tying a silk ligature around it.

sero-. Combining form pertaining to serum.

seroalbuminuria (sē'rō-ăl-bū-mĭn-ū'rĭ-ă). Serum albumin in the urine.

serobacterin (sē'rō-băk'ter-ĭn). Bacterial vaccine sensitized with serum from an animal partially immunized against the same microörganism. SEE: vaccine.

serochrome (sē'rō-krōm). The pigment which colors the normal serum. SYN: lipochrome, lutein.

serocolitis (sē'rō-kō-lī'tĭs). Inflammation of serous coat of the colon. SYN: pericolitis.

seroculture (sē'rō-kŭl-chūr). A bacterial culture on blood serum.

serocystic (sē'rō-sĭs'tĭk). Composed of cysts containing serous fluid.

serodermatosis (sē'rō-der-mă-tō'sĭs). Skin disease with serous effusion into tissues of the epidermis.

serodiagnosis (sē'rō-dī-ăg-nō'sĭs). Diagnosis by observing the reactions of blood serum.

seroenteritis (sē'rō-ĕn-ter-ī'tĭs). Inflammation of serous covering of the intestine.

seroenzyme (sē'rō-ĕn'zīm). Any enzyme in the blood serum.

serofibrinous (sē'rō-fīb'rĭn-ŭs). 1. Composed of both serum and fibrin. 2. Denoting a serofibrinous exudate.

seroglobulin (sē'rō-glŏb'ū-lĭn). The globulin contained in the blood serum.

serohemorrhagic (sē'rō-hem-or-răj'ĭk). Consisting of both serum and blood.

serohepatitis (sē'rō-hĕp-ă-tī'tĭs). Inflammation of the peritoneal covering of the liver.

seroimmunity (sē'rō-ĭm-mū'nĭ-tĭ). Immunity conferred by antitoxins or vaccines. SYN: passive immunity.

serolactescent (sē'rō-lăk-tĕs'ĕnt). Resembling serum and milk, as the secretion of Montgomery's glands.

serolemma (sē'rō-lĕm'ă). External layer of the embryonic false amnion.

serolin (sē'rō-lĭn). A neutral fatty constituent of blood containing cholesterol, the nature of which is unknown.

serolipase (sē'rō-lĭp'ās). Lipase found in blood serum.

serologic, serological (sē-rō-lŏj'ĭk, -ăl). Pert. to or the study of sera.

serologist (sē-rŏl'ō-jĭst). One versed in serology.

serology (sē-rŏl'ō-jĭ). The science of serum reactions, diagnosis, and treatment.

serolysin (sē-rŏl'ĭs-ĭn). A bactericidal substance or lysin found in the blood serum.

seromembranous (sē'rō-mĕm'brăn-ŭs). Both serous and membranous; relating to a serous membrane.

seromucoid (sē'rō-mū'koyd). A substance resembling serum and mucus sometimes found in urine.

seromucous (sē'rō-mū'kŭs). Composed of serum and mucus.

seromuscular (sē'rō-mŭs'kū-lar). Referring to the serous and muscular intestinal coats.

seroperitoneum (sē'rō-pĕr-ĭ-tō-nē'ŭm). Fluid in the peritoneum. SYN: ascites, hydroperitoneum.

serophysiology (sē'rō-fīz-ĭ-ŏl'ō-jĭ). The study of the physiology of serum action.

serophyte (sē'rō-fīt). A microörganism which can grow readily in the body fluids.

seroplastic (sē'rō-plăs'tĭk). Containing serum and fibrin. SYN: serofibrinous.

seropneumothorax (sē'rō-nū-mō-thō'răks). Effusion of serum and air in the pleural cavity.

seroprevention (sē'rō-prē-vĕn'shŭn). Prevention by the injection of serum.

seroprognosis (sē'rō-prŏg-nō'sĭs). Prognosis of disease determined by seroreactions.

seroprophylaxis (sē'rō-prō-fī-lăks'ĭs). Prevention of a disease by injection of serum. SYN: seroprevention.

seropurulent (sē'rō-pū'rū-lĕnt). Composed of serum and pus, as an exudate.

seropus (sē'rō-pus). A fluid consisting of serum and pus.

seroreaction (sē'rō-rē-ăk'shŭn). 1. Any reaction taking place in serum. SEE: deviation of complement, fixation of complement. 2. Reaction to an injection of serum marked by rash, fever, pain, etc. SYN: serum sickness.

serosa (sē-rō'să). A serous membrane.

serosamucin (sē-rō'să-mū'sĭn). Mucoid in serous fluids.

serosanguineous (sē'rō-săn-gwĭn'ē-ŭs). Containing or of the nature of serum and blood.

seroscopy (sē-rŏs'kō-pĭ). Examination of serum for diagnostic purposes.

seroserous (sē'rō-sē'rŭs). Pert. to 2 serous surfaces.

serositis (sē'rō-sī'tĭs). Inflamed condition of a serous membrane.

serosity (sē-rŏs'ĭ-tĭ). 1. The quality of being serous. 2. A thin, watery, serous fluid, not the real secretion of serous membranes.

serosynovitis (sē'rō-sĭn-ō-vī'tĭs). Synovitis with increase of synovial fluid.

serotaxis (sē'rō-tăks'ĭs). The drawing of blood serum to the skin surface by application of a solution of caustic potash for diagnostic or therapeutic purposes.

serotherapy (sē'rō-thĕr'ă-pĭ). Injection of a specific serum or antitoxin in the treatment of an infectious disease.

serothorax (sē'rō-thō'răks). Fluid in the pleural cavity. SYN: hydrothorax.

serotina (sĕr-ō-tī'nă). Part of decidua that becomes maternal portion of the placenta. SYN: *decidua serotina.*

serotoxin (sē-rō-toks'ĭn). A toxin in the blood serum.

serous (sē'rŭs). Having the nature of serum.

  s. cavity. A large lymph space.

  s. effusion. One of serum.

  s. exudate. One consisting mostly of serum.

  s. fluids. Liquids of the body, similar to blood serum, which are in part secreted by serous membranes.

  s. glands. Certain glands secreting a watery fluid, as those found in the digestive tract.

  s. inflammation. One with a serous exudate or inflammation of a serous membrane.

  s. membrane. One with 2 layers of flat endothelial cells lining closed cavities.

serovaccination (sē'rō-văk-sĭn-ā'shŭn). Injection of a serum to secure passive immunity and also to secure active immunization.

serozyme (sē'rō-zīm). Substance in the blood which is converted into thrombin. SYN: *thrombogen.*

serpiginous (ser-pĭj'ĭn-ŭs). Creeping from one part to another.

  s. ulcer. One extending in one direction, while healing in another direction.

serpigo (ser-pī'gō). A creeping eruption, esp. ringworm. SYN: *herpes, ringworm.*

serrate (sĕr'rāt). Notched; toothed. SYN: *dentate.*

serration (ser-ā'shŭn). 1. Formation with sharp projections like the teeth of a saw. 2. Notch resembling one bet. teeth of a saw.

serratus muscle (sĕr-ā'tŭs). Any of several muscles arising from the ribs or vertebrae by separate slips.

serrefine (săr-fēn'). A small, spring wire forceps for compressing bleeding vessels.

serrenoeud (săr-nōōd'). Device employed for constricting uterus near *os internum* with strong steel wire, used for ligating.

serrulate (ser'ū-lāt). Minutely notched.

Sertoli's cells (sĕr-tō'lē). Supporting, elongated, striated cells of seminiferous tubules which nourish spermatids.

  S.'s column. Elongated cell in a seminiferous tubule giving support to spermatogenic cells.

serum (sē'rum) (pl. *serums, sera*). 1. Any serous fluid, esp. the fluid which moistens the surfaces of serous membranes. 2. The watery portion of the blood after coagulation; a fluid found when clotted blood is left standing long enough for the clot to shrink. 3. Serum from an animal rendered immune against a pathogenic organism, to be injected into a patient with the disease resulting from the same organism. SEE: *plasma, blood.* 4. Whey of milk.

  s. albumin. A protein found in blood serum. For properties, see *proteins;* for amount, see *blood.*

  s., anticrotalus. Serum to overcome the effect of rattlesnake poison.

  s., antidiphtheritic. One used to overcome the effects of diphtheria.

  s., antimeningococcus. Serum antagonistic to meningococcus infection.

  s., antiophidic. Serum antagonistic to snake poisons.

  s., antipneumococcus. Serum for pneumococcus infection.

  s., antitetanic. Serum given to overcome tetanus toxin.

  s., antitoxic. One containing the antitoxin of the microörganism against which it is supposed to be protective.

  s., antityphoid. A sterilized culture of typhoid bacilli administered by vaccination against typhoid fever.

  s., bactericidal. One having no effect on toxins but which destroys bacteria.

  s., bacteriolytic. A serum containing a lysin that destroys certain bacteria.

  s., Behring's. An antidiphtheritic one.

  s., blood. The liquid clear portion of blood without its fibrin and corpuscles.

  s., cerebrospinal. The cerebrospinal fluid.

  s. coagulation reaction. Weltmann's reaction for differential diagnosis bet. exudative, necrotic processes and proliferative, fibrotic processes.

  s., convalescent. Blood serum from one convalescent from an infection to be used on others having the same disease.

  s., foreign. Serum from one animal injected into another animal of another species, or into man.

  s. globulin. A protein found in blood serum.

  It contains 15.85% of nitrogen, 1.11% of sulfur, 52.71% of carbon, 7.01% of hydrogen, and 23.32% of oxygen. SEE: *blood, protein.*

  s., immune. A serum containing many amboceptors having a special affinity for a given bacterium. SYN: *specific serum.*

  s., inorganic. A solution of various salts in same proportion as in the human blood.

  s. lutein. Yellow pigment from serum.

  s., Maragliano's. A serum that is antitubercular.

  s., Marmorek's. The antitoxin of *Streptococcus pyogenes* and the tubercle bacillus.

  s. pains. Joint pains accompanying serum reaction.

  s., pooled. Blood serum from several persons, which has been mixed.

  s., pregnancy. Blood serum from pregnant women given to premature infants in food.   [serum.

  s. protein. Any protein in blood Serum protein forms weak acids mixed with alkali salts and this increases the buffer effects of the blood but to a lesser extent than cell protein.

  s., Quéry's. An antisyphilitic serum from inoculated monkeys.

  s. rash. One first seen at site of an injection of serum.

s. reaction. SEE: *serum sickness.*

s., salvarsanized. One used in cerebrospinal syphilis, taken from a patient half an hour after an intravenous injection of salvarsan.

s. sickness. An eruption of purpuric spots, with pain in limbs and joints, following administration of serum, such as streptococcic serum.

s., specific. SEE: *immune serum.*

s. test for typhoid fever. SEE: *Widal's serum test.*

s. therapy. Therapeutic use of animal serums. SYN: *serotherapy, q.v.*

s., Trunecek's. Same as *inorganic serum.*

s., Widal's, test. One for typhoid fever. SEE: *Widal.*

serumal (sē-rū′măl). Relating to serum.

s. calculus. One formed about the teeth from serous exudate.

serumuria (sē-rūm-ū′rĭ-ă). Albumen in the urine. SYN: *albuminuria.*

sesamoid (ses′am-oyd). Resembling in size or shape a grain of sesame.

s. bone. An oval nodule of bone or fibrocartilage in a tendon playing over a bony surface.

The patella is the largest one.

s. cartilages. Small ones in the side of the wing of the nose.

sesqui-. Prefix meaning *one and a half.*

sessile (sĕs′ĭl). Having no peduncle but attached directly by a broad base.

setaceous (sē-tā′shŭs). Resembling a bristle; bristly, hairy.

seton (sē′tŏn). A thread or threads drawn through a fold of skin to act as a counterirritant, or a fistulous tract so produced.

setose (sē′tōs). Having bristlelike appendages.

Setchenoff's or **Sechenoff's inhibitory centers** (sĕtsh′ĕn-ŏf, sē-cha′nof). Centers in the spinal cord and oblongata for inhibiting reflex movement.

seventh cranial nerve. Facial nerve*; *nervus facialis.*

s. sense. Perception of normal functioning of internal organs. SEE: *visceral sense.*

sevum (sē′vŭm). Tallow or suet.

sewer gas. Foul air of a sewer. SEE: *carbon monoxide gas.*

sex (sĕks). 1. The distinctive quality which differentiates bet. male and female. 2. Males or females, collectively.

s. chromosomes. Chromosomes in a cell determining sex.

sexdigital (sĕks-ĭ-dĭj′ĭ-tăl). Having 6 fingers or toes.

sexivalent (sĕks-ĭ-vā′lĕnt, -ĭv′ăl-ĕnt). Capable of combining with 6 atoms of hydrogen.

sexo-aesthetic inversion (sĕk″o-ĕs-thĕt′ĭk). Inclination to dress as one of the opp. sex. SYN: *eonism, transvestism.*

sextan (sĕks′tăn). Occurring every 6th day.

sextigravida (sĕks-tĭ-grăv′ĭd-ă). A woman pregnant for the 6th time.

sextipara (sĕks-tĭp′ă-ră). A woman who has borne 6 children at different pregnancies.

sextuplet (sĕks′tū-plĕt). One of 6 children born of a single gestation.

sexual (sĕks′ū-ăl). 1. Pert. to sex. 2. Having sex.

s. bondage. An abnormal phenomenon (not perverse) of dependence of one person upon another of the opposite sex, one dominating the other.

s. intercourse. Sexual congress bet. a male and a female. SYN: *coition, coitus, concubitus, copulation.*

s. inversion. A perversion in which an abnormal affection for one of the same sex is experienced.

s. involution. The menopause.

s. metamorphosis. A perversion in which one adopts the habits and dress of the opposite sex.

s. psychopathy. A term for the group in which exist perversions of sex, such as *bestiality,* coprolagnism,* exhibitionism,* fetishism,* frottage,* homosexualism,* lesbianism,* masochism,* masturbation,* onanism,* pedophilia,* renifleurs,* sadism,* sodomy,* transvestism,* voyeur.*

s. reflex. Erection and ejaculation resulting from genital stimulation or indirectly from emotion whether asleep or awake.

sexuality (sĕks-ū-ăl′ĭ-tĭ). 1. State of having sex; the collective characteristics which mark the differences bet. the male and the female. 2. Undue concern with what is sexual. 3. Constitution and life of individual as related to sex; all the dispositions related to the love life whether associated with the sex organs or not.

shadowgram, shadowgraph (shăd′ō-grăm, -grăf). A print on a photographic plate exposed to x-rays. SYN: *skiagraph.*

shakes (shāks). Shivering caused by a chill, esp. in an intermittent fever.

shaking (shāk′ĭng). A passive movement in Swedish massage.

s. cure. Vibratory movements for treatment of paralysis agitans.

s. palsy. A basal ganglion disease with progressive rigid tremulousness, peculiar gait, muscular contraction, and weakness. SYN: *paralysis agitans.*

shampoo (shăm-poo′). 1. A thorough cleansing of the entire body or hair and scalp with thick soap lather applied with friction and followed by an affusion with clear water. 2. To thoroughly wash the hair or body.

shank (shăngk). The tibia or leg from knee to ankle. SYN: *shin.*

shape (shāp). 1. To mold to a particular form. 2. Outward form; contour.

Sharpey's intercrossing fibers (shar′pē). Fibers forming the lamellae constituting the walls of the haversian canals in bone.

S. perforating fibers. Those which connect the lamellae in walls of the haversian canals.

sheath (shēth). A covering structure of

connective tissue, usually of an elongated part, such as the membrane covering a muscle, etc.

s., arachnoid or **arachnoidean.** Delicate partition between pial sheath and dural one of the optic nerve.

s., crural. The femoral sheath.

s., dentinal. One lining the dental canals.

s., dural. A fibrous membrane or ext. investment of the optic nerve.

s., femoral. The fascial covering of femoral vessels.

s. of Henle. An extension of perineurium investing fibers composing nerve trunk funiculi.

s., lamellar. Connective tissue sheath covering bundle of nerve fibers. SYN: *perineurium.*

s., medullary. Myelin sheath surrounding the axis cylinder.

s., myelin. A fatty, semifluid covering of a nerve fiber; also called the *medulla*. It may insulate the nerve fiber and prevent the escape of the nerve impulse.

s., nerve. SEE: *lamellar sheath.*

s., perivascular. Lymphatic tube around the smallest blood vessels.

s., pial. Extension of the pia, closely investing surface of the optic nerve.

s. of Schwann. Membranous covering of myelin sheath of a nerve fiber. SYN: *neurilemma.*

s., synovial. Sheath membrane lining cavity of a bone through which a tendon glides.

sheet (shēt). Linen or cotton bedcovering next to the sleeper.

s., draw. One folded under patient so it may be withdrawn without lifting the patient.

shell shock. PSY: Any one of the disorders of motor, sensory and special sense centers; a form of psychoneurosis which occurs during military service and in training camps, but not as a result of exploding shells. SYN: *war neurosis.*

shield (shēld). 1. Any protecting device. 2. BIOL: A protective plate.

s. bone. The scapula.

s., Buller's. A watch glass to be worn over the eye to protect it from gonorrheal or ophthalmic infection.

s., embryonic. An area of proliferating cells in the ovum in which the primitive streak appears.

s., nipple. A protective covering to protect sore nipples.

s., phallic. An antiseptic covering for the male genitals during operations.

Shiga's bacillus (shē′gă). The bacillus causing a form of dysentery.

Shigella (shĭ-jel′lă, -gĕl′ă). A genus or the family *Bacteriaceae* containing the dysentery organisms.

shin (shĭn). Anterior edge of tibia. Also, leg bet. ankle and knee. SYN: *shank.*

shingles (shĭng′lz). Eruption of acute, inflammatory, herpetic vesicles on the trunk of the body along a peripheral nerve; occasionally elsewhere. SYN: *herpes zoster, q.v.*

ship fever. A fever due to unhygienic conditions aboard ship, usually typhus fever or yellow fever occasionally.

shiver (shĭv′ĕr). 1. A slight tremor of the skin, as from cold, or from fear. 2. To tremble or shake, as from fear or cold

shock (shŏk). A depression or cessation of the influences of the nervous system over various important body functions principally the circulation and respiration.

s., aerial. Condition in soldiers from exposure to bursting shells.

s., anaphylactic. Reaction from injection of protein substance to which patient is sensitized.

s., anesthesia. This is not surgical shock, but is due to an overdosage of anesthetic and calls for the immediate cessation of anesthesia.

s., apoplectic. Sudden attack of paralysis and coma with hemorrhage into brain and spinal cord. SYN: *apoplexy.*

s., barium. One caused by intravenous injection of barium causing destruction of red blood corpuscles.

s., cardiac. Shock caused by overexertion.

s., colloid. One causing symptoms of anaphylaxis when colloids are injected.

s., deferred or **delayed.** Late manifestation following injury or burns.
May appear in 3 to 30 hours and may be due to transportation, emotional stress, hemorrhage, dehydration, acidosis, or toxemia.

s., electric. The result of passage of electric current.

s., epigastric. Result of a blow or other trauma (surgery) in upper abdomen.

s., erethismic. Excitement, toxic or traumatic delirium following shock.

s., faradic. The result of faradization.

s., heart. Heart failure due to overexertion.

s., hemoclastic. Shock resulting from destruction of blood cells.

s., hypoglycemic. SEE: *insulin shock.*

s., injection. Shock resulting from injection of various medicaments or foreign proteins.

s., insulin. Condition resulting from overdosages of insulin.

s., mental. SEE: *psychic shock.* Due to emotional stress or seeing injury, accidents, etc.

s., metabalodispersion. The result of change in colloidal dispersion in the body.

s., peptone or **protein.** Reaction resulting from parenteral administration of a protein.

s., phenolic. Shock caused by intravenous injection of phenol.

s., pleural. Shock sometimes following thoracentesis.

s., pneumothorax acute. Acute shock resulting upon entrance of air into pleural cavity by perforation from disease or trauma.

s., psychic. Shock due to excessive fear, joy, anger, grief.   [accident.

s., railway. One caused by a railroad

s., secondary. Same as *deferred shock.*

s., sense. A mild nightmare.

s., serum. One occurring as part of reaction to injection of serum.

s., sexual. Prostration or heart failure following coition or rape.

s., shell. An indefinite nervous condition found in soldiers.

s., surgical. Following operations and including traumatic shock, *q.v.*

s., testicular. Result of blow to or torsion of testicles.

s., traumatic (broad interpretation). Shock due to injury or surgery.

s., wound. Same as *traumatic shock.*

shod'dy fever. A condition caused by the inhalation of dust among workers in shoddy factories.

shoe'makers' cramp or spasm. Spasm of muscles of hand and arm occurring in shoemakers.

shortsightedness (short-sīt'ĕd-nĕs). A condition of not being able to see very far. Due to light rays coming to a focus in front of the retina. SYN: *myopia, near-sightedness.*

shot'gun prescrip'tion. One containing many drugs given with hope that one of them may prove effective.

shoulder (shōl'dĕr). The junction of the clavicle and scapula where the arm meets the trunk.

s., blade. The scapula.

s., dislocation of. Displacement of shoulder joint.

s., girdle. The 2 scapulae and 2 clavicles attaching the bones of the upper extremities to the axial skeleton.

s., joint. Formed by humerus and glenoid cavity of scapula.

show (shō). The sanguinoserous discharge from the vagina during the first stage of labor or just preceding menstruation.

Shrapnell's membrane (shrăp'nĕl). A small, triangular area of membrane of the eardrum fitting in the notch of Rivinus.

shunt (shŭnt). 1. Conductor connecting 2 points in a circuit to form a parallel or derived circuit through which a portion of the current may pass. 2. Conductor providing a low-resistance path for the flow of current.

Si. Symb. of *silicon.*

siagonantritis (sī″ăg-ŏn-ăn-trī'tĭs). Inflammation within the antrum of Highmore.

sialaden (sī-ăl'ăd-ĕn). A salivary gland.

sialadenitis (sī-ăl-ăd-ĕn-ī'tĭs). Inflamed condition of a salivary gland.

sialadenoncus (sī-ăl-ăd-ĕn-ŏng'kŭs). Tumor of salivary gland.

sialogogue (sī-ăl'ă-gŏg). Agent increasing flow of saliva.

sialaporia (sī″ăl-ap-ō'rĭ-ă). Deficiency in secretion of saliva.

sialemesis (sī″ăl-ĕm'ĕs-ĭs). Vomiting of saliva or vomiting caused by an excessive secretion of it.

sialine (sī-ăl-īn). Concerning the saliva.

sialism, sialismus (sī'ăl-ĭzm, sī-ăl-ĭz'mŭs). An excessive secretion of saliva. SYN: *ptyalism, salivation.*

sialoadenitis (sī″ăl-ō-ăd-ĕn-ī'tĭs). Inflammation of a salivary gland. SYN: *sialadenitis.*

sialoaerophagy (sī″ăl-ō-ā-ĕr-ŏf'ă-jī). Constant swallowing, thus taking saliva and air into the stomach.

sialoangitis (sī″ăl-ō-ăn-jī'tĭs). Inflamed condition of the salivary ducts.

sialodochitis (sī″ăl-ō-dō-kī'tĭs). Inflamed condition of salivary ducts.

s. fibrinosa. Sialodochitis with duct obstructed by a fibrinous exudate.

sialoductitis (sī″ăl-ō-dŭk-tī'tĭs). Inflamed condition of Stensen's duct.   [liva.

sialogenous (si-al-ŏj'en-us). Forming sa-

sialogogic, sialogogue (sī-ăl-ō-gŏj'ĭk, -ăl'ō-gŏg). Producing or promoting a secretion of saliva; or that which stimulates its secretion.

sialography (sī-ăl-ŏg'ră-fī). Examination of salivary ducts and glands with x-rays. SYN: *ptyalography.*

sialolith (sī-ăl'ō-lĭth). A salivary concretion or calculus.

sialolithiasis (sī-ăl-ō-lĭth-ī'ăs-ĭs). Presence of salivary calculi.

sialolithotomy (sī″ăl-ō-lĭth-ŏt'ō-mī). Removal of a calculus from a salivary gland or duct.

sialoncus (sī-ăl-ŏng'kŭs). A tumor under the tongue caused by obstruction of a salivary gland or duct.

sialoporia (sī″ăl-ō-pō'rĭ-ă). Deficient secretion of saliva.

sialorrhea (sī-ăl-or-ē'ă). Excessive flow of saliva. SYN: *sialism.*

sialoschesis (sī-ăl-ŏs'kĕs-ĭs). Suppression or retention of saliva.

sialosemeiology (sī″ăl-ō-sē-mī-ŏl'ō-jī). Diagnosis based upon examination of the saliva.

sialosis (sī-ăl-ō'sĭs). The flow of saliva.

sialostenosis (sī″ăl-ō-stĕn-ō'sĭs). Closure of a salivary duct.

sialosyrinx (sī″ăl-ō-sī'rĭnks). 1. Fistula into the salivary gland. 2. A syringe for washing out salivary ducts. 3. Drainage tube for a salivary duct.

sialotic (sī-ăl-ŏt'ĭk). Concerning the flow of saliva.

sialozemia (sī″ăl-ō-zē'mĭ-ă). Involuntary loss of saliva. SYN: *salivation.*

Siamese twins (sī-ă-mēz'). Congenitally united twins, usually at the hips or buttocks, the members being capable of activity.

sibilant (sĭb'ĭl-ănt). Hissing or whistling, as a sound heard in a certain râle, *q.v.*

sibilus (sĭb'ĭl-ŭs). A hissing râle.

sibling (sĭb'lĭng). One of 2 or more children of same parents.

siccant (sĭk'ănt). Drying.

siccative (sĭk'ă-tĭv). Drying or that which dries. SYN: *siccant.*

siccus (sĭk'ŭs). Not moist; dry.

sick (sĭk). 1. Not well. SYN: *ill.* 2. Nauseated or "sick at the stomach." 3. Menstruating.

s. headache. One with nausea, vomiting, anorexia, etc. SYN: *migraine, q.v.*

s. at the stomach. Inclined to vomit. SYN: *nauseated.*

sick'le cell. Abnormal red blood corpuscle of crescent shape.

s. c. anemia. A form of anemia in which are present abnormal sickle or crescent-shaped erythrocytes. SEE: *anemia.*

sicklemia (sĭk-lē'mĭ-ă). Sickle cells in the blood.

sick'ness. State of being unwell. SYN: *illness.*

s., bleeding. Abnormal tendency to bleed. SYN: *hemophilia.*

s., car. Nausea and malaise from riding in street cars, on elevated railroads and railroads.

s., falling. Epilepsy.

s., green. Form of anemia with greenish pallor. SYN: *chlorosis.*

s., monthly. Menstruation.

s., morning. Nausea of early pregnancy.

s., mountain. Nausea and dyspnea caused by being on great elevations.

s., sea. Sickness caused by motion of a vessel while at sea.

s., serum. Sickness following injection of serum.

s., sleeping. 1. Infection with genus of Trypanosomes with involvement of central nervous system and ultimately continuous sleeping. SYN: *trypanosomiasis.* 2. Acute infectious disease with increasing lethargy. SYN: *lethargic encephalitis.*

Siddall test (sĭd'al). A hormone test for pregnancy in early or late stage.

side (sīd). 1. Left or right part of wall of trunk of body. 2. An outer portion considered as facing in a particular direction.

s.-chain theory. Theory concerning cell dissolution and immunity; complex molecules react with one another through their side chains when they have definite correspondence in structure. SEE: *Ehrlich's theory.*

s. position. Lying on one side, thighs flexed, with underarm behind back. SYN: *Sims' position, q.v.*

sideration (sĭd-ĕr-ā'shŭn). 1. Therapeutic application of electric sparks. 2. A sudden stroke of disease, as in apoplexy. 3. Lightning stroke.

siderism, siderismus (sĭd'ĕr-ĭzm, -ĭz'mŭs). Therapeutic application of metals to the skin. SYN: *metallotherapy.*

sidero-. Combining form meaning *iron* or *steel,* as *siderosis.*

sideroderma (sĭd''ĕr-ō-der'mă). Bronzed coloration of the skin from disordered hemoglobin disintegration.

siderodromophobia (sĭd''ĕr-ō-drō''mō-fō'bĭ-ă). Morbid fear of railway travel.

siderofibrosis (sĭd''ĕr-ō-fĭ-brō'sĭs). Fibrosis associated with deposits of iron.

siderogenous (sĭd-ĕr-ŏj'ĕn-ŭs). Producing or forming iron.

siderophilous (sĭd-ĕr-of'ĭl-ŭs). Having a tendency to absorb iron, as the red blood corpuscles.

sideroscope (sĭd'ĕr-ō-skōp). Instrument for finding metal particles in the eye.

siderosis (sĭd-ĕr-ō'sĭs). 1. Disease of lungs caused by inhalation of metallic dust. SYN: *pneumonoconiosis.* 2. Deposit of iron pigments in a tissue or in the blood.

s. bulbi. Iron pigment deposits in the eyeball.

s., hepatic. Condition in which there is an abnormal amt. of iron in the liver.

Sigault's operation (sē-go'). Division of the symphysis pubis to aid delivery. SYN: *symphyseotomy.*

sight (sīt). 1. Power or faculty of seeing. SYN: *vision.* 2. Range of sight. 3. A thing or view seen.   *[talopia.*

s., day. Night blindness. SYN: *nyc-*

s., far-. Rays of light focusing behind the retina. SYN: *hyperopia.*

s. meter. Device for measuring intensity of light in foot candles.

s., near-. Rays of light focusing before the retina. SYN: *myopia.*

s., night. Day blindness. SYN: *hemeralopia.*

s., old. Loss of accommodation of near point. SYN: *presbyopia.*

s., second. Improvement of vision in the aged usually due to incipient cataract.

sigmatism (sĭg'mă-tĭzm). Excessive or defective use of *s* sounds in speech.

sigmoid (sĭg'moyd). Shaped like the Greek letter *sigma, s.*

s. flexure. The lower part of descending colon bet. iliac crest and the rectum, shaped like the letter S.

sigmoidectomy (sĭg-moy-dĕk'tō-mĭ). Removal of all or part of the sigmoid flexure.

sigmoiditis (sĭg-moy-dī'tĭs). Inflammation of the sigmoid flexure of the colon.

sigmoidopexy (sĭg-moyd'ō-pĕks''ĭ). Fixation of the sigmoid to an abdominal incision for prolapse of the rectum.

sigmoidoproctostomy (sĭg-moyd''ō-prŏk-tos'tō-mĭ). Establishment of artificial passage by anastomosis of the sigmoid flexure with the rectum.

sigmoidorectostomy (sĭg-moyd''ō-rĕk-tŏs'tō-mĭ). Anastomosis of sigmoid flexure with the rectum to establish an artificial passage. SYN: *sigmoidoproctostomy.*

sigmoidoscope (sĭg-moy'dō-skōp). Tubular speculum for examination of sigmoid flexure.

sigmoidostomy (sĭg-moyd-ŏs'tō-mĭ). Creation of an artificial anus in the sigmoid flexure.

sign (sīn). 1. Symbol or abbreviation, esp. one used in pharmacy. 2. Any objective evidence of an abnormal nature in the body or its organs.

s., objective. One recognized by an observer. SYN: *physical sign.*

s., physical. One revealed by auscultation, percussion, inspection, etc.

signa (sĭg'nă). A term used in writing prescriptions,* meaning mark. Usually designated S or sig.

signature (sĭg'nă-tŭr). The part of a prescription giving instructions to the patient.

sig'natures, doctrine of. Obsolete belief that medicinal uses of plants can be determined from peculiar visible characters.

silica (sĭl'ĭ-kă). Silicon dioxide, SiO_2.

silicate (sĭl'ĭ-kāt). A salt of silicic acid.

silicic (sĭl-ĭs'ĭk). Pert. to silica or silicon.

   s. acid. One of a number of colloid acids.

silicon (sĭl'ĭ-kon). SYMB: Si. A nonmetallic element found in the soil. At. wt. 28.06. Sp. gr. 2.48.

silicosis (sĭl-ĭ-kō'sĭs). A condition caused by the inhalation of small particles of stone or stone dust.

   SEE: *pneumonoconiosis, -is.*

silicotic (sĭl-ĭ-kŏt'ĭk). 1. Relating to silicosis. 2. One affected with silicosis.

silicotuberculosis (sĭl''ĭ-kō-tū-bĕr-kū-lō'sĭs). Silicosis associated with pulmonary tuberculosis.

siliqua olivae (sĭl'ĭk-wă ō-lī'vē). Nerve fibers encircling the inf. olive of the brain.

siliquose (sĭl'ĭ-kwōs). Resembling a 2-valve capsule.

   s. cataract. Cataract with a dry, wrinkled capsule.

   s. desquamation. Shedding of dried vesicles from the skin.

silver (sĭl'ver). SYMB: Ag. A white metal widely used in medicine.

   s. arsphenamine. A brownish black arsphenamine derivative, containing 19% arsenic and 14% silver.

   DOSAGE (adult): From 0.1 Gm. to 0.3 Gm. given with caution.

   s. nitrate. USP. A toxic preparation made from silver. Most of its former uses have passed out of vogue, but it remains important as a germicide and local astringent.

   DOSAGE: As an antiseptic in the eyes of newly born, 1%; topically as an astringent to the mucous membrane of the throat, from 5 to 10%.

   s. picrate. A compound of silver and picric acid, containing 30% silver. Useful as an antiseptic, similar to other preparations of silver.

   DOSAGE: Dilutions from 1 to 2%.

   s. protein. USP. A combination of silver and protein, containing from 7 to 19% silver. Two strengths are official, the strong and mild.

sil'ver-fork deformity or **fracture.** Deformity in Colles' fracture of wrist and hand resembling curve on back of a fork.

Silves'ter's method. A method of artificial respiration consisting of constant movements of the patient's arms. Useless in asphyxia neonatorum.

silvol (sĭl'vol). USP. A commercial brand of mild silver protein.

simesthesia (sĭm-ĕs-thē'zĭ-ă). Sensibility felt in a bone.

similia similibus curantur (sĭm-ĭl'ĭ-ă sĭm-ĭl'-ĭ-bŭs kū-rahn'tŭr). The homeopathic doctrine that a drug producing pathological symptoms in those who are well will cure such symptoms in disease states.

Simmond's disease or **syndrome** (sĭm'-mond). Condition in which complete atrophy of the pituitary body causes premature senility and psychic symptoms.

   SYN: *pituitary cachexia, q.v.*

Simon's position (zē'mon). An exaggerated lithotomy position in which the hips are somewhat elevated with thighs strongly abducted. Employed in operations on the vagina.

simple (sĭm'pl). 1. Not complex; not compound. 2. Deficient in intellect. 3. A medicinal plant.

   s. fracture. Fracture without rupture of ligaments and skin.

   s. inflammation. Inflammation without pus or other inflammatory exudates.

   s. mixed enema. A soapsuds enema to which is added 1 dram of salt and ½ oz. of molasses.   [muscle.

   s. reflex. One acting upon a single

simples (sĭm'plz). Medicinal plants.

Sims' position (sĭmz). A semiprone position; the patient lies on the left side, and the right knee and thigh are drawn up well above the left lower limb. The patient may present an anterior or posterior view. The left arm is placed back of the patient or projecting over the side of the table or bed. The chest is inclined forward so that the patient rests upon it.

simul (sī'mŭl). At once or at the same time.

simulation (sĭm-ū-lā'shŭn). Pretense of having a disease; feigning of illness. Imitation of symptoms of 1 disease by another. SEE: *malingering.*

Sinapis (sĭn-ā'pĭs). Mustard.

sinapiscopy (sĭn-ăp-ĭs'kō-pĭ). Use of mustard in testing for sensory disturbance.

sinapism (sĭn'ăp-ĭzm). A mustard plaster.

sinapized (sĭn'ăp-īzd). Containing mustard.

sincipital (sĭn-sĭp'ĭ-tăl). Concerning the sinciput.

sinciput (sĭn'sĭp-ŭt). 1. Fore and upper part of the cranium. 2. Upper half of the skull. SYN: *calvaria.*

sinew (sĭn'ū). 1. A tendon. 2. Chiefly in the plural, strength; nervous energy; muscular power.

sing. Abbr. of *singulorum,* meaning *of each.*

singer's node or **nodule** (sĭn'gerz nōd, nŏd'-ūl). A swelling bet. the arytenoid cartilages of singers. SYN: *chorditis nodosa.*

singultus (sĭng-gŭl'tŭs). Hiccups, *q.v.*

sinistrad (sĭn'ĭs-trăd). Toward the left.

sinistral (sĭn'ĭs-trăl). 1. Pert. to or showing preference for the left hand, eye, or foot in certain actions. 2. On the left side.

sinistrality (sĭn''ĭs-trăl'ĭ-tĭ). Left-handedness.

sinistraural (sĭn-ĭs-traw'răl). Having better hearing with the left ear.

sinistro- (sĭn'ĭs-trō). Prefix meaning *left.*

sinistrocardia (sĭn-ĭs-trō-kar'dĭ-ă). Displacement of the heart to left of the medial line; opp. of *dextrocardia.*

sinistrocerebral (sĭn-ĭs-trō-ser′ē-brăl). Located in the left cerebral hemisphere.

sinistrocular (sĭn-ĭs-trok′ū-lar). Having stronger vision in the left eye.

sinistrocularity (sĭn-ĭs-trŏk-ū-lăr′ĭ-tĭ). Condition of having better vision in the left eye.

sinistrogyration (sĭn-ĭs-trō-jī-rā′shŭn). Inclination to the left.

sinistromanual (sĭn-ĭs-trō-măn′ū-ăl). Left-handed.

sinistropedal (sĭn-ĭs-trŏp′ĕd-ăl). Left-footed.

sinistrosis (sĭn-ĭs-trō′sĭs). Shell shock.

sinistrotorsion (sĭn-ĭs-trō-tor′shŭn). A twisting or turning toward the left.

sinoauricular (sī″nō-aw-rĭk′ū-lar). Pert. to the right cardiac auricle and the sinus venosus.

   s. node. One at entrance of the sup. vena cava into right auricle, regarded as starting point of the heartbeat. Syn: *sinuauricular node.*

sinuauricular (sī″nu-aw-rĭk′ū-lar). Concerning the sinus venosus and the right cardiac auricle.

   s. node. Node at junction of sup. vena cava with right cardiac auricle, regarded as starting point of the heartbeat.

sinuitis (sĭ-nū-ī′tĭs). Inflammation of a sinus. Syn: *sinusitis.*

sinuotomy (sĭn-ū-ŏt′ō-mĭ). Surgical incision into a sinus.

sinuous (sĭn′ū-ŭs). Winding; wavy; tortuous.

sinus (sī′nŭs) (pl. *sinuses, sinūs*). 1. A canal or passage leading to an abscess. 2. A cavity within a bone. 3. Dilated channel for venous blood. 4. Any cavity having a relatively narrow opening.

   s's., accessory nasal. Frontal, maxillary, ethmoidal, and sphenoidal. *Anterior group:* Frontal, maxillary, and anterior ethmoids. *Posterior group:* Posterior ethmoids and sphenoid.

   s., aortic. Saclike dilatation of the aorta.

   s., arrhythmia. Irregularity of heartbeat due to interference with impulses from the sinoauricular node.

   s., basilar. See: *transverse sinus.*

   s., cavernous. A large sinus from sphenoidal fissure to apex of petrous portion of temporal bone.

   s., circular. A venous sinus around the pituitary body, communicating on each side with the cavernous sinus.

   s's., circular, of the placenta. A plexus of veins in the maternal portion of placenta.

   s., clinoid. See: *circular sinus.*

   s., coronary, of the heart. A vein in transverse groove bet. left cardiac auricle and ventricle.

   s's., cranial. Venous canals bet. folds of the dura.

   s's., ethmoidal. Air cavities in the ethmoid bone.

   s., frontal. An irregular cavity in frontal bone on each side of midline above the nasal bridge. One may be larger than the other. A duct carries secretions to upper part of nostrils.

   s., genital. The cleft of the vulva.

   s., genitourinary. See: *urogenital sinus.*

   s., great, of the aorta. A dilatation on right side of ascending portion of the aorta.

   s., inferior longitudinal. A venous sinus along post. half of lower border of the falx cerebri.

   s., inferior petrosal. A large venous sinus from cavernous sinus, running along lower margin of the petrous portion of the temporal bone.

   s's., intercavernous. The ant. and post. halves of the circular sinus.

   s., lateral. One of 2 large venous sinuses in inner side of skull passing near the mastoid antrum, emptying into the jugular vein.

   s's., lymph. Small spaces throughout the parenchyma of a lymphatic gland.

   s's., mastoid. Cells within mastoid portion of the temporal bone.

   s., maxillary. A cavity in the maxillary bone opening at upper part of antrum into the nose. Syn: *antrum* or *antrum of Highmore.*

   s., occipital. A small venous sinus in attached margin of the falx cerebelli extending to margin of the foramen magnum.

   s., placental. A venous passage around edge of the placenta.

   s's., pleural. Spaces in pleural sac along the lower and inf. portions of lung which the lung does not occupy.

   s. pocularis. Lacuna in prostatic part of the urethra.

   s. prostaticus. See: *sinus pocularis.*

   s. pulmonalis. Atrium of the left auricle of the heart.

   s., rhomboid. The 4th cranial ventricle.

   s. rhythm. Normal cardiac rhythm commencing at the sinoauricular node.

   s's., sphenoidal. Air sinuses which occupy the body of sphenoid bone and connect with nasal cavity.

   s., sphenoparietal. 1. A vein uniting the cavernous sinus and a meningeal vein. 2. The portion of the cavernous sinus below the ensiform process.

   s., straight. One which is continuous with the inf. longitudinal sinus and running along junction of the falx cerebri and tentorium.

   s., superior longitudinal. A triangular one along upper edge of the falx cerebri.

   s., superior petrosal. A venous canal running in a groove in the petrous portion of the temporal bone.

   s. tachycardia. Uncomplicated rapid heartbeat.

   s., terminal. A vein encircling the vascular area of the blastoderm.

   s., transverse. 1. Sinus that unites the 2 inf. petrosal sinuses. 2. Venous network in the dura over basilar process of occipital bone.

s., urinogenital or **urogenital.** 1. Duct into which, in the embryo, the wolffian ducts and bladder empty and which opens into the cloaca. 2. The common receptacle of genital and urinary ducts.

s's., uteroplacental. Slanting venous channels from the placenta serving to convey the maternal blood from the intervillous lacunae back into the uterine veins.

s. of Valsalva. A dilatation of the aorta or pulmonary artery opp. segment of the semilunar valve. SYN: *aortic sinus.*

s., venous. One conveying venous blood.

s's., vertebral. Veins within the vertebrae.

sinusitis (sī-nū-sī′tĭs). Inflammation of a sinus, esp. the accessory nasal ones.

s., acute catarrhal. Inflammation accompanying a similar process in the nose.

s., acute suppurative. Purulent inflammation with symptoms of pain over the sinus, fever, chills, headache, etc.

s., chronic hyperplastic. Polypi present in sinuses and nose and underlying osteitis of sinus walls.

s., chronic hypertrophic. Inflammation found in conjunction with chronic hypertrophic rhinitis.

Ideal treatment in these cases is change of climate where the temperature fluctuations are not extreme.

sinusoid (sī′nŭs-oyd). 1. Resembling a sinus. 2. A minute terminal, endothelium-lined space, or passage for blood in tissues of an organ, as the liver.

sinusoidal (sī-nŭs-oyd′ăl). Pert. to a sinusoid.

s. current. Alternating induced electric current, the 2 strokes of which are equal.

sinusoidalization (sī-nŭs-oyd-al-ĭ-zā′shŭn). Use of a sinusoidal current.

sinusotomy (sī-nū-sŏt′ō-mĭ). The operation of incising a sinus.

SiO₂. Silicon dioxide.

siphon (sī′fŏn). A tube bent at an angle to form 2 unequal lengths for removing liquids by atmospheric pressure.

siphonoma (sī-fon-ō′mă). A tumor made up of fine tubes.

Sippy diet (sĭp′ē). Treatment of gastric ulcer by diet checking acidity of gastric juice.

Small amounts of milk and cream every hour and alkaline powders every ½ hr.

siriasis (sĭ-rī′ă-sĭs). Sunstroke, *q.v.*

sismotherapy (sĭs-mō-ther′ă-pĭ). Therapeutic employment of vibration. SYN: *seismotherapy, vibrotherapeutics.*

sissorexia (sĭs-ō-rĕk′sĭ-ă). Accumulation of blood corpuscles in the spleen.

sistomensin (sĭs-tō-mĕn′sĭn). Commercial preparation containing the luteolipoid of the corpus luteum and used to check excessive menstrual flow.

sitieirgia (sĭt-ĭ-ĭr′jĭ-ă). Hysterical refusal to take food.

sitio-, sito-. Combining forms meaning *bread,* or *made from grain; food,* as *sitomania.*

sitiology (sĭt-ĭ-ŏl′ō-jĭ). Science of nutrition. SYN: *sitology.*

sitiomania (sĭt-ĭ-ō-mā′nĭ-ă). Periodic abnormal appetite or craving for food. SYN: *sitomania.*

sitology (sī-tŏl′ō-jĭ). Science of nutrition and food. SYN: *sitiology.*

sitomania (sī″tō-mā′nĭ-ă). 1. Periodic abnormal craving for food. SYN: *sitiomania.* 2. Periodic abnormality of appetite.

sitophobia (sī″tō-fō′bĭ-ă). Psychoneurotic abhorrence of food, or morbid dread of, or repugnance to food, whether generally or only to specific dishes.

sitotherapy (sī″tō-ther′ă-pĭ). The therapeutic use of food.

sitotoxism (sī″tō-tŏks′ĭzm). Poisoning by vegetable foods infested with molds or bacteria.

sitotropism (sī-tŏt′rō-pĭzm). Response of cells to the attraction or repusion of food elements.

situs (sī′tŭs). A position.

s. inversus viscerum. Displacement of viscera abnormally to opposite side of the body.

s. perversus. Malposition of any visceral structure.

sitz bath (sĭtz bath). Bath to sit in with water above and covering the hips. SYN: *hip bath, q.v.* SEE: *bath.*

sixth cranial nerve (sĭksth). Abducens nerve which supplies the external rectus of the eye. SEE: *cranial nerves.*

skatol(e (skăt′ōl). Beta-methyl indole, C₉H₉N, a malodorous, solid, heterocyclic nitrogen compound found in feces, formed by protein decomposition in the intestines and giving them their odor.

skein (skān). Coiled thread of chromatin seen in the earlier stages of mitosis. SYN: *spireme.*

skelalgia (skĕ-lăl′jĭ-ă). Pain in the leg.

skeletal (skĕl′ĕ-tăl). Pert. to the skeleton.

s. muscle. One attached to, or one moving some structure.

s. tissue. Bony, cartilaginous, fibrous, or ligamentous tissues forming the framework of the body.

skeletization (skĕl-ĕt-ĭ-zā′shŭn). 1. Excessive emaciation. 2. Removal of soft parts of the body leaving only the skeleton.

skeleto-. Prefix meaning *skeleton.*

skeletogenous (skĕl-ĕt-ŏj′ĕn-ŭs). Forming skeletal structures or tissues.

skeletology (skĕl-ē-tŏl′ō-jĭ). The study of the skeleton.

skeleton (skĕl′ĕt-ŏn). The bony framework of the body, consisting of 206 bones, as follows:

AXIAL GROUP (80 Bones)

8 cerebral cranials.
14 visceral cranials.
1 os hyoideum (hyoid).
6 ossicula auditus (ossicles, ear bones).

26 columna vertebralis (vertebrae).
24 costae (ribs).
1 sternum (chest).
80 Total

APPENDICULAR GROUP (126 Bones)
64 extremitas sup. (32 in each upper extremity).
62 extremitas inf. (31 in each lower extremity).
126 Total

TRUNK (51 Bones)
Columna vertebralis (vertebrae), 26 Bones
7 cervicales (cervicals).
12 thoraces (dorsals).
5 lumbales (lumbar).
1 os sacrum.
1 os coccygis.
26 Total

Ribs (24 Bones)
14 costae verae (true ribs).
6 costae spuriae (false ribs).
4 costae vertebrales (floating ribs).
24 Total
1 sternum (chest bone).

HEAD (28 Bones)
Cerebral cranials (8 Bones)
1 os frontale (frontal).
2 ossa parietalia (parietals).
1 ossa occipitale (occipital).
2 ossa temporales (temporal).
1 os sphenoidale (sphenoid).
1 os ethmoidale (ethmoid).
8 Total

Visceral cranials (facial) (14 Bones)
2 ossa maxillae (sup. maxillary).
1 os mandibula (inf. maxillary).
2 ossa zygomatica (malar).
2 ossa lacrimales (lacrimal).
2 ossa nasalia (nasal).
2 conchae nasales inferiores (turbinates).
1 os vomer.
2 ossa palatina (palate).
14 Total
1 os hyoideum (hyoid).

EAR: Ossicula auditus (ossicles of the tympanum).
2 malleus.
2 incus.
2 stapes.
6 Total

EXTREMITAS SUPERIOR (upper extremities)
(64 Bones)
(Arm, 5 bones, 10 in both arms)
2 clavicula (clavicle).
2 scapula (shoulder blade).
2 humerus (arm bone).
2 radius (forearm).
2 ulna (elbow bone).
10 Total

Ossa carpi (wrist bones, 16)
2 os naviculare manus (scaphoid).
2 os lunatum (semilunar).
2 os triquetrum (cuneiform).
2 os pisiforme (pisiform).

2 os multangulum majus (trapezium).
2 os multangulum minus (trapezoid—like a trapezium).
2 os capitatum (os magnum).
2 os hamatum (unciform).
16 Total

Hands (38 Bones)
10 metacarpalia (metacarpus).
28 phalanges digitorum manus.
38 Total
10 both arms.
16 ossi carpi.
64 Total

EXTREMITAS INFERIOR (lower extremities)
(62 Bones)
(Leg, 5 bones each, or total of 10)
2 os coxae (hipbone).
2 femur.
2 tibia.
2 fibula.
2 patella (kneepan).
10 Total

Ossa tarsi (ankle, 7 bones each, total 14)
2 talus (astragalus).
2 calcaneus (os calis, heel bone).
2 os naviculare pedis (scaphoid).
2 os cuboideum (cuboid).
2 os cuneiforme primus (int. cuneiform).
2 os cuneiforme secundum (middle cuneiform).
2 os cuneiforme tertium (ext. cuneiform).
14 Total

14 ossa tarsi (as above).
10 ossa metatarsalia (metatarsal).
28 phalanges digitorum pedis.
10 leg and hip.
62 Total

SUMMARY
28 Head.
1 Hyoid.
51 Trunk.
64 Extremitas superior.
62 Extremitas inferior.
206 Total bones in skeleton.

s., appendicular. The bones of the limbs.
s., axial. Bones of the head and trunk.
s., cartilaginous. Structure from which the bones have been formed through ossification.
s., visceral. That part of the skeleton that protects the viscera.
Skene's glands (skēn). Glands lying just inside of and on the post. floor of the urethra, in the female.
skenitis (skē-nī'tĭs). Inflamed condition of Skene's glands.
skeocytosis (skē-ō-sī-tō'sĭs). Immature white corpuscles in the peripheral blood. SYN: neocytosis.
skiagram (skī'ă-grăm). An x-ray picture. SEE: roentgenogram.

skiagraph (skĭ′ă-grăf). An x-ray picture. SYN: *roentgenograph.*

skiagraphy (skĭ-ăg′ră-fĭ). Process of taking pictures with roentgen rays. SYN: *radiography, roentgenography.*

skiameter (skĭ-ăm′ĕt-ĕr). Device for determining differences in density and penetration of x-rays.

skiascope (skĭ′ă-skōp). 1. Device for examination by the fluoroscope. 2. Examination of the eye employing movement of shadow and light.

skiascopy (skĭ-ăs′kō-pĭ). 1. Retinoscopy or shadow test used in determining the refractive error of an eye. 2. Fluoroscopic inspection of the body.

skin (skĭn). The integument or external covering of the body.

s., alligator. Severe scaling of the skin with formation of thick plates resembling hide of an alligator.

s., deciduous. Shedding of the epidermis. SYN: *heratolysis.*

s., elastic. Skin which has property of great elasticity.

s., glossy. Shining atrophy of the skin.

s. grafting. Grafting of skin from another part of body to repair a defect or trauma. SEE: *Thiersch's graft.*

s., loose. Hypertrophy of the skin.

s., parchment. Atrophy of the skin with stretching.

s., scarf; s., scurf. Cuticle, epidermis, the outer layer of the skin.

s., true. Corium or inner layer of the skin, *q.v., above.*

skleriasis (sklē-rī′ăs-ĭs). Progressive hardening of the skin in patches. SYN: *scleroderma.*

sklero-. See words beginning with *sclero-.*

Skoda's râles (skō′dă). Bronchial ones heard through consolidated tissue of the lungs in pneumonia.

S.'s resonance, S.'s tympany. Tympanic resonance above the line of fluid in pleuritic effusion, or above consolidation in pneumonia.

S.'s sign. Same as *Skoda's resonance.*

skotogram, skotograph (skō′tō-grăm, -grăf). A roentgen ray picture. SYN: *skiagram.*

skotography (skō-tŏg′ră-fĭ). Photography by x-rays. SYN: *skiagraphy.*

skull (skŭl). The bony framework of the head, composed of 8 cranial bones and the 14 bones of the face. SYN: *calvaria, cranium.* SEE: *skeleton.*

s. cap. Upper round portion of skull covering the brain.

s., fractured. Fractures of the skull can be classified according to whether the fracture is in the vault or the base, but from the point of view of treatment a more useful classification is as follows:

(1) *Simple Uncomplicated Fractures:* Not common.

(2) *Compound Fractures:* If in vault of skull, the bone is depressed and driven inwards with possible damage to brain. Treatment is operative.

sleep (slēp). A normal (more or less periodic) loss of consciousness, apparently favoring recuperation following the exhaustion entailed in conscious activity.

s., crescendo. Normal sleep with increased movement during the night.

s. drunkenness. The stupor of sleep in drunkenness. SYN: *somnolentia.*

s. epilepsy. Uncontrollable desire to sleep at periodic intervals. SYN: *narcolepsy.*

s., hypnotic. Sleep induced by hypnotic suggestion.

s. paralysis. Temporary paralysis of a part due to pressure during sleep.

s., paroxysmal. SEE: *sleep epilepsy.*

s., pathologic. A term used in encephalitis lethargica (sleeping sickness); here sleep reasserts itself excessively and under conditions not to the best interests of the patient.

s., twilight. A procedure of spinal injection of scopolamine and morphine to abolish the subsequent memory of pain felt during childbirth, but it does not abolish pain at the time. The patient is delivered in deliriumlike state.

s. walking. Walking in one's sleep. SYN: *somnambulism.*

sleep′ing sick′ness. 1. Acute, infectious disease marked by increasing lethargy, drowsiness, muscular weakness, and cerebral symptoms. SYN: *encephalitis lethargica, q.v.* 2. African trypanosomiasis caused by a protozoan introduced into the blood and cerebrospinal fluid by the bite of a tsetse fly; characterized by fever, protracted lethargy, weakness, tremors, and wasting.

slide (slīd). A glass plate, usually 3 x 1 in., on which objects are placed for examination under a microscope.

slimy (slīm′ĭ). Resembling slime or a viscid substance; of a growth, adhering to needle so it can be drawn out as a long thread.

sling (slĭng). A support for an injured upper extremity.

s., clove hitch. Make clove hitch in center of roller bandage. Fit to hand and carry ends over shoulder. Tie beside neck with square knot, making longer ends. They may be carried over the shoulder, brought under each axilla and tied over chest.

s., cravat. The center of cravat is placed under wrist or forearm and ends tied around neck.

s., folded cravat (lesser arm sling). Place broad fold in position on chest with one end over affected shoulder and other hanging down in front of chest. Flex arm as desired across sling. Bring lower end up over sound shoulder. Knot with other end on affected shoulder.

s., open. The point of the triangle is placed at tip of elbow. The ends brought around at back of neck and tied. The point should be brought forward and pinned or tied in a single knot, forming a cup to prevent elbow from slipping out.

s., simple figure-of-eight roller arm. Flex arm on chest in desired position, then fix bandage with single turn toward uninjured side around arm and chest, crossing elbow just above external epicondyle of humerus. Make 2nd turn overlapping 2/3 of 1st and bring bandage forward under tip of elbow, then upwards, along flexed forearm to root of neck of sound side. Then bring downward over scapula and cross chest and arm horizontally, overlapping, turn above and continue as in progressive figure-of-eight.

s., St. John's. Apply triangle with point downwards under elbow, upper end over sound shoulder. Flex arm acutely on chest. Bring lower end under affected arm and around back to knot with upper end on sound shoulder. Bring point up over elbow and fasten to base. Support is wholly for injured shoulder.

s., swathe arm or cravat. (Use wide cravat or folded muslin band.) Place center under acutely flexed elbow, carry front and upwards across the forearm and over affected shoulder. Proceed obliquely across back to sound axilla. Bring other end around front of arm and across body to sound axilla, where it is pinned to other end, continuing around back to part of sling surrounding affected elbow and pinned again.

s., triangular. With suspension from uninjured side (brachioscapular sling). Place triangle on chest with one end over sound shoulder, the point under affected extremity, fold the base. Flex injured arm outside of triangle. Carry lower end upward under axilla of injured side, back of shoulder and tie with upper end behind back. Bring point of triangle anteriorly and medially around back of elbow and fasten to body of bandage. (This bandage changes point of carrying and also relieves clavicle of injured side of a load.)

s., triangular, reversed (reversed brachiocervical sling). Apply with one end over injured shoulder, point toward the sound side, base vertical under injured elbow. Flex arm acutely over triangle. Lower end is brought upwards over front of arm and over sound shoulder. Pull ends taut and tie over sound shoulder. The point is pulled taut over forearm and fixed to anterior and posterior layers between forearm and arm. (Holds elbow more acutely flexed—the weight is supported by the elbow.)

slough (slŭf). 1. Dead matter or necrosed tissue separated from living tissue or an ulceration. 2. To separate in the form of dead or necrosed parts from living tissue. 3. To cast off, as dead tissue. SEE: *eschar, scab.*

sloughing (slŭf'ĭng). The formation of a slough; separation of dead from living tissue.

s. phagedena. Hospital gangrene.

slow (slō). 1. Mentally dull. 2. Exhibiting retarded speed, as the pulse. 3. Of a morbid condition or fever, not acute. SEE: *"brady-" words.*

slows (slōz). An infectious disease of cattle transmitted to man through milk or butter, marked by severe neural symptoms, constipation, vomiting; frequently fatal. SYN: *milk sickness, trembles.*

sludge (slŭj). The semisolid matter deposited in sewage.

s., activated. Sludge from well-aerated sewage, exposed to oxidizing bacteria, supplying oxidizing organisms sufficient to activate another supply of sewage.

s., dewatered. Sludge that has been dried.

smallpox (smawl'pŏks). An acute, contagious, febrile disease, the constitutional symptoms of which are followed by successive stages of eruptions. SYN: *variola, q.v.*

smear, smear culture (smēr). 1. BACT: Material spread on a surface, as a microscopic slide or a culture medium. 2. One obtained from infected matter spread over a solidified medium.

Smee's battery or cell (smē). A form of electric battery.

smegma (smĕg'mă). Secretion of sebaceous glands, specifically, the thick, cheesy, ill-smelling secretion found under the labia minora about the glans clitoridis and under the male prepuce from Tyson's glands. SYN: *sebum.*

s. clitoridis. BNA. Odoriferous secretion of the glands of the clitoris.

s. praeputii. BNA. Cheesy odoriferous substance collecting under prepuce in the male, secreted by Tyson's glands.

smegmatic (smĕg-măt'ĭk). Pert. to or made up of smegma.

smegmolith (smĕg'mō-lĭth). Calcareous mass in the smegma.

smell (smĕl). 1. To perceive by stimulation of the olfactory nerves. 2. To emit an odor, pleasant or offensive. 3. A chemical sense dependent upon end organs on the surface of the upper part of the nasal septum and the superior nasal conch. 4. Property of a thing affecting the olfactory organs, pleasant or unpleasant. SYN: *odor, scent, stench.*

smiths' spasm. An occupational neurosis in form of a spasm of the arm and hand in blacksmiths.

smok'er's can'cer or tongue. Cancer of the lip or throat due to irritation from a pipe stem or excessive smoking.

Sn. Symb. of tin.

snake bite (snăk bīt). All snakes should be considered poisonous, although there are only a few that secrete an amount of venom sufficient to inoculate poison deeply into the tissues.

snap'ping hip. Slipping of the hip joint with a snap due to displacement over great trochanter of a tendinous band.

snare (snăr). Device for excision of polypi, tumors, etc., by tightening wire loops around them.

sneeze (snēz). 1. To expel air forcibly through the nose and mouth by spasmodic contraction of muscles of expiration due to irritation of nasal mucosa. 2. The act of sneezing.

Snellen's reflex (sněl'ěn). Congestion of ear on same side resulting when distal end of the divided auriculocervical nerve is stimulated.

snore (snōr). 1. To breathe noisily during sleep, due to vibration of the uvula and soft palate. 2. Noisy breathing in sleep or coma. SYN: *rhonchus, stertor.*

snoring râle (snōr'ing rahl). A sonorous râle, low in pitch, resembling a snore.

snow blind'ness. Irritation of the conjunctiva caused by reflection of the sun on the snow.

snuffles (snŭf'ls). Obstructed nasal breathing with discharge from the nasal mucosa, esp. in infants, chiefly in congenital syphilis.

soap (sōp). A cleansing chemical compound formed by an alkali acting on a fatty acid; example: sodium stearate, $NaC_{18}H_{35}O_2$. SEE: *saponification.*
    Castile soap is made by saponifying olive oil with sodium hydroxide, and contains mainly sodium oleate, $NaC_{18}H_{33}O_2$.

   s. liniment. USP. Liquid opodeldoc. A solution of soap and camphor in alcohol and water.

   s. suds enema. One given so that the irritating action of the soap will start bowel motion. SEE: *enema.*

sobisminol (so-bĭs'mĭn-ōl). An antisyphilitic for intramuscular injection on solution, and orally in mass.

socia parotidis (sō'shē-ă pă-rŏt'ĭd-ĭs). An accessory parotid gland sometimes detached at beginning of Stenson's duct.

sociology (sō-sĭ-ŏl'ō-jĭ). Science of the forms, institutions, and functions of human groups.

socket (sŏk'ĕt). A hollow in a joint or part for another corresponding organ, as a bone socket or an eye socket. SEE: *ambon.*

soda (sō'dă). 1. Term loosely applied to various salts of sodium, esp. to caustic soda (sodium hydroxide) and baking soda (sodium bicarbonate). SEE: *sodium.* 2. Short for soda water, which is water charged with carbon dioxide.

sodic (sō'dĭk). Relating to or containing soda or sodium.

sodio-. Prefix denoting a *compound containing sodium.*

sodium (sō'dĭ-ŭm). SYMB: Na. At. wt. 23.00. Sp. gr. 0.97. Melting point 97.5. A metallic element of the alkali group.

   s. acetate. USP. Colorless, odorless, translucent crystals, saline in taste and soluble in water.
     DOSAGE: 25 gr. (1.5 Gm.).

   s. aleurate. The monosodium salt of allyl isopropyl barbituric acid.
     DOSAGE: 1 gr. for each 15 lb. of body weight (10 mg. per Kg.).

   s. amytal. The monosodium salt of isoamylethylbarbituric acid.
     DOSAGE: 3 gr. (0.2 Gm.) as sedative or hypnotic. 3-9 gr. (0.2-0.6 Gm.) as preliminary anesthetic, depending upon many factors.

   s. barbital. SEE: *barbital.*

   s. benzoate. USP. A white, odorless powder with sweet taste.
     DOSAGE: Internally, 15 gr. (1 Gm.).

   s. bicarbonate. USP. White, odorless power with saline taste.
     DOSAGE: 15 gr. (1 Gm.).

   s. biphosphate. USP. Sodium acid phosphate.
     DOSAGE: 10 gr. (0.6 Gm.).

   s. bisulfite. Granular or crystalline powder, sulfurous taste and odor, soluble in water.
     DOSAGE: 10-20 gr. (0.6-1/3 Gm.).

   s. borate. USP. Borax.
     DOSAGE: 1 to 2% solution used as an eyewash.

   s. bromide. USP. NaBr. White crystalline powder with saline taste.
     DOSAGE: 15 gr. (1 Gm.).

   s. cacodylate. USP. The sodium salt of cacodylic acid.
     DOSAGE: Hypodermically, 1 gr. (0.06 Gm.).

   s. carbonate. USP. Na_2CO_3. White crystalline powder (washing soda).
     DOSAGE: 5-20 gr. (0.33-1.333 Gm.).

   s. chloride. USP. NaCl. Common salt.
     DOSAGE: 10-60 gr. (0.666-4 Gm.).

   s. citrate. White granular powder, saline in taste and soluble in water.
     DOSAGE: 10-20 gr. (0.6-2.0 Gm.).

   s. fluoride. White crystalline powder, saline in taste, soluble in 25 parts of water.
     DOSAGE: 1/12-1/6 gr. (0.005-0.01 Gm.).

   s. hexametaphosphate. A salt of metaphosphoric acid.
     DOSAGE: 1-2% solution.

   s. hydroxide. A whitish solid; soluble in water, making a clear solution.
     DOSAGE: 15♏ (1 cc.).   [sulfate.

   s. hyposulfite. Same as sodium thiosulfate.

   s. iodide. USP. NaI. A salt resembling in appearance and action potassium iodide.
     DOSAGE: 5 gr. (0.3 Gm.).

   s. morrhuate. The sodium salt of the fatty acids, found in cod liver oil.
     DOSAGE: 0.5-1 cc. of 5% solution.

   s. nitrate. SEE: *Chile saltpeter.*

   s. nitrite. USP. $NaNO_3$. White crystalline powder, characteristic properties of nitroglycerine, but effects more lasting.
     DOSAGE: 1 gr. (0.06 Gm.).

   s. oleate. A white, soft mass; sodium salt of oleic acid.
     DOSAGE: 1-3 gr. (0.6-1 Gm.).

   s. phosphate. USP. $Na_2HPO_4.12H_2O$. White crystalline powder.
     DOSAGE: 1 dram (4 Gm.).

   s. phosphate effervescent. USP. A mixture of sodium phosphate, sodium bicarbonate, and tartaric acid.
     DOSAGE: 2½ drams (10 Gm.).

   s. salicylate. USP. White powder or scales with sweet saline taste.
     DOSAGE: 15 gr. (1 Gm.).

   s. sulfate (Glauber's salt). USP. Resembles magnesium sulfate in appearance and action.
     DOSAGE: 4 drams (15 Gm.).

s. tartrate. $Na_2C_4H_4O_6$—2 H_2O. White soluble crystals.
DOSAGE: 15-30 gr. (1-2 Gm.); 4-8 drams (15-30 Gm.).

s. taurocholate. Extract of bile from carnivora; a yellowish gray powder soluble in water.
DOSAGE: 2-6 gr. (0.13-0.4 Gm.).

s. thiocyanate. NaSCN. A sodium salt.
DOSAGE: 5 gr. (0.3 Gm.).

s. thiosulfate. USP. White crystalline substance, having a cooling taste.
DOSAGE: 15 gr. (1 Gm.).

s. valerianate. White crystalline powder with faint odor and taste of valerian. Soluble in water and of unctuous feel.
DOSAGE: 2-5 gr. (0.13-0.3 Gm.).

sodokosis (sŏd-ō-kō'sĭs). Infectious febrile disease caused by infection from bite of a rat. SYN: *rat-bite fever, sodoku*.

sodoku (sō-do'koo). Infectious febrile disease due to rat bite. SYN: *rat-bite fever, sodokosis*.

sodomy (sŏd'ō-mĭ). Anal coitus, usually bet. males; bestiality (*concubitus cum bestia*), and pederasty,* (*concubitus cum persona ejusdem sexus*).

Soemmering's foramen (sĕm'ĕr-ĭng). Marginal process of the malar bone. SYN: *fovea centralis*.

S.'s spot. The macula lutea of the retina.

S.'s yellow spot. Same as *Soemmering's spot*.

soft or convalescent diet. Fish, egg, and cheese dishes; chicken; cereals; bread; toast; butter; nothing not soft, semisolid or liquid. No red meats, vegetables, or fruits having seeds or thick skins. No cellulose, raw fruits, or salads.

s. diet, cold. Suitable for tonsillectomies. All forms of milk and cream, iced cocoa, coffee and tea iced, gelatin, junket, custard, strained cereals and fruits if not seeded, such as berries. No fruit juices unless ordered.

s. d., light. Medical liquids; cream soups, strained; toast; cream; poached or coddled eggs; mashed potatoes; carrots, peas, and spinach purées; gelatins; junkets; custards; stewed fruits; souffles; jellies; gruels; cereals if strained; ice cream; sherbets.

s. d., l., surgical. Fluids plus thick water gruels, toast, stewed fruits if strained but no seeded fruits.

s. d., modified. Small meals, frequent feedings, gradual additions to full liquid diet—crackers, baked potato, soft cooked egg, cream of wheat, farina, strained oatmeal, applesauce, puréed pears, jelly, simple desserts; later, cottage cheese, puréed vegetables, minced tender meat.

soft (sŏft). Not hard, firm, or solid.

s. palate. The soft post. part of the palate. SYN: *palatum molle, velum pendulum palati*.

s. sore. A venereal sore, not due to syphilis, caused by Ducrey's bacillus. SYN: *chancroid*.

softening (sŏf'ĕn-ĭng). Process of becoming soft. SYN: *malacia, mollities*.

s., anemic. White softening of the brain from lack of blood.

s. of the brain. Paresis with progressive dementia. SYN: *encephalomalacia*.

s., gray. Softening of the brain with absorption of fat following yellow softening.

s., hemorrhagic. Red softening, q.v.

s., mucoid. Myxomatous degeneration.

s., red. Softening of the brain with bleeding into necrosed portions.

s., white. Same as anemic softening.

s., yellow. Softening of brain in a late stage with deposit of changing pigment and fatty degeneration of cells.

sol (sŏl, sōl). In the chemistry of colloids, a fluid mixture of a colloid and a liquid.

solanine (sō'län-ĭn). A poisonous narcotic alkaloid obtained from potatoes.

solar (sō'lar). Pert. to the sun or its rays.

s. fever. An infectious febrile disease. SYN: *dengue, q.v.*

s. ganglion. Ganglion on 5th cranial nerve. SYN: *gasserian ganglion*.

s. plexus. The celiac plexus behind the stomach and bet. the suprarenal glands, and consisting of 2 large ganglia.

s. therapy. Treatment with the sun's rays. SYN: *heliotherapy*.

solargentum (sol-ar-jĕn'tŭm). A brand of mild silver protein, containing 19-23% colloidal silver.

solarium (sō-lā'rĭ-ŭm). A room designed for heliotherapy or for the application of artificial light.

solation (sō-lā'shŭn). In colloidal chemistry, the transformation of a gel into a sol.

solbisminol (sŏl-bĭz'mĭn-ōl). An antisyphilitic drug which can be taken by mouth.

sole (sōl). Underpart of the foot. SYN: *planta, plantar surface*. SEE: *antithenar, thenar*.

s. plate. Flattened nucleated mass in which motor nerve endings rest.

s. reflex. Contraction of muscles when tickling the sole.

solenoid (sō'lē-noyd). Tubular coil used in producing a magnetic field.

solepism (so'le-pizm). The theory that nothing may be known objectively, because only may one's own mental processes be known.   [calf of leg.

soleus (sō'lē-ŭs). A flat, broad muscle of

solid (sŏl'ĭd). 1. Not gaseous, hollow, or liquid. 2. A substance not gaseous, liquid, or hollow.

s. carbon dioxide therapy. Therapeutic application of solid carbon dioxide. SEE: *refrigeration*.

solitary glands or follicles (sol'i-tar-ĭ). Lymphatic glands in mucous membrane of small intestines not included in Peyer's* patches.

solubility (sŏl''ū-bĭl'ĭ-tĭ). Capability of being dissolved.

soluble (sŏl'ū-bl). Able to be dissolved.

solute (sŏl'ūt). The substance that is dissolved in a solution.

solution (sō-lū'shŭn). 1. Liquid containing dissolved substance. 2. Process by which a solid is homogeneously mixed with a fluid, or a solid or gas, so that the dissolved substances cannot be distinguished from the resultant fluid. 3. Mixture so formed. 4. Termination of a disease.

s., colloidal. That in which the solute is suspended and not dissolved, such as gelatin, albumin.

s., dilute. One containing a small amount of a dissolved material in proportion to the amount that could be dissolved.

s., inorganic. Watery solution of substances such as alkalies and acids and their salts having such properties as ionization and osmosis.

s., saline; s., salt. Sodium chloride (0.6 to 0.75%) in distilled water. It may be *isotonic*, having the same salt concentration as the blood and the same osmotic power, or *hypotonic*, having a lesser concentration of salt than the blood, thus affecting the integrity of the cells or tissues.

s., saturated. A solution that contains all the solute it can dissolve. This limit is called the *saturation* point.

s., supersaturation. Solution in which the saturation point is reached, but when heated it is possible to dissolve more of the solute.

solv. Abbr. of *solve*, meaning *dissolve*.

solvent (sŏl'vĕnt). 1. Producing a solution; dissolving. 2. A liquid holding another substance in solution.

soma (sō'mǎ). 1. The body without its appendages. 2. Psy: The body as differentiated from the psyche.

somacule (sō'măk-ūl). A physiological unit; the smallest possible division of protoplasm.

somal (sō'măl). Concerning the body.

somasthenia (sō-mǎs-thē'nĭ-ǎ). A condition of chronic bodily weakness. Syn: *somatasthenia*.

somatalgia (sō-mǎt-ǎl'jĭ-ǎ). Bodily pain.

somatasthenia (sō-mǎt-ǎs-thē'nĭ-ǎ). Chronic bodily weakness usually with low blood pressure, but *not* neurasthenia. Syn: *somasthenia*.

somatesthesia (sō-mǎt-ĕs-thē'zĭ-ǎ). The consciousness of the body; bodily sensation.

somatic (sō-mǎt'ĭk). Concerning the body as distinguished from the viscera or mind; physical.

s. death. Death of the entire body.

s. tissue. All tissue other than the reproductive tissue.

somatoblast (sō-mat'ō-blăst). Any plastidule from which cell material is developed.

somatochrome (sō-mat'ō-krōm). A nerve cell or group which stains readily.

somatogenetic (sō-mat'ō-jĕn-ĕt'ĭk). Facilitating the reproduction of the body.

somatology (sō-mǎt-ŏl'ō-jĭ). Comparative study of structure, functions, and development of the human body.

somatopathic (sō-mǎt-ō-păth'ĭk). Organically ill, as distinguished from neuropathic or psychopathic diseases.

somatoplasm (sō-mǎt'ō-plăzm). The protoplasmic substance of the body.

somatopleure (sō-mat'ō-plūr). The embryonic outer layer together with the epiblast after the mesoderm splits into 2 layers.

somatopsychic (sō-mǎt-ō-sī'kĭk). Pert. to both body and mind.

somatopsychosis (sō'mǎ-tō-sī-kō'sĭs). Any mental disorder which is a symptom of a bodily disease.

somatoschisis (sō-mǎt-ōs'kĭs-ĭs). Splitting of the vertebral bodies.

somatoscopy (sō-mǎt-ōs'kō-pĭ). Physical examination of the body.

somatotomy (sō-mǎ-tŏt'ō-mĭ). Anatomy of the human body.

somatotropic (sō'mǎt-ō-trŏp'ĭk). 1. Having selective attraction for, or influencing body cells. 2. Stimulating growth.

somatropin (sō-mǎt'rō-pĭn). The anterior pituitary lobe's growth-stimulating principle.

somesthesia (som-es-the'sĭ-ǎ). Awareness of bodily sensations. Syn: *somatesthesia*.

somesthetic (sō-mĕs-thĕt'ĭk). Pert. to sensations and sensory structures of the body.

s. area. The region in the cortex in which lie the terminations of the axons of general sensory conduction-paths.

s. path. General sensory conduction-path leading to the cortex.

somite (sō'mĭt). 1. Embryonic blocklike segment formed on either side of the neural tube and its underlying notochord. 2. Any one of the embryonic segments.

somnambulism (sŏm-năm'bŭ-lĭzm). 1. A form of hysteria in which behavior and purposeful actions are not subsequently remembered. 2. Sleepwalking, an affection that prompts the sleeping person to perform, unconsciously, acts that naturally belong to the waking state. Syn: *noctambulism, q.v.*

somnarium (sŏm-nā'rĭ-ŭm). A sanitarium in which sleep therapy is employed in the treatment of neuroses.

somnifacient (sŏm-nĭ-fā'shĕnt). 1. Producing sleep. Syn: *hypnotic*. 2. A medicine producing sleep. Syn: *soporific, q.v.*

somniferous (sŏm-nĭf'ĕr-ŭs). Sleep-producing; pert. to that which promotes sleep.

somnific (sŏm-nĭf'ĭk). Producing sleep. Syn: *somnifacient*.

somniloquy (sŏm-nĭl'ō-kwĭ). Act of talking during sleep or in a hypnotic condition.

somnipathy (sŏm-nĭp'ǎ-thĭ). 1. Any disorder of sleep. 2. Hypnotism.

somnocinematograph (sŏm-nō-sĭn-ĕ-mǎt'ō-grǎf). Device for recording motions of those who are asleep. Syn: *hypnocinetograph*.

somnolence (sŏm'nō-lĕns). Prolonged drowsiness or a condition resembling trance which may continue for a number of days; sleepiness.

somnolent (sŏm'nō-lĕnt). Sleepy; drowsy.

somnolentia (sŏm-nō-lĕn'shĭ-ǎ). 1. Drowsiness. 2. The sleep of drunkenness in which the faculties are only partially in repose. SEE: *sleep*.

somopsychosis (sŏm″ō-sī-kō′sĭs). A psychosis in which symptoms are mostly of a bodily nature.

sonitus (sŏn′ĭ-tŭs). Subjective noises in the ear. SYN: *tinnitus aurium, q.v.*

sonometer (sō-nŏm′ĕt-ĕr). Device for testing the hearing.

sonorous (sō-nō′rŭs). Giving forth a loud and rounded sound. SYN: *resonant*.

   s. râle. A dry or low pitched râle often caused by vibration of mucous secretion in a bronchus.

soot cancer, soot wart (sŏŏt). Epithelioma of the scrotum found in chimney sweepers.

soothing syrups. Syrups used to induce sleep in infants.

sophistication (sō-fĭs-tĭ-kā′shŭn). Adulteration of any substances.

sopor (sō′por). Deep, lethargic sleep. SYN: *stupor*.

soporific (sō-por-ĭf′ĭk). 1. Inducing sleep. 2. Narcotic; a drug producing sleep.

soporose, soporous (sō′por-ōs, -ŭs). Marked by or resembling sound sleep or coma. Causing or that which causes or promotes absorption.

sorbefacient (sor″bē-fā′shĕnt). Causing or that which causes or promotes absorption.

sordes (sor′dēz). 1. Foul, brown crusts or accumulations on the teeth and about the lips from foul stomach or secretions of the mouth in low forms of fever. 2. Filth.

sore (sōr). 1. Causing physical pain. 2. A tender or painful ulcer or lesion of the skin.

   s., bed. Gangrene of skin due to pressure. SYN: *decubitus, q.v.; pressure sore*.

   s., cold. Blister on the lips. SYN: *herpes* facialis*.

   s., fungating. A granulating chancroid.

   s., hard. Syphilitic chancre,* primary lesion of syphilis.

   s., pressure. A bedsore, *q.v.*

   s., soft venereal. Soft, nonsyphilitic, venereal sore occurring on the genitalia. SYN: *chancroid.**

   s. throat. Any inflammation of the tonsils, pharynx, or larynx.

   s. t., clergyman's. Granular pharyngitis with dysphonia.

   s. t., diphtheritic. Croupous tonsillitis.

   s. t., hospital. Superficial septic inflammation of fauces and pharynx.

   s. t., septic. Severe, epidemic, pseudomembranous inflammation of fauces and tonsils caused by the hemolytic streptococcus.

   s. t., spotted. Follicular tonsillitis.

   s. t., ulcerated. Pharyngitis with formation of gangrenous patches.

   s., venereal. SEE: *soft venereal sore*.

sororiation (so-ror-ĭ-ā′shŭn). Growth of the breasts at puberty.

soterocyte (sō′ter-ō-sīt). A blood platelet.

souffle (soof′fl). A soft blowing sound heard in auscultation; a bruit; an auscultatory murmur.

   s., cardiac. Heart murmur.

   s., fetal. The soft blowing sound heard over the location of the umbilical cord of the fetus *in utero* and synchronous with the fetal heartbeat during late pregnancy.

   s., funic; s., funicular; s., umbilical. Same as fetal souffle. [in malaria.

   s., splenic. Sound heard over spleen

   s., uterine. Sound caused by blood entering dilated arteries of uterus in last months of pregnancy; synchronous with maternal pulse. It is more frequent than the fetal souffle and is heard as a loud blowing murmur along left side of uterus, and frequently all over it. An enlarged uterus may cause it. That of pregnancy is variable, whereas other forms are constant.

sound (sownd). 1. Auditory sensations produced by vibrations; noise. 2. Healthy, not diseased. 3. Heart sounds. 4. Instrument for introduction into a cavity or canal for diagnosis or treatment. SEE: *diastole, systole*.

   s., blowing. Organic murmur as of air from an aperture expelled with moderate force.

   s., bottle. Noise as of fluid in a bottle. SYN: *amphoric* murmur*.

   s., cracked-pot. A tympanic resonance heard over pulmonary cavities.

   s., fetal heart. One made by the fetal heart.

   s., friction. One produced by rubbing together of 2 inflamed mucous surfaces.

   s's., heart. The "lub" "dub" sounds of the heart.

   s., to and fro. Rasping friction sounds of pericarditis.

sozalbumin (sō-zăl-bū′mĭn). A defensive proteid normally in the body. SYN: *mycosozin, toxosozin*.

sozin (sō′zĭn). A protein in the body which destroys microörganisms (a mycosozin) or which counteracts bacterial poisons (toxosozin).

space (spās). An area, region, or segment.

   s., arachnoid. Space beneath the arachnoid membrane.

   s., axillary. The axilla or space beneath the arm.

   s., epidural. Space bet. the dura mater and vertebral periosteum, or bet. the bones of the cranium and the dura mater, assumed to be lymph spaces.

   s's. of Fontana. Spaces bet. the processes of the *ligamentum pectinatum*.

   s. nerves. Auditory nerve fibers carrying impulses to the semicircular canals.

   s., Nuel's. Space bet. outer hair cells and rods in the organ of Corti.

   s., perforated. Space pierced by blood vessels at base of brain. SYN: *substantia perforata*.

   s., plantar. Space (1 of 4) bet. fascial layers of the foot. When the foot is infected, pus may be found here.

   s., popliteal. Space back of knee joint containing the popliteal artery and vein, and small sciatic and popliteal nerves.

s., Prussak's. Space in tympanum behind Shrapnell's membrane.

s., subarachnoid. Space bet. the pia mater and arachnoid containing the spinal fluid.

s., Tenon's. Lymph space bet. the sclera and Tenon's capsule.

spanemia (spăn-ē'mĭ-ă). Poverty of blood —diminution of supply of red blood corpuscles. SYN: *anemia.*

Spanish fly (spăn'ĭsh flī). A strong rubefacient and blistering agent, diuretic stimulant to reproductive and urinary organs. SYN: *cantharides.*

spanogyny (spăn-ŏj'ĭ-nĭ). More males than females; decrease in female births.

spanomenorrhea (spăn″ō-mĕn-ō-rē'ă). Scanty menstruation.

spanopnea (spăn-ŏp-nē'ă). Infrequent respiratory functioning; slow and shallow respiration.

sparadrap (spăr'ă-drăp). A medicated adhesive plaster.

sparer (spăr'er). A substance destroyed by catabolism, but which, nevertheless, lessens catabolic action upon other substances.

sparganosis (spar-gă-nō'sĭs). Infestation with a variety of *Sparganum.*

spargosis (spar-gō'sĭs). 1. Distention of the female breasts with milk. 2. Swelling or thickening of the skin. SYN: *elephantiasis.*

spark coil. Coil consisting of primary and secondary coils with an interrupted current passing through them. SYN: *induction coil.*

s. gaps. Arrangement of opposed points or surfaces, between which an electric spark may jump.

An adjustable gap between needle points or between spheres is used to measure high potentials. For sparkover voltages see American Institute of Electrical Engineers Standardization Rules.

s., g., quenched. A multiple spark gap with numerous electrodes about 0.3 mm. apart and equipped with a copper air-cooling device.

sparteine sulfate (spar'tēn). The salt of an alkaloid obtained from Scoparius.
DOSAGE: 1/6 gr. (0.01 Gm.).

spasm (spăzm). An involuntary, sudden movement or convulsive muscular contraction.

s., Bell's. Convulsive tic of the face.

s. center. Point in the oblongata where it meets the pons.

s., choreiform. Spasmodic movements resembling chorea.

s., clonic. Intermittent contractions and relaxation of muscles.

s. of esophagus. Paroxysmal dysphagia (inability to swallow), often associated with a sense of constriction in the chest. Little or no loss of flesh.

s. of glottis. Spasm of laryngeal adductors.

s., habit. Spasms due to habit.

s., nodding. A psychogenic condition in adults, causing nodding of the head from clonic spasms of the sternomastoid muscles. A similar nodding in babies with head turning from side to side.

s., saltatory. Term employed to designate a condition allied to hysteria, in which a violent spasm seizes the muscles of the leg as soon as the feet touch the ground and as a result patient is thrown violently in the air.

s., tetanic. Spasm in which contractions continue for a time without interruption.

s., tonic. Continued involuntary contractions.

s., toxic. Spasm due to poison.

spasmatic, spasmodic (spăz-măt'ĭk, -mŏd'ĭk). Pert. to, like, or marked by, spasm. SEE: *cholepathia spastica.*

s. asthma. Asthma caused by spasm of the bronchioles.

s. croup. Laryngismus stridulus.

s. stricture. Temporary narrowing of any canal, as the urethra, due to localized spasmodic muscular contraction of its coat.

spasmodermia (spăz-mō-der'mĭ-ă). A spasmodic skin disorder.

spasmodism (spăz'mō-dĭzm). Medullary excitation causing various intermittent nervous conditions.

spasmology (spăz-mŏl'ō-jĭ). The study of spasms, their nature and cause.

spasmolygmus (spăz-mō-lĭg'mŭs). 1. Spasmodic hiccup. 2. Spasmodic sobbing.

spasmolysis (spăz-mŏl'ĭs-ĭs). The arrest of a spasm or convulsion.

spasmolytic (spăz-mō-lĭt'ĭk). Checking or that which checks spasms.

spasmomyxorrhea (spăz″mō-mĭks-or-re'ă). Excessive secretion of intestinal mucus. SYN: *myxorrhea intestinalis.*

spasmophemia (spăz-mō-fē'mĭ-ă). A spasmodic disorder of speech. SYN: *stuttering.*

spasmophilia (spăz-mō-fĭl'ĭ-ă). A tendency to tetany and convulsions; almost always associated with rickets.

spasmotin (spăz'mō-tĭn). Poisonous ecbolic principle obtained from ergot.

spasmous (spăz'mŭs). Of the nature of a spasm.

spasmus (spăz'mŭs). A spasm.

s. agitans. Paralysis agitans, q.v.

s. bronchialis. Bronchial asthma.

s. caninus. Spasm of face causing a constant grin. SYN: *risus sardonicus.*

s. coordinatus. Imitative or compulsive movements, as mimic tics or festination.

s. cynicus. Spasmodic contraction of muscles on both sides of the mouth.

s. Dubini. Rhythmic contractions, in rapid succession, of a group or groups of muscles, starting at an extremity or half of the face, and covering a large part or all of the body. SYN: *electric chorea.*

s. glottidis. Spasm of larynx. SYN: *laryngismus stridulus.*

s. intestinorum. Pain in intestines. SYN: *enteralgia.*

s. nictitans. A winking movement of the eyelid.

s. nutans. Nodding spasm.

spastic (spăs'tĭk). Resembling or of the nature of spasms or convulsions.

s. gait. A stiff movement with toes seeming to catch together and to drag.

s. hemiplegia. Partial hemiplegia with spasmodic muscular contractions.

s. paralysis. Muscular rigidity accompanying partial paralysis.

s. paraplegia. Paraplegia due to transverse lesions of the cord or sclerosis.

spasticity (spăs-tĭs'ĭ-tĭ). Hypertension of muscles causing stiff and awkward movements; the result of upper motor neuron lesion.

spatula (spăt'ū-lă). Instrument for spreading or mixing semisolids.

s., eye. Blades for separating lips of corneal wounds, arresting hemorrhage or for making pressure; sheet metal or rubber.

s., nasal. Device for holding mucous flaps in place or to guard against burning from cautery.

spay (spā). Surgical removal of ovaries, usually said of animals. See: *castration.*

specialist (spĕsh'ăl-ĭst). A physician who treats a special type of diseases.

species (spē'shēz). Biol: Category of classification, a subdivision between a genus and a variety in which all the individuals are almost identical.

specific (spē-sĭf'ĭk). 1. A remedy having a curative effect on a particular disease or symptom. 2. Pert. to a species. 3. A disease always caused by the same organism.

s. gravity. Weight of a substance compared with an equal volume of water. Water is represented by 1.000.

specificity (spē-sĭ-fĭs'ĭ-tĭ). State of being specific; having a relation to a definite result, or to a particular cause.

specillum (spē-sĭl'lŭm). 1. Lens. 2. Button-shaped silver probe.

specimen (spĕs'ĭ-mĕn). A part of a thing intended to show kind and quality of the whole, as a specimen of urine.

spectacles (spĕk'tăk-lz). Two lenses supported by a nose bridge and side pieces passing over the ears, to aid vision or protect the eyes.

spectro-. Combining form meaning *appearance, image, form, spectrum.*

spectrocolorimeter (spĕk-trō-kŭl-or-ĭm'ĕt-ĕr). Device for detecting color blindness by isolating a single spectral color.

spectrograph (spĕk'trō-grăf). An instrument designed to photograph spectra on a sensitive photographic plate.

spectrometer (spĕk-trŏm'ĕt-ĕr). A spectroscope so constructed that angular deviation of a ray of light produced by a prism or by a diffraction grating thus indicates the wave length.

spectrophotometer (spĕk"trō-fō-tŏm'ĕt-ĕr). Device for measuring amt. of color in a solution by comparison with the spectrum.

spectrophotometry (spĕk"trō-fō-tŏm'ĕt-rĭ). Estimation of coloring matter in a solution by use of the spectroscope, or spectrophotometer.

spectropyrheliometer (spĕk"trō-pĭr-hē-lĭ-ŏm'ĕ-tĕr). Instrument to measure solar radiation.

spectroscope (spĕk'trō-skōp). An instrument for separating radiant energy into its component frequencies or wave lengths by means of a prism or grating to form a correct spectrum for inspection.

spectroscopy (spĕk-trŏs'kō-pĭ). The branch of physical science that treats of the phenomena observed with the spectroscope, or those principles on which its action is based; also, the art of using the spectroscope.

spectrum (spĕk'trŭm). Charted band of wave lengths of electromagnetic vibrations obtained by refraction and diffraction of ray of white light.

s., invisible. Spectral portion either below the red (infrared) or above the violet (ultraviolet), which is invisible to the eye, the waves being too long or too short to affect the retina.

s., visible. Seven colors from red to violet.

speculum (spĕk'ū-lŭm) (pl. *specula*). 1. Instrument for examination of canals. 2. Membrane separating ant. cornua of lateral ventricles of brain. Syn: *septum pellucidum.*

s., ear. Short, funnel-shaped tubes, tubular or bivalve; former preferable.

s., eye. Device for separating eyelids. Plated steel wire, plain, Von Graefe's, Steven's or Luer's most common.

speech. Verbal expression of one's thought.

s. abnormalities. These are numerous as would be expected from so highly complicated a series of mechanisms underlying language. Primitively, certain crude sounds served as warnings or threats in much the same way as did facial and bodily expressions. As sounds became highly differentiated, each became associated, and gradually identified with a certain idea.

s. center. The 3rd frontal convolution of the brain which controls speech.

s., clipped. Same as scamping speech.

s., echo. Parrotlike repetition of words spoken by others. Syn: *echolalia.*

s., mirror. Reversing the order of syllables of a word.

s., scamping. Omission of consonants or syllables when unable to pronounce them.

s., scanning. A staccatolike speech with pauses bet. syllables.

s., slurring. Slovenly articulation of letters difficult to pronounce.

s., staccato. Slow and laborious speech with each syllable pronounced separately, as in multiple sclerosis.

spend (spĕnd). To ejaculate semen in coitus or masturbate, or during sleep.

sperm (spĕrm). 1. The male germ cell. 2. Male fertilizing secretion. Syn: *semen.*

s. cell. A spermatozoon or spermatid.

sperma (sper'mä). 1. Testicular secretion containing the male reproductive cells. Syn: *semen.* 2. Individual male germ cell.

spermacrasia (spĕr"mäk-rā'zĭ-ă). Lack of spermatozoa in the semen.

spermatemphraxis (sper-mät-ĕm-frăks'ĭs). An obstruction to emission of semen.

spermatid (sper'mät-ĭd). A cell derived from fission of a secondary spermatocyte which develops into a spermatozoon.

spermatin (sperm'ă-tĭn). A mucilaginous substance in the semen.   [sperm.

spermatic (sper-mät'ĭk). Pert. to semen or

   s. arteries. Two long, slender vessels, branches of the abdominal aorta, following each spermatic cord to the testes.

   s. cord. The cord suspending the testis composed of *veins, arteries, lymphatics, nerves,* and the *vas deferens.* See: *cord, infundibuloform, varicocele.*

   s. duct. Canal for passage of semen.

spermatid (sper'mä-tĭd). A cell arising by division of the secondary spermatocyte to become a spermatozoon.

spermatism (sper'mä-tĭzm). Ejaculation of semen, voluntarily or otherwise.

spermatitis (sper"mä-tī'tĭs). Inflammation of the spermatic cord or of the vas deferens. Syn: *deferentitis, funiculitis.*

spermato-. Combining form meaning *sperm, to sow seed.*

spermatoblast (sper-mät'ō-blăst). The rudimentary spermatozoon. Syn: *spermatid.*

spermatocele (sper-mät'ō-sēl). A cystic tumor of the epididymis containing spermatozoa.

spermatocidal (sper"mä-tō-sī'dăl). Destroying spermatozoa.

spermatocyst (sper-mät'ō-sĭst). 1. A seminal vesicle. 2. Tumor of epididymis containing semen. Syn: *spermatocele.*

spermatocystectomy (sper"mät-ō-sĭs-tĕk'tō-mĭ). Removal of the seminal vesicles.

spermatocystitis (sper"mät-ō-sĭs-tī'tĭs). Inflammation of a seminal vesicle. Syn: *seminal vesiculitis.*

spermatocystotomy (sper"mät-ō-sĭs-tŏt'ō-mĭ). Incision into a seminal vesicle for drainage.

spermatocyte (sper-mät'ō-sīt). A cell originating from a spermatogonium, and which forms by division the spermatids which give rise to spermatozoa.

spermatogenesis, spermatogeny (sper-mät-ō-jĕn'ĕ-sĭs, -ŏj'ĕ-nĭ). The formation of spermatozoa.

spermatogonium (sper-mät-ō-gō'nĭ-ŭm). A seminal cell in its formative state; a mass of spermatoblasts.

spermatoid (sper'mät-oyd). 1. Resembling semen. 2. A male germ cell. Syn: *spermatozoid, spermatozoon.*

spermatology (sper-mä-tŏl'ō-jĭ). The study of the seminal fluid.

spermatolysin (sper-mät-ŏl'ĭ-sĭn). A lysin destroying spermatozoa.

spermatolysis (sper-mät-ŏl'ĭ-sĭs). Dissolution or destruction of spermatozoa.

spermatolytic (sper-mät-ō-lĭt'ĭk). Destroying spermatozoa.

spermatomere (sper'mä-tō-mēr, sper"mä-tō-mē'rīt). One of the particles of the nucleus of the spermatozoon into which it divides after fertilization of the ovum.

spermatopathia, spermatopathy (sper"mä-tō-păth'ĭ-ă, sper-mät-ŏp'ă-thĭ). Disease of sperm cells or their secreting glands or ducts.

spermatophobia (sper-mät-ō-fō'bĭ-ă). Abnormal fear of being afflicted with spermatorrhea, involuntary loss of semen.

spermatophore (sper-mät'ō-fōr). 1. A capsule surrounding a mass of spermatozoa. 2. Rudimentary undifferentiated male germ cell. Syn: *spermatogonium.*

spermatoplania (sper"mät-ō-plā'nĭ-ă). An assumed metastasis of semen.

spermatopoietic (sper-mät-ō-poy-ĕt'ĭk). Promoting the formation and secretion of semen.

spermatorrhea (sper-mät-or-ē'ă). Abnormally frequent, involuntary loss of semen without orgasm.

spermatoschesis (sper-mät-ŏs'kĕ-sĭs). Suppression of the seminal fluid.

spermatospore (sper-mat'ō-spōr). A primitive cell from which spermatozoa arise. Syn: *spermatogonium.*

spermatotoxin (sper-mät-ō-tŏks'ĭn). A toxin which destroys spermatozoa. Syn: *spermatoxin.*

spermatovum (sper-mät-ō'vŭm). A fecundated or impregnated ovum.

spermatoxin (sper-mä-tŏks'ĭn). A toxin which causes destruction of spermatozoa. It is formed by injecting spermatozoa from animal of another species.

spermatozoa (sper"mät-ō-zō'ă) (sing. *spermatozoon*). Male germ cells.

spermatozoid (sper'mät-ō-zoyd). 1. Like semen. 2. Male germ cell. Syn: *spermatoid.*

spermatozoon (sper"mät-ō-zō-ŏn) (pl. *spermatozoa*). The basic or fecundating nature element of the semen.

spermaturia (sper-mät-ū'rĭ-ă). Semen discharged with the urine.

spermectomy (sper-mĕk'tō-mĭ). Resection of a portion of the spermatic cord and duct.

spermic (sper'mĭk). Concerning sperm, male reproductive cells.

spermicidal (sper"mĭ-sī'dăl). Killing spermatozoa.

spermicide (sper'mĭ-sīd). An agent which kills spermatozoa.

spermiduct (sper'mĭ-dŭkt). The ejaculatory duct and vas deferens considered as one.

spermoblast (sper'mō-blăst). A cell developing into a spermatozoon. Syn: *spermatoblast* or *spermatid.*

spermolith (sper'mō-lĭth). A calculus in the seminal vesicle or spermatic duct.

spermolytic (sper-mō-lĭt'ĭk). Causing the destruction of spermatozoa.

spermoneuralgia (sper"mō-nū-răl'jĭ-ă). Neuralgic pain in the testicles and spermatic cord.

spermophlebectasia (sper″mō-flē-bĕk-tā′-zĭ-ă). Varicosity of the spermatic veins.

spermoplasm (sper′mō-plăzm). The protoplasm of a male germ cell.

spermosphere (sper′mō-sfēr). Mass of spermatoblasts derived from spermatogonia.

spermospore (sper′mō-spōr). A primitive cell from which spermatozoa originate. SYN: *spermatogonium, spermatospore.*

sp. gr. Abbr. for *specific gravity.*

spes phthisica (spēz′ tĭz′ĭk-ă). A sense of well-being, happiness, and hopefulness in patients ill with tuberculosis.

sphacelate (sfăs′ĕl-āt). 1. To affect with gangrene. 2. Gangrenous. SYN: *mortified, necrosed.*

sphacelation (sfăs-ĕl-ā′shŭn). Mortification; formation of a mass of gangrenous tissue. SYN: *gangrene, necrosis.*

sphacelism (sfăs′ĕl-ĭzm). Condition of being affected with sphacelus, or gangrene. SYN: *necrosis.*

sphaceloderma (sfăs″ĕl-ō-der′mă). Gangrene of the skin, esp. when symmetrical. SEE: *Raynaud's disease.*

sphacelotoxin (sfăs″ĕl-ō-tŏks′ĭn). Poisonous principle obtained from ergot used as an ecbolic. SYN: *spasmotin.*

sphacelous (sfăs′ĕl-ŭs). Pert. to a slough or patch of gangrene. SYN: *gangrenous, necrosed, necrotic.*

sphacelus (sfăs′ĕl-ŭs). 1. A necrosed mass of tissue. SYN: *slough.* 2. Process of becoming gangrenous. SYN: *gangrene, mortification, necrosis.*

sphenion (sfē′nĭ-ŏn). Point at apex of the sphenoidal angle of the parietal bone.

spheno-. Combining form meaning a *wedge,* the *sphenoid bone.*

sphenoethmoid (sfē″nō-ĕth′moyd). Pert. to the sphenoid and the ethmoid bones.

    s. recess. Groove back and above the sup. concha, or turbinate bone.

sphenoid (sfē′noyd). Cuneiform, or wedge-shaped.

    s. bone. Large bone at base of skull bet. *occipital* and *ethmoid* in front, and the *parietals* and *temporal* bones at the side.

    s. fissure. Fissure in sphenoid and frontal bones for nerves and blood vessels.

sphenoiditis (sfē-noy-dī′tĭs). 1. Inflammation of the sphenoidal sinus. 2. Necrosis of the sphenoid bone.

●**sphenomaxillary** (sfē″nō-măks′ĭl-lă-rĭ). Concerning sphenoid and maxilla.

sphenopalatine (sfē″nō-păl′ăt-ēn). Concerning the sphenoid and palatine bones.

sphenotresia (sfē-nō-trē′zĭ-ă). Perforating of the basal part of the fetal skull in craniotomy.

sphenotribe (sfē′nō-trīb). Instrument for breaking up basal part of fetal cranium.

sphere (sfēr). 1. A ball or globelike structure. 2. The limited space of one's action, esp. that in which one is most capable.

    s., hearing. Portions of temporal cranial lobes supposed to be seats of sense of hearing.

    s., motor. Region ant. to fissure of Rolando that originates movements when stimulated.

    s., segmentation. 1. Cellular mass developed by segmentation of ovum's nucleus. SYN: *morula.* 2. A cell formed by segmentation of nucleus of an ovum.

    s., sensory. Region of the central nervous system that perceives sensory impressions. It is post. to the fissure of Rolando.

    s., vitelline. SEE: *segmentation sphere, 1.*

spheresthesia (sfē-rĕs-thē′zĭ-ă). A morbid sensation, as of swallowing a globe in the throat.

spherical (sfĕr′ĭ-kăl). Having the form of, or pert. to, a sphere. SYN: *globular.*

spherobacteria (sfē″rō-băk-tē′rĭ-ă). A class of organisms to which the micrococci belong.

spheroid (sfē′royd). 1. A body shaped like a sphere. 2. Sphere-shaped.

spherolith (sfē′rō-lĭth). A minute concretion in the kidney of the newly born.

spheroma (sfē-ro′mă). A tumor of spherical form.

spherometer (sfē-rŏm′ĕt-ẽr). Device to ascertain curvature of a surface.

spherospermia (sfē″rō-sper′mĭ-ă). Round spermatozoa without tails.

spherule (sfĕr′ŭl). A very small sphere.

sphincter (sfĭngk′tẽr). Circular muscle constricting an orifice. SEE: *tenesmus.*

    s. ani. Sphincter that closes the anus, the *external* one being of striated muscle, the *internal* one, of plain muscle.

    s., bladder. Plain muscle about opening of bladder into the urethra.

    s., cardiac. Plain muscle about the esophagus at cardiac opening into the stomach.

    s., ileocecal. Plain muscle about the ileum at its opening into the cecum.

    s. of Oddi. Contracted region in common bile duct at ampulla of Vater.

    s., pyloric. A thickening of the muscular wall around the pyloric orifice.

sphincteralgia (sfĭngk-tẽr-ăl′jĭ-ă). Pain in the sphincter ani muscles.

sphincterectomy (sfĭngk-tẽr-ĕk′tō-mĭ). 1. Dissection of any sphincter muscle. 2. Excision of part of the iris' pupillary border; oblique blepharotomy.

sphincterismus (sfĭngk-tẽr-ĭz′mŭs). Spasm of sphincter ani muscles.

sphincteritis (sfĭngk-tẽr-ī′tĭs). Inflammation of any sphincter muscle.

sphincterolysis (sfĭngk-tẽr-ŏl′ĭ-sĭs). Freeing of the iris from the cornea in anterior synechia affecting only the pupillary border.

sphincteroplasty (sfĭngk′tẽr-ō-plăs″tĭ). Plastic operation upon any sphincter muscle.

sphincteroscope (sfĭngk′tẽr-o-skŏp). Instrument for inspection of a sphincter.

sphincteroscopy (sfĭngk-tẽr-ŏs′kō-pĭ). Inspection of the internal anal sphincter.

sphincterotomy (sfĭngk-tẽr-ŏt′ō-mĭ). Cutting of a sphincter muscle.

sphygmic (sfĭg′mĭk). Relating to the pulse.

sphygmo-. Combining form meaning the pulse.

sphygmobolometer (sfĭg"mō-bō-lŏm'ĕ-tĕr). Device to measure force of the pulse rather than the blood pressure.

sphygmocardiogram (sfĭg"mō-kar'dĭ-ō-grăm). A tracing made by a sphygmocardiograph of the heartbeat and radial pulse.

sphygmocardiograph (sfĭg"mō-kar'dĭ-ō-grăf). Device for recording the radial pulse and the heartbeat.

sphygmocardioscope (sfĭg"mō-kar'dĭ-ō-skōp). Device for recording the action of the pulse and heart. SYN: *sphygmocardiograph*.

sphygmochronograph (sfĭg"mō-krō'nō-grăf). A sphygmograph recording graphically time bet. the heartbeat and the pulse.

sphygmogenin (sfĭg-mŏj'ĕn-ĭn). Active principle derived from the suprarenal capsule. SYN: *epinephrine*.

sphygmogram (sfĭg'mō-grăm). A tracing of the pulse made by using the sphygmograph.

sphygmograph (sfĭg'mō-grăf). Instrument for recording differences of pulse beat in disease and health.

sphygmoid (sfĭg'moyd). Resembling the pulse.

sphygmology (sfĭg-mŏl'ō-jĭ). The study of the pulse.

sphygmomanometer (sfĭg"mō-măn-ŏm'ĕt-ĕr). Instrument for determining arterial pressure.

sphygmometer (sfĭg-mŏm'ĕt-ĕr). Instrument for measuring the pulse. SYN: *sphygmograph*.

sphygmometroscope (sfĭg"mō-mĕt'rō-skōp). Instrument for auscultating the pulse by reading diastolic blood pressure.

sphygmophone (sfĭg'mō-fōn). Instrument for hearing the pulse beat.

sphygmoplethysmograph (sfĭg"mō-plĕth-ĭz'mō-grăf). Device which traces the pulse with its curve of fluctuation in volume.

sphygmoscope (sfĭg'mō-skōp). Instrument for showing the heart's movements or pulsations of arteries and veins.

sphygmosystole (sfĭg"mō-sĭs'tō-lē). The segment of the pulse wave that corresponds to the heart's systole.

sphygmotonograph (sfĭg"mō-tō'nō-grăf). An instrument for recording both blood pressure and pulse pressure.

sphygmotonometer (sfĭg"mō-tō-nŏm'ĕt-ĕr). Instrument for ascertaining elasticity of walls of an artery.

sphyrectomy (sfī-rĕk'tō-mĭ). Surgical excision of the malleus.

sphyrotomy (sfī-rŏt'ō-mĭ). Partial excision of the malleus.

spica (spī'kă). A reverse spiral bandage, the turn of which crosses like letter V. SEE: *bandage*.

spicular (spĭk'ū-lar). Pert. to, or resembling, a spicule; dartlike.

spicule (spĭk'ūl). A small, needle-shaped body.

  s., bony. A needle-shaped fragment of bone.

spiculum (spĭk'ū-lŭm) (pl. *spicula*). A sharp, small spike. SYN: *spicule*.

spider bites or **poisoning** (spī'der). All spider bites are not dangerous.

  s. cancer. SEE: *spider nevus*.

  s. cells. Branching cells in neuroglia. SEE: *Deiter's cell, neuroglia cell*.

  s. fingers. Abnormally long phalanges of the fingers. SYN: *arachnodactyly*.

  s. nevus. A branched growth on the skin of dilated capillaries, resembling a spider. SYN: *nevus araneus*.

Spies' diet. One for pellagra.

  Brewer's yeast, milk, eggs, lean meat and perhaps calves' liver, all in greater abundance than in Goldberger's* diet.

spigelian line (spī-jē'lĭ-ăn, spē-gă'lĭ-ăn). One marking musculotendinous junction of transversus abdominis muscle.

  s. lobe. A small lobe behind right lobe of liver. SYN: *lobus caudatus of liver*.

spill (spĭl). An overflow.

  s., cellular. Dissemination of cells through lymph or the blood resulting in metastasis.

spiloma, spilus (spī-lō'mă, spī'lŭs). A birthmark. SYN: *nevus*.

spiloplaxia (spī"lō-plăks'ĭ-ă). A red spot appearing in leprosy.

spina (spī'nă) (pl. *spinae*). 1. Any spine-like protuberance. 2. The spine.

  s. bifida. Congenital defect in walls of spinal canal caused by lack of union bet. the laminae of the vertebrae.

  s. ventosa. Absorption of bone bordering the medulla, appearing to be inflated with air. Seen in cancer or tuberculosis of bone.

spinal (spī'năl). Pert. to the spine or spinal cord.

  s. anesthesia. An anesthetic injected into the spinal canal.

  s. canal. Canal of the vertebral column.

  s. column. The vertebral column enclosing spinal cord. Thirty-three bones in all, 7 cervical, 12 dorsal or thoracic, 5 lumbar, 5 sacral vertebrae forming 1 bone and 4 coccygeal vertebrae which, with the sacrum, are fused into 1 bone.

  s. cord. An ovoid column of nervous tissue about 44 cm. long, flattened anteroposteriorly, extending from the medulla to the 2nd lumbar vertebra in the spinal canal.

  s. curvature. Abnormal curvature of the spine, frequently constitutional in children.

  It may be *angular* (caries), or *lateral* (scoliosis), or *anteroposterior* (kyphosis,* lordosis*).

  s. c., angular. Caries of the spine. SYN: *Pott's disease, q.v.*

  s. c., lateral. Deviation of spine to one or other side causing a twist of the spine.

  s. fluid. The fluid contained within the spinal canal.

  s. nerves. Those arising from the spinal cord; 31 pairs, consisting of 8 *cervical*, 12 *dorsal*, 5 *lumbar*, 5 *sacral*, and 1 *coccygeal,* corresponding with the spinal vertebrae. SEE: *skeleton.*

s. puncture. Puncture of the spinal cavity with a needle to extract the spinal fluid for diagnostic purposes, or to relieve tension aroused by pressure of the fluid, or to induce anesthesia, or to prevent an excess of fluid when a liquid is to be injected.

s. reflex. Any reflex centering in the spinal cord.

spinalgia (spī-nǎl'jǐ-ǎ). Pain in a vertebra under pressure.

spinalis (spī-nā'lǐs). A muscle attached to the spinal process of a vertebra.

spinant (spī'nǎnt). Any agent which increases spinal cord excitability.

spinate (spī'nāt). Having spines or shaped like a thorn.

spindle (spǐn'dl). A fusiform-shaped body, esp. one in cell nucleus during karyokinesis.

s. cells. Fusiform cells.

s. legged. Having long, thin legs.

s., nuclear. Cone-shaped nucleus during a stage of karyokinesis.

spine (spīn). 1. A sharp process of bone. 2. The spinal column, consisting of 33 vertebrae. Cervical 7, dorsal 12, lumbar 5, sacral 5, coccygeal 4. The bones of the sacrum and coccyx are ankylosed in adult life and counted as one each. SYN: *backbone.*

s., alar; s., angular. Spinous process of the sphenoid bone. SYN: *spina angularis.* [column.

s., dorsal. The backbone or spinal

s., hemal. That part of the hemal arch of a typical vertebra that closes it in.

s., Henle's. SEE: *suprameatal spine.*

s., ischiatic. Spine of the ischium, a pointed eminence on its post. border.

s., mental. Four prominent tubercles on int. surface of lower jaw.

s., nasal. A sharp process descending in middle line from inf. surface of frontal bone bet. the sup. maxillae.

s., neural. Spinous process of a vertebra.

s., palatine. Same as nasal spine.

s., pharyngeal. Ridge under basilar process of the occipital bone.

s. of the pubes. A prominent tubercle on upper border of the pubis.

s. railway. 1. Chronic meningomyelitis resulting from shock in a railway accident. 2. Traumatic neurasthenia.

s. of the scapula. An osseous plate projecting from the post. surface of the scapula.

s., sciatic. Same as ischiatic spine.

s. of the sphenoid. Spinous process of greater sphenoid wing.

s., suprameatal. A small spine at junction of sup. and post. walls of the ext. auditory meatus. SYN: *Henle's spine.*

s. of the tibia. Eminence projecting upward from the head of the tibia.

s., typhoid. Acute arthritis due to infection causing spinal ankylosis during or following typhoid fever.

spinifugal (spī-nǐf'ū-gǎl). Moving away from the spinal cord.

spinipetal (spī-nǐp'ět-ǎl). Moving toward the spinal cord.

spinitis (spī-nī'tǐs). Inflammation of the spinal cord. SYN: *myelitis.*

spinobulbar (spī"nō-bŭl'bar). Concerning the spinal cord and medulla oblongata.

spinocellular (spī"nō-sěl'ū-lar). Pert. to or like prickle cells.

spinocerebellar (spī"nō-sěr-ē-běl'ar). Concerning spinal cord and cerebellum.

spinocortical (spī"nō-kor'tǐ-kǎl). Pert. to the spinal cord and cerebral cortex. SYN: *corticospinal.*

spinoglenoid (spī"nō-glen'oyd). Relating to the spine of scapula and glenoid cavity.

s. ligament. Ligament joining spine of the scapula to the border of the glenoid cavity.

spinomuscular (spī"nō-mŭs'kū-lar). Pert. to the spinal cord and muscles.

s. segment. Motor cells and nerves in the medulla and spinal cord.

spinoneural (spī"nō-nū'ral). Pert. to the peripheral nerves and spinal cord.

spinous (spī'nŭs). Pert. to or. resembling a spine.

s. point. Spot over a spinous process very sensitive to pressure.

s. process. Prominence at post. part of each vertebra.

spinthariscope (spǐn-thǎr'ǐ-skōp). Apparatus for examining the emanations of radium.

spintherism (spǐn'ther-ǐzm). Sensation of sparks before the eyes.

spintheropia (spǐn-thěr-ō'pǐ-ǎ). Subjective sensation of sparks before the eyes.

spiradenitis (spi-ra-den-i'tis). A funiculus beginning in coil of a sweat gland. SYN: *hidrosadenitis phlegmonous.*

spiradenoma (spī-rǎd-en-ō'mǎ). Tumor of the sweat glands.

spiral (spī'rǎl). Coiling like the thread of a screw.

s. bandage. Roller bandage to be applied spirally.

s. canal of the cochlea. One that runs spirally around the modiolus.

s. lamina. A thin plate in the ear. SYN: *lamina spiralis.*

spirem, spireme (spī'rēm, spī-rēm'). First stage in karyokinesis or mitotic division in which a wreath of chromatin fibrils forms. SYN: *skein.*

spirilla (spī-rǐl'ǎ). Plural of *spirillum.*

spirillicidal (spī-rǐl"ǐ-sīd'ǎl). Destroying spirochetes or spirilla.

spirillicide (spī-rǐl'ǐs-īd). Destructive to spirilla.

spirillicidin (spī-rǐl-lǐ-sī'dǐn). A substance developed in blood of patients immunized against spirilla which has the power to destroy them.

spirillolysis (spī-rǐl-lōl'ǐ-sǐs). The destruction of spirilla.

spirillosis (spī-rǐl-ō'sǐs). A disease caused by presence of spirilla in the blood.

spirillotropic (spī-rǐl-lō-trōp'ǐk). Having an attraction to spirilla.

spirillotropism (spĭ-rĭl-lŏt'rō-pĭzm). The ability to attract spirilla.

Spirillum (spĭ-rĭl'ŭm) (pl. *Spirilla*). A group of more or less spiral-shaped, motile microörganisms, one of which (comma bacillus) causes cholera.

    S. buccale. Spirillum from tartar of teeth.

    S. cholerae asiaticae. Comma bacillus of epidemic cholera.   [teeth.

    S. Milleri. Spirillum from carious

    S. Obermeieri. Spirillum found in relapsing fever.

    S. sputigenum. Spirillum in saliva.

    S. tyrogenum. Spirillum found in very old cheese resembling that of Asiatic cholera.

    S., Vincent's. Spirillum found in Vincent's angina.

spirit (spĭr'ĭt). 1. Any distilled or volatile liquor or a solution of volatile liquid in alcohol. 2. Alcohol.

    s., rectified. Alcohol with 16% water.

spir'itual ther'apy. The application of spiritual knowledge in the treatment of all mental and physical disorders, based upon the assumption that man is a spiritual being living in a spiritual universe; that in proportion to his acceptance of this idea, and in proportion to his success in demonstrating it, he may control the body and the material elements in harmony with a Divine plan.

spirituous (spĭr'ĭt-ū-ŭs). Alcoholic; pert. to alcohol.

spiritus (spĭr'ĭt-ŭs). Alcoholic solution of a volatile substance.   .

    Usually, 5-10% strength. Thirteen are official. SYN: *spirit*.

    s. frumenti. Whisky.

    s. juniperi. Gin.

    s. myrciae. Bay rum.

    s. vini gallici. Brandy.

spirobacteria (spī"rō-băk-tē'rĭ-ă). Curved bacteria, including spirilla, spirochetes, and vibrios.

Spirochaeta (spī"rō-kē'tă). A genus of slender, nonflagellated bacteria with spiral filaments.

    S. bronchialis. A species in sputum in some nontuberculous forms of bronchitis.

    S. icterohaemorrhagiae. Species found in Weil's disease or acute febrile jaundice.

    S. morsus muris. The microörganism of rat-bite fever.

    S. nodosa. Assumed pathogenic organism of Weil's disease.

    S. pallida. Species which is the cause of syphilis. SYN: *Treponema pallidum.*

    S. refringens. A species found in gonorrhea and balanitis and in healthy genital organs; apparently nonpathogenic.

    S. vincenti. Variety found in Vincent's angina or ulcerative disease of the tonsils.

spirochetal (spī"rō-kē'tăl). Pert. to spirochetes, esp. infections caused by them.

spirochetalytic (spī"rō-kē-tă-lĭt'ĭk). Destructive of spirochetes.

spirochete (spī'rō-kēt). Any member of the genus *Spirochaeta.*

spirochetemia (spī"rō-kē-tē'mĭ-ă). Spirochetes in the blood.

spirocheticidal (spī"rō-kē-tĭ-sī'dăl). Destructive to spirochetes.

spirocheticide (spī"rō-kē'tĭs-īd). Anything which destroys spirochetes.

spirochetolysis (spī"rō-kē-tŏl'ĭ-sĭs). The destruction of spirochetes by specific antibodies.

spirochetosis (spī"rō-kē-tō'sĭs). Any infection caused by spirochetes.

spirochetotic (snī"rō-kē-tŏt'ĭk). Pert. to or marked by spirochetosis.

spirocheturia (spī"rō-kē-tū'rĭ-ă). Spirochetes in the urine.

spirogram (spī'rō-grăm). A tracing made by a spirograph of respiratory movements.

spirograph (spī'rō-grăf). Device for recording graphically respiratory movements.

spiroid (spī'royd). Resembling a spiral.

spiroindex (spī"rō-ĭn'děks). The quotient obtained by dividing vital capacity by height.

spiroma (spī-rō'mă). Multiple, benign, cystic epithelioma of the sweat glands. SYN: *spiradenoma.*

spirometer (spī-rŏm'ĕt-ĕr). An apparatus consisting of a cylindrical bell immersed in water and so equipped with outlets that gases can be exhaled into it or inhaled out of it while measurements of volume are made.

spirometry (spī-rŏm'ē-trĭ). Measurement of air capacity of the lungs.

Spironema (spī-rō-nē'mă). Another name for a genus of spirochetes. SYN: *Borrelia.*

    S. pallida. Causative organism of syphilis. SYN: *Spirochaeta pallida.*

spirophore (spī'rō-fōr). Device for artificial respiration. SYN: *iron lung.*

spirosal (spī'rō-săl). An acid derivative of salicylic acid.

    DOSAGE: Diluted with 3 parts alcohol, or 8 parts olive oil, or equal parts by weight of petrolatum.

spiroscope (spī'rō-skōp). Device for measuring air capacity of the lungs.

spiroscopy (spī-rŏs'kō-pĭ). The use of the spiroscope to measure respiratory capacity of the lungs.

spirulina (spī'rū-lī'nă). A microörganism coiled and twisted.   [*inspissated.*

spissated (spĭs'ă-ted). Thickened. SYN:

spissitude (spĭs'ĭ-tūd). Condition of being inspissated, as a fluid thickened by evaporation almost to a solid; thickness.

spit (spĭt). 1. Saliva. SYN: *expectoration, sputum, spittle.* 2. To expectorate spittle.

spit'tle. The digestive fluid of the mouth. SYN: *saliva.*

splanchnapophysis (splăngk-nă-pŏf'ĭ-sĭs). 1. Any skeletal element connected with the alimentary canal, as the hyoid bone. 2. Outgrowth of a vertebra on opp. side of a vertebral axis, enclosing some viscus.

splanchnectopia (splăngk-něk-tō'pĭ-ă). Dislocation of a viscus or of the viscera.

splanchnemphraxis (splăngk-něm-frăks′ĭs). Obstruction of any internal organ, particularly of the intestine.

splanchnesthesia (splăngk-něs-thē′zĭ-ă). Visceral sensation.

splanchnesthetic (splăngk-něs-thět′ĭk). Relation to visceral consciousness or sensation. [cera.

splanchnic (splăngk′nĭk). Pert. to the vis-
  s. nerves. Three nerves from the thoracic sympathetic ganglia distributed to the viscera.

splanchnicotomy (splăngk-nĭ-kŏt′ō-mĭ). Section of a splanchnic nerve.

splanchnoblast (splăngk′nō-blăst). Incipient rudiment of a viscus. SEE: *anlage*, *proton*.

splanchnocele (splăngk′nō-sēl) 1. That part of the celom persisting in the adult, giving rise to the visceral cavities. SYN: *splanchnocoele*. 2. Protrusion of any abdominal viscus.

splanchnocoele (splăngk′nō-sēl). Rudimentary embryonic cavity from which the visceral cavities arise.

splanchnodiastasis (splăngk-nō-dī-ăs′tăs-ĭs). Displacement or dislocation of a viscus.

splanchnodynia (splăngk-nō-dĭn′ĭ-ă). Pain in the abdominal region.

splanchnography (splăngk-nŏg′ră-fĭ). Descriptive treatise on anatomy of the viscera.

splanchnolith (splăngk′nō-lĭth). An intestinal calculus.

splanchnology (splăngk-nŏl′ō-jĭ). The study of the viscera.

splanchnopathia (splăngk-nō-păth′ĭ-ă). Pathological conditions of the viscera.

splanchnopleure (splăngk′nō-plŭr). The embryonic layer formed by the union of the visceral layer of the mesoderm with the entoderm. SEE: *somatopleure*.

splanchnoptosia, splanchnoptosis (splăngk-nŏp-tō′sĭ-ă, -sĭs). Prolapse of the viscera. SYN: *abdominal ptosis, enteroptosia, visceroptosia, Glénard's disease*.

splanchnosclerosis (splăngk-nō-sklē-rō′sĭs). Hardening of any of the viscera through overgrowth of connective tissue.

splanchnoscopy (splăngk-nŏs′kō-pĭ). Examination of the viscera with aid of roentgen rays or transillumination.

splanchnoskeleton (splăngk″nō-skěl′ě-tŏn). 1. Any osseous structure in an organ, or the cartilaginous rings of the bronchi and trachea. 2. The visceral skeleton, i. e., the *ribs, sternum, innominate bones*, etc., protecting the viscera.

splanchnotomy (splăngk-nŏt′ō-mĭ). Dissection of the viscera.

splanchnotribe (splăngk′nō-trīb). An instrument for obliterating the lumen of the intestine temporarily before resection.

splayfoot (splā′foot). A flatfoot or the deformity flatfoot. SYN: *pes planus*, *talipes valgus*.

spleen (splēn). An oval, vascular, ductless gland situated below the diaphragm in the upper abdominal quarter to the left of the cardiac end of the stomach.

s., accessory. Splenic tissue nodules near the spleen.

s., floating or wandering. An enlarged movable one not protected by the ribs.

s., lardaceous. Enlargement of spleen from lardaceous matter. SEE: *amyloid degeneration*.

s. pulp. The spleen's soft parenchyma.

s., sago. One having appearance of sago* grains.

splenadenoma (splē′nad-en-ō′mă). Enlargement of the spleen caused by hyperplasia of its pulp.

splenalgia (splē-năl′jĭ-ă). Pain in the spleen. SYN: *splenodynia*.

splenauxe (splē-nawk′sē). Enlarged condition or hypertrophy of the spleen. SYN: *splenomegaly*.

splenceratosis (splěn-sěr-ă-tō′sĭs). Induration of the spleen.

splenculus (splěn′kū-lŭs). An accessory spleen. SYN: *splenulus*.

splenectasia (splē-něk-tā′zĭ-ă). Enlargement of the spleen.

splenectasis (splē-něk′tă-sĭs). Enlargement of the spleen. SYN: *splenectasia*.

splenectomy (splē-něk′tō-mĭ). Surgical excision of the spleen.

splenectopia, splenectopy (splē-něk-tō′pĭ-ă, -něk′tō-pĭ). Displacement or mobility of the spleen. SYN: *spleen, floating*.

splenelcosis (splē-něl-kō′sĭs). Ulceration or abscess of the spleen.

splenemia (splē-nē′mĭ-ă). 1. Leukemia with splenic hypertrophy. 2. Splenic congestion.

splenemphraxis (splē″něm-frăks′ĭs). Congested condition of the spleen.

splenepatitis (splěn-ēp-ă-tī′tĭs). Inflammation of both spleen and liver.

splenetic, splenic (splē-nět′ĭk, splěn′ĭk). 1. Pert. to the spleen. 2. Suffering with chronic disease of the spleen. 3. Surly, fretful, impatient.

s. flexure. Junction of transverse and descending colon, making a bend on the left side near the spleen.

s. vein. One carrying blood from spleen to the portal vein.

splenicterus (splē-nĭk′těr-ŭs). Inflammation of spleen associated with jaundice.

splenification (splěn-ĭf-ĭ-kā′shŭn). Change in a structure whereby it resembles splenic tissue. SYN: *splenization*.

splenitis (splē-nī′tĭs). Inflamed condition of the spleen.

splenium (splē′nĭ-ŭm). 1. A compress or bandage. 2. A structure resembling a bandaged part.

s. corporis callosi. The thickened post. end of the corpus callosum.

splenius (splē′nĭ-ŭs). A flat muscle on either side of back of neck and upper thoracic area.

splenization (splěn-ĭ-zā′shŭn). The change in a tissue, as of the lung, when it resembles splenic tissue.

splenoblast (splē′nō-blăst). The mother cell of a splenocyte.

splenocele (splē′nō-sēl). 1. A hernia of the spleen. 2 A splenic tumor.

splenoceratosis (splē″nŏ-sĕr-ă-tō′sĭs). Induration of the spleen.

splenocleisis (splē″nŏ-klī′sĭs). Friction on the surface of the spleen or wrapping with gauze to induce the formation of fibrous tissue.

splenocolic (splē″nŏ-kŏl′ĭk). Pert. to the spleen and colon or reference to a fold of peritoneum bet. the two viscera.

splenocyte (splē″nŏ-sīt). A unicellular leukocyte or lymphocyte of the spleen, which probably originates elsewhere in the body.

splenodiagnosis (splē″nŏ-dī-ăg-nō′sĭs). Injection of typhoid bacilli extract in the spleen to diagnose typhoid fever.

splenodynia (splē″nŏ-dĭn′ĭ-ă). Pain in the spleen. SYN: *splenalgia.*

splenogenic, splenogenous (splē″nŏ-jĕn′ĭk, splē-nŏj′ĕn-ŭs). Originating or found in the spleen.

splenography (splē-nog′ră-fĭ). A treatise on or a description of the spleen.

splenohemia (splē″nŏ-hē′mĭ-ă). Congestion of the spleen. SYN: *splenemia,* 2.

splenohepatomegaly (splē″nŏ-hĕp″ă-tŏ-mĕg′ă-lĭ). Enlargement of both spleen and liver.

splenoid (splē′noyd). Resembling the spleen.

splenokeratosis (splē″nŏ-kĕr-ă-tŏ′sĭs). Induration of the spleen.

splenology (splē-nŏl′ŏ-jĭ). The study of the spleen, its functions and diseases.

splenolysin (splē-nŏl′ĭ-sĭn). An antibody which destroys splenic tissue.

splenolysis (splē-nŏl′ĭ-sĭs). Destruction of splenic tissue.

splenoma (splē-nō′mă). A tumor of the spleen. SYN: *splenocele.*

splenomalacia (splē″nŏ-măl-ā′sĭ-ă). Softening of the spleen.

splenomedullary (splē″nŏ-mĕd′ŭ-la-rĭ). Concerning, or formed by, bone marrow and spleen.

   s. leukemia. A disease associated with a great increase in leukocytes per cubic millimeter, hemorrhage into skin and from mucous membranes, enlargement of spleen, and changes in bone marrow. SEE: *leukemia.*

splenomegalia, splenomegaly (splē″nŏ-mĕg-ă′lĭ-ă, -mĕg′ă-lĭ). Enlargement of the spleen.

splenomyelogenous (splē″nŏ-mī-ĕl-ŏj′ĕn-ŭs). Originating in the spleen and bone marrow, said of a form of leukemia. SYN: *splenomedullary.*

splenomyelomalacia (splē″nŏ-mī″ĕl-ŏ-mă-lā′sĭ-ă). Abnormal softening of the spleen and the bone marrow.

splenoncus (splē-nŏng′kŭs). A splenic tumor or hernia. SYN: *splenocele, splenoma.*

splenonephric (splē″nŏ-nĕf′rĭk). Relating to the spleen and the kidney. SYN: *lienorenal.*

splenonephroptosis (splē″nŏ-nĕf-rŏp-tō′sĭs). Displacement of the spleen and kidney downward.

splenopancreatic (splē″nŏ-păn-krē-ăt′ĭk). Relating to the spleen and pancreas.

splenoparectasis (splē″nŏ-pă-rĕk′tă-sĭs). Abnormal enlargement of the spleen.

splenopathy (splē-nŏp′ă-thĭ). Any disorder of the spleen.

splenopexy (splē″no-pĕks-ĭ). Artificial fixation of a movable spleen.

splenophrenic ligament (splē″nŏ-frĕn′ĭk). 1. Pert. to the spleen and diaphragm. 2. Peritoneal fold extending bet. the spleen and diaphragm.

splenopneumonia (splē″nŏ-nū-mō′nĭ-ă). Pneumonia with splenization of the lung.

splenoptosis (splē″nŏ-nop-tō′sĭs). Displacement of the spleen downward.

splenorrhagia (splē″nŏ-rā′jĭ-ă). Hemorrhage from a ruptured spleen.

splenorrhaphy (splē-nor′ăf-ĭ). Suture of wound of the spleen.

splenotherapy (splē″nŏ-thĕr′ă-pĭ). Therapeutic administration of splenic tissue or extract.

splenotomy (splē-nŏt′ō-mĭ). Incision of spleen.

splenulus (splĕn′ū-lŭs). A rudimentary or accessory spleen.

splint (splĭnt). An appliance made of bone, wood, metal, and/or plaster of Paris, used for the fixation, union, or protection of an injured part of the body.

   s., aeroplane. An appliance usually used on ambulatory patients in the treatment of fractures of the humerus, and it takes its name from the elevated (abducted) position in which it holds the arm suspended in air.

   s., Agnew's. A splint for fracture of the patella and metacarpus.

   s., anchor. A splint for fracture of the jaw, with metal loops fitting over the teeth and held together by a rod.

   s., Ashhurst's. A bracketed splint of wire with a footpiece to cover the thigh and leg after excision of the knee joint.

   s., Balkan. One for extension in fracture of the femur.

   s., banjo traction. Made out of a steel rod bent to resemble the shape of a banjo, and is used for the treatment of contractures and fractures of the fingers.

   s., Bavarian. An immovable dressing in which the plaster is applied bet. 2 layers of flannel.

   s., Bond's. A splint for fracture of the lower end of the radius.

   s., Bowlby's. One for fracture of shaft of humerus.

   s., bracketed. A splint composed of 2 pieces of metal or wood united by brackets.

   s., Cabot's. A posterior wire splint.

   s., Carter's intranasal. A steel bridge with wings connected by a hinge; used for operation of depressed nasal bridge.

   s., coaptation. Small splint adjusted about a fractured limb to produce coaptation of fragments.

   s., Dupuytren's. A splint to prevent eversion in Pott's fracture.

   s., Fox's. A splint for fractured clavicle.

   s., Gibson walking. Modification of Thomas' splint.

s., Gordon's. A side splint for the arm and hand in Colles' fracture.

s., Jones' nasal. A splint for fracture of the nasal bones.

s., Kanavel. One for stiff hands.

s., Levis'. A splint of perforated metal extending from below the elbow to the end of the palm; shaped to fit the arm and hand.

s., McIntire's. A post. splint for the leg and thigh like a double inclined plane.

s., Sayre's. One of 3 varieties of splint, for the ankle, for the knee, and for use in hip joint disease.

s., Stromeyer's. A splint of 2 hinged portions which can be fixed at any angle.

s. technology. The scientific study of splints.

s., Thomas' knee. A splint for removing the pressure of the body weight from the knee joint by transferring it to the ischium and perineum.

s., Thomas' posterior. A splint used in hip joint disease.

s., Volkmann's. One for fracture of lower extremity.

splinter (splĭn'ter). 1. A fragment from a fractured bone. 2. A slender, sharp piece of wood piercing the skin.

splinting (splĭnt'ĭng). Fixation of a fracture or dislocation with a splint.

split (splĭt). 1. A longitudinal fissure. 2. Characterized by a deep fissure.

s. foot. Congenital deformity, the division of the toes extending into the metatarsal region.

s. hand. Congenital deformity, the division bet. the fingers extending into the metacarpal region. SYN: *cleft hand.*

s. pelvis. Congenital failure of pubic bones to form a union at the symphysis.

s. tongue. Furrowed tongue. SYN: *cleft tongue.*

splitting (splĭt'ĭng). A change in a complex substance whereby more simple products are produced chemically. SYN: *hydrolysis, q.v.*

spodiomyelitis (spō″dĭ-ō-mī-ō-lī'tĭs). Inflammation of spinal cord's anterior cornua. SYN: *poliomyelitis.*

spodogenous (spō-dŏj'ĕn-ŭs). Caused by waste material.

s. splenomegaly. Enlargement of the spleen due to degenerated red blood cells.

spodophagous (spō-dŏf'ă-gŭs). Destroying the waste matters in the body; said of scavenger cells.

spondylalgia (spŏn″dĭl-ăl'jĭ-ă). Painful condition of a vertebra.

spondylarthritis (spŏn″dĭl-ar-thrī'tĭs). Inflammation of a vertebra.

spondylarthrocace (spŏn″dĭl-ar-thrŏk'ă-sē). Tuberculous condition of the vertebrae.

spondyle (spŏn'dĭl). A vertebra.

spondylexarthrosis (spŏn″dĭl-ĕks″ar-thrō'sĭs). Displacement of a vertebra.

spondylitis (spŏn-dĭl-ī'tĭs). Inflammation of one or more vertebrae; esp. tuberculous disease of the vertebrae, Pott's disease.

s. deformans. Inflammation of the vertebral joints resulting in the outgrowth of bonylike deposits on the vertebrae which may fuse and cause rigid and distorted spine.

s., Kummell's. Traumatic spondylitis in which the symptoms do not appear until some time after the injury.

s. rhizomelica. Progressive rigidity of the spine caused by ankylosis of the vertebrae from below upward.

s. tuberculosa. Tuberculosis of the vertebral joints. SYN: *vertebral caries, Pott's disease.*

spondylizema (spŏn″dĭl-ĭ-zē'mă). Downward settlement of a vertebra caused by the disintegration of the one below it.

spondylo-. Combining form meaning a *vertebra.*

spondylocace (spŏn-dĭ-lŏk'ă-sē). Tuberculosis of the vertebrae. SYN: *spondylarthrocace.*

spondylodiagnosis (spŏn″dĭ-lō-dī-ăg-nō'sĭs). Diagnosis by means of visceral reflexes obtained by percussion of the vertebrae.

spondylodynia (spŏn″dĭl-ō-dĭn'ĭ-ă). Pain in a vertebra. SYN: *spondylalgia.*

spondylolisthesis (spŏn″dĭl-ō-lĭs-thē'sĭs). Forward subluxation of the lower lumbar vertebrae, usually on the sacrum, with consequent pelvic deformity.

spondylolysis (spŏn-dĭ-lŏl'ĭ-sĭs). The breaking down of a vertebral structure.

spondylopathy (spŏn″dĭl-ŏp'ă-thĭ). Any disorder of the vertebrae.

spondylopyosis (spŏn″dĭl-ō-pī-ō'sĭs). Suppuration with inflammation of a vertebra.

spondyloschisis (spŏn-dĭl-ŏs'kĭ-sĭs). Congenital fissure of one or more of the vertebral arches. SYN: *rhachioschisis.*

spondylosis (spŏn-dĭ-lō'sĭs). Vertebral ankylosis.

s., rhizomelic. Ankylosis interfering with movements of hips and shoulders.

spondylosyndesis (spŏn″dĭ-lō-sĭn'dē-sĭs). Surgical formation of an ankylosis bet. vertebrae.

spondylotherapy (spŏn″dĭl-ō-thĕr'ă-pĭ). Spinal therapeutics; spinal manipulation in the treatment of disease.

spondylotomy (spŏn-dĭl-ŏt'ō-mĭ). Removal of part of the vertebral column to correct a deformity or facilitate delivery of a fetus.

sponge (spŭnj). 1. Elastic, porous mass forming internal skeleton of certain marine animals used in surgery to mop up fluids and in bathing. 2. An absorbent pad made of gauze and cotton. 3. Short for sponge bath.

s., abdominal. Flat sponges from ½ to 1 in. thick, 3 to 6 in. in diameter, used as packing, to prevent closing or obstruction by intrusion of viscera, as covering to prevent tissue injury, and as absorbents.

s., artificial. Constructed of antiseptic gauze.

s. bath. Bathing of the body with a wet sponge.

s. graft. Sponge placed in an ulcer to cause granulation.

s. sterilization. Should be chemical, not by steam or boiling water. Clean or soak in cold water, wrap in linen towel or sack, immerse in 1% hot soda solution, 20 to 30 minutes. Remove, immerse in sack in sterilized water, then preserve in an antiseptic solution.

s. tent. One impregnated with mucilage of acacia, dried in desired shape, to dilate the os uteri or sinuses by absorbing moisture and expanding.

spongiform (spŭn'jĭ-form). Having the appearance or quality of a sponge.

spongioblast (spŭn'jĭ-ō-blăst). 1. An embryonic neuroglia cell of the layer of columnar cells in the neural tube. 2. A modified nerve cell process.

spongiocyte (spŭn'jĭ-ō-sīt). A neuroglia cell.

spongioid (spŭn'jĭ-oyd). Resembling a sponge. SYN: *spongiform.*

spongiopilin (spŭn-jĭ-ō-pī'lĭn). A loosely woven cotton fabric containing bits of sponge and coated on one side with India rubber, used as a poultice.

spongioplasm (spŭn-jĭ-ō-plăzm). Fibrillar network supporting protoplasm. SYN: *cytoreticulum.*

spongy (spŭn'jĭ). Resembling a sponge in texture.

s. body. Spongy portion of the penis surrounding the urethra. SYN: *corpus spongiosum.*

s. bone. 1. A turbinate bone. 2. Cancellous bone of a spongy texture.

s. portion. That part of the urethra within the corpus spongiosum.

spontaneous (spŏn-tā'nē-ŭs). Occurring unaided or without apparent cause; voluntary.

s. evolution. A rare method by which the fetus is expelled from the uterus while lying in the transverse position. Only possible (a) when the fetus is very small and pelvis large, (b) when fetus is dead.

s. fracture. Fracture due to the state of the bone and causing little or no injury.

s. version. The unaided conversion of a transverse presentation into a vertex or breech presentation.

spoon (spōōn). Instrument consisting of a small bowl on a handle, used in scooping out tissues, tumors, etc., or in measuring quantities.

s. nail. A nail having a concave outer surface.

sporadic (spō-răd'ĭk). Occurring occasionally or in scattered instances, as a disease.

sporadoneure (spō-răd'ō-nūr). A nerve cell occurring outside of the ganglia or nerve centers in any tissue.

sporangiophore (spō-răn'jĭ-ō-fōr). BACT: The supporting stalk for a spore sac of certain fungi.

sporangium (spō-răn'jĭ-ŭm). A sac enclosing spores, seen in certain fungi.

spore (spōr). Any germ or reproductive element of a plant or protozoan less organized than a true cell.

sporicidal (spor-ĭs-ī'dăl). Destructive to spores.

sporicide (spor'ĭs-īd). An agent which destroys spores.

sporidium (spor-ĭd'ĭ-ŭm). An embryonic protozoan organism.

sporiferous (spor-ĭf'ĕr-ŭs). Producing spores.

sporoblast (spor'ō-blăst). A secondary cyst within the oöcyst, giving rise to the sporozoite, in certain protozoans.

sporocyst (spor'ō-sĭst). 1. Sac secreted by certain protozoans prior to spore production. 2. A stage in development of trematode worms in which the int. lining gives off cells, which develop in the cavity.

sporogenesis (spor″ō-jĕn'ē-sĭs). Reproduction by spores. SYN: *sporogony.*

sporogenic (spor″ō-jĕn'ĭk). Having the ability of developing into spores.

sporogony (spor-ŏg'ō-nĭ). Reproducing by development of spores. SYN: *sporogenesis.*

sporont (spor'ŏnt). A sexually mature protozoan detached from its host in its sexual cycle.

sporophore (spor'ō-fōr). Part of a plant which bears the seeds.

sporophyte (spor'ō-fīt). The spore-bearing stage of a plant exhibiting alternation of generation.

sporoplasm (spor'ō-plăzm). Protoplasm of the ovum.

sporotrichosis (spor″ō-trī-kō'sĭs). Infection or mycosis caused by sporotricha affecting the skin and mucosa of the mouth and pharynx.

Sporotrichum (spō-rŏt'rĭ-kŭm) (pl. *Sporotricha*). A yeastlike genus of microorganisms.

Of the pathogenic species, one is the causative agent of sporotrichosis.*

Sporozoa (spor″ō-zō'ă). A class of protozoa, some of which are parasitic and which reproduce by spore formation.

sporozoite (spor″ō-zō'ĭt). An elongated, sickle-shaped body formed by division of an oöcyst after fertilization.

In malaria, it is introduced by the bite of a mosquito into an erythrocyte.

sport (spōrt). An individual organism which spontaneously differs from its parents or from type. SYN: *mutation.*

sporulation (spor-ū-lā'shŭn). Production of spores or method of reproduction of unicellular organisms.

sporule (spor'ŭl). A spore, or a small one.

spot (spŏt). A small area of surface differing from surrounding parts in appearance. SYN: *loculus, macula, papule, pustule.*

s., blind. The optic disk where optic nerve enters the retina.

s., embryonic. Nucleolus of the ovum.

s's., Filatow's; s's., Flindt's. SEE: *Koplik's spots.*

s., germinal. Same as embryonic spot.

s., hectic. Bright red spot on cheek from hectic fever.

s., hypnogenic. A point which, when pressed, will throw a susceptible person into hypnosis or sleep.

s., hysterogenic. A point which, upon pressure, will induce in a susceptible subject an attack of hysteroepilepsy.

s., Koplik's. Minute white spots or bluish-white ones on mucous membrane of mouth before appearance of the rash of measles.

s's., rose. Rose-colored maculae of eruption in typhoid fever.

s., yellow. Area surrounding and including the *fovea centralis* in the retina. SYN: *macula lutea.*

spot'ted fe'ver. Popular name for various eruptive fevers: 1. Typhus. 2. Tick fever. 3. Cerebrospinal meningitis.

sprain (sprān). 1. To wrench a joint. 2. The forcible wrenching of a joint, with partial rupture or other injury of its attachments, and without luxation of bones.

s. of back. Overstretching of muscles, ligaments, or other structures of spinal mechanism, often associated with small fractures.

s. of foot. Usually a fracture or tearing of the ligaments of the foot or ankle.

s. fracture. The separation of a tendon or ligament from its insertion, taking with it a piece of the bone.

s., riders'. Sprain of the adductor longus muscles of the thigh, resulting from strain in riding horseback.

spray (sprā). 1. A jet of fine medicated vapor applied to a diseased part or discharged into the air. 2. An instrument for applying such a spray. SYN: *atomizer.* 3. To discharge fluid in a fine stream.

s. tube. Device for converting liquid into a spray.

spreading (sprĕd'ĭng). BACT: Noting a growth extending much (several mm. or more) beyond the site of inoculation.

spring (sprĭng). 1. The 1st of the 4 annular seasons. SYN: *vernal season.* 2. A flying back of a body to its original position through its elasticity.

s. conjunctivitis. A form recurring each year in the spring but disappearing with the first frost. SYN: *vernal catarrh.*

s.-finger. Arrested movement of a finger in flexion or extension followed by a jerk. SYN: *trigger finger.*

s. ligament. Int. calcaneoscaphoid ligament of the sole of the foot.

It joins the os calcis to the scaphoid bone.

sprue (sprū). 1. A form of stomatitis with ulcers, due to a fungus. SYN: *thrush.* 2. Tropical disease with chronic diarrhea and digestive disturbances, accompanied by chronic inflammation of the bowel, atrophy of its wall, and ulceration of the mouth. SYN: *psilosis.*

spud (spŭd). Short, flattened, spadelike blade to dislodge a foreign substance.

spur (spŭr). A projecting sliver of bone, tissue, or horny outgrowth from the skin.

spurious (spū'rĭ-ŭs). Not true or genuine; adulterated; false.

sputum (spū'tŭm) (pl. *sputa*). Substance ejected from the mouth containing saliva and mucus, and sometimes pus.

s., bloody. This is seen, of course, in hemorrhages. If the blood is mixed with the sputum the hemorrhage is in the finer bronchioles. Large quantities of blood indicate rupture of larger vessel.

s., currant jelly or **raspberry.** Indicates tumor of a lung. If of a fetid odor, bronchitis.

s., fruity. This precedes rupture of an echinococcus cyst.

s., nummular. Round, coin-shaped, flat forms which sink in water; seen in bronchiectasis and advanced pulmonary tuberculosis.

s., prune juice. Thin, reddish, bloody sputum in gangrene, cancer of the lung and certain pneumonias.

s., rusty. This is seen in lobar pneumonia.

s., septicemia. Sputum acquired from inoculation with organisms in saliva or sputum.

squama (sqwā'mă) (pl. *squamae*). 1. A thin plate of bone. 2. A scale from the epidermis.

squamoparietal (skwă″mō-pă-rī'ĕ-tăl). Relating to the squamous and parietal bones.

squamosa (skwă-mō'să). The squamous part of temporal bone.

squamous (skwā'mŭs). Scalelike.

s. bone. Upper anterior portion of temporal bone.

s. cell. Flat, scaly, epithelial cell.

s. epithelium. Flat form of epithelial cells.

s. suture. Line uniting squamosa and parietal bone.

square knot (skwăr). Double knot in which ends and standing parts are together and parallel to each other.

s. lobe. 1. The quadrate lobe of the liver. SYN: *lobus quadratus.* 2. A lobe on upper surface of the cerebellum.

squarrose, squarrous (skwăr'ōs, -ŭs). Scurfy or scaly; full of scabs or scales.

squat'ting position. One in which patient stoops with knees pressed on abdomen. SYN: *kneeling-squatting position.*

squill (skwĭl). USP. A drug once popular as an expectorant and diuretic.

s., syrup and **s., compound syrup.** Used to some extent at present.

DOSAGE: 30 ℳ (2 cc.).

squint (skwĭnt). 1. Abnormality in which both the visual axes do not bear toward an objective point simultaneously. SYN: *strabismus.* 2. To close the eyes partly, as in excess light. 3. To be unable to direct both eyes simultaneously toward an objective point.

s., convergent. Condition existing when eyes are turned toward the medial line. SYN: *esotropia.*

s., divergent. Condition existing when eyes are turned outwards. SYN: *exotropia.*

s., external. Same as *divergent.*

s., internal. Same as *convergent.*

Sr. Symb. of *strontium.*

ss. Abbr. for *semis,* half.

s. s. & p. enema. A mixture of 1 dram of peppermint added to a soapsuds solution given to relieve flatulence. SEE: *enema.*

s. s. & t. enema. Compound cleaning enema using a mixture of thick liquid soap. SEE: *enema.*

ST. 37. Proprietary germicide and disinfectant. SYN: *caprokol, hexylresorcinal, q.v.*

stab (stăb). 1. To pierce with a knife. 2. Inoculum plunged deeply into a solid culture medium with a wire or needle, also, the culture so produced.

s. culture. Bacterial culture in which organism is introduced into a solid gelatin medium with a wire or needle.

stabile (stā'bĭl). Not moving; fixed.

s. current. An electric current generated by holding stationary electrodes in a fixed position.

stable (stā'bl). Firm; steady.

s. element. Tissue cells which no longer multiply by mitosis.

staccato speech or **utterance** (stah-kah'tō). Jerky pronunciation with words and syllables separated by pauses. SYN: *scanning speech.* SEE: *speech.*

stactometer (stăk-tŏm'ĕt-ēr). Instrument for counting drops.

stadium (stā'dĭ-ŭm). A stage or period, as of a disease.

s. acmes. The height of a disease.

s. augmenti. Period of rising temperature or other symptoms.

s. decrementi. Period of defervescence or decrease of symptoms.

s. florescentiae. Stage of eruption in an exanthematous disease.

s. frigoris. Cold stage in intermittent fevers, as malaria.

s. incrementi. Period of increase of fever or symptoms.

s. invasionis. Incubative stage of an infectious disease.

s. sudoris. Sweating stage of a paroxysm of malaria.

staff (stăf). 1. An instrument to be introduced into the urethra and bladder as a guide to a surgical knife. 2. The medical corps attached to a hospital.

s., attending. Attending physicians and surgeons of a hospital.

s., consulting. Physicians and surgeons attached to a hospital who may be consulted by members of the attending staff.

s. of Wrisberg. Prominence of the cuneiform cartilage seen in the normal larynx during examination.

stage (stāj). 1. A period in the course of a disease. SYN: *stadium.* 2. The platform of a microscope.

s., algid. The cold stage or stage of collapse in cholera.

s., amphibolic. Stage which intervenes bet. acme of a disease and its outcome.

s., asphyxial. Preliminary stage of Asiatic cholera.

s., cold. Chill or rigor of a malarial paroxysm.

s., eruptive. Period in which an exanthem appears.

s., expulsive. Stage of dilatation of the cervix uteri during which the child is expelled from uterus.

s., first. Period when the fetal head is molded and the cervix dilated.

s., hot. Febrile stage in a malarial paroxysm.

s. of invasion. Period in which a morbific influence precedes the onset of a disease.

s. of latency. The incubation period of an infectious disease.

s., preëruptive. Stage following infection and before appearance of eruption.

s., pyrogenetic. Stage of invasion in a febrile disease.

s., sweating. The 3rd or terminal stage of malaria during which sweating occurs.

stagnation (stăg-nā'shŭn). 1. Cessation of motion. 2. PATH: A stoppage of motion of any fluid in the body, as blood. SYN: *stasis.*

stagnin (stăg'nĭn). A commercial preparation from the spleen of horses, causing coagulation of the blood.

stain (stān). 1. Any discoloration. 2. A pigment used in coloring microscopic objects and tissues. 3. To apply pigment to a tissue or microscopic object.

s., acid. Stain produced by an acid.

s., basic. A nonacid (aniline salt) stain.

s., contrast. One used to color one part of a tissue or cell unaffected when another part is stained by another color.

s., green. A greenish fungous deposit on the teeth.

s., neutral. A combination of an acid and a basic stain.

s., nuclear. A basic stain affecting nuclei.

s., plasmatic, s., plasmic. One which colors uniformly.

s's., removal from linen. SEE: *antistain formulary.*

staining (stān'ĭng). Process of impregnating a substance, esp. a tissue, with pigments so that its component parts may be visible under a microscope.

staircase (stăr'kās). A continuous series of reactions of progressive intensity, a phenomenon seen when a muscle, particularly that of the heart, is stimulated rapidly at regular intervals after a period of rest.

stalagmometer (stă-lăg-mŏm'ĕ-tēr). Instrument for measuring number of drops in a given amount of fluid.

stamina (stăm'ĭn-ă). Inherent force; constitutional energy; strength; endurance.

stammering (stăm'ēr-ĭng). Hesitant or faltering speech disorder.

s. of bladder. Interrupted and irregular flow of urine, the muscles acting spasmodically.

standard (stăn′dard). That which is established by custom or authority as a model, criterion or rule for comparison of measurement.

s. solution. A solution of fixed strength, used as a reagent.

stannum (stăn′ŭm). Tin; a metallic element. SYMB: Sn. At. wt. 119.

stapedectomy (stā-pē-dĕk′tō-mĭ). Excision of the stapes in the ear.

stapedial (stā-pē′dĭ-ăl). Relating to the stapes.

stapediotenotomy (stā-pē″dĭ-ō-tĕn-ŏt′ō-mĭ). Division of the tendon of the stapedius muscle.

stapediovestibular (stā-pē″dĭ-ō-vĕs-tĭb′ū-lar). Relating to the stapes and vestibule of the ear.

stapedius (stā-pē′dĭ-ŭs). A small muscle of the middle ear inserted in the stapes.

stapes (stā′pēz). Ossicle in middle ear which articulates with the incus.

staphyle (stăf′ĭ-lē). Pendulous, fleshy mass hanging from the soft palate. SYN: *uvula, q.v.*

staphylectomy (stăf-ĭl-ĕk′tō-mĭ). Amputation of the uvula. SYN: *staphylotomy, uvulotomy.*

staphyledema (stăf-ĭl-ē-dē′mă). Swelling of the uvula.

staphyline (stăf′ĭ-lĭn). 1. Relating to the uvula. SYN: *uvular.* 2. Resembling a bunch of grapes. SYN: *botryoid.*

staphylinopharyngeus (stăf-ĭ-lī″nō-făr-ĭn′jē-ŭs). Muscle in undersurface of soft palate which contracts the fauces and elevates back of the tongue.

staphylinus (stăf-ĭ-lī′nŭs). One of 2 muscles which elevate the soft palate and make it tense.

staphylion (stăf-ĭl′ĭ-ŏn). Craniometric point at median line of posterior border of hard palate.

staphylitis (stăf-ĭl-ī′tĭs). Inflammation of uvula.

staphylo-. Combining form meaning the *uvula.*

staphyloangina (stăf″ĭl-ō-ăn-jī′nă). Sore throat due to staphylococcus.

staphylobacterin (stăf″ĭl-ō-băk′tĕr-ĭn). A staphylococcic bacterial vaccine.

staphylococcemia (stăf″ĭl-ō-kŏk-sē′mĭ-ă). The presence of staphylococcus in the blood. SEE: *staphylomycosis.*

Staphylococcus (stăf-ĭl-ō-kŏk′ŭs). A class of minute, round organisms found in clusters like bunches of grapes.

  S. albus. Mild form in boils, abscesses, etc.

  S. aureus. Species found in boils, on mucous membranes, in abscesses, and on the skin; also in other suppurative inflammations.

  S. cereus aureus. Species found in nasal mucus in coryza.

  S. cereus flavus. Species found in pus causing yellow color.

  S. pyogenes albus. Form causing suppuration.

  S. pyogenes aureus. A pus-producing form.

  S. viridis flavescens. Species found in lesions of varicella, causing greenish-yellow color.

staphylodialysis (stăf-ĭ-lō-dĭ-ăl′ĭ-sĭs). Relaxation of the uvula.

staphylohemia (stăf-ĭ-lō-hē′mĭ-ă). Staphylococci in the blood. SYN: *staphylococcemia.*

staphylolysin (stăf-ĭ-lol′ĭ-sĭn). 1. The hemolysin thrown off by a staphylococcus. 2. An antibody producing lysis of staphylococci.

staphyloma (stăf-ĭl-ō′mă). Protrusion of cornea produced by a perforating keratitis.

  s. anterior. Globular enlargement of ant. part of the eye. SYN: *keratoglobus.* [the cornea.

  s. corneae. Thinning and bulging of

  s. partial. Extends in one direction displacing the pupil; the remainder of the cornea is clear.

  s. posterior, s. posticum. Bulging of sclera backward.

  s. total. Opaque protuberant, cicatrix found in place of cornea.

staphylomycosis (stăf″ĭl-ō-mĭ-kō′sĭs). The systemic condition resulting from staphylococci in blood. SYN: *staphylococcemia.*

staphyloncus (stăf-ĭ-long′kŭs). A tumor or enlargement of the uvula.

staphylopharyngeus (stăf″ĭl-ō-far-ĭn′jē-ŭs). Muscle of soft palate narrowing fauces and occluding nasopharynx.

staphyloplasty (stăf′ĭ-lō-plăs-tĭ). Plastic surgery of the uvula or soft palate.

staphyloptosia, staphyloptosis (stăf″ĭ-lŏp-tō′sĭ-ă, -sĭs). Relaxation or elongation of the uvula. SYN: *staphylodialysis.*

staphylorrhaphy (stăf-ĭl-or′ă-fĭ). Suture of a cleft palate.

staphyloschisis (stăf-ĭ-los′kĭ-sĭs). Fissure of the uvula. SYN: *cleft palate.*

staphylotomy (stăf-ĭl-lŏt′ō-mĭ). Amputation of the uvula.

star. Any structure resembling a star. SYN: *aster.*

  s. daughter. A figure forming the disaster in mitosis.

  s's. of Verheyen. Star-shaped masses of veins in renal cortex. SYN: *venae stellatae.*

starch. Noncrystalline carbohydrate of the polysaccharose* group found in plants.

stare (stăr). To gaze fixedly at anyone or anything.

starvation (star-vā′shŭn). The condition of being without food for a long period of time.

stasibasiphobia (stă″sĭ-bā″sĭ-fō′bĭ-ă). Delusion of one's inability to stand or walk or fear to make the attempt.

stasimorphy (stăs′ĭ-mor-fĭ). Deformity resulting from arrested development of a part.

stasiphobia (stă-sĭ-fō′bĭ-ă). Delusion of one's inability to stand erect or to make the attempt.

stasis (stā′sĭs). Stagnation of normal flow of fluids, as of the blood, urine, or of the intestinal mechanism.

s., diffusion. Stasis with diffusion of lymph or serum.

s., venous. Stasis of blood caused by venous congestion.

stat. Abbr. of *statim*, immediately.

static (stăt'ĭk). At rest; in equilibrium; not in motion.

s. breeze. The brush discharge as used in therapy.

s. brush. SEE: *static breeze*.

s. electricity. Electricity produced by friction.

s. induced current. The charging and discharging current of a pair of Leyden jars or other condensers which is passed through a patient.

s. machine. Term applied to certain type of machine for producing high tension direct current.

s. reflex. One occurring without stimulation.

s. wave current. The current resulting from the sudden periodic discharge from a patient who has been raised to a high potential by means of an electrostatic generator.

statics (stăt'ĭks). Study of matter at rest and forces bringing about equilibrium. SEE: *dynamics*.

statim (stăt'ĭm). Immediately; at once.

station (stā'shŭn). 1. The manner of standing. 2. A stopping place.

s., aid. One in the army for collecting the wounded in battle.

s., dressing. A temporary one for wounded soldiers in the field.

s., rest. A temporary relief station for the sick on a military road or railway.

stationary (stā'shŭn-ar-ĭ). Not moving.

s. air. Air in lungs after normal expiration.

statometer (stăt-ŏm'ĕt-ĕr). Instrument for measuring amount of abnormal protrusion of eyeball.   [body.

stature (stăt'ŭr). Natural height of the

status (sta'tŭs) (pl. *statuses*). An abnormal state or condition.

s. arthriticus. Predisposition toward having attacks of gout.

s. epilepticus. Rapid succession of epileptic attacks without regaining consciousness during the intervals.

s. lymphaticus. A hyperplastic condition of all lymphatic tissue, the spleen, bone marrow, and thymus, resulting in lowered vitality.

s. praesens. The state of a patient under observation.

s. thymicolymphaticus. Condition resembling *status lymphaticus*, but with enlarged thymus as primary factor.

s. thymicus. Same as *status thymicolymphaticus*.

s. typhosus. Condition in wasting fevers in which symptoms are stupor; great prostration; coma; vigil or muttering delirium; feeble, frequent pulse; involuntary discharge of urine and feces; sordes, and dry, brownish tongue.

s. verminosus. Condition due to infestation by worms.

s. vertiginosus. Persistent condition of vertigo.*

staurion (staw'rĭ-ŏn). Croniometric point where transverse palatine suture crosses the median one.

stauroplegia (staw-rō-plē'jĭ-ă). Hemiplegia of a part on one side of the body and another part on the other side. SYN: *hemiplegia, crossed*.

steam (stēm). 1. Invisible vapor into which water is converted at boiling point by heat. 2. Mist formed by condensation of water vapor. 3. Any vaporous exhalation.

s. tent. A device for inhalation of vapors.

steapsin (stē-ăp'sĭn). A ferment or proteolytic enzyme in the pancreatic juice that splits neutral fat into glycerin and fatty acids.

stearic acid (stē-ăr'ĭk). A white, fatty acid found in solid animal fats and a few vegetable fats.

steariform (stē-ăr'ĭ-form). Resembling fat.

stearin (stē'ăr-ĭn). $C_3H_5(C_{18}H_{35}O_2)_3$. A white, crystalline solid in animal and vegetable fats; any of the esters of glycerol and stearic acid, specifically glyceryl tristearate.

stearoconotum (stē''ăr-ō-kŏn-ō'tŭm). An insoluble yellowish fat in brain tissue.

stearodermia (stē''ăr-ō-der'mĭ-ă). Disease of the sebaceous glands of the skin.

stearopten(e (stē-ăr-ŏp'tēn). A concrete or solid substance obtained from a volatile oil.

stearrhea (stē-ăr-ē'ă). Excessive secretion of sebum or fat. SYN: *seborrhea, steatorrhea*.

s. flavescens. Stearrhea with yellow sebaceous matter deposited on the skin.

s. nigricans. Stearrhea with black sweat due to presence of indican. SEE: *chromidrosis, chromodermatosis*.

s. simplex. Excessive discharge of sebum.

steatadenoma (stē-ăt-ăd-en-ō'mă). Tumor of the sebaceous glands.

steatitis (stē-ă-tī'tĭs). Inflammation of adipose tissue.

steato- (stē'ăt-ō). Prefix meaning *fatty*.

steatocele (stē-ăt'ō-sēl, stē'ăt-ō-sēl). Fatty tumor within the scrotum.

steatocryptosis (stē''ăt-ō-krĭp-tō'sĭs). Any disease of sebaceous glands. SEE: *stearodermia*.

steatogenous (stē-ă-tŏj'ĕn-ŭs). Causing fatty degeneration or any sebaceous gland disease.

steatolysis (stē-ă-tŏl'ĭs-ĭs). Process by which fats are prepared by emulsification into glycerol and free fatty acids for absorption and assimilation.

steatolytic (stē''ăt-ō-lĭt'ĭk). Concerning steatolysis.

steatoma (stē-ăt-ō'mă). 1. Sebaceous cyst. SYN: *wen*. 2. Benign tumor composed of fat cells. SYN: *lipoma*.

s., Mueller's. Tumor composed of fibrous and fatty tissue. SYN: *lipofibroma*.

steatonecrosis (stē''ăt-ō-nē-krō'sĭs). Necrosis of fatty tissue in small patches.

steatopathy (stē-ă-tŏp′ă-thĭ). Disease of the sebaceous glands of the skin.

steatopygia (stē-ăt-ō-pī′jĭ-ă, -pĭj′ĭ-ă). Abnormal fatness of the buttocks.

steatorrhea (stē-ăt-or-rē′ă). 1. Increased secretion of sebaceous glands. SYN: *seborrhea.* * 2. Fatty stools, as seen in pancreatic diseases.

steatosis (stē-ăt-ō′sĭs). 1. Fatty degeneration. 2. Disease of the sebaceous glands. 3. Excessive accumulation of fat in the body. SYN: *adiposis,* * *obesity.*

steatozoon (stē″ăt-ō-zō′ŏn). A mite found in comedones.

stechiology (stē-kĭ-ŏl′ō-jĭ). Sum of what is known of elements and of elementary principles of any branch of science.

stechiometry (stē-kĭ-ŏm′ĕt-rĭ). 1. The mathematics of chemistry. 2. Measurement of proportion in which elements combine to form compounds.

stegano-. Combining form meaning *covered.*

stege (stē′jē). The inner layer of rods of Corti.

stegnosis (stĕg-nō′sĭs). 1. Checking of a secretion or discharge. 2. Closing of a passage. SYN: *stenosis.* 3. Constipation. SYN: *costiveness.*

stegnotic (stĕg-nŏt′ĭk). Bringing about stegnosis. SYN: *astringent, constipating.*

stellate (stĕl′āt). Star-shaped; arranged with parts radiating from a center.

   s. bandage. One wound on the back, crossways.

   s. cells. Nerve cells in the cortex cerebri.

   s. fracture. One with numerous fissures radiating from central point of injury.

   s. ligament. One of the ant. costovertebral ligaments.

   s. veins. Venous plexuses beneath the kidney's capsule. SYN: *stars of Verheyen.*

Stellwag's sign (stĕl′vahg). Widening of palpebral aperture with absence or lessened frequency of winking, seen in Graves' disease.

stem (stĕm). 1. Any stalklike structure. 2. Offspring. 3. To derive from. 4. To check.

   s., brain. The brain without its fissured portion and cerebrum.

stenion (stĕn′ĭ-ŏn). Craniometric point at extremities of the smallest transverse diameter in the temporal region.

steno-. Combining form meaning *narrow, short,* as stenosis, stenography.

stenocardia (stĕn-ō-kar′dĭ-ă). Angina* pectoris.

stenocephaly (stĕn-ō-sĕf′ăl-ĭ). Narrowness of the cranium in one or more diameters.

stenochoria (stĕn-ō-kō′rĭ-ă). Partial constriction, esp. of the lacrimal duct. SYN: *stenosis.*

stenocompressor (stĕn-ō-kŏm-prĕs′or). An instrument for compressing Stensen's ducts to stop the flow of saliva.

stenocoriasis (stĕn-ō-kō-rī′ăs-ĭs). Narrowing of pupil of the eye.

Stenon's or Steno's duct (stē′nŏn. stē′nō).

Excretory duct of the parotid gland. SYN: *Stensen's duct.*

stenopaic, stenopeic (sten-o-pā′ĭk, -pē′ĭk). Having a narrow opening.

stenosed (stē-nōst′, stĕn′ōzd). Characterized by stenosis; constricted.

stenosis (stĕn-ō′sĭs, stē-nō′sĭs). Constriction or narrowing of a passage or orifice. SYN: *stricture.*

   s., aortic. Constriction of the aortic orifice at cardiac base or narrowing of the aorta.

   s., cardiac. Lessened diameter of the *conus arteriosus* on either side of heart with obstruction to free flow of blood from ventricle into corresponding artery.

   s., cicatricial. Stenosis resulting from any contracted cicatrix.

   s., mitral. Stenosis of mitral valve or orifice of heart, or of both.

   s., pyloric. Obstruction caused by hypertrophy of walls of the pyloric orifice.

stenostegnosis (stē″nō-stĕg-nō′sĭs). Stenosis or stricture of Stensen's duct.

stenostenosis (stē″nō-stĕn-ō′sĭs). Constriction of Stensen's duct. SYN: *stenostegnosis.*

stenostomia (stĕn″ō-stō′mĭ-ă). Narrowing of the mouth.

stenothermal (stĕn″ō-ther′măl). Resisting only a small change of temperature.

stenothorax (stĕn″ō-thō′răks). An unusually narrow thorax.

stenotic (stĕn-ŏt′ĭk). Produced by or characterized by stenosis.

Stensen's duct (stĕn′sĕn). The excretory duct of parotid gland.

   S.'s foramina. Incisive foramina of sup. maxillary bone transmitting ant. branches of descending palatine vessels.

step-down transformer. A transformer in which the number of turns of wire in the primary and secondary windings are in such relation as to reduce voltage.

   s.-up t. A transformer in which the number of turns of wire in the primary and secondary windings are in such relation as to increase voltage. SEE: *transformer.*

stephanion (stē-fă′nĭ-ŏn). Point at intersection of sup. temporal ridge and coronal suture.

step′page gait. The high-stepping gait seen in diabetic neuritis of the peroneal nerve and in tabes dorsalis.

   Patient lifts the foot very high in walking to raise the drooping toes from the ground or floor.

sterco-. Combining form meaning *dung,* as *stercobilin.*

stercobilin (stĕr″kō-bī′lĭn). A brown pigment derived from the bile giving the characteristic color to feces. SEE: *urobilin.*

stercoraceous (stĕr-kō-rā′shŭs). Having the nature of, pert. to or containing, feces.

stercoral (ster′kō-ral). Pert. to feces. SYN: *stercoraceous.*

stercoremia (ster-kō-rē′mĭ-ă). Toxic state from absorption of poisons in retained feces.

stercorin (ster'kō-rĭn). Crystallizable reduction product of cholesterol in feces.

stercorolith (ster'kō-rō-lĭth). A fecal concretion. SYN: *coprolith, fecalith.*

stercoroma (ster-kō-rō'mă). A fecal tumorlike mass in the rectum. SYN: *coproma, fecaloma, scotoma.*

stercorous (ster'kōr-ŭs). Resembling excrement. SYN: *stercoral, stercoraceous.*

stercus (ster'kŭs). Feces. SYN: *excreta, excrement.*

stere (stēr, stär). A measure of capacity. SYN: *cubic meter, kiloliter.*

stereo-. Combining form meaning *solid.*

stereoanesthesia (stēr"ē-ō-ăn-ĕs-thē'zĭ-ă). Inability to recognize objects by feeling their form.

stereoarthrolysis (stēr"ē-ō-ar-thrŏl'ĭ-sĭs). Surgical formation of a movable new joint in bony ankylosis.

stereochemical (stēr"ē-ō-kĕm'ĭ-kăl). Concerning stereochemistry.

stereochemistry (stēr"ē-ō-kĕm'is-trĭ). That branch of chemistry dealing with atoms in their space relation.

stereognosis (stēr-ē-ō-ŏg-nō'sĭs). Ability to recognize form of solid objects by touch.

stereometry (stēr-ē-ō-ŏm'ĕt-rĭ). The measurement of a solid body or the cubic contents of a hollow body.

stereoörthopter (stēr"ē-ō-ōr-thŏp'ter). A mirror-reflecting device for treatment of strabismus.

stereophantoscope (stēr"ē-ō-făn'tō-skōp). A stereoscopical device with rotating disks for testing vision.

stereophorometer (stēr"ē-ō-for-ŏm'ē-ter). A prism-refracting device for use in correcting defective vision.

stereophotography (stēr"ē-ō-fō-tŏg'ră-fĭ). Photography which produces effect of solidity or depth of pictures.

stereophotomicrograph (stēr"ē-ō-fō"tō-mī'krō-grăf). A photograph showing solidity or depth of a microscopical subject.

stereoplasm (ster'ē-ō-plăzm). The solid portion of cell protoplasm.

stereoscope (ster'ē-ō-skōp). Instrument which creates an impression of solidity or depth of objects seen by combining images of 2 pictures.

stereoscopic, stereoscopical (ster-ē-ō-skōp'ĭk, -ĭ-kăl). Pert. to the stereoscope or its use.

   s. vision. Vision in which things have the appearance of solidity and relief as though seen in 3 dimensions.

stereotypy (stēr-ē-ō-tī'pĭ). Repetition of words, posture, or movement without meaning; seen in catatonic partial stupors.

sterile (stěr'ĭl). 1. Free from living microorganisms. SYN: *aseptic.* 2. Not fertile; unable to reproduce young. SYN: *barren.*

sterility (stěr-ĭl'ĭ-tĭ). Absence of reproductive power.

   s., absolute. After 5 years of married life without the use of contraceptives with no ensuing pregnancy.

   s., acquired (secondary sterility). The failure of further conception after once having given birth to a child.

   s., female. Inability to give birth to living young.

   s., primary. Condition in which woman has never become pregnant.

   s., relative. Sterility due to causes other than defect of sex organs.

sterilization (ster"ĭl-ĭ-zā'shŭn). 1. Process of destruction of all microörganisms on a substance by exposure to chemical or physical agents. 2. Process of rendering barren.

   s., discontinuous. Exposure for about an hour on several successive days to 212° F. (100° C.).

   s., fractional. Sterilization in which heating is done at separated intervals, so that spores can develop into bacteria and be destroyed.

   s., steam, by flowing. Exposure at 212° F. (100° C.) to steam in an unsealed receptacle.

   s., steam under pressure. Exposure to steam in an autoclave.

sterilize (ster'ĭl-īz). 1. To free from microörganisms. 2. To make barren.

sterilizer (ster'ĭl-ĭ-zer). Oven or appliance for sterilizing.

sterilometer (stěr-ĭl-ŏm'ē-ter). An apparatus to test the degree of sterilization of any material.

sternal (ster'năl). Relating to the sternum or breastbone.

sternalgia (stěr-năl'jĭ-ă). Pain in the sternum. SYN: *sternodynia.*

sternebra (ster'nē-bră). Segment of the sternum.

sterno-. Combining form meaning *sternum.*

sternoclavicular (ster"nō-klă-vĭk'ū-lar). Concerning the sternum and clavicle.

sternocleidomastoid (ster"nō-klī-dō-măs'toyd). One of 2 muscles arising from sternum and inner part of clavicle.

sternocostal (ster"nō-kŏs'tăl). Relating to sternum and ribs.

sternodynia (ster"nō-dĭn'ĭ-ă). Pain in the sternum. SYN: *sternalgia.*

sternohyoid (ster"nō-hī'oyd). Muscle from medial end of clavicle and sternum to hyoid bone.

sternoid (ster'noyd). Resembling the breastbone.

sternopericardial (ster"nō-per"ĭ-kar'dĭ-al). Concerning the sternum and pericardium.

sternothyroid (ster"nō-thī'royd). Muscle extending beneath the sternohyoid which depresses the larynx.

sternotomy (ster-nŏt'ō-mĭ). The operation of cutting the sternum.

sternotrypesis (ster"nō-trī-pē'sĭs). Surgical perforation of the sternum.

sternum (ster'nŭm). The narrow, flat bone in the median line of the thorax in front. SYN: *breastbone.*

   s., cleft. Congenital fissure of the sternum.

sternutament (ster-nū'tăm-ĕnt). A substance causing sneezing.

sternutatio (stěr-nū-tā'shē-ō). Sneezing.

   s. convulsiva. Paroxysmal sneezing, as in hay fever.

sternutation (ster-nū-tā'shŭn). Act of sneezing.

   s., convulsive. Spasmodic or paroxysmal sneezing with profusion of watery secretion from the nose.

sternutatory (ster-nū'tă-tō"rĭ). 1. Causing sneezing. 2. An agent causing sneezing. Ex: *quillaja, salicylic acid.*

sterol (stēr'ŏl). Any of a class of solid higher alcohols in plants and animals.

stertor (stēr'tŏr). Snoring or laborious breathing due to obstruction of air passages in the head, seen in certain diseases, as apoplexy.

stertorous (stēr'tō-rŭs). Pert. to laborious breathing provoking a snoring sound.

sterule (stēr'ūl). A glass capsule containing a sterile solution. SYN: *ampoule.*

stetho-. Combining form meaning the *chest.*

stethogoniometer (steth"ō-gō-nĭ-ŏm'ĕt-ĕr). Device for measuring the curvature of the chest.

stethograph (stĕth'ō-grăf). Device to record chest movements in respiration.

stethokyrtograph (stĕth"o-kir'tō-grăf). Device for measuring and recording the dimensions and amount of curves of the chest.

stethometer (stĕth-ŏm'ĕt-ĕr). Device for measuring the chest's expansion during respiration.

stethophonometer (stĕth"ō-fō-nŏm'ĕt-ĕr). Instrument for determining intensity of sound emitted in auscultation.

stethoscope (stĕth'ō-skōp). Instrument used in auscultation to convey to the ear the sounds produced in the body.

   s., binaural. Stethoscope designed for use with both ears.

   s., compound. More than 1 set attached to the same fork and chest piece.

   s., double. Stethoscope with 2 earpieces and tubes.

   s., percussion. Solid cylinder of wood, 1 end wedge-shaped, other enlarged into an earpiece adapted for intercostal use.

   s., single or **monaural.** For 1 ear only; rigid or flexible.

stethoscopy (stĕth-ŏs'kō-pĭ). Examination by means of the stethoscope.

stethospasm (stĕth'ō-spăzm). Spasm of the pectoral or chest muscles.

sthenia (sthē'nĭ-ă). Normal or unusual strength, the opp. of *asthenia.*

sthenic (sthĕn'ĭk). Active; strong.

   s. fever. One with high temperature; tense, quick pulse, and highly colored urine.

sthenometer (sthĕn-ŏm'ĕ-tĕr). Device for measuring muscular strength.

sthenometry (sthĕn-ŏm'ĕ-trĭ). Determination of bodily strength.

sthenopyra (sthĕn"ō-pī'ră). Fever with a strong, bounding pulse; active delirium, and high temperature. SYN: *sthenic fever.*   [soning.

stibialism (stĭb'ĭ-ăl-ĭzm). Antimonial poisoning.

stibium (stĭb'ĭ-ŭm). Antimony.

stichochrome (stĭk'ō-krōm). A nerve cell in which the stainable bodies (tigroid mass) are arranged in parallel rows.

stictacne (stĭk-tăk'nē). Acne with red base and black pointed comedo at apex. SYN: *acne punctata.*

stiff neck. Rigidity of neck due to rheumatism or contraction of cervical muscles. SYN: *torticollis, wryneck.*

   s.-n. fever. 1. Dengue. 2. Cerebrospinal meningitis.

stigma (stĭg'mă) (pl. *stigmata*). 1. A mark or spot on the skin. 2. Spot on ovarian surface where rupture of a graafian follicle will occur. 3. Intercellular cleft in endothelial cells in a capillary. 4. Red spot due to extravasation of blood produced by nervous influence. 5. Mark characterizing a specific disease.

   s. of degeneration. Any of the bodily variations from the normal found in numerous instances in degenerate individuals.

   s., hysterical. Spot on skin due to nervous influence.

stigmatic (stĭg-măt'ĭk). Pert. to or marked with a stigma.

stigmatization (stĭg"măt-ĭ-zā'shŭn). The formation of stigmata, esp. hysterical stigmata on the skin.

stigmatodermia (stĭg"măt-ō-der'mĭ-ă). Disease of skin's prickle cell layer.

stigmatometer (stĭg-mă-tŏm'ĕ-tĕr). Device for testing eye refraction. SYN: *astigmatometer.*

stigmatosis (stĭg-mă-tō'sĭs). A skin disease marked by superficial spots of inflammation.

stilet, stilette (stĭl-ĕt'). 1. Small, sharp-pointed instrument for probing. 2. Wire used to pass through or stiffen a flexible catheter.

stillbirth (stĭl'birth). Birth of a dead fetus.

stillborn (stĭl'born). Dead at birth.

stillicidium (stĭl-ĭ-sĭd'ĭ-ŭm). A dribbling or flowing, drop by drop.

   s. lacrimarum. Watering of the eye. SYN: *epiphora.*

   s. narium. Watery mucus discharged at onset of coryza.

   s. urinae. Urinary incontinence from a distended bladder. SYN: *strangury.*

Stilling's canal (stĭl'ĭng). The hyaloid canal of the vitreous in the eye.

   S.'s nucleus. 1. Nucleus containing red ganglion cells found in tegmental region of crus cerebri. 2. Origin of hypoglossal nerve in 4th ventricle.

stimulant (stĭm'ū-lănt). Any agent temporarily increasing functional activity.

stimulate (stĭm'ū-lāt). To increase functional activity of an organ or structure.

stimulating en'ema. One given to excite activity in shock or unconscious state. SEE: *enema.*

stimulation (stĭm"ū-lā'shŭn). 1. Process of being stimulated. 2. Irritating action of agents on muscles, nerves, or sensory end-organs by which activity in a part is evoked.

stimulin (stĭm'ū-lĭn). 1. Substance in fresh gastric juice stimulating gastric glands. 2. A substance in blood serum that increases phagocytic activity.

stimulus (stĭm'ū-lŭs) (pl. *stimuli*). Any agent or factor able to influence directly living protoplasm, as one capable of causing muscular contraction or secretion in a gland, or of initiating an impulse in a nerve.

  s., adequate. One which acts upon nerve terminations in any special organ.

  s., chemical. A stimulus acting by a chemical process.

  s., electric. Stimulus resulting from application of electricity.

  s., heterologous. One acting upon any part of a sensory organ or nerve tract.

  s., homologous. Same as adequate stimulus.

  s., mechanical. Stimulus caused by mechanical means.

  s., thermal. Stimulus caused by application of heat.

sting (stĭng). 1. Sharp, smarting sensation, as of a wound or astringent. 2. Wound made by a sting; the sharp offensive weapon of an insect, esp. a painful or poisonous wound. SEE: *insect bite.*

stippling (stĭp'lĭng). A spotted condition, as in retina in certain ocular diseases or in basophilic red corpuscles.

stirpiculture (ster'pĭ-kŭl'tūr). Scientific breeding of stock or race to improve it.

stirrup, stirrup bone (stir'ŭp). Stapes of the ears.

stitch (stĭch). 1. A local, sharp, lancinating, or spasmodic pain. 2. A single loop of suture material passed through skin or flesh by a needle, to facilitate healing of a wound. 3. To unite skin or flesh with a needle and suture material.

  s. abscess. One developing in a suture due to infection.

stock (stŏk). The race or line of a family.

  s. culture. Permanent culture of a microörganism reinforced from time to time by fresh media.

  s. vaccine. Vaccine prepared from any strain of the species, but not from patient himself.

Stokes-Adams syndrome (stŏks-ăd'ăms). A series of symptoms in those suffering from heart block. Onset is sudden, resembling epilepsy, for which it is sometimes mistaken.

Stokes' law (stŏks). A muscle is frequently a seat of paralysis if lying above an inflamed serous or mucous membrane.

  S.'s lens. Device used to diagnose astigmatism.

stoma (stō'mä) (pl. *stomata*). 1. A mouth or small opening or a pore. 2. Artificially created opening bet. 2 passages or body cavities or bet. a cavity or passage and the body's surface.

stomach (stŭm'ăk). A dilated, saclike, distensible portion of the alimentary canal below the esophagus, 12x4 in., below the diaphragm to right of spleen, partly under the liver.

  s.-ache. Pain in the stomach. SYN: *gastralgia, gastrodynia, stomachalgia, stomachodynia.*

  s., bilocular. SEE: *hourglass stomach.*

  s., cardiac. Fundus of the stomach.

  s. cough. One caused by reflex action from the stomach.

  s., hourglass. One resembling an hourglass, caused by constriction from a band of fibrous exudate.

  s., leather bottle. One caused by hypertrophy of the stomach walls.

  s. pump. Device for removing contents of the stomach by mouth.

  s. tooth. A lower canine one during first dentition.

  s. tube. One for washing out or feeding the stomach.

  s., water-trap. One with the pylorus unusually high, causing slow emptying.

stomachal (stŭm'ăk-ăl). 1. Relating to the stomach. 2. A gastric tonic.

stomachalgia (stŭm-ăk-ăl'jĭ-ä). Pain in the stomach.

stomachic (stō-măk'ĭk). 1. Concerning the stomach. 2. Medicine exciting action of the stomach. SYN: *stomachal.*

stomachoscopy (stŭm-ăk-os'kō-pĭ). Examination of the stomach. SYN: *gastroscopy.*

stomatalgia (stō-măt-ăl'jĭ-ä). Pain in the mouth. SYN: *stomatodynia.*

stomatitis (stō-măt-ī'tĭs). Inflammation of the mouth.

  s., aphthous. Formation of tiny ulcers on mucosa of the mouth.

  s., catarrhal. Simple stomatitis.

  s., corrosive. Stomatitis resulting from use of corrosive substances.

  s., diphtheritic. Diphtheria of mucous membranes of the gums or cheeks. SYN: *buccal diphtheria.*

  s., follicular. SEE: *aphthous stomatitis.*

  s., gangrenous. This form seen in debilitated children from 2 to 6 years; usually follows one of the specific fevers, esp. measles and whooping cough.

  s. materna. Stomatitis during pregnancy or lactation.

  s., mercurial. This form is seen in artisans who work in mercury; after the administration of very large doses of mercurials, and after small doses where there has been unnatural susceptibility.

  s., parasitic. Stomatitis caused by a fungus. *Saccharomyces albicans.* SYN: *thrush.*

  s., simple. Erythematous inflammation of the mouth occurring in patches on the mucous membranes.

  s., ulcerative. Thought by some to be an infectious disease, as it often occurs in epidemics and attacks both children and adults when congregated and subjected to bad hygienic conditions.

  s., vesicular. SEE: *aphthous stomatitis.*

stomato-. Combining form meaning *mouth.*

stomatodynia (stō"mä-tō-dĭn'ĭ-ä). Pain in the mouth. SYN: *stomatalgia.*

stomatodysodia (stō"mä-tō-dĭs-ō'dĭ-ä). Foul odor from the mouth.

stomatogastric (stō"mä-tō-găs'trĭk). Concerning the stomach and mouth.

stomatography (stō″mă-tŏg′ră-fĭ). A treatise on the mouth.

stomatologist (stō″mă-tŏl′ō-jĭst). Specialist in treatment of diseases of the mouth.

stomatology (stō″mă-tol′ō-jĭ). Science of the mouth and teeth and their diseases.

stomatomalacia (stō″mă-tō-mă-lā′sĭ-ă). Pathological softening of any structures of the mouth.

stomatomy (stō-măt′ō-mĭ). Surgical nicking of the edges of the os uteri to facilitate delivery.

stomatomycosis (stō″mă-tō-mĭ-kō′sĭs). Any mouth disease resulting from fungi.

stomatonecrosis, stomatonoma (stō″mă-tō-nē-krō′sĭs, -nō-mă). Gangrenous, ulcerative inflammation of the mouth. SYN: *cancrum oris, noma.*

stomatopathy (stō-mă-tŏp′ă-thĭ). Any mouth disease.

stomatoplasty (stō-măt′ō-plăs″tĭ). Plastic operation upon the mouth.

stomatorrhagia (stō″mă-tor-rā′jĭ-ă). Hemorrhage from the mouth or gums.

stomatoscope (stō′măt-ō-skōp). Instrument for examining the mouth.

stomodaeum, stomodeum (stō″mō-dē′ŭm). An invagination of the ectoderm or outer layer of the embryo that forms the mouth cavity.

stone (stōn). Hardened mineral matter, as *gallstones.* SYN: *calculus, q.v.*

stool (stōōl). 1. Evacuation of the bowels. 2. Waste matter discharged from the bowels. SYN: *feces, q.v.*

s., bilious. Yellowish or yellowish-brown discharges in diarrhea becoming darker on exposure.

s., fatty. Fat in the feces, as in pancreatic diseases.

s., pea soup. Liquid stools of typhoid.

s., rice water. Watery serum stools with detached epithelium, as in cholera.

stop needle. One with eye at tip and a disk to prevent penetration deeper than desired.

stoppage (stŏp′ăj). Obstruction of an organ. SEE: *cholestasia.*   [*corpulent.*

stout (stowt). Having a bulky body. SYN:

stovaine (stō-vā′ĭn). Local anesthetic less toxic than cocaine.

DOSAGE: ⅓-¾ gr. (0.02-0.05 Gm.).

stovainization (stō-vă-ĭn-ĭ-zā′shŭn). Induction of local anesthesia with stovaine.

stovarsol (stō′var-sol). A commercial brand of acetarsone* used in spirochetal infections.

DOSAGE: 4 gr. (0.25 Gm.).

strabismic (stră-bĭz′mĭk). Pert. to or afflicted with strabismus.

strabismometer (stră-bĭz-mŏm′ĕt-ĕr). Instrument for determining amount of strabismus.

strabismus (stră-bĭz′mŭs). Disorder of eye in which optic axes cannot be directed to same object, due to lack of muscular coördination. SYN: *squint.*

s., accommodative. Strabismus due to disorder of ocular accommodation.

s., alternating. Strabismus affecting either eye alternately.

s., bilateral. Same as accommodative strabismus.

s., concomitant. Form in which 2 eyes move freely, but retain false relation to each other.

s., convergent (internal squint). The deviating eye turns inwards.

s., deorsum vergens. Vertical strabismus downwards. SYN: *hypotropia.*

s., divergent. Deviating eye turns outwards.

s., intermittent. One recurring at intervals.

s., monocular. When the same eye habitually deviates.

s., monolateral. When the squinting eye is always the same.

s., paralytic. That which is due to paralysis of a muscle. The deviation is present only in the sphere of action of the paralyzed muscle. In paralytic squint the secondary deviation is greater than the primary.

s., spastic. Strabismus due to contraction of an ocular muscle.

s., sursum vergens. Vertical squint upwards. SYN: *hypertropia.*

s., vertical. Eye turns upward. The vision is double (diplopia), unless there is unconscious suppression of the image in squinting eye, and expression of face is bizarre and sometimes malign. It is usually the result in childhood of ametropia, or in adult life of central nervous disease.

strabometer (stră-bŏm′ĕt-ĕr). Instrument to ascertain the degree of strabismus.

strabotomy (stră-bŏt′ō-mĭ). Operation for strabismus.

strain (strān). 1. A stock, said of bacteria or protozoa from a specific source and maintained in successive cultures or animal inoculation. 2. Hereditary streak or tendency. 3. To pass through, as a filter. 4. To injure by making too strong an effort or by excessive use. 5. Excessive use of a part of the body so that it is injured. 6. Injury to muscles from tension due to overuse or misuse. SYN: *sprain.*

strainer (strān′er). Device used for retaining solid pieces while liquid passes through. SYN: *filter.*

strait (strāt). A constricted or narrow passage.

s., inferior. The lower outlet of the pelvic canal.

s.-jacket. Shirt with long sleeves laced on patient and fastened to restrain the arms. SYN: *camisole.*

s's. of the pelvis. The inferior and superior openings of the true pelvis.

s., superior. The upper opening or inlet of the pelvic canal.

stramonium (stră-mō′nĭ-ŭm). USP. Jamestown weed, Jimson weed. The dried leaves of *Datura stramonium.*

DOSAGE: 1.25 gr. (0.075 Gm.).

strangalesthesia (strang″ăl-ĕs-thē′zĭ-ă). A girdlelike sensation of constriction. SYN: *zonesthesia.*

strangle (strang′gl). To choke or suffocate or be choked from compression of the trachea.

strangulated (străng'ū-lā″tĕd). Constricted so that air or blood supply is cut off, as strangulated hernia.

strangulation (străng-ū-lā'shŭn). Compression or constriction of a part, as the bowel or throat, such as causes suspension of breathing or of passage of contents; congestion accompanies condition.

s., *internal.* Slipping of a coil of the intestine through the diaphragm or an abnormal opening.

strangury (străng'ū-rĭ). Painful and interrupted urination in drops, produced by spasmodic muscular contraction of urethra and bladder.

strap (străp). 1. A band, as one of adhesive plaster, used to hold dressings in place or to approximate surfaces of a wound. 2. To bind with strips of adhesive plaster.

strapping (străp'ĭng). 1. Adhesive plaster or other substance used to bind surfaces together or hold dressings in place. 2. Application of adhesive plaster strips on a part so as to give it support or compress it.

stratified (străt'ĭ-fīd). In strata or in the form of layers.

s. *epithelium.* Epithelium in superimposed layers with differently shaped cells in the various layers.

stratiform (străt'ĭ-form). Arranged in layers, as manner of liquefaction of gelatin stab culture, in which there is liquefaction to the walls of the tube at the top and then downward horizontally.

stratum (strā'tŭm, străt'ŭm) (pl. *strata*). A layer.

s. *corneum.* BNA. Horny layer of the skin.

s. *germinativum.* Innermost layer of epidermis, a row of columnar cells, which divide to replace rest of the epidermis as it wears away. SEE: *prickle cell.*

s. *granulosum.* A layer of very small cells, or cells containing granules, as that in the skin.

s. *granulosum epidermidis.* Lozenge-shaped or trapezoid-shaped cells covering the *rete mucosum* and covered by the stratum lucidum in the skin.

s. *lucidum.* A translucent layer of the epidermis.

s. *malpighii.* Inner layer of the epidermis. SYN: *rete mucosum, stratum germinativum.*

s. *mucosum.* Same as *stratum malpighii.*

s. *spinsosum.* Same as *stratum malpighii.*

s. *spongiosum.* 1. Spongy layer of the urethra. 2. Medial layer of decidua.

straw'berry tongue. The peculiar, redly papillated tongue of scarlatina, *q.v.* SEE: *tongue.*

straw itch (strau). A skin condition accompanied by itching due to working in straw or sleeping on a straw mattress.

streak (strēk). A line or stripe. SYN: *stria.*

s. *culture.* A bacterial culture in streaks.

s., *medullary.* Deep longitudinal groove on dorsal surface of the embryo which becomes the medullary tube. SYN: *dorsal groove.*

s., *meningitic.* A red line across the skin formed by drawing a pointed article across it; seen in meningitis and nerve center affections. SYN: *tache cérébrale.*

s., *primitive.* An opaque band at end of germinal area forming the first signs of the blastoderm in the fertilized ovum.

s. *reflex.* A white, shining streak along center of retinal vessels.

strephotome (strĕf'ō-tōm). Instrument for invagination of a hernial sac.

strepitus (strĕp'ĭt-ŭs). A sound or noise, as that heard on auscultation.

strepticemia (strĕp-tĭ-sē'mĭ-ă). Streptococci present in the blood stream causing infection. SYN: *streptococcemia.*

strepto-. Combining form meaning *twisted.*

streptoangina (strĕp″tō-ăn-jī'nă). Sore throat with membranous formation due to streptococci.

streptobacteria (strĕp″tō-băk-tē'rĭ-ă). Those bacteria which are arranged in chains.

streptobacterin (strĕp″tō-băk'tĕr-ĭn). A vaccine made from streptococci.

streptococcal (strĕp″tō-kŏk'ăl). Caused by or pert. to streptococci.

streptococcemia (strĕp″tō-kŏk-sē'mĭ-ă). Presence of streptococci in the blood causing infection.

streptococcic (strĕp″tō-kŏk'sĭk). Resembling, produced by, or pert. to streptococci.

s. *sore throat.* Severe epidemic form with membranous formation caused by *Streptococcus haemolyticus.*

streptococcicosis (strĕp″tō-kŏk-sĭ-kō'sĭs). Any streptococcal infection.

streptococcolysin (strĕp″tō-kŏk-ŏl'ĭ-sĭn). A lysin produced by streptococci.

Streptococcus (strĕp″tō-kŏk'ŭs) (pl. *Streptococci*). A genus of spherical organisms occurring in chains of various lengths.

Str. anginosus. Hemolytic variety found in acute pharyngitis.

Str. cardioarthritidis. Variety found in blood and throat secretion cultures in cases of rheumatic fever.

Str. epidemicus. Hemolytic variety seen in throat cultures in cases of epidemic sore throat.

Str. erysipelatis. Organism causing erysipelas, which resembles *Streptococcus pyogenes.*

Str. haemolyticus, Str., hemolytic. Any of the streptococci causing complete hemolysis of erythrocytes; majority of pathogenic varieties are in this group.

Str. mixtos. SEE: *Streptococcus haemolyticus.*

Str. morbilli. Variety found in cases of measles, the probable cause of that disease.

Str. puerperalis. Species found in puerperal septicemia, which resembles *Streptococcus pyogenes*.

Str. pyogenes. Any of the hemolytic streptococci causing suppurative processes.

Str. scarlatinae. Probable causative agent of scarlet fever.

Str. viridans. Nonhemolytic form producing green colonies on blood agar which frequently is the cause of focal infection, which in turn leads to symptoms of arthritis, neuritis, endocarditis, etc.

streptocolysin (strĕp″tō-kŏl′ĭ-sĭn). A hemolysin produced by streptococci.

streptodermatitis (strĕp″tō-der-mă-tī′tĭs). Inflammation of the skin caused by streptococci.

streptoleukocidin (strĕp″tō-lū-kō-sĭ′dĭn). A toxin produced by streptococci destructive to leukocytes.

streptolysin (strĕp-tŏl′ĭ-sĭn). A hemolysin excreted by a streptococcus. SYN: *streptococcolysin, streptocolysin*.

streptomycosis (strĕp″tō-mī-kō′sĭs). Infection caused by streptococci.

streptosepticemia (strĕp″tō-sĕp-tĭ-sē′mĭ-ă). Septicemia resulting from streptococcus infection. SYN: *streptococcemia, streptomycosis*.

streptothricosis (strĕp-tō-thrĭ-kō′sĭs). Infection caused by a species of Streptothrix.

Streptothrix (strĕp′tō-thrĭks). A genus of Chlamydobacteriaceae, of which one form is the cause of actinomycosis and another is assumed to be cause of rat-bite fever.

stretcher (strĕch′er). A litter for carrying the sick, injured, or dead.

stretch'ing of contrac'tures. Process performed to loosen contracted ligaments, muscles, and adhesions in stiff joints.

stria (strī′a) (pl. *striae*). A line or band elevated above or depressed below surrounding tissue, or differing in color and texture.

s., acoustic; s., auditory. One of the horizontal white stripes on floor of the 4th ventricle of the brain.

s. acustica. Same as *stria medullaris*.

s. atrophica. Whitish cicatricial line on the skin caused by stretching, as in pregnancy or obesity.

s. gravidarum. Same as *stria atrophica*.

s. longitudinalis lateralis. One of the longitudinal bands of gray matter, slightly elevated on upper part of the corpus callosum.

s. medullaris. Same as *stria, acoustic; stria acustica; s. pinealis*.

s. pinealis. Longitudinal strand of fibers along walls of the 3rd ventricle below the taenia thalami.

s. terminalis. A band of fibers in roof of inf. horn running to floor of body of the lateral ventricle.

striate, striated (strī′āt, strī′āt-ĕd). Striped; marked by streaks or striae.

s. body. Mass of gray and white bands in each cerebral hemisphere. SYN: *corpus striatum*.

striation (strī-ā′shŭn). 1. State of being striped or streaked. 2. One of a series of streaks. SYN: *stria*.

striatum (strī-ā′tŭm). The caudate and lentiform nuclei of the brain considered as one. SYN: *corpus striatum*.

stricture (strĭk′chŭr). A localized contraction of a tube or canal due to pressure or changes in the wall tissue; may affect the esophagus, ureters, and urethra. SEE: *arctation, stenosis*.

s., bridle. One caused by a band across the tube, partially occluding it.

s., cicatricial. One resulting from a scar or wound.

s., functional. One due to muscular spasm.

s., impermeable. One closing the lumen of a tube or canal.

s., irritable. One causing pain when an instrument is passed.

s., spasmodic. Same as *functional stricture*.

s. of urethra. Most common in men. May be partial or complete.

stricturotome (strĭk′chŭr-ō-tōm). Instrument for cutting strictures.

stricturotomy (strĭk-chŭr-ŏt′ō-mĭ). Operation of cutting strictures.

stridor (strī′dŏr). Harsh sound during respiration; high-pitched and like the blowing of the wind due to obstruction of air passages.

s., congenital or **laryngeal.** Inspiration at birth or during first 3 weeks giving forth a crowing sound.

s. dentium. Noise from grinding of the teeth.

s. serraticus. Sound of respiration like that of sawing, when heard through a tracheotomy tube.

stridulous (strĭd′ū-lŭs). Making a shrill grating sound.

strip (strĭp). To remove all contents from, esp. by gentle pressure, as to strip the seminal vesicles.

strobila (strō-bī′lă). Consecutive segments of body of a tapeworm.

stroke (strōk). 1. A sudden, severe attack of affliction, as apoplexy; a sharp blow. 2. To rub gently in one direction, as in massage. 3. Gentle movement of the hand across a surface.

s., back. Ventricular recoil of the heart during systole. SYN: *basculation, 2*.

s. culture. One made by spreading inoculum on surface of the medium. SYN: *smear culture*.

stroma (strō′mă) (pl. *stromata*). 1. Foundation supporting tissues of an organ. 2. Spongy, colorless framework of an erythrocyte.

s. plexus. Ramification of nerves of the cornea.

s. vitreum. Delicate framework of the vitreous body of the eye.

stromal, stromatic (strō′măl, strō-măt′ĭk). Concerning or resembling the stroma of an organ.

stromatolysis (strō″mă-tŏl′ĭ-sĭs). Destruction of the enveloping membrane of a cell without affecting the cell body.

Stromeyer's splint (strō′mī-ĕr). A hinged splint for a joint, which can be fixed at any angle.

stromuhr (strō′moor). Device for measuring velocity of blood flow. SYN: *rheometer*.

Strongyloides (strŏn-jī-loy′dēz). A genus of roundworms frequently found in the intestines.

  S. intestinalis. An intestinal roundworm.

strongyloidosis (strŏn″jĭ-loy-dō′sĭs). Infestation with Strongyloides.

strongylosis (strŏn-jĭ-lō′sĭs). Infestation with Strongylus.

Strongylus (strŏn′jĭ-lŭs). A genus of parasitic roundworms.

strontium (strŏn′shĭ-ŭm). A dark, yellowish metal, some of its salts being medicinal.

Strophanthus (strō-făn′thŭs). USP. Plant yielding a poisonous, white, crystalline glucoside; used chiefly in the form of alkaloid; strophanthin.

  DOSAGE: 1 gr. (0.06 Gm.).

strophulus (strŏf′ū-lŭs). An infantile red eruption. SYN: *gum rash, red rash, tooth rash.*

  s. albidus. Small, white nodule below the epidermis. SYN: *milium.*

  s. infantum. Urticaria in infants.

  s. pruriginosus. A form with itching papules.

structural (strŭk′tū-răl). Pert. to organic structure.

  s. disease. A disease effecting changes in any structure.

struma (strū′mă). 1. Tuberculosis of the lymphatics. SYN: *scrofula*. 2. Enlargement of the thyroid gland. SYN: *goiter.*

  s. maligna. Carcinoma of the thyroid gland. [the suprarenals.]

  s. suprarenalis. Fatty tissue tumor of

  s. vasculosa. Enlargement of the thyroid gland due to dilatation of the blood vessels.

strumectomy (strū-mĕk′tō-mĭ). Excision of scrofulous glands or of a goiter.

strumiprivous (strū″mĭ-prī′vŭs). Referring to or caused by removal of the thyroid gland. SEE: *cachexia.*

strumitis (strū-mī′tĭs). Inflammation of a thyroid gland with goiter. SYN: *thyroiditis.*

strumoderma (strū″mō-der′mă). Any tuberculous skin disease. SYN: *scrofuloderma.*

strumous (strū′mŭs). 1. Affected with scrofula. SYN: *scrofulous.* 2. Affected with goiter.

Strumpell's reflex (strŭm′pĕl). Stroking of thigh and abdomen results in movement of leg on same side accompanied by adduction of corresponding foot.

strychnine (strĭk′nĭn, -nĕn, -nīn). A poisonous alkaloid obtained from plants, as nux vomica.

  s. nitrate. USP. The nitrate of the alkaloid strychnine.

  DOSAGE: Same as strychnine sulfate.

  s. sulfate. USP. The sulfate of an alkaloid obtained from nux vomica.

  DOSAGE: 1/300 gr. (0.002 Gm.).

strychninism (strĭk′nĭn-ĭzm). Chronic strychnine poisoning. SYN: *strychnism.*

strychninomania (strĭk″nĭ-nō-mā′nĭ-ă). Insanity resulting from continued use of strychnine.

strychnism (strĭk′nĭzm). Poisoning from use of strychnine. SYN: *strychninism.*

student's placenta (stū′dĕnt). Retention of the placenta in childbirth because of unskillful manipulation by the obstetrician or midwife.

stump (stŭmp). Basal part of limb left after amputation.

  s. hallucination. Consciousness of still being possessed of a limb or arm after its amputation.

stun (stŭn). To render unconscious or stupified by a blow.

stupe (stūp). Cloth of flannel wrung out of hot water for a fomentation, often saturated with a counterirritant such as turpentine. SEE: *fomentation.*

  s., opium. 30-60 minims of opium sprinkled over stupe after it has been wrung out.

  s., turpentine. 1-2 drams of turpentine sprinkled evenly over dry flannel before water is poured on.

stupefacient (stū-pē-fā′shĕnt). Causing or that which causes stupor. SYN: *narcotic; soporific.*

stupemania (stū-pē-mā′nĭ-ă). Insanity with symptoms of stupor.

stupor (stū′por). 1. Condition of unconsciousness, torpor, or lethargy with suppression of sense or feeling. 2. PSY: A state of lessened responsiveness.

stupration, stuprum (stū-prā′shŭn, stū′prŭm). Sexual intercourse with a woman without her consent and by overpowering force, or intimidation. SYN: *rape.*

sturine (stū′rĭn). Protamine obtained from sperm of sturgeon which has bactericidal action.

stutter (stŭt′er). To hesitate and repeat or stumble spasmodically in speaking, due to difficulty in pronouncing initial consonants caused by spasm of lingual and palatal muscles.

stuttering (stŭt′er-ĭng). Defect in speech in which there is stumbling and spasmodic repetition of same syllable.

  s., urinary. Irregular, spasmodic urination. SYN: *stammering* of the bladder.*

stye (stī) (pl. **styes** or **sties**). A circumscribed inflammation of a sebaceous gland near edge of eyelid ending in suppuration. SYN: *hordeolum.*

  s., meibomian. Inflammation of a meibomian gland.

  s., Zeissian. Inflammation of one of Zeiss' glands.

styles, stylet (stīles, stī′lĕt). 1. A slender, solid or hollow plug of metal for making permanent a canal after operation or for stiffening or clearing a cannula or catheter. 2. A thin probe.

styliscus (stī-lĭs′kŭs). A slender, cylindrical plug for dilating a channel or for keeping a wound open. SEE: *tent.*

styloglossus (stī-lō-glŏs′ŭs). A muscle connecting the tongue and styloid process which raises and retracts the tongue.

styloid (stī′loyd). Resembling a stylus or pointed instrument.

   s. process. 1. A pointed process of the temporal bone, projecting downward, and to which some of the muscles of the tongue are attached. 2. A pointed projection behind the head of the fibula. 3. A protuberance on distal end of radius' outer portion. 4. An ulnar projection on inner side of the distal end.

styloiditis (stī-loyd-ī′tĭs). Inflammation of a styloid process.

stylomastoid (stī′lō-măs′toyd). Concerning the styloid and mastoid processes of the temporal bone.

stylomaxillary (stī′lō-măks′ĭ-lă-rĭ). Concerning the styloid process of the temporal bone and the mandible.

stylopharyngeus (stī′lō-far-ĭn′jē-ŭs). Muscle connecting the styloid process and pharynx which elevates and dilates the pharynx.

stylus (stī′lŭs). 1. A probe or slender wire for stiffening or clearing a canal or catheter. 2. Pointed medicinal preparation in stick form for external application.

stype (stīp). A pledget or tampon of cotton or other material.

stypsis (stĭp′sĭs). Astringency or the use of an astringent.

styptic (stĭp′tĭk). 1. Contracting a blood vessel; stopping a hemorrhage by astringent action. 2. Anything that checks a hemorrhage. SYN: *astringent, hemostat.*

stypticin (stĭp′tĭ-sĭn). Proprietary preparation of cotarnine hydrochloride, a yellow, odorless, crystalline powder.

   DOSAGE: ½-4 gr. (0.03-0.25 Gm.).

stypven (stĭp′vĕn). Commercial preparation of Russell's viper venom.

   The results of recent investigation have proven this to be of value as a hemostatic, used topically to stop bleeding in dental surgery, etc.

sub-. Combining form meaning *under, beneath, in small quantity.*

subabdominal (sŭb-ăb-dŏm′ĭ-năl). Below the abdomen.

subacetate (sŭb-ăs′ĕt-āt). A basic acetate.

subacromial (sŭb-ă-krō′mĭ-ă). Under the acromion process.

subacute (sŭb-ă-kūt′). Bet. acute and chronic, but with some acute features, said of the course of a disease.

subalimentation (sŭb-ăl-ĭ-mĕn-tā′shŭn). A state of insufficient nourishment.

subanconeus (sŭb-ăn-kō′nē-ŭs). 1. Below the elbow. 2. Muscle beneath the elbow which contracts its post. ligament.

subaponeurotic (sŭb″ap-ō-nū-rŏt′ĭk). Below an aponeurosis.

subarachnoid (sŭb-ă-răk′noyd). Below the arachnoid membrane.

   s. space. Space between the pia proper and arachnoid containing the cerebrospinal fluid.

subarcuate (sŭb-ar′kū-āt). Slightly arched.

   s. fossa. Depression beneath the arcuate eminence.

subastragalar (sŭb-ăs-trăg′ă-lar). Beneath the astragalus.

subastringent (sŭb-ăs-trĭn′jĕnt). Mildly astringent.

subaural (sŭb-aw′răl). Below the ear.

subcapsular (sŭb-kăp′sū-lar). Below any capsule, especially the capsule of the brain, or a capsular ligament.

subcarbonate (sŭb-kar′bŏn-āt). A basic carbonate; one having less carbonic acid radical than the normal carbonate.

subcartilaginous (sŭb-kar-tĭl-ăj′ĭn-ŭs). 1. Beneath a cartilage. 2. Cartilaginous in part.

subchronic (sŭb-krŏn′ĭk). Noting a condition bet. subacute and chronic; almost chronic.

subclavian (sŭb-klā′vĭ-ăn). Under the clavicle or collarbone. SYN: *subclavicular.*   [neck.

   s. artery. Large artery at base of

   s. triangle. One of the neck formed by the clavicle, and the omohyoid and sternomastoid muscles.

subclavicular (sŭb-klăv-ĭk′ū-lar). Beneath the clavicle. SYN: *subclavian.*

subclavius (sŭb-klā′vĭ-ŭs). A tiny muscle from the 1st rib to the undersurface of the clavicle.

subclinical (sŭb-klĭn′ĭ-kal). Pert. to a period before appearance of typical symptoms of a disease.

subcollateral (sŭb-kō-lăt′ĕr-ăl). Below the collateral fissure, indicating a cerebral convolution.

subconjunctival (sŭb-kŏn-jŭnk-tī′văl). Beneath the conjunctiva.

subconscious (sŭb-kŏn′shŭs). Not clearly conscious; pert. to activities of which the mind is not aware or to that which is not cognized through the physical senses; below the threshold of objective consciousness; that which is activated by involuntary processes; intuitional.

subconsciousness (sŭb-kŏn′shŭs-nĕs). 1. The state of being partially unconscious. 2. Noting of impressions and ideas without conscious knowledge of them. 3. The seat of a hypothetical subconscious mind in which are buried past impressions of objective knowledge. SEE: *subconscious.*

subcontinuous (sŭb-kŏn-tĭn′ū-ŭs). Almost continuous; with periods of abatement, but no interruptions to continuity.

   s. fever. Fever with periods of remission and exacerbation. SYN: *remittent fever.*

subcoracoid (sŭb-kor′ă-koyd). Beneath the coracoid process.

subcortex (sŭb-kor′tĕks). White substance of the brain underlying the cortex.

subcortical (sŭb-kor′tĭ-kal). Pert. to the region beneath the cerebral cortex.

subcostal (sŭb-kŏs′tăl). Beneath the ribs.

subcostalgia (sŭb-kŏs-tăl′jĭ-ă). Pain in region over the subcostal nerve.

subcranial (sŭb-krā′nĭ-ăl). Beneath or below the cranium.

subcrepitant (sŭb-krep′ĭ-tănt). Partially crepitant or crackling in character; noting a râle.

subcrureus (sŭb-krū-rē′ŭs). Small muscle bet. ant. surface of femoral shaft and synovial membrane of knee joint.

subculture (sŭb-kŭl′chŭr). 1. To make a culture of bacteria with material derived from another culture. 2. One made by transferring bacteria from a previous culture to a fresh medium.

subcutaneous (sŭb-kū-tā′nē-ŭs). Beneath or to be introduced beneath the skin. Syn: *hypodermic*.

   s. surgery. Operation performed through a small opening in the skin.

   s. wound. A wound with only a small opening through the skin.

subcuticular (sŭb-kū-tĭk′ū-lar). Beneath the cuticle or epidermis. Syn: *subepidermal*.

subdelirium (sŭb-dē-lir′ĭ-ŭm). A mild or not continuous delirium.

subdiaphragmatic (sŭb-dī-ă-frăg-măt′ĭk). Beneath the diaphragm.

subdural (sŭb-dū′răl). Beneath the dura mater.

   s. space. Space bet. the arachnoid and dura mater.

subencephalon (sŭb-ĕn-sef′ă-lŏn). The pons, medulla oblongata, and corpora quadrigemina together. Syn: *hypencephalon*.

subendocardial (sŭb″ĕn-dō-kar′dĭ-ăl). Below the endocardium.

subendothelial (sŭb″ĕn-dō-thē′lĭ-ăl). Beneath endothelium.

subendothelium (sŭb″ĕn-dō-thē′lĭ-ŭm). A layer bet. the epithelium and basement membrane of the mucosa of the bronchi and intestines. Syn: *Débove's membrane*.

subepidermal (sŭb″ĕp-ĭ-der′măl). Beneath the epidermis. Syn: *subcuticular*.

subepithelial (sŭb″ĕp-ĭ-thē′lĭ-ăl). Beneath the epithelium.

subfascial (sŭb-făsh′ĭ-ăl). Beneath a fascia.

subfebrile (sŭb-fē′brĭl). Somewhat feverish.

subflavous (sŭb-flā′vŭs). Yellowish.

   s. ligament. Yellowish ligament connecting the laminae of the vertebrae. Syn: *ligamentum subflavum*.

subfrontal (sŭb-frŭn′tăl). Below a frontal convolution or lobe of the brain.

subglenoid (sŭb-glē′noyd). Below the glenoid fossa or glenoid cavity.

subglossal (sŭb-glos′ăl). Under the tongue. Syn: *hypoglossal, sublingual*.

subglossitis (sŭb-glos-sī′tĭs). Inflammation of the undersurface or tissues of the tongue.

subgrondation, subgrundation (sŭb-grondā′shŭn, -grŭn-dā′shŭn). Depression of one fragment of a broken bone beneath the other, as of the cranium.

subhyoid (sŭb-hī′oyd). Beneath the hyoid bone.

subiculum (sū-bĭk′ū-lŭm). A division of

hippocampal convolution, composed of a thick layer of myelinated fibers on its surface, and containing the olfactory association centers. Syn: *convolution, uncinate; uncus gyri hippocampi*.

subiliac (sŭb-ĭl′ĭ-ăk). 1. Below the ilium. 2. Pert. to the subilium.

subilium (sŭb-ĭl′ĭ-ŭm). The lowest part of the ilium.

subimbibitional (sŭb-ĭm-bĭb-ĭsh′ŭn-ăl). Pert. to a condition due to deficient fluid intake.

subinfection (sŭb-ĭn-fĕk′shŭn). 1. Mild infection because of the weakening of the resisting power of the cells against toxic conditions. 2. Condition caused by toxins liberated from bacteria undergoing lysis.

subinflammation (sŭb″ĭn-flăm-ā′shŭn). Very mild inflammation. Syn: *irritation*.

subinflammatory (sŭb″ĭn-flăm′ă-tō-rĭ). Very mildly inflammatory.

subintrant (sŭb-ĭn′trănt). Having cycles or paroxysms in such rapid succession that they intermingle.

   s. fever. Intermittent fever in which the paroxysms occur so rapidly that one comes on before the previous one has disappeared.

subinvolution (sŭb″ĭn-vō-lū′shŭn). Imperfect involution; incomplete return of a part to normal dimensions after physiological hypertrophy, as when the uterus following childbirth fails to reduce to normal size. See: *uterus*.

subject (sŭb′jĕkt). 1. A patient undergoing treatment, observation, or experiment. 2. A body used for dissection.

subjective (sŭb-jĕk′tĭv). Arising from or concerned with the individual; not perceptible to an observer. Opp: *objective*.

   s. sensation. A sensation occurring when stimuli due to internal causes excite the nervous system; one not of objective origin.

   s. symptoms. Those which are of internal origin and evident only to the patient.

subjugal (sŭb-jū′găl). Below the malar bone or *os zygomaticum*.

sublatio (sŭb-lā′shĭ-ō). Removal or detachment of a part.

   s. retinae. Detachment of the retina.

sublethal (sŭb-lē′thăl). A little less than lethal; almost fatal.

   s. dose. Dose containing not quite enough toxin to cause death.

sublimate (sŭb′lĭ-māt). 1. A substance obtained or prepared by sublimation. 2. To vaporize a solid substance by heat and condense it again without liquefying, for purification. 3. Psy: To overcome the libido by diverting it into nonsexual or higher activities.

sublimation (sŭb-lĭ-mā′shŭn). 1. Chem: To convert a solid into a vapor and condense it again without liquefying to purify it. 2. Psy: Conversion of the libido into nonsexual channels.

sublime (sŭb-lĭm′). Chem: To evaporate a substance directly from the solid into the vapor state and condense it again.

Thus, metallic iodine on heating does not liquefy, but forms directly a violet gas.

subliminal (sŭb-lĭm'ĭn-ăl). 1. Below the threshold of sensation; too weak to arouse sensation or muscular contraction. 2. Below the normal consciousness. SYN: *subconscious*.

s. self. PSY: Part of a normal individual's personality in which his mental processes function without consciousness under normal waking conditions.

sublingual (sŭb-lĭng'gwăl). Beneath or concerning the area beneath the tongue.

s. gland. The smallest of the salivary glands, located bet. side of tongue and the mandible, one on each side.

It has about 20 ducts opening for the most part directly above the gland.

sublinguitis (sŭb"lĭng-gwī'tĭs). Inflammation of the sublingual gland.

sublobular (sŭb-lŏb'ū-lar). Beneath a lobule.

sublumbar (sŭb-lŭm'bar). Below the lumbar region.

subluxation (sŭb"lŭks-ā'shŭn). A partial or incomplete dislocation.

sublymphemia (sŭb-lĭm-fē'mĭ-ă). Abnormal decrease in lymphocytes in the blood with number of white cells being normal. SYN: *hypolymphemia*.

submammary (sŭb-mam'ă-rĭ). Below the mammary gland.

submaxilla (sŭb-măks-ĭl'ă). The lower jaw or mandible. SYN: *maxilla, inferior.*

submaxillaritis (sŭb-măks-ĭl-ar-ī'tĭs). 1. Pert. to the mandible. 2. Inflammation or mumps of the submaxillary gland.

submaxillary (sŭb-măks'ĭl-a-rĭ). Beneath the lower jaw or inferior maxilla.

s. gland. A salivary racemose gland below the angle of the jaw discharging into the mouth, 1/3 the size of the parotid gland.

submaxillitis (sŭb-măks-ĭl-lī'tĭs). Inflammation of or mumps affecting the submaxillary gland.

submental (sŭb-mĕn'tăl). Under the chin.

submicron (sŭb-mī'krŏn). A tiny particle invisible except with the ultramicroscope. SYN: *ultramicron.*

submicroscopical (sŭb"mī-krō-skŏp'ĭ-kal). Too minute to be visible under the microscope.

submorphous (sŭb-mor'fŭs). Neither completely amorphous nor crystalline, as some calculi.

submucosa (sŭb-mū-kō'să). The layer of areolar connective tissue under a mucous membrane.

submucous (sŭb-mū'kŭs). Beneath a mucous membrane.

subnarcotic (sŭb-nar-kŏt'ĭk). Mildly narcotic.

subnasal (sŭb-nā'zăl). Under the nose.

s. point. Craniometric point at base of nasal spine.

subneural (sŭb-nū'răl). Beneath the neural axis or the central nervous system.

subnormal (sŭb-nor'măl). Below normal.

subnucleus (sŭb-nū'klē-ŭs). 1. One of the secondary nuclei into which the nucleus of a nerve cell divides. 2. An accessory nucleus.

suboccipital (sŭb-ŏk-sĭp'ĭ-tăl). Situated below the occiput or occipital bone.

suboperculum (sŭb-ō-per'kū-lŭm). Portion of occipital convolution overlapping the insula. SEE: *operculum.*

suborbital (sŭb-or'bĭ-tăl). Beneath the orbit.

subpapular (sŭb-păp'ū-lar). Very slightly papular, as papules elevated being scarcely more than macules.

subpatellar (sŭb-pă-tĕl'ar). Beneath the patella.

subpeduncular (sŭb"pē-dŭn'kū-lar). Below a peduncle.

s. lobe. Tiny lobe on undersurface of either cerebellar hemisphere. SYN: *flocculus.*

subpericardial (sŭb"pĕr-ĭ-kar'dĭ-ăl). Beneath the pericardium.

subperiosteal (sŭb"pĕr-ĭ-ŏs'tē-ăl). Beneath the periosteum.

s. operation. Bone surgery without removal of the periosteum.

subperitoneal (sŭb"pĕr-ĭ-tō-nē'ăl). Beneath the peritoneum.

subpharyngeal (sŭb-făr-ĭn'jē-ăl). Beneath the pharynx.

subphrenic (sŭb-frĕn'ĭk). Beneath the diaphragm. SYN: *subdiaphragmatic.*

s. abscess. Collection of pus beneath the diaphragm.

subplacenta (sŭb-plă-sĕn'tă). Part of the decidua directly lining the uterus. SYN: *decidua vera.*

subpleural (sŭb-plū'răl). Beneath the pleura.

subpontine (sŭb-pŏn'tĭn, -tīn). Below the pons Varolii.

subpreputial (sŭb"prē-pū'shăl). Under the prepuce.

subpubic (sŭb-pū'bĭk). Beneath the pubic arch, as a ligament.

subpulmonary (sŭb-pŭl'mō-na-rĭ). Below the lung.

subretinal (sŭb-rĕt'ĭ-năl). Beneath the retina.

subscapular (sŭb-skăp'ū-lar). Below the scapula.

subscription (sŭb-skrĭp'shŭn). Part of a prescription containing direction to a pharmacist.

subserous (sŭb-sē'rŭs). Beneath a serous membrane.

subspinous (sŭb-spī'nŭs). 1. Beneath any spine. 2. Anterior to or beneath the spinal column.

s. dislocation. Dislocation with head of the humerus resting below spine of the scapula.

substage (sŭb'stāj). Attachment to the microscope beneath the stage by which attachments are held in place.

substance (sŭb'stăns). That of which any material thing is composed; matter.

s., agglutinable. Substance in red blood corpuscles and bacteria which unites with agglutinin producing specific agglutination.

s., alible. That portion of chyme that nourishes the body.

s., alimentary. Any article of food.

s., alpha. Reticular substance.

s., beta. Tiny body in erythrocytes after staining with azure I.

s., black. Grayish substance in crus cerebri. SYN: *substantia nigra.*

s., chromophilic. Elements of a cell which stain easily.

s., colloid. Jellylike substance in colloid degeneration.

s., cytotoxin. The specific amboceptor and complement in serum which dissolves special cells.

s., depressor. A substance secreted by the pituitary gland which lowers blood pressure.

s., gray. Gray matter of the brain and spinal cord.

s., hemolytic. Substance in serum that destroys red blood cells in an added serum. SYN: *alexin.*

s., medullary. 1. White matter of central nervous system. 2. Marrowlike substance of organs, as the kidney.

s., parietal. The matrix of cartilage.

s., prelipoid. Nerve tissue degenerated but not converted into fat.

s., reticular. Threadlike mass in red blood corpuscles after staining. SYN: *alpha substance.*

s., sarcous. Substance of sarcous elements of a muscle.

s., supporting. Neuroglia, connective tissue, etc., supporting a structure.

s., white. White matter of brain and spinal cord.

s., w., of Schwann. A nerve fiber's medullary sheath.

s., zymoplastic. Substance that hastens coagulation of the blood. SYN: *coagulin.*

substantia (sŭb-stăn'shĭ-ă). Substance.

s. alba. White substance of the brain.

s. cinerea. Gray substance of brain and spinal cord.

s. ferruginea. Elongated mass of pigmented cells in the locus caeruleus.

s. gelatinosa. Gray matter of the cord surrounding central canal and capping head of post. horns of spinal cord.

s. grisea. BNA. Gray matter of the spinal cord.

s. nigra. BNA. Black substance in a section of the crus cerebri. SYN: *locus niger.*

s. perforata anterior. BNA. Area on either side of optic chiasm in the olfactory trigone.

s. perforata posterior. BNA. Gray area at base of brain.

s. propria membranae tympani. Fibrous middle layer of drum membrane.

substernal (sŭb-ster'năl). Situated beneath the sternum.

substitution (sŭb-stĭ-tū'shŭn). 1. CHEM: Displacing an atom (or more than one) of an element in a compound by atoms of another element, equivalently. 2. PSY: The turning from an obstructed desire to one whose gratification is socially acceptable. 3. The turning from an obstructed form of behavior to a more primitive one, as a substitution neurosis.

s. products. Compounds formed by an element or a radical replacing another element or radical in a compound.

s. therapy. Administration of hormone or glandular extract to counteract the deficiency of that gland. SYN: *organotherapy.*

substitutive (sŭb-stĭ-tū-tĭv). Causing a change or substitution of characteristics.

s. therapy. Treatment to overcome an inflammation of a specific character by exciting an acute nonspecific inflammation.

substrate, substratum (sŭb'străt, sŭb-strā'tŭm). 1. An underlying layer or foundation. 2. A base, as of a pigment. 3. The substance acted upon, as by an enzyme. SYN: *zymolyte.* SEE: *enzyme.*

subsultus (sŭb-sŭl'tŭs). Any morbid tremor or twitching, as of the tendons; a grave symptom in certain fevers.

s. clonus, s. tendinum. Involuntary twitchings of muscles, esp. of arms and feet, causing movement of tendons, observed in certain febrile conditions.

subsylvian (sŭb-sĭl'vĭ-ăn). Below the fissure of Sylvius.

subtarsal (sŭb-tar'săl). Below the tarsus.

subthalamic (sŭb-thă-lăm'ĭk). Located below the thalamus.

s. nucleus. A small ganglion beneath the optic layer. SYN: *Luy's body, hypothalamic nucleus.*

subthalamus (sŭb-thăl'ă-mŭs). Prominences and ganglia on ventral side below the thalamus. SYN: *hypothalamus.*

subthyroidism (sŭb-thī'royd-ĭzm). Condition due to lack of activity of the thyroid gland. SYN: *hypothyroidism.*

subtile, subtle (sŭb'tĭl, sŭt'l). 1. Very fine or delicate. 2. Very acute. 3. Mentally acute or crafty or piercing, as sharp. 4. Operating without attracting attention, as subtle poisons.

subtotal (sŭb-tō'tăl). Just less than total, as subtotal removal of a gland.

subtrochanteric (sŭb-trō-kăn-ter'ĭk). Below a trochanter.

subtuberal (sŭb-tū'bĕr-ăl). Located under a tuber.

subtympanic (sŭb-tĭm-păn'ĭk). Below the tympanum.   [dren.

subures (sŭb-ū'ber-ēz). Suckling chil-

subumbilical (sŭb-ŭm-bĭl'ĭ-kăl). Below the umbilicus.

s. space. Space within the body cavity below the navel resembling a triangle in shape.

subungual, subunguial (sŭb-ŭng'gwăl, -gwĭ-ăl). Situated beneath nail of a finger or toe. SEE: *hyponychium.*

suburethral (sŭb-ū-rē'thrăl). Below the urethra.

s. gland. One on either side of the ant. portion of the vagina. SYN: *Bartholin's or Duverney's glands, vulvovaginal gland.*

subvaginal (sŭb-văj'ĭn-ăl). 1. Below the vagina. 2. On inner side of any tubular sheathing membrane.

subvertebral (sŭb-ver'tĕ-brăl). Beneath or on ventral side of the vertebral column or of a vertebra. SYN: *subspinal*.

subvirile (sŭb-vĭr'ĭl, -vĭ'rĭl). Of lowered or inferior virility.

subvitrinal (sŭb-vĭt'rĭn-ăl). Located beneath the vitreous body.

subvolution (sŭb-vō-lū'shŭn). Method of surgically turning over a flap to prevent adhesions.

subzonal (sŭb-zō'năl). Below any zone, such as the *zona pellucida*.

succagogue (sŭk'ăg-ōg). Anything inducing glandular secretion, or which stimulates secretion of a gland or of the digestive juice.

succedaneous (sŭk-sē-da'nē-ŭs). Acting as a substitute or relating to one.

succedaneum (sŭk-sē-dā'nē-ŭm). A substitute for anything; a remedy used as a substitute.

  s., caput. Serosanguineous infiltration of connective tissue upon presenting part of head of a fetus.

succenturiate (sŭk-sĕn-tū'rĭ-āt). Serving as a substitute or accessory.

  s. kidney. A suprarenal or adrenal body.

  s. placenta. A supernumerary or accessory one.

succorrhea (sŭk-kor-rē'ă). Unnatural increase in secretion of any juice, esp. of a digestive fluid.

succus (sŭk'kŭs). A juice or fluid secretion.

  s. entericus. The intestinal juice of the body. It is alkaline. Sp. gr. 1.010. The secretion of the minute glands lining the small intestine.

  s. gastricus. The gastric juice.

  s. pyloricus. An alkaline secretion by the pyloric end of the stomach.

succussion (sŭk-ŭs'shŭn). Shaking of a person to detect the presence of fluid in the bodily cavities by listening for a splashing sound, esp. in the thorax.

suck (sŭk). 1. To draw fluid into the mouth, as from the breast. 2. To exhaust air from a tube and thus siphon fluid from a container. 3. That which is drawn into the mouth by sucking.

suck'ing pad. Mass of fat in cheeks, esp. well developed in an infant, aiding it to suck. SEE: *myzesis*.

sucrase (sū'krās). An enzyme in the intestinal juice which splits cane sugar into glucose and fructose, which are absorbed into the portal circulation. SYN: *invertin*.

sucroclastic (sū-krō-klăs'tĭk). Splitting up or hydrolyzing a sugar.

sucrose (sū'krōs). Saccharose or cane sugar. $C_{12}H_{22}O_{11}$, a disaccharose giving dextrose and levulose on inversion.

sucrosemia (sū-krō-sē'mĭ-ă). Sucrose or cane sugar in the blood serum.

sucrosuria (sū-krō-sū'rĭ-ă). Sugar in the urine.

suction (sŭk'shŭn). The act of or capacity for sucking up by reduction of air pressure over part of the surface of a substance.

  s., post-tussive. Suction sound over a lung cavity heard on auscultation after a cough.

sudamen (sū-dā'mĕn) (pl. *sudamina*). Noninflammatory eruption from sweat glands characterized by whitish vesicles caused by the retention of sweat in corneous layer of the skin, appearing after profuse sweating or in certain febrile diseases, disappearing by absorption.

sudamina (sū-dăm'ĭn-ă). Plural of sudamen,* an eruption of vesicles due to retention of sweat in corneous layer of the skin.

sudan (sū'dăn'). A term given to several fat dyes used as stains.

  s. III, s. red III. A powder that colors fatty tissues red, and which stains the fatty covering of the tubercle bacilli.

  s. yellow G. A dye staining fat cells yellow.

sudanophil, sudanophilous (sū-dăn'ō-fĭl, -of'ĭ-lŭs). Staining readily with sudan.

sudanophilia (sū-dăn-ō-fĭl'ĭ-ă). A condition in which minute fat droplets contained in the leukocytes take a brilliant red stain, probably indicative of suppuration.

sudation (sū-dā'shŭn). 1. The act of sweating. 2. Excessive perspiration.

sudatoria (sū-dă-to'rĭ-ă). Excessive sweating. SYN: *ephidrosis, hyperidrosis*.

sudatorium (sū-dă-tō'rĭ-ŭm). 1. A hot air bath or any bath to induce perspiration. 2. A room used to induce sweat baths.

sudokeratosis (sū''dō-ker-ă-tō'sĭs). Circumscribed, horny overgrowths obstructing the sweat ducts.

sudomotor (sū''dō-mō'tŏr). Pert. to stimulating the secretion of sweat; noting certain nerves.

sudor (sū'dŏr). Secretion from the sweat glands. SYN: *perspiration, sweat*.

  s. cruentus. Sweating of blood. SYN: *hematidrosis*.

sudoral (sū'dŏr-ăl). Pert. to, caused by, or marked by, perspiration.

sudoresis (sū-dō-rē'sĭs). Profuse sweating. SYN: *diaphoresis*.

sudoriferous (sū-dor-if'ĕr-ŭs). Conveying or producing sweat. [the skin.

  s. glands. Sweat-secreting glands of

sudorific (sū-dŏr-ĭf'ĭk). 1. Secreting or promoting the secretion of sweat. 2. Agent which produces sweating. SYN: *diaphoretic*.

sudoriparous (sū-dor-ĭp'ă-rŭs). Secreting sweat. SYN: *sudoriferous*.

suet (sū'ĕt). Hard fat from the ox or sheep's kidneys and loins, used as the base of certain ointments and as an emollient.

suffocation (sŭf''ō-kā'shŭn). 1. State of being choked by obstruction of air passages by drowning, smothering, throttling, or inhalation of noxious gases. SYN: *asphyxia.* Generally from gases. 2. Act of obstructing the air passages.

suffumigation (sŭf-ū''mĭ-gā'shŭn). 1. Treatment by application of medicated vapors from below. 2. A vapor so used.

suffusion (sŭf-ū'zhŭn). 1. Spreading of a bodily fluid into surrounding tissues. SYN: *extravasation*. 2. Pouring of a fluid over the body as treatment.

sugar (shu'gar). A sweet-tasting carbohydrate belonging to the monosaccharose and disaccharose groups. Crystalline carbohydrates of comparatively low molecular weight and generally having a sweet taste.

   s., beet. A saccharine from beets.

   s., cane. Sugar from sugar cane.

   s., diabetic. Glucose.

   s., fruit. Levulose.

   s., grape. Dextrose, glucose.

   s., invert. One consisting of 1 molecule of glucose and 1 of fructose.

   s., liver. Glycogen.

   s., malt. Maltose.

   s., milk. Lactose.

   s., muscle. Inosite.

suggestibility (sŭg-jĕs''tĭ-bĭl'ĭ-tĭ). A condition in which a person responds readily to suggestions or opinions of another.

suggestible (sŭg-jĕs'tĭ-bl). Very susceptible to the opinions or suggestions of others.

suggestion (sŭg-jĕs'chŭn). 1. Imparting of an idea in any indirect way. 2. The idea so conveyed. 3. The acceptance or the effect of the statements or actions of one person upon another, depending on the emotional set-up of the recipient and his psychic relationship to the other person.

   s., auto-. Self-suggestion as distinguished from that coming from another person, esp. in hypnotic state.

   May produce or cure functional disturbances.

suggestive (sŭg-jĕs'tĭv). Stimulating or pert. to suggestion.

   s. medicine. Therapy by suggestion either during consciousness or hypnosis.

   s. therapeutics. The practice of treating disease by suggestion or hypnotism.

suggillation (sŭg-jĭl-ā'shŭn). A bruise or black and blue mark. SYN: *ecchymosis*.

suicide (sū'ĭ-sīd). 1. Act or instance of taking one's own life voluntarily. 2. One who attempts or commits self-murder.

sulcal (sŭl'kăl). Pert. to a sulcus.

   s. artery. A tiny branch of ant. spinal artery.

sulcate, sulcated (sŭl'kăt, -ĕd). Furrowed or grooved.

sulcus (sŭl'kŭs) (pl. *sulci*). A furrow or groove, or slight depression or fissure, esp. of the brain.

   s. centralis. BNA. Fissure dividing the frontal and parietal lobes of each cerebral hemisphere. SYN: *fissure of Rolando.*

   s., intraparietal. One that separates the inf. from the sup. parietal bones and lobes.

   s. praecentra'lis. BNA. An interrupted one generally parallel with the fissure of Rolando and ant. to it.

   s. pulmona'lis. Depression on either side of the vertebral column.

   s. spira'lis cochleae. Groove bet. the labium tympanicum and labium vestibulare.

   s. tympanicus. Furrow in bony tympanic ring which receives the margin of the tympanic membrane. [*tralis.*

   s., vertical. Same as *sulcus praecen-*

sulf-, sulfo-. Prefix showing that a compound with this prefix contains sulfurous anhydride or the group SO_2.

sulfacetimide (sŭl-fă-sĕt'ĭ-mĭd). A sulfonamide used in treatment of *B. coli*, gonorrhea, and infections of the urinary tract, esp. when resistant to sulfanilamide and sulfathiazole.

sulfadiazine (sŭl''fă-dī-ā'zēn). A synthetic compound of sulfanilamide and vitamin B_1 which is destructive to streptococci, staphylococci, and pneumococci.

sulfamethylthiazol (sŭl''fă-mĕth''ĭl-thī-ā'zŏl). A sulfanilamide derivative which is less toxic than sulfapyridine; effective against staphylococcic organisms.

sulfanilamide (sŭl''fă-ĭl'ă-mĭd) (para-amino-benzene-sulfonamide). A white, slightly bitter, crystalline substance from coal tar, the parent of the azo dyes, which has come into use within the past few years, and is regarded by many as an important contribution to our list of effective medicines; however, far too potent to be used indiscriminately.

   DOSAGE: Calculated on the basis of body weight: 15 gr. (1 Gm.) for each 20 lb. up to 100 lb. The maximum dose seems to have been 75 gr. (5 Gm.) given over a period of 24 hours to a person of average weight, but average dose is 15 gr. every 4 hours for 48 hours, after which dose is lowered.

sulfanilylguanidine (sŭl-făn-ĭl''ĭl-gwan'ĭ-dĭn). Derivative of sulfanilamide having antibacterial activity useful in treating intestinal infections.

sulfanilyl-sulfanilamide (sŭl-făn-ĭl-ĭl-sŭl''făn-ĭl'ă-mĭd). A sulfanilamide derivative which is less toxic and more effective in the treatment of gonorrhea.

sulfapyridine (sŭl''fă-pĭr'ĭ-dĕn). A sulfanilamide derivative which differs in its chemical structure in that 1 hydrogen atom in the sulfonamide group has been replaced by a basic pyridine group, and is less toxic.

sulfapyr'idine so'dium monohy'drate. A soluble salt of sulfapyridine for intravenous use only, as an emergency treatment in pneumonia, where response has not been sufficient by oral administration, or where it is imperative to administer adequate medication at once.

   DOSAGE: Calculated on the basis of 0.06 Gm. per kilogram of body weight, and given as a 5% solution in sterile distilled water.

sulfarsphenamine (sŭlf''ars-fĕn'ă-mēn). An arsenic compound containing 19% arsenic.

   DOSAGE: Intramuscularly, 0.4-0.5 Gm.

sulfate (sŭl'fāt). A salt or ester of sulfuric acid.

sulfathiazole (sŭl″fă-thī-ā′zōl). A sulfanilamide derivative which is less toxic and which can be given in smaller doses.

sulfhemoglobin (sŭlf″hĕm-ō-glō′bĭn). Substance formed by action of hydrogen sulfide on blood.

sulfhemoglobinemia (sŭlf″hĕm-ō-glō″bĭn-ē′-mĭ-ă). Persistent cyanotic condition due to sulfhemoglobin in blood.

sulfonal (sŭl′fō-năl). A proprietary hypnotic and sedative.
 DOSAGE: 12 gr. (0.75 Gm.).

sulfonalism (sŭl′fō-năl-ĭzm). 1. Sulfonal poisoning and its symptoms. 2. Addiction to sulfonal.

sulfonamides. A family of drugs, including sulfanilamide, sulfapyridine, sulfathiazole, etc.

sulfonethylmethane (sŭl″fŏn-ĕth″ĭl-mĕth′-ān). USP. Trional. White powder or crystalline substance with a bitter taste.
 DOSAGE: 12 gr. (0.75 Gm.).

sulfonmethane (sŭl″fŏn-mĕth′ān). USP. Crystalline compound with hypnotic and sedative properties. SYN: *sulfonal.*

sulfourea (sŭl″fō-ū-rē′ă). Urea with oxygen replaced with sulfur. SYN: *thiourea.*

sulfugator (sŭl′fū-gā″tor). A roll of cloth impregnated with sulfur to be ignited for fumigation.

sulfur (sŭl′fŭr). SYMB: S. At. wt. 32.064. Sp. gr. 2.07. It is a pale, yellow, crystalline element which burns with a blue flame, producing sulfur dioxide.

 s. dioxide. An irritating gas used in industries to manufacture acids, also used in electrical refrigerators. A bactericide and important disinfectant.

sulfurated, sulfureted (sŭl′fū-rā-ted, -rĕt-ĕd). Combined or impregnated with sulfur.

 s. hydrogen. A colorless, inflammable gas of disagreeable odor resulting from decomposition of organic matter containing sulfur; used as a chemical reagent. SYN: *hydrogen sulfide.* H_2S.

sulfuric acid (sŭl-fū′rĭk). H_2SO_4. A heavy, corrosive, oily, poisonous acid used as an astringent in colic and diarrhea, and in manufacturing processes, as in cleaning metals, batteries.
 DOSAGE: (Arom.) 8 gr. (0.5 Gm.); (dil. 10%) 15 gr. (1.0 Gm.).

summation (sŭm-ā′shŭn). Cumulative action or effect, as of stimuli.   [year.

summer (sŭm′ẽr). The hot season of the
 s. catarrh. Allergic reaction to grass pollen in early summer. SYN: *rose cold.*
 s. cholera, s. complaint, s. diarrhea. Acute form of gastroenteritis with diarrhea, cramps and vomiting. SYN: *cholera morbus, q.v.*
 s. itch. Severe bullous eruption occurring in summer.
 s. rash. Rash due to perspiration. SYN: *lichen tropicus, prickly heat.*

sunburn (sŭn′bŭrn). Dermatitis due to exposure to the actinic rays of the sun. SEE: *burn.*

Sun′day or Mon′day morn′ing paralysis. A musculospiral paralysis following excessive use of alcohol.

sunstroke (sŭn′strōk). An affection from undue exposure to rays of the sun or excessive heat.

super-. Combining form meaning *above, beyond, superior.*

superalimentation (sūp″er-ăl-ĭ-mĕn-tā′-shŭn). Therapeutic forcing of food in excess of body needs or appetite.

superalkalinity (sūp″er-ăl-kă-lĭn′ĭ-tĭ) Excessive alkalinity.

superciliary (sūp-er-sĭl′ĭ-ă-rĭ). Pert. to or in the region of an eyebrow.

supercilium (sū-pĕr-sĭl′ĭ-ŭm). 1. Eyebrow. 2. A hair of the eyebrow.

super-ego (sūp″er-ē′gō). An inner, subconscious censor. SEE: *ego.*

superfecundation (sū″pĕr-fē-kŭn-dā′shŭn). Successive fertilization by more than 1 coitus of 2 or more ova formed at the same menstrual period.

superfetation (sū″pĕr-fē-tā′shŭn). Supposed fertilization of 2 ova in the same uterus at different menstrual periods within a short interval.

superficial (sū-pĕr-fĭsh′ăl). 1. Confined to the surface. 2. Not thorough; cursory.
 s. reflex. One induced by very light stimulus such as stroking skin lightly with soft cotton wad.

superficialis (sū″pĕr-fĭsh-I-ā′lĭs). Superficial; noting a superficial artery, vein, or nerve, or structure near the surface.

superimpregnation (sū″pĕr-ĭm″prĕg-nā′-shŭn). Conception during pregnancy; fertilization from 2 different ovulations. SYN: *superfecundation, superfetation.*

superinduce (sū″pĕr-ĭn-dūs′). To bring in over or above that already existing condition or situation.

superinfection (sū″pĕr-ĭn-fĕk′shŭn). A new infection by the same organism, in addition to a similar one already existing.

superinvolution (sū″pĕr-ĭn-vō-lū′shŭn). Excessive reduction of the uterus following childbirth to less than its normal size. SYN: *hyperinvolution.*

superior (sū-pē′rĭ-or). 1. Higher than; situated above something else. 2. Better than. 3. One in charge of others.

superior′ity com′plex. An exaggerated conviction of one's own superiority; a pretense of superiority in order to compensate for supposed inferiority.

superlactation (sū-pĕr-lăk-tā′shŭn). Oversecretion of milk, or continuance of lactation beyond normal time.

superlethal (sū″pĕr-lē′thăl). Beyond a fatal limit, as a dose that will probably kill.

supermoron (sū″pĕr-mō′rŏn). One slightly subnormal but above a moron mentally.

supermotility (sū″pĕr-mō-tĭl′ĭ-tĭ). Excessive motility in any part. SYN: *hypercinesia.*

supernatant (sū″pĕr-nā′tănt). Floating on surface, as oil on water.

supernate (sū-pĕr-nāt′). A supernatant fluid.

supernumerary (sū″pĕr-nū′mĕr-a-rĭ). Exceeding the regular number.

supernutrition (sū″pĕr-nū-trĭ′shŭn). More than normal nutrition.

supersaturated solution (sū″pĕr-săt′ū-rāt′-ĕd). One containing more salt or other substance than it can dissolve at normal temperature.

superscription (sū″pĕr-skrĭp′shŭn). The beginning of a prescription noted by the sign ℞, signifying L. *recipe*, take.

supersecretion (sū″pĕr-sē-krē′shŭn). An excess of any secretion.

supersedent (sū″pĕr-sē′dĕnt). A remedy which partially cures or prevents a disease.

supersensitiveness (sū″-per-sĕn′sĭ-tĭv″nĕs). Excessive susceptibility to a foreign protein or pollen. SYN: *hypersensitiveness*.

supersoft (sū″pĕr-sŏft′). Exceptionally soft; noting roentgen rays of extremely long wave length and low penetrating power.

supersphenoid (sū″pĕr-sfē′noyd). Over the sphenoid bone.

supertemporal (sū″pĕr-tĕm′pō-răl). In the upper part above the temporal bone, region, or lobe.

   s. convolution. Convolution bet. sylvian and sup. temporal fissures.

   s. fissure. One ant. and parallel to the sylvian fissure.

supertension (sū″pĕr-tĕn′shŭn). Extremely high tension. SYN: *hypertension*.

supervenosity (sū″pĕr-vē-nŏs′ĭ-tĭ). Incomplete oxidation of the blood; a condition of excessive venosity.

supervention (sū″pĕr-vĕn′shŭn). Additional condition developing besides something already existing, as a complication to an existing disease.

supervirulent (sū″pĕr-vĭr′ū-lĕnt). More virulent than usual.

supinate (sū′pĭ-nāt). 1. To turn the forearm or hand so that the palm faces upward. 2. To rotate the foot and leg outward. 3. To cause to assume, or to assume, a position of supination.

supination (sū-pĭn-ā′shŭn). 1. Turning of the palm or foot upward. 2. Act of lying flat upon the back. 3. Condition of being on the back or having the foot or palm facing upward.

supinator (sū″pĭn-ā′tor). A muscle producing the motion of supination of the forearm.

   s. longus reflex. Flexion of the forearm caused by tapping of the tendon of the supinator longus.

supine (sū-pīn′). 1. Of position, lying on the back or with the face upward. 2. Of the hand or foot noting position with the palm or foot facing upward. OPP: *prone*. SEE: *position*.

supplemental (sŭp-lē-mĕn′tăl). Referring to something added to supply a need or to reinforce.

   s. air. The *residual* air of the lungs which, after *tidal* air has been expelled in normal respiration, may be driven out by forced inspiration. SEE: *air*.

suppository (sŭp-pŏz′ĭ-tō-rĭ) (pl. *suppositories*). A semisolid, fusible, medicated substance for introduction into the rectum, vagina, or urethra, where it dissolves and is absorbed.

   s., r., anodyne. For local or general effects to reduce pain.

   s., rectal, astringent. To contract blood vessels and tissues.

   s., r., evacuant. To cause evacuation.

   s., r., specific. Used when specifics cannot be taken by mouth.

suppression (sŭ-prĕsh′ŭn). 1. Repression of the ext. manifestation of a morbid condition. 2. Complete failure of a natural secretion or excretion. OPP: *retention*. 3. PSY: Conscious inhibition of an idea or desire as distinguished from repression which is considered an unconscious process.

   s. of menses. 1. Amenorrhea in which menstruation ceases after once being established and from some cause other than pregnancy or the climacteric. 2. Any suppression of the menses.

   s. of urine. Suppression of urine resulting from renal conditions.

suppurant (sŭp′ū-rănt). 1. Producing, tending to produce, or characterized by pus formation. 2. Agent causing pus formation. SYN: *suppurative*.

suppurate (sŭp′pū-rāt). To form or generate pus.

suppuration (sŭp-ū-rā′shŭn). 1. The process of pus formation. 2. The discharge produced by suppuration. SYN: *pus*.

suppurative (sŭp′ū-rā″tĭv, -rā-tĭv). 1. Producing or associated with generation of pus. 2. Agent producing pus formation.

   s. fever. Pus in the blood causing fever; a form of septicemia. SYN: *pyemia*.

supra-. Combining form meaning *above*.

supra-acromial (sū-prä-ăk-rō′mĭ-ăl). Located above the acromion.

supra-auricular (sū″prä-aw-rĭk′ū-lar). Located above an auricle.

supracapsulin (sū″prä-kăp′sū-lĭn). Commercial preparation of active principle of medulla of the suprarenals. SYN: *epinephrine*.

supracerebellar (sū″prä-sĕr-ē-bĕl′ar). On or above the upper surface of the cerebellum.

suprachoroid (sū″prä-kō′royd). Upon the outer side of the choroid of the eye.

   s. lam′ina. Connective tissue bet. the sclerotic coats of the eye and the choroid. SYN: *suprachoroidea*.

suprachoroidea (sū″prä-ko-roy′dē-ă). Outermost layer of the choroid. SYN: *suprachoroid lamina*.

supraclavicular (sū″prä-klä-vĭk′ū-lar). Located above the clavicle.

   s. fossa. Depression on either side of neck reaching down behind the clavicle.

   s. point. A stimulation point over the clavicle at which contraction of arm muscles may be produced.

supracommissure (sū″prä-kŏm′mĭ-shūr). A cerebral commissure ant. to the stalk of the pineal body.

supracondylar (sū″prä-kŏn′dĭl-ar). Above a condyle.

supracostal (sū″prä-kŏs′tăl). Above or beyond the ribs.

supracotyloid (sū″pră-kŏt′ĭ-loyd). Above the acetabulum or cotyloid body.

supracranial (sū″pră-krā′nĭ-ăl). On the upper surface of the skull.

supradiaphragmatic (sū″pră-dī″ă-frăg-mat′ĭk). Above the diaphragm.

supra-epicondylar (sū″pră-ĕp″ĭ-kŏn′dĭ-lar). Above an epicondyle.

supraglenoid (sū″pră-glē′noyd). Above the glenoid cavity or fossa.

s. tubercle. A rough surface of the scapula above glenoid cavity to which is attached the large head of the biceps muscle.

suprahyoid (sū″pră-hī′oyd). Located above the hyoid bone; denoting accessory thyroid glands within the geniohyoid muscle.

s. muscles. The digastric, geniohyoid, mylohyoid, and stylohyoid muscles.

suprainguinal (sū″pră-ĭn′gwĭn-ăl). Above the groin.

supraliminal (sū″pră-lĭm′ĭ-năl). Psy: 1. Above the threshold of consciousness; conscious. 2. Exceeding the stimulus threshold. See: subliminal.

supralumbar (sū″pră-lŭm′bar). Above the lumbar region.

supramalleolar (sū″pră-mal-lē′ō-lar). Located above either malleolus.

supramarginal (sū″pră-mar′jĭn-ăl). Above any border.

s. convolution, s. gyrus. A cerebral convolution on lateral surface of the parietal lobe above post. part of sylvian fissure.

supramastoid (sū″pră-măs′toyd). Above the mastoid process of the temporal bone.

s. crest. A ridge on the temporal bone.

supramaxilla (sū″pră-măks-ĭl′lă). The upper jawbone. Syn: maxilla.

supramaxillary (sū″pră-măks′ĭl-lă-rĭ). 1. Relating to the upper jaw. 2. Located above the upper jaw.

suprameatal (sū″pră-mē-ā′tăl). Above a meatus, esp. the ext. auditory meatus, noting the spine of Henle, a small, bony projection at post. sup. margin of ext. auditory meatus.

s. triangle. Triangular space bordered by upper half of post. wall of ext. auditory meatus, and the supramastoid crest used to locate the mastoid antrum.

supraoccipital bone (sū″pră-ŏk-sĭp′ĭ-tăl). Situated above the occiput, noting a portion of occipital bone above the foramen magnum forming part of occipital bone in the adult but distinct in early childhood.

supraorbital (sū″pră-or′bĭ-tăl). Located above the orbit.

s. neuralgia. Neuralgia of the supraorbital nerve. Syn: hemicrania.

s. reflex. Contraction of orbicularis palpebrarum with closure of lids resulting from percussion above supraorbital nerve.

s. ridge. Prominence on frontal bone over eye caused by projection of frontal air sinuses.

suprapelvic (sū″pră-pĕl′vĭk). Located above the pelvis.

suprapontine (sū″pră-pŏn′tĭn). Located above the pons Varolii.

suprapubic (sū″pră-pū′bĭk). Above the pubic arch.

s. cystotomy. Surgical opening of the bladder from just above the symphysis pubis.

s. reflex. Deflection of linea alba toward stroked side when abdomen is stroked above Poupart's ligament.

suprarenal (sū″pră-rē′năl). 1. Above the kidney. 2. Tiny gland above each kidney. Syn: adrenal, suprarenal body, suprarenal capsule, suprarenal gland. 3. Pert. to the suprarenal gland.

s. body, s. capsule, s. gland. Small, flat body above each kidney, the left one larger than the right, composed of a cortex and a medulla differing in function and secreting epinephrine. See: medulla, below.

suprarenalemia (sū″pră-rē-năl-ē′mĭ-ă). Undue amt. of adrenalin, the suprarenal secretion, in the blood.

suprarenalism (sū″pră-rē′năl-ĭzm). The condition resulting from overactivity of the suprarenal glands.

suprarenalopathy (sū″pră-rē-năl-ŏp′ă-thĭ). A disorder due to abnormal functioning of the suprarenal glands.

suprarenogenic (sū″pră-rē″no-jĕn′ĭk). Of suprarenal origin.

s. syndrome. Suprarenalism characterized by adiposity; hirsuties, and pigmentation, and amenorrhea in women.

suprarenoma (sū″pră-rē-nō′mă). Suprarenal tissue tumor.

suprarenopathy (sū″pră-rē-nŏp′ă-thĭ). Any disorder of the suprarenal glands.

suprarenotropic (sū″pră-rē-nō-trŏp′ĭk). 1. Having an influence on the suprarenal secretion; said of an ant. pituitary hormone. 2. Characterized by suprarenal influence on development.

suprascapular (sū″pră-skăp′ū-lar). Located above the scapula.

suprasellar (sū″pră-sĕl′ar). Above or over the sella turcica.

suprasonic (sū″pră-sŏn′ĭk). Noting sound with frequencies of vibration above 34,-000 per second, probably heard by some animals.

supraspinal (sū″pră-spī′năl). Above a spine or the spinal column.

supraspinous (sū″pră-spī′nŭs). Above any spine.

s. fossa. A groove above the spine of the scapula.

suprasternal (sū″pră-ster′năl). Above the sternum. Syn: episternal.

suprasylvian (sū″pră-sĭl′vĭ-ăn). Above the fissure of Sylvius.

s. convolution. One above the post. limb of the sylvian fissure. Syn: supramarginal convolution.

supratrochlear (sū″pră-trŏk′lē-ar). Above a trochlea, esp. that of the humerus.

supravaginal (sū″pră-văj′ĭ-năl). Above the vagina or any sheathing membrane.

sura (sū′ră). The calf of the leg.

sural (sū′răl). Relating to the calf of the leg.

suralimentation (sŭr-ăl-ĭm-ĕn-tā′shŭn). Treatment by overfeeding. SYN: *gavage, superalimentation*.

surdity (sŭr′dĭ-tĭ). Inability to hear. SYN: *deafness*.

surdomute (sŭr′dō-mūt″). 1. A deaf-mute. 2. Deaf and dumb.

surface (sur′făs). The outer integument of any body.

   s. tension. Intramolecular attraction inward at the surface of a liquid.

surgeon (sŭr′jŭn). A medical practitioner who specializes in surgery.

   s., dental. A dentist authorized to operate on the mouth and teeth. SYN: *stomatologist*.

   s., house. The chief surgical intern in a hospital.

surgery (sur′jur-ĭ). 1. Branch of medicine dealing with manual and operative procedures for correction of deformities and defects, repair of injuries, diagnosis and cure of disease, relief of suffering and prolongation of life. SYN: *chirurgery, chirurgia*. 2. Surgeon's operating room.

   s., major. Important and serious operations involving risk to life.

   s., minor. Simple, less serious operations.

   s., orificial. Treatment of orifices of the body based on theory that many disorders are due to reflexes at the anus and other orifices.

   s., orthopedic. Surgery for correction of deformities.

   s., plastic. Repair of parts by transference.

surgical (sur′jĭk-ăl). Of the nature of or pert. to surgery.

   s. diathermy. The use of high-frequency electrical oscillations in such a way that animal tissues are destroyed.

   s. dressing. Sterile protective covering of gauze or other substance applied to an operative wound. SEE: *chemise*.

   s. fever. Fever following an operation or injury.

   s. kidney. Suppuration of the kidney subsequent to surgery on the genitourinary tract.

   s. neck. Constricted part of shaft of humerus below the tuberosities; commonly the seat of fracture.

surgiology (sŭr-jĭ-ŏl′ō-jĭ). Surgery for experimental purposes in physiology.

surrogate (sŭr′rō-gāt). Something that replaces another; a substitute.

sursumduction (sŭr″sŭm-dŭk′shŭn). Elevation, as the power or act of turning an eye upward independently of the other one.

sursumvergence (sŭr″sŭm-vĕr′jĕns). An upward turning, as of the eyeballs.

sursumversion (sŭr″sŭm-vĕr′shŭn). Process of turning upward; simultaneous movement of both eyes upward.

susceptible (sŭs-sĕp′tĭ-bl). 1. Having little resistance to a disease or foreign protein. 2. An individual with little re-

sistance to an infectious disease or who is not known to have become immune to one. 3. Easily impressed or influenced.

suscitate (sŭs′sĭ-tăt). To arouse to increased activity; to stimulate.

suscitation (sŭs″sĭ-tā′shŭn). Act of stimulating to greater activity. SYN: *excitation*.

suspended (sŭs-pĕnd′ĕd). 1. Hanging. 2. Temporarily inactive.

   s. animation. A cessation of the vital functions temporarily.

suspension (sŭs-pĕn′shŭn). 1. A condition of temporary cessation, as of any vital process. 2. Treatment by immobilization of a part or whole of a patient by hanging in desired position. 3. State of a solid when its particles are mixed with, but not dissolved in, a fluid or another solid; also a substance in this state.

   s., cephalic. Suspension of a patient by the head to extend the vertebral column.

   s. colloid. Solution containing very tiny, solid, dispersed particles. SYN: *suspensoid*.

   s. stability. Degree of speed with which erythrocytes sink to bottom in a mass of citrated blood. SYN: *sedimentation rate*.

   s. of the uterus. The operation of attaching the uterus to the abdominal wall.

suspensoid (sŭs-pĕn′soyd). A colloid solution in which the dispersed particles are solid, as distinguished from *emulsoid*. SYN: *suspension colloid*.

suspensory (sŭs-pĕn′sōr-ĭ). 1. Supporting a part, as a muscle, ligament, or bone. 2. A structure of the body which supports a part. 3. Bandage or sac for supporting or compressing a part, esp. the scrotum.   [the testicles.

   s. bandage. A sling for support of

suspirious (sŭs-pī′rĭ-ŭs). Breathing with apparent effort; sighing.

sustentacular (sŭs-tĕn-tăk′ū-lar). Supporting; upholding.

   s. cell. A supporting cell, esp. a branching connective tissue cell of the spleen.

sustentaculum (sŭs-tĕn-tăk′ū-lŭm). A supporting structure.

   s. lieni. Phrenocolic ligament which apparently supports the spleen.

   s. tali. A process of the calcaneum which supports part of the astragalus.

susurrus (sū-sŭr′ŭs). A murmur.

sutura (sū-tū′ră) (pl. *suturae*). Suture.

   s. denta′ta. One with interlocking of bones by toothlike processes.

   s. harmo′nia. Simple apposition of 2 contiguous bones.

   s. limbo′sa. Bevelled suture in which opposing margins fit in parallel ridges, as the interparietal surfaces.

   s. no′tha. A false suture with ill-defined projections.

   s. serra′ta. One with deeper and more irregular indentations than a dental sutura.

s. squamo'sa. A scalelike suture.

sutural (sū'tū-răl). Relating to a suture.

s. joint. Articulation bet. 2 bones.

s. ligament. Fibers uniting opposed bones forming a cranial suture.

suturation (sū″tū-rā'shŭn). Application of sutures; stitching.

suture (sū'tūr). 1. Line of union in an immovable articulation, as those bet. the skull bones; also such an articulation itself. SYN: *synarthrosis.* 2. Operation of uniting parts by stitching them together. 3. The thread or wire or other material used in the operation of stitching parts of the body together. 4. The seam or line of union formed by surgical stitches. 5. To unite by stitching, as *to suture a wound.* SEE: *raphe.*

s., absorbable. Suture undergoing liquefaction or replaced by living tissue.

s., basilar. The one bet. the occipital bone and sphenoid bone.

s., bifrontal. SEE: *coronal suture.*

s., biparietal. SEE: *sagittal suture.*

s's., buried. Those completely covered by skin and not involving that structure at all.

s., button. One in which the threads are passed through buttons on the surface and tied to prevent the thread from cutting.

s., coaptation. One uniting as distinguished from one intended to relieve tension.

s., cobbler's. A suture in which the thread has a needle at each end.

s., continuous. The closure of a wound by means of 1 continuous thread, usually by transfixing first 1 lip and then the other, alternately, from within outward.

s., coronal. The junction of the frontal and parietal bones.

s's., cranial. Those sutures bet. the bones of the skull.

s., dentate. An articulation of long and toothlike processes.

s., ethmoidofrontal. The one bet. the ethmoid and frontal bones.

s., ethmoidolacrimal. The one bet. the ethmoid and lacrimal bones.

s., ethmosphenoid. The one bet. the ethmoid and sphenoid bones.

s., false. Any form of suture in which one surface is smooth.

s., figure-of-eight. SEE: *twisted suture.*

s., frontal. An occasional one in the frontal bone from the sagittal suture to root of nose.

s., frontolacrimal. The one bet. the frontal and lacrimal bones.

s., frontomalar. The one bet. the frontal and malar bones.

s., frontomaxillary. The one bet. the frontal bone and sup. maxilla.

s., frontonasal. The one bet. the frontal bone and the alae of the sphenoid bone.

s., frontoparietal. The coronoid suture.

s., frontotemporal. The one bet. the frontal and temporal bones.

s., Glover's. A continuous suture in which the needle is, after each stitch, passed through the loop of the preceding stitch.

s., harelip. SEE: *twisted suture.*

s., harmonic. One in which there is simple apposition of bone.

s., horsehair. Suture adapted for light, superficial sutures, alternated with heavier ones and for exposed places like the face, where scar tissue is to be avoided. *Dry,* 100 strands in a bunch. *Sterilized,* 50 in a bottle.

s., implanted. A suture formed by placing pins opposite each other on the 2 sides of a wound, and approximating the lips by winding thread or other similar material about the pins.

s., intermaxillary. The suture bet. the sup. maxillae.

s., internasal. The one bet. the nasal bones.

s., interparietal. SEE: *sagittal suture.*

s., interrupted. A suture formed by single stitches inserted separately, the needle being usually passed through 1 lip from without inward, and through the other from within outward.

s., jugal. SEE: *sagittal suture.*

s., lambdoid. The one bet. the parietal bones and the 2 sup. borders of the occipital bone.

s., Lembert's. An intestinal suture.

s., longitudinal. SEE: *sagittal suture.*

s., mattress. A continuous suture in which a stitch is taken with a needle, the thread tied, and then needle inserted upon the same side as that from which it emerged and passed in opposite direction through both lips of the wound, the direction of the needle being reversed at each stitch.

s., maxillolacrimal. The one bet. the maxilla and lacrimal bone.

s., maxillopremaxillary. One bet. the premaxillary portion of sup. maxilla and rest of the bone.

s., mediofrontal. SEE: *frontal suture.*

s., metopic. SEE: *frontal suture.*

s., nasomaxillary. The one bet. the nasal bone and sup. maxilla.

s., nonabsorbable. Silk, silkworm gut, horsehair, and wire.

s., occipital. SEE: *lambdoid suture.*

s., occipitomastoid. The one bet. the occipital bone and mastoid portion of temporal bone.   [*ture.*

s., occipitoparietal. SEE: *lambdoid suture.*

s., palatine. One bet. the palate bones.

s., palatine transverse. One bet. the palate processes of palate bone and sup. maxilla.

s., parietal. SEE: *sagittal suture.*

s., parietomastoid. The one bet. the parietal bone and mastoid portion of the temporal bone.

s., petroöccipital. The one bet. the petrous portion of the temporal bone and occipital bone.

s., petrosphenoidal. The one bet. petrous portion of the temporal bone and ala magna of sphenoid bone.

s., quilled; s., quill. An interrupted suture in which a double thread is passed deep into the tissues, even quite below the bottom of the wound, needle being so withdrawn as to leave a loop hanging from 1 lip and the 2 free ends of the thread from the other. A quill, or, more commonly, a piece of bougie, is passed through the loops, which are tightened upon it and the free ends of each separate thread are then tied together over a second quill. The object is to bring the deep parts into firm coaptation and to relieve tension.

s., relaxation. A suture that may be loosened if the tension of the wound becomes excessive.

s., relief. A row of supplementary sutures including the tissues to the extent of 1 or 1½ in. on each side of a fistula or a deep wound, for the purpose of lessening the strain on the coaptation sutures.

s., right-angled. A suture used in sewing intestine. The needle is passed in the same direction as the long axis of the incision and the process repeated on the opposite side of the incision, the suture being continuous.

s., Sabatier's. Approximation of an intestinal wound by using cardboard soaked in turpentine oil.

s., sagittal. The suture bet. upper margins of parietal bones.

s., serrated. An articulation by suture in which there is an interlocking of bones by small, fine, and delicate projections and indentations.

s., shotted. A suture in which both ends of a wire or silkworm gut are passed through a perforated shot that is then compressed tightly over them.

s., silk. Does not produce suppuration if sterilized. Twisted, braided, and floss.

s., silkworm gut. Causes little friction, pliable, does not curl or twist, less liable to produce irritation, and sterilizable. Should always be soaked in a sterile solution 30 minutes.

s., sphenoparietal. The one bet. the parietal bone and ala magna of the sphenoid bone.

s., sphenosquamous. Articulation of the large wing of the sphenoid with the squamous portion of the temporal bone.

s., sphenotemporal. The one bet. the sphenoid and temporal bones.

s., squamoparietal; s., squamosal. The one bet. the parietal and squamous portion of the temporal bone.

s., squamosphenoidal. One bet. the squamous portion of the temporal bone and great wing of sphenoid.

s., subcuticular. A buried continuous suture in which needle is passed horizontally under epidermis into cutis vera emerging at angle of wound, then in a similar manner passed through cutis vera of opposite side of wound, and so on until other angle of wound is reached.

s., temporoöccipital. SEE: *occipito-mastoid suture*

s., temporoparietal. One bet. the temporal and parietal bones.

s., twisted. A suture in which pins are passed through the opposite lips of a wound, at right angles to direction of wound, and material is wound about the pins, crossing them first at one end and then at the other in a figure-of-eight fashion, thus holding the lips of the wound firmly together.

s., uninterrupted. SEE: *continuous suture.*

s., wire. Usually silver. Adapted for cases where there is much tension, ends of bones, resection, etc.

s., zygomatic. One bet. the zygomatic process of sup. maxilla and temporal bone.

Suzanne's gland (sū-zanz′). A small mucous gland in floor of the mouth, below the alveolingual groove.

swab (swŏb). 1. Cotton or gauze on end of slender stick used for cleansing cavities, applying remedies or for obtaining a piece of tissue or secretion for bacteriological examination. 2. To wipe with a swab, as to *swab a wound.*

s., test tube. For cleansing tubes, etc.

s., urethral. Slender rod for holding cotton, used in examinations with speculum, in treating ulcers, removing secretions, etc.

s., u., male. About 7 in. long.

s., uterine. For absorbing or wiping away discharges. Slender, flattened wire, plain rod or one with coarse thread on distal end.

swallow (swŏl′ō). To pass into the stomach through the mouth and throat.

swallowing (swŏl′ō-ĭng). 1. A complicated act usually initiated voluntarily but always completely reflexly whereby food is moved from the mouth through the pharynx and esophagus to the stomach. 2. Performance of motions characteristic of swallowing, as in emotion. Movements of the tongue must first get the material into the back of the mouth. Further muscular activity prevents it from returning; the post. nares are closed; the glottis is closed and protected by special mechanisms, and the contraction of the musculi constrictores pharyngis forces the food into the esophagus.

s. reflex. Swallowing induced by stimulation of soft palate.

swallow's nest (swŏl′ōz). Cerebral depression bet. the uvula and the post. velum. SYN: *nidus hirundinis.*

sweat (swĕt). 1. The secretion of the sudoriparous glands of the skin. SYN: *perspiration, sudor.* SEE: *glands, Moll's.* 2. Condition of perspiring or of being made to perspire freely, as to order a sweat for a patient. 3. To emit moisture through the skin's pores. SYN: *perspire.* 4. To cause to emit moisture through the pores.

s., bloody. Sweat tinged with blood. SYN: *hematidrosis.*

s. center. Medullary area controlling sweating.

s., colored. Sweat tinged with a pigment. SYN: *chromidrosis.*

s., fetid. Sweat with foul odor. SYN: *bromidrosis.*

s. glands. These are invaginated, epithelial, tubular, coil glands which penetrate the corium* into the subcutaneous fatty tissue and which secrete sweat.

s., night. Sweating during the night, a symptom of pulmonary tuberculosis.

s., profuse. Excessive perspiration. SYN: *hyperidrosis.*

s., scanty. Abnormally small amount or lack of sweat. SYN: *anidrosis.*

sweating (swĕt′ĭng). 1. Act of exuding sweat. 2. Emitting sweat. 3. Causing profuse sweating.

Swedish gymnastics, movements. System of active and passive exercise of the various muscles and joints of the body without using apparatus.

S. massage. Massage combined with Swedish gymnastics.

sweet (swēt). 1. Pleasant to the taste or smell. SEE: *taste,* 2. Free from excess of acid, sulfur, or corrosive salts.

swelling (swĕl′ĭng). A morbid enlargement, esp. one appearing on the surface of the body.

s., albuminous. Same as cloudy swelling.

s., cloudy. Degeneration of tissues marked by cloudy appearance, swelling, and appearance of tiny albuminoid granules in the cells.

s., glassy. Starchy degeneration of tissue. SYN: *amyloid degeneration.*

s., white. Swelling seen in tuberculous arthritis, esp. of the knee.

Swift's disease (swĭft). Condition occurring in very young children characterized by irritability and restlessness; redness and swelling of the hands and feet, esp. on the palms and soles; desquamation; a sensation of tingling or burning; loss of appetite, and the appearance of a rash, mainly on the trunk, and loss of muscle tone. SYN: *acrodynia.*

switch, foot. In the application of surgical, high-frequency currents where both hands of the operator are needed, the current is started and cut off by a foot switch.

s., pole-changing. P.T. A switch by which the polarity of a circuit may be reversed.

swoon (swōōn). 1. A syncope* or fainting fit. 2. To sink into a fainting fit.

sycoma (sī-kō′mǎ). A large, soft wart. SYN: *condyloma.*

sycophancy (sĭk′ō-făn-sĭ). PSY: Characteristics of one maturely intelligent who has not developed a sense of responsibility and who is more or less dependent upon others.

sycophant (sĭk′ō-fănt). An adult who, though mature intellectually, lacks a sense of responsibility.

sycosiform (sī-kō′sĭ-form). Resembling sycosis.

sycosis (sī-kō′sĭs). Chronic inflammation of hair follicles.

s. barbae. Sycosis of the beard, marked by papules and pustules perforated by hairs, and surrounded by infiltrated skin. SYN: *folliculitis barbae.*

s. tinea. A form due to infection with ringworm commonly affecting the beard.

s. vulgaris. Same as sycosis.

Sydenham's chorea (sĭd′ĕn-hăm). Simple chorea with only mild convulsive movements.

S.'s cough. Cough produced in hysteria by spasm of respiratory muscles.

syllabic utterance (sĭl-ab′ĭk). A staccato accentuation of syllables, slowly but separately, observed in multiple *sclerosis.* SYN: *scanning speech.*

syllable stumbling (sĭl′ă-bl). Hesitating utterance (dysphasia) with difficulty in pronouncing certain syllables.

syllabus (sĭl′ă-bŭs). Abstract of a lecture or outline of a course of study or of a book.

syllepsiology (sĭl-lĕp-sĭ-ol′ō-jĭ). The study of conception and pregnancy.

syllepsis (sĭl-ĕp′sĭs). Conception; impregnation, or pregnancy.

Sylvester's method. Method of artificial respiration by drawing arms of a supine patient out above head, and then bringing them down folded onto the chest, with pressure on the abdomen and ribs to cause expiration.

sylvian aqueduct (sĭl′vĭ-ăn). A narrow canal from 3rd to 4th ventricle. SYN: *aqueduct of Sylvius.*

s. artery. Middle cerebral artery in the fissure of Sylvius.

s. fissure. The fissure separating the temporal lobe from the frontal and parietal lobes.

s. line. One on ext. of cranium marking direction of the sylvian fissure.

sym-, syn-. Combining form meaning *with, along, together with, beside.*

symbion, symbiont (sĭm′bĭ-ŏn, -ŏnt). An organism which lives with another to their mutual advantage. SYN: *commensal.*

symbiosis (sĭm-bĭ-ō′sĭs). 1. The association of 2 diverse nonparasitic organisms dependent upon each other for existence or where the association is advantageous. 2. PSY: Incorporation of a symptom as a part of one's personality, as delusions of grandeur, seen in paranoia.

symblepharon (sĭm-blĕf′ă-rŏn). Adhesion bet. conjunctivae of lid and eyeball due to injuries, esp. burns from lime, acids, etc.

symbol (sĭm′bŏl). 1. A representation of an idea or quality in the form of an object or that which stands for something beside itself.

2. PSY: An object used as an unconscious substitute and which is not connected consciously with the libido, but into which the libido is concentrated.

3. CHEM: A mark or letter representing an atom of an element.

symbolism (sĭm′bŏl-ĭzm). PSY: 1. Unconscious substitutive expression of subconscious thoughts of sexual significance in terms recognized by the objective consciousness.

2. An abnormal condition in which everything that occurs is interpreted as a symbol of the patient's own thoughts.

symbolophobia (sĭm-bō-lō-fō'bĭ-ă). Fear of expressing one's self in words or action that may be interpreted as possessing a symbolic meaning.

Syme's operation (sīm). 1. Amputation of the foot at the ankle joint with removal of the malleoli. 2. Excision of the tongue. 3. External urethrotomy.

symmetric, symmetrical (sĭm-ĕt'rĭk, -rĭ-kl). 1. Exhibiting correspondence in size and shape of parts. 2. CHEM: Denoting an atomic arrangement in a molecule at equal relative intervals.

s. gangrene. Gangrene affecting corresponding parts simultaneously and similarly. SYN: *Raynaud's disease, q.v.*

symmetromania (sĭm″ĕ-trō-mā'nĭ-ă). An abnormal impulse to make symmetrical motions with the arms.

symmetry (sĭm'ĕt-rĭ). Correspondence in shape, size, and relative position of parts on opposite sides of a body.

sympathectomy (sĭm-pă-thek'tō-mĭ). Partial excision of sympathetic nerve.

s., chemical. The use of chemicals to destroy part of the sympathetic nerve.

s., periarterial. Removal of sheath of an artery in which are the sympathetic nerve fibers, used in trophic disturbances.

sympatheoneuritis (sĭm-păth″ē-ō-nū-rī'tĭs). Inflammation of the sympathetic nerve.

sympathesis (sĭm-păth'ē-sĭs). The morbid tendencies of the organism as a whole.

sympathetic (sĭm-pă-thĕt'ĭk). 1. Pert. to a special set of nerves and ganglia, uniting all parts of the body and subjecting them to a common involuntary nerve impulse. SEE: *autonomic system.* 2. Caused by or pert. to sympathy.

s. irritation. Irritation of a structure caused by irritation of another related structure.

s. nerves, s. nervous system. A division of the autonomic* nervous system consisting of a pair of ganglionated cords, 1 on each side of the entire vertebral column, connected with the thoracic and lumbar parts of spinal cord by means of *rami communicantes,* and communicating visceral, sensory, and preganglionic fibers, distributing to the viscera of the abdomen, and pelvis, the heart and lungs, the peripheral blood vessels, glands and smooth muscles of the skin.

s. ophthalmia. Inflammation of the uveal tract in one eye due to similar inflammation in the other eye.

s. plexuses. Plexuses formed at intervals by the sympathetic nerves and ganglia.

sympatheticalgia (sĭm-pă-thĕt-ĭ-kal'jĭ-ă). Pain in the cervical sympathetic ganglion.

sympatheticless (sĭm-pă-thĕt'ĭk-lĕs). Noting absence of the abdominal sympathetic chain.

sympatheticoparalytic (sĭm-pă-thĕt″ĭk-ō-par-ăl-ĭt'ĭk). Resulting from paralysis of the sympathetic nervous system.

sympatheticopathy (sĭm-pă-thĕt-ĭ-kŏp'ă-thĭ). Any condition resulting from disorder of the sympathetic nervous system.

sympatheticotonia (sĭm-pă-thĕt″ĭk-ō-tō'nĭ-ă). Condition characterized by excessive tone of the sympathetic nervous system with unusually high blood pressure and tendency to vascular spasm. SYN: *sympathicotonia.*

sympatheticotonic (sĭm-păth-ĕt″ĭk-ō-ton'ĭk). Marked by increased arterial tone or vasoconstriction due to overaction of the sympathetic nervous system.

sympatheticotripsy (sĭm-pă-thĕt″ĭk-ō-trĭp'sĭ). Surgical crushing of the sup. cervical ganglion in treatment of mental diseases.

sympathicectomy (sĭm-păth-ĭs-ĕk'tō-mĭ). Excision of part of the sympathetic nerve. SYN: *sympathectomy.*

sympathicoblast (sĭm-păth'ĭ-kō-blăst). A primitive sympathetic nerve cell. SEE: *sympathoblast.*

sympathicoblastoma (sĭm-păth″ĭk-ō-blăs-tō'mă). A tumor made up of sympathicoblasts.

sympathicomimetic (sĭm-păth″ĭk-ō-mĭm-ĕt'ĭk). Simulating action of adrenalin, said of stimulants of the sympathetic nervous system. SYN: *adrenergic.*

sympathiconeuritis (sĭm-păth″ĭk-ō-nū-rī'tĭs). Inflammation of the sympathetic nerves.

sympathicotonia (sĭm-păth″ĭ-kō-tō'nĭ-ă). Increased tonus of the sympathetic system with marked tendency to vascular spasm and heightened blood pressure. OPP: *vagotonia.*

sympathicotripsy (sĭm-păth″ĭk-ō-trĭp'sĭ). Crushing of the sup. cervical ganglion in treatment of mental diseases. SYN: *sympatheticotripsy.*

sympathicotropic (sĭm-păth″ĭ-kō-trop'ĭk). Having a special affinity for the sympathetic nerve.

sympathicus (sĭm-păth'ĭ-kŭs). The sympathetic nervous system. SYN: *systema nervorum sympathicum.*

sympathin (sĭm'păth-ĭn). An assumed hormone produced in the body by the sympathetic nerves which stimulates cardiac action and parts controlled by impulses of sympathetic nervous system.

sympathism (sĭm'păth-ĭzm). Condition of susceptibility to suggestion. SYN: *suggestibility.*

sympathoblast (sĭm-păth'ō-blăst). A primitive cell from which arises a sympathetic ganglion cell.

sympathoblastoma (sĭm″păth-ō-blăs-tō'mă). A malignant tumor made up of sympathetic nerve cells.

sympathoglioblastoma (sĭm″păth-ō-glī'ō-blăs-tō'mă). A tumor made up primarily of sympathoblasts, with scattered neuroblasts and spongioblasts.

sympathogonia (sĭm″păth-ō-gō′nĭ-ă). Primitive cells from which sympathetic cells are derived.

sympathogonioma (sĭm″păth-ō-gō-nĭ-ō′-mă). A tumor containing sympathogonia.

sympathoma (sĭm-păth-ō′mă). A tumor composed of tissue similar to that of the sympathetic nervous system.

sympathomimetic (sĭm″păth-ō-mĭm-ĕt′ĭk). Capable of stimulating or inhibiting sympathetic nerve endings. SYN: *adrenergic.*

sympathy (sĭm′pă-thĭ). 1. Relationship bet. 2 organs or parts through which 1 unaffected part is affected or becomes disordered from disease in the other part without actual transmission of morbific cause. 2. Mental influence exerted by one person on another, as in yawning or transmission of hysterical symptoms from one to another.

sympexion (sĭm-pĕks′ĭ-on). A concretion in the seminal vessels, the thyroid and lymphatic glands.

sympexis (sĭm-pĕks′ĭs). Term for arrangement of red blood cells in harmony with the laws of surface tension.

symphalangism (sĭm-făl′ăn-jĭzm). 1. Ankylosis of joints of the fingers or toes. 2. Web-fingered or web-toed condition.

symphyseal (sĭm-fĭz′ē-ăl). Pert. to symphysis.

symphyseotomy (sĭm-fĭz-ē-ŏt′ō-mĭ). Section of symphysis pubis to enlarge the pelvic diameters during delivery.

symphysiectomy (sĭm-fĭz-ĭ-ĕk′tō-mĭ). Section of the symphysis pubis to facilitate delivery.

symphysion (sĭm-fĭz′ĭ-ŏn). Most ant. point of the alveolar process of the lower jaw.

symphysiotomy (sĭm″fĭz-ĭ-ŏt′ō-mĭ). Section of symphysis pubis to facilitate delivery by enlarging pelvic diameters.

symphysis (sĭm′fĭz-ĭs) (pl. *symphyses*). 1. The joint or point of junction and fusion by fibrocartilage bet. bones originally distinct. 2. Union of any 2 structures. 3. A morbid adhesion.

 s., cardiac. The adhesion of the parietal and visceral layers of the pericardium. SEE: *intervertebral disk.*

 s. of jaw. An ant., median, vertical ridge upon outer surface of lower jaw representing line of union of its 2 halves.

 s. mandibulae. The central line of union of the 2 halves of the mandible.

 s. pubis. The junction of the pubic bones on midline in front; bony eminence under the pubic hair. SEE: *disk, interpubic.*

sympodia (sĭm-pō′dĭ-ă). Condition in which lower extremities are united.

symptom (sĭmp′tŭm). Any perceptible change in the body or its functions which indicates disease or the kind or phases of disease.

 s's., cardinal. Those pert. to pulse, respiration, and temperature.

 s. complex. The entire group of symptoms presenting a clear picture of a disease. SYN: *syndrome.**

 s., constitutional; s., general. One caused by or indicating disease of the whole body.

 s. of Magendi. Deviation of 1 eye up and out, and the other down, produced by division of the restiform body.

 s's., objective. Those that are manifested externally and which are apparent to the observer.

 s., pathognomonic. One which unmistakably points out presence of a particular disease.

 s's., prodromal. Those which indicate an approaching disease. SYN: *prodrome.**

 s's., subjective. Those that have an internal origin and are perceptible to the patient only, including mental symptoms.

 s's., withdrawal. Those following sudden withdrawal of a stimulant from an addict, generally excitement and collapse.

symptomatic (sĭmp-tō-măt′ĭk). Of the nature of or concerning a symptom.

symptomatology (sĭmp-tō-mă-tŏl′ō-jĭ). 1. Science of symptoms and indications. SYN: *semeiology.* 2. All of the symptoms of a given disease as a whole.

symptomatolytic (sĭmp″tō-măt″ō-lĭt′ĭk). Causing the removal of symptoms.

symp′tom com′plex. All of the symptoms of a disease forming together a picture of it. SYN: *syndrome.*

symptomolytic (sĭmp-tō-mō-lĭt′ĭk). Pert. to the removal of symptoms. SYN: *symptomatolytic.*

syn-. Prefix meaning *joined, together.* SEE: *prefix con.*

synalgia (sĭn-ăl′jĭ-ă). Referred or reflex pain felt in a part distant from the site of its origin.

synalgic (sĭn-ăl′jĭk). Pert. to or characterized by referred pain.

synanastomosis (sĭn″an-as″tō-mō′sĭs). The connection of several vessels.

synanthema (sĭn-ăn-thē′mă). Exanthem made up of several different forms of eruption.

synapse, synapsis (sĭn′ăps, sĭn-ăp′sĭs). 1. The minute space or apparent meeting point bet. the terminal arborization of the axon of 1 neuron and the dendrites of another. There is no actual communication, but the synapse functions possibly by either modifying or intensifying the nerve impulse as it passes through. SEE: *nerve.* 2. Process of pairing off of chromosomes from the male and female pronuclei in the ovum. SYN: *syndesis.*

synaptase (sĭn-ăp′tās). A hydrolyzing enzyme found in almonds and certain fungi. SYN: *emulsin.*

synarthrodia (sĭn-ăr-thrō′dĭ-ă). Type of immovable cartilaginous joint without a joint cavity in which bones are separated by only a connective tissue membrane; a fixed articulation. SYN: *synarthrosis.* SEE: *joint.*

synarthrodial (sĭn-ar-thrō′dĭ-ăl). Pert. to an immovable articulation bet. bones.

synarthrosis (sĭn″ar-thrō′sĭs) (pl. *synar-*

throses). An immovable joint in which there is no disk of intervening tissue bet. the bones.

syncanthus (sĭn-kăn'thŭs). Adhesion of eyeball to the structures of the orbit.

synchilia (sĭn-kĭ'lĭ-ă). Adhesion or imperforation (*atresia*) of the lips.

synchiria (sĭn-kĭ'rĭ-ă). Disorder of sensibility in which stimulus is referred to the opposite side of the body from that to which it was applied. SYN: *allochiria.*

synchondroseotomy (sĭn-kŏn-drŏ-sē-ŏt'ō-mĭ). An operation of cutting through the sacroiliac ligaments and closing the arch of the pubes in congenital absence of the ant. wall of the bladder (*exstrophy*).

synchondrosis (sĭn-kŏn-drŏ'sĭs). An immovable joint having the surfaces bet. the bones connected by cartilages.

synchondrotomy (sĭn-kŏn-drŏt'ō-mĭ). 1. Division of articulating cartilage. 2. Section of the symphysis pubis to facilitate childbirth. SEE: *symphyseotomy.*

synchronism (sĭn'krō-nĭzm). Occurrence of acts or events simultaneously.

synchronous (sĭn'krŏn-ŭs). Occurring simultaneously.

synchysis (sĭn'kĭs-ĭs). Fluid state of vitreous of the eye.

  s. *scintil'lans.* Abnormally fluid vitreous, with presence of floating cholesterin crystals.

syncinesis (sĭn-sĭn-ē'sĭs). An involuntary movement produced in association with a voluntary one.

  s., *imitative.* Occurs on sound side when movement is attempted on paralyzed side.

  s., *spasmodic.* Occurs on hemiplegic side when msucles of opp. side are voluntarily moved.

synciput (sĭn'sĭp-ŭt). Ant. upper half of the cranium. SYN: *sinciput.*

synclitism (sĭn'klĭt-ĭzm). Parallelism bet. the planes of the fetal head and those of the maternal pelvis.

synclonus (sĭn'klō-nŭs). 1. Clonic contraction of several muscles together. 2. A disease marked by muscular spasms.

syncopal (sĭn'kō-păl). Relating to or marked by syncope.

syncope (sĭn'kō-pē). A transient form of unconsciousness, during which the person slumps to the ground. SYN: *fainting, swoon.*

  s. *angio'sa.* Cardiac spasm due to occlusion of coronary arteries.

  s., *laryngeal.* Brief unconsciousness following coughing and tickling in the throat. SYN: *vertigo, laryngeal.*

  s., *local.* Numbness of a part with sudden blanching, as of the fingers; a symptom of Raynaud's disease or of local asphyxia.

syncytiolysin (sĭn-sĭt-ĭ-ol'ĭ-sĭn). A cytolysin that is formed from injections of emulsions of placental tissue.

syncytioma (sĭn-sĭt-ĭ-ō'mă). A tumor of the chorion. SYN: *chorioma, deciduoma.*

  s. *benig'num.* A mole.

  s. *malig'num.* A tumor formed of cells from the syncytium and chorion, occurring frequently after abortion or in the puerperium at site of placenta.

syncytium (sĭn-sĭt'ĭ-ŭm). 1. Multinucleated protoplasmic aggregation of cells without apparent cell outlines. 2. A multinucleated protoplasmic membrane forming outer layer of early chorionic villi.

syndactylism (sĭn-dăk'tĭl-ĭzm). A fusion of 2 or more toes or fingers, usually congenital.

syndectomy (sĭn-dĕk'tō-mĭ). Excision of a circular strip of the conjunctiva around cornea to relieve *pannus.* SYN: *peritomy.*

syndesis (sĭn-dē'sĭs). 1. Surgical fixation of a joint. 2. Pairing of chromosomes in pronuclei of ovum. SYN: *synapse, 2.*

syndesmectomy (sĭn-dĕs-mĕk'tō-mĭ). Excision of a section of a ligament.

syndesmectopia (sĭn″dĕs-mĕk-tō'pĭ-ă). Abnormal position of a ligament.

syndesmitis (sĭn-dĕs-mī'tĭs). 1. Inflammation of a ligament or ligaments. 2. Inflammation of the conjunctiva.

syndesmography (sĭn-dĕs-mŏg'ră-fĭ). Treatise on the ligaments.

syndesmology (sĭn-dĕs-mŏl'ō-jĭ). Study of the ligaments and their disorders.

syndesmoma (sĭn-dĕs-mō'mă). A connective tissue tumor.

syndesmopexy (sĭn-dĕs'mō-pĕks-ĭ). Joining of 2 ligaments or fixation of a ligament in a new place, used in correction of a dislocation.

syndesmoplasty (sĭn-dĕs'mō-plăs-tĭ). Plastic surgery on a ligament.

syndesmorrhaphy (sĭn-dĕs-mor'ăf-ĭ). Repair or suture of a ligament.

syndesmosis (sĭn-dĕs-mō'sĭs) (pl. *syndesmoses*). Articulation in which the bones are united by ligaments. SEE: *joint.*

syndesmotomy (sĭn-dĕs-mŏt'ō-mĭ). Surgical section of ligaments.

syndrome (sĭn'drōm, -drō-mē). A complexus of symptoms. All the symptoms of a disease considered as a whole. The complete picture of a disease.

  s., *Adams-Stokes.* Bradycardia and intermittent convulsive seizures with loss of consciousness due to organic obstruction of the bundle of His.

  s., *Angelucci's.* Palpitation, excitable temperament and vasomotor disturbance in spring conjunctivitis.

  s., *Fröhlich's.* Increase in fat, atrophy of the genitals, transition to feminine type due to lesions of the hypophysis.

  s., *Gradenigo's.* External rectus paralysis, temporoparietal pain and suppurative otitis media on same side.

  s. *of Horner.* Contracted pupil, ptosis, enophthalmos and dry, cool face on affected side produced by paralysis of sympathetics.

  s., *Korsakoff's.* A psychosis, ordinarily due to chronic alcoholism, with polyneuritis, disorientation, insomnia, muttering delirium, hallucinations, and a bilateral wrist or foot drop.

s., Weber's. Paralysis of hypoglossal nerve on one side and of oculomotor nerve on other with paralysis of limbs due to lesion of a cerebral peduncle.

syndromic (sĭn-drom'ĭk). Pert. to or occurring as a syndrome.

synechia (sĭn-ē-kĭ-ă). Adhesion of parts, esp. adhesion of iris to lens and cornea.

s., annular. Adhesion of the iris to the lens throughout its entire pupillary margin.

s., anterior. Adhesion of iris to cornea.

s., posterior. Adhesion of iris to capsule of lens.

s., total. Adhesion of entire surface of the iris to the lens.

synechotomy (sĭn-ĕk-ŏt'ō-mĭ). Division of a synechia or adhesion.

synecology (sĭn-ē-kŏl'ō-jĭ). The study of organisms in relation to their environment in group form.

syneresis (sĭn-ĕr'ĕs-ĭs). Contraction of a gel resulting in its separation from the liquid, as a shrinkage by fibrin and other colloidal gels.

synergenesis (sĭn-ĕr-jĕn'ĕ-sĭs). The theory that each cell contains the protoplasm of every generation of cells derived therefrom.

synergetic (sĭn-ĕr-jĕt'ĭk). Exhibiting co-operative action, said of certain muscles; working together. SYN: *synergic.*

synergic (sĭn-ĕr'jĭk). Relating to or exhibiting coöperation, as certain muscles.

synergist (sĭn'ĕr-jĭst). 1. A remedy that stimulates the action of another. SYN: *adjuvant.* 2. A muscle or organ functioning in coöperation with another, as the flexor muscles.

synergy (sĭn'ĕr-jĭ). Action of 2 or more agents or organs coöperating with each other; coöperation. Combined action; coördinated action.

synesthesia (sĭn-ĕs-thē'zĭ-ă). 1. A sensation in an area from a stimulus applied to another part. 2. A subjective sensation of another sense than the one being stimulated. SEE: *chromatism, phonism.*

s. al'gica. Painful synesthesia.

synesthesialgia (sĭn″ĕs-thē-zĭ-ăl'jĭ-ă). A painful sensation giving rise to a subjective one of different character. SEE: *synesthesia.*

synezesis (sĭn-ĕ-zē'sĭs). Closure of the pupil.

syngamy (sĭn'gă-mĭ). Sexual reproduction; cell union, as of gametes in fertilization.

syngenesis (sĭn-jĕn'ĕ-sĭs). 1. Reproduction sexually. 2. Doctrine that each sexual cell contains the germs from which all future cells will be derived.

syngignocism (sĭn-jĭg'nō-sĭzm). Hypnotism and its results.

synizesis (sĭn-ĭz-ē'sĭs). 1. A closure or shutting. 2. Massing of nuclear chromatin prior to maturation division.

s. pupillae. Closure of the pupil of the eye with loss of vision.

synkaryon (sĭn-kar'ĭ-ŏn). A nucleus resulting from fusion of 2 pronuclei.

synkinesis (sĭn-kĭ-nē'sĭs). Involuntary movements in a part when another part is voluntarily moved, as in a paralyzed limb following movements made in an opposite limb.

synneurosis (sĭn-ū-rō'sĭs). Synarthrosis in which fibrous connective tissue unites opposing surfaces. SYN: *syndesmosis.*

synocha, synochus (sĭn'ō-kă, -kŭs). A fever that is continued.

synococcus (sĭn-ō-kŏk'ŭs). A coccus often associated with the gonococcus.

synonym (sĭn'ō-nĭm). A word which has the same or very similar meaning as another word.

synoptophore (sĭn-ŏp'tō-for). Apparatus for diagnosing and treating strabismus.

synoptoscope (sĭn-ŏp'tō-skōp). An instrument for diagnosis and treatment of strabismus. SYN: *synoptophore.*

synorchidism, synorchism (sĭn-or'kĭd-ĭzm, -kĭzm). Union or partial fusion of the testicles.

synosteology (sĭn″ŏs-tē-ŏl'ō-jĭ). The science of joints and articulations.

synosteosis, synostosis (sĭn″ŏs-tē-ō'sĭs, -tō'sĭs). 1. Articulation by osseous tissue of adjacent bones. 2. Union of separate bones by osseous tissue.

synosteotomy (sĭn-ŏs-tē-ŏt'ō-mĭ). Dissection of joints.

synovectomy (sĭn-ō-vĕk'tō-mĭ). Excision of synovial membrane.

synovia (sĭn-ō'vĭ-ă). A colorless, viscid, lubricating fluid of joints, bursae, and tendon sheaths secreted within synovial membranes.

It contains mucin, albumin, fat, and mineral salts. SEE: *asynovia.*

synovial (sĭn-ō'vĭ-ăl). Pert. to synovia, the joint lubricating fluid.

s. bursa. The mucosa of a bursa.

s. crypt. Diverticulum of a synovial membrane of a joint.

s. cyst. Accumulation of synovia in a bursa, synovial crypt, or sac of a synovial hernia, causing a tumor.

s. fluid. Lubricating, clear fluid secreted by the synovial membrane of a joint. SYN: *synovia.*

s. glands. Folds on synovial membrane secreting synovia. SYN: *haversian glands.*

s. hernia. Protrusion of a portion of synovial membrane through a tear in the stratum fibrosum of a joint capsule.

s. ligament. A large synovial fold in a joint.

s. membrane. One lining the capsule of a joint.

s. sheath. The mucosa of a tendon sheath.

synovin (sĭn'ō-vĭn). A form of mucin found in synovia.

synovioma (sĭn″ō-vĭ-ō'mă). A tumor arising from a synovial membrane.

synoviparous (sĭn-ō-vĭp'ă-rŭs). Producing or secreting synovia.

synovitis (sĭn-ō-vī'tĭs). Inflammation of a synovial membrane.

s., chronic. The active congestion largely disappears, but there is an undue amount of fluid in the cavity and the membrane itself is edematous. Later, if the disease does not subside, membrane and articular structures become irregularly thickened by plastic exudation and formation of fibrous tissue.

s., dendritic. Synovitis with villous growths developing in the sac.

s., dry. Synovitis without much effusion or no effusion.

s., fungous. Tuberculosis of a joint. SYN: *arthritis fungosa.*

s., pannous. Is rarely met with; occurs in tubercular arthritis. The great serous accumulation in the synovial sac will almost certainly be regarded as nontubercular until after aspiration and examination of the fluid.

s., purulent. Synovitis with purulent effusion within the sac.

s., serous. Synovitis with nonpurulent, copious effusion.

s. sicca. Same as *dry* synovitis.*

s., simple. Synovitis with effusion only slightly turbid if not clear.

s., tendinous. Inflammation of a tendon sheath.

s., vaginal. Same as *tendinous* synovitis.*

s., vibration. Synovitis resulting from a wound near a joint.

synpneumonic (sĭn-nū-mŏn'ĭk). Concurrent with pneumonia; complicating pneumonia.

synreflexia (sĭn″rē-flĕks'ĭ-ă). The relationship existing bet. various reflexes.

syntaxis (sĭn-tăks'ĭs). A junction bet. 2 bones. SYN: *articulation.*

syntenosis (sĭn-tĕn-ō'sĭs). A hinge joint protected by tendons, as a *phalangeal articulation.*

synthermal (sĭn-thĕr'măl). Having the same temperature.

synthesis (sĭn'thĕs-ĭs). 1. CHEM: The union of elements to produce compounds; the process of building up; the opposite of analysis or decomposition. 2. Reuniting of broken or separated structures.

synthetic (sĭn-thĕt'ĭk). Relating to or made by synthesis; artificially prepared.

syntone (sĭn'tōn). An individual temperamentally responsive to his environment and its social demands. SEE: *syntonic.*

syntonic (sĭn-tŏn'ĭk). Pert. to a reaction type in which the subject responds strongly to emotional stimuli in harmony with the situation.

syntonin (sĭn'tō-nĭn). An acid albumin; esp. one formed by the action of dilute hydrochloric acid on muscle during gastric digestion.

syntoxoid (sĭn-tŏks'oyd). A toxoid having the same degree of affinity for an antitoxin as the toxin has.

syntripsis (sĭn-trĭp'sĭs). A comminuted fracture or act causing it.

syntropan (sĭn'trō-păn). A synthetic compound resembling in effects those of atropine.

DOSAGE: 50 mg.

syntropic (sĭn-trŏp'ĭk). 1. Turned in the same direction, as the ribs. 2. Noting a

type characterized by mixing well and easily. SYN: *koinotropic, q.v.*

synulotic (sĭn-ū-lot'ĭk). 1. An agent stimulating cicatrization. 2. Promoting cicatrization.

syphilelcosis (sĭf-ĭl-ĕl-kō'sĭs). Syphilitic ulceration.

syphilelcus (sĭf-ĭl-ĕl'kŭs). A syphilitic ulcer.

syphilide (sĭf'ĭl-ĭd). Any cutaneous affection of syphilitic origin. SYN: *syphiloderm.*

syphilimetry (sĭf-ĭl-ĭm'ĕt-rĭ). Determination of a syphilitic infection's intensity.

syphilionthus (sĭf-ĭl-ĭ-ŏn'thŭs). A copper-colored, branny-scaled syphilide.

syphiliphobia (sĭf-ĭl-ĭ-fō'bĭ-ă). Morbid fear of syphilis. SYN: *syphilophobia.*

syphilis (sĭf'ĭl-ĭs). An infectious, chronic venereal disease resulting in various lesions of structural and cutaneous nature.

s., congenital. Syphilis present at birth.

s. innocen'tium, s. inson'tium. Syphilis not contracted through coition.

s., visceral. Due to pressure of gummata may affect brain, cord, lungs, liver, rectum, heart, kidneys, testicles, or arteries.

syphilitic (sĭf-ĭl-ĭt'ĭk). Related to, caused by, or affected with syphilis.

s. fever. Rise in temperature in early stage of secondary syphilis.

s. macules. Small red eruptions manifested in secondary syphilis which often cover the entire body.

syphilization (sĭf-ĭl-ĭ-zā'shŭn). Inoculation with the exudate of a chancre to immunize against syphilis.

syphilized (sĭf'ĭl-īzd). Infected with syphilis.

syphilocerebrosis (sĭf″ĭl-ō-sĕr-ē-brō'sĭs). Syphilis of the brain.

syphiloderm, syphiloderma (sĭf'ĭl-ō-derm, sĭf″ĭl-ō-der'mă). A syphilitic cutaneous disorder. SYN: *syphilide.*

syphilogenesis, syphilogeny (sĭf″ĭl-ō-jĕn'ē-sĭs, sĭf-ĭl-ŏj'ĕn-ĭ). The development or origin of syphilis.

syphilographer (sĭf-ĭl-ŏg'ră-fer). One who writes about syphilis.

syphilography (sĭf-ĭl-ŏg'ră-fĭ). A treatise on syphilis.

syphiloid (sĭf'ĭl-oyd). 1. Resembling syphilis. 2. A disease akin to syphilis.

syphilologist (sĭf-ĭl-ŏl'ō-jĭst). A specialist in treatment of syphilis.

syphilology (sĭf-ĭl-ŏl'ō-jĭ). The study of syphilis and its treatment.

syphiloma (sĭf-ĭl-ō'mă). A syphilitic tumor.

syphilomania (sĭf-ĭl-ō-mā'nĭ-ă). Morbid fear of syphilis or inference that one is suffering with it. SYN: *syphilophobia.*

syphilopathy (sĭf-ĭl-ŏp'ă-thĭ). Any syphilitic disorder.

syphilophobia (sĭf-ĭl-ō-fō'bĭ-ă). Morbid fear of syphilis or delusion of having the disease.

syphilophobic (sĭf″ĭl-ō-fō'bĭk). Pert. to or affected with syphilophobia.

syphilophyma (sĭf″ĭl-ō-fī'mă). 1. Any

growth or excrescence due to syphilis.
2. Syphiloma of the epidermis.

syphilopsychosis (sĭf″ĭl-ō-sĭ-kō′sĭs). Any mental disease caused by syphilis.

syphilosis (sĭf-ĭ-lō′sĭs). Generalized syphilitic disease.

syphilotropic (sĭf-ĭl-ō-trŏp′ĭk). Especially susceptible to syphilis.

syphilous (sĭf′ĭl-ŭs). Of the nature of or pert. to syphilis. SYN: *syphilitic.*

syphionthus (sĭf-ĭ-ŏn′thŭs). The copper-colored patches seen in syphilis. SYN: *syphilionthus.*

syphitoxin (sĭf-ĭ-tŏks′ĭn). Antisyphilitic serum.

syrigmophonia (sĭr″ĭg-mō-fō′nĭ-ă). 1. A sibilant râle. 2. A whistling sound in pronunciation of *s* due to a denture peculiarity.

syringadenoma (sĭr-ĭng-ăd-en-ō′mă). Tumor of a sweat gland.

syringe (sĭr-ĭnj′, sĭr′ĭnj). 1. Instrument for injecting fluids into cavities or vessel. 2. To wash out or introduce fluid with a syringe.

syringectomy (sĭr-ĭn-jĕk′tō-mĭ). Removal of the walls of a fistula.

syringitis (sĭr-ĭn-jī′tĭs). Inflammation of the eustachian tube.

syringo-. Combining form meaning *pipe* or *tube.*

syringobulbia (sĭr-ĭn-gō-bul′bĭ-ă). Presence of pores in the medulla oblongata, resembling *syringomyelia.*

syringocele (sĭr-ĭn′gō-sēl). The central canal of the myelon or spinal cord.

syringocystadenoma (sĭr-ĭn″gō-sĭs-tad-ĕn-ō′mă). Adenoma of sweat glands characterized by tiny, hard, papular formations.

syringocystoma (sĭr-ĭn″gō-sĭs-tō′mă). Cystic tumor having its origin in ducts of the sweat gland.

syringoid (sĭr-ĭng′oyd). Resembling a tube.

syringoma (sĭr-ĭn-gō′mă). Tumor of the sweat glands.

syringomeningocele (sĭr-ĭn″gō-men-ĭn′gō-sēl). Meningocele which is similar to a syringomyelocele.

syringomyelia (sĭr-ĭn″gō-mī-ē′lĭ-ă). The development of cavities within the spinal cord.

syringomyelitis (sĭr-ĭn″gō-mī-ĕ-lī′tĭs). Inflammation coincident with abnormal dilation of the central canal of spinal cord.

syringomyelocele (sĭr-ĭn″gō-mī′ĕl-ō-sēl). A form of spina bifida in which the cavity of the projecting portion communicates with the central canal of the spinal cord.

syringomyelus (sĭr-ĭn″gō-mī′ĕl-ŭs). Abnormal dilatation of central canal of spinal cord.

syringopontia (sĭr-ĭn″gō-pŏn′shĭ-ă). Cavities in the pons Varolii similar to *syringomyelia.*

syringosystrophy (sĭr-ĭn″gō-sĭs′trō-fĭ). Twisting of the oviduct.

syringotome (sĭr-ĭng′ō-tōm). Instrument for incision of a fistula.

syringotomy (sĭr-ĭn-gŏt′ō-mĭ). Operation for cure of fistula by cutting.

syrinx (sĭr′ĭnks). 1. The eustachian tube. 2. Pathological cavity in the spinal cord or brain. 3. A fistula.

syrup (sĭr′ŭp). Concentrated solution of sugar in water or aqueous liquid.

syssarcosis (sĭs-ar-kō′sĭs). The union of bones by means of muscles; muscular articulation, as of the *hyoid* and *patella.*

systaltic (sĭs-tăl′tĭk). Contracting and dilating; having a systole. SYN: *pulsating.*

system (sĭs′tĕm). 1. A grouping of related structures; the whole organism. 2. An interrelationship of organs because of their function.

   s., alimentary. The digestive system.

   s., autonomic nervous. Part of peripheral nervous system regulating involuntary impulses controlling function of ductless glands, blood vessels, and viscera.

   s., central nervous. The brain and spinal cord.

   s., circulatory. SEE: *vascular system.*

   s., digestive. That of the alimentary tract, its glands and organs.

   s., endocrine. That of the ductless glands and their hormones.

   s., genitourinary. That of the genitals and urinary organs.

   s., muscular. That of the muscles, ligaments, and tendons.

   s., nervous. That of the nerves.

   s., osseous. That of the bones and cartilages.

   s., portal. That of the portal circulation.

   s., pulmonary. That of the lungs and air passages.

   s., respiratory. SEE: *pulmonary system.*

   s., urinary. That of the kidneys, bladder, and appendages.

   s., vascular. That of the heart, blood vessels, and lymphatics.

systema (sĭs-tē′mă). System.

   s. nervorum sympath′icum. BNA. The sympathetic nervous system.

systemic (sĭs-tĕm′ĭk). Pert. to a whole body rather than to one of its parts; somatic.

   s. circulation. Course of the blood through the general system from left ventricle to right atrium.

   s. death. Death of the body as a whole. SYN: *somatic death.*

   s. remedies. Remedies which will act on the body as a whole, as a tonic.

systemoid (sĭs′tē-moyd). 1. Resembling a system. 2. Pert. to tumors made up of several types of tissues.

systole (sĭs′tō-lē). That part of the heart cycle in which the heart is in contraction, *i. e.,* the myocardial fibers are tightening and shortening.

   s., aborted. One which fails to increase arterial pressure because of mitral regurgitation or insufficient energy.

   s., anticipated. One that is aborted because it occurs before the ventricle is filled.

   s., arterial. Arterial retraction after a cardiac systole.

s., auricular. An auricular contraction.

s., extra. A premature one occurring in addition to the fundamental rhythm.

s., hemic. One independent and separate systole of one of the ventricles.

s., ventricular. Ventricular contraction.

systolic (sĭs-tŏl'ĭk). Pert. to the systole.

s. murmur. A cardiac one during systole. One heard in both systole and diastole.

s. pressure. Blood pressure is expressed in terms of the systolic pressure; the greatest force exerted by the heart and the highest degree of resistance put forth by the arterial walls.

systolometer (sĭs-tō-lŏm'ĕt-ĕr). Device for determining quality and character of cardiac murmurs.

systremma (sĭs-trĕm'ă). Cramp in calf of the leg, the muscles assuming form of a hard ball.

syzygial (sĭz-ĭj'ĭ-ăl). Pert. to a syzygium.

syzygiology (sĭz-ĭ-jĭ-ŏl'ō-jĭ). Interdependence or interrelationships of the whole as opposed to isolated functions or separate parts.

syzygium (sĭ-zĭj'ĭ-ŭm). Partial fusion of 2 structures.

syzygy (sĭz'ĭj-ĭ). Fusion of organs, each remaining distinct.

s. bone. An S-shaped bone, such as the *episternum*.   [chloric acid.

Szabo's test (sah'bō). A test for hydro-

T

T. Abbr. for *temperature* and for *tension*. T + indicates increased tension; T—, diminished tension.

t. Abbr. for *temporal,* and for Latin, *ter, three times.*

T-bandage. Bandage resembling the letter T. SEE: *bandage.*

T-fiber. One given off at right angles from the axis-cylinder process of a nerve cell.

T-wave. One of the waves or elevations in an electrocardiogram due to ventricular activity.

TA. Abbr. for alkaline tuberculin.*

T. A. Abbr. for *toxin-antitoxin.*

tabacism (tăb'ă-sĭzm). Chronic tobacco poisoning. SYN: *tabacosis.*

tabacosis (tăb-ă-kō'sĭs). Chronic tobacco poisoning, esp. from inhaling tobacco dust.

tabacum (tăb-ăk'ŭm). Tobacco.

tabagism (tăb'ăj-ĭzm). Tobacco poisoning. SYN: *tabacosis.*

tabatière anatomique (tah-bah-tē-air' ahn-ah-tō-mēk'). Depression at back of hand at base of thumb.

tabefaction (tă-bē-făk'shŭn). A wasting away of the body gradually.

tabella (tă-bĕl'ă) (pl. *tabellae*). A medicated mass of material formed into a small disk.

tabes (tā'bēz). 1. A gradual, progressive wasting in any chronic disease. 2. The final manifestation of syphilis involving particularly the posterior columns of the spinal cord. SYN: *locomotor ataxia.*

  t., cerebral. Chronic degenerative brain disease with physical and mental deterioration. SYN: *paresis, general.*

  t., cervical. Tabes first affecting the upper extremities.

  t., diabetic. Peripheral neuritis, affecting diabetics. May affect spinal cord and simulate tabes dorsalis.

  t. dorsalis. Degeneration of posterior columns of the spinal cord. SYN: *locomotor ataxia, tabes.*

  t., marantic. Tabes with great emaciation.

  t. mesenterica. Emaciation and general disorder of the functions of nutrition due to engorgement and tubercular degeneration of the mesenteric glands.

  t., spasmodic. Lateral sclerosis of spinal cord. SYN: *Little's disease.*

tabetic (tă-bĕt'ĭk). Pert. to or afflicted with tabes or tabes dorsalis.

  t. ataxia. Occurs when there are lesions of first order of sensory neurons.

  t. crises. Paroxysms of pain or other acute manifestations of episodic character in tabes dorsalis.

  t. foot. Twisted foot in locomotor ataxia.

tabetiform (tăb-ĕt'ĭ-form). Resembling or characteristic of tabes.

tabic (tăb'ĭk). Pert. to or affected with tabes or tabes dorsalis. SYN: *tabetic.*

tabid (tăb'ĭd). Pert. to tabes. SYN: *tabetic, tabic.*

table (tā'bl). 1. A flat-topped structure, as an operating table. 2. A thin, flat plate, as of bone.

  t's. of skull. Inner and outer condensed layers of the cranial bone separated by diploe (cancellous bony tissue).

  t., vitreous. The inner cranial table.

tablespoon (tā'bl-spoon). A large spoon containing about 15 cc. or 4 fluidrams.

tablet (tăb'lĕt). A small, disklike mass of medicinal powder.

  t., coated. Usually made by coating compressed tablets with sugar, chocolate, etc.

  t., compressed. Made by forcibly compressing the powdered substances into the desired shape; usually made to contain from 1 to 10 gr. of the active drug.

  t., dispensing. Those that contain a comparatively large amount of the active drug, as 1 gr. of strychnine sulfate.

  t., hypodermic. Usually made as are tablet triturates, frequently containing, in addition, some agents that produce chemical action when water is added, thus causing a rapid disintegration of the mass.

  t. triturates. Made by moistening the powder with a volatile liquid, as alcohol, and then molding into shape and allowing the liquid to evaporate.

taboparalysis (ta″bō-păr-ăl'ĭs-ĭs). Tabes associated concurrently with general paralysis.

taboparesis (ta″bō-păr-ē'sĭs, -par'ĕ-sĭs). General paralysis in combination with tabes. SYN: *taboparalysis.*

tabophobia (tā″bō-fō'bĭ-ă). A morbid fear of being afflicted with tabes, a common symptom of neurasthenia.

tabular (tăb'ū-lar). 1. Resembling a table. 2. Set up in columns, as a *tabulation*

  t. bone. A flat one, or one with 2 compact, bonelike parts with cancellous tissue bet. them.

tabule (tăb'ūl). A medicated tablet.

tache (tahsh). A colored spot or macule on the skin, as a freckle.

  t. blanche. A white spot seen on liver in some infectious diseases.

  t. bleuâtre (blu-ăhtr'). A blue spot on skin usually due to bite of cutaneous parasites. SYN: *macula caerulea.*

  t. cérébrale. The red line which occurs in meningitis and other nervous disorders, when the fingernail is drawn across the skin, *q.v.*

  t. de feu. Reddish area on skin caused by hypertrophy of cutaneous capillaries. SYN: *nevus vascularis.*

tachetic (tăk-ĕt'ĭk). Marked by purple or reddish blue patches (*taches*).

tachogram (tăk'ō-grăm). A graphic tracing of rate of flow of blood current.

tachography (tăk-ŏg'ră-fĭ). The recording of the speed of the blood circulation.

tachy-. Combining form meaning *swift*.

tachycardia (tăk″ĭ-kar'dĭ-ă). Abnormal rapidity of heart action.

t., constant. Occurs in some valvular affections, fatty degeneration, compensation failure, pregnancy, nervous disorders, exhaustive diseases, exophthalmic goiter.

t., essential. Rapid, persistent heart action due to functional disturbance.

t., extrinsic. Tachycardia caused by factors outside of the heart, as increased metabolism or instability of the nervous system.

t., intrinsic. Tachycardia caused by infection, as from rheumatism.

t., paroxysmal. Sudden and abrupt acceleration of cardiac rate, ceasing abruptly.

t., sinus. Uncomplicated tachycardia when sinus rhythm is faster than 100 beats per minute, as that due to exercise.

tachycardiac (tăk-ĭ-kar'dĭ-ăk). Pert. to or afflicted with tachycardia.

tachylalia (tăk″ĭ-lā'lĭ-ă). Rapid speech.

tachymeter (tăk-ĭm'ĕ-ter). Instrument for estimating the rapidity of any body in motion.

tachyphagia (tăk″ĭ-fā'jĭ-ă). Rapid eating.

tachyphasia (tăk″ĭ-fā'zĭ-ă). Very rapid or voluble speech. SYN: *tachyphrasia*.

tachyphrasia (tăk″ĭ-frā'zĭ-ă). Excessive volubility or rapidity of speech, as seen in mental disorders. SYN: *tachyphasia*.

tachyphrenia (tăk″ĭ-frē'nĭ-ă). Abnormally rapid mental activity.

tachyphylaxis (tăk″ĭ-fĭl-ăk'sĭs). Rapid immunization to a toxic dose of a substance by previously injecting tiny doses of the same substance.

tachypnea (tăk-ĭp-nē'ă). Abnormal rapidity of respiration.

t., nervous. Forty or more respirations per minute. It occurs in hysteria, neurasthenia, etc.

tachypragia (tăk″ĭ-prā'jĭ-ă). Rapidity of action.

tachypsychia (tăk-ĭ-sī'kĭ-ă). Rapid action of psychic processes.

tachyrythmia (tăk-ĭ-rĭth'mĭ-ă). Rapid heart action. SYN: *tachycardia*.

t., auricular. Condition in which auricular contractions are extremely rapid, causing impulses to arise in a place other than the sinuauricular node. SYN: *auricular flutter*.

tachysterol(e (tăk'ĭ-stē-rōl). One of the isomers of ergosterol* obtained by irradiation.

tachysystole (tăk″ĭ-sĭs'tō-lē). Abnormally rapid systole. SEE: *extrasystole*.

tachytrophism (tăk″ĭ-trō-fĭzm). Accelerated metabolism.

tactile (tăk'tĭl). 1. Perceptible to the touch. 2. Pert. to the sense of touch.

t. cell or **corpuscle.** One in which a sensory nerve fibril terminates.

t. papilla. One of the skin containing a tactile cell or corpuscle.

tactometer (tăk-tŏm'ĕt-ēr). Instrument for determining acuity of tactile sensitiveness.

tactor (tăk'tor). A tactile organ, specifically a tactile corpuscle.

tactual (tăk'tū-al). Relating to the sense of touch. SYN: *tactile*.

tactus (tăk'tus). Touch.

e. eruditus, t. expertus. Sensitiveness of touch acquired by long practice, as by a diagnostician or surgeon.

taenia (tē'nĭ-ă). 1. Any bandlike structure. 2. A tapeworm.

t. coli. BNA. One of 3 bands of the large intestines into which muscular fibers are collected, *i. e., taenia mesocolica* (mesenteric insertion), *taenia libera* (opp. mesocolic band), and *taenia omentalis* (at place of adhesion of omentum to transverse colon).

t. for'nicis. One of the upper peduncles of the pineal gland.

t. hippocam'pi. 1. Band on edge of the cornu inferius of lateral ventricle of brain. 2. Outer end of the oviduct. SYN: *corpus fimbriatum*.

t. semicircula'ris. Band on wall of lateral ventricle bet. the corpus striatum and thalamus.

Taenia (tē'nĭ-ă). A genus of tapeworms.

T. echinococcus. Species found in dogs' intestines.

Infection from food containing the eggs of this worm from having contaminated hands. It results in hydatid cysts. SEE: *echinococcus*.

T. saginata. Is derived from beef and is 5 or 6 yards in length.

T. solium. Pork tapeworm derived from the hog. Is 2 to 3 yards in length.

T. vulgaris. A broad tapeworm.

tagliacotian operation (tăl-yă-kō'shăn). Plastic operation on the nose in which skin is used from another part of the body. SYN: *rhinoplasty*.

tagma (tăg'mă) (pl. *tagmas, tagmatas*). An aggregate of molecules; protoplasm.

tail (tāl). Posterior, long, flexible terminus, as the extremity of the spinal column. SEE: *cauda*.

t. bone. Bone at caudal end of spine. SYN: *coccyx*.

t. fold. An embryonic one enveloping the hindgut.

t. gut. Prolongation of the archenteron in the embryonic caudal extremity.

tailors' cramp or **spasm** (tā'lor). Spasmodic occupational neurosis affecting muscles of the forearm and hand.

Tait's law (tāt). Exploratory laparotomy should be made in every case of obscure abdominal or pelvic disease which is a threat to health or life.

T.'s operation. Repair of a torn perineum. SYN: *perineorrhaphy*.

talalgia (tăl-ăl'jĭ-ă). Pain in the heel. SYN: *pternalgia*.

Talbot's law (tăl'but). If visual stimuli

from a revolving disk are fused and if sensation is uniform, then the intensity is the same as would occur were the same amount of light spread uniformly over the disk.

talc, talcum (tălk, tălk'ŭm). Powdered soapstone; a soft, soapy powder; native hydrous magnesium silicate used as a dusting powder and as a filter.

talipes (tăl'ĭ-pēz). A nontraumatic deviation of the foot in the direction of 1 or the other of the 4 lines of movement, or of 2 of these combined. Syn: *clubfoot.*

  t. arcua'tus. Exaggerated normal arch of the foot. Syn: *talipes cavus.*

  t. calcaneus (flexion). Heel alone touching the ground, the patient walking on inner side of heel. Often follows infantile paralysis of muscle of tendo Achillis.

  t. cavus. Same as *talipes arcuatus.*

  t. equinus (extension). Form with walking on the toes.

  t. planus. Flatfoot, splayfoot.

  t. valgus (abduction). Form with everted foot.

  t. varus (adduction). With inverted foot.

talipomanus (tăl-ĭp-ŏm'ăn-ŭs). Deformity of the hand in which it is twisted out of shape. Syn: *clubhand.*

talocalcanean (tă″lō-kăl-kā′nē-ăn). Relating to the astragalus and calcaneum. Syn: *astragalocalcanean.*

talocrural (tă″lō-krū′răl). Relating to the astragalus and leg bones.

talonid (tal′ō-nĭd). The crushing region; the post. part of a lower molar tooth.

talus (tā′lŭs). 1. BNA. The anklebone articulating with the tibia and fibula, and forming the ankle joint. 2. The entire ankle. Syn: *astragalus.*

tambour (tam′boor). A shallow, drum-shaped appliance used in transmitting and registering arterial pulsations, blood pressure, respiratory movements, peristaltic contractions and other slight movements.

tampon (tam′pon). 1. A plug, usually of lint or cotton, for closing a wound or cavity, to absorb secretions, or to arrest hemorrhage. 2. To plug up a wound or cavity with a tampon, as to stop hemorrhage.

  t., nasal. Soft rubber bulb, dilated with compressed air, for plugging nostrils to stop hemorrhage from the nose.

tamponade, tamponage (t̮ăm-pŏn-ād′, tăm′pŏn-āj). To use or make use of a tampon.

tannic acid (tăn′ĭk). Acid extracted from gallnuts. Syn: *tannin, q.v.*

tannigen (tăn′ĭ-jĕn). A brand of acetyltannic acid, which is a diacetic ester of tannic acid.

  Dosage: 3-10 gr. (0.2-0.6 Gm.).

tannin (tăn′ĭn). 1. Acid substance found in bark of certain plants and trees or their products, usually from nutgall. Found in coffee and to a greater extent in tea. 2. Any of several substances containing tannin.

  Dosage: As an antidote, 15 gr. (1.0 Gm.); locally, 1-5% solution; as an ointment, 20%.

tanning (tăn′ĭng). Exposure of face or body surface to the rays of the sun, thus acquiring a "coat of tan."

tap (tăp). 1. To puncture or to empty of fluid by paracentesis. 2. A slight blow.

tapetum (tă-pē′tŭm). BNA. A layer of fibers from the corpus callosum to each lateral ventricle of the brain and to the temporal lobe.

tapeworm (tāp′wôrm). *Tenia, q.v.* See: *cestode, Cestoidea.*

  t., armed. The pork tapeworm, *Taenia solinan.*

  t., beef. Common tapeworm found in beef. Syn: *Taenia saginata.*

taphephobia, taphophobia (tăf″ĕ-fō′bĭ-ă, -ō-fō′bĭ-ă). Abnormal fear of being buried alive.

tapinocephalic (tăp″ĭn-ō-sĕf-al′ĭk). Pert. to flatness of top of cranium.

tapinocephaly (tăp″ĭn-ō-sĕf′ă-lĭ). Flatness of top of the skull.

tapiroid (tă′pĭr-oyd). Resembling a tapir's snout; said of an elongated cervix uteri.

tapotement (tă-pōt-mon′). Percussion in massage.

tapping (tăp′ĭng). 1. Percussion in massage. Syn: *tapotement.* 2. Removal of fluid from a cavity. Syn: *paracentesis.* See: *thoracentesis.*

tarantism (tăr′ăn-tĭzm). A nervous affection marked by stupor, melancholy and uncontrollable dancing mania.

taran'tula bite. Treatment the same as for black widow spider* bite, *q.v.*

Tardieu's ecchymoses or spots (tar-dyu′). Subpleural spots of ecchymosis following death by strangulation.

target (tar′gĕt). 1. PT: The electrode on which cathode rays within an x-ray tube are focused and from which roentgen rays are emitted; usually of a heavy metal such as tungsten. 2. A tiny figure on an ophthalmometer's arm whose image is used to determine the amount of corneal astᵢgmatᵢsm. Syn: *mire, q.v.*

Tarnier's sign (tahr-ne-ā′). A sign of coming abortion; the disappearance of angle bet. upper and lower uterine segments in pregnancy.

tarsal (tar′săl). Pert. to the framework of the eyelid or to the instep.

  t. arches. Those above and below the tarsal cartilages.

  t. bones. The 7 bones of the instep.

  t. cartilages. Layers of cartilage in free edge of each eyelid.

  t. cyst. Small tumor on border of eyelid. Syn: *chalazion.*

  t. glands. Tiny sebaceous follicles at edge of the eyelid. Syn: *meibomian glands.*

tarsalgia (tar-săl′jĭ-ă). Pain in a tarsus due to flatfoot or shortening of Achilles' tendon. Syn: *podalgia, policeman's disease.*

tarsalia (tar-sā′lĭ-ă) (sing. *tarsale*). The tarsal bones.

tarsalis (tar-sā′lĭs). One of the tarsal muscles.

tarsectomy (tar-sĕk′tō-mĭ). 1. Excision of tarsus or a tarsal bone. 2. Removal of tarsal plate of an eyelid.

tarsitis (tar-sī′tĭs). 1. Inflammation of tarsus of the foot. 2. Inflammation of eyelid's border. SYN: *blepharitis.*

tarso-. Combining form meaning the *flat of the foot, edge of the eyelid.*

tarsocheiloplasty (tar″sō-kī′lō-plăs-tĭ). Plastic surgery of borders of the eyelid.

tarsoclasia, tarsoclasis (tar″sō-klā′sĭ-ă, tar-sŏk′lăs-ĭs). Surgical fracture of the tarsus for correction of clubfoot.

tarsomalacia (tar″sō-mă-lā′sĭ-ă). Softening of the tarsal cartilages of the eyes.

tarsometatarsal (tar″sō-mĕt-ă-tar′săl). Pert. to the tarsus and the metatarsus.

tarsophyma (tar″sō-fī′mă). Any tarsal tumor of the eyelid. SYN: *hordoleum, sty.*

tarsoplasia, tarsoplasty (tar″sō-plā′zĭ-ă, tar′sō-plăs″tĭ). Plastic surgery of margin of the eyelid. SYN: *blepharoplasty.*

tarsoptosis (tars-ŏp-tō′sĭs). Falling of the tarsus. SYN: *flatfoot.*

tarsorrhaphy (tar-sor′ă-fĭ). The operation of uniting the edges of the lids at the outer commissure for the purpose of reducing the width of the palpebral fissure.

tarsotomy (tar-sŏt′ō-mĭ). 1. Incision of tarsal cartilage of an eyelid. 2. Any surgical incision of the tarsus of the foot.

tarsus (tar′sŭs) (pl. *tarsi*). 1. The instep proper with its 7 bones, bet. the tibia and the metatarsus. 2. The condensed connective tissue framework of the eyelids.

tartar (tar′ter). Calcareous matter deposited upon the teeth.

   t., cream of. Potassium bitartrate.

   t. emetic. A poisonous, white, crystalline salt, the tartrate of potassium and antimony, used in medicine as a diaphoretic, emetic, expectorant, and counterirritant.

   DOSAGE: As *expectorant*, 1/20 gr. (0.003 Gm.); as *emetic*, ½ gr. (0.03 Gm.).

tartaric acid (tar-tar′ĭk). An acid derived from lees of wine and certain plants, occurring in 4 forms. Sometimes used in artificial lemonades or in effervescent drinks and is rarely toxic unless taken in large doses.

tartarization (tar″tar-ĭ-zā′shŭn). Treatment with tartar emetic, esp. in syphilis.

tartarized (tar′tar-īzd). Impregnated with tartaric acid.

taste (tāst). 1. To try or perceive by touch of the tongue. 2. A chemical sense dependent upon sense organs on the surface of the tongue when they are in contact with a substance to ascertain its attributes, the nervous impulses being carried to the brain by the lingual (from the anterior two-thirds of the surface) and the glossopharyngeal (from the posterior third) nerves.

   t. buds. Oval nerve end organ with hairlike processes that project through the central taste pores, principally on the surface of the tongue, but also in various parts of the mouth and throat upon which flavors have an effect.

   t. cells. Internal cells of a taste bud.

T. A. T. Abbr. for toxin-antitoxin.

taurocholemia (taw″rō-kō-lē′mĭ-ă). Taurocholic acid in the blood.

tauto-. Combining form meaning *the same.*

tautomeral, tautomeric (taw-tŏm′ĕr-ăl, -to-mĕr′ĭk). Noting certain neurons which send processes to the white matter on the same side of the spinal cord.

tautomerism (taw-tŏm′ĕr-ĭzm). Phenomenon in which 2 formulae are possible but only one stable substance is obtainable.

tautorotation (taw″tō-rō-tā′shŭn). A change in specific rotation which occurs when a solution of certain sugars stands a while.

Tawara's node (tah-wah′rah). One near the coronary sinus in the right atrium forming beginning of the bundle of His. SYN: *Aschoff's node.*

taxis (tăks′ĭs). Manual replacement of displaced structures.

   t., bipolar. Replacing of a retroverted uterus by drawing down the cervix in the vagina and pressing upward through the rectum.

taxonomy (tăks-ŏn′ō-mĭ). Laws and principles of classification of animals and plants.   [*tuberculosis.*]

T. b. Abbr. for *tubercle bacillus* and for

t. d. s. Abbr. meaning *take 3 times a day.*

Te. Symb. of *tellurium.*

tea (tē). 1. An infusion of a medicinal plant. 2. Leaves of plant *Thea chinensis*, from which a beverage is made

   t., Paraguay. A tea made from the leaves and stems of the *Ilex paraguaiensis.* It is a stimulating drink and contains volatile oil, tannin, and caffeine.

Teale's amputation. Amputation with short ant. and long post. rectangular flaps used in excision of the lower half of forearm, the leg, or the thigh.

   Length of flaps in amputation of the leg may be reversed.

tear (tēr). A drop of the saline fluid normally secreted by the lacrimal glands to moisten the parts.

   t. ducts. The 2 lacrimal● ducts. SEE: *lacrimal.*

   t. sac. Upper part of the nasolacrimal duct into which the 2 lacrimal ducts empty. SYN: *saccus lacrimalis.*

tease (tēz). To separate a tissue into minute parts with a needle to prepare it for the microscope.

teat (tēt). 1. The nipple of the mammary gland. SYN: *papilla mammilla.* 2. Any protuberance resembling a nipple.

teatulation (tēt″ū-lā′shŭn). The development of a nipplelike elevation.

technic (tĕk-nēk′). Details of a procedure or of an operation.

technical (těk'nĭ-kal). Requiring technic or special skill.

technician (těk-nĭsh'ǎn). One skilled in a special art.

techno-. Combining form meaning *art, skill.*

tecno-. Combining form meaning *child.*

tectocephaly (těk-tō-sěf'ǎl-ĭ). Possession of a boat-shaped cranium. Syn: *scaphocephalism.*

tectonic (těk-tŏn'ĭk). Relating to plastic surgery.

tectorial (těk-tō'rĭ-ǎl). Pert. to a roof or covering. Syn: *tegmental.*

tectorium (těk-tō'rĭ-ŭm). 1. Any rooflike structure. 2. Corti's membrane. Syn: *membrana tectoria.*

tectospinal (těk'tō-spī'nǎl). From the tectum mesencephali to the spinal cord.

    t. tract. A tract of white fibers of the spinal cord passing from the tectum of midbrain on 1 side, crossing, and going down through the medulla to the spinal cord.

tectum (těk'tŭm). Any structure serving as, or resembling, a roof.

    t. mesencephali. Roof of the midbrain including the corpora quadrigemina.

teeth (tēth) (sing. *tooth*). Hard, bony projections in jaws serving as organs of mastication, there being 32 permanent teeth, 16 in each jaw. See: *dentition, tooth.*

teething (tēth'ĭng). Eruption of the teeth. Syn: *dentition.*

tegmen (těg'měn) (pl. *tegmina*). A structure that covers a part.

    t. mastoideum. Bony roof of mastoid cells.

    t. tympani. BNA. Roof of tympanum separating middle ear from cranial cavity.

tegmental (těg-měn'tǎl). Relating to a tegument or tegmentum; covering.

    t. nucleus. Nucleus of gray substance containing red ganglion cells in the cover of the crus cerebri. Syn: *red nucleus.*

tegmentum (těg-měn'tŭm). Dorsal portion of crus cerebri above the substantia nigra, with fibers running to the cortex.

    t. auris. Membrane bet. middle and external ear. Syn: *membrana tympani.*

tegument (těg'ū-měnt). 1. The skin; the covering of the body. Syn: *integument.* 2. A covering structure.

tegumental, tegumentary (těg"ū-měn'tǎl, -tǎ-rĭ). Concerning a tegument; covering. Syn: *cutaneous.*

Teichmann's crystals (tīk'mahn). Brownish-red crystalline form of hematin hydrochloride. Syn: *hematin hydrochloride, hemin.*

teichopsia (tī-kŏp'sĭ-ǎ). Zigzag lines bounding a luminous area appearing in the visual field causing a temporary blindness in that portion of the eye, sometimes accompanying severe sick headaches and mental or physical strain. Syn: *scotoma, scintillating.*

teinodynia (tī"nō-dĭn'ĭ-ǎ). Pain in the tendons. Syn: *tenodynia.*

tela (tē'lǎ). Any weblike structure.

    t. cellulo'sa. Connective tissue.

    t. choroi'dea. Part of the pia mater covering roof of the 3rd and 4th cerebral ventricles.

telalgia (tēl-ǎl'jĭ-ǎ). Pain felt at a distance from its stimulus. Syn: *pain, referred.*

telangiectasia, telangiectasis (tel-ǎn"jĭ-ěk-tā'zhĭ-ǎ, -ěk'tǎ-sĭs). Dilatation of capillaries and sometimes of terminal arteries producing an angioma of maculalike appearance, or hyperemic spot.

    t. lymphat'ica. Tumor composed of dilated lymph vessels.

telangiectoma (tel-ǎn-jĭ-ěk-tō'mǎ). Angioma from dilatation of capillaries or arterioles. Syn: *telangioma.*

telangiitis (tēl-ǎn-jĭ-ī'tĭs). Inflammation of the capillaries.

telangioma (těl"ǎn-jĭ-ō'mǎ). A tumor made up of dilated capillaries or arterioles.

telangiosis (tel-ǎn-jĭ-ō'sĭs). Disease of capillary vessels. See: *telangiectasis.*

tele-, tel-. Combining forms meaning *at a distance, far off.*

telecardiogram (tel"ě-kar'dĭ-ō-grǎm). A cardiogram which records at a distance from the patient. Syn: *telelectrocardiogram.*

telecardiography (těl"ě-kar"dĭ-og'rǎ-fĭ). Process of taking telecardiograms.

telecardiophone (těl"ě-kar'dĭ-ō-fōn). A stethoscope that will magnify heart sounds so that they may be heard at a distance from the patient.

teleceptive (tēl-ē-sěp'tĭv). Relating to a teleceptor.

teleceptor (tēl'ě-sěp-tor). A device that receives stimuli from a distance.

telecinesia (tēl"ě-sīn-ē'zĭ-ǎ). Apparent automatic movement of an object produced without contact with any stimulus or power.

teleo-, tele-. Combining forms meaning *perfect, complete.*

telecurietherapy (tēl-ě-kū-rĭ-thěr'ǎ-pĭ). Application of radium rays from a distance from a patient.

teledendrite, teledendron (tēl-ē-děn'drĭt, -děn'drŏn). A terminal dendron. Syn: *telodendron.*

telediastolic (te"lē-dĭ-as-tol'ĭk). Concerning the last phase of the diastole.

telegony (tēl-ěg'ō-nĭ). An alleged theory that the male sperm from a dam's first sexual contact modifies the blood of the female, thus influencing the offspring resulting from mating with another sire.

telelectrocardiogram (těl"ē-lěk"trō-kar'dĭ-ō-grǎm). One taken with a galvanometer attached to the patient by a wire some distance from the instrument. Syn: *telecardiogram.*

telencephalic (tēl-ěn-sěf-al'ĭk). Pert. to the endbrain (telencephalon).

telencephalon (tēl-ěn-sěf'ǎ-lŏn). The embryonic endbrain or ant. division of the prosencephalon from which the cerebral hemispheres are developed.

teleneurite (tĕl-ē-nū'rīt). The terminal arborization of an axis cylinder.

teleneuron (tĕl-ē-nū'rŏn). A nerve ending at which an impulse terminates.

teleology (tĕl-ē-ŏl'ō-jĭ). The belief that everything has a final purpose.

teleomitosis (tĕl"ē-ō-mĭ-tō'sĭs). Completed indirect cell division. SEE: *karyokinesis, mitosis.*

teleorganic (tĕl"ē-or-găn'ĭk). Necessary to organic life. SYN: *vital.*

teleotherapeutics (tĕl"ē-ō-ther-ă-pū'tĭks). The use of hypnotic suggestion in the treatment of disease. SYN: *suggestive therapeutics.*

telepathist (tĕl-ĕp'ă-thĭst). One who claims the ability to read the mind of others.

telepathy (tĕl-ĕp'ă-thĭ). Supposed communication of one mind with another at a distance without any means known to physical or psychological science. SYN: *thought transference.*

telephase (tĕl'ē-fāz). Final stage of mitosis in which the cytoplasm divides.

teleradiography (tĕl"ē-rā-dĭ-og'ră-fĭ). Radiography with the tube about 2 meters (6½ ft.) from the body.

teleroentgenography (tĕl"ē-rĕnt"gĕn-ŏg'-răf-ĭ). Radiography in which the tube is about 2 meters (6½ ft.) from the body. SYN: *teleradiography.*

telergy (tĕl'er-jĭ). 1. Action without conscious exercise of the will. SYN: *automatism.* 2. Hypothetical action of one individual's thoughts upon brain of another by transmission of some unknown form of energy.

telesthesia (tĕl-ĕs-thē'zĭ-ă). An impression received at a distance without normal operation of organs of sense. SYN: *telepathy.*

telesyphilis (tĕl-ĕ-sĭf'ĭl-ĭs). 1. Congenital syphilis without lesions. SYN: *metasyphilis.* 2. Any nonsyphilitic condition due to syphilis. SEE: *parasyphilitic.*

telesystolic (tĕl"ē-sĭs-tol'ĭk). Pert. to the termination of the cardiac systole.

teletherapy (tĕl-ē-thĕr'ă-pĭ). Absent treatment; treatment of disease by telepathy*; method of mental healers.

tellurism (tĕl'ū-rĭzm). Morbific influence of the soil.

tellurium (tĕl-ū'rĭ-ŭm). SYMB: *Te.* A nonmetallic element used as an electric rectifier and in coloring glass.

teloblast (tĕl-ō-blăst). A segmentation cell at the growing end of a germinal band.

telodendron (tĕl-ō-dĕn'drŏn). Terminal arborization of the axis cylinder process of a neuron.

telophase (tĕl'ō-fāz). The last stage of karyokinesis in which the cytoplasm divides into 2 daughter cells; the last stage in mitosis.*

telotism (tĕl'ō-tĭzm). The entire performance of a function, as that of one of the senses.

temperament (tĕm'per-ă-mĕnt). Individual peculiarity of physical and mental organization.

 t., bilious. One in which the nutritive system is predominant; usually characterized by dark complexion, muscular activity, energy of action, firmness of purpose, and passionate disposition.

 t., choleric. Same as *bilious temperament.*

 t., equal. An equable disposition.

 t., lymphatic. Same as *phlegmatic temperament.*

 t., melancholic. One characterized by brooding thoughtfulness, irritability, tenacity of purpose, and obstinacy of disposition.

 t., nervous. One in which the nervous organization is exceedingly sensitive, characterized by quick mental action and vivid emotions.

 t., phlegmatic. One in which the lymphatic system is supposed to predominate, characterized by mental sluggishness, pale complexion, flabby muscles, and dullness of passionate emotions.

 t., sanguine. A temperament characterized by marked physical vitality, irritability, energy of action and liability to nervous exhaustion, light hair, eyes and complexion, good digestion.

temperature (tĕm'per-ă-tūr). 1. Degree of heat of a living body; loosely, body heat above normal. 2. Degree of hotness or coldness of a substance.

Temperature Indications

107° F.	Generally fatal except in intermittent fever.
106° F.	Intense fever.
105° F.	High fever, dangerous.
104° F.	Severe fever.
102° F.	Moderate fever.
101° F.	Slight fever.
98.6° F.	Normal.
98° F.	Subnormal.
96° F.	Collapse.
94° F.	Algid collapse.
93° F.	Fatal collapse except in cholera.

 t., absolute. Temperature measured from absolute zero, —273° C.

 t., animal. Normal temperature of the healthy adult.

 t., body. The temperature of the body.

 t., critical. The temperature below which a gas may be converted to liquid form by pressure.

 t. curve. Line indicating the fluctuations of temperature for a given period.

 t., fall of. Extreme weakness.

 t., high. More alarming with wet skin than with dry skin.

 t., maximum. BACT: Temperature above which growth will not take place.

 t., mean. The average temperature for a stated period in a given locality.

 t., minimum. BACT: Temperature below which growth will not take place.

 t., normal. Temperature of the body in health, 98.6° F. (37° C.) in man.

 t., optimum. Temperature at which an operation is best carried out, as the culture of a given organism.

t., rectal. The thermometer should be inserted at least 1½ in. and allowed to remain 3-5 minutes. Do not take following rectal operation or if rectum is diseased.

t., room. Temperature bet. 65-80° F.

t. sense. Sense responding to heat and cold.

t., subnormal. Temperature below the normal of 98.6° F.

t., zero. Temperature at which heat and cold are not felt by a sensory end organ.

temple (tĕm′pl). The region of head in front of ear and over the zygoma.

tempolabile (tĕm″pō-lā′bl). Becoming altered spontaneously within a definite time.

temporal (tĕm′por-ăl). 1. Pert. to or limited in time. 2. Relating to the temples.

t. bone. A bone on both sides of the skull at its base. SYN: *os temporale*. SEE: *Arnold's canal, mastoid, petrosa, petrosal, squamous, styloid process.*

t. crest. The ridge on frontal bone attaching the temporalis muscle. SYN: *crista temporalis.*

t. fissure. One on lateral surface of the temporal lobe.

t. ganglion. A sympathetic one on the ext. carotid artery.

t. ramus. A branch of the facial nerve in the temporal region.

temporalis (tĕm″pō-rā′lĭs). Muscle in temporal fossa which elevates the mandible.

temporo-. Combining form meaning *temples of the head.*

temporomaxillary (tĕm″por-ō-măks′ĭl-lā-rĭ). Pert. to the temporal and maxillary bones.

temporoöccipital (tĕm″por-ō-ŏk-sĭp′ĭ-tăl). Pert. to the temporal and occipital bones or their regions.

temporosphenoid (tĕm″por-ō-sfē′noyd). Pert. to the temporal and sphenoid bones.

tempostabile, tempostable (tĕm″pō-stā′bl). Not subject to change chemically in course of time.

temulence (tĕm′ū-lĕns). Drunkenness; intoxication.

tenacious (tē-nā′shŭs). Adhering to; adhesive; retentive.

tenaculum (tĕn-ăk′ū-lŭm). Sharp, hooklike, pointed instrument with slender shank for grasping and holding a part, as an artery.

t., abdominal. Longer than others with smaller hook. *Sim's, Emmet's, Kelly's,* etc.

t., uterine. Heavier and shorter hook used for manipulating uterus.

tenalgia (tĕn-ăl′jĭ-ă). Pain in a tendon. SYN: *tenodynia.*

t. crepitans. Inflammation of a tendon sheath which on movement results in a crackling sound. SYN: *tendosynovitis crepitans.*

tenderness (tĕn′dĕr-nĕs). Sensitiveness to pain upon pressure, usually cutaneous.

tendinitis (tĕn-dĭn-ī′tĭs). Inflammation of a tendon. SYN: *tenonitis, 1; tenontitis.*

tendinoplasty (tĕn′dĭ-nō-plăs″tĭ). Plastic surgery of tendons. SYN: *tenontoplasty, tenoplasty.*

tendinosuture (tĕn″dĭn-ō-sū′tūr). The suturing of a divided tendon. SYN: *tenorrhaphy.*

tendinous (tĕn′dĭn-ŭs). Pert. to, composed of, or resembling tendons.

t. spot. A white thickening of a serous membrane.

t. synovitis. Inflammation of a tendon's synovial sheath.

tendo (tĕn′dō) (pl. *tendines*). A tendon.

t. Achil′lis. The tendon of the soleus and gastrocnemius muscles inserted into tuberosity of the os calcis.

t. calca′neus. BNA. Same as *tendo Achillis.*

tendolysis (tĕn-dŏl′ĭ-sĭs). The process of freeing a tendon from adhesions.

tendon (tĕn′dŭn). Fibrous connective tissue serving for the attachment of muscles to bones and other parts. SYN: *sinew.*

t., Achilles′. The large tendon at lower end of gastrocnemius muscle, inserted into the *os calcis.*
It is the strongest and thickest one in the body.

t., calcaneous. Achilles* tendon.

t. cells. Certain flat ones in white tissue fiber of tendons.

t. reflex. Reflex act in which a muscle contracts when its tendon is percussed.

t. r., patella. Response to tapping of the quadriceps muscle tendon when patient is sitting with toes pressing on the floor.

t. spindle. Fusiform nerve ending in a tendon.

tendoplasty (tĕn′dō-plăs″tĭ). Reparative surgery of an injured tendon. SYN: *tenoplasty, tenontoplasty.*

tendosynovitis (tĕn″dō-sĭn″ō-vī′tĭs). Inflammation of a sheath of a tendon or the tendon. SYN: *tendovaginitis, tenontothecitis.*

t. crepitans. Tendosynovitis accompanied on movement by a crackling sound.

tendotome (tĕn′dō-tōm). Instrument for severing a tendon. SYN: *tenotome.*

tendotomy (tĕn-dŏt′ō-mĭ). Division of a tendon. SYN: *tenotomy.*

tendovaginal (tĕn″dō-văj′ĭ-năl). Relating to a tendon and its sheath.

tendovaginitis (tĕn″dō-văj″ĭn-ī′tĭs). Inflamed condition of a tendon and its sheath. SYN: *tenontothecitis.*

tenesmic (tĕn-ĕz′mĭk). Pert. to or like tenesmus.

tenesmus (tē-nĕz′mŭs). Spasmodic contraction of anal or vesical sphincter with pain and persistent desire to empty the bowel or bladder, with involuntary, ineffectual straining efforts.

tenia (tē′nĭ-ă). 1. A flat band of tissue. 2. A genus of tapeworm. SYN: *taenia, q.v.*

teniacide (tē'nĭ-ăs-ĭd). Destroying or that which destroys tapeworms.

teniafuge (tē'nĭ-ả-fūj). Expelling or a drug that expels tapeworms. Ex: *oleoresin of male fern, pelctierine tannat.* SYN: *tenifuge.*

teniasis (tē-nī'ás-ĭs). Presence of tapeworms in the body.

tenifuge (tĕn'ĭf-ūj). Causing or that which causes expulsion of tapeworms. SYN: *teniafuge.*

ten'nis el'bow. An obscure, insidious, distressing complaint after playing tennis following a period of muscular inactivity of the arm or following a long duration of play.

teno-. Combining form meaning *tendon.*

tenodesis (tĕn-od'e-sĭs). Suturing of the end of a tendon to a point of attachment.

tenodynia (tĕn-ō-dĭn'ĭ-ă). Pain in a tendon. SYN: *tenalgia.*

tenomyoplasty (tĕn″ō-mĭ'ō-plăs″tĭ). Reparative operation upon a tendon and muscle. SYN: *tenontomyoplasty.*

tenomyotomy (tĕn″ō-mī-ŏt'ō-mĭ). Excision of lateral portion of a tendon or muscle.

tenonitis (tĕn-ō-nī'tĭs). 1. Inflammation of a tendon. SYN: *tenontitis.* 2. Inflammation of Tenon's capsule.

tenonometer (tē″nō-nŏm'ĕ-ter). Device for measuring amount of intraocular tension.

Tenon's capsule (tē-non'). A thin connective tissue envelope of the eyeball behind the conjunctiva.

   T.'s space. One bet. the post. surface of the eyeball and Tenon's capsule.

tenontagra (tĕn-ŏn-tă'gră, -tăg'ra). A gouty inflammation of the tendons.

tenontitis (tĕn-ŏn-tī'tĭs). Inflammation of a tendon. SYN: *tendinitis, tenositis.*

tenontodynia (tĕn-ŏn-tō-dĭn'ĭ-ă). Pain in a tendon. SYN: *tenalgia, tenodynia.*

tenontography (tĕn-ŏn-tog'ră-fĭ). A treatise on the tendons.

tenontology (tĕn-ŏn-tŏl'ō-jĭ). The study of the tendons.

tenontomyoplasty (tĕn-ŏn″tō-mĭ'ō-plăs″tĭ). Plastic surgery, including muscle and tendon repair, in treatment of hernia. SYN: *tenomyoplasty.*

tenontomyotomy (tĕn-ŏn″tō-mĭ-ŏt'ō-mĭ). Cutting of the principal tendon of a muscle, with excision of the muscle in part or in whole. SYN: *myotenotomy.*

tenontoplasty (tĕn-ŏn″tō-plăs″tĭ). Plastic surgery of defective or injured tendons. SYN: *tenoplasty.*

tenontothecitis (tĕn-ŏn-tō-thē-sī'tĭs). Inflammation of a tendon and its sheath. SYN: *tendosynovitis, tendovaginitis, tenosynovitis.*

   t. steno'sans. A chronic form of tenontothecitis with narrowing of the sheath.

tenophyte (tĕn'ō-fīt). A cartilaginous or osseous growth on a tendon.

tenoplasty (tĕn'ō-plăs″tĭ). Reparative surgery of tendons. SYN: *tenontoplasty.*

tenorrhaphy (tĕn-or'ă-fĭ). Suturing of a tendon.

tenositis (tĕn-ō-sī'tĭs). Inflammation of a tendon. SYN: *tenontitis.*

tenostosis (tĕn-ōs-tō'sĭs). Conversion of a tendon into bony tissue.

tenosuspension (ten-o-sus-pen'shun). Suspension of the humerus by a layer of a tendon to the acromion process.

tenosuture (tĕn'ō-sū'tūr). Reunion of a divided tendon. SYN: *tenorrhaphy.*

tenosynovitis (tĕn″ō-sĭn-ō-vī'tĭs). 1. Inflammation of a tendon and its sheath. 2. Inflammation of a tendon sheath.

   t. crepitans. Inflammation of a tendon sheath in which a crackling sound is heard on motion.

   t. hyperplastica. Painless swelling of extensor tendons over the wrist joint.

tenotome (tĕn'ō-tōm). Instrument for section of a tendon.

tenotomist (tĕn-ŏt'ō-mĭst). Specialist in tenotomy.

tenotomy (tĕn-ŏt'ō-mĭ). Section of a tendon.

tenovaginitis (tĕn″ō-văj-ĭn-ī'tĭs). Inflammation of a tendon or a tendon and its sheath. SYN: *tenontothecitis.*

tension (tĕn'shŭn). 1. Process or act of stretching; state of being strained or stretched. 2. Pressure, as arterial tension. 3. Expansive force of a gas or vapor. 4. PT: A synonym for voltage; thus high tension would mean high voltage.

   t., arterial. That of an artery at height of the pulse wave in pressing against the walls.

   t. of gases. Gas pressure measured in percentages of atmospheric pressure.

   t., intraocular. Internal pressure of liquid within eyeball.

   t., surface. Molecular property of film on surface of a liquid to resist rupture, the particles tending to pull inward.

   t. suture. One used to reduce pull of the edges of a wound.

tensiophone (tĕn'sĭ-ō-fōn). Device for obtaining blood pressure readings by auscultation and palpation.

tensor (tĕn'sor). A muscle making a part tense.

tent (tĕnt). 1. To keep open with a tent. 2. Cylindrical rod of absorbable material used to dilate the mouth of any hollow organ or canal, to keep the orifices of a wound open, or to absorb discharges.

tentative (tĕn'tă-tĭv). Noting a diagnosis subject to change because of insufficient data; experimental.

tenth cranial nerve. Nerve supplying most of the abdominal viscera, the heart, lungs, and esophagus. SYN: *pneumogastric nerve, q.v.*

tentigo (tĕn-tī'gō). Abnormal sexual desire. SYN: *lasciviousness, lust, nymphomania, satyriasis.*

tentorium (tĕn-tō'rĭ-ŭm). A tentlike structure or part.

   t. cerebelli. BNA. The process of the dura mater bet. the cerebrum and cerebellum supporting the occipital lobes.

tentum (tĕn'tŭm). The penis.

tephromalacia (tĕf″rō-măl-ă'sĭ-ă). Softening of the gray substance of brain or spinal cord.

tephromyelitis (tĕf″rō-mī-ĕl-ī′tĭs). Inflammation of the gray matter of the spinal cord. SYN: *poliomyelitis.*

tephrosis (tĕf′rō′sĭs). Incineration; cremation.

tephrylometer (tĕf-rĭ-lom′ĕ-ter). Device for measuring the thickness of the cerebral cortex, the gray matter of brain.

tepid (tĕp′ĭd). Slightly warm; lukewarm.
  t. bath. One about 86° F. (30° C.).

tepidarium (tĕp-ĭd-ā′rĭ-ŭm). A place for a warm bath.

ter-. Combining form meaning *thrice.*

teratic (tĕr-ăt′ĭk). Pert. to a monster.

terato-. Combining form meaning a *marvel, prodigy, monster.*

teratoblastoma (tĕr″ă-tō-blăs-tō′mă). A tumor containing embryonic material but which is not representative of all 3 germinal layers. SEE: *teratoma.*

teratoid (tĕr′ă-toyd). Resembling a monster.
  t. tumor. Tumor of embryonic remains from all of the germinal layers. SYN: *teratoma.*

teratology (tĕr-ăt-ŏl′ō-jĭ). Branch of science dealing with the study of monsters.

teratoma (tĕr-ă-tō′mă). Congenital tumor containing embryonic elements of all 3 primary germ layers, as hair, teeth, etc. SYN: *dermoid.*

teratomatous (ter-ă-tō′mă-tus). Pert. to or resembling a teratoma.

teratophobia (tĕr″ă-tō-fō′bĭ-ă). Abnormal fear of giving birth to a monster or of being in contact with one.

teratosis (tĕr-ă-tō′sĭs). A monstrosity.

tere (te′re). Rub.

terebinthinate (tĕr″ē-bĭn′thĭ-nāt). Containing or agent containing turpentine.

terebrant, terebrating (ter′ē-brant, -brāt-ing). Boring or piercing, said of pain.

terebration (tĕr-ē-brā′shŭn). 1. The act of boring. SYN: *trephining.* 2. A boring pain.

teres (tē′rēz). 1. Round and smooth; cylindrical. 2. A rounded muscle.
  t. major. A muscle that draws the arm down and back.
  t. minor. A muscle inserted in the great tuberosity of the humerus, which rotates the humerus outward and abducts it.

tereti-. Combining form meaning *round.*

tergo-. Combining form meaning *the back.*

tergum (ter′gŭm). The back.

ter in die. Three times a day.

term (term). 1. A limit or boundary. 2. A definite period. 3. Gestation at the normal period.

terma (ter′mă). A thin plate in front of the optic chiasm. SYN: *lamina terminalis.*

terminal (ter′mĭn-ăl). 1. An end or extremity. 2. Pert. to or placed at the end.
  t. alveolus. A pulmonary vesicle or air sac.
  t. artery. One with no branches, but which splits into capillaries.

t. dementia. Dementia following mania or melancholia or other acute attacks of insanity.
  t. filum. Slender end of the spinal cord. SYN: *filum terminale.*
  t. infection. One appearing in the late stage of another disease; often fatal.

terminology (ter-mĭn-ŏl′ō-jĭ). The special terms used in any field, as an art or science. SYN: *nomenclature.*

ternary (ter′na-rĭ). 1. Threefold; triple; third. 2. Composed of 3 elements.
  t. acid. An inorganic acid containing hydrogen and 2 other elements.
  t. bodies. The fats, proteins, and carbohydrates of any food.

ter′pin hy′drate. USP. White crystalline substance with a turpentine taste made by the interaction of rectified spirits of turpentine, alcohol, and nitric acid.
  DOSAGE (average): 4 gr. (0.25 Gm.).

terra (tĕr′ă). Earth; soil.
  t. al′ba. White clay.
  t. fullon′ica. Fuller's earth.

terracing (ter′ăs-ĭng). Suturing in several rows through thick tissues in closing a wound.

terror (ter′or). Very great fear.
  t., night. Nightmare or night terror, esp. of children.

tertian (ter′shŭn). Occurring every 3rd day.
  t. fever. A malarial fever with paroxysms every other day.
  t. fever, double. The paroxysms occur every day, being similar on alternate days. SEE: *quotidian fever.*

tertiarism, tertiarismus (ter′shĭ-ar-ĭzm, -ĭz′mŭs). All the symptoms, collectively, of tertiary syphilis.

tertiary (ter′shĭ-a-rĭ). Third in order or stage.
  t. alcohol. One containing the trivalent group. COH.
  t. syphilis. Third and most advanced stage of syphilis.

tertipara (ter-tĭp′ă-ră). A woman who has given birth to 3 children.

tessellated (tĕs′ĕl-ā-tĕd). Composed of little squares; checkered.
  t. epithelium. Pavement epithelium* composed of overlapping squamous cells.

test (test). 1. An examination. 2. Method to determine the presence or nature of a substance, or the presence of a disease. 3. A chemical reaction. 4. A reagent or substance used in making a test.
  t., acetone. Test for presence of acetone in the urine; made by adding a few drops of sodium nitroprusside to the urine along with strong ammonia water. Presence of acetone causes formation of a magenta ring at outline of contacts.
  t., Allen-Doisy. Test to determine amount of estrogen content in female blood serum by its reaction on secretions of mice.
  t., Aschheim-Zondek. Test for pregnancy by injecting the patient's urine subcutaneously in immature female mice.
  t., Binet-Simon. Method of ascertaining the mental capacity of children by

asking a series of suitable questions. SEE: *Binet age.*

t., bluret. Test for the presence of proteins or urea.

t., Brouha. Test for pregnancy by injecting the urine of the patient into male mice for 8 to 10 days. Positive reaction indicated by hypertrophy and hyperemia of the seminal vesicles.

t., Chrobak. Cancer is present if probing an eroded cervix produces bleeding and crumbling of the tissue.

t., Friedman. Test for pregnancy by injecting urine of the patient into unmated mature female rabbits, a positive reaction being indicated by formation of corpora lutea and corpora haemorrhagica.

t., Gelle's. Test for lesions of the ear by employing rubber tubing and a tuning fork.

t., Huhner. Aspiration of vagina within an hour after coitus, to investigate sperm activity.

t., Kahn's. Precipitation test for syphilis.

t., paper. Paper used in making tests, as litmus paper.

t., pregnancy. Test to determine pregnancy.

t., Rubin. Test for patency of the fallopian tubes by insufflation with carbon dioxide; used to determine cause of sterility.

t., Schiller's. Test for cancer of the cervix by painting with iodine solution; since cancer cells do not stain with iodine, they turn white or yellow.

t., Schneider's. A pregnancy test using female rabbits.

t., Schwabach's. Test for hearing using tuning forks.

t. solution. A standard solution used in making a test.

t. tube. A plain tube of thin glass, closed at 1 end, used for simple tests.

t., urea balance. Test of the kidney function by measuring intake and output of urea.

t., Wassermann. Diagnostic test for syphilis based on principle of fixation of complement.

testectomy (těs-těk'tō-mǐ). 1. Removal of a testicle. SYN: *castration.* 2. Removal of a corpus quadrigeminum.

testes (těs'tēs) (sing. *testis*). Two glandular bodies in the scrotum of the male. The producers of the male germinative cell. SYN: *testicles.*

testicle (těs'tǐ-kl). One of the 2 ovoid male gonads situated in the scrotum which produce spermatozoa and some of the fluid elements of the semen. SYN: *testis, q.v.*

t. compression reflex. Contraction of abdominal muscles following moderate compression of testicle.

t., displaced. A testicle within (abnormally) the inguinal canal, or pelvis.

t., inverted. One reversed in the scrotum so that the epididymis attaches to the ant. instead of post. part of gland.

t., undescended. One or both remain in the inguinal canal or abdominal cavity at birth.

testicond (tes'tǐ-kŏnd). Having the testicles undescended.

testicular (těs-tǐk'ū-lar). Relating to a testicle.

t. cord. The spermatic cord. SYN: *funiculus spermaticus.*

t. duct. Excretory duct of the testicle. SYN: *vas deferens.*

t. fluid. Semen.

t. therapy. 1. The injections of testicular fluid or extracts. 2. Testicular substances administered by inunction.

testis (tes'tǐs) (pl. *testes*). 1. A testicle, the male reproductive gland in the scrotum. 2. One of the 2 post. tubercles of the corpus quadrigeminum. SYN: *colliculus inferior.*

t., descent of. Change in position of the testis from abdominal cavity to scrotum during fetal life.

testitis (těs-tī'tǐs). Inflammation of a testis. SYN: *orchitis.*

testitoxicosis (těs''tǐ-tŏks-ǐ-kō'sǐs). A toxic state sometimes following ligation of the vas deferens.

test meal. A meal, usually small, of definite quality and composition, given to stimulate gastric secretion and thus furnish material to be withdrawn for examination.

testosterone (těs''tō-stē'rŏn). A hormonal crystalline substance isolated from bull's testes and prepared synthetically from cholesterol.

t. propionate. The propionic acid ester of testosterone, a much more potent form.

DOSAGE: Minimum effective 3/8 gr. (25 mg.) intramuscularly, 3 times weekly.

tetanic (tē-tǎn'ǐk). 1. Pert. to or producing tetanus. 2. Any agent producing tetanic spasms.

t. convulsion. A tonic one with constant muscular contraction.

tetaniform (tē-tǎn'ǐ-form). Resembling tetanus.

tetanilla (tět-ǎn-ǐl'lǎ). 1. Mild form of tetany* without rigidity. 2. Twitchings of a limited group of muscular fibers with clonic paroxysmal contractions.

tetanism (tět'ǎn-ǐzm). Persistent muscular hypertonicity resembling tetanus, esp. in infants.

tetanization (tět-ǎn-ǐ-zā'shŭn). The production or condition of tetanic convulsions or symptoms.

tetanize (tět'ǎn-īz). To induce tonic muscular spasms.

tetanode (tět'ǎ-nŏd). 1. Resembling tetanus. SYN: *tetanoid.* 2. Noting interval bet. recurrent tonic spasms in tetany.

tetanoid (tět'ǎ-noyd). Resembling tetanus. SYN: *tetaniform.*

t. fever. Inflamed condition of membrane of spinal cord and brain. SYN: *cerebrospinal meningitis.*

t. paraplegia. Paralysis of lower extremities due to lateral sclerosis of spinal cord. SYN: *spastic paraplegia.*

tetanomotor (tĕt″ăn-o-mō′tor). Appliance for the production of tetanic motor spasms mechanically by shocking a nerve.

tetanophil, tetanophilic (tĕt′ăn-ō-fĭl, tĕt″-ăn-ō-fĭl′ĭk). Possessing an affinity for tetanus toxin.

tetanus (tĕt′ă-nŭs). 1. An infectious, acute disease due to the toxin of *Bacillus tetani,* in which there is a state of more or less persistent, painful tonic spasm of some of the voluntary muscles. 2. Continuous tonic spasm of a muscle.

t., anticus. Form in which the body is bowed forward.

t., artificial. Form produced by a drug like strychnine or by mechanical appliance.

t., cephalic. Same as *kopf tetanus.*

t., cerebral. A form produced by inoculating the brain of animals with tetanus antitoxin, marked by epileptiform convulsions and excitement.

t. dorsalis. Tetanus in which the body is bent backward.

t., extensor. That which affects the extensors especially.

t., head. Same as *kopf tetanus.*

t., hydrophobic. Kopf tetanus.

t., idiopathic. That which occurs without any visible lesion.

t., imitative. Hysteria which simulates tetanus.

t., impf. Inoculated tetanus; cultures afford a special form of pathogenic bacillus.

t. infantum. Tetanus of young infants, due to infection of umbilicus.

t., intermittent. A disease characterized by painful tonic and symmetric spasm of muscles of extremities. Occurs after typhoid fever, diarrhea, exposure to cold, rickets, after ingestion of alkaline salts, deficiency of calcium, and excision of the parathyroid gland. May continue for several weeks; usually ends in recovery. SYN: *tetany.*

t., kopf. Form due to a wound of the head, esp. one near the eyebrow. It is marked by trismus, facial paralysis on one side, and pronounced dysphagia; resembles rabies; often fatal. Called also *cephalic tetanus, head tetanus, hydrophobic tetanus.*

t. lateralis. Form in which the body is bent sideways.

t., localized. Tetanic spasm of a single part.

t., neonatorum. Tetanus of very young infants, usually due to infection of navel.

t. paradoxus. Cephalic tetanus in which condition is combined with paralysis of the facial or other cranial nerve.

t., partial. Tetany.

t. posticus. Same as *tetanus dorsalis.*

t., postoperative. Tetanus which follows an operation.

t., puerperal. Tetanus which occurs in childbed.

t., rheumatic. Form due to exposure to cold and wet.

t., Ritter's. Tetanic contractions at opening of a constant current which has been passing along a nerve for some time; seen in tetany.

t., toxic. Produced by overdose of nux vomica or strychnine.

t., traumatic. Tetanus which follows wound poisoning.

tetany (tĕt′ă-nĭ). A nervous affection, characterized by intermittent tonic spasms, which are usually paroxysmal and involve the extremities; most frequent in the young; frequently associated with pregnancy or lactation.

t., duration. Continuous contraction. esp. in degenerated muscles, in response to a continuous electric current.

t., gastric. Severe tetany from stomach disorders accompanied by tonic, painful spasms of extremities.

t., hyperventilation. Tetany caused by continued forced respiration.

t., latent. Tetany caused by stimulation.

t., parathyroid. Tetany due to excision of the parathyroid gland.

t., thyroprival. Tetany resulting from suspended thyroid function.

tetarcone (tĕt′ar-kōn). Fourth or distolingual cusp of an upper molar tooth. SYN: *tetartocone.*

tetartanopia, tetartanopsia (tĕt″ar-tăn-ō′pĭ-ă, -ŏp′sĭ-ă). Symmetrical blindness in the same quadrant of each visual field. SYN: *hemianopsia, quadrant.*

tetartocone (tĕt-ar′tō-kōn). The distolingual cusp of an upper molar tooth. SYN: *tetarcone.*

tethelin (tĕth′ĕ-lĭn). A substance derived from the ant. lobe of the pituitary having an accelerating effect on growth.

tetmil (tĕt′mĭl). Ten millimeters; a unit of measurement. [*four.*

tetra-, tetr-. Combining forms meaning **tetrabasic** (tĕt″ră-bā′sĭk). Having 4 replaceable hydrogen atoms, said of an acid or acid salt.

tetrablastic (tĕt″ră-blăs′tĭk). Having 4 germinal layers, the *ectoderm, endoderm,* and 2 *mesodermic* layers.

tetrabromofluorescein (tĕt″ră-brŏm″ō-flū-or-ĕs′ĭn, -ē-ĭn). A dye, $C_{20}H_8Br_4O_5$, obtained from action of bromine on fluorescein, used as a stain in microscopy. SYN: *eosin.*

tetrachlorethylene (tĕt″ră-klor-ĕth′ĭl-ēn). A clear, colorless liquid with a characteristic odor.

DOSAGE: 15-45 ♏ (1-3 cc.), followed by saline cathartic.

tetracid (tĕ-trăs′ĭd). 1. Able to react with 4 molecules of a monoacid or 2 of a diacid to form a salt or ester, said of a base or alcohol; term disapproved by some authorities. 2. Having 4 hydrogen atoms replaceable by basic atoms or radicals, said of acids. 3. An acid containing 4 acid hydrogen atoms.

Tetracoccus (tĕt″rā-kŏk′ŭs). Genus of micrococcus arranged in groups of 4 by division into 2 planes.

tetracrotic (tĕt″rā-krŏt′ĭk). Noting a pulse or pulse tracing with 4 upward strokes in the descending limb of the wave. Syn: *catatricrotic*.

tetrad (tĕt′răd). 1. A group of 4 things with something in common. 2. An element having a valency or combining power of 4. 3. Group of 4 similar bodies. 4. Group of 4 parts, said of cells produced by division in 2 planes, or of a chromosome in 4 parts in preparation for 2 mitotic divisions in maturation.

tetragenous (tĕt-răj′ĕn-ŭs). Dividing into groups of 4; noting bacteria, as *Micrococcus tetragenus*.

tetragonum (tĕt″rā-gō′nŭm). Quadrangle.
　　t. lumba′le. A lumbar quadrangle surrounded by 4 muscles.

tetramastia (tĕt″rā-măs′tĭ-ă). Condition characterized by presence of 4 breasts. Syn: *tetramazia*.

tetramazia (tĕt″rā-mā′zĭ-ă). Condition of having 4 breasts. Syn: *tetramastia*.

tetrameric, tetramerous (tĕt″rā-mĕr′ĭk, tĕt-răm′ĕr-ŭs). Having 4 parts, or arranged in groups of 4 parts.

tetranopsia (tĕt-rā-nŏp′sĭ-ă). Obliteration of visual field by one-quarter.

tetraplegia (tĕt-rā-plē′jĭ-ă). Paralysis of both arms and legs.

tetraster (tĕt-răs′tẽr). A figure in which there are 4 asters, instead of more commonly 2; occurring abnormally in mitosis.

Tetrastoma (tĕt-răs′tō-mă). A genus of trematode worms found in urine occasionally, having 4 suckers.

tetter (tĕt′ẽr). 1. Any of various vesicular cutaneous diseases, as herpes, ringworm, or eczema. 2. A pimple or blister.
　　t., blister. Disease with bullae formation and pigmented spots. Syn: *pemphigus*.
　　t., brawny. Excessive discharge from oil glands of scalp. Syn: *seborrhea capitis*.
　　t., crusted. Inflammatory skin disease with pustule formation. Syn: *impetigo*.
　　t., dry. Inflammatory skin disease with vesiculation and shedding of dry scales. Syn: *eczema, scaly*.
　　t., eating. Tuberculous disease of the skin. Syn: *lupus*.
　　t., honeycomb. Contagious skin disease with honeycomblike crust formation. Syn: *favus*.
　　t., milky. Brawny tetter in infants. Syn: *crusta lactea*.

textiform (tĕks′tĭ-form). Resembling a network, web or mesh.

textoblastic (tĕks″tō-blăs′tĭk). Forming adult tissue; regenerative; noting cells.

textoma (tĕks-tō′mă). A tumor made up of completely differentiated tissue cells.

textural (tĕks′tū-răl). Concerning the texture or constitution of a tissue.

T fracture. One in which bone splits both longitudinally and transversely.

thalamencephalon (thăl″ăm-ĕn-sĕf′ăl-ŏn). The interbrain; an embryonic structure produced from the post. part of the anterior cerebral vesicle composed of the epithalamus, hypothalamus, and the thalamus. Syn: *diencephalon*.

thalamic (thăl-ăm′ĭk). Pert. to the thalamus.
　　t. epilepsy. Epilepsy resulting from disease of the thalamus.
　　t. syndrome. Sensory disturbances and pain in conjunction with mild hemiplegia.

thalamo-. Combining form meaning *chamber, part of brain at which a nerve originates*.

thalamocele, thalamocoele (thăl′ăm-ō-sēl). The 3rd ventricle of the brain.

thalamocortical (thăl″ăm-ō-kor′tĭ-kăl). Pert. to the optic thalamus and the cerebral cortex.

thalamolenticular (thăl″ăm-ō-lĕn-tĭk′ū-lar). Concerning the optic thalamus and the lenticular nucleus.

thalamus (thăl′ă-mŭs) (pl. *thalami*). BNA. The largest subdivision of the diencephalon on either side, consisting chiefly of an ovoid, gray nuclear mass in the lateral wall of the 3rd ventricle.
　　t. opticus. Same as *thalamus*.

thalassophobia (thăl-ăs″sō-fō′bĭ-ă). Abnormal fear of the sea.

thalassotherapy (thăl-ăs″sō-ther′ă-pĭ). Treatment of disease by living at the seaside, by sea bathing, sea voyages, or sea air.

thallinization (thăl-lĕn-ĭ-zā′shŭn). Treatment with doses of thalline or its salts.

thallium (thăl′lĭ-ŭm). A rare, lustrous, white metal. Symb: Tl. At. wt. 204.39.

thamuria (thă-mū′rĭ-ă). Abnormally frequent urination. Syn: *pollakiuria*.

thanato-. Combining form meaning *death*.

thanatobiological (thăn″ă-tō-bī-ō-lŏj′ĭk-ăl). Relating to the processes of life and death.

thanatognomonic (thăn″ăt-ŏg-nō-mŏn′ĭk). Indicative of the approach of death.

thanatoid (thăn′ă-toyd). Resembling death.

thanatology (thăn″ă-tol′ō-jĭ). The science of death.

thanatomania (thăn″ă-tō-mā′nĭ-ă). Condition of homicidal or suicidal mania.

thanatometer (thăn-ă-tŏm′ĕt-ẽr). Instrument for determining occurrence of death by internal temperature.

thanatophobia (thăn″ă-tō-fō′bĭ-ă). Morbid fear of death.

thanatopsia, thanatopsy (thăn″ă-top′sĭ-ă, thăn′ăt-ŏp″sĭ). Examination of a dead body to determine cause of death. Syn: *autopsy, necropsy*.

thaumato-. Combining form meaning *wonder, marvel*.

theaism (thē′ă-ĭzm). Chronic poisoning from excess of tea drinking. Syn: *themism, theism*.

thebaism (thē′bă-ĭzm). Condition produced by opium.

Thebesius' foramina (thē-bē′zĭ-ŭs). Orifices of the Thebesius' veins, opening into the right auricle of the heart.

T.'s valve. An endocardial fold at entrance of the coronary sinus into right auricle.

T.'s veins. Venules conveying blood from the myocardium to the auricles or ventricles.

theca (thē'kǎ). A sheath of investing membrane, esp. the synovial sheath of a tendon.

   t. cor'dis. Pericardium, which sheathes the heart.

   t. follic'uli. Outer wall of a graafian follicle. [tendon.

   t. ten'dinis. Synovial sheath of a

   t. vertebra'lis. Dura mater of the spinal cord.

thecal (thē'kǎl). Pert. to a sheath.

   t. abscess. One of the theca of a tendon.

   t. puncture. Puncture of the meningeal sac. SEE: *spinal puncture*.

thecitis (thē-sī'tĭs). Inflammation of the sheath of a tendon.

theco-. Combining form meaning *sheath, case, receptacle*.

thecodont (thē'kō-dont). Having teeth which are inserted in sockets.

thecostegnosis, thecostegnosis (thē"kō-stĕg-nō'sĭ-ǎ, -nō'sĭs). Constriction of a tendon sheath.

theelin (thē'lĭn). Crystalline estrogenic hormone secreted by the placenta and ovarian follicles and found in the blood and urine of pregnant women.

   DOSAGE: 0.1-1.0 mg. (1000-10,000 internal units).

   SYN: *estrin, estrone, female sex hormone, folliculin, progynon*.

theelol (thē'lōl). An estrus-exciting hormone similar to but more active than theelin, found in urine of pregnant women. SYN: *estriol*.

theism (thē'ĭzm). Chronic poisoning from excess of tea drinking.

thelalgia (thē-lǎl'jǐ-ǎ). Pain in the nipples.

theleplasty (thĕl'ĕ-plǎs"tǐ). Plastic surgery of the nipple.

thelerethism (thĕl-ĕr'ĕ-thĭzm). Erection of the nipple.

thelitis (thē-lī'tǐs). Inflammation of the nipples.

thelium (thē'lǐ-ŭm). 1. A papilla. 2. A nipple. 3. A cellular layer.

thelyblast (thĕl'ǐ-blǎst). Nucleus of ovum immediately following fertilization. SYN: *feminonucleus*. SEE: *arsenoblast*.

thenad (thē'nǎd). Toward the palm or thenar eminence.

thenal (thē'nǎl). Pert. to the palm or thenar prominence.

   t. aspect. Outer side of the palm.

   t. eminence. Ball of the thumb. SYN: *thenar*.

thenar (thē'nar). 1. Palm of hand or sole of foot. 2. Fleshy eminence at base of thumb. 3. Concerning the palm.

   t. eminence. One at the base of the thumb.

   t. muscles. Abductor and flexor muscles of the thumb.

Theobroma (thē"ō-brō'mǎ). Plant yielding cacao butter.

theobromine (thē-ō-brō'mēn). A white powder obtained from Theobroma cacao.

   DOSAGE: 5-8 gr. (0.3-0.5 Gm.).

   t. with sodium salicylate. USP. Diuretin. Combination of sodium salicylate and theobromine.

   DOSAGE: 5-10 gr. (0.3-0.6 Gm.).

theocalcin (thē"ō-kǎl'sĭn). A double salt or mixture of calcium theobromine and calcium salicylate.

   DOSAGE: 7-15 gr. (0.5-1 Gm.).

theocin (thē'ō-sĭn). A brand of theophylline. USP.

   DOSAGE: 1½ gr. (0.1 Gm.).

   t. soluble (theocin-sodium acetate).

   DOSAGE: 2½ gr. (0.16 Gm.).

theomania (thē-ō-mā'nǐ-ǎ). Religious insanity; esp. that in which patient thinks he is the Deity or is inspired.

theophobia (thē"ō-fō'bǐ-ǎ). Abnormal fear of the wrath of God.

theophylline (thē"ō-fĭl'ĕn, -ĭn). USP. A white crystalline powder with action resembling caffeine and theobromine.

   DOSAGE: 4 gr. (0.25 Gm.).

theotherapy (thē"ō-thĕr'a-pǐ). Treatment of disease by spiritual and religious methods.

therapeutic (thĕr-ă-pū'tĭk). 1. Pert. to results obtained from treatment. 2. Having medicinal or healing properties. 3. A healing agent.

   t. carbons. PT: Carbon electrodes cored or filled with various materials. When burning they emit radiation of various intensities and qualities of ultraviolet, visual, and infrared energy.

   t. exercise. Scientific supervision of bodily movements for curative purposes. SEE: *exercise*.

therapeutics (thĕr"ă-pū'tĭks). That branch of medicine concerned with the application of remedies and the treatment of disease. SYN: *therapy, q.v.*

   t., suggestive. Treatment of a condition by using hypnotic suggestion.

therapeutist (thĕr-ă-pū'tĭst). One who practices therapeutics.

therapia sterilisans magna (thĕr"ă-pī'ă stē-rĭl'ĭ-sǎns mǎg'nǎ). Ehrlich's method of administering chemical agent which will destroy in 1 large dose all the parasites in the body of a patient without causing serious injury to the patient.

therapy (thĕr'ă-pǐ). Application of remedies in the treatment of disease. SYN: *therapeutics*.

   t., light. Treatment with radiation from the visible spectrum.

   t., maggot. Use of maggots in suppurating wounds of bones and soft tissues to remove necrotic areas.

   t., mental. The use of suggestion in the treatment of disease.

   t., nonspecific. Use of injections of foreign proteins, bacterial vaccines, etc., in treatment of infection to stimulate general cellular activity. SEE: *specific therapy*.

   t., opsonic. Use of bacterial vaccines to elevate the opsonic index of the blood.

t., physical. Use of physical agents in the treatment of disease, as massage, heat, hydrotherapy, radiation, electricity, and exercise.

t., serum. Use of injections of blood serum from immunized animals or persons in the treatment of disease. SYN: *serotherapy.*

t., specific. Administration of a remedy acting directly against the cause of a disease, as arsphenamine or mercury for syphilis, or quinine for malaria.

t., spiritual. The application of spiritual knowledge in the treatment of disease. SEE: *spiritual therapy.*

t., substitution. Use of glandular extracts to balance the deficiency of secretion of a gland.

t., vaccine. Injection of bacteria or their products to produce active immunization against a disease. SYN: *opsonic therapy.*

t., zone. Mechanical manipulation or stimulation of an area in the same longitudinal zone as disorder causing distress.

theriac, theriaca (thē'rǐ-ăk, thē-rī'ǎ-kǎ). 1. An antidote to poison of venomous animals, esp. a mixture of about 70 drugs pulverized and mixed with honey into an electuary. 2. An opium confection. 3. Molasses.

therm (therm). A small calory, the amt. of heat required to raise 1 Gm. of water 1° C.

thermacogenesis (thẽr''mǎ-kō-jĕn'ĕs-ĭs). Production of an increase of body temperature by drug therapy.

thermaerotherapy (thẽr-mā''er-ō-ther'ǎ-pǐ). Therapeutic application of hot air.

thermal (ther'mǎl). Pert. to heat.

t. capacity. Heat necessary to raise any body from 0° to 1° C.

t. death point. Degree of heat that will kill a fluid culture in 10 minutes.

t. radiation. Heat radiation.

t. sense. Capacity for recognition of heat and cold. SYN: *thermesthesia.*

thermalgia (thẽr-mǎl'jǐ-ǎ). Neuralgia accompanied by intense burning sensation, pain, redness, and sweating of the area involved. SYN: *causalgia.*

thermanalgesia (thẽr''măn-ăl-jē'zǐ-ǎ). Inability to experience reaction to heat because of cerebral lesion.

thermanesthesia (thẽr''măn-ĕs-thē'zǐ-ǎ). Inability to recognize sensations of heat and cold; insensibility to heat changes. It sometimes occurs in syringomyelia. SYN: *thermoanesthesia.*

thermatology (thẽr-mǎ-tŏl'ō-jǐ). The study of heat in treatment of disease.

thermelometer (thẽr-mĕl-ŏm'ĕt-ẽr). An electric thermometer used to indicate temperature changes too slight to be measured on an ordinary thermometer.

thermesthesia (thẽr-mĕs-thē'zǐ-ǎ). Sensitiveness to heat; temperature sense. SYN: *thermoesthesia.*

thermesthesiometer (thẽr''mĕs-thē-zǐ-ŏm'ĕt-ẽr). Device for determining sensibility to heat.

thermhypesthesia (thẽrm-hī-pĕs-thē'zǐ-ǎ). Lessened sensibility of the temperature sense. SYN: *thermohypesthesia.*

thermic (thẽr'mǐk). Pert. to heat.

t. fever. Sunstroke, collapse and high cutaneous temperature after long exposure to the sun. SYN: *insolation, siriasis.*

t. sense. The temperature sense; ability to react to heat stimuli. SYN: *thermesthesia, thermoesthesia.*

thermionic rectifier (thẽr''mǐ-ŏn'ĭk). PT: A device that converts alternating current into direct current; an electric valve in which electrons are supplied by a heated electrode. [*heat.*

thermo-. Combining form meaning *hot.*

thermoalgesia (thẽr''mō-ăl-jē'zǐ-ǎ). Condition in which pain is caused by application of moderate heat. SYN: *thermalgesia.*

thermoanalgesia (thẽr''mō-ăn-ăl-jē'zǐ-ǎ). Loss of heat sensation. SYN: *thermanalgesia.*

thermoanesthesia (thẽr''mō-ăn-ĕs-thē'zǐ-ǎ). 1. Inability to distinguish bet. heat and cold. 2. Insensibility to heat or temperature changes.

thermobiosis (thẽr-mō-bī-ō'sǐs). Ability to withstand high temperature.

thermobiotic (thẽr''mō-bī-ot'ǐk). Able to exist at high temperature.

thermocauterectomy (thẽr''mō-kaw-tẽr-ĕk'tō-mǐ). Excision by thermocautery.

thermocautery(thẽr''mō-kaw'tẽr-ǐ). 1. Cautery by application of heat. 2. Cauterizing iron. SEE: *cautery, actual.*

thermocoagulation (thẽr''mō-kō-ăg-ū-lǎ'shŭn). The use of high frequency currents to produce coagulation in checking growths.

thermocouple (thẽr'mō-kŭp-ĕl). Device for measuring slight temperature changes. SYN: *thermopile.*

thermocurrent (thẽr''mō-kŭr'ĕnt). Current developed or set in motion by heat; specifically, an electric current. SEE: *thermoelectricity.*

thermodiffusion (thẽr''mō-dǐ-fū'zhŭn). Diffusion of substances by heat.

thermoduric (thẽr''mō-dū'rǐk). Able to live in high temperatures. SEE: *thermophylic.*

thermoelectricity (thẽr''mō-ē-lĕk-trǐs'ǐ-tǐ). Electricity generated by heat, as by unequal heating of a circuit of 2 dissimilar metals.

thermoesthesia (thẽr''mō-ĕs-thē'zǐ-ǎ). Ability to recognize temperature differences. SYN: *thermesthesia.*

thermoexcitory (thẽr''mō-ĕk-sī'tō-rǐ). Exciting the production of heat in the body.

thermogen (thẽr'mō-jĕn). Device for maintaining the temperature of the body during operation.

thermogenesis (thẽr''mō-jĕn'ĕ-sǐs). The production of heat, esp. in the body.

thermograph (thẽr'mō-grǎf). Device for registering variations of heat.

thermohale (thẽr'mō-hǎl). An electric device for giving inhalations of warmed or medicated air in congestion of the respiratory tract.

thermohyperalgesia (thĕr″mō-hī″pĕr-ăl-gē′zĭ-ă). Unbearable pain upon the application of heat.

thermohyperesthesia (thĕr″mō-hī″pĕr-ĕs-thē′zĭ-ă). Exceptional sensitiveness to heat.

thermohypesthesia (thĕr″mō-hī″pĕs-thē′zĭ-ă). Diminished perception of heat.

thermoinhibitory (thĕr″mō-ĭn-hĭb′ĭ-tō″rĭ). Arresting or impeding the generation of bodily heat.

thermolabile (thĕr″mō-lā′bĭl). Destroyed or changed easily by heat; unstable. SEE: *heat, latent heat.*

thermolite (thĕr′mō-līt). A large, carbon, high-power filament lamp used for infrared radiation.

thermology (thĕr-mŏl′ō-jĭ). The science of heat.

thermolysis (thĕr-mŏl′ĭs-ĭs). 1. Loss of heat from the body, as by evaporation. 2. Chemical decomposition by heat.

thermometer (thĕr-mŏm′ĕ-tĕr). An instrument for registering heat or cold.

   t., air or gas. One filled with air or gas, the expansion of which registers high temperatures.

   t., alcohol. One containing alcohol.

   t., Celsius. Centigrade thermometer.

   t., centigrade. Temperature of boiling water at sea level 100° and freezing point 0°, with 100° bet. Generally used in Latin America and in Europe, and in scientific work.

   t., clinical. One for measuring temperature of body and in which the mercury remains stationary at registration point until shaken down.

   t., differential. One recording slight variations.

   t., Fahrenheit. Boiling point 212°, freezing point 32°. Used in English-speaking countries and in Holland.

   t., mercury. One containing mercury.

   t., Reaumur. Used in some parts of Germany and in Russia. Zero is same as 0° C. or same as 32° F., having 80° instead of 100° like the Centigrade thermometer.

   t., spirit. One filled with alcohol instead of mercury for registering low temperatures.

   t. scale. Graduated device on a thermometer to register the temperature.

   t., self-registering. One recording variations of temperature.

   t., surface. One for showing temperature of the body's surface.

thermometric (thĕr″mō-mĕt′rĭk). Pert. to heat measurement or a thermometer.

thermometry (thĕr-mŏm′ĕt-rĭ). Measurement of temperature.

   t., clinical. Temperature of body in a state of health ranges between 97.8° and 98.6° F.

thermoneurosis (thĕr″mō-nū-rō′sĭs). Elevation of body temperature in hysteria and other nervous conditions.

thermopalpation (thĕr″mō-păl-pā′shŭn). Estimation of temperature of the body

by palpation at different parts of the body.

thermopenetration (thĕr″mō-pĕn-ĕ-trā′shŭn). Application of heat to the deeper tissues of the body by diathermy.

thermophilic (thĕr″mō-fĭl′ĭk). Preferring or thriving best under high temperature, said of bacteria.

thermophobia (thĕr″mō-fō′bĭ-ă). Abnormal dread of heat.

thermophore (thĕr″mō-fōr). Apparatus for applying heat to a part, consisting of water heater and tubes conveying water to a coil and returning to heater, or salts which produce heat when moistened.

thermophylic (thĕr″mō-fī′lĭk). Resistant to destruction by heat, noting certain bacteria.

thermopile (thĕr′mō-pīl). PT: A thermo-electric battery used in measuring small variations in the degree of heat.

thermoplegia (thĕr″mō-plē′jĭ-ă). Heat-stroke; sunstroke. SYN: *insolation, siriasis.*

thermopolypnea (thĕr″mō-pŏl-ĭp-nē′ă). Quickened breathing caused by high fever or great heat.

thermoradiotherapy (thĕr″mō-rā″dĭ-ō-thĕr′ă-pĭ). Application of heat to deep tissues by diathermy. SYN: *thermo-penetration.*

thermoresistant (thĕr″mō-rē-zĭs′tănt). Able to resist high temperature, but not develop in it, noting bacteria.

thermostabile (thĕr″mō-stā′bl). Not changed or destroyed by heat.

thermostat (thĕr″mō-stăt). An automatic device for regulating the temperature.

thermosteresis (thĕr″mō-stĕ-rē′sĭs). The deprivation or loss of heat.

thermosystaltic (thĕr″mō-sĭs-tăl′tĭk). Pert. to contraction of the muscles under stimulus of heat.

thermotactic, thermotaxic (thĕr″mō-tăk′tĭk, -tăks′ĭk). Relating to regulation of the bodily temperature.

thermotaxis (thĕr″mō-tăks′ĭs). 1. Regulation of bodily temperature. 2. Reaction of organisms or of protoplasm in the living body to heat.

thermotherapeutics (thĕr″mō-thĕr-ă-pū′tĭks). Use of heat in treatment of disease. SYN: *thermotherapy.*

thermotherapy (thĕr″mō-ther′ă-pĭ). PT: The therapeutic application of heat.

thermotolerant (thĕr″mō-tŏl′ĕr-ănt). Able to live normally in high temperature.

thermotonometer (thĕr″mō-tō-nŏm′ĕt-ĕr). Device for measuring degree of muscular contraction when under influence of heat.

thermotoxin (thĕr″mō-toks′ĭn). A poison formed in the tissues by excessive heat.

thesis (thē′sĭs). An essay on a given subject offered by a candidate for a collegiate degree.

thiamin chloride (thī′ă-mĭn). Crystalline vitamin B₁ hydrochloride, which may be prepared from rice polishings, yeast, or synthetically.

DOSAGE: For infants, 50 to 75 international units per day; for adults, 200 to 300 international units per day. Carbohydrates increase the need for it.

thiemia (thī-ē'mĭ-ă). Sulfur in the blood.

Thiersch's graft or **method** (tērsh). A method of skin grafting using epidermis and a portion of the dermis.

thigh (thī). The upper leg above the knee and below the hip. SEE: *hip, pectineus, sartorius.*

   t. bone. The femur.

   t. joint. The hip joint. SYN: *articulatio coxae.*

thigmesthesia (thĭg-mĕs-thē'zĭ-ă). The sense of touch.

thigmocyte (thĭg'mō-sīt). A blood platelet.

thigmotaxis (thĭg″mō-tăks'ĭs). Arrangement in which some cells are attracted by contact with solids. SYN: *thigmotropism.*

thigmotropism (thĭg-mŏt'rō-pĭzm). The attraction exerted by contact with solids over certain cells. SEE: *thigmotaxis.*

thio-. Prefix denoting *presence of sulfur replacing oxygen.*

thiobismol (thī'ō-bĭz'mol). A compound containing 38% bismuth. [larly.]

   DOSAGE: 3 gr. (0.2 Gm.) intramuscu-

thiocol (thī'ō-kol). A derivative of guaiacol, but less toxic, tasteless, and does not disturb digestion.

   DOSAGE: 5-20 gr. (0.3-1.3 Gm.).

thiogenic (thī-ō-jĕn'ĭk). Able to convert hydrogen sulfide into higher sulfur compounds, said of bacteria in the water of some mineral springs.

thioneine (thī-ō'nē-ēn). Crystalline sulfur-containing compound found in ergot and blood.

thiopectic, thiopexic (thī-ō-pĕk'tĭk, -pĕks'ĭk). Pert. to the fixation of sulfur.

thiopexy (thī'ō-pĕks-ĭ). The fixation of sulfur.

thiophil, thiophilic (thī'ō-fĭl, thī-ō-fĭl'ĭk). Thriving in the presence of sulfur or its compounds, as some bacteria.

thiourea (thī″ō-ū-rē'ă). Colorless crystalline compound of urea in which sulfur replaces the oxygen.

third cranial nerve. Oculomotor nerve.

   t. corpuscle. A blood plate.

   t. intention. Healing of a wound by filling with granulations. SEE: *resolution.*

   t. ventricle. Third ventricle of the brain, a narrow cavity bet. the 2 optic thalami. SYN: *ventriculus tertius.*

thirst. Desire for fluid, esp. for water. This may obtain in fevers and certain other maladies, or it may be entirely lacking in some conditions. The nurse should note whether the intake of fluids allays the patient's thirst.

   t., absence of. Adipsia, aposia.

   t., excessive. Polydipsia.

   t., morbid. Dipsosis.

Thiry's fistula (tē'rē). An artificial fistula in a dog's intestines for obtaining intestinal juice for experimental purposes.

Thoma-Zeiss hemocytometer (tō'mă-tsīs hem″ō-sī-tom'ē-ter). Device for counting the blood cells.

Thomsen's disease (thŏm'sĕn). A disease confined to certain families, characterized by tonic spasms of the muscles induced by voluntary movements; usually congenital and transmitted from one generation to another; several of same family commonly affected.

thomsonianism (tŏm-sō'nĭ-ăn'ĭzm). An empiric system assuming that only vegetable remedies are of value in treatment.

thoracalgia (thō-răk-ăl'jĭ-ă). Pain in the chest wall. SYN: *pleurodynia.*

thoracectomy (thō-ră-sĕk'tō-mĭ). Incision of the chest wall with resection of a portion of rib.

thoracentesis (thō″răs-ĕn-tē'sĭs). Tapping through the chest wall for removal of fluids. SYN: *pleurocentesis, q.v.*

thoracic (thōr-ăs'ĭk). Pert. to the chest or thorax.

   t. cavity. The pleural cavity, the chest. It contains the trachea, esophagus, lungs and bronchi, the heart and its vessels. It is separated from the abdominal cavity by the diaphragm.

   t. duct. Passage bet. receptaculum chyli and meeting point of left int. jugular and left subclavian veins.

   t. girdle. One formed by the clavicles and scapulae.

   t. limbs. Upper extremities.

   t. spine. The spinal column.

thoraco-. Combining form meaning *chest, chest wall.*

thoracobronchotomy (thō″răk-ō-brŏn-kŏt'ō-mĭ). Incision through the thoracic wall into the bronchus.

thoracocautery (thō″răk-ō-kaw'tĕr-ĭ). The use of cautery in breaking up pulmonary adhesions to collapse the lung.

thoracoceloschisis (thō″răk-ō-sē-lŏs'kĭ-sĭs). Congenital fissure of the thoracic and abdominal cavities.

thoracocentesis (thō″răk-ō-sĕn-tē'sĭs). Tapping of the thorax. SYN: *thoracentesis.*

thoracocyllosis (thō″răk-ō-sĭl-ō'sĭs). Deformity of the chest.

thoracocyrtosis (thō″răk-ō-sĭr-tō'sĭs). Excessive curvature of the chest.

thoracodynia (thō″răk-ō-dĭn'ĭ-ă). Pain in the thorax.

thoracogastroschisis (thō″răk-ō-găs-trŏs'kĭs-ĭs). Congenital fissure of abdomen and thorax.

thoracograph (thō-răk'ō-grăf). Device for recording diagrams of the chest outlines and movements.

thoracolumbar (thō″răk-ō-lŭm'bar). Pert. to the thoracic and lumbar parts of the spine; noting their ganglia and the fibers of the sympathetic nervous system.

thoracolysis (thō″răk-ŏl'ĭs-ĭs). The freeing of a lung by severing abnormal adhesions bet. it and the chest wall.

thoracometer (thō-răk-ŏm'ĕt-ĕr). Device for recording variations in respiration of circumference of the chest or abdomen. SYN: *stethometer.*

thoracomyodynia (thō″ră-kō-mī″ō-dĭn'ĭ-ă). Pain in muscles of the chest wall.

thoracopathy (thō″răk-ŏp′ăth-ĭ). Any disease of the thorax, thoracic organs, or tissues.

thoracoplasty (thō′ră-kō-plăs″tĭ, thō-ră′-kō-plăs″tĭ). A plastic operation upon the thorax; removal of portions of the ribs in stages to collapse diseased areas of the lung. SEE: *empyema.*

thoracopneumoplasty (thō″ră-kō-nū′mō-plăs-tĭ). Plastic surgery involving the chest and lung.

thoracoschisis (thō-ră-kŏs′kĭ-sĭs). Congenital fissure of the chest wall.

thoracoscope (thō-ră′kō-skōp, -răk′ō-skōp). 1. An instrument used in auscultation to convey the sounds of the chest to the ear. SYN: *stethoscope.* 2. Instrument for inspecting the thoracic cavity which has an electric light and is inserted through an intercostal space.

thoracoscopy (thō″ră-kŏs′kō-pĭ). Diagnostic examination of the pleural cavity with an endoscope.

thoracostenosis (thō″ră-kō-stĕn-ō′sĭs). Narrowness of the thorax. SYN: *waspwaist.*

thoracostomy (thō-răk-ŏs′tō-mĭ). Resection of chest wall to allow room for enlarged heart or for drainage.

thoracotomy (thō″răk-ŏt′ō-mĭ). Surgical incision of the chest wall.

thorax (thō′răks) (pl. *thoraces* or *thoraxes*). That part of the body bet. the base of the neck superiorly and the diaphragm inferiorly. SYN: *chest.*

  t., Amazon. A chest with only 1 breast.

  t., barrel-shaped. A malformed chest rounded like a barrel seen in pulmonary emphysema.

  t., fusiform. A chest deformed by long continued tight lacing.

  t. paralyticus. The long, flat chest of patients with constitutional visceroptosis.

  t., Peyrot's. A chest that has an obliquely oval, deformed shape; seen in large pleural effusions.

  t., pigeon. One in which the sternum and ribs anteriorly form a prominent edge or ridge resembling the breastbone of a pigeon.

thorium (thō′rĭ-ŭm). SYMB: Th. A metallic element occurring in combination, at. wt. 232.12.

Thornwaldt's disease (torn′vahlt). Inflammation of crypt of the pharyngeal tonsil with formation of a pus-containing cyst and nasopharyngeal stenosis.

thoron (thō′rŏn). A gaseous, radioactive element; an emanation or transformation product of thorium.

three-day fever. An epidemic, infectious, eruptive fever due to a parasite transmitted by a mosquito. SYN: *breakbone fever, dandy fever, dengue.*

thremmatology (thrĕm-ă-tŏl′ō-jĭ). Science of breeding according to the laws of heredity and variation.

threpsology (thrĕp-sŏl′ō-jĭ). Science of nutrition.

threshold (thrĕsh′ōld). 1. Point at which

a psychological or physiological effect begins to be produced. 2. A measure of the sensitivity of an organ or function which is obtained by finding the limiting value of the appropriate stimulus that will give the response.

  t., auditory. Minimum audible sound.

  t. of consciousness. PSY: Point at which a stimulus is hardly perceived.

  t., erythe′ma. Stage in which erythema of the skin due to radiation just begins.

  t. point. One at which the concentration of glucose begins to pass from the blood into the urine.

  t., stim′ulus. Minimal point at which a sensation is aroused.

  t. of visual sensation. Threshold of the minimum vision of an object.

thrill (thrĭl). 1. Abnormal tremor accompanying a vascular or cardiac murmur felt on palpation. SYN: *fremitus.* 2. A tingling or shivering sensation of tremulous excitement, as from pain, pleasure, or horror.

  t., aortic. One heard over aortic aperture in lesions of valves.

  t., arterial. One heard over an artery.

  t., hydatid. Peculiar tremor felt on palpation of a hydatid cyst.

  t., presystolic. One sometimes felt over apex of the heart preceding ventricular contraction.

throat (thrōt). 1. Cavity from arch of palate to glottis and sup. opening of the esophagus. 2. The front of the neck. SYN: *jugulum.* 3. Any narrow orifice.

  t., sore. Inflammation of tonsils, larynx, or pharynx. SYN: *odynphagia.*

throb (thrŏb). 1. A beat or pulsation, as of the heart. 2. To pulsate.

throbbing (thrŏb′ĭng). Pulsation; a beating; rhythmic movement.

Throckmorton's reflex (thrŏk′mor″tŭn). Extension of great toe and flexion of others when dorsum of foot is percussed in metatarsophalangeal region.

throe (thrō). A severe pain or pang, esp. one in childbirth.

thromballosis (thrŏm-băl-ō′sĭs). Condition due to coagulation of venous blood.

thrombase (thrŏm′bās). An unstable chemical substance formed in the blood after it is shed and capable of causing the prompt clotting of additional blood by converting fibrinogen into fibrin. SYN: *thrombin.*

thrombasthenia (thrŏm-băs-thē′nĭ-ă). Deficiency of the blood platelets.

thrombectomy (thrŏm-bĕk′tō-mĭ). Excision of a thrombus.

thrombin (thrŏm′bĭn). Substance present in blood after it is shed which unites with fibrinogen to form fibrin in blood clotting. SYN: *thrombase.*

thrombo-. Combining form meaning *clot of blood, curd of milk, lump, piece, pert. to a thrombus.*

thromboangiitis (thrŏm-bō-ăn-jĭ-ī′tĭs). Inflammation of inner coat of a blood vessel with clot formation. SEE: *thrombosis.*

t. obliterans. Obliteration by thrombi of the larger veins and arteries of a limb, resulting in gangrene. SYN: *Buerger's disease.*

thromboarteritis (thrŏm″bō-ar-tĕ-rī′tĭs). Inflammation of an artery in connection with thrombosis.

thromboblast (thrŏm′bō-blăst). A small basophilic cell, said to be the mother cell of the blood platelet.

thromboclasis (thrŏm-bŏk′lă-sĭs). The breaking up of a thrombus. SYN: *thrombolysis.*

thromboclastic (thrŏm-bō-klăs′tĭk). Pert. to or producing the dissolution of a thrombus. SYN: *thrombolytic.*

thrombocyst, thrombocystis (thrŏm′bō-sĭst, -sĭs′tĭs). A membranous sac enveloping a thrombus.

thrombocyte (thrŏm′bō-sīt). One of the pale disks found in normal blood, 200,-000 to 400,000 per c.mm., which aid in coagulation. SYN: *platelet.*

thrombocytocrit (thrŏm″bō-sī′tō-krĭt). Device for estimating the platelet content of the blood.

thrombocytolysis (thrŏm″bō-sī-tŏl′ĭ-sĭs). Dissolution of thrombocytes.

thrombocytopenia (thrŏm″bō-sī″tō-pē′nĭ-ă). Abnormal decrease in number of the blood platelets. SYN: *thrombopenia.*

thrombocytopoiesis(thrŏm″bō-sī″tō-poy-ē′sĭs). The development of blood platelets.

thrombocytozyme (thrŏm-bō-sī′tō-zīm). An activating substance from thrombocytes which aids in the formation of thrombin.

thrombogen (thrŏm′bō-jĕn). A substance believed to be present in blood plasma which is the precursor of thrombin. SYN: *prothrombin.*

thrombogenesis (thrŏm″bō-jĕn′ĕs-ĭs). The formation of a blood clot.

thrombogenic (thrŏm″bō-jĕn′ĭk). Producing or tending to produce a clot.

thromboid (thrŏm′boyd). Resembling a thrombus or clot.

thrombokinase (thrŏm-bō-kīn′ās). A substance liberated from tissues capable of initiating the clotting of blood.

thrombokinesis (thrŏm″bō-kĭn-ē′sĭs). The coagulation of the blood.

thrombolymphangitis (thrŏm″bō-lĭm-făn-jī′tĭs). Inflammation of a lymphatic vessel due to obstruction by thrombus formation.

thrombolysis (thrŏm-bŏl′ĭ-sĭs). The breaking up of a thrombus. SYN: *thromboclasis.*

thrombolytic (thrŏm″bō-lĭt′ĭk). Pert. to or causing the breaking up of a thrombus.

thrombopathy (thrŏm-bŏp′ăth-ĭ). A defect in the coagulation apparatus of the blood. SYN: *hemophilia, q.v.*

thrombopenia (thrŏm-bō-pē′nĭ-ă). Lessening of the number of blood platelets.

thrombophilia (thrŏm-bō-fĭl′ĭ-ă). A tendency to the occurrence of clot formation.

thrombophlebitis (thrŏm-bō-flē-bī′tĭs). In-

flammation of a vein associated with formation of a thrombus.

t. migrans. Slowly advancing thrombophlebitis which recurs.

t. saltans. Thrombophlebitis occurring in the same vein or in a distant one, but not near the original lesion.

thromboplastic (thrŏm″bō-plăs′tĭk). Pert. to or causing acceleration of clot formation in the blood.

thromboplastin (thrŏm″bō-plăs′tĭn). 1. A substance found in the tissues which accelerates clotting of the blood. 2. Proprietary extract of thromboplastin from cattle brain in physiological salt solution.

thrombopoiesis (thrŏm″bō-poy-ē′sĭs). The formation of blood platelets.

thrombosed (thrŏm′bōzd). 1. Coagulated; clotted. 2. Denoting a vessel containing a thrombus.

thrombosin (thrŏm-bō′sĭn). A substance derived from the cleavage of fibrinogen which can be converted into fibrin.

thrombosinusitis (thrŏm″bō-sī-nū-sī′tĭs). Thrombus formation of a dural sinus.

thrombosis (thrŏm-bō′sĭs). The formation of a blood clot or *thrombus.*

t., atrophic. Marasmic thrombosis.

t., cardiac. Thrombosis of the heart.

t., coagulation. Thrombosis due to coagulation of fibrin in a blood vessel.

t., compression. Thrombosis due to compression bet. a thrombus and the heart.

t., coronary. Thrombosis of the coronary arteries.

t., dilatation. Thrombosis due to dilatation of a vein.

t., embolic. Thrombosis due to an embolus obstructing a vessel.

t., infective. Thrombosis due to bacterial infection.

t., marasmic. Thrombosis due to wasting diseases of infancy and old age.

t., placental. Thrombi in the placenta and veins of the uterus.

t., plate. Thrombus formed from an accumulation of blood platelets.

t., puerperal. Coagulation in veins following labor.

t., sinus. Thrombosis of a venous sinus.

t., traumatic. Thrombosis due to a wound or injury of a part.

t., venous. Thrombosis of a vein.

thrombostasis (thrŏm-bŏs′tă-sĭs). Stasis of blood in a part causing or due to formation of thrombus.

thrombotic (thrŏm-bŏt′ĭk). Related to, caused by, or of the nature of, a thrombus.

thrombus (thrŏm′bŭs). A blood clot obstructing a blood vessel or a cavity of the heart.

t., agony. Heart clot formed after prolonged heart failure occurring while patient is dying.

t., antemortem. A clot formed before death in heart or large vessels.

t., ball. A round clot in the heart, esp. in the auricles.

t., lateral. A clot attached to the wall of a vessel, without obstructing its lumen completely.

t., milk. A curdled milk tumor in the female breast due to obstruction in a lactiferous duct.

t., mural. Thrombus which is located on a diseased area of endocardium.

through drainage (thrū). Drainage by tube passing through a cavity from one surface to another. SEE: *drainage.*

t. illumina'tion. Passage of light through the walls of an organ or cavity, for medical examination. SYN: *transillumination.*

thrush (thrŭsh). Mycotic infection of mouth or throat, esp. in infants and young children, characterized by formation of white patches, ulcer formation, and frequently fever and gastrointestinal inflammation. SYN: *aphtha, sprue, stomatitis, q.v.*

thrypsis (thrĭp'sĭs). A comminuted fracture.

thulium (thū'lĭ-ŭm). A rare metallic element found in combination with minerals. SYMB: *Tm.* At. wt. 169.4.

thumb (thŭm). The short, thick, first finger on radial side of the hand, having but 2 phalanges and greater freedom of movement than other fingers. SYN: *pollex.*

thylacitis (thī''lă-sī'tĭs). Inflammation of the sebaceous glands of the skin.

thymectomy (thī-měk'tō-mĭ). Surgical removal of the thymus gland.

thymelcosis (thī-měl-kō'sĭs). Ulceration of the thymus gland.

thymergastic reaction (thī-měr-găs'tĭk). Name for psychic disorders most equivalent to manic-depressive or affect psychosis.*   [gland.

thymic (thī'mĭk). Relating to the thymus

t. acid. 1. Acid obtained by heating nucleic acid of thymus gland with water. 2. Thymol, *q.v.*

t. asthma. Spasmodic closing of the glottis followed by a pronounced inspiration. SYN: *laryngismus stridulus.*

t. death. Sudden death in status lymphaticus and thymic asthma.

t. stridor. Thymic asthma.

thymion (thĭm'ĭ-ŏn). A wart.

thymitis (thī-mī'tĭs). Inflammation of the thymus gland.

thymo-. Combining form meaning *thymus.*

thymocyte (thī'mō-sīt). A lymphocyte having origin in the thymus gland.

thymokesis (thī''mō-kē'sĭs). Abnormal enlargement and persistence of the thymus in the adult.

thymol (thī'mōl). USP. White crystals obtained from oil of thyme.

DOSAGE: Antiseptic, 0.1-3 gr. (0.06-0.2 Gm.). Anthelmintic, 15-30 gr. (1-2 Gm.).

t. iodide. USP. A reddish-brown powder.

thymolysis (thī-mōl'ĭ-sĭs). Dissolution of thymus tissue.

thymolytic (thī''mō-lĭt'ĭk). Destructive to thymus tissue.

thymoma (thī-mō'mă). A tumor originating in epithelial tissues of the thymus gland.

thymopathy (thī-mŏp'ă-thĭ). 1. Any disease of the thymus gland. 2. Any mental disorder.

thymotoxic (thī''mō-tŏks'ĭk). Poisonous to thymus tissue.

thymotrope (thī'mō-trōp). A person exhibiting thymotropism.

thymotropic (thī''mō-trōp'ĭk). Relating to thymotropism.

thymotropism (thī-mŏt'rō-pĭzm). The endocrine type in which the thymus influence predominates.

thymus (thī'mŭs). A lymphoid or ductless glandular organ in the neck and upper part of the thorax behind the manubrium of the sternum, which is included in the endocrine system although it produces no known hormone.

t., accessory. A lobule isolated from the mass of the thymus gland.

t. persistens hyperplastica. A thymus persisting into adulthood, sometimes hypertrophying.

thymusectomy (thī''mŭs-ěk'tō-mĭ). Surgical excision of the thymus.

thypar (thī'păr). Lacking the thyroid and parathyroid glands.

thyrasthenia (thī-răs-thē'nĭ-ă). Neurasthenic condition resulting from deficient thyroid secretion.

thyremphraxis (thī-rěm-frăks'ĭs). Arrested function of the thyroid gland.

thyreocele (thī're-ō-sēl). Enlargement of the thyroid gland. SYN: *goiter.*

thyreoid (thī're-oyd). Thyroid.

thyreoitis (thī-rē-ō-ī'tĭs). Inflammation of the thyroid gland. SYN: *thyroiditis.*

thyrin(e (thī'rĭn). The active principle of the thyroid gland's secretion.

thyro-, thyreo-. Combining forms meaning *oblong, shield, thyroid.*

thyroadenitis (thī''rō-ăd-en-ī'tĭs). Inflammation of thyroid gland.

thyroaplasia (thī''rō-ă-plā'zĭ-ă). Imperfect development of the thyroid gland.

thyroarytenoid (thī''rō-ă-rĭt'en-oyd). Relating to the thyroid and arytenoid cartilages.

thyrocardiac (thī''rō-kar'dĭ-ăk). 1. Pert. to the heart and thyroid gland. 2. A person suffering from thyroid disease complicated by heart disorder.

thyrocarditis (thī''rō-kar-dī'tĭs). Any affection of heart muscle occurring with hyperthyroidism, such as auricular fibrillation, tachycardia, etc.

thyrocele (thī'rō-sēl). Enlarged condition of the thyroid gland. SYN: *goiter.*

thyrochondrotomy (thī''rō-kŏn-drŏt'ō-mĭ). Surgical incision of thyroid cartilage. SYN: *laryngotomy.*

thyrocricotomy (thī-rō-krī-kot'ō-mĭ). Tracheotomy; division of the cricothyroid membrane.

thyroepiglottic (thī''rō-ěp-ĭ-glŏt'ĭk). Relating to the thyroid and epiglottis.

thyroepiglottideus (thī''rō-ěp'ĭ-glŏt-ĭd'ěŭs). Muscle in the thyroid cartilage that depresses the epiglottis.

thyrogenic, thyrogenous (thī″rō-jĕn′ĭk, thī-rŏj′ĕn-ŭs). Having origin in the thyroid gland.

thyroglobulin (thī″rō-glŏb′ū-lĭn). A protein derived from the thyroid gland which contains iodine.

thyrohyal (thī″rō-hī′ăl). 1. Concerning thyroid gland and hyoid bone. 2. Greater cornu of hyoid bone. 3. Embryonic skeletal remnant which becomes one of the major cornu of the hyoid.

thyrohyoid (thī″rō-hī′oyd). Rel. to thyroid cartilage and hyoid bone. SYN: *hyothyroid*.

thyroid (thī′royd). 1. Thyroid extract, *q.v.* 2. A gland of internal secretion in the neck, ant. to and partially surrounding the thyroid cartilage and upper rings of the trachea.
   DOSAGE: 1 gr. (0.06 Gm.).
   t. cachexia. Exophthalmic goiter.
   t. cartilage. Cartilage of the larynx shaped like a shield.
   t. extract. USP. The dried thyroid glands of the ox or sheep.
   DOSAGE: 1-5 gr. (0.06-0.32 Gm.).
   t. therapy. Thyroid extract treatment.

thyroidectomized (thī-roy-dĕk′tō-mīzd). With the thyroid gland removed.

thyroidectomy (thī-royd-ĕk′tō-mĭ). Excision of the thyroid gland.

thyroidism (thī′roy-dĭzm). 1. Poisoning from overdose of thyroid extract or increased secretion of the thyroid gland. 2. Deficiency of thyroid function, as in removal of the gland.

thyroiditis (thī″roy-dī′tĭs). Inflammation of the thyroid gland.

thyroidization (thī″roy-dĭ-zā′shŭn). Thyroid extract therapy.

thyroidotomy (thī-royd-ŏt′ō-mĭ). Incision of thyroid gland.

thyrointoxication (thī″rō-ĭn-tŏks-ĭ-kā′-shŭn). Poisoning from excessive use of thyroid extract or hypersecretion of the thyroid gland.

thyrolytic (thī″rō-lĭt′ĭk). Causing destruction of thyroid tissue.

thyroncus (thī-rŏng′kŭs). Enlarged thyroid gland. SYN: *goiter, struma, thyrocele.*

thyroparathyroidectomy (thī″rō-par-ă-thī-roy-dĕk′tō-mĭ). Surgical removal of the thyroid and parathyroid glands.

thyropenia (thī″rō-pē′nĭ-ă). Defective thyroid secretion with no clinical symptoms.

thyrophyma (thī″rō-fī′mă). Neoplasm of the thyroid gland.

thyroprival (thī-rō-prī′văl). Pert. to a condition resulting from loss of function or removal of the thyroid gland.

thyroptosis (thī-rŏp-tō′sĭs). Downward displacement of a goitrous thyroid into the thorax.

thyrosis (thī-rō′sĭs). Any condition due to abnormal thyroid action.

thyrotherapy (thī″rō-ther′ă-pĭ). Treatment with thyroid gland extracts.

thyrotome (thī′rō-tōm). Knife for cutting the thyroid cartilage.

thyrotomy (thī-rŏt′ō-mĭ). 1. The splitting of the thyroid cartilage anteriorly in midline in order to expose laryngeal structures. SYN: *laryngofissure.* 2. Surgery on the thyroid gland.

thyrotoxic (thī″rō-tŏks′ĭk). Pert. to, affected by, or marked by toxic activity of the thyroid gland.

thyrotoxicosis (thī″rō-tŏks-ĭ-kō′sĭs). The condition of intoxication due to excessive thyroid secretion. SYN: *exophthalmic goiter, q.v.*

thyrotrope (thī′rō-trōp). One with tendency to thyroid disorders or thyroid influence of the endocrine system.

thyrotropic (thī″rō-trŏp′ĭk). Pert. to or characterized by thyrotropism.

thyrotropin (thī-ro-trō′pĭn). The anterior pituitary element which influences the thyroid gland.

thyrotropism (thī-rŏt′rō-pĭzm). That type of endocrine constitution dominated by the effects of thyroid secretion.

thyroxin (thī-rŏks′ĭn). USP. Thyroid glands of animals which are used for food by man, dried, powdered, and containing not less than 0.17 or more than 0.23 per cent of iodine.
   DOSAGE: Average 1 gr. (0.06 Gm.).

thyroxine (thī-rŏks′ēn). The crystalline, active iodine principle (an amino acid derivative) of the thyroid secretion which stimulates the rate of oxidation.

tibia (tĭb′ĭ-ă). The inner and larger bone of the leg bet. the knee and ankle articulating with the femur above and with the astragalus below.
   t., Lannelongue's. A syphilitic tibia.
   t., saber-shaped. A deformity of the tibia due to gummatous periostitis (syphilitic) in which it curves outward.

tibial (tĭb′ĭ-ăl). Pert. to the tibia.

tibialis (tĭb-ĭ-ā′lĭs). One of 2 muscles of the calf of the leg.

tibioadductor reflex (tĭb″ĭ-ō-ăd-dŭk′tor). Lateral or crossed adduction of leg when tibia is percussed on its inner side.

tibiofemoral (tĭb″ĭ-ō-fem′ō-răl). Relating to the tibia and femur.

tibiofibular (tĭb″ĭ-ō-fĭb′ū-lar). Relating to the tibia and fibula.

tibiotarsal (tĭb″ĭ-ō-tar′săl). Relating to the tibia and tarsus.

tic (tĭk). A spasmodic muscular contraction, most commonly involving the face, head, neck, or shoulder muscles. SYN: *habit spasm.*
   t., convulsive. Spasm of the facial muscles.
   t. douloureux (doo-loo-ru′). Degeneration of the trigeminal nerve resulting in neuralgia of that nerve. SEE: *neuralgia.*
   t., facial. Same as *convulsive tic.*
   t., habit. Habitual repetition of a grimace or muscular action.
   t., spasmodic. Tonic contractions and paralysis of muscles of one or both sides of the face.

tick (tĭk). Any of the numerous blood-sucking arachnids of the order Acarida. Ixodidae is the hard tick family and Argas the soft.

　　t. fever. 1. Any infectious disease transmitted by the bite of a tick. 2. African relapsing fever. 3. Specifically, an acute infectious disease transmitted by the bite of a wood tick in the Rocky Mountain region. SYN: *Rocky Mountain spotted fever, spotted fever.*

tickle (tĭk′l). 1. Peculiar sensation caused by titillation or touching, esp. in certain regions, resulting in reflex muscular movements, laughter, or hysteria. 2. To arouse such a sensation by touching a surface lightly.

tickling (tĭk′ling). Gentle stimulation of a sensitive surface and its reflex effect, such as involuntary laughter, etc. SYN: *titillation.*

tictology (tĭk-tŏl′ō-jĭ). Science of managing pregnancy and childbirth. SYN: *obstetrics.*

t. i. d. Three times a day.

tidal air (tī′dăl). That which is inhaled and exhaled during normal, quiet breathing. SEE: *air, respiration.*

　　t. respiration. Cycles of respiratory movements of varying intensity with pauses between them. SYN: *Cheyne-Stokes respiration, q.v.*

tide. Alternate rise and fall; a space of time.

　　t., acid. Temporary acidity of urine following fasting.

　　t., alkaline. Temporary decrease in acid of urine after eating.

tigretier (tē-grĕt-ē-ā′). A dancing mania or form of tarantism due to bite of a poisonous spider occurring in Tigré, Abyssinia.

tigroid (tī′groyd). Marked like a tiger, a term applied to chromophil corpuscles.

　　t. bodies, t. masses. Chromophilic bodies in protoplasm of a nerve cell. SYN: *Nissl bodies.*

tigrolysis (tī-grŏl′ĭs-ĭs). Disintegration of tigroid masses in a cell.

tilmus (tĭl′mŭs). Delirious picking at the bedclothes by the patient. SYN: *carphology.*

timbre (tĭm′ber, tahn′br). Resonance quality of a sound by which it is distinguished, other than pitch or intensity, depending upon the number and character of vibrating body's overtones.

time (tīm). Interval bet. beginning and ending; measured duration. SEE: *biduous, bis in die.*

　　t. bleeding. Three minutes or less.

　　t. coagulation. Time taken by coagulation of a drop of blood.

　　t. reaction. Period bet. application of a stimulus and the response.

tin (tĭn). SYMB: *Sn.* At. wt. 118.70. A metallic element, forms of which are used in medicine.

tinctorial (tĭnk-tō′rĭ-al). Relating to staining or color.

tincture (tĭngk′tŭr). Diluted alcoholic solutions of nonvolatile substances (tinc-

ture of iodine being an exception), 10% being standard strength for powerful drugs and 20% for weaker ones.

　　t. iodine. POISONING: This commonly used antiseptic is sometimes taken by mouth.

　　DOSAGE: 1½ ℳ (0.1 cc.).

tinea (tĭn′ē-ă). Any fungous skin disease, esp. ringworm, occurring in various parts of the body, names indicating the part affected, as *Tinea barbae, Tinea corporis, Tinea tonsurans,* etc.

　　t. circinata. On the body—red, slight, elevated, scaly patches, which on examination reveal minute vesicles or papules. New patches spring from the periphery while central portion clears up. Often considerable itching.

　　t. circinata cruris. Tinea about the genitals, esp. on inside of thighs.

　　t. cruris. Same as *tinea circinata cruris.*

　　t. favosa. An infectious disease of skin, typically on scalp, due to a specific fungus; characterized by peculiar saucer-shaped, sulfur yellow crusts. The fungus is *Achorion schönleinii.* SYN: *favus.*

　　t. furfuracea. Tinea with whitish, greasy scales or crusts.

　　t. inguinalis. SEE: *tinea cruris.*

　　t. intersecto. A rare condition beginning as small, roundish, slightly elevated, itching spots on arms, chest, and back which become brown, with a smooth, tense surface, increasing in size, and coalesce.

　　t. kerion. A form of *tinea tonsurans.*

　　t. nodosa. Sheathlike, nodular masses in hair of beard and mustache from growth of an unknown fungus. They surround the hairs, which become brittle, and hair may be penetrated by fungus and thus split.

　　t. sycosis. Begins as a red, scaly patch involving the bearded region; purplish tubercles and pustules form around the opening of the hair follicles and hairs become lusterless, brittle and loose. Considerable itching.

　　t. tonsurans. Observed almost exclusively on scalp of children. Characterized by 1 or more rounded, scaly, elevated, grayish-colored patches through which project dry, brittle, lusterless, broken-off hairs.

　　t. trichophytina. Local infectious disease of skin, produced by the trichophyton fungus. The organism grows in the horny epithelium. The lesions vary according to part of body attacked, and whether the hairs are involved. SYN: *ringworm.*

　　t. versicolor. A chronic disease excited by a vegetable parasite, the *Microsporon furfur.*

tingible (tĭn′jĭ-bl). Capable of being stained.

tinnitus (tĭn-ī′tŭs). A ringing or tinkling sound that is purely subjective.

　　t. aurium. Ringing, tinkling, buzzing, or other sounds in the ear.

　　t. cere′bri. Noises in the head.

t., nervous. A neurosis; a subjective humming or buzzing sound in nervous people due to disturbance of otic nerve.

t., telephone. Tinnitus resulting from excessive use of the telephone.

tintometer (tĭn-tŏm'ĕ-ter). A scale of different shades of color to determine by comparison the intensity of color of the blood or other fluid.

tintometric (tĭn″tō-mĕt'rĭk). Relating to tintometry.

tintometry (tĭn-tŏm'ĕ-trĭ). Estimation of a color by comparison with a scale of colors.

-tion. O.E. and L. suffix forming abstract names.

-tious. O.E. suffix forming adjective.

tiqueur (tē-kur'). One afflicted with a tic.

tire (tīr). 1. Exhaustion; fatigue. 2. To exhaust or fatigue. 3. To become fatigued.

tirefond (tēr-fon'). Appliance like a corkscrew for raising depressed portions of bone or for removing foreign bodies.

tires (tīrz). Condition marked by constipation, vomiting, muscular tremors, and pain. SYN: *milk sickness, trembles.*

tisic (tĭz'ĭk). Pert. to wasting away or emaciation. SYN: *phthisic.*

tissue (tĭsh'ū). A collection of similar cells and fibers forming a definite fabric or structure in plants and animals, such as: (a) *Connective tissue;* (b) *muscular tissue;* (c) *nerve tissue;* (d) *epithelial tissue,* etc.

t., adenoid. Reticular tissue or lymphoid tissue, which holds lymph cells in the meshes of its network.

t., adipose. Areolar tissue filled with fat cells.

t., areolar. It forms sheaths, insulates and connects. The cells are separated by an irregular network of white and yellow fibers.

t., chromophil. Those tissues which give a chromophil reaction; found in the medulla and sympathetic ganglia.

t., connective. Tissue which supports and connects other tissues and parts.

t., elastic. Part of connective tissue consisting of elastic fibers, or membranes.

t., embryonic. Found in the embryo; a connective tissue in which the cells unite and form a network with closely packed nuclei.

t., epithelial. Cells held together by collagen or a cell cement, arranged to form a membrane or skin covering external surfaces and lining internal ones. It is called *boundary tissue.* It may be squamous, columnar, or modified.

t., erectile. Spongy tissue, the spaces of which fill with blood, causing it to harden and expand. Found in the penis, clitoris, and nipples.

t., fibrous. Connective tissue consisting of white or yellow fibers, arranged side by side in bundles; part of the body's supporting framework, and found in the ligaments, tendons, aponeuroses, fascias, and membranes.

t., interstitial. Connective tissue forming a network with the cellular elements of the body. SYN: *stroma.*

t., liquid. Connective tissue with the cells in a liquid intercellular fluid of blood and lymph.

t., lymphoid. Same as *adenoid tissue.*

t., muscular (*voluntary*). Striped or striated tissue principally connected with the bony framework. In animals it is known as "lean meat" or "flesh." It is a cross-striped, muscular tissue, the fibers like a long cylinder with flattened sides and conical ends, enveloped in a delicate sheath, the *sarcolemma.* (*Involuntary*): Smooth or unstriped, or nonstriated, not under control of the will. Principally found in walls of hollow organs, tubes, arteries, and veins.

t., nervous. A mass of nerve cells and their processes supported by neuroglia.

t., neuroglia. Connective tissue containing *glia cells* with many processes intertwining among the cells and nerves of the brain and cord.

t., osseous or bone. Connective tissue with intercellular substance impregnated with phosphate and carbonate of calcium, the mineral substances being 2/3 of the bone's weight.

t., reticular or retiform. Connective tissue resembling areolar tissue with a network of white fibers, the cells being broad and flat, and wrapped about the fibers.

t., simple. Tissue made up of 1 structural element or slight admixture of others.

t., skeletal. Fibrous, adenoid, adipose, osseous, and cartilaginous tissue.

t., subarachnoid. Trabeculae of fibrous tissue bet. arachnoid and pia, covered with endothelia.

t., subcutaneous. Areolar tissue beneath the corium and becoming part of it.

t., s. adipose. Adipose tissue within subcutaneous tissue. ·

t., s. areolar. Areolar tissue beneath a mucous membrane connecting it with other parts.

t., subserous areolar. Areolar tissue attaching serous membranes to parts they invest.

t., trabecular. Tissue, esp. connective tissue, in form of trabeculae often forming a network.

t., white fibrous. Connective tissue with white, inelastic, fibers, forming tendons, ligaments, and resistant membranes.

t., w. nervous. Nervous tissue of medullated nerve fibers.   [*tissue.*

t., yellow elastic. Same as *elastic*

tissue extract (tĭsh'ū). An insulin-free extract of the pancreas.

DOSAGE: 2-5 cc. subcutaneously or intramuscularly.

titanium (tĭ-tā'nĭ-ŭm). A metallic element found in combination in minerals. SYMB: Ti.

titillation (tĭt-ĭl-ā'shŭn). 1. Act of tickling, as in the throat. 2. State of being tickled. 3. Sensation produced by tickling.

ti'ter. Standard of strength per volume of volumetric test solution.

titration (tī-trā'shŭn). Determining strength of a solution by use of solutions of known strength.

titrimetric (tī"trĭ-mĕt'rĭk). Employing the process of titration.

titubation (tĭt-ū-bā'shŭn). A staggering gait, seen in diseases of the cerebellum.
  t., lingual. Stuttering, stammering.

Tl. Symb. of *thallium.*

Tn. Symb. of *normal intraocular tension.*

toadstool (tŏd'stool). Any of various fungi with an umbrella-shaped cap; popularly a poisonous mushroom.

tobacco (tō-băk'ō). Dried leaves of *Nicotiana tabacum* and other species.
  t. heart. Disturbance of function of heart from use of tobacco.
  t., Indian. Lobelia.

tobaccoism (tō-băk'ō-ĭzm). Morbid state due to excessive use of tobacco.

tocodynamometer (tō"kō-dī-năm-ŏm'ĕter). Device for estimating expulsive force of uterine contractions in childbirth.

tocogony (tō-kŏg'ō-nĭ). Parental generation as opposed to abiogenesis.

tocograph (tŏk'ō-graf). A device for estimating and recording the force of uterine contractions.

tocology (tō-kŏl'ō-jĭ). Science of parturition and obstetrics.

tocomania (to"kō-mā'nĭ-ă). Puerperal insanity.

tocometer (tō-kŏm'ĕt-ĕr). Device for estimating expulsive force of the uterus in labor. SYN: *tocodynamometer.*

tocophobia (tō"kō-fō'bĭ-ă). Abnormal fear of childbirth.

tocus (tō'kŭs). Parturition; childbirth.

toe (tō). A digit of the foot.
  t. clonus. Contraction of the big toe in sudden extension of the first phalanx.
  t., dislocations of. These are treated essentially same as dislocations of the fingers, *q.v.*
  t. drop. Inability to lift the toes.
  t. reflex. When great toe is strongly flexed all muscles below knee become tense.

toilet (toy'lĕt). Cleansing of a wound after operation or of an obstetrical patient.

toko-. Combining form meaning *birth.*

tolerance (tol'ĕr-ăns). Capacity for enduring a poison, or a food or drug which may be harmful if taken in excess; power of resistance to such, or point at which such resistance ends; amount of a drug or food which may be so tolerated.
  t. test. Master's exercise tolerance test for circulatory efficiency consists in ascending and descending 2 steps a variable number of times and in a given period. Blood pressure and pulse readings are estimated for age and weight.

tolu balsam (tō-loo'). USP. A resinlike substance obtained from a tree grown in South America. [cc.].
  DOSAGE: Of the syrup, 1-2 drams (4-8

-tome. Combining form meaning *a cutting, a cutting instrument.*

tomentum, tomentum cerebri (tō-men'tum ser'ē-brī). Network of numerous minute blood vessels bet. the cerebral surface of the pia mater and cortex cerebri.

Tomes' fibers, fibrils (tōmz). Processes from the odontoblasts which enter the tubules of dentine.

tomomania (tō"mō-mā'nĭ-ă). 1. Tendency of a surgeon to resort to unnecessary surgical operations. 2. Abnormal desire to be operated upon.

tomotocia (tō"mō-tō'sĭ-ă). Cesarean section delivery by incising the uterus.

tonaphasia (tō-nă-fā'zhĭ-ă). Inability to remember a tune due to cerebral lesion. SYN: *amusia, vocal.*

tone (tōn). 1. PHYS: That state of a body or any of its organs or parts in which the functions are healthy and performed with due vigor. 2. Normal tension or responsiveness to stimuli, as of arteries or muscles, seen particularly in involuntary muscle (such as the sphincter of the urinary bladder). 3. A musical or vocal sound.
  t. deafness. Inability to detect differences in musical sounds. SYN: *amusia.*
  t., muscle. Contractile tension in muscle. SEE: *tonus.*

tongue (tŭng). The organ of speech and taste.
  t., smoker's. Disease with white patch and fissure formation on tongue. SYN: *leukoplakia.*

tongue tie (tŭng' tī). This is a congenital shortening of the frenum.

tonic (tŏn'ĭk). 1. Pert. to or characterized by tension or contraction, esp. muscular tension. 2. Restoring tone. 3. A medicine that increases strength and tone.
  t. spasm. A persistent, involuntary, firm or violent muscular contraction. SEE: *clonic.*

tonicity (tō-nĭs'ĭ-tĭ). 1. Property of possessing tone, esp. muscular tone. 2. State of normal tension or partial contraction of muscle fibers while at rest. SYN: *tone.*

tonisator (tō"nĭ-sa'tor). Instrument giving both the interrupted galvanic and faradic current with a sinusoidal wave superimposed.

tonoclonic (tŏn"ō-klŏn'ĭk). Both tonic and clonic; said of muscular spasms.

tonofibrils (tŏn-ō-fī'brĭls). Fibrils seen in cells, particularly in epithelial cells.

tonograph (tŏn'ō-grăf). Device for recording blood pressure.

tonometer (tŏn-ŏm'ĕ-tẽr). Instrument for measuring the intraocular tension or blood pressure.

tonometry (tŏn-ŏm'ĕ-trĭ). The measurement of tension of a part, as intraocular tension.

tonophant (tŏn'ō-fănt). Device for visualizing sound waves.

tonoplast (tŏn'ō-plăst). An intracellular body. SYN: *vacuole*.

tonoscope (tŏn'ō-skōp). A device for examining interior of the skull or brain by means of sound.

tonsil (tŏn'sĭl). 1. Any mass of lymphoid tissue. 2. Either of a pair of masses of lymphoid tissue bet. anterior and posterior pillars of the fauces.

t., cerebellar. One of a pair of cerebellar lobules on either side of the uvula* projecting from inf. surface of cerebellum.

t., laryngeal. Lymphoid tissue on the ventricular band.

t., Luschka's. Same as *pharyngeal tonsil.*

t., pharyngeal. Lymphoid tissue on post. sup. wall of pharynx. SEE: *adenoid.*

t., nasal. Lymphoid tissue on the nasal septum.

t., sublingual. One behind the faucial pillars.

tonsilla (ton-sĭl'ă). Tonsil.

t. pharyngea. BNA. Lymphoid mass on post. wall of the nasopharynx.

tonsillar (tŏn'sĭ-lar). Pert. to a tonsil, esp. the faucial or palatine tonsils.

tonsillectomy (tŏn-sĭl-ĕk'tō-mĭ). Surgical removal of the tonsils.

tonsillitis (tŏn-sĭl-ī'tĭs). Inflammation of faucial tonsils.

t., acute catarrhal. Associated with an acute nasopharyngitis. Tonsils reddened and enlarged. Posterior pillars edematous and injected.

t., acute follicular. Inflammation of tonsils with islands of exudate on the surface of the tonsils representing crypts filled with débris and pus.

t., herpetic. Herpes on the tonsil.

t., mycotic. Tonsillitis due to fungi.

t., parenchymatous. Inflammation of all of the faucial tonsil.

t., pustular. Tonsillitis with pustular formations.

t., superficial. Inflammation of membrane covering the tonsil.

t., suppurative. Tonsillitis with high fever, suppuration, pain, etc. SYN: *quinsy, q.v.*

t., ulcerative. Plaut-Vincent's angina, syphilis, tuberculosis, agranulocytic angina, blood dyscrasias, fungi, as Leptothrix.

tonsillolith (tŏn'sĭl-ō-lĭth). A concretion within a tonsil. SYN: *amygdalolith.*

tonsillomycosis (tŏn"sĭl-lō-mĭ-kō'sĭs). A fungous infection of the tonsil.

tonsillooidiosis (tŏn"sĭl-lō-oy-dĭ-ō'sĭs). Infection of a tonsil with the fungus Oidium.

tonsilloscopy (tŏn"sĭl-los'kō-pĭ). Inspection of the tonsils.

tonsillotome (tŏn'sĭl-ō-tōm). Sliding knife for excision of enclosed soft tissue.

tonsillotomy (tŏn-sĭl-ŏt'ō-mĭ). Excision of the tonsils. SEE: *amygdalotomy.*

tonus (tō'nŭs). That partial, steady contraction of muscle which determines tonicity or firmness. SYN: *tone, tonicity.*

t., neurogenic. Tonic muscular contraction caused by constant sensory impulses into the cord and brain.

t., reflex. Assumption that muscular tonus is due to reflex from flow of sensory impulses into the central nervous system.

tooth (tooth) (pl. *teeth*). One of the conical hard structures in the upper and lower jaws used for mastication.

t. ache. Neuralgic pain in a tooth.

topesthesia (to-pes-the'zĭ-ă). Ability through tactile sense to determine any part that is touched.

tophaceous (tō-fā'shŭs). 1. Relating to a tophus. 2. Sandy, gritty.

tophus (tō'fŭs) (pl. *tophi*). 1. Deposit of sodium biurate in tissues near a joint in gout. 2. A salivary calculus. 3. Tartar on the teeth.

t. syphilit'icus. A syphilitic node on the tibia or periosteum of the cranium.

tophyperidrosis (tŏf"ĭp-ĕr-ĭd-rō'sĭs). Excessive sweating in local areas.

top'ical. Pert. to a definite area; local.

topoalgia (tō-pō-ăl'jĭ-ă). Localized pain; common in neurasthenia following emotional upsets.

topoanesthesia (tō"pō-ăn-ĕs-the'zĭ-ă). Loss of ability to recognize the location of a tactile sensation.

topognosia, topognosis (tō-pŏg-nō'sĭ-ă, -sĭs). Recognition of the location of a tactile sensation. SYN: *topesthesia.*

topographic (top-ō-grăf'ĭk). Pert. to description of special regions.

topography (tō-pŏg'ră-fĭ). Description of a part of the body.

toponarcosis (tō"pō-nar-kō'sĭs). Local anesthesia.

toponeurosis (tō"pō-nū-rō'sĭs). Neurosis of a limited area.

topophobia (tō-pō-fō'bĭ-ă). A fear of psychoneurotic origin in relation to a particular locality.

topothermesthesiometer (top"ō-ther-mĕs-the-zhĭ-ŏm'ĕ-ter). Device for measuring local temperature sense.

torantil (tō-răn'tĭl). A biologically standardized histamine destroying enzyme, obtained from the mucosa of the small intestines and kidneys of hogs.

DOSAGE: Varies according to the condition, from 10 to 20 units 3 times a day.

torcular Herophili (tor'kū-lar her-of'ĭl-ī). Expanded end of the sup. longitudinal sinus in a depression on inner surface of the occipital bone.

tormen (tor'mĕn) (pl. *tormina*). Griping pain in the bowels.

tormina (tor'mĭn-ă) (sing. *tormen*). Intestinal colic with griping pains.

Tornwald's disease (torn'valdt). Purulent inflammation of Luschka's tonsil.

torose, torous (tō'rōs, -rŭs). Knobby or bulging; tubercular.

torpent (tor'pĕnt). 1. Medicine which modifies irritation. 2. Not capable of active functioning; dormant.

torpid (tor'pĭd). Not acting vigorously; sluggish.

torpidity (tor-pĭd'ĭ-tĭ). Sluggishness; inactivity.

torpor (tor'por). Abnormal inactivity; dormancy; numbness; apathy.

   t. intestino'rum. Constipation.

   t. peristal'ticus. Atonic constipation.

torrefaction (tor-e-fǎk'shŭn). The act of drying or parching.

torrefy (tor'ĕ-fī). To parch or dry by heat.

torsion (tor'shŭn). 1. Act of twisting or condition of being twisted. 2. Formerly, a griping pain. SEE: *ileus*. 3. Rotation of the vertical meridians of the eye.

torsive (tor'sīv). Twisted, as in a spiral.

torso (tor'sō). The trunk of the body.

torsoclusion (tor-sŏk-lū'zhun). 1. Acupressure in combination with torsion to stop a bleeding vessel. 2. Malocclusion characterized by rotation of a tooth on its long axis.

torticollis tor-tĭk-ŏl'ĭs). Stiff neck caused by spasmodic contraction of neck muscles drawing the head to one side with chin pointing to the other side. Congenital or acquired. SYN: *wryneck.*

   t., fixed. Abnormal position of head due to organic shortening of the muscles.

   t., intermittent. Same as *spasmodic torticollis.*

   t., ocular. Torticollis from inequality in sight of the two eyes.

   t., rheumatic. Same as *symptomatic torticollis.*

   t., spasmodic. Torticollis with recurrent but transient contractions of muscles of neck and esp. of the sternocleidomastoid.

   t., spurious. Torticollis from caries of the cervical vertebrae.

   t., symptomatic. Rheumatic stiff neck.

tortipelvis (tor''tĭ-pĕl'vĭs). Muscular contractions distorting the spine and hip. SYN: *dystonia musculorum deformans.*

toruloid (tor'ū-loyd). BACT: Beaded; noting an aggregate of colonies like those seen in the budding of yeast.

torulosis (tor-ū-lō'sĭs). Infestation with Torula or yeast cells.

torulus (tor'ū-lŭs). A very small elevation. SYN: *papilla.*

   t. tac'tilis. A tactile cutaneous elevation on palms and soles.

touch (tŭtsh). 1. To perceive by the tactile sense; to feel with the hands, to palpate. 2. The sense by which pressure on the skin or mucosa is perceived; the tactile sense. 3. Examination with the hand. SYN: *palpation.*

   t., abdominal. Palpation of the abdomen.

   t., double. Vaginal and rectal examination made at same time.

   t., rectal. Digital exploration of the rectum.

   t., vaginal. Digital exploration of the vagina.   [bladder.

   t., vesical. Digital exploration of the

tour de maître (toor deh mātr). A method of introducing a catheter or sound into the male bladder or into the uterus.

Tourette's disease (too-rĕt'). Convulsive tic, with echolalia and coprolalia, associated with motor incoördination.

Tournay's sign (toor-nā'). Dilatation of the pupil of the eye on unusually strong lateral fixation.

tourniquet (tūr'nĭ-kĕt). Any constrictor used on an extremity to make pressure over an artery and to control bleeding; also used to distend veins for aspiration or intravenous injections.

Tousey method (tow'zē). Painless removal of cutaneous tumors without anesthesia by electrocoagulation.

tow (tō). Coarse fibers of flax, used for surgical dressings.

towelette (tow-ĕl-ĕt'). A small towel for surgical or obstetrical use.

toweling, towelling (tow'ĕl-ĭng). Friction with a coarse towel.

toxalbumin (tŏks''ăl-bū'mĭn). A poisonous albumin or protein.

toxalbumose (tŏks-ăl'bū-mōs). A poisonous albumose.

toxamin (tŏks'ăm-ĭn). One of a class of injurious substances said to be present in grain food, which are harmful unless counteracted by vitamins.

toxanemia (tŏks''ă-nē-mĭ-ă). Anemia due to a hemolytic poison.

toxemia (tŏks-ē'mĭ-ă). Distribution throughout body of poisonous products of bacteria growing in a focal or local site, thus producing generalized symptoms.

   t. of pregnancy. Series of conditions affecting women in pregnancy.

toxenzyme (tŏks-ĕn'zīm). A poisonous enzyme.

toxic (tŏks'ĭk). Pert. to, resembling or caused by poison. SYN: *poisonous.*

   t. unit. Smallest dose of a toxin fatal to a guinea pig of standard weight in 3-4 days. Also, smallest amount of scarlet fever toxin necessary to produce a positive skin test reaction in a susceptible person.

toxicant (tŏks'ĭ-kănt). 1. Poisonous; toxic. 2. Any poison, esp. one from alcohol.

toxicide (tŏks'ĭ-sīd). 1. Destructive to toxins. 2. A chemical antidote for poisons.

toxicity (tŏks-ĭs'ĭ-tĭ). The condition of being poisonous.

toxico-. Combining form meaning *poison.*

toxicoderma (tŏks''ĭ-kō-der'mă). Any skin disease resulting from a poison.

toxicogenic (tŏks''ĭk-ō-jĕn'ĭk). Caused by, or producing, a poison.

toxicohemia (tŏks''ĭ-ko-hē'mĭ-ă). Blood poisoning. SYN: *toxemia.*

toxicoid (tŏks'ĭ-koyd). Of the nature of a poison.

toxicology (tŏks-ĭ-kŏl'ō-jĭ). The science of poisons, their nature, effects and antidotes.

toxicomania (tŏks''ĭ-kō-mā'nĭ-ă). Abnormal craving for narcotics, intoxicants, or poisons.

toxicopathic (tŏks''ĭ-kō-păth'ĭk). Pert. to any condition caused by a poison.

toxicopathy (tŏks''ĭ-kop'ă-thĭ). Any disease caused by a poison.

toxicopexic (tŏks''ĭ-kō-pĕks'ĭk). Relating to neutralization of poison.

toxicophobia (tŏks''ĭk-ō-fō'bĭ-ă). Abnormal fear of being poisoned by any medium: food, gas, water, drugs, etc.

toxicophylaxin (tŏks″ĭ-kō-fĭ-lăks′ĭn). Any antitoxin which contracts bacterial poisons.

toxicosis (tŏks″ĭ-kō′sĭs). A diseased condition resulting from poisoning. SYN: *toxicopathy*.

t., endogen′ic. Disease due to poisons generated within the body. SYN: *autointoxication*.

t., exogen′ic. Any disease resulting from a poison not generated in the body.

t., retention. Toxicosis from retained products which normally are excreted as formed.

toxidermitis (tŏks″ĭ-der-mī′tĭs). Any inflammatory skin disease due to poisoning. SYN: *toxicodermatitis*.

toxiferous (tŏks-ĭf′ĕr-ŭs). Containing a poison. SYN: *poisonous*.

toxigenic (tŏks″ĭ-jĕn′ĭk). Producing toxins or poisons.

toxignomic (tŏks-ĭg-nŏm′ĭk). Having the toxic action peculiar to a poison.

toxin (tŏks′ĭn). Poisonous substance or compound of vegetable, animal, or bacterial origin.

t., bacterial. Toxin produced by bacteria.

t., endo-. Toxin produced in the body of the bacterium and freed only after its destruction.

t., exo-. Toxin excreted during life of the bacterium.

t., extracellular. Same as *exotoxin*.

t., fatigue. Substance deposited by body fluids in tissues after muscular exertion, said to be the cause of fatigue.

t., intracellular. Same as *endotoxin*.

toxin-antitoxin (tŏks′ĭn-ăn″tĭ-tŏks′ĭn). Diphtheria toxin with its antitoxin in a nearly neutral mixture, the diphtheria toxin being about 85% neutralized.

toxinemia (tŏks″ĭn-ē′mĭ-ă). Blood poisoning. SYN: *toxemia*.

toxinfection (tŏks-ĭn-fĕk′shŭn). Infection caused by toxins or other poisons.

toxinicide (tŏks-ĭn′ĭs-ĭd). That which is destructive to toxins.

toxinosis (tŏks-ĭn-ō′sĭs). Disease due to a toxin.

toxipathy (tŏks-ĭp′ă-thĭ). Any disease due to poison.

toxiphobia (tŏks″ĭ-fō′bĭ-ă). Abnormal fear of being poisoned.

toxiphoric (tŏks-ĭ-for′ĭk). Having affinity for or carrying a toxin.

toxis (tŏks′ĭs). Condition of being poisoned; poisoning. SYN: *toxicosis*.

toxitabellae (tŏks-ĭ-tăb-ĕl′ē). Poisonous tablets.

toxitherapy (tŏks″ĭ-ther′ă-pĭ). Use of toxins in treatment of disease.

toxoalexin (tŏks″ō-ăl-ĕks′ĭn). An alexin which counteracts bacterial toxins.

toxogenin (tŏks″ŏj′ĕn-ĭn). Hypothetical substance in the blood caused by injection of antigens, innocuous in itself, but causing anaphylaxis upon addition of fresh antigen.

toxoid (tŏks′oyd). A toxin treated so as

to destroy its toxicity, but still capable of inducing formation of antibodies on injection. SEE: *Ehrlich's side-chain theory*.

t., alum-precipitated. Toxoid of diphtheria or tetanus precipitated with potash-alum.

t., diphtheria. Diphtheria toxin detoxified by formaldehyde treatment.

toxolysin (tŏks-ŏl′ĭ-sĭn). Substance destroying toxins. SYN: *antitoxin, toxicide*.

toxomucin (tŏks″ō-mū′sĭn). Specific toxic albuminoid from cultures of tubercle bacilli.

toxon, toxone (tŏks′ŏn, -ōn). A bacterial toxin with lessened activity, producing paralysis and delayed death.

toxonoid (tŏks′ō-noyd). A nontoxic substance with a weak affinity for antitoxin.

toxonosis (tŏks-ō-nō′sĭs). A disease caused by poisoning. SYN: *toxicosis, toxinosis*.

toxopeptone (tŏks-ō-pĕp′tōn). A protein derivative produced by action of a toxin on peptones.

toxopexic (tŏks″ō-pĕks′ĭk). Pert. to the neutralization of a toxin.

toxophil(e (tŏks-ō-fĭl, -fīl). Having a special affinity for toxins, said of certain haptophore groups.

toxophore group (tŏks′ō-for). Poison-bearing group of a toxin. SEE: *Ehrlich's side-chain theory*.

toxophore, toxophorous (tŏks′ō-fōr, tŏks-ŏf′ō-rŭs). Producing the combination of a toxin with the cells of an organism. SEE: *Ehrlich's side-chain theory*.

toxophylaxin (tŏks-ō-fĭ-lăks′ĭn). A defensive protein that neutralizes bacterial poisons. SYN: *toxicophylaxin*.

toxosozin (tŏks″ō-sō′zĭn). A normal defensive protein that neutralizes bacterial poisons. SEE: *sozin*.

trabecula (tră-bĕk′ū-lă) (pl. *trabeculae*). Fibrous cord of connective tissue, serving as supporting fiber by forming septum extending into an organ from its wall or capsule.

t. carneae. BNA. Thick muscular tissue bands attached to inner walls of the ventricles of the heart.

trabs, trabs cerebri (trăbz ser′ē-brī). Arched band of white fibers connecting the cerebral hemispheres. SYN: *corpus callosum*.   [2. A mark.

trace (trās). 1. A very small quantity.

t., primitive. Pale white streak in germinal area indicating beginning of development of the blastoderm. SYN: *primitive streak*.

trachea (tră′kē-ă) (pl. *tracheae*). A cylindrical cartilaginous tube, 4½ inches long, from the larynx to the bronchial tubes. SYN: *windpipe*.

tracheaectasy (tră′kē-ă-ĕk′tă-sĭ). Dilatation of the trachea.

tracheal (tră′kē-ăl). Pertaining to the trachea.

t. tugging. Pulsation of the larynx or downward pull of the trachea, symptomatic of thoracic aneurysm. SYN: *Cardarelli's sign*.

trachealgia (trā″kē-ăl′jĭ-ă). Pain in the trachea.

trachealis (trā-kē-ā′lĭs). Unstriped muscular fibrous membrane connecting with the tracheal rings.

tracheitis (trā-kē-ī′tĭs). An inflammation of the trachea.

trachelagra (trā-kĕl-ăg′ră). Rheumatic condition of neck muscles resulting in torticollis.

trachelectomopexy (trā″kĕl-ĕk-tom″o-peks′ĭ). Fixation of uterine neck with partial excision.

trachelectomy (trā-kĕl-ĕk′tō-mĭ). Amputation of the cervix uteri.

trachelematoma (trā″kĕl-ē-mă-tō′mă). A hematoma situated on the neck.

trachelism, trachelismus (trā′ke-lĭzm, trā-ke-lĭz′mŭs). Backward spasm of the neck, sometimes preceding an epileptic attack.

trachelitis (trā-kē-lī′tĭs). Inflammation of mucous membrane of the cervix uteri. SYN: *cervicitis*.

trachelo-. Combining form, meaning *neck*.

trachelobregmatic (trā″kē-lō-brĕg-măt′ĭk). Pert. to the neck and the bregma.

trachelocystitis (trā″kĕl-ō-sĭs-tī′tĭs). Inflammation of neck of bladder.

trachelodynia (trā″kē-lō-dĭn′ĭ-ă). Pain in the neck.

trachelology (trā″ke-lŏl′ō-jĭ). Scientific study of the neck, its diseases and injuries.   [muscle of the neck.

trachelomastoid (trā″ke-lō-măs′toyd). A

trachelomyitis (trā″ke-lō-mĭ-ī′tĭs). Inflammation of muscles of neck.

trachelopexy (trā-kĕl-ō-pĕks′ĭ). Surgical fixation of the cervix uteri to an adjacent part.

tracheloplasty (trā′kel-ō-plas″tĭ). Plastic surgery of the cervix uteri.

trachelorrhaphy (trā-kel-or′ă-fĭ). Suturing of a torn cervix uteri.

trachelos (tra′ke-lŏs). Neck.

trachelotomy (trā-kel-ŏt′ō-mĭ). Incision of the cervix of the uterus.

tracheo-. Combining form meaning *trachea, windpipe*.

tracheoaerocele (trā″kē-ō-ā′er-ō-sēl). Hernia or cyst of trachea containing air.

tracheobronchoscopy (trā″kē-ō-brŏng-kŏs′kō-pĭ). Inspection of the trachea and bronchi through a bronchoscope.

tracheocele (trā′kē-ō-sēl). 1. Protrusion of mucous membrane through the wall of the trachea. 2. Enlargement of the thyroid gland. SYN: *goiter*.

tracheoesophageal (trā″kē-ō-ē-so-faj′ē-ăl). Pert. to the trachea and esophagus.

tracheolaryngotomy (trā″kē-ō-lăr-ĭn-gŏt′ō-mĭ). Incision into larynx and trachea.

tracheopathia, tracheopathy (trā″kē-ō-păth′ĭ-a, -op′ă-thĭ). Diseased condition of the trachea.

tracheopharyngeal (trā″kē-ō-far-ĭn′jē-ăl). Pert. to both the trachea and pharynx.

tracheophonesia (trā″kē-ō-fŏn-ē′zhĭ-ă). Cardiac auscultation at the sternal notch.

tracheophony (trā-kē-ŏf′ō-nĭ). Sound heard over the trachea in auscultation.

tracheoplasty (trā′kē-ō-plăs-tĭ). Plastic operation on the trachea.

tracheopyosis (trā″kē-ō-pī-ō′sĭs). Tracheitis with suppuration.

tracheorrhagia (trā-kē-or-ā′jĭ-ă). Tracheal hemorrhage.

tracheoschisis (trā-kē-ŏs′kĭs-ĭs). Fissure of the trachea.

tracheoscopy (trā-kē-ŏs′kō-pĭ). Inspection of interior of trachea, by means of reflected light.

tracheotome (trā′kē-ō-tōm). Instrument used in opening of trachea.

tracheostenosis (trā″kē-ō-sten-ō′sĭs). Contraction or narrowing of lumen of the trachea.

tracheotomy (trā-kē-ŏt′ō-mĭ). Operation of cutting into the trachea usually for insertion of tube to overcome tracheal obstruction.

　　t. tube. Tube to insert into opening made in tracheotomy.

trachitis (trā-kī′tĭs). Inflammation of the trachea. SYN: *tracheitis*.

trachoma (trā-kō′mă). A chronic contagious form of conjunctivitis, noted by hypertrophy of conjunctiva, formation of follicles with subsequent cicatricial changes.

　　t., brawny. Trachoma with general lymphoid infiltration without granulation of the conjunctiva.

　　t. deformans. Vulvitis with cicatricial contractions.

　　t., diffuse. Trachoma with large granulations.

trachychromatic (trā″kĭ-krō-mat′ĭk). Pert. to a nucleus with very deeply staining chromatin.

trachyphonia (trā-kĭ-fō′nĭ-ă). Roughness of the voice.

tract (trăkt). A region or area longer than its breadth, serving a special purpose.

　　t., alimentary. The canal or passage from the mouth to the anus.

　　t., ascending. Afferent white fibers in spinal cord.

　　t., descending. Efferent fibers in the spinal cord.

　　t., digestive. SEE: *alimentary tract*.

　　t., genitourinary. The genital and urinary organs.

　　t., habenular. White fibers from the habenula to the red nucleus.

　　t., intermediolateral. Olivospinal tracts of the spinal cord.   [*tract*.

　　t., Monakow's. Same as *rubrospinal*

　　t., motor. Descending tract of an impulse from the brain to a muscle.

　　t., olfactory. Central portion of the olfactory lobe of the brain.

　　t., ophthalmic, t., optic. Fibers bet. the visual centers and optic chiasm.

　　t., pyramidal. Any of columns of motor fibers in the spinal cord which are continuations of pyramids in the medulla.

　　t., respiratory. The respiratory organs in continuity.

　　t., rubrospinal. Fibers from the red nucleus to the gray matter of the spinal cord.

t., sensory. Any tract of fibers conducting sensation to the brain.

tractellum (trăk-tel'lŭm). An ant. locomotor protozoan flagellum.

traction (trăk'shŭn). 1. Process of drawing or pulling. 2. Contraction, as of a muscle.

t., axis. Traction in line with the long axis of a course through which a body (fetus) is to be drawn.

tractus (trăk'tŭs) (pl. *tractūs*). A tract or path.

tragacanth (trăg'ă-kănth). USP. The dried gummy exudation from a plant grown in Asia, used in the form of mucilage as a greaseless lubricant, and as an application for chapped skin.

tragal (trā'găl). Relating to the tragus.

tragicus (trăj'ĭk-ŭs). Muscle on the outer surface of the tragus.

tragomaschalia (trăg"ō-măs-kăl'ĭ-ă). Odorous perspiration (bromidrosis) of the axilla.

tragophonia, tragophony (trăg"ō-fō'nĭ-ă, -of'ō-nĭ). A bleating sound heard in auscultation at level of fluid in hydrothorax. SYN: *egophony*.

tragopodia (trăg-ō-pō'dĭ-ă). Knock-knee.

tragus (trā'gŭs). 1. Cartilaginous tonguelike projection in front of the ext. meatus of the ear. 2. One of the hairs at the entrance of the ext. auditory meatus.

trajector (tra-jĕk'tor). Device for determining approximate location of a bullet in a wound.

trance (trăns). A sleeplike state, as in deep hypnosis, appearing also in hysteria and in some spiritualistic mediums, with limited sensory and motor contact with the ordinary surroundings, and with subsequent amnesia of what has occurred during the state.

t., coma. Hypnotic lethargy.

t., death. Trance simulating death.

t., induced. Hypnotic or somnambulistic trance.

t., somnambulistic. Trance with anesthesia, or catalepsy, or paralysis induced by hypnotism.

trans-. Prefix meaning *across, over, beyond, through.*

transanimation (trans"ăn-ĭ-mā'shŭn). Resuscitation of a stillborn infant.

transaudient (trăns"aw'dĭ-ent). Permeable to sound waves.

transcalent (trăns-kā'lĕnt). Permeable to heat rays. SYN: *diathermanous.*

transection (trăn-sĕk'shŭn). A cutting made across a long axis; a cross section.

transfer, transference (trans'fer, transfer'ĕns). 1. PSY: Transmission of any affect from one idea to another, or from one object or person to another, unconscious identifications being the activating motive. 2. State in which the symptoms of one area are transmitted to a similar area on the other side, as in hysteria.

t. neuroses. Compulsion neuroses and hysteria.

t. situation. The emotional state of a patient existing bet. him and his physician during psychoanalysis.

Either affection or distrust is transferred by the patient to the physician, although such feelings are not related to reality.

t., thought. Transference of one's thoughts to another. SYN: *telepathy.*

transfix (trăns-fĭks'). To pierce through or impale with a sharp instrument.

transfixion (trăns-fĭk'shŭn). Maneuver in performing an amputation.

transforation (trăns"for-ā'shŭn). The perforation of the fetal skull at the base in craniotomy.

transforator (trăns'fo-rā-tor). Instrument for perforating fetal skull.

transformation (trăns"for-mā'shŭn). 1. Change of shape or form. SYN: *metamorphosis*. 2. Change of one tissue into another. 3. Degeneration.

transformer (trăns-form'er). PT: A stationary induction apparatus to change electrical energy at one voltage and current to electrical energy at another voltage and current through the medium of magnetic energy, without mechanical motion.

transfusion (trăns-fū'zhŭn). 1. Injection of the blood of one person into the blood vessels of another. SEE: *blood transfusion*. 2. Injection of saline or other solutions into a vein for a therapeutic purpose. SEE: *donor.*

t., direct. Transfer of blood directly from one person to another.

t., indirect. Transfusion of blood from a vessel to the patient.

t., subcutaneous. Infusion of saline solution or other fluid beneath the skin.

t., venous. Transfusion direct from a vein of a donor into a vein of patient.

transic (trăn'sĭk). Relating to a trance.

transiliac (trăns-ĭl'ĭ-ăk). Extending bet. the 2 ilia.

transillumination (trăns"ĭl-lŭ"mĭ-nā'shŭn). Inspection of a cavity or organ by passing a light through its walls.

transition (trănz-ĭ'shŭn). Passage from one state or position to another, or from one part to another form. SEE: *transitional.*

transitional (trănz-ĭsh'ŭn-ăl). Marked by or relating to a transition.

t. douche. One using alternately hot and cold water.

t. tumor. A benign one which, if it recurs after removal, may become malignant.

transitionals (trănz-ĭsh'ŭn-ăls). Mononuclear leukocytes, characterized by their large size, often 3 times as large as a red cell.

translucent (trăns-lū'sĕnt). Not transparent but permitting passage of light.

transmigration (trăns"mĭ-grā'shŭn). The passage of cells, as of the blood, through a membranous septum. SYN: *diapedesis.*

t., external. Transfer of an ovum from an ovary to an opp. tube through the pelvic cavity.

t., internal. Transfer of an ovum through the uterus to the opposite oviduct.

transmissible (trăns-mĭs′ĭ-bl). Capable of being carried from one person to another, as an infectious disease.

transmission (trăns-mĭsh′ŭn). Transfer of anything, as a disease or hereditary characteristics.

t., duplex. Passage of impulses through a nerve trunk in both directions.

transmutation (trăns-mū-tā′shŭn). A transformation or change, as of one species into another.

transparent (trăns-păr′ĕnt). 1. Transmitting light rays so that objects are visible through the substance. 2. Pervious to radiant energy. SEE: *clearing agent.*

transpirable (trăns-pī′ră-bl). Permitting excretion through the skin or membranes, as perspiration.

transpiration (trăns-pī-rā′shŭn). 1. Act of exhaling water, gas, or vapor through the skin or a membrane. SEE: *perspiration.* 2. Substance exhaled.

t., cutaneous. Giving off sweat from pores of the skin. SYN: *perspiration.*

t., pulmonary. Escape of watery vapor from the blood to the air in the lungs.

transplantation (trăns-plăn-tā-shŭn). The taking of a portion of living tissue from its normal position in the body or from the body of another person and uniting it with like tissue in another place, to lessen defect or remedy deformity or injury. SEE: *autotransplantation, graft.*

transposition (trăns-pō-zĭ′shŭn). 1. A transfer of position from one spot to another. SEE: *metathesis.* 2. Displacement of an organ, esp. a viscus, to the opposite side. 3. Transplantation of a flap of tissue without severing it entirely from its original position until it has united in the new position.

transsegmental (trăns″sĕg-mĕn′tăl). Extending across or beyond a segment as of a limb.

transseptal (trăns-sĕp′tăl). Across a septum.

transtemporal (trăns-tĕm′pō-ral). Crossing the temporal lobe of the cerebrum.

transthalamic (trăns″thăl-ăm′ĭk). Passing across the optic thalamus.

transthermia (trăns-thĕr′mĭ-ă). Production of heat in the deep tissues by electric currents. SYN: *diathermy, medical, thermopenetration.*

transthoracic (trăns-thō-răs′ĭk). Across the thorax.

transthoracotomy (trăns″thō-răk-ŏt′ō-mĭ). The operation of incising across the thorax.

transudate (trăns′ū-dāt). A substance which has passed through the pores of tissues or textures, as blood serum.

transudation (trăns-ū-dā′shŭn). 1. Oozing of a fluid through pores or interstices, as of a membrane. 2. The substance so passed.

A transudate has a low specific gravity, very few cells, and traces of albumin.

transurethral (trăns″ū-rē′thrăl). Pert. to an operation performed through the urethra.

transvaginal (trăns-văj′ĭn-ăl). Through the vagina.

transverse (trăns-vĕrs′). Lying across; crosswise.

t. fora′men. Canal in each transverse process of a cervical vertebra for the arteries and veins.

transversectomy (trăns-vĕr-sĕk′tō-mĭ). Excision of a transverse vertebral process.

transversospinalis (trăns-vĕr″sō-spī-nā′lĭs). Semispinalis capitus, semispinalis cervicis.

transversus (trăns-vĕr′sŭs). 1. Any of several small muscles. 2. Lying across the long axis of a part or organ.

transvestism (trăns-vĕst′ĭzm). A sexual perversion in which men prefer to dress as women, or women dress like men. SYN: *eonism, q.v.*

transvestitism (trăns-vĕs′tĭt-ĭzm). Sexual perversion in which person dresses in clothing of opposite sex. SYN: *eonism.*

trapezium (tră-pē′zĭ-ŭm). 1. First bone of the second carpal row. SYN: *os multangulum majus.* 2. A bundle of transverse fibers in dorsal part of pons Varolii.

trapezius (tră-pē′zĭ-ŭs). Large muscle of back and neck.

trapezoid (trăp′ĕ-zoyd). Shaped like a table.

t. bone. One of the carpal bones of the wrist, bet. the trapezium and magnum. SYN: *os multangulum minus.*

Trapp-Hässer formula (trăp-hä′sĕr). To estimate the grains of solids in urine, multiply last 2 figures of the sp. gr. by 2.33, which gives the solids in 1000 cc.

tras′entin. Spasmolytic agent similar to atropine, but lacking its undesirable properties. Sometimes used in small intestinal intubation.

trauma (traw′mă) (pl. *traumata* or *traumas*). An injury or a wound.

t., psychic. A painful, emotional experience, which may cause a neurosis.

traumatic (traw-măt′ĭk). 1. Caused by or relating to an injury. 2. Causing the healing of wounds. SYN: *vulnerary.* 3. A drug promoting healing.

t. fever. One following an injury.

traumatin (traw′măt-ĭn). Plant substance which helps the healing of injured tissues. SYN: *hormone, wound.*

traumatism (traw′mă-tĭzm). 1. Morbid condition of system due to an injury or wound. 2. Incorrectly, a trauma.

traumatology (traw-mă-tŏl′ō-jĭ). The science of wounds and their care.

traumatopnea (traw″mă-tŏp-nē′ă). Passage of air in and out of a wound in the chest wall.

treatment (trēt′mĕnt). Management, medical or surgical care of a patient. SYN: *therapeutics, therapy.*

t., active. Treatment directed specifically toward cure of a disease.

t., expectant. Relief of symptoms as they arise.

t., hygienic. Application of the laws of health.

t., preventive, prophylactic. Treatment directed to prevention of disease.

t., specific. Treatment directed to the cause of a disease.

t., surgical. Treatment by means of operation.

trematode (trĕm'ăt-ōd). 1. A parasitic worm, a fluke. 2. Pert. to a parasitic worm. SEE: *cercaria.*

tremelloid, tremellose (trĕm'el-oyd, -ĕl-ōs). Gelatinous.

tremogram (trĕm'ō-grăm). Graphic representation made by a tremograph.

tremograph (trĕm'ō-grăf). Device for recording tremors.

tremolabile (trĕ″mō-lā'bĭl). Easily destroyed or inactivated by shaking; said of a ferment.

tremophobia (trĕm″ō-fō'bĭ-ă). Abnormal fear of trembling.

tremor (trĕm'or, trē'mor). A quivering or shaking, esp. continuous quivering of a convulsive nature.

t., alcoholic. The visible tremor exhibited by alcoholics.

t., continuous. One that resembles tremors of paralysis agitans.

t., fibrillary. One caused by consecutive contractions of separate muscular fibrillae, rather than of a muscle or muscles.

t., forced. Tremors continuing after voluntary motion has ceased.

t., hysterical. Due to the instability of nervous impulse seen in hysteria.

t., intention. Tremor when voluntary motion is attempted.

t., intermittent. One common to paralyzed muscles in hemiplegia when attempting voluntary movement.

t., mercurial. One seen in chronic mercury poisoning.

t., muscular. Slight oscillating muscular contractions following in rhythmical order.

t., volitional. Trembling of limbs or of body when making a voluntary effort; in connection with multiple sclerosis and other nervous diseases.

tremulous (trĕm'ū-lŭs). Trembling or shaking.

trench mouth. Infection of tonsils and floor of the mouth with Vincent's bacillus, characterized by inflammation, ulceration, and painful swelling. SYN: *ulceromembranous angina, Vincent's angina, q.v.*

trend, psychiatric. Benign or malignant emotional interests and urges, revealed by postures, gestures, actions, and speech.

Trendelenburg position (trĕn-dĕl'ĕn-burg). The bed or table is raised from the foot, greatly elevating the knees, the legs projecting on an extended leg rest.

trepan (trē-păn'). 1. To perforate the skull with a trepan to relieve brain from pressure. 2. An instrument resembling a carpenter's bit for incision of the skull. SYN: *trephine.*

trephination (trĕf-ĭn-ā'shŭn). Process of cutting out a piece of bone with the trephine.

trephine (trē-fīn'). 1. To perforate with a trephine. 2. A cylindrical saw for cutting circular piece of bone out of skull. SEE: *trepan.*

trephocyte (trĕf'ō-sīt). Any cell supplying nutritive substances to the tissues.

trephone (trĕf'ōn). Hypothetical growth-promoting substance in the blood serum, used by cells as food material.

trepidant (trĕp'ĭ-dănt). Marked by tremor.

trepidation (trĕp-ĭ-dā'shŭn). 1. Fear, anxiety. 2. Trembling movement, esp. when involuntary.

Treponema (trĕp-ō-nē'mă). A genus of spirochetes, parasitic in man, with undulating or rigid bodies.

T. pallidum. Causative organism of syphilis. SYN: *Spirochaeta pallida.*

treponemiasis (trĕp″ō-nē-mī'ă-sĭs). Infestation with Treponema.

treponemicidal (trĕp″ō-nē-mī-sī'dăl). Destructive to Treponema.

treppe (trĕp'eh). Increase in height of contractions when the heart or a muscle is stimulated rapidly at regular intervals. SYN: *staircase effect, q.v.*

tresis (trē'sĭs). Perforation.

tri-. Combining form meaning *three.*

triad (trī'ăd). 1. Any 3 things having something in common. 2. A trivalent element. 3. Trivalent.

triakaidekaphobia (trī″ăk-ī-dĕk-ă-fō'bĭ-ă). Superstition regarding the number 13.

trial case (trī'ăl kās). An optician's box containing trial lenses.

t. frame. Spectacle frame for holding lenses for testing one's vision.

triangle (trī'ăng-l). A figure or area formed by 3 angles and 3 sides.

t., anterior, of the neck. The space bounded by the middle line of the neck, the ant. border of the sternocleidomastoid, and a line running along the lower border of the mandible and continued to the mastoid process of the occipital bone.

t., carotid, inferior. The space bounded by the middle line of the neck, the sternomastoid and the ant. belly of the omohyoid muscle.

t., carotid, superior. The space bounded by the ant. belly of the omohyoid muscle, the post. belly of the digastricus and the sternomastoid.

t., cephalic. A triangle on the antero-posterior plane of the skull formed by lines joining the occiput and forehead and chin, and 1 uniting the 2 latter.

t., facial. A triangle bounded by lines uniting the basion and the alveolar and nasal points, and 1 uniting the 2 latter.

t., femoral. Triangle on the inner part of the thigh, bounded by the sartorius and adductor longus muscle, and above by inguinal ligament.

t., frontal. A triangle bounded by the maximum frontal diameter and lines joining its extremities and the glabella.

t., Hesselbach's. The interval in the groin bounded by Poupart's ligament, edge of rectus muscle, and deep epigastric artery.

t., inferior occipital. Of Welcker, a triangle having the bimastoid diameter for its base and the inion for its apex.

t., inguinal. SEE: *femoral triangle.*

t., lumbocostoabdominal. The space bounded in front by the obliquus abdominis externus, above by the lower border of the serratus posticus inferior and the point of the 12th rib, behind by the outer edge of the erector spinae, and below by the obliquus abdominis internus.

t., muscular. SEE: *inferior carotid triangle.*

t., mylohyoid. The triangular space formed by the mylohyoid muscle and the 2 bellies of the digastric muscle.

t., occipital, of the neck. The space bounded by the sternocleidomastoid, the trapezius, and the omohyoid.

t., omoclavicular. SEE: *subclavian triangle.*

t., omohyoid. SEE: *superior carotid triangle.*

t. of Petit. The space above the hipbone, bet. the ext. oblique muscle, the latissimus dorsi, and int. oblique muscle.

t., posterior cervical; t., posterior, of the neck. The space bounded by the upper border of the clavicle, the posterior border of the sternocleidomastoid muscle, and the anterior border of the trapezius muscle.

t., pubourethral. A triangular space in the perineum, bounded externally by the ischiocavernous muscle, internally by the bulbocavernous muscle, and posteriorly by the transversus perinei muscle.

t., subclavian. A space bounded by the post. belly of the omohyoid, the upper border of the clavicle, and the post. margin of the sternocleidomastoid.

t., submaxillary. The space between the lower border of the inf. maxilla, the parotid gland, and the mastoid process of the temporal bone above, the post. belly of the digastric and the stylohyoid below, and the middle line of the neck in front.

t., supraclavicular. SEE: *subclavian triangle.*   [ally.

triangular bandage. One folded diagonWhen folded the several thicknesses afford some support.

t. ligament. 1. Ligament having 3 sides or angles. 2. One of the urethra attached to Poupart's ligament.

t. nucleus. Upper part of the cuneate fasciculus in the medulla oblongata. SYN: *nucleus, cuneate.*

triangularis (trī-ăng-ū-lā'rĭs). A muscle of the chin.

tribadism (trĭb'ăd-ĭzm). A form of perversion in which women seek sexual gratification from one of their own sex.

triceps (trī'sĕps). A muscle arising by 3 heads with a single insertion.

t. reflex. Sharp extension of forearm resulting from tapping of triceps tendon while arm is held loosely in bent position.

trichangiectasia, trichangiectasis (trĭk″ăn-jĭ-ĕk-ta'zĭ-ă, -ĕk'tă-sĭs). Dilatation of capillaries. SYN: *telangiectasia.*

trichauxe, trichauxis (trĭk-awk'sē, -sĭs). Excessive growth of hair. SYN: *hypertrichosis.*

trichi-, tricho-. Combining forms meaning *hair.*

trichiasis (trĭk-ī'ăs-ĭs). 1. Presence of hairlike filaments in the urine. 2. Inversion of eyelashes so that they rub against the cornea, causing a continual irritation of the eyeball.

Trichina (trĭk-ī'nă). A nematoid, parasitic worm usually found in the intestinal tract of certain lower animals and man.

Trichinella (trĭk-ĭn-ĕl'ă). A genus of nematode worms. SYN: *Trichina.*

T. spira'lis. The adult nematode causing trichinosis.

trichinellosis (trĭ-kĭ-nel-lo'sĭs). Disease caused by *Trichinella spiralis.* SYN: *trichinosis, q.v.*

trichinization (trĭk″ĭn-ĭ-zā'shŭn). Infestation with trichinae.

trichinophobia (trĭk″ĭn-ō-fō'bĭ-ă). Abnormal fear of developing trichiniasis.

trichinoscope (trĭk-ī'nō-skōp). Magnifying glass used to discover trichinae in meat.

trichinosis (trĭk-ĭn-ō'sĭs). Disease caused by the ingestion of *Trichina spiralis* into the system through eating raw or insufficiently cooked pork.

trichinous (trĭk'ĭn-ŭs). Infested with trichinae.

trichitis (trĭk-ī'tĭs). Inflammation of hair bulbs.

trichlorethylene (trī″klor-ĕth'ĭl-ēn). A colorless liquid ($CHCl:CCl_2$).

DOSAGE: 20-25 drops by inhalation, 6 or 7 breaths.

trichobacteria (trĭk″ō-băk-tē'rĭ-ă). Filamentous or flagellate bacteria.

trichobezoar (trĭk″ō-bē'zō-ar). A hair ball or concretion in the intestine or stomach.

trichocardia (trĭk-ō-kar'dĭ-ă). Pericardial inflammation with elevations resembling hair. SYN: *cor hirsutum, hairy heart, shaggy pericardium.*

trichocephaliasis (trĭk″ō-sĕf-ăl-ī'ă-sĭs). Infestation with Trichocephalus.

Trichocephalus (trĭk-ō-sĕf'ăl-ŭs). A genus of parasitic worms infesting the colon.

T. dis'par. A common, harmless, intestinal parasite of the cecum.

trichoclasia, trichoclasis (trĭk″ō-klā'zĭ-ă, -ok'lăs-ĭs). Brittleness of the hair. SYN: *trichorrhexis.*

trichocryptosis (trĭk″ō-krĭp-tō'sĭs). Any disease of the hair follicles.

trichoepithelioma (trĭk″ō-ĕp″ĭ-thē-lĭ-ō'mă). A benign skin tumor originating in the hair follicles.

trichoesthesia (trĭk″ō-ĕs-thē'zĭ-ă). 1. Sensation felt when a hair is touched. 2. A paresthesia causing a sensation of the presence of a hair on a mucous membrane or on the skin.

trichoesthesiometer (trĭk″ō-ĕs-thē-zĭ-ŏm′-ĕ-ter). Device for testing sensibility of the scalp by means of the hair.

trichogen (trĭk′ō-jĕn). An agent stimulating growth of hair.

trichogenous (trĭk-ŏj′ĕn-ŭs). Promoting hair growth.

trichoglossia (trĭk-ō-glŏs′sĭ-ă). Hairy condition of the tongue.

trichoid (trĭk′oyd). Hairlike.

trichokyptomania (trĭk″ō-kĭp″tō-mā′nĭ-ă). Abnormal desire to break off the hair or beard with the fingernail. SYN: *trichorrhexomania.*

trichology (trĭk-ŏl′ō-jĭ). Study of the hair and its care and treatment.

trichoma (trĭk-ō′mă). 1. Inversion of 1 or more eyelashes. SYN: *entropion.* 2. Matted, verminous, encrusted state of the hair. SYN: *plica polonica.*

trichomatosis (trĭk-ō-mă-tō′sĭs). Entangled, matted hair due to fungous disease of scalp and want of cleanliness. SYN: *plica polonica.*

trichomatous (trĭk-ō′mă-tŭs). Of the nature of, or affected with trichoma.

Trichomonas (trĭk-ŏm′ō-năs). Genus of flagellate parasitic protozoa.

   T. **hom′inis.** Species in human intestines sometimes causing diarrhea and bacillary dysentery.

   T. **vaginalis.** Vaginitis caused by a species of Trichomonas in secretions of the vagina; sometimes found in the male urethra. SEE: *colpitis.*

trichomoniasis (trĭk″ō-mō-nī′ăs-ĭs). Infestation with a parasite of genus Trichomonas.

trichomycosis (trĭk-ō-mī-kō′sĭs). Any disease of the hair due to a fungus.

   t. **nodosa.** Disease marked by nodule formations on the hair shafts. SYN: *piedra.*

trichonosis, trichonosus (trĭk-ō-nō′sĭs, -ŏn′-ō-sŭs). Any diseased condition of the hair.

trichopathophobia (trĭk″ō-păth-ō-fō′bĭ-ă). Morbid fear of hair on the face experienced by women, or any abnormal anxiety regarding hair.

trichopathy (trĭk-ŏp′ăth-ĭ). Any disease of the hair.

trichophagia, trichophagy (trĭk-ō-fā′jĭ-ă, -ŏf′ă-jĭ). The habit of swallowing hair.

trichophobia (trĭk-ō-fō′bĭ-ă). Abnormal dread of hair or of touching it.

trichophytic (trĭk″ō-fĭt′ĭk). 1. Relating to Trichophyton. 2. Promoting hair growth.

Trichophyton (trĭk-ŏf′ĭt-ŏn). A parasitic fungus on the hair causing ringworm.

   T. **ton′surans.** The fungus responsible for ringworm.

trichophytosis (trĭk″ō-fī-tō′sĭs). Infestation with trichophyton fungi; mostly in children.

trichoptilosis (trĭk″ŏp-tĭl-ō′sĭs). 1. The splitting of hairs at their ends, giving them a featherlike appearance. 2. Disease of hair marked by development of nodules along the hair shaft at which

point it splits off. SYN: *trichorrhexis nodosa.*

trichorrhea (trĭk-or-ē′ă). Rapid falling of the hair.

trichorrhexis (trĭk″ō-rĕks′ĭs). Condition in which the hair splits. SYN: *fragilitas crinium, trichoschisis.*

   t. **nodo′sa.** Longitudinal splitting of hair at nodules formed on the shaft. SYN: *clastothrix, trichoclasia.*

trichorrhexomania (trĭk″ō-rĕks″ō-mā′nĭ-ă). The abnormal habit of breaking off the hair with the fingernails.

trichoschisis (tri-kos′kis-is). Splitting of the hairs.

trichoscopy (trĭk-ŏs′kō-pĭ). Inspection of the hair.

trichosis (trĭ-kō′sĭs). Any disease of the hair or its abnormal growth or development in an abnormal place.

   t. **dec′olor.** Any abnormal coloring or lack of coloring of the hair. SYN: *canities.*

   t. **seto′sa.** Coarse hair.

Trichosporon (trĭ-kŏs′pō-rŏn). A genus of fungi causing trichomycosis nodosa.

trichosporosis (trĭk″ō-spō-rō′sĭs). Infestation of the hair with Trichosporon.

trichosyphilis, trichosyphilosis (trĭk″ō-sĭf′-ĭ-lĭs, -sĭf″ĭl-ō′sĭs). Any hair disease arising from a syphilitic condition.

Trichothecium (trĭk″ō-thē′sĭ-ŭm). A genus of mold fungi causing disease of the hair.

   T. **ro′seum.** A species of mold fungus found in certain cases of inflammation of the eardrum (mycomyringitis).

trichotillomania (tri-ko-til-ō-ma′nĭ-ă). The unnatural impulse to pull out one's own hair.

trichotomy (trĭ-kŏt′ō-mĭ). Division into three parts.

trichotoxin (trĭk″ō-tŏks′ĭn). An antibody or cytotoxin which destroys ciliated epithelial cells.

trichotrophy (trĭ-kŏt′rō-fĭ). Nutrition of the hair.

trichroic (trĭ-krō′ĭk). Presenting 3 different colors from 3 different aspects.

trichroism (trĭ′krō-ĭzm). Quality of showing a different color from each of 3 positions.

trichromatic (trĭ″krō-măt′ĭk). Relating to or able to see the 3 primary colors; noting normal color vision.

trichromic (trĭ-krō′mĭk). Pert. to normal color vision or ability to see the 3 primary colors. SYN: *trichromatic.*

trichuriasis (trĭk″ū-rī′ă-sĭs). Presence of worms of genus Trichuris in the colon, or in the ileum. SYN: *trichocephaliasis.*

Trichuris (trĭ-kū′rĭs). A genus of Trematoda.

   T. **trichiur′ia.** The whipworm. SYN: *Trichocephalus dispar.*

tricipital (trĭ-sĭp′ĭ-tăl). Three-headed, as the triceps muscle.

tricornic, tricornute (trĭ-kor′nĭk, -nūt). Having 3 horns or cornua.

tricrotic (trĭ-krŏt′ĭk). Having 3 beats, as the downward stroke of the sphygmographic tracing.

tricrotism (trī'krŏt-ĭzm). Condition of being tricrotic.

tricuspid (trī-kŭs'pĭd). 1. Pert. to the tricuspid valve. 2. Having 3 points or cusps. 3. A tooth having 3 cusps.

   t. area. Lower portion of body of sternum where sounds of right atrioventricular orifice are best heard.

   t. murmur. One caused by stenosis of the tricuspid valve or by its incompetency.

   t. orifice. Right atrioventricular cardiac aperture.

   t. tooth. One with a crown having three cusps.

   t. valve. Right atrioventricular valve. SYN: *valvula tricuspidalis.*

trident, tridentate (trī'dĕnt, trī-dĕn'tāt). Having three prongs.

tridermic (trī-der'mĭk). Developed from the ectoderm, endoderm, and mesoderm.

tridermoma (trī''der-mō'mä). A teratoid growth containing all three germ layers.

trielcon (trī-ĕl'kŏn). Instrument with 3 branches for removing foreign substances from wounds.

trifacial (trī-fā'shăl). Pert. to the 5th pair of cranial nerves. SYN: *trigeminal.*

   t. neuralgia. Neuralgia of 1 of the branches of the 5th cranial nerve; often severe. SYN: *tic douloureux.*

trifid (trī'fĭd). Split into 3; having 3 clefts.

trigeminal (trī-jĕm'ĭn-ăl). Pert. to the trigeminus or 5th cranial nerve.

   t. cough. A reflex cough from irritation of the trigeminal nerve terminations in respiratory upper passages.

   t. neuralgia. Facial neuralgia. SYN: *tic* douloureux.

   t. pulse. One with longer or shorter interval after each 3 beats because the 3rd beat is an extra systole. SYN: *pulsus trigeminus.*

trigeminus (trī-jĕm'ĭ-nŭs). The 5th cranial nerve or trifacial nerve.

trig'ger finger. State in which flexion or extension is arrested temporarily, but finally completed with a jerk.

trigonal (trĭg'ō-năl). Triganular; pert. to a trigone.

trigone (trī'gŏn). A triangular space, esp. one at the base of the bladder. SYN: *trigonum.*

trigonitis (trī-gō-nī'tĭs). Inflammation of trigone of bladder confined to its mucous membrane.

trigonocephalic (trī''gō-nō-sef-ăl'ĭk). Having a head shaped like a triangle.

trigonum (trī-gō'nŭm). Any triangular area. SYN: *trigone.*

trilabe (trī'lāb). Three-pronged forceps for removing foreign substances from the bladder. SEE: *lithotrite.*

trill (trĭl). A tremulous sound, esp. in vocal music, made by vibration of 1 speech organ against another.

trimanual (trī-măn'ū-ăl). Performed with three hands, as an obstetrical maneuver.

trimensual (trī-mĕn'shū-ăl). Occurring quarterly or every 3 months.

trimorphous (trī-mor'fŭs). Having 3 different forms, as the larva, pupa, and image of certain insects, or certain crystals.   [inders.

trineuric (trī-nū'rĭk). Having 3 axis cylinders.

trinitrophenol (trī-nī-trō-fē'nŏl). USP. Picric acid, a yellow crystalline powder, explosive when heated.

triorchid, triorchis (trī-or'kĭd, -kĭs). One having 3 testicles.

triorchidism (trī-or'kĭd-ĭzm). The condition of having 3 testicles.

tripara (trĭp'ä-rä). A woman who has had 3 children in separate pregnancies. SYN: *tertipara.*

tripeptide (trī-pĕp'tĭd). Product of combination of 3 amino acids formed during proteolytic digestion.

triphalangia (trī-fä-lan'jĭ-ä). Deformity marked by presence of 3 phalanges in a thumb or great toe.

triphasic (trī-fā'sĭk). Consisting of 3 phases or stages, said of electric currents.

triphthemia (trĭf-thē'mĭ-ä). Waste products in the blood.

Tripier's amputation (trĭp-ē-ā'). Amputation of a foot with part of the calcaneus removed.

triplegia (trī-plē'jĭ-ä). Hemiplegia with paralysis of 1 limb on the other side of the body.

triplet (trĭp'lĕt). 1. One of 3 persons born of the same mother from 1 pregnancy. SEE: *Hellin's law.* 2. A combination of 3 of a kind.

triplex (trī'plĕks, trĭp'lĕks). Triple; threefold.

triplopia (trĭp-lō'pĭ-ä). Condition in which 3 images are visioned of the same object.

triquetrous (trī-kwē'trŭs). Triangular.

   t. bone. 1. A wormian bone. 2. The Cuneiform bone of the carpus.

triradial, triradiate (trī-rā'dĭ-ăl, -ra'dĭ-āt). Radiating in 3 directions.

   t. lines. The embryonic stars of the lens.

   t. sulcus. The orbital fissure. SYN: *sulcus orbitalis.*

trismoid (trĭz'moyd). 1. Of the nature of trismus. 2. A form of trismus nascentium; once thought to be due to pressure on occiput during delivery.

trismus (trĭz'mŭs). Tonic spasm of muscles of the jaw seen in inflammation of the mouth at the angle of the jaw. SYN: *lockjaw.*

   t. capistra'tus. Adhesion of cheeks to the gums; congenital.

   t. nascentium. A form attacking infants within 2 weeks of birth, due to infection through the navel. Generally fatal. Also called 9-day fits. SEE: *tetanus.*

   t. neonatorum. SEE: *trismus nascentium.*

   t. sardon'icus. Facial muscle spasm producing a grinning expression.

trisodarsin (tri-sō-dar'sĭn). An antisyphilitic drug esp. good in congenital cases. DOSAGE: 0.45-0.6 Gm.

trisplanchnic (trī-splănk'nĭk). Pert. to the 3 visceral cavities, the *skull, thorax,* and *abdomen.*

t. nervous system. Sympathetic nervous system.

tristichia (trĭ-stĭk′ĭ-ă). The presence of 3 rows of eyelashes.

tristimania (trĭs-tĭm-ā′nĭ-ă). Melancholia.

trisulcate (trī-sŭl′kāt). Having 3 grooves or furrows.

tritanopia (trĭ-tăn-ō′pĭ-ă). Color blindness in which blue and yellow appear gray.

triticeous (trĭt-ĭsh′ŭs). Shaped like a grain of wheat.

t. cartilage, t. nodule. A cartilaginous nodule in the thyrohyoid ligament.

triticeum (trĭt-ĭs′ē-ŭm). A nodule in the thyrohyoid ligament.

tritium (trĭsh′ĭ-ŭm). The mass 3 isotope of hydrogen; triple-weight hydrogen.

tritotoxin (trī″tō-tŏks′ĭn). A toxin, according to Ehrlich, which is the 3rd or lowest in order of toxicity.

triturable (trĭt′ū-ră-bl). Susceptible of being powdered.

triturate (trĭt′ū-rāt). 1. To reduce to a fine powder by rubbing. 2. A finely divided substance made by rubbing.

trituration (trĭt-ū-rā′shŭn). Powdered preparation containing 10% of the active drug and 90% of sugar of milk. None are official.

trivalent (trī-vā′lĕnt, trĭv′ăl-ĕnt). Combining with or replacing 3 hydrogen atoms.

trocar (trō′kar). Instrument with a triangular tip used for aspiration or removal of fluids from cavities.

trochanter (trō-kăn′ter). Either of the 2 bony processes below the neck of the femur.

t. major. BNA. A thick process at upper end of the femur projecting upward externally to union of neck and shaft.

t. minor. BNA. A conical tuberosity upon inner and post. surface of upper end of femur, at junction of shaft and neck.

t. tertius. The gluteal ridge of the femur when it is unusually prominent.

trochanterian, trochanteric (trō″kăn-tē′rĭ-ăn, trō-kăn-ter′ĭk). Relating to a trochanter.

troche (trō′kē). Solid, discoid, or cylindrical mass consisting chiefly of medicinal powder, sugar, and mucilage.

trochin (trō′kĭn). The lesser tuberosity of the head of the humerus. SYN: *tuberculum minus.*

trochiter (trŏk′ĭt-er). Greater tuberosity of the head of the humerus.

trochlea (trok′lē-ă) (pl. *trochleae*). 1. A structure having the function of a pulley; a ring or hook through which a tendon or muscle projects. 2. The articular smooth surface of a bone upon which glides another bone.

trochlear nerve. Patheticus or 4th cranial nerve.

trochlearis (trō-klē-ā′rĭs). Sup. oblique muscle of the eye.

trochocardia (trō″kō-kar′dĭ-ă). Rotary displacement of the heart on its axis.

trochocephalia, trochocephaly (trō″kō-se-fā′lĭ-ă, -sĕf′ă-lĭ). Roundheadedness, a deformity due to premature union of frontal and parietal bones.

trochoid (trō′koyd). Rotating or revolving, noting an articulation.

trochoides (trō-koy′dēz). A pivot or rotary joint.

trombidiiasis, trombidiosis (trŏm-bĭ-dī-ī′ă-sĭs, -bĭd-ĭ-ō′sĭs). Infestation with the *Trombidium irritans.*

Trombidium (trŏm-bĭd′ĭ-ŭm). A genus of red mites, some of which attack man.

T. irritans. The harvest mite which is a semiparasite.

Trommer's test (trŏm′er). Test for sugar in the urine.

tromomania (trŏm″ō-mā′nĭ-ă). Delirium tremens.

tropesis (trō-pē′sĭs). An inclination to action possessed by all substances.

troph-, tropho-. Combining forms meaning *nourishment.*

trophedema (trō-fĕ-dē′mă). A permanent, localized edema of the extremities.

trophema (trō-fē′mă). Nutrient blood of the uterine mucosa.

trophesy (trof′ĕ-sĭ). Deficient nutrition of a part from failure of nerve regulating nutrition. SYN: *trophoneurosis.*

trophic (trŏf′ĭk). Concerned with nourishment.

t. center. One of the centers of the sympathetic system whence the nutrition of nerve fiber is supposed to be controlled.

t. nerve. One regulating nutritive functions of a part.

t. neurosis. Disorder due to injury of the trophic nerves of a part. SYN: *trophoneurosis.*

trophoblast (trŏf′ō-blăst). The outer epiblastic layer that establishes relations with the uterus and is supposedly concerned with nutrition.

trophoblastoma (trof″ō-blăs-tō′mă). A neoplasm due to excessive proliferation of chorionic epithelium. SYN: *chorioepithelioma.*

trophoderm (trŏf′ō-derm). A layer of cells on the ext. surface of the ectoderm of the blastodermic vesicle which brings about ovular implantation in the uterus and nourishment.

trophology (tro-fŏl′ō-jĭ). The science of nutrition.

trophoneurosis (trŏf″ō-nū-rō′sĭs). Any trophic disorder due to defective function of the nerves concerned with nutrition of the part.

t., disseminated. Thickening and hardening of the skin. SYN: *sclerema, scleroderma.*

t., facial. Progressive facial atrophy.

t., muscular. Muscular changes in connection with nervous disorders.

trophoneurotic (trŏf″ō-nū-rŏt′ĭk). Relating to a trophoneurosis.

trophonosis (trŏf″ō-nō′sĭs). Any disease of metabolism or nutrition, or condition resulting from them.

trophonucleus (trŏf″ō-nū′klē-ŭs). Protozoan nucleus concerned with vegetative functions in metabolism and not reproduction. SYN: *macronucleus*.

trophopathia, trophopathy (trŏf″ō-path′-ĭ-ă, trof-op′ă-thĭ). 1. Any disorder of the nutrition. 2. A trophic disease.

trophoplast (trŏf′ō-plăst). A granular body of specialized protoplasm in a cell. SYN: *plastid*.

trophospongia (trŏf″ō-spŭn′jĭ-ă). 1. A deeply staining, delicate, intracellular network of certain cells which is probably instrumental in nutritive circulation. 2. The outer layer of the trophoblast which is a vascular, spongy, mucous membrane.

trophotaxis (trŏf″ō-tăks′ĭs). The adaptation or selectivity and repulsion to nutrients by organic cells. SYN: *trophotropism*.

trophotherapy (trŏf″o-ther′ă-pĭ). The therapeutic use of foods. SYN: *dietotherapy*.

trophotonos (trŏf-ŏt′ōn-ŏs). A rigid state of contractile tissue resulting from trophic disorder.

trophotropism (trŏf-ot′rō-pĭzm). Attraction and repulsion of cells to nutritive substances. SYN: *trophotaxis*.

trophozoite (trŏf″ō-zō′ĭt). A sporozoan nourished by its host during its growth stage.

tropical (trŏp′ĭ-kăl). Pert. to the tropics.

t. **anemia.** Anemia, or merely pallor without blood changes, in northerners traveling in the tropics.

t. **lichen.** Prickly heat, acute inflammation of the sweat glands.

tropism (trō′pĭzm). Reaction of living organisms involuntarily toward or away from light, darkness, heat, cold, or other stimuli.

tropistic action (trō-pĭs′tĭk). Directional response of an organism to certain ext. influences. SYN: *tropism*.

t. a., **chemio-.** Influence of chemicals on the organism.

tropometer (trŏp-om′ĕ-ter). 1. Device for measuring the rotation of the eyeballs. 2. Instrument for measuring torsion in long bones.

Trousseau's disease (trū-sō′). 1. Generalized hypertrophy of lymphatic glands. 2. Gastric vertigo.

T's. **spots.** Streaking of the skin with the fingernail, seen in meningitis and other cerebral diseases. SYN: *meningitic streak*.

T's. **symptom.** Spasmodic muscular contractions indicative of tetany, on pressing the principle vessel and nerve of the limb.

troy weight (troi). A system of weighing gold, silver, precious metals, and jewels, and in making philosophical experiments. 5,760 gr. equal 1 lb.

24 grains (gr.) equal	1 pennyweight
20 pennyweights equal	1 ounce (oz.)
12 oz. equal	1 pound (lb.)

true (trū). Not false; real; genuine.

t. **pelvis.** Portion below the iliopectineal line.

t. **ribs.** The 7 upper ones on each side with cartilages articulating directly with the sternum. SYN: *costa vera*. SEE: *ribs*.

truncal (trŭng′kăl). Relating to the trunk.

truncate (trŭng′kāt). 1. Cut across at right angles to the long axis. 2. To cut off; to amputate.

trunk (trŭnk). 1. The body exclusive of the head and limbs. SYN: *torso*. 2. Main stem of a lymphatic, nerve, or blood vessel.

truss (trŭs). Device for holding a hernia in its place.

trypanocide, trypanocidal (trĭp″ăn-ō-sīd, trĭp″ăn-ō-sī′dăl). 1. Destructive to trypanosomes. 2. An agent which kills trypanosomes. SYN: *trypanosomicide*.

trypanolysis (trĭp-an-ōl′ĭ-sĭs). The dissolution of trypanosomes.

Trypanoplasmia (tri″păn-ō-plăz′mă). A genus of protozoan parasites resembling trypanosomes.

Trypanosoma (trī″păn-ō-sō′mă). A genus of parasite, flagellate protozoa found in the blood. [disease.

T. **bru′cel.** The cause of tsetse fly

T. **gambien′se.** The parasite of sleeping sickness.

trypanosomal (trĭp-ăn-ō-sō′măl). Pert. to trypanosomata.

trypanosome (trī-pan′ō-sōm). Any protozoan of the Trypanosoma genus.

t. **fever.** Sleeping sickness.

trypanosomiasis (tri-pan-o-sō-mī′ă-sĭs). A disease caused by trypanosomes.

trypanosomic (trī-păn-ō-sō′mĭk). Pert. to trypanosomes.

trypanosomicide (trī-păn-ō-so′mĭ-sīd). Destructive to trypanosomes.

trypanosomid(e (trī-pan′ō-sō-mĭd). A skin eruption in any disease caused by a trypanosome.

tryparsamide (trĭp-ars′ă-mĭd, -mĭd). An arsenic compound containing about 25% arsenic.

DOSAGE: 15-45 gr. (1-3 Gm.) intravenously preferably.

trypesis (trĭp-ē′sĭs). An incision of the skull to reduce pressure by removing a disk of bone. SYN: *trephining*.

trypsin (trĭp′sĭn). A proteolytic ferment of pancreatic fluid.

DOSAGE: *Intracut.*, 3-10 ṃ (0.2-0.6 cc.).

trypsinized (trĭp′sĭ-nīzd). Subjected to action of trypsin, thus having antitryptic power abolished.

trypsinogen (trĭp-sĭn′ō-jĕn). The proenzyme, or inactive form of trypsin found in pancreatic juice, believed to be activated when mixed in the intestine with the enterokinase of the *succus entericus*.

tryptic (trĭp′tĭk). Relating to trypsin.

tryptolysis (trĭp-tol′ĭ-sĭs). The splitting up of tryptone.

tryptone (trĭp′tōn). Peptone formed by action of trypsin.

tryptonemia (trĭp″tō-nē′mĭ-ă). Tryptones in the blood.

tryptophan(e (trĭp′tō-fān). An amino acid in proteins needed for tissue repair and growth; a product of tryptic digestion.

t. **test.** One to determine presence of tryptophan in gastric juice, the presence of which indicates cancer.

tryptophanuria (trĭp-tō-fă-nū'rĭ-ă). Tryptophan in the urine.

tsetse fly (tsĕt'sĕ). One that carries the infective protozoan of trypanosomiasis.

tub (tŭb). 1. A receptacle for bathing. 2. The use of the cold bath. 3. To treat by using a cold bath.

tubal (tū'băl). Pert. to a tube, esp, the fallopian tube.

t. **nephritis.** Inflammation of kidney tubules.

t. **pregnancy.** Pregnancy in one of the oviducts.

tubatorsion (tū''bă-tor'shŭn). The twisting of an oviduct.

tube (tūb). A long, hollow, cylindrical structure.

t., **cathode-ray.** A vacuum tube with a thin window at the end opposite the cathode to allow the cathode rays to pass outside. More generally, any discharge tube in which the vacuum is fairly high.

t., **Coolidge.** A kind of hot cathode tube, which is so highly exhausted that the residual gas plays no part in the production of the cathode stream, and which is regulated by variable heating of the cathode filament.

t., **Crookes'.** One with an exhausted vacuum, used in obtaining roentgen rays.

t., **drainage.** A glass or rubber tube which, when inserted into a cavity, drains away its fluid contents.

t., **electric.** Hollow glass or metal receptacles wired for electricity.

t., **esophageal.** Same as *stomach tube.*

t., **eustachian.** The tube passing from the throat to the middle ear.

t., **fallopian.** One of 2 oviducts.

t., **hot-cathode.** A vacuum tube in which the cathode is electrically heated to incandescence and in which the supply of electrons depends on the temperature of the cathode.

t., **h.-c. roentgen-ray.** A vacuum roentgen-ray tube in which the electron stream is supplied by a heated cathode. The cathode stream may be regulated by varying the current through the cathode filament.

t., **intubation.** A tube for passing into the larynx to facilitate breathing.

t., **Leonard.** SEE: *cathode-ray tube.*

t., **oscillator vacuum.** Method of producing alternating current. Current produced by this is a continuous sine wave current in contradistinction to the damped harmonic wave of spark gap diathermy machine.

t., **stomach.** A rubber tube, 16 in. in length, for introducing food or other fluid into the stomach.

t., **tracheotomy.** A tube for inserting into the trachea.

tube feeding diet. Milk, cream, eggs, glucose, orange juice or tomato juice, strained spinach, vitamin concentrates, other constituents added when ordered.

tuber (tū'ber) (pl. *tubers, tubera*). A swelling or enlargement.

tubercle (tū'ber-kl). 1. The lesion of tuberculosis. 2. Elevation of a bone for the attachment of a ligament or muscle. 3. Large, circumscribed, solid elevation of skin or mucosa from size of a large pea to that of a hazelnut.

t., **adductor.** That part of femur to which is attached the tendon of the adductor magnus.

t. **bacillus.** Organism causing tuberculosis.

t., **deltoid.** One in clavicle for attachment of deltoid muscle.

t., **genial.** One on either side of lower jawbone.

t., **genital.** The fetal structure that becomes the clitoris, or the penis.

t., **lacrimal.** One on upper jawbone.

t., **laminated.** The cerebellar nodule.

t., **Lisfranc's.** Tubercle for scalenus anticus muscle on the 1st rib.

t., **miliary.** A small tubercle resembling a millet seed; the lesion of tuberculosis.

t., **zygomatic.** One on the zygoma at junction of ant. root.

tubercular (tū-ber'kū-lar). 1. Relating to or marked by nodules. 2. Incorrectly pert. to tuberculosis. 3. Person with tuberculosis. SEE: *torose.*

t. **syphilide.** Cutaneous gummata.

tuberculase (tū-ber'kū-lās). An extract of tubercle bacilli used for immunizing against tuberculosis.

tuberculate, tuberculated (tū-ber'kū-lāt, -lāt''ed). Covered with nodules. SYN: *tubercular.*

tuberculation (tū-ber''kū-lā'shŭn). The formation of tubercles.

tuberculid(e (tū-ber'kū-lĭd, -lĭd). A tuberculous cutaneous eruption due to toxins of tuberculosis.

tuberculigenous (tū-ber-kū-lĭj'ĕn-ŭs). Causing or predisposing to tuberculosis.

tuberculin (tū-ber'kū-lĭn). A culture of tubercle bacillus to be used for active immunization or for diagnostic purposes in tuberculosis. SEE: *anticutin, antiphthisin, autotuberculin.*

t., **alkaline.** Substance obtained from tubercle bacilli by extracting with 1/10 normal soda solution.

tuberculinization (tū-ber''kū-lĭ-nĭ-zā'shŭn). Treatment or diagnosis with tuberculin.

tuberculinose (tū-ber'kū-lĭn-ōs). A form of tuberculin.

tuberculitis (tū-ber''kū-lī'tĭs). Inflammation of any tubercle.

tuberculization (tū-ber''kū-lĭ-zā'shŭn). 1. The formation of tubercles. 2. Therapeutic use of tuberculin. SYN: *tuberculinization.*

tuberculocele (tū-ber'kū-lō-sēl). Tuberculosis of a testicle.

tuberculocide (tū-ber'kū-lō-sīd). Destroying tubercle bacilli.

tuberculoderma (tū-ber''kū-lō-der'mă). A tuberculous lesion of the skin. SYN: *tuberculide.*

tuberculofibroid (tū-ber''kū-lō-fī'broyd).

Denoting fibroid degeneration of tubercles.

tuberculofibrosis (tū-ber″kū-lō-fī-brō′sĭs).
1. Chronic pulmonary inflammation with formation of fibrous tissue. 2. Interstitial pneumonia.

tuberculoid (tū-ber′kū-loyd). Resembling tuberculosis or a tubercle.

tuberculoidin (tū-ber-kū-loy′dĭn). A form of tuberculin treated with alcohol.

tuberculol (tū-ber′kū-lol). Tuberculin which is free from secondary products.

tuberculoma (tū-ber-kū-lō′mă). 1. A tuberculous abscess. 2. Any tuberculous neoplasm.

tuberculomania (tū-ber″kū-lō-mā′nĭ-ă). Abnormal certainty that one has tuberculosis.

tuberculomucin (tū-ber″kū-lō-mū′sĭn). A mucinlike substance prepared from old cultures of tubercle bacilli.

tuberculopsonic index (tū-ber″kū-lō-ŏp-sŏn′ĭk). Opsonic index in tuberculous infection.

tuberculophobia (tū-ber″kū-lō-fō′bĭ-ă). An abnormal fear of becoming affected with tuberculosis.

tuberculosis (tū-ber″kū-lō′sĭs). An infectious disease marked by the formation of tubercles in any tissue, due to the presence of the tubercle bacillus.

   t., acute general. An acute infectious disease excited by the tubercle bacillus, characterized anatomically by the simultaneous formation of miliary tubercles in many parts of the body.

   t. cutis. Tuberculosis of the skin of various forms marked by warty growths, pustules, and brownish patches. SYN: *scrofuloderma.*

   t. c. orificialis. Secondary to tuberculosis of internal organs and attacks integument contiguous to mucous outlet, beginning with yellowish miliary tubercles which break down to form rounded or oval, sluggish, granulating, painless ulcers.

   t. c. vulgosa. Patches of soft, "apple-butterlike" tubercles which ultimately undergo absorption but which may break down and ulcerate, healing with more or less scarring. Progresses slowly by formation of more patches. Deformity may be great from scarring and cicatrization.

   t., pulmonary. A specific, inflammatory disease of the lungs, caused by the tubercle bacillus, characterized anatomically by a cellular infiltration, which subsequently caseates, softens and leads to ulceration of lung tissues. Manifested clinically by wasting, exhaustion, fever, and cough.

tuberculotherapy (tū-ber″kū-lō-ther′ă-pī). The treatment of tuberculosis, esp. with meat of cattle affected with tuberculosis in an attempt at immunization.

tuberculotoxoidin (tū-ber″kū-lō-tŏks-oy′dĭn). A preparation of nontoxic, immunizing tubercle bacilli.

tuberculotropic (tū-ber″kū-lō-trop′ĭk). Combining with tubercle bacilli.

tuberculous (tū-ber′kū-lŭs). Relating to

or affected with tuberculosis, or conditions marked by infiltration of a specific tubercle, as opposed to the term tubercular, referring to nonspecific tubercle.

tuberculum (tū-ber′kū-lŭm) (pl. *tubercula*). A small knot or nodule.

   t. acus′ticum. Dorsal nucleus of the cochlear nerve.

   t. majus humeri. BNA. Larger tuberosity of the humerus at upper end of its lateral surface giving attachment to infraspinatus, supraspinatus, and teres minor muscles.

   t. minus humeri. BNA. The projection at proximal end of humerus' ant. surface giving attachment to subscapularis muscle.

tuberin (tu′ber-ĭn). A simple protein; a globulin in potatoes.

tuberositas (tū-ber-ŏs′ĭt-ăs) (pl. *tuberositates*). A projection, nodule, or prominence.

tuberosity (tū-ber-ŏs′ĭ-tĭ). 1. An elevated round process of a bone. 2. A tubercle or nodule.

tuberous (tū′ber-ŭs). Resembling a nodular or knotty mass.

   t. root. A thickened primary root.

   t. sclero′sis. A localized or diffuse fibrosis of the brain often associated with grave mental deterioration and epilepsy, showing adenoma sebaceum, esp. about the face, and often tumors elsewhere in the body, notably the kidneys and viscera. SEE: *sclerosis.*

tubo-. Combining form meaning *tube.*

tuboabdominal (tū″bō-ăb-dŏm′ĭn-ăl). Pert. to the fallopian tubes and the abdomen.

   t. pregnancy. Ectopic gestation with embryo partly in tube and partly in the abdominal cavity.

tuboligamentous (tū″bō-lĭg-ă-měn′tŭs). Pert. to the fallopian tube and broad ligament of the uterus.

tuboövarian (tū″bō-ō-vā′rĭ-ăn). Pert. to the fallopian tube and the ovary.

tuboövariotomy (tū″bō-ō-vā-rĭ-ŏt′ō-mĭ). Excision of ovaries and oviducts. SYN: *salpingo-oöthecotomy.*

tuboperitoneal (tū″bō-pěr-ĭ-tō-nē′ăl). Relating to the oviduct and peritoneum.

tuborrhea (tū-bor-rē′ă). Discharge from the eustachian tube.

tubotympanal (tū″bō-tĭm′pă-năl). Relating to the tympanum of the ear and the eustachian tube.

tubouterine (tū″bō-ū′těr-ĭn). Relating to the oviduct and the uterus.

tubular (tū′bū-lar). Relating to or having the form of a tube or tubule.

   t. breathing. Bronchial breathing.

   t. gestation. Ectopic pregnancy in the fallopian tube.

   t. membrane. Connective tissue sheath of a primary bundle of nerve fibers or of a funiculus. SYN: *perineurium.*

tubule (tū′bŭl). A small tube or canal.

   t., collecting. Tubule in renal medulla which is part of the discharging tubule.

   t., excretory. The uriniferous tubules in medullary portion of kidneys.

t., junctional. Short part of a uriniferous tubule connecting with a collecting tubule.

t's., seminal. Epithelial lined tubes (1/150-1/200 in. in diam.) forming the major portion of the testis.

t., uriniferous. Minute canals forming the glandular substance of the kidney, originating in Bowman's capsules and emptying into pelvis of kidney.

tubulodermoid (tū″bū-lō-der′moyd). A dermoid tumor due to the persistent embryonic tubular structure.

tubulus (tū′bū-lŭs) (pl. *tubuli*). A tubule; a small tube.

Tufnell's method (tŭf′nĕl). The treatment of int. aneurysm by low diet, with little liquid, rest, and potassium iodide.

tug′ging. A dragging or pulling.

t., tracheal. An indication of thoracic aneurysm.

tularemia (too-lăr-ē′mĭ-ă). Deer fly fever transmitted to man from rodents and rabbits bitten by a blood-sucking insect infected with *Pasteurella tularensis* or by direct contact.

tulase (tū′lās). Von Behring's tuberculin for treatment of tuberculosis.

tumefacient (tū-mĕ-fā′shĕnt). Producing or tending to produce swelling; swollen.

tumefaction (tū″mĕ-făk′shŭn). 1. A swelling. 2. Act of swelling or the state of being swollen.

tumor (tū′mor). 1. A swelling or enlargement. 2. A neoplasm, abnormal prominence of a part not due to inflammation with no physiological function.

t., connective tissue (chondroma). Composed of some variety of connective tissue, forming hard, elastic, slowly growing tumors, often nodular or lobulated. Occurs on bones, salivary glands, testicle, etc.

t., fatty (lipoma). Consists of adipose tissue, identical with normal fat. Innocent—grows slowly. May reach large size. Adults—do not recur after removal. Occur on shoulders, back, nates. Diffuse form, under chin.

t., fibrous (fibroma). Consisting of fibrous tissue. May be dense and firm as a tendon, or soft as areola tissue. Innocent—commonly possess distinct capsule. May occur wherever fibrous tissue is found in any of its forms.

Classification of Tumors

Benign	Malignant
Generally encapsulated (not invasive).	Not encapsulated (invasive).
Slow growing.	Rapidly growing.
Do not metastasize.	Metastasize.
Do not interfere with health.	Detrimental to health and life.

I. Connective Tissue Tumors

A. Benign:
    (a) Fibroma, composed of fibrous tissue.
    (b) Chondroma, composed of cartilage.
    (c) Osteoma, composed of bone.
    (d) Lipoma, composed of fat.

B. Malignant:
    Sarcoma, a cellular tumor composed of any connective tissue cells in disorderly arrangement

II. Muscle Tissue Tumors

Benign
    Myoma, composed of smooth muscle tissue.

III. Epithelial Tumors

A. Benign:
    (a) Papilloma, composed of surface epithelium.
    (b) Adenoma, composed of glandular epithelium.

B. Malignant:
    (a) Epithelioma, composed of squamous epithelial cells in disorderly arrangement.
    (b) Carcinoma, composed of glandular epithelial cells in disorderly arrangement.

IV. Endothelial Tumors

A. Benign:
    (a) Hemangioma, composed of blood vessels.
    (b) Lymphangioma, composed of lymph vessels.

B. Malignant:
    Endothelioma, composed of endothelial cells in disorderly arrangement.

V. Pigmented Tumors

A. Benign:
    Nevus, a pigmented mole.

B. Malignant:
    Melanoma, pigmented tumor derived from moles.

t., glandular (adenoma). Innocent growths originate only from preëxisting glandular tissue which they imitate. Two forms: Acinous and tubular. Do not infiltrate the connective tissue. Acinous occur in mammae, lip, ovary, testes, prostate, thyroid, parotid, lacrimal gland, cutaneous and sebaceous glands. Tubular, in intestine, esp. in rectum.

t., lymphatic (vessel) (lymphangioma). Lymphatic vessels are subject to dilatations and varicosities of every degree and extent. To such dilatations in general the term lymphangiectasis is applied, but when by their size, confluence and aggregation they form tumors the term lymphangiomata may be substituted. Occurs on inside of thigh, genitals, ant. wall of abdomen.

t., mucous (myxomata). Resemble the whartonian jelly of the umbilical cord and vitreous humor of the eye. Grows slowly; large size; innocent, not returning if completely removed. Mucoid softening may attack other forms of tumors. Occurs most frequently in nasal cavities, mammary gland, intermuscular spaces, and submucous and subserous spaces.

t., muscular (myomata). Only those of congenital muscle origin are composed of striated muscle elements (rhabdomyoma), but even in these, the bulk of tumor not composed of muscle cells — new growths made up in part of smooth, nonstriated muscle cells. Occurs in uterus and in prostate, in combination with fibromata.

t., nerve (neuromata). True neuromata other than the bulbous ends of cut nerves, made up of nerve fibers themselves, are rare. Usually made up of amyelenic fibers, *i. e.*, fibers that have no myelin within the sheath.

t., osseous (osteomata). Formed of true bone—almost solely of either cancellous or compact bone. Occurs on tibia, fibula, humerus, great toe, cranial and nasal sinuses. Compact form grows from cranium; great density, scarcely be cut by any instrument.

t., vascular (angiomata). Neoplasms composed of blood vessels, either arteries, veins, or capillaries, or in which blood is contained in cavernous spaces, not true blood vessels. Angiomata of nose are rare — must be distinguished from simple varicose condition of mucous membrane which is common. Occurs mostly in males during adolescence. Epistaxis frequent, profuse, and persistent. SEE: *nevus* and *varix.*

tumoraffin (tū'mor-ăf-ĭn). Having an affinity for tumor cells. SYN: *oncotropic.*

tumultus (tū-mŭl'tŭs). Over or disturbed action.   [palpitation.

t. cordis. Irregular heart action with

t. sermo'nis. Extreme stuttering due to pathologic cause.

tungsten arc (tŭng'stĕn). Lamp with tungsten electrodes for production of ultraviolet radiation. SEE: *lamp, tungsten.*

tunic (tū'nĭk). An investing membrane.

tunica (tū'nĭ-kă) (pl. *tunicae*). An enveloping or covering membrane.

t. adnata. The conjunctival lining of the eyeball.

t. adventitia. BNA. Outer coat of an artery or any tubular structure.

t. albuginea. The white fibrous coat of the eye, testicle, ovary, or spleen.

t. externa. Outer coat of an artery.

t. interna. SEE: tunica intima.

t. intima. Lining coat of an artery.

t. media. Middle muscular coat of an artery.

t. propria. BNA. Deep portion of the corium containing blood vessels, nerves, glands, and hair follicles.

t. vaginalis. Serous lining of the testicles.

tunnel anemia (tŭn'ĕl). A disease due to ankylostoma, and resembling idiopathic anemia.

t. disease. Paralytic and apoplectic symptoms in those working under high atmospheric pressure. SYN: *caisson disease.*

turbidimeter (tŭr-bĭ-dĭm'ē-ter). Device for estimating degree of turbidity of a fluid.

turbidimetry (tŭr-bĭ-dĭm'ē-trĭ). Estimation of the turbidity of a liquid.

turbidity (tŭr-bĭd'ĭ-tĭ). 1. BACT: Quality of not having translucent appearance of liquid due to growth of microorganisms. 2. Having flaky or granular particles suspended in a clear liquid giving it a cloudy appearance. SEE: *clarificant.*

turbinal (tŭr'bĭ-năl). 1. Spiral; scroll-like. 2. A turbinated bone; any 1 of the 3 bones situated in the lateral wall of the nose. *Inferior, middle,* and *superior* turbinates.   [shaped.

turbinated (tŭr'bĭ-nā''tĕd). Top- or cone-

t. bones. The 3 spiral, bony projections upon the outer walls of each nasal fossa.

turbinectomy (tŭr-bĭn-ĕk'tō-mĭ). Excision of a turbinated bone.

turbinotome (tŭr-bĭn'ō-tōm). Instrument for excision of a turbinated bone.

turbinotomy (tŭr-bĭn-ŏt'ō-mĭ). Surgical incision of a turbinated bone.

Türck's zone (tŭrk). One in intestinal wall in which microörganisms penetrating from the lumen are destroyed.

turgescence (tur-jĕs'ĕns). Swelling or enlargement of a part.

turgescent (tur-jĕs'ĕnt). Swelling; inflated.

turgid (tur'jĭd). Swollen; bloated.

turgor (tur'gor). 1. Normal tension in a cell. 2. Distention, swelling.

t. vita'lis. Normal fullness of the capillaries and blood vessels.

turning (turn'ĭng). Process of manually changing position of fetus in utero to permit normal delivery. SYN: *version.*

turpentine (tur'pĕn-tĭn). Oleoresin obtained from the pine tree.

DOSAGE: Internally, of the rectified oil, 5 minims (0.3 cc.).

turunda (tu-run'dă). 1. A surgical tent, drain, or tampon. 2. A suppository.

tussal (tŭs′ăl). Relating to a cough. SYN: *tussive*.

tussis (tŭs′ĭs). A cough, as bronchial tussis, senile tussis, etc.

  t. convulsi′va. Pertussis* or whooping cough.

  t. stomacha′lis. Reflex cough from irritation of the mucosa of the stomach.

tussive (tŭs′ĭv). Relating to a cough. SYN: *tussal*.

tutamen (tū-tā′mĕn) (pl. *tutamina*). Any protective structure.

  t. cerebri. The scalp, cranium, and cerebral meninges. [eyelashes.

  t. oculi. The eyebrows, eyelids, and

tutocain (tū′tō-kān). A local anesthetic used both locally and hypodermically.

twelfth cranial nerve. One of a pair of cranial nerves distributing to the base of the tongue. SEE: *hypoglossal nerve.*

twilight sleep (twī′lĭt slēp). A state of partial anesthesia and hypoconsciousness in which pain sense has been greatly reduced by the injection of morphine and scopolamine.

  t. state. PSY: One in which consciousness is disordered, making possible actions subsequently forgotten.

twin (twĭn). One of 2 children developed within the uterus at the same time from the same impregnation. SEE: *Hellin's law.*

  t′s. dizygotic. Those from 2 separate ova fertilized at the same time.

  t′s. identical. Twins of the same sex developed from the same ovum having 2 nuclei, both of which have been impregnated, or resulting from a splitting of the blastodermic vesicle, thus forming two embryos.

twinge (twĭnj). A sudden, keen pain.

twitch (twĭch). 1. A simple, quick, spasmodic contraction of a muscle. 2. To jerk convulsively. SEE: *myokymia, myopalmus.*

two-four-six enema. An enema with a double portion of the ingredients of the one-two-three enema; often given for flatulence as well as evacuation.

tylion (tĭl′ĭ-ŏn). Point at middle of ant. edge of the sulcus chiasmatis.

tyloma (tī-lō′mă). A callosity.

tylosis (tī-lō′sĭs). 1. A callosity. SYN: *tyloma.* 2. Formation of a callus.

tympanal (tĭm′păn-ăl). Relating to the tympanum. SYN: *tympanic.*

tympanectomy (tĭm-păn-ĕk′tō-mĭ). Excision of the tympanic membrane.

tympanic (tĭm-păn′ĭk). 1. Pert. to the tympanum. 2. Resonant.

  t. bone, ring, or **plate.** The wall surrounding the tympanum and supporting tympanic membrane.

  t. membrane. Membrane closing cavity of the middle ear. SEE: *tympanum.*

tympanism (tĭm′păn-ĭzm). Abdominal inflation from gas. SYN: *tympanites.*

tympanites (tĭm-păn-ī′tēz). Gaseous distention of the abdomen.

tympanitic (tĭm-păn-ĭt′ĭk). 1. Pert to or characterized by tympanites. 2. Resonant. SYN: *tympanic.*

  t. resonance. A sound produced by percussion over an air- or gas-filled cavity.

tympanitis (tĭm-păn-ī′tĭs). Inflammation of the middle ear. SYN: *otitis media.*

tympano-. Combining form meaning *eardrum, tympanum of the ear.*

tympanohyal (tĭm″păn-ō-hī′ăl). 1. Pert. to the hyoid arch and the tympanum. 2. A small, fetal cartilage, part of the hyoid arch, which later fuses with the styloid process.

tympanomastoiditis (tĭm″păn-ō-măs-toy-dī′tĭs). Inflammation of the tympanum and mastoid cells.

tympanotomy (tĭm″păn-ŏt′ō-mĭ). Incision of the membrana tympani. SYN: *myringotomy.*

tympanous (tĭm′păn-ŭs). Marked by abdominal distention with gas.

tympanum (tĭm′păn-ŭm). The eardrum; the cavity of the middle ear containing the ossicular chain, *epitympanum, mesotympanum,* and *hypotympanum.*

tympany (tĭm′pă-nĭ). 1. Abdominal distention with gas. 2. Tympanic resonance on percussion.

type (tīp). The general character of a person, a disease, or substance.

  t., asthenic. One who is slender with a long chest that is flat and who has poor muscular development.

  t., pyknic. One with a rounded body, thick shoulders, large chest, short neck, and broad head.

  t., vagotonic. One with deficient adrenal stimulus, slow pulse, low blood pressure, and high sugar tolerance.

  t., vesanic. Functional insanity due to no evident external cause.

typembryo (tī-pĕm′brĭ-ō). An embryo in that stage of development when its structural type may be recognized.

typhemia (tī-fē′mĭ-ă). Typhoid bacilli in the blood. SYN: *typhoid bacillemia.*

typh fever (tĭf). Name for all low fevers of typhus and typhoid type.

typhinia (tī-fĭn′ĭ-ă). Disease marked by recurrent periods of fever, chills, vomiting, and neuromuscular pains. SYN: *relapsing fever.*

typhization (tī-fī-zā′shŭn). 1. Typhus or typhoid infection. 2. Inoculation with typhoid vaccine.

typhlatonia, typhlatony (tĭf-lă-tō′nĭ-ă, -lăt′ō-nĭ). Deficient motor activity of the cecum.

typhlectasis (tĭf-lĕk′tă-sĭs). Cecal distention.

typhlectomy (tĭf-lĕk′tō-mĭ). Excision of the cecum. SYN: *cecectomy.*

typhlenteritis (tĭf-ĕn-ter-ī′tĭs). Inflammation of the cecum. SYN: *typhlitis.*

typhlitis (tĭf-lī′tĭs). Inflammation of the cecum.

  Clinically cannot be distinguished from appendicitis. Treatment similar.

typhlodiclidentis (tĭf″lō-dĭk-lĭ-dī′tĭs). Inflammation of the ileocecal valve.

typhloempyema (tĭf″lō-ĕm-pī-ē′mă). An abdominal abscess following typhlitis.

typhloenteritis (tĭf″lō-ĕn-ter-ī′tĭs). Inflammation of the cecum. Syn: *typhlenteritis, typhlitis.*

typhlolexia (tĭf″lō-lĕks′ĭ-ă). Inability to recognize written words. Syn: *word blindness.*

typhlology (tĭf-lŏl′ō-jĭ). Study of blindness, its causes and effects.

typhlopexy (tĭf′lo-pĕks″ĭ). Suturing of a movable cecum to the abdominal wall.

typhlosis (tĭf-lō′sĭs). Blindness.

typhlostenosis (tĭf-lō-stĕn-ō′sĭs). Stenosis or stricture of the cecum.

typhlostomy (tĭf-lŏs′tō-mĭ). Establishment of a permanent cecal fistula.

typhlotomy (tĭf-lŏt′ō-mĭ). Incision of the cecum.

typhloureterostomy (tĭf″lō-ū-rē″ter-ŏs′tō-mĭ). Implantation of a ureter in the cecum.

typho-. Combining form *pert. to fever, typhoid.*

typhobacillosis (tĭ″fō-băs-ĭl-ō′sĭs). Poisoning due to toxins produced by the *Bacillus typhosus.*

typhogenic (tĭ″fō-jĕn′ĭk). Causing typhus or typhoid fever.

typhohemia (tĭ″fō-hē′mĭ-ă). Degeneration of the blood due to presence of bacilli.

typhoid (tĭ′foyd). Resembling typhus.

    t. fever. An acute, infectious disease characterized by definite lesions in Peyer's patches, mesenteric glands, and spleen accompanied by fever, headache, and abdominal symptoms.

    t. state. Condition in many diseases marked by profound prostration and other symptoms like those of typhus or typhoid fever.

    t., walking. Typhoid fever with mild general constitutional symptoms, the patient being able to be up and to walk. Syn: *ambulatory typhoid.*

typhoidal (tĭ-foy′dăl). Resembling typhoid.

typhoidette (tĭ-foy-dĕt′). A mild form of typhoid fever.

typhoin (tĭ′fō-ĭn). A preparation of dead typhoid bacilli introduced hypodermically in typhoid fever as a vaccine.

typholysin (tĭ-fŏl′ĭ-sĭn). A lysin destructive to typhoid bacilli.

typhomalarial (tĭ″fō-mă-lā′rĭ-ăl). Having symptoms of both typhoid and malarial fever.

typhomania (tĭ-fō-mā′nĭ-ă). Muttering delirium characteristic of typhoid fever and typhus.

typhonia (tĭ-fō′nĭ-ă). The delirium in typhoid or typhus fever.

typhophor (tĭ′fō-fōr). A typhoid carrier.*

typhopneumonia (tĭ″fō-nū-mō′nĭ-ă). 1. Pneumonia occurring in typhoid fever. 2. Pneumonia with typhoid symptoms.

typhose (tĭ′fōs). Having the appearance of typhoid fever, esp. when its symptoms appear in some forms of syphilis with pyrexia.

typhosepsis (tĭ″fō-sĕp′sĭs). The general poisoning which occurs in typhoid fever.

typhosis (tĭ-fō′sĭs). A morbid condition with symptoms similar to those of typhoid or typhus fever.

typhosus (tĭ-fō′sŭs). Pert. to typhoid or typhus fever.

typhous (tĭ′fŭs). Pert. to typhus fever.

typhus, typhus fever (tĭ′fŭs). An acute, contagious disease manifested by great prostration, a petechial rash, marked by nervous symptoms and high fever. Syn: *jail fever, ship fever.*

    t., petechial. True typhus fever.

    t. recur'rens. Relapsing fever.

    t. sid'erans. Malignant typhus, quickly fatal.

typical (tĭp′ĭ-kăl). Having the characteristics of, pert. to, or conforming to, a type or condition or group.

typ′ing of blood. Determination of agglutination in the blood of donor and recipient before blood transfusion. See: *blood transfusion.*

typo-. Combining form meaning a *type.*

typology (tĭ-pŏl′ō-jĭ). The study of types, as of blood or constitutional types.

typoscope (tĭ′pō-skōp). Device to aid patients with amblyopia and cataract in reading.

tyrannism (tĭr′ăn-ĭzm). Abnormal tendency to exercise cruelty. Syn: *sadism, q.v.*

ty reflex (tĭ). Sudden reflex grasping of mother's body by infant when startled.

tyremesis (tĭ-rĕm′ĕ-sĭs). Infant vomiting of curdy or cheesy substances.

tyriasis (tĭr-ĭ′ăs-ĭs). 1. Hypertrophy of skin and connective tissue with induration due to obstruction of the lymphatics. Syn: *elephantiasis.* 2. Baldness. Syn: *alopecia.*

tyrogenous (tĭ-rŏj′ĕn-ŭs). Having origin in cheese or produced by it.

tyroid (tĭ′royd). Caseous; cheesy.

tyroma (tĭ-rō′mă). A caseous tumor.

tyromatosis (tĭ-rō-mă-tō′sĭs). Cheesy degeneration. Syn: *caseation.*

tyrosinase (tĭ-rō′sĭn-ās). A ferment that acts on tyrosine.

tyrosine (tĭ′rō-sēn). An amino acid formed in decomposition of protein.

tyrosinuria (tĭ-rō-sĭn-ū′rĭ-ă). Tyrosine in the urine.

tyrosis (tĭ-rō′sĭs). 1. Curdling of milk. 2. Vomiting of cheesy substance by infants. Syn: *tyremesis.* 3. Cheesy degeneration. Syn: *tyromatosis.*

Tyrothrix (tĭ′rō-thrĭks). A genus of bacteria (Schizomycetes) causing coagulation of casein.

tyrotoxin (tĭ″rō-tŏks′ĭn). Any toxic product of milk or cheese due to a bacillus.

tyrotoxism (tĭ-rō-tŏks′ĭzm). Poisoning produced by a milk product or by cheese.

tyroxin (tĭ-rŏks′ĭn). A decomposition product of albumin.

Tyrrel's fascia (tĭr′ĕl). An illy-defined ilbromuscular layer from the middle aponeurosis of the perineum, behind the prostate gland. Syn: *rectovesical fascia.*

    T's. hook. Blunt, slender hook for operations on the eye.

Tyson's glands (tĭ′sŭn). Sebaceous glands at base of glans penis which secrete a sebaceous substance, *smegma.**

U

U. 1. Chem. symbol of *uranium*. 2. Abbr. for *unit*.

uarthritis (ū″ar-thrī′tĭs). Gout supposed to result from excess of uric acid. SYN: *arthritis urica*.

uaterium (wă-tē′rĭ-ŭm). A medical preparation to be used in the ear. [tile.

uberous (ū′bĕr-ŭs). Prolific; fruitful; fer-

uberty (ū′bĕr-tĭ). Fruitfulness; fertility.

Uffelmann's test (oof′ĕl-mahn). Gastric test for hydrochloric acid or lactic acid.

Uhthoff's sign (oot′hof). The nystagmus which occurs in multiple disseminated sclerosis.

ulalgia (ū-lăl′jĭ-ă). Pain in the gums.

ulatrophia (ū″lăt-rō′fĭ-ă). Shrinking of gums; recession of the gums.

ulcer (ŭl′ser). An open lesion upon the skin or mucous membrane of the body, with loss of substance, accompanied by formation of pus.

  u., amputating. One which destroys tissue to the bone by encircling the part.

  u., atonic. A chronic ulcer.

  u., callous. A chronic ulcer with indurated, elevated edges and no granulations, which does not heal.

  u., duodenal. An ulcer on the mucosa of the duodenum, due to the action of the gastric juice.

  u., erethistic. One with an inflamed, red, painful surface.

  u., follicular. A tiny ulcer having its origin in a lymph follicle and affecting a mucous membrane.

  u., fungous. One in which the granulations protrude above edges of wound and bleed easily.

  u., gastric. SEE: *peptic ulcer*.

  u., healthy. An ulcer which tends toward healing, its surface being soft and smooth with tiny red granulations.

  u., indolent. Nearly painless ulcer usually found on leg, characterized by indurated and elevated edge, and nongranulating base.

  u., peptic. An ulcer of the mucosa of the duodenum or stomach.

  u., perforating. An ulcer which permeates the entire thickness of the part, as the foot.

  u., phagedenic. An ulcer which sloughs particles, spreading rapidly and disintegrating the tissues.

  u., rodent. A deeply infiltrating ulcer which slowly eats away the bones and soft tissues; commonly affects the upper part of the face.

  u., round. SEE: *peptic ulcer*.

  u., serpiginous. A creeping ulcer which heals in 1 part and extends to another.

  u., simple. A local ulcer with no severe inflammation or pain.

  u., specific. An ulcer which is caused by a specific disease, as syphilis or lupus.

  u., stercoral. 1. Ulcer caused by pressure from impacted feces. 2. Ulcer through which feces escapes.

ulcerate (ŭl′sĕr-āt). To produce or become affected with an ulcer.

ulcerated (ŭl′sĕr-ā″tĕd). Of the nature of an ulcer or affected with one.

  u. sore throat. Putrid sore throat, a gangrenous inflammation.

  u. tooth. Suppuration of the alveolar periosteum with ulceration of gum surrounding the decaying root of a tooth.

ulceration (ŭl″sĕr-ā′shŭn). Suppuration taking place on a free surface, as on the skin or on a mucous membrane. A termination of inflammation.

ulcerative (ŭl′sĕr-ă-tĭv). Pert. to or causing ulceration.

  u. scrofuloderma. Progressive fatal skin disease with hard, red, ulcerating tumors.

ulceromembranous (ŭl″sĕr-ō-mĕm′brăn-ŭs). Pert. to ulceration and formation of a membrane.

  u. tonsillitis. Tonsillitis that ulcerates and develops a membranous film.

ulcerous (ŭl′sĕr-ŭs). Pert. to or affected with an ulcer.

ulcus (ŭl′kŭs) (pl. *ulcera*). Ulcer.

  u. cancrosum. 1. Cancerous ulcer which eats away the tissues. SYN: *rodent ulcer*. 2. Same as *ulcus durum*.

  u. durum. Lesion of syphilis. SYN: *chancre*.

  u. induratum. Same as *ulcus durum*.

  u. tuberculosum. Tuberculosis of the skin. SYN: *lupus*.

  u. ventriculi. Gastric ulceration.

  u. vulvae acutum. Nonvenereal, rapidly spreading ulceration of the vulva of about 2 weeks' duration associated with presence of *Bacillus crassus*.

ulectomy (ū-lĕk′tō-mĭ). 1. Excision of scar tissue, esp. in secondary iridectomy. 2. Removal of gum tissue, as in pyorrhea alveolaris. SYN: *gingivectomy*.

ulemorrhagia (ū-lē-mor-ā′jĭ-ă). Bleeding from the gums.

ulerythema (ū-lĕr-ĭ-thē′mă). An erythematous disorder with atrophic scar formation. SEE: *lupus erythematosus*.

  u. ophryogenes. Folliculitis of eyebrows.

uletic (ū-lĕt′ĭk). Pert. to the gums.

uletomy (ū-lĕt′ō-mĭ). Incision of a scar to relieve tension. SEE: *cicatricotomy*.

uliginous (ū-lĭj′ĭn-ŭs). Muddy; slimy.

ulilampe (ū′lĭ-lămp). Low pressure glow tube used in uviol glass tube used abroad for therapeutic purposes. SEE: *uviol*.

ulitis (ū-lī′tĭs). Inflammation of the gums.

  u., interstitial. Inflammation of connective tissue of gums about the necks of the teeth.

U-1

ulna (ŭl′nă). The inner and larger bone of the forearm, bet. the wrist and the elbow, on the side opposite that of the thumb. [ulna.

ulnad (ŭl′năd). In the direction of the ulna.

ulnar (ŭl′nar). 1. Relating to the ulna, or to nerve or artery named from it. 2. Cuneiform carpal bone. SYN: *ulnare.*

ulnare (ŭl-nā′rē). The 3rd or cuneiform bone of the carpus.

ulnaris (ŭl-nā′rĭs). A muscle on ulnar side of the forearm.

ulnocarpal (ŭl″nō-kar′păl). Relating to the carpus and ulna, or to the ulnar side of the wrist.

ulnoradial (ŭl″nō-rā′dĭ-ăl). Relating to the ulna and radius, as their ligaments and articulations.

ulocace (ū-lŏk′ă-sē). Ulcerative inflammation of the gums.

ulocarcinoma (ū″lō-kar-sĭn-ō′mă). Carcinoma of the gums.

uloglossitis (ū″lō-glos-ī′tĭs). Inflammation of the gums and tongue.

uloid (ū′loyd). 1. Scarlike. 2. A scarlike lesion caused by subcutaneous degeneration.

  u. cicatrix. Same as *uloid, 2.*

uloncus (ū-lŏn′kŭs). Swelling or tumor of the gums. SEE: *epulis.*

ulorrhagia (ū-lor-ā′jĭ-ă). Bleeding from the gums.

ulorrhea (ū-lor-rē′ă). Slow bleeding from the gums.

ulosis (ū-lō′sĭs). Formation of scar tissue. SYN: *cicatrization.*

ulotic (ū-lŏt′ĭk). Causing cicatrization. SYN: *cicatricial.*

ulotomy (ū-lŏt′ō-mĭ). 1. The cutting of scar tissue to relieve deformity or tension. 2. Incision of the gums.

ulotrichous (ū-lŏt′rĭk-ŭs). Having short, woolly hair, as a negro.

ulotropsis (ū″lō-trop′sĭs). Revitalization of the gums by massage.

ultex (ŭl′tĕks). A bifocal glass in which the near section is ground with the spherical curve.

ultimate (ŭl′tĭm-ăt). Final or last.

  u. analysis. Resolution of a substance into its constituent elements.

ultimum moriens (ŭl′tĭ-mŭm mō′rĭ-ĕns). 1. The right auricle, last part of the body to die, said to contract after the heart has ceased to beat. 2. Upper portion of the trapezius muscle, which frequently is not involved in progressive muscular atrophy.

ultra-. Prefix meaning *beyond, excess.*

ultrabrachycephalic (ŭl″tră-brăk″ĭ-sē-făl′-ĭk). Having a cephalic index of 90 or over.

ultrafiltration (ŭl″tră-fĭl-trā′shŭn). Filtration of a colloidal substance in which the dispersed particles, but not the liquid, are held back.

ultraligation (ŭl″tră-lĭ-gā′shŭn). Ligation of a blood vessel beyond the origin of a branch.

ultramicrobe (ŭl″tră-mī′krōb). A microorganism too small to be visible by the ordinary microscope.

ultramicroscope (ŭl″tră-mī′krō-skōp). Microscope by which objects invisible through an ordinary microscope may be seen by means of powerful side illumination.

ultramicron (ŭl″tră-mī′krŏn). A particle so tiny that it can be seen only through the ultramicroscope. SYN: *submicron.*

ultramicroscopical (ŭl″tră-mĭk-rō-skŏp′ĭ-kăl). Too small to be seen with aid of an ordinary microscope.

ultramicroscopy (ŭl″tră-mī-krŏs′kō-pĭ). The use of the ultramicroscope for scientific purposes.

ultraprophylaxis (ŭl″tră-prō-fĭl-ăks′ĭs). Prevention of diseased or abnormal offspring by regulating the marriage of the unfit.

ultratherm (ŭl′tră-therm). A short wave diathermy machine.

ultratoxon (ŭl″tră-tŏks′ŏn). A toxon of a very low degree of toxicity.

ultraviolet (ŭl″tră-vī′ō-lĕt). Beyond the visible spectrum at its violet end, said of rays. SEE: *infrared.*

  u. therapy. Treatment with ultraviolet radiation. SEE: *heliotherapy, light therapy.*

ultravirus (ŭl″tră-vī′rŭs). A virus which is filtrable but which can be demonstrated by inoculation test. SEE: *filtrable virus.*

Ultzmann's test (oolts′mahn). A solution test for bile pigments in the urine.

  The fluid will show bright green if bile pigments are present.

umbilical (ŭm-bĭl′ĭ-kăl). Pert. to the umbilicus.

  u. cord. The attachment connecting the fetus with the placenta, artificially severed at birth of the child.

  u. fissure. Portion of hepatic longitudinal fissure in which the umbilical vein is lodged.

  u. hernia. A hernia in the region of the umbilicus.

  u. souffle. A hissing sound said to arise from the umbilical cord.

  u. vesicle. That part of the embryonic yolk sac leading from the umbilicus.

umbilicate (ŭm-bĭl′ĭ-kāt). Pert. to or shaped like the navel, noting a bacterial colony with a central depression resembling an umbilicus.

umbilication (ŭm-bĭl-ĭ-kā′shŭn). 1. A depression resembling a navel. 2. Formation at apex of a pustule or vesicle of a pit or depression.

umbilicus (ŭm-bĭ-lī′kŭs, -bĭl′ĭ-kŭs) (pl. *umbilici*). A depressed point in the middle of the abdomen; the scar which marks the former attachment of the umbilical cord to the fetus.

umbo (ŭm′bō). Projecting center of a round surface.

  u. tympani. Shallow, funnel-shaped area on drum membrane at the tip of the manubrium where malleus is attached.

umbrascopy (ŭm-brăs′kō-pĭ). Use of shadows in refraction of the eye or use of roentgen rays. SYN: *skiascopy.*

un-. Prefix meaning *back*, *reversal*, *annulment of*, *not*.

uncia (ŭn′sĭ-ă). An ounce, or an inch.

unciform (ŭn′sĭ-form). Hook-shaped.

    u. **bone.** Hook-shaped bone on ulnar side of distal row of the carpus. SYN: *os hamatum.*

    u. **fasciculus.** Bundle of fibers connecting frontal cerebral lobes with the temporosphenoid ones.

    u. **process.** 1. Long, thin lamina of bone from orbital plate of the ethmoid articulating with the inf. turbinate. 2. Hook at ant. end of hippocampal gyrus. 3. Hooked end of unciform bone.

uncinariasis (ŭn-sĭ-na-rī′ă-sĭs). Hookworm disease. SYN: *ankylostomiasis, q.v.*

    u. **of skin.** Vesicular dermatitis generally of the feet from invasion by the *Uncinaria duodenale.*

Uncinaria (ŭn-sĭn-ā′rĭ-ă). A genus of nematode worms infesting man and lower animals. [hooked.]

uncinate (ŭn′sĭn-āt). Hook-shaped;

    u. **convolution.** An occipital lobe convolution near temporal lobe.

    u. **epilepsy.** Form of epilepsy occurring in disease of uncinate area of the temporal lobe.

    u. **gyrus.** SEE: *uncinate convolution.*

uncinatum (ŭn-sĭn-ā′tŭm). The unciform bone of the hand. SYN: *os hamatum.*

uncipressure (ŭn′sĭ-prĕsh-ur). Pressure by means of hooks to arrest hemorrhage.

un″condi′tioned re′flex. Any reflex not the result of special training.

unconscious (ŭn-kŏn′shŭs). 1. In a state unaccompanied by conscious experience, as in a faint. PSY: Excluded from consciousness by repression. 3. Repository of previous experiences in life of the individual and of the historical past of the race.

unconsciousness (ŭn-kŏn′shŭs-nĕs). State of being insensible or without conscious experiences.

unction (ŭnk′shŭn). 1. The application of an ointment. 2. Substance used for anointing. SYN: *unguent.*

unctuous (ŭnk′chū-ŭs). Oily; greasy.

uncus (ŭn′kŭs). Any structure that is hook-shaped.

    u. **gyri hippocampi.** BNA. Hooked ant. end of the hippocampal gyrus.

undertoe (ŭn′dĕr-tō). Condition of displacement of the great toe underneath the others.

undifferentiation (ŭn-dĭf-ĕr-ĕn-shĭ-ā′shŭn). Alteration in cell character to a more embryonic type or toward a malignant state. SYN: *anaplasia.*

undine (ŭn′dĭn). A small glass flask used for irrigating the conjunctiva and in removal of a cataract.

undinism (ŭn′dĭn-ĭzm). Awakening of the libido by running water, as by urination or at sight of urine.

undulant (ŭn′dū-lănt). Rising and falling like waves, or moving like them.

    u. **fever.** One of long duration due to the *Brucella melitensis.*

undulate (ŭn′dū-lāt). Wavy; having a wavy border with shallow sinuses, said of bacterial colonies.

undulation (ŭn-dū-lā′shŭn). A continuous wavelike motion or pulsation.

un′finished cough. A cough frequently caused by, and typical of, aneurysm of the aortic arch.

ung. Abbr. of *unguentum*, ointment.

ungual (ŭng′gwăl). Pert. to or resembling the nails. SYN: *unguinal.*

    u. **bone.** The thin, platelike lacrimal bone.

    u. **phalanx.** Terminal phalanx of each finger and toe.

    u. **tuberosity.** Spatula-shaped extremity of the terminal phalanx which supports the nails of fingers and toes.

unguent (ŭng′gwĕnt). A lubricant or salve for sores, burns, etc. SYN: *ointment.*

unguentum (ŭn-gwĕn′tŭm). 1. Fatty, soft, solid preparation intended to be applied to the skin by inunction. Sixteen ointments are official. 2. Simple ointment, usually a compound of lard and yellow wax or occasionally wool fat, white wax, and white petroleum. SYN: *ointment, q.v.*

ungues (ŭng′gwēz) (sing. *unguis*). The nails. SEE: *unguis.*

unguinal (ŭng′gwĭn-ăl). Relating to or resembling a nail or an unguis.

unguis (ŭng′gwĭs) (pl. *ungues*). 1. A finger- or toenail. SYN: *onyx*. 2. The lacrimal bone. 3. Pus mass in cornea. 4. A white prominence on floor of the lateral ventricle's post. horn. SYN: *hippocampus minor.*

ungula (ŭn′gū-lă). Instrument for removal of dead fetus.

uni-. Combining form meaning *one*.

unicellular (ū″nĭ-sĕl′ū-lar). Having only 1 cell.

uniceptor (ū′nĭ-sĕp″tor). A receptor occurring in blood serum having only a single combining group.

unicorn (ū′nĭ-korn). Having a single cornu or horn.

    u. **uterus.** A uterus with but 1 horn perfectly formed.

unicornous (ū-nĭ-kor′nŭs). Having but 1 horn or cornu.

unidirectional (ū″nĭ-dĭ-rĕk′shŭn-ăl). Flowing in only one direction, as an electric current in a circuit.

uniglandular (ū″nĭ-glăn′dū-lar). Pert. to or having only one gland.

unigravida (ū″nĭ-grăv′ĭ-dă). Woman who is pregnant for the first time.

unilateral (ū″nĭ-lăt′ĕr-al). Affecting or occurring on only one side.

unilocular (ū″nĭ-lŏk′ū-lar). Having but one cavity.

uninuclear, uninucleate(d (ū″nĭ-nū′klē-ar, -ăt, -ā-tĕd). Having only one nucleus.

uniocular (ū″nĭ-ok′ū-lar). Pert. to or having only one eye.

union (ūn′yŭn). 1. Act of joining 2 or more things into 1 part, or state of being so united. 2. Growing together of severed or broken parts, as of bones or lips of a wound. SEE: *healing.*

u. of granulations. A healing by third* intention with wound filling up with granulations.

u., non-. Failure to unite, as a fractured bone.

u., secondary. A healing by second* intention with adhesion of granulating surfaces.

u., vicious. Union of ends of a broken bone in such a way as to cause deformity.

unioval (ū″nĭ-ō′văl). Developed from 1 ovum, as identical twins.

unipara (ū-nĭp′ă-rä). A woman who has had only 1 child.

uniparous (ū-nĭp′ă-rŭs). 1. Having produced but 1 child. 2. Giving birth to 1 offspring at a time.

unipolar (ū″nĭ-pō′lar). 1. Having, produced by, or acting by, only 1 pole, as a nerve cell, the branches of which project from only 1 side. 2. At 1 extremity of a cell only. SEE: *monoterminal.*

unipotent (ū-nĭp′ō-tent). Having power in 1 way only, as a cell capable of producing cells of only 1 order. SYN: *unipotential.*

unipotential (ū″nĭ-pō-tĕn′shăl). Able in 1 way only, as able to give rise to cells of 1 order only; said of certain cells.

unit (ū′nĭt). 1. One of anything. 2. A determined amount adopted as a standard of measurement.

u., Allen-Doisy. SEE: *mouse and rat unit.*

u., amboceptor. The smallest amount of amboceptor required in the presence of which a given quantity of red blood corpuscles will be dissolved by an excess of complement.

u., Angström's. An internationally adopted unit of measurement of wave length, 1/10,000,000 of a millimeter, or 1/254,000,000 of an inch.

u., antigen. Smallest quantity of antigen required to fix 1 unit of complement, preventing hemolysis.

u., antitoxic. The amt. of antitoxon needed to neutralize 100 times the least fatal dose of standard toxin that will kill a guinea pig weighing 250 Gm.

u., British thermal. The amt. of heat necessary to raise 1 pound of water at 39° F. one degree.

u., candlepower. SEE: *light unit.*

u. of capacity. Capacity of a condenser which gives a difference of potential of 1 volt when charged with 1 coulomb. SYN: *curie; farad; unit, zlumen.*

u., cat. The amount of a drug per kg. of weight of animal just sufficient to kill a cat when injected intravenously slowly and continuously.

u., complement. Smallest quantity of complement required for hemolysis of a given amount of red blood corpuscles with 1 amboceptor unit present.

u., electrical. SEE: *ampere, ohm, volt, watt, etc.*

u., Hampson. An x-ray unit of measurement, ¼ the erythema dose.

u., hemolytic. The amount of inactivated immune serum which causes complete hemolysis of 1 cc. of a 5% emulsion of washed red blood corpuscles, in the presence of complement.

u., Holzknecht. An x-ray unit of measurement, 1/5 the erythema dose. ABBR: *H.*

u., immunizing. SEE: *antitoxic unit.*

u., international, of vitamin A. The vitamin activity of 0.6 mg. of the international standard carotene.

u., i., of vitamin B. The vitamin activity of 10 mg. of the international standard absorption product.

u., i., of vitamin C. The vitamin activity of 0.05 mg. of the international standard levo-ascorbic acid.

u., i., of vitamin D. The vitamin activity of 1 mg. of the international standard solution of irradiated ergosterol (0.025 mg. crystalline vitamin D).

u., Kienböck. Measurement of x-ray dosage, 1/10 the erythema dose.

u., light. A foot-candle, or the amount of light 1 ft. from a standard candle.

u., Mache. Unit of measurement of radium emanation. ABBR: *M. u.*

u., mouse. Least amount of estrus-producing hormone which induces, in a spayed mouse, a characteristic desquamation of the vaginal epithelium.

u., physical. SEE: *coulomb, erg, dyne, household measures, metric system, apothecaries' system, avoirdupois system, Troy weight.*

u., radiation. SEE: *Angrström unit, Mache unit.*

u., rat. Greatest dilution of an estrus-producing hormone which will cause desquamation and cornification of vaginal epithelium during 1st day, if given to a mature spayed rat in 3 injections, 1 every 4 hours.

u., toxic. 1. Lowest dose of diphtheria toxin which in 3-4 days will kill a guinea pig weighing 250 Gm. 2. The amount of scarlet fever toxin that gives a positive reaction in susceptible persons when injected intradermally or no reaction in immune individuals.

u., X-radiation. The international unit is the quantity of X-radiation which, when the secondary electrons are fully utilized, and the wall effect of the chamber is avoided, produces in 1 cc. of atmospheric air at 0° C. and 76 cm. mercury pressure, such degree of conductivity that 1 electrostatic unit of charge is measured at saturation current. Designated by the small letter "r."

u., x-ray. SEE: *Kienböck unit.*

unitarian (ū-nĭ-tā′rĭ-an). Composed of a single unit.

u. theory. That of Bordet that assumes only 1 alexin or complement in the serum of an animal, despite the fact that the alexins in different species differ.

unitary (ū′nĭ-tā-rĭ). Relating to a unit. SYN: *unitarian.*

uniterminal (ū″nĭ-ter′mĭn-ăl). Having only 1 terminal. SEE: *monoterminal.*

univalent (ū″nĭ-vā′lĕnt, ū-nĭv′ă-lĕnt). 1. Possessing the power of combining or replacing 1 atom of hydrogen. 2. Single, noting a chromosome which lacks or fails to unite with a synaptic mate.

universal (ū″nĭ-ver′săl). General.

u. joint. One movable in any direction, as a ball and socket joint.

unofficial (ŭn-of-ĭsh′ăl). Not listed by the pharmacopoeia.

unorganized (ŭn-or′găn-īzd). 1. Not organized into an organic structure. 2. Without the characteristics of a living organism; inorganic.

u. ferment. A chemical ferment, one that is not a living organism. SYN: *enzyme.* SEE: *ferment.*

unsaturated (ŭn-săt′ū-rāt″ĕd). 1. Capable of dissolving or absorbing to a greater degree. 2. Not combined to the greatest possible extent.

u. compound. One capable of combining with additional elements or compounds, as any member of the hydrocarbon series. SEE: *saturated compound.*

Unschuld's sign (oon′shoolt). Cramps frequently felt in the calves of the legs, an early sign in diabetes.

unsex (ŭn-sĕks′). To castrate; to spay or excise the ovaries.

unstriated (ŭn-strī′āt-ĕd). Unstriped, as smooth muscle fiber.

unwell (ŭn-wĕl′). 1. Sick; ill; indisposed. 2. Menstruating.

upsiloid (ŭp′sĭ-loyd). Shaped like the letter U or V.

urachal (ū′ră-kăl). Relating to the urachus.

urachus (ū′răk-ŭs). Fibrous cord from the bladder to umbilicus, the remnant of part of the duct of the allantois of the embryo.

uracrasia (ū-ră-krā′sĭ-ă). 1. A disordered condition of urine. 2. Inability to retain the urine. SYN: *enuresis.*

uracratia (ū-ră-krā′shĭ-ă). Incontinence of the urine. SYN: *enuresis.*

uragogue (ū′ră-gog). Increasing the secretion of urine. SYN: *diuretic.*

uranalysis (ū″răn-ăl′ĭs-ĭs). Chemical analysis of the urine.

uranisconitis (ū-răn-ĭs″kon-ī′tĭs). Inflammation of the palate.

uraniscoplasty (ū-răn-ĭs′kō-plăs″tĭ). Operation for repair of cleft palate. SYN: *uranoplasty, uranorrhaphy.*

uraniscorrhaphy (ū-răn-ĭs-kor′ră-fĭ). Operation for suturing of a cleft palate. SYN: *uraniscoplasty.*

uraniscus (ū-răn-ĭs′kŭs). Palate, or roof of mouth.

uranism (ū′răn-ĭzm). Unnatural sex relations bet. males. SYN: *urningism, q.v.*

uranist (ū′răn-ĭst). A male homosexual. SYN: *urning.**

uranium (ū-rā′nĭ-ŭm). SYMB: U. Primary radioactive element, the parent of radium and other radio-elements.

u. unit. A measure of radioactivity, uranium being taken as 1.

uranoplasty (ū′răn-ō-plăs″tĭ). Operation cleft palate. SYN: *uraniscoplasty.*

uranorrhaphy (ū-răn-or′ră-fĭ). Operation for suture of a cleft palate. SYN: *uraniscorrhaphy.*

uranoschisis (ū-răn-ŏs′kĭs-ĭs). Cleft palate.

uranostaphyloplasty (ū″răn-ō-stăf′ĭl-ō-plăs″tĭ). Operation for correction of a defect of the soft and hard palates.

uranostaphylorrhaphy (ū″răn-ō-stăf-ĭl-or′ă-fĭ). Operation for repair of cleft of hard and soft palates.

uraroma (ū-ră-rō′mă). Aromatic, spicy odor of the urine.

urarthritis (ū″rar-thrĭ′tĭs). Gouty inflammation of the joints.

urate (ū′rāt). Combination of uric acid with a base; a salt of uric acid.

Urates in urine insignificant unless excessive. Urates can be dispersed by boiling the urine. SEE: *antiuratic.*

uratemia (ū″ră-tē′mĭ-ă). Urates, esp. sodium urate, in the blood.

uratic (ū-răt′ĭk). Relating or made up of urates.

uratolysis (ū-ră-tŏl′ĭ-sĭs). Decomposition of urates.

uratolytic (ū-ră-tō-lĭt′ĭk). Capable of dissolving urates.

uratoma (ū-ră-tō′mă). A concretion composed of urates. SYN: *tophus.*

uratosis (ū-ră-tō′sĭs). Morbid condition of the body, due to the deposit of urates in the tissues and circulating fluids.

uraturia (ū-ră-tū-rĭ′ă). Excess of urates in the urine. SYN: *lithuria.*

urceiform (ŭr-sē′ĭ-form). Shaped like a pitcher.

urea (ū-rē′ă). The diamide of carbonic acid, a crystalline solid having the formula $CO(NH_2)_2$; found in blood, lymph, and urine.

DOSAGE: 8-60 gr. (0.5-4.0 Gm.).

ureagenetic (ū-rē″ă-jĕn-ĕt′ĭk). Pert. to or producing urea.

ureal (ū-rē′ăl). Relating to or containing urea.

ureameter (ū-rē-ăm′et-er). Device for determining amount of urea in urine.

ureametry (ū-rē-ăm′ĕt-rĭ). Determination of amt. of urea in urine.

ureapoiesis (ū-rē″ă-poy-ē′sĭs). Formation of urea.

urease (ū′rē-ās). An enzyme which accelerates hydrolysis of urea into ammonium carbonate and hippuric acid into glycocoll and benzoic acid.

urecchysis (ū-rĕk′ĭs-ĭs). Effusion of urine into areolar tissue.

uredema (ū-re-dē′mă). Urine in the subcutaneous tissues distending them.

uredo (ū-rē′dō). 1. Burning sensation in the skin. 2. Skin disorder marked by smooth, white elevations which itch severely. SYN: *hives, urticaria, q.v.*

ureide (ū′rē-īd). Any compound of urea in which acid radicals have taken the place of 1 or more of its hydrogen atoms.

urein(e (ū-rē′ĭn). An oily substance isolated from urine supposed to cause symptoms of uremia.

urelcosis (ū-rĕl-kō′sĭs). Ulceration of the urinary organs.

uremia (ū-rē'mĭ-ă). Toxic condition produced by the presence of urinary constituents in the blood.

u., chronic. Visual disturbance, headache, dizziness, anorexia, low heart action, vomiting, scanty urine, retention of nitrogenous products in the blood.

uremic (ū-rē'mĭk). Pert. to or caused by uremia.

uremide (ū're-mīd). The skin lesions of uric acid poisoning.

uremigenic (ū-rē-mĭ-jĕn'ĭk). Caused by uremia or producing it.

ureometer (ū"rē-ŏm'ĕt-ĕr). Appliance used to determine the amt. of urea in urine. SYN: *ureameter*.

ureometry (ū-rē-ŏm'ĕt-rĭ). Estimation of amt. of urea in urine.

ureopoiesis (ū-rē"ō-poy-ē'sĭs). Formation of urea. SYN: *ureapoiesis*.

ureosecretory (ū-rē-ō-sē'kre-tōr-ĭ). Relating to the secretion of urea.

urerythrin (ūr-er'ĭ-thrĭn). A red pigment in the urine in rheumatic and certain other fevers. SYN: *uroerythrin*.

uresiesthesia, uresiesthesis (ū-rē"sĭ-ĕs-thē'zĭ-ă, -sĭs). The normal inclination to void urine.

uresis (ū-rē'sĭs). The excretion of urine. SYN: *urination*.

ureter (u're-ter, ū-rē'tĕr). One of 2 tubes carrying urine from the kidney to the bladder, beginning with the pelvis of the kidney, and emptying into the base of the bladder.

ureteralgia (ū-rē-ter-ăl'jĭ-ă). Pain in the ureter.

uretercystoscope (ū-rē"tĕr-sĭs'tō-skōp). A cystoscope combined with a ureteral catheter.

ureterectasis (ū-rē"ter-ĕk-tă'sĭs). Dilatation of the ureter.

ureterectomy (ū-rē"ter-ĕk'tō-mĭ). Excision of a ureter.

ureteritis (ū-rē"tĕr-ī'tĭs). Inflammation of the ureters.

ureterocele (ū-rē'tĕr-ō-sēl). Hernia of the ureter or hernia containing the ureter.

ureterocolostomy (ū-rē"tĕr-ō-kō-lŏs'tō-mĭ). The implantation of the ureter into the colon.

ureterocystoneostomy (ū-rē"tĕr-ō-sĭst"ō-nē-ŏs'tō-mĭ). Formation of a passage bet. a ureter and the bladder. SYN: *ureterocystostomy, ureteroneocystostomy*.

ureterocystostomy (ū-rē"tĕr-ō-sĭs-tŏs'tō-mĭ). Artificial formation of a passage bet. a ureter and the bladder.

ureterodialysis (ū-rē"tĕr-ō-dī-ăl'ĭ-sĭs). Rupture of one of the ureters.

ureteroenterostomy (ū-rē"tĕr-ō-ĕn-ter-ŏs'tō-mĭ). Formation of a passage bet. a ureter and the intestine.

ureterography (ū-rē"tĕr-ŏg'ră-fĭ). X-ray photography of the ureter after injection of some opaque substance into it.

ureterolith (ū-rē'ter-ō-lĭth). A stone or calculus in the ureter.

ureterolithiasis (ū-rē"ter-ō-lĭth-ī'ăs-ĭs). Development of a calculus in the ureter.

ureterolithotomy (ū-rē"ter-ō-lĭth-ŏt'ō-mĭ). Surgical incision for removal of a calculus from ureter.

ureterolysis (ū-rē"ter-ŏl'ĭ-sĭs). 1. Rupture of the ureter. SYN: *ureterodialysis*. 2. Paralysis of the ureter. 3. The process of loosening adhesions around the ureter.

ureteroneocystostomy (ū-rē"ter-ō-nē"ō-sĭs-tŏs'tō-mĭ). Surgical formation of a passage bet. the ureter and the bladder. SYN: *ureterocystostomy*.

ureteroneopyelostomy (ū-rē"ter-ō-nē"ō-pī-ĕ-lŏs'tō-mĭ). Excision of a portion of the ureter with attachment of the ureter to a new aperture in the renal pelvis.

ureteronephrectomy (ū-rē"ter-o-nef-rĕk'tō-mĭ). Removal of a kidney and its ureter.

ureteropathy (ū-rē-ter-ŏp'ă-thĭ). Any diseased condition of the ureter.

ureterophlegma (ū-rē"ter-ō-flĕg'mă). Mucous accumulation in the ureter.

ureteroplasty (ū-rē'ter-ō-plăs"tĭ). Plastic surgery of the ureter.

ureteroproctostomy (ū-rē"ter-ō-prŏk-tŏs'tō-mĭ). Formation of a passage from the ureter to the anus.

ureteropyelitis (ū-rē"ter-ō-pī-ĕl-ī'tĭs). Inflammation of the pelvis of the kidney and a ureter.

ureteropyeloneostomy (ū-rē"ter-ō-pī"ĕl-ō-nē-ŏs'tō-mĭ). Artificial formation of a new passage from pelvis of kidney to ureter. SYN: *ureteroneopyelostomy*.

ureteropyelonephritis (ū-rē"ter-ō-pī"ĕl-ō-nef-rī'tĭs). Inflammation of the renal pelvis and the ureter.

ureteropyeloplasty (ū-rē"ter-ō-pī'ĕl-ō-plăs"tĭ). Plastic surgery of the ureter and renal pelvis.

ureteropyosis (ū-rē"tĕr-ō-pī-ō'sĭs). Suppurative inflammation within a ureter.

ureterorrhagia (ū-rē"ter-or-rā'jĭ-ă). Hemorrhage from the ureter.

ureterorrhaphy (ū-rē"ter-or'ră-fĭ). Suture of the ureter, as for fistula.

ureterosigmoidostomy (ū-rē"ter-ō-sĭg-moyd-ŏs'tō-mĭ). Surgical implantation of the ureter into the sigmoid flexure.

ureterostenosis (ū-rē"ter-ō-stĕn-ō'sĭs). Stricture of a ureter.

ureterostomy (ū-rē"ter-ŏs'tō-mĭ). Formation of a permanent fistula for drainage of a ureter.

ureterotomy (ū-rē"ter-ŏt'ō-mĭ). Incision or surgery of the ureter.

ureteroureterostomy (ū-rē"ter-ō-ū-rē"ter-ŏs'tō-mĭ). 1. Formation of a connection from 1 ureter to the other. 2. Reëstablishment of a passage bet. the ends of a divided ureter.

ureterovaginal (ū-rē"ter-ō-văj'ĭ-năl). Relating to a ureter and the vagina, noting a fistula connecting them.

ureterovesical (ū-rē"ter-ō-vĕs'ĭ-kăl). Pert. to a connection bet. the ureter and the bladder.

ureterovesicostomy (ū-rē"ter-ō-vĕs"ĭ-kŏs'tō-mĭ). Reimplantation of a ureter into the bladder.

urethra (ū-rē'thră). A membranous canal for the external discharge of urine from the bladder to the *meatus urinarius* and in the male also for an outlet for the seminal fluids.

u. mulie'bris. BNA. The female urethra.

u. viri'lis. BNA. The male urethra.

urethral (ū-rē'thrăl). Relating to the urethra.

    u. caruncle. Small, fleshy growth from wall of the urethra. Very sensitive.

urethralgia (ū-rē-thrăl'jĭ-ă). Urethral pain; pain in the urethra.

urethratresia (ū-rē-thră-trē'zĭ-ă). Occlusion, or imperforation of the urethra.

urethrectomy (ū-rē-thrĕk'tō-mĭ). Surgical excision of the urethra or part of it.

urethremphraxis (ū-rē-thrĕm-frăks'ĭs). Urethral obstruction. SYN: *urethrophraxis.*

urethreurynter (ū-rē-thrū-rĭn'tĕr). Appliance for dilating the urethra.

urethrism, urethrismus (ū're-thrĭzm, ū''rē-thrĭz'mŭs). Irritability or spasm of the urethra.

urethritis (ū-re-thrī'tĭs). Inflammation of the urethra.

    u., anterior. Inflammation of that portion of the urethra ant. to the ant. layer of the triangular ligament.

    u., gonococcal. Urethritis caused by gonococcus.

    u., posterior. Inflammation of membranous and prostatic portions of the urethra.

    u., simple. Catarrhal inflammation of the urethra. SYN: *blennorrhea.*

    u., specific. Urethritis occurring in gonorrhea.

    u. vene'rea. SEE: *urethritis, specific.*

urethro-. Combining form meaning *urethra.*

urethrocele (ū-rē'thrō-sēl). 1. Pouchlike protrusion of the urethral wall in the female. 2. Thickening of connective tissue around the urethra in the female.

urethrocystitis (ū-rē''thrō-sĭs-tī'tĭs). Inflammation of urethra and bladder.

urethrography (ū-rē-thrŏg'ră-fĭ). X-ray photography of the urethra, after the injection of an opaque medium.

urethrometer (ū-rē-thrŏm'et-er). Instrument for measuring diameter of urethra or lumen of a stricture.

urethropenile (ū-rē''thrō-pē'nĭl). Relating to the urethra and penis.

urethroperineal (ū-rē''thrō-pĕr-ĭ-nē'ăl). Relating to the urethra and perineum.

urethroperineoscrotal (ū-rē''thrō-pĕr-ĭ-nē''ō-skrō'tăl). Relating to the urethra, perineum, and scrotum.

urethrophraxis (ū-rē-thrō-frăks'ĭs). Urethral obstruction. SYN: *urethremphraxis.*

urethrophyma (ū-rē-thrō-fī'mă). A neoplasm in the urethra.

urethroplasty (ū-rē'thrō-plăs''tĭ). Reparative surgery of the urethra.

urethrorectal (ū-rē''thrō-rĕk'tăl). Relating to the urethra and the rectum.

urethrorrhagia (ū-rē''thror-ā'jĭ-ă). Hemorrhage from urethra.

urethrorrhaphy (ū-rē-thror'ăf-ĭ). Suture of the urethra, as a urethral fistula.

urethrorrhea (ū-rē''thror-ē'ă). Morbid discharge from the urethra.

urethroscope (ū-rē'thrō-skōp). Device for examining interior of urethra.

urethroscopic (ū-rē''thrō-skōp'ĭk). Relating to the urethroscope or urethroscopy.

urethroscopy (ū-rē-thrŏs'kō-pĭ). An examination of the mucous membrane of the urethra with a urethroscope.

urethrospasm (ū-rē'thrō-spăzm). Spasmodic stricture of the urethra.

urethrostaxis (ū-rē''thrō-staks'ĭs). Oozing of blood from the urethral mucous membrane.

urethrostenosis (ū-rē''thrō-sten-ō'sĭs). Stricture of the urethra.

urethrostomy (ū-rē-thrŏs'tō-mĭ). Formation of a permanent fistula opening into the urethra by perineal section and fixation of membranous urethra in perineum.

urethrotome (ū-rē'thrō-tōm). An instrument for incision of urethral stricture.

urethrotomy (ū-rē-thrŏt'ō-mĭ). Incision of a urethral stricture.

urethrovaginal (ū-rē''thrō-văj'ĭ-năl). Pert. to the urethra and vagina.

uretic (ū-ret'ĭk). 1. Pert. to urine. 2. Pert. to or stimulating the flow of urine. 3. That which stimulates the flow of the urine. SYN: *diuretic.*

urginin (ŭr'jĭn-ĭn). A proprietary mixture of 2 glucosides derived from squill.

    DOSAGE: From 1-3 mg. per day, depending on the severity.

uric (ū'rĭk). Of or pert. to urine.

    u. acid. A crystalline acid in the urine, a metabolism product of nuclein. It is a common constituent of urinary and renal calculi, and gouty concretions.

    u. a., endogenous. Uric acid derived from purines undergoing metabolism from the nucleoprotein of body tissues.

    u. a., exogenous. Uric acid derived from those purines from food made up of free purines and nucleoproteins.

    SEE: *urate, uratosis, uraturia.*

uricacidemia (ū''rĭk-ăs-ĭd-ē'mĭ-ă). Excess uric acid in the blood and the condition produced thereby.

uricaciduria (ū''rĭk-ăs-ĭd-ū'rĭ-ă). Excessive amount of uric acid in the urine.

uricase (ū'rĭ-kāz). A hydrolytic enzyme capable of changing uric acid into allantoin.

uricemia (ū-rĭ-sē'mĭ-ă). Uric acid in the blood. SYN: *uricacidemia.*

uricocholia (ū''rĭk-ō-kō'lĭ-ă). Uric acid in the bile.

uricolysis (ū-rĭk-ŏl'ĭs-ĭs). The decomposition of uric acid.

uricolytic (ū''rĭk-ō-lĭt'ĭk). Decomposing uric acid into urea.

    u. index. The amt. of uric acid converted into allantoin.

uricometer (ū-rĭk-ŏm'ĕ-tĕr). Apparatus for quantitative estimation of uric acid in the urine.

uricopoiesis (ū''rĭk-ō-poy-ē'sĭs). The development of uric acid.

uricoxydase (ū''rĭk-oks'ĭ-dās). An enzyme capable of oxidizing uric acid.

uridrosis (ū-rĭd-rō′sĭs). The presence of urea in the sweat.

Evaporation may show white scales, the crystals of urinary solids.

u. crystalli′na. White powder of uric acid deposited on the skin.

uriesthesis (ū-re-ĕs-thē′sĭs). Normal desire to void urine.

urina (ū-rī′nă). Urine.

u. cibi. Urine voided after a full meal.

u. cruenta. Bloody urine.

u. galactodes. Urine of a milky color.

u. hysterica. Watery, pale urine following hysteria.

u. jumentosa. Cloudy urine.

u. potus. Urina voided after drinking.

u. sanguinis. Urina on arising in morning uninfluenced by food or drink.

urinal (ū′rĭn-ăl). 1. A vessel for the urine. 2. A toilet for the male consisting of a vessel attached to a wall.

urinalysis (ū-rĭn-ăl′ĭs-ĭs). Analysis of the urine.

urinary (ū′rĭn-a″rĭ). Pert. to secreting, or containing urine.

u. bladder. Receptacle for urine before it is voided. SEE: *bladder.*

u. calculi. Concretions formed in the urinary passages.

They contain urates, calcium oxalate, calcium carbonate, phosphates, and cystine.

u. casts. Casts of kidney tubules passed in the urine.

u. organs. The structures concerned with the secretion and excretion of urinary products, consisting of the 2 *kidneys,* 2 *ureters,* the *bladder,* and the *urethra.*

u. pigments. Urochrome, urobilin, uroerythrin, and hematoporphyrin.

u. reflex. Desire to void resulting from accumulation of urine in bladder.

u. sediments. Substances found in standing urine, *i. e.,* water, phosphates, uric acid, calcium oxalate, calcium carbonate, calcium phosphate, magnesium and ammonium phosphate; more rarely, crystine, tyrosine, xanthine, hippuric acid, hematoidin.

u. stammering. Temporary interruptions in voiding urine.

u. stuttering. Same as *urinary stammering.* [and urethra.

u. system. Kidneys, ureters, bladder,

urinate (ū′rĭn-āt). To discharge the urine.

urination (ū-rĭn-ā′shŭn). The act of voiding urine.

urine (ū′rĭn). The fluid secreted from the blood by the kidneys, stored in the bladder, and discharged, usually voluntarily, by the urethra.

urinemia (ū-rĭn-ē′mĭ-ă). Contamination of the blood with urinary constituents. SYN: *uremia, q.v.*

uriniferous (ū-rĭn-ĭf′ĕr-ŭs). Carrying urine.

u. tubules. Small tubes of the kidneys for passage of kidney products.

uriniparous (ū-rĭn-ĭp′ăr-ŭs). Producing or secreting urine.

urinogenital (ū″rĭn-ō-jĕn′ĭt-ăl). Pert. to the genital and urinary organs. SYN: *urogenital.*

urinogenous (ū″rĭn-ŏj′ĕn-ŭs). 1. Producing urine. 2. Originating in urine. SYN: *urogenous.*

urinoglucosometer (ū″rĭn-ō-glū″kŏs-ŏm′ĕ-tĕr). Apparatus for estimating amt. of glucose in the urine.

urinology (ū-rĭn-ŏl′ō-jĭ). Scientific study of the urine. SYN: *urology.*

urinoma (ū″rĭn-ō′mă). A cyst containing urine.

urinometer (ū-rĭn-ŏm′ĕt-ĕr). Device for determining urine's specific gravity.

urinometry (ū″rĭn-ŏm′ĕt-rĭ). Determination of specific gravity of the urine.

urinophil (ū′rĭn-ō-fĭl). Capable of existing in the urine.

urinoscopy (ū-rĭn-ŏs′kŏ-pĭ). Examination of the urine.

urinose, urinous (ū′rĭn-ōs, ū′rĭn-ŭs). Having the characteristics of, or containing urine.

urisolvent (ū″rĭ-sŏl′vĕnt). Dissolving uric acid or causing it to be dissolved.

urning (oorn′ĭng). One exhibiting and conscious of sexual inversion. SYN: *homosexual, uranist.* SEE: *urningism.*

urningism, urnism (oorn′ĭng-ĭzm, oorn′ĭzm). Perversion in which sexual desire is only for one of the same sex. SYN: *lesbianism, sapphism, tribadism, amor lesbicus, homosexualism, q.v.*

uro-. Combining form meaning, *pert. to urine.*

uroacidimeter (ū″rō-ăs-ĭ-dĭm′ĕ-tĕr). An apparatus for measuring the degree of acidity of the urine.

Urobacillus (ū″rō-bă-sĭl′ŭs). A rod-shaped organism found in urine of decomposing urine.

urobilin (ū″rō-bī′lĭn). A derivative of the bile pigments of yellow color found in urine.

u. jaundice. Jaundice said to be result of urobilin in the blood.

urobilinemia (ū″rō-bī″lĭn-ē′mĭ-ă). Urobilin in blood.

urobilinicterus (ū″rō-bĭ-lĭn-ĭk′tĕr-ŭs). Jaundice resulting from urobilinemia. SYN: *urobilin-jaundice.*

urobilinogen (ū-rō-bī-lĭn′ō-jĕn). A chromogen in urine which gives rise to urobilin on oxidation.

urobilinogenemia (ū″rō-bī″lĭn-ō-jĕn-ē′mĭ-ă). Urobilinogen in the blood.

urobilinuria (ū″rō-bī″lĭn-ū′rĭ-ă). Excess of urobilin in the urine.

urocele (ū′rō-sēl). Effusion of urine into the scrotum.

urocheras (ū-rŏk′ĕr-ăs). Sand in the urine. SYN: *uropsammus.*

urochesia (ū-rō-kē′zĭ-ă). A discharge of urine through the anus.

urochrome (ū′rō-krōm). A yellow coloring matter in urine, assumed to be closely related to urobilin, which probably gives urine its color.

uroclepsia (ū-rō-klĕp′sĭ-ă). Involuntary and unconscious discharge of urine.

urocrisia (ū″rō-krĭz′ĭ-ă). 1. A diagnosis

by inspection of the urine. 2. Change (generally favorable) which supervenes in the crisis of a disease accompanied by copious urination.

urocrisis (ū-rŏk'rĭs-ĭs). 1. A crisis marked by excessive urination. 2. Examination of the urine. 3. Pain in bladder in locomotor ataxia.

urocriterion (ū″rō-krī-tē′rĭ-ŏn). A symptom observed in the inspection of urine which indicates the diagnosis.

urocyanogen (ū″rō-sī-ăn′ō-jĕn). A blue pigment in urine, esp. in cholera patients.

urocyanosis (ū″rō-sī-ăn-ō′sĭs). Blue discoloration of the urine. SYN: *indicanuria*.

urocyst (ū′rō-sĭst). The urinary bladder.

urocystitis (ū″rō-sĭs-tī′tĭs). Inflammation of the urinary bladder.

urodialysis (ū″rō-dī-ăl′ĭs-ĭs). A partial and temporary suppression of the urine.

    u. neonatorum. Urodialysis when occurring in children.

    u. senum. Urodialysis in the aged.

uroedema (ū″rō-ē-dē′mă). Extravasation of urine distending the tissues. SYN: *uredema*.

uroerythrin (ū-rō-ĕr′ĭth-rĭn). A reddish pigment of urine with acid reaction found in rheumatism and other diseases.

urofuscohematin (ū″rō-fŭs″kō-hĕm′ăt-ĭn). A red-brown pigment in urine in some diseases.

urogaster (ū″rō-găs′tĕr). The urinary intestine or urinary tract of the embryo.

urogenital (ū″rō-jĕn′ĭ-tăl). Pert. to the urinary organs and the genitalia.

    u. ducts. Embryonic ducts of the mesonephron; the wolffian duct and duct of Müller.

    u. sinus. Ant. part of the cloaca into which the urogenital ducts open in the embryo.

urogenous (ū-rŏj′ĕn-ŭs). 1. Producing urine. 2. Originating in urine.

uroglaucin (ū″rō-glaw′sĭn). Indigo blue, a pigment sometimes occurring in the urine, assumed to be result of chromogen oxidation, as in *scarlatina*.

urogram (ū′rō-grăm). An x-ray photograph of any part of the urinary tract.

urography (ū-rŏg′ră-fĭ). Roentgenography of any part of the urinary tract, after introduction of an opaque medium.

urogravimeter (ū″rō-grăv-ĭm′ĕt-ĕr). Apparatus for estimating sp. gr. of urine. SYN: *urinometer.*

urohematin (ū″rō-hĕm′ăt-ĭn). Pigment in urine, considered as identical with hematin,* which alters color of urine in proportion to degree of oxidation.

urohematoporphyrin (ū″rō-hĕm″ăt-ō-por′fĭr-ĭn). Iron-free hematin in urine when hemolysis occurs.

urolith (ū′rō-lĭth). A concretion in the urine.

urolithiasis (ū″rō-lĭth-ī′ăs-ĭs). Formation of urinary calculi. SEE: *calculus, renal.*

urolithology (ū″rō-lĭth-ŏl′ō-jĭ). Science dealing with urinary calculi.

urologic (ū-rō-lŏj′ĭk). Pert. to urology.

urologist (ū-rŏl′ō-jĭst). One who specializes in the practice of urology.

urology (ū-rŏl′ō-jĭ). The science dealing with the urine and diseases of the urinogenital organs.

urolutein (ū″rō-lū′tē-ĭn). A yellow pigment seen in the urine.

uromancy (ū′rō-măn-sĭ). Diagnosis of disease by inspection of urine.

urometer (ū-rŏm′ĕt-ĕr). Instrument for determining specific gravity of urine. SYN: *urinometer.*

uroncus (ū-rŏn′kŭs). A swelling or cyst containing urine.

uronephrosis (ū″rō-nĕf-rō′sĭs). Dilatation of renal structures from obstruction of urinary flow. Distention of renal pelvis and tubules with urine. SYN: *hydronephrosis.*

uronology (ū-rŏn-ŏl′ō-jĭ). The science of urine and genitourinary diseases. SYN: *urology.*

urononcometry (ū″rŏn-ŏn-kŏm′ĕ-trĭ). Measurement of amt. of urine voided in 24 hours.

uronophile (ū-rŏn′ō-fīl). Developing best in a culture containing urine, noting a microörganism.

uropathy (ū-rŏp′ă-thĭ). Any disease affecting the urinary tract.

    u., obstructive. Any disease resulting from obstruction of the urinary tract.

uropenia (ū-rō-pē′nĭ-ă). Lack of urinary secretion.

urophanic (ū-rō-făn′ĭk). Appearing in the urine.

urophein, urophaein (ū″rō-fē′ĭn). Gray pigment in urine said to cause its characteristic odor.

urophosphometer (ū″rō-fŏs-fŏm′ĕ-tĕr). Device for estimating amt. of phosphorus in the urine.

uroplania (ū″rō-plā′nĭ-ă). Condition in which urine is present or discharged from parts other than the urinary organs.

uropoiesis (ū″rō-poy-ē′sĭs). Secretion of urine by the kidneys.

uropoietic (ū″rō-poy-ĕt-ĭk). Concerned in the formation of urine, or uropoiesis.

uropsammus (ū″rō-săm′ŭs). Gravel in urine.

uroptysis (ū-rŏp′tĭs-ĭs). Urination through the mouth.

uropyonephrosis (ū″rō-pī-ō-nĕf-rō′sĭs). Urine and pus in the renal pelvis.

uropyoureter (ū″rō-pī″ō-ū-rē′tĕr). Mass of urine and pus in the ureter.

urorosein (ū″rō-rō′zē-ĭn). A rose-colored pigment in urine, which is increased in certain diseases. SYN: *urorrhodin.*

urorrhagia (ū-ror-ā′jĭ-ă). Excessive secretion of urine. SYN: *polyuria.*

urorrhea (ū-ror-ē′ă). Involuntary flow of urine. SYN: *enuresis.*

urorrhodin (ū-rō-rō′dĭn). A rose-colored pigment in the urine. SYN: *urorosein, q.v.*

urorrhodinogen (ū-rō-rō-dĭn′ō-jĕn). A chromogen of the urine which, when decomposed, forms urorrhodin.

urorubin (ū-rō-rū′bĭn). A red pigment ob

tained from urine, by treatment with hydrochloric acid.

urorubrohematin (ū″rō-rū″brō-hĕm′ă-tĭn). A reddish pigment occasionally found in the urine in some chronic diseases.

urosaccharometry (ū″rō-săk-ăr-ŏm′ĕ-trĭ). Determination of amt. of sugar in the urine.

urosacin (ū-rō′sa-sĭn). A red pigment in the urine. SYN: *urorrhodin.*

uroscheocele (ū-rŏs′kē-ō-sēl). Swelling of scrotum from extravasation of urine into scrotal sac. SYN: *urocele.*

uroschesis (ū-rŏs′kĕs-ĭs). 1. Suppression of urine. 2. Retention of the urine.

uroscopy (ū-rŏs′kō-pĭ). 1. Examination of the urine. 2. Diagnosis by examination of the urine.

uroselectan (ū″rō-sĕ-lĕk′tăn). A pyridine derivative for intravenous pyelography.

urosemiology (ū″rō-sē-mĭ-ŏl′ō-jĭ). Examination of the urine as an aid to diagnosis.

urosepsin (ū-rō-sĕp′sĭn). A septic poison formed from decomposition of urine in the tissues.

urosepsis (ū-rō-sĕp′sĭs). Septic poisoning due to retention and absorption of urinary products in the tissues.

urosin (ū′rō-sĭn). A proprietary uric acid solvent.

urosis (ū-rō′sĭs). Any disease of the urinary organs.

urospectrin (ū-rō-spĕk′trĭn). A pigment derived from normal urine when shaken with acetic ether.

urostealith (ū″rō-stē′ă-lĭth). A fatty substance in some urinary calculi.

urotherapy (ū″rō-ther′ă-pĭ). Therapeutic subcutaneous injection of the patient's urine.

urotoxia (ū-rō-tŏks′ĭ-ă). 1. Urinary systemic poisoning. 2. Toxicity of the urine. 3. The toxic unit of urine which is amt. needed to kill 1 kilogram of living matter. SYN: *urotoxy.*

urotoxic (ū″rō-tŏks′ĭk). Pert. to poisonous substances in the urine or poisoning by urine.

u. coefficient. Number of urotoxias (in 24 hr.) formed by a person, about 0.4 for each kilogram of body weight.

urotoxicity (ū″rō-tŏks-ĭs′ĭ-tĭ). The toxic character of the urine.

urotoxin (ū″rō-tŏks′ĭn). The toxic principle of the urine.

urotoxy (ū′rō-tŏks″ĭ). Amount of urine required to kill an animal weighing 1 kilogram; unit of toxicity of urine. SYN: *urotoxia.*

urotropin (ū-rŏt′rō-pĭn). A proprietary uric acid solvent.

DOSAGE: 5 gr. (0.3 Gm.).

uroureter (ū″rō-ū-rē-tĕr, -ū-rē′tĕr). Distention of the ureter with urine, due to stricture or obstruction. SYN: *hydroureter.*

urous (ū′rŭs). Having the nature of urine.

uroxanthin (ū″rō-zăn′thĭn). Yellow coloring matter of the urine; an indigo-forming substance. [loxan.*

uroxin (ū-rŏk′sĭn). A derivative of al-

urticaria (ŭr-tĭ-kā′rĭ-ă). An inflammatory affection, characterized by the eruption of pale, evanescent wheals, which are associated with severe itching. SYN: *hives, nettle rash.* SEE: *allergy.*

u. bullo′sa. Eruption of temporary vesicles with infusion of fluid under the epidermis.

u. confer′ta. Urticaria with lesions in groups.

u. endem′ica, u. epidem′ica. Urticaria caused by caterpillar hairs.

u. facti′tia. Wheals following slight irritation of the skin. SYN: *autographism.*

u. gigan′tea. Urticaria with very large wheals. SYN: *angioneurotic edema.*

u. haemorrhagica. Urticaria with lesions infiltrated with blood.

u. maculo′sa. A chronic form of urticaria with red-colored lesions.

u. mariti′ma. Urticaria due to salt water bathing.

u. medicamento′sa. Urticaria due to certain drugs.

u. papulosa. In this form the wheal is followed by a lingering papule which is attended by considerable itching. Most commonly observed in debilitated children. [wheals remain.

u. per′stans. Urticaria in which

u. pigmentosa. An eruption of wheals which are itchy and persistent and which leave behind a yellowish or brownish pigmentation. Observed in young children. Runs a chronic course of months or years.

u. subcuta′nea. Urticaria without wheals but persistent itching.

u. vesiculo′sa. Same as *urticaria bullosa.*

urticarial, urticarious (ŭr-tĭk-ā-rĭ-ăl, ŭr-tĭk-ā′rĭ-ŭs). Pert. to urticaria.

urtication (ŭr-tĭk-ā′shŭn). 1. Flogging of a part with nettles to induce counter-irritation. 2. Burning or itching sensation. 3. Eruption of itching wheals. SYN: *urticaria.*

U. S. P., U. S. Phar. Abbr. for *United States Pharmacopeia.*

U. S. P. H. S. Abbr. for *United States Public Health Service.*

ustilaginism (ŭs-tĭl-ăj′ĭn-ĭzm). Poisoning caused by Ustilago, a moldlike fungus.

ustion (ŭs′chŭn). 1. Cauterization with actual cautery. 2. Incineration.

ustulation (ŭs-tū-lā′shŭn). Roasting, parching, or drying of a moist substance.

ustus (ŭs′tŭs). Burned. SEE: *calcination.*

uteralgia (ū-tĕr-ăl′jĭ-ă). Uterine pain.

uterectomy (ū-tĕr-ĕk′tō-mĭ). Removal of uterus through the abdomen or vagina. SYN: *hysterectomy, q.v.*

uterine (ū′tĕr-ĭn, -ĭn). Pert. to the uterus.

u. cake. The placenta.

u. glands. The tubular glands in the endometrium.

u. milk. A milky, white substance bet. the gravid uterus and the placental villi.

u. souffle (soof'fl). Vascular sound in the pregnant uterus heard with stethoscope.

u. tubes. Small tubes attached to either side of the uterus, and leading from the region of the ovary. SYN: *fallopian tubes.*

uteritis (ū-tĕr-ī'tĭs). Inflammation of the uterus.

uteroabdominal (ū″tĕr-ō-ăb-dŏm'ĭn-ăl). Pert. to both the uterus and abdomen.

uterocele (ū-tĕr'ō-sēl). Hernia containing the uterus.

uterocervical (ū″tĕr-ō-sĕr'vĭ-kăl). Relating to the uterus and the cervix.

uterocystostomy (ū″tĕr-ō-sĭs-tŏs'tō-mĭ). Formation of a passage bet. the uterine cervix and the bladder.

uterofixation (ū″tĕr-ō-fĭks-ā'shŭn). Fixation of a displaced uterus. SYN: *hysteropexy.*

uterogenic (ū″tĕr-ō-jĕn'ĭk). Developed in the uterus.

uterogestation (ū-tĕr-ō-jĕs-tā'shŭn). Pregnancy in the uterus, normal pregnancy.

uterography (ū″tĕr-ŏg'ră-fĭ). Roentgenography of the uterus.

uterolith (ū'tĕr-ō-lĭth). A uterine concretion.

uterologist (ū″tĕr-ŏl'ō-jĭst). One who specializes in the practice of gynecology and obstetrics.

uterology (ū-tĕr-ŏl'ō-jĭ). Gynecology combined with obstetrics.

uteromania (ū″tĕr-ō-mā'nĭ-ă). Pathological sexual desire in a woman. SYN: *nymphomania.*

uterometer (ū″tĕr-ŏm'ĕt-ĕr). Device for measuring the uterus and for determining its position.

uteroövarian (ū″tĕr-ō-ō-vā'rĭ-ăn). Relating to the uterus and ovary.

uteropexia, uteropexy (ū″tĕr-ō-pĕks'ĭ-ă, ū'tĕr-ō-pĕks-ĭ). Fixation of the uterus to the abdominal wall. SYN: *hysteropexy.*

uteroplacental (ū″tĕr-ō-plă-sen'tăl). Relating to the placenta and uterus.

uteroplasty (ū″tĕr-ō-plăs'tĭ). Reparative operation upon the uterus.

uterosacral (ū″tĕr-ō-sā'krăl). Relating to the uterus and sacrum.

uterosalpingography (ū″tĕr-ō-săl-pĭng-ŏg'ră-fĭ). Visualization of the interior of the uterus and fallopian tubes by x-ray.

uterosclerosis (ū″tĕr-ō-sklē-rō'sĭs). Uterine sclerosis.

uteroscope (ū'tĕr-ō-skōp). Device for viewing the uterine cavity.

uterotome (ū'tĕr-ō-tōm). An instrument used for uterotomy. SYN: *hysterotome.*

uterotomy (ū-tĕr-ŏt'ō-mĭ). Incisions of the uterus.

uterotonic (ū″tĕr-ō-tŏn'ĭk). Giving muscular tone to the uterus.

uterotractor (ū″tĕr-ō-trăk'tor). An instrument for making traction on the cervix uteri.

uterotubal (ū″tĕr-ō-tū'băl). Relating to the uterus and the oviducts.

uterovaginal (ū″tĕr-ō-văj'ĭ-năl). Relating to the uterus and vagina.

uterovesical (ū″tĕr-ō-vĕs'ĭ-kăl). Relating to the uterus and bladder.

uterus (ū'tĕr-ŭs). The organ of gestation. SYN: *womb.*
  ANAT: A muscular, hollow, pear-shaped structure of the female. It is partly covered by peritoneum, the cavity lined by mucous membrane which is the *endometrium.*

u. acollis. Uterus without a cervix.

u. arcuatus. Uterus with a depressed arched fundus.

u. bicornis. Uterus in which the fundus is divided into 2 parts.

u. biforis. Uterus in which the ext. os is divided into 2 parts by a septum.

u. bilocularis. Uterus in which the cavity is divided into 2 parts by partition.

u. cordiformis. A heart-shaped uterus.

u. didelphys. Double uterus.

u. gravid. Pregnant uterus.

u. septus. SEE: *uterus bilocularis.*

u. unicornis. Uterus that is only one-half developed and has only 1 horn.

utricle (ū'trĭk-l). One of 2 sacs of the membranous labyrinth in the bony vestibule of the inner ear.

u. of the urethra. The prostatic vesicle of the male.

u. of vestibule. Vestibular cavity connecting with the semicircular canals.

utricular (ū-trĭk'ū-lar). 1. Pert. to the utricle. 2. Uterine; pert. to the uterus. 3. Like a bladder.

utriculitis (ū-trĭk-ū-lī'tĭs). Inflammation of the internal ear, or of the utriculus prostaticus.

utriculoplasty (ū-trĭk'ū-lō-plăs'tĭ). Reduction of the uterus by excision of a longitudinal, wedge-shaped section.

utriculosaccular (ū-trĭk″ū-lō-săk'ū-lar). Pert. to the utricle and saccule of the labyrinth.

u. duct. A duct uniting the utricle and saccule.

utriculus (ū-trĭk'ū-lŭs). 1. The larger membranous sac in the vestibule of the labyrinth (in the *recessus ellipticus*), from which the semicircular duct arises. 2. Same as *utriculus prostaticus.* SYN: *utricle.*

u. masculi'nus, u. prostat'icus. BNA. Very small pouch in the prostate gland opening into the urethra, the analogue of the vagina and uterus.

utriform (ū'trĭ-form). Having a shape like a leather bottle.

uvea (ū've-ă). The 2nd or vascular coat of the eye lying immediately beneath the sclera.

uveal (ū've-ăl). Pert. to the middle coat of the eye, or uvea.

u. tract. Pigmented layer of the eye. SYN: *uvea.*

uveitic (ū-ve-ĭt'ĭk). Marked by or pert. to uveitis.

uveitis (ū-ve-ī'tĭs). Inflammation of the iris, ciliary body, and choroid, the entire uveal tract.

uveoplasty (ū've-ō-plăs'tĭ). Reparative operation on the uvea.

uveoparotitis (ū″vē-ō-păr-ō-tī′tĭs). Parotitis with uveitis.

uviarc (ū′vĭ-ark). Trade name of a mercury quartz lamp, *q.v.*

uviform (ū′vĭ-form). Shaped like or resembling a bunch of grapes, or a grape.

uviofast (ū′vĭ-ō-făst). Unaffected by ultraviolet radiation.

uviol (ū′vĭ-ŏl). Glass which is unusually transparent to ultraviolet rays.
 u. lamp. Electric light with uviol glass globe.

uviolize (ū′vē-ō-līz). To use ultraviolet rays therapeutically.

uvioresistant (ū″vĭ-ō-rē-zĭs′tănt). Resistant to effects of ultraviolet rays. SYN: *uviofast.*

uviosensitive (ū″vĭ-ō-sĕn′sĭ-tĭv). Sensitive to effects of ultraviolet rays.

uvula (ū′vū-lă). 1. Tiny projection on inf. vermiform cerebellar process bet. the amygdalae. 2. Small, soft structure hanging from free edge of soft palate in midline above the root of the tongue. It is composed of muscle, connective tissue and mucous membrane.

 u. of cerebellum. Projection on inf. vermiform process of cerebellum in front of pyramid and bet. the amygdalae.

 u. vesicae. BNA. Post. portion of *caput galli* projecting into the prostatic urethra, or into the bladder in old men, marking the prostatic middle lobe.

uvulaptosis (ū″vū-lăp-tō′sĭs). A relaxed condition of the uvula. SYN: *uvuloptosis.*

uvular (ū′vū-lar). Pert. to the uvula.

uvularis (ū-vū-lā′rĭs). The azygos uvulae muscle.

uvulatome (ū′vū-lă-tōm). Instrument for removal of uvula.

uvulatomy (ū-vū-lăt′ō-mĭ). Excision of the uvula.

uvulitis (ū″vū-lī′tĭs). Inflammation of the uvula.

uvuloptosis (ū-vū-lŏp-tō′sĭs). Relaxed condition of the uvula.

uvulotome (ū′vū-lo-tōm). Instrument for performing uvulotomy. SYN: *uvulatome.*

uvulotomy (ū-vū-lŏt′ō-mĭ). Amputation of the uvula.

V

V. Abbr. of *vision, visual acuity, Vibrio*, and for *volt*. SYMB. for *vanadium*.

vaccigenous (văk-sĭj'ĕn-ŭs). Producing vaccine. SYN: *vaccinogenous*.

vaccin (văk'sĭn). Any substance for inoculation against disease. SYN: *vaccine*.

vaccina (văk-sī'nă). A disease resulting from inoculation with cowpox virus.

vaccinal (văk'sĭn-ăl). Relating to vaccine or to vaccination.

v. fever. A mild fever that may follow vaccination.

vaccinate (văk'sĭn-āt). 1. To inoculate with cowpox vaccine to prevent or mitigate an attack of smallpox. 2. To inoculate with any vaccine to produce immunity against disease.

vaccination (văk-sĭn-ā'shŭn). 1. Inoculation against smallpox. 2. Inoculation with bacterial vaccine as a preventive measure.

v., arm-to-arm. Vaccination in which virus is taken from arm of one person and injected into arm of another.

v., bovine. Vaccination with vaccine lymph of a calf.

v. rash. One sometimes following vaccination.

vaccinationist (văk"sĭn-ā'shŭn-ĭst). One who upholds the efficacy of vaccination.

vaccinator (văk'sĭn-ā"tor). 1. One who vaccinates. 2. An instrument for vaccinating.

vaccine (văk'sēn). 1. Pert. to vaccine or vaccination. 2. Substance containing virus of cowpox in a form for vaccination against smallpox. 3. Any substance for preventive inoculation, esp. a bacterial preparation. SEE: *bacterine*.

v., aqueous. Vaccine employing physiological salt solution as the vehicle.

v., autogenous. Bacterial vaccine taken from the individual to be inoculated.

v., bacterial. Preparation of bacteria in saline solution or in oil injected into the body to induce immunity to same species of bacteria or their toxins.

v., BCG (Calmette - Guérin bacillus). Substance used in prophylactic vaccination of infants against tuberculosis with virulence reduced by repeated cultures on glycerinated ox bile.

v., corresponding. SEE: *stock vaccine*.

v., humanized. Vaccine obtained from vaccinia vesicles in human beings.

v., oil. Vaccine prepared with oil as the vehicle. SEE: *aqueous vaccine*.

v. point. A bone or quill coated with vaccine lymph at its tip.

v., polyvalent. Vaccine made from several strains of the same species of bacterium.

v. rash. One due to vaccination.

v., sensitized. Vaccine made more active by treatment of the bacteria with their specific immune serum. SYN: *serobacterin*.

v., stock. Bacterial vaccine made from same species as that causing the infection, but not autogenous.

v. therapy. Treatment of a disease by inoculation with a vaccine specific for that disease.

v. virus. An emulsion containing substance from pustules of vaccinia used for inoculation.

vaccinella (văk-sĭn-ĕl'ă). A secondary eruption sometimes following vaccination, but not conferring immunity.

vaccinia (văk-sĭn'ĭ-ă). A contagious disease resulting from inoculation with cowpox virus.

vacciniform (văk-sĭn'ĭ-form). Of the nature of vaccinia or cowpox.

vaccinin (văk'sĭn-ĭn). The inoculable element by which cowpox is transmitted.

vacciniola (văk-sĭn-ĭ-ō'lă). Secondary general eruption after local eruption from vaccine.

vaccinization (văk"sĭn-ĭ-zā'shŭn). Vaccination by repeated inoculations until the virus has no effect.

vaccinogenous (văk"sĭn-ŏj'ĕn-ŭs). Producing vaccine or pert. to its production.

vaccinosyphilis (văk"sĭn-ō-sĭf'ĭl-ĭs). Syphilis following inoculation conveyed by impure vaccine or a contaminated instrument.

vaccinotherapeutics, vaccinotherapy (văk"-sĭn-ō-thĕr-ă-pū'tĭks, -thĕr'ă-pĭ). Treatment by injection of bacterial vaccines.

vacuolation (văk-ū-ō-lā'shŭn). Formation of vacuoles.

vacuole (văk'ū-ōl). 1. A clear space in cell protoplasm filled with fluid or air. 2. A very small space in any tissue; source of a lymphatic vessel. SEE: *cytoplasm*.

vacuolization (văk"ū-ō-lĭz-ā'shŭn). The formation of vacuoles. SYN: *vacuolation*.

vacuum (văk'ū-ŭm). A space exhausted of its air content.

v. treatment. Insertion of a limb in a partial vacuum.

v. tube. A vessel of insulating material (usually glass) provided with metal electrodes, which has been so highly evacuated that the residual gas does not affect the current passing bet. metal electrodes projecting from the outside.

vag'abond's disease. Discoloration of skin caused by exposure and scratching due to presence of lice.

vagal (vā'găl). Pert. to the vagus nerve.

v. attack. A condition of dyspnea, cardiac distress, a fear of impending death, and a sinking sensation assumed to be the result of vasomotor spasm.

v. nervous system. The autonomic* nervous system, which controls the viscera, ductless glands, blood vessels, and organs containing involuntary muscle.

vagina (vă-jī'nă) (pl. *vaginae, vaginas*). 1. A sheathlike part. 2. A musculomembranous tube which forms passageway bet. uterus and external orifice.

v., bulb of. Small erectile body on each side of the vaginal vestibule. SYN: *bulbi vestibuli.*

v. cordis. Sac investing the heart. SYN: *pericardium.*

v. femoris. Fascia lata of the thigh.

v. oculi. Sheath investing the eyeball forming its socket. SYN: *Tenon's capsule.*

vaginal (văj'ĭn-ăl). Pert. to the vagina or to any enveloping sheath.

v. hysterectomy. Excision of uterus. through vagina.

vaginalectomy (văj'ĭn-ăl-ĕk'tō-mĭ). Excision of the tunica vaginalis. SYN: *vaginectomy.*

vaginalitis (văj-ĭn-ăl-ī'tĭs). Inflammation of *tunica vaginalis testis.*

vaginate (văj'ĭn-āt). Sheathed.

vaginectomy (văj-ĭn-ĕk'tō-mĭ). Resection of tunica vaginalis.

vaginicoline (văj-ĭn-ĭk'ō-līn). Living in the vagina, as microörganisms.

vaginismus (văj-ĭn-ĭz'mŭs). Painful spasm of vagina from contraction of the vaginal walls preventing coitus.

v., mental. Vaginismus resulting from repugnance to cohabitation.

v., posterior. Vaginismus due to contraction of the levator ani muscle.

vaginitis (văj-ĭn-ī'tĭs). 1. Inflammation of a sheath. 2. Inflammation of vagina.

v. adhaesiva. Inflammation with mucous membrane exfoliation causing adhesions and partial obliteration of the vaginal lumen.

v., diphtheritic. Vaginitis with membranous exudate.

v., emphysematous. Vaginitis with gas in connective tissues.

v., glandular. Vaginitis when the follicles alone seem affected, when mucous membrane shows no traces of change and when secretion appears more copious and of a yellowish-white or grayish color.

v., granular. Vaginitis with infiltrated cells and enlarged papillae. The most common form of vaginitis.

v., papulous. Vagina and neck of womb covered with papulae or follicles more or less developed or resembling fleshy granulations.

v., pustulous. May result from appearance of pustules in persons affected with pustulous affections of the skin.

v. senilis. Same as *vaginitis adhaesiva, q.v.*

v. testis. Inflammation of the tunica vaginalis of the testis.

v., trichomonas. Vaginitis due to infection with Trichomonas.

v., vesicular. Vaginitis from extension of eczema from vulva to the vagina.

vaginoabdominal (văj'ĭn-ō-ăb-dŏm'ĭn-ăl). Relating to the vagina and abdomen.

vaginocele (văj'ĭn-ō-sēl). Vaginal hernia. SYN: *colpocele.*

vaginodynia (văj'ĭn-ō-dĭn'ĭ-ă). Pain in the vagina.

vaginofixation (văj'ĭn-ō-fĭks-ā'shŭn). 1. Process of rendering the vagina immovable. 2. Attachment of uterus to vaginal peritoneum.

vaginogenic (văj'ĭn-ō-jĕn'ĭk). Developed in the vagina.

vaginography (văj'ĭn-ŏg'ră-fĭ). The taking of x-ray pictures of the vagina.

vaginolabial (văj'ĭn-ō-lā'bĭ-ăl). Relating to the vagina and the labia. SYN: *vaginolulvar, vulvovaginal.*

vaginometer (văj-ĭn-ŏm'ĕ-tĕr). Device for measuring the length and expansion of the vagina.

vaginomycosis (văj'ĭn-ō-mĭ-kō'sĭs). A fungous infection (mycosis) of the vagina.

vaginoperineal (văj'ĭn-ō-pĕr-ĭ-nē'ăl). Relating to the vagina and perineum.

vaginoperineorrhaphy (văj'ĭn-ō-pĕr-ĭ-nē-or'ăf-ĭ). Repair of a perineal laceration in the vagina. SYN: *colpoperineorrhaphy.*

vaginoperineotomy (văj'ĭn-ō-pĕr-ĭn-ē-ŏt'-ō-mĭ). Separation of the vagina and perineum.

vaginoperitoneal (văj'ĭn-ō-pĕr-ĭ-tō-nē'ăl). Relating to the vagina and peritoneum.

vaginopexy (vă-jĭ'nō-pĕk"sĭ). Fixation of the vagina. SYN: *colpopexy.*

vaginoplasty (vă-jĭ'nō-plăs"tĭ). Reparative surgery on the vagina.

vaginoscope (văj'ĭn-ō-skōp). Instrument for inspection of the vagina.

vaginoscopy (văj-ĭn-ŏs'kō-pĭ). Visual examination of the vagina.

vaginotome (văj-ĭ'nō-tōm). An instrument for making an incision in the vaginal walls.

vaginotomy (văj-ĭn-ŏt'ō-mĭ). Incision of vagina.

vaginovesical (văj'ĭn-ō-vĕs'ĭk-ăl). Relating to the vagina and the bladder. SYN: *vesicovaginal.*

vaginovulvar (văj'ĭn-ō-vŭl'var). Pert. to the vulva and vagina.

vagitis (văj-ī'tĭs). Inflammation of the vagus, the 10th cranial nerve.

vagitus (vă-jī'tŭs). First cry of newly-born infant.

v. uterinus. Crying of the fetus before birth when membrane has been ruptured permitting passage of air into the uterus.

v. vaginalis. Cry of a child or infant with head still in the vagina.

vagogram (vă'gō-grăm). Tracing of variations of the vagus nerve made by an electrical device.

vagolysis (vă-gŏl'ĭ-sĭs). Process of loosening the esophageal branches of the vagus nerve for relief of cardiospasm.

vagomimetic (vă"gō-mĭm-ĕt'ĭk). Resembling action of stimulated vagus nerve.

vagosympathetic (vă″gō-sĭm-pă-thĕt′ĭk). The cervical sympathetic and the vagus nerves considered together.

vagotomy (vă-gŏt′ō-mĭ). Section of the vagus nerve.

vagotonia (vă-gō-tō′nĭ-ă). Hyperirritability of vagus nerve resulting in a condition marked by spastic tendency in smooth muscles, fatigue, nervousness, and vasomotor instability.

vagotonic (vă′gō-tŏn′ĭk). Pertaining to vagotonia.

v. type. Type characterized by deficient suprarenal activity.

vagotropic (vă″gō-trŏp′ĭk). Acting upon the vagus nerve.

vagotropism (vă-gŏt′rō-pĭzm). Affinity for the vagus nerve, as a drug.

vagrant (vă′grănt). 1. Wandering from place to place, as the leukocytes. 2. A vagabond.

v's. disease. Cutaneous discoloration and irritation caused by filth and body lice. SYN: vagabond's disease.

vagus (vă′gŭs) (pl. vagi). The pneumogastric or 10th cranial nerve.

v. pneumonia. Pneumonia caused by trauma of the pneumogastric nerve.

v. pulse. A slow pulse caused by the slowing action of the heart due to inhibition of the vagus nerve. SEE: vagotomy, vagotonia.

valence, valency (vă′lĕns, -lĕn-sĭ). 1. Property of an element or radical combining with or replacing other elements or radicals in definite proportion. 2. Degree of the combining power or replacing power of an element or radical, the hydrogen atom being unit of comparison.

SEE: artiad, atomicity.

valetudinarian (văl-e-tū-dĭn-ă′rĭ-ăn). 1. Sickly; ailing. 2. One subject to frequent illness, or feebleness. SYN: invalid.

valgus (văl′gŭs). 1. Clubfoot in which the foot is bent outward. 2. Bowlegged or knock-kneed. 3. One with knock-knees or bowlegs. SYN: talipes* valgus.

valine (văl′ēn, vă′lēn). An amino acid derived from protein decomposition. $C_5H_{11}NO_2$.

vallate (văl′āt). Having a rim around a depression.   [crevice.

vallecula (văl-lĕk′ŭ-lă). A depression or

v. cerebel′li. BNA. A deep fissure on inf. surface of the cerebellum.

v. ova′ta. A depression in the liver in which rests the gallbladder.

v. syl′vii. A depression marking beginning of the fissure of Sylvius.

v. un′guis. Fold of skin in which the proximal and lateral edges of the nails are imbedded.

Vallet's mass (văl-ā′). Mass of ferrous carbonate, containing 36% ferrous carbonate.

DOSAGE: 3-5 gr. (0.2-0.3 Gm.).

valley of the cerebellum (văl′ē). Hollow on inf. surface of cerebellum. SYN: vallecula cerebelli.

vallum unguis (văl′um ŭng′gwĭs). BNA. Fold of skin overlapping the nail.

Valsalva's sinuses (văl-săl′vă). Pouches of the aortic and pulmonary arteries behind the flaps of the semilunar valves.

valvate (văl′vāt). Pert. to or provided with valves. SYN: valvular.

valvotomy (văl-vŏt′ō-mĭ). Surgical cutting of a valve, esp. one of the rectum.

valve (vălv). Any one of various structures for temporarily closing an orifice or passage, or for allowing movement of fluid in 1 direction only.

v., aortic. The semilunar valve preventing regurgitation at the entrance of the aorta to the heart, composed of 3 segments.

v., bicuspid. Valve closing orifice bet. left cardiac auricle and ventricle.

v., ileocecal. Valve bet. ileum and large intestine to prevent regurgitation of intestinal contents; composed of 2 membranous folds.

v., mitral. Cardiac valve bet. the left auricle and ventricle. SYN: bicuspid valve.

v., pulmonary. Valve composed of 3 cusps separating pulmonary artery and right ventricle.

v., pyloric. Prominent circular membranous fold at pyloric orifice of the stomach.

v., semilunar. Valve bet. heart and the aorta and valve bet. the heart and the pulmonary artery.

v., tricuspid. Valve bet. the right cardiac auricle and ventricle.

v. tube. An electric valve consisting of a vacuum tube having for 1 electrode a hot filament.

v. of Varolius. SEE: ileocecal valve.

valvula (văl′vū-lă). A valve, specifically a small valve.

v. bicuspidalis. BNA. Valve bet. left cardiac auricle and ventricle.

v. coli. BNA. Valve bet. ileum and large intestine.

v. pylori. BNA. Prominent mucosal fold at pyloric entrance of the stomach.

v. semilunaris. BNA. Valve separating heart and aorta and heart and pulmonary artery.

v. tricuspidalis. BNA. Valve bet. the right auricle and ventricle of the heart.

valculae conniventes (văl′vū-lē kon-nĭ-vĕn′tēs). Circular membranous folds projecting into lumen of small intestine; they do not disappear on distention of bowel, and act by retarding passage of the food along the bowel; they also provide a greater absorbing area. SYN: plicae circulares.

valvular (văl′vū-lar). Relating to or having a valve. SYN: valvate.

valvulitis (văl-vū-lī′tĭs). Inflammation of a valve, especially a cardiac valve. SYN: dicliditis.

valvulotome (văl′vū-lō-tōm). An instrument for incising a valve.

valvulotomy (văl-vū-lŏt′ō-mĭ). Process of cutting through a valve, as a too rigid rectal fold. SYN: valvotomy.

vanadium (văn-ā′dĭ-ŭm). A light gray metallic element. SYMB: V. At. wt. 50.95.

van Buren's disease (văn bū'rĕn). Induration of the corpora cavernosa.

van den Bergh's test. A direct or indirect test to detect the presence of bilirubin in blood serum in assumed cases of obstructive jaundice or impaired liver functioning.

vanillism (văn-ĭl'lĭzm). Irritation of the skin, mucous membranes and conjunctiva sometimes experienced by workers handling vanilla.

van Swieten's solution (văn swē'ten). Mercuric chloride 1, alcohol 100, distilled water 900.

vapor (vā'por). 1. Gaseous state of any substance. 2. Medicinal substance for administration in form of inhaled vapor.

    v. bath. Exposure of body to hot vapor.   [vapor baths.

    v. cabinet. Cabinet in which to give

    v. douche. Treatment with a jet of hot vapor.

    SEE: *halitus, nebulization.*

vaporium (vā-pō'rĭ-ŭm). Apparatus for applying hot or cold or medicated vapors.

vaporization (vā"por-ĭ-zā'shŭn). 1. The conversion of a liquid or solid into vapor. 2. Therapeutic use of a vapor.

vaporizer (vā'por-ĭz-ĕr). Device for converting liquids into a vapor spray.

vaporole (vā'pō-rōl). 1. An ampule or capsule of glass containing a single dose of a volatile drug for inhalation. 2. Trade name of a glass ampule.

vaporous (vā'por-ŭs). Consisting of, pert. to, or producing vapors.

Vaquez's disease (vă-kā'). Continuous excessive erythrocyte formation by the diseased bone marrow with enlargement of the spleen.

varicella (var-ĭ-sel'ă). An acute, highly contagious disease characterized by an eruption that makes its appearance in crops and passes through successive stages of macules, papules, vesicles, and crusts. SYN: *chickenpox.*

varices (var'ĭs-ēz) (Sing. *varix*). Enlarged twisted veins.

variciform (văr-ĭs'ĭ-form). Resembling a varix. SYN: *varicose.*

varicoblepharon (văr-ĭ-kō-blĕf'ă-ron). Varicose tumor of the eyelid.

varicocele (văr'ĭ-kō-sēl). Enlargement of the veins of the spermatic cord (spermatic plexus), occurring in adolescents and young men, most commonly on the left side. SYN: *cirsocele.*

varicocelectomy (văr-ĭ-kō-sē-lĕk'tō-mĭ). Excision of portion of scrotal sac with ligation of the dilated veins to relieve varicocele.

varicography (văr-ĭ-kŏg'ră-fĭ). X-ray photography of varicose veins.

varicomphalus (văr-ĭk-ŏm'făl-ŭs). Varicose tumor of the navel.

varicophlebitis (văr"ĭ-kō-flē-bī'tĭs). Phlebitis combined with varicose veins.

varicose (văr'ĭ-kōs). Pert. to varices; distended, swollen, noting veins.

    v. veins. Enlarged twisted veins most commonly found on leg and thigh.

varicosity (văr-ĭ-kŏs'ĭ-tĭ). 1. Condition of being varicose. 2. A swollen, twisted vein. SYN: *varix.*

varicotomy (văr-ĭ-kŏt'ō-mĭ). Excision of a varicose vein.

varicula (văr-ĭk'ū-lă). A small varix, esp. a varicose dilation of the veins of mucous membrane covering ant. surface of the eye.

varietism (vă-rī'ĕt-ĭzm). Plural love relations; generally on the part of the male. SEE: *polyandry.*

variola (vă-rī'ō-lă). An acute contagious disease characterized by a prodromal stage during which the constitutional symptoms are usually severe, and followed by an eruption which passes through the successive stages of macules, papules, vesicles, pustules, and crusts. SYN: *smallpox.*

    v., black. Same as *hemorrhagic variola.*

    v., coherent. Variola in which pustules are not confluent,* but coalesce at edges.

    v., confluent. Variola in which pustules run together. In confluent smallpox, the onset may be no different than in the discrete variety.

    v., discrete. Variola when pustules are distinct.

    v., hemorrhagic. Variola with hemorrhage into the vesicles.

    v., malignant. A fatal form of hemorrhagic variola, *q.v.*

    v., modified. Type of the disease commonly called varioloid. Case of modified smallpox seen in patients who have been vaccinated some years previously, but have not retained a complete immunity to the disease.

variolate (văr'ĭ-ō-lāt). 1. To vaccinate with smallpox virus. 2. Having lesions like those of smallpox.

variolation, variolization (văr-ĭ-ō-lā'shŭn, văr-ĭ-ō-lĭ-zā'shŭn). Inoculation with smallpox.

varioloid (văr'ĭ-ō-loyd). 1. Resembling smallpox. 2. Pert. to varioloid. 3. A mild but contagious type of smallpox in those who have had smallpox or have been vaccinated.

variolous (văr-ĭ'ō-lŭs). Relating to smallpox.

varix (vă'rĭks). 1. A tortuous dilatation of a vein. 2. Less commonly, dilatation of an artery or lymph vessel.

    v., aneurysmal. A direct communication bet. an artery and a varicose vein without an intervening sac.

    v. lymphaticus. Dilatation of lymphatic vessel.

    v., turbinal. Permanent dilatation of veins of turbinate bodies.

varolian (vă-rō'lĭ-ăn). Relating to the pons Varolii.

    v. bend. Ant. extension of hindgut on its ventral surface in the fetus.

varus (vă'rŭs). 1. Turned inward; bow-legged. 2. A condition in which a club-footed person walks on outer border of the foot. SYN: *talipes varus.* 3. Any eruption of papules on the face. SYN: *acne*.

v. com'edo. A blackhead.

vas (văs) (pl. *vasa*). A vessel or duct.

v. aberrans. 1. A narrow tube varying in length from 1½ to 14 inches, occasionally found connected with the lower part of the canal of the epididymis or with the commencement of the vas deferens. 2. Vestige of the biliary ducts sometimes found in the liver.

v. capillare. BNA. A capillary blood vessel.

v. deferens. The excretory duct of the testis, the continuation of the epididymis, terminating at *ductus ejaculatorius* at prostatic urethra. SYN: *ductus deferens*.

v. lymphaticum. BNA. One of the vessels carrying the lymph.

v. prominens. BNA. Blood vessel on the cochlea's accessory spiral ligament.

v. spirale. A large blood vessel beneath the tunnel of corti in the basilar membrane.

vasa (vā'să) (sing. *vas*).

v. afferen'tia. 1. Arteries carrying blood to a structure. 2. The lymphatic vessels entering a gland.

v. bre'via. Branches of the splenic artery going to greater curvature of the stomach.

v. efferen'tia. 1. Lymphatics which leave a gland. 2. Veins carrying blood away from a part. 3. Excretory ducts of the testis.

v. prae'via. The blood vessels of the cord presenting before the fetus.

v. rec'ta. 1. Tubules which become straight prior to entering the mediastinum testis. 2. Straight collecting tubules of the kidney.

v. vaso'rum. BNA. Tiny blood vessels which are distributed to walls of larger veins and arteries.

v. vortico'sa. Stellate veins of the choroid, carrying blood to the sup. ophthalmic vein.

vasal (vā'săl). Relating to a vas or vessel.

vasalium (văs-ā'lĭ-ŭm) (pl. *vasalia*). Tissue peculiar to vascular organs.

vascular (văs'kū-lăr). Pert. to or composed of blood vessels.

v. reflex. Constriction or dilation of vascular trunk or area resulting from mental or physical irritation.

v. system. The heart, blood vessels, lymphatics and their parts considered collectively. [systems.

It includes the pulmonary and portal

v. tuft. One of the vascular processes on the chorion in the fetus at an early stage of development. SYN: *villi, chorionic*.

v. tumor. One containing dilated blood vessels. SYN: *angioma, telangioma*.

vascularization (văs″kū-lă-rĭ-zā'shŭn). Development of new blood vessels in a structure.

vascularize (văs'kū-lă-rīz). To become vascular by development of new blood vessels.

vasculitis (văs-kū-lī'tĭs). Inflammation of a vessel. SYN: *angeitis*.

vasculum (văs'kū-lŭm). A tiny vessel.

v. aber'rans. A tube with a blind end occasionally connected with the vas deferens or the epididymis. SYN: *vas aberrans*.

vasectomy (văs-ĕk'tō-mĭ). Removal of all or a segment of the vas deferens.

vasifactive (văs-ĭ-făk'tĭv). Forming new vessels. [lar structure or vas.

vasiform (văs'ĭ-form). Resembling a tubu-

vaso-. Combining form meaning *a vessel*, as a blood vessel.

vasoconstrictive (văs″ō-kŏn-strĭk'tĭv). Causing constriction of the blood vessels.

vasoconstrictor (văs″ō-kŏn-strĭk'tor). 1. Causing constriction of blood vessels. 2. That which constricts or narrows the caliber of blood vessels, as a drug or a nerve.

vasocorona (văs″ō-kor-ō'nă). The system of peripheral vessels of the spinal cord sending branches inward.

vasodentin(e (văs″ō-dĕn-tēn). Modified dentine provided with blood capillaries.

vasodepression (văs″ō-dē-prĕsh'ŭn). Vasomotor depression or collapse.

vasodepressor (văs″ō-dē-prĕs'or). 1. Having a depressing influence on the circulation. 2. An agent which depresses circulation.

vasodilatation (văs″ō-dĭl-ă-tā'shŭn). Dilatation of lumen of blood vessels.

v., reflex. Formation of a red mark on the skin, which turns white quickly when rubbed firmly by a penholder.

vasodilatin (văs″ō-dĭ-lā'tĭn). A vasodilator substance said to be present in organic extracts, which depresses nerves and blood vessels.

vasodilator (văs″ō-dĭ-lā'tor). 1. Causing relaxation of the blood vessels. 2. A nerve or drug which dilates the blood vessels.

vaso-epididymostomy (văs″ō-ĕp″ĭ-dĭd-ĭ-mŏs'tō-mĭ). Formation of a passage bet. the vas deferens and the epididymis.

vasofactive (văs″ō-făk'tĭv). Forming new blood vessels. SYN: *vasifactive, vasoformative*.

vasoformative (văs″ō-for'mă-tĭv). Forming new blood vessels. SYN: *vasofactive*.

vasoganglion (văs″ō-găng'glĭ-ŏn). Mass of blood vessels. SYN: *rete*.

vasogen (văs'ō-jĕn). Commercial ointment base used as a vehicle for remedies for skin diseases.

vasography (văs-ŏg-ră-fĭ). X-ray photography of the blood vessels.

vasohypertonic (văs″ō-hī-pĕr-tŏn'ĭk). Causing or that which causes constriction of blood vessels. SYN: *vasoconstrictor*.

vasohypotonic (văs″ō-hī-pō-tŏn'ĭk). Relaxing or that which relaxes blood vessels. SYN: *vasodilator*.

vasoinhibitor (văs″ō-ĭn-hĭb'ĭ-tor). An agent that depresses vasomotor nerves.

vasoinhibitory (văs″ō-ĭn-hĭb'ĭ-tor-ĭ). Restricting vasomotor activity.

vasoligation (văs″ō-lǐ-gā′shŭn). Ligation of a vessel, specifically the vas deferens.

vasomotion (văs″ō-mō′shŭn). Change in caliber of a blood vessel.

vasomotor (văs″ō-mō′tor). 1. Pert. to the nerves having muscular control of the blood vessel walls.

   v. catarrh. An allergic acute nasal catarrh. SYN: *hay fever.*

   v. epilepsy. Epilepsy with vasomotor changes in the skin.

   v. nerves. Those which cause either contraction or dilation of blood vessels.

   v. spasm. Spasm of smaller arteries.

vasomotory (văs″ō-mō′tor-ǐ). Controlling changes in the size of the blood vessels. SYN: *vasomotor.*

vasoneurosis (văs″ō-nū-rō′sǐs). A neurosis affecting blood vessels; a disorder of the vasomotor system. SEE: *angioneurosis.*

vasoörchidostomy (văs″ō-or-kǐd-ŏs′tō-mǐ). Surgical connection of the epididymis to the severed end of the vas deferens.

vasoparesis (văs″ō-păr′ē-sǐs, -păr-ē′sǐs). Partial paralysis or weakness of the vasomotor nerves.

vasopressin (văs″ō-prĕs′ǐn). A post. pituitary lobe hormone.

   It stimulates intestinal muscles and raises blood pressure. SEE: *oxytocin, pitressin.*

vasopuncture (văs″ō-pŭnk-chūr). Puncture of the vas deferens.

vasorelaxation (văs″ō-rē-lăks-ā′shŭn). Lessening of vascular pressure.

vasorrhaphy (văs-or′ă-fǐ). Surgical suture of the vas deferens.

vasosection (văs″ō-sĕk′shŭn). Surgical division of the vasa deferentia.

vasosensory (văs″ō-sen′sō-rǐ). Distributing sensory filaments to the blood vessels.

vasospasm (văs″ō-spăzm). Spasm of any vessel, esp. of a blood vessel. SYN: *angiospasm, vasoconstriction.*

vasostimulant (văs″ō-stǐm′ū-lănt). Exciting vasomotor action.

vasostomy (va-zos′to-mǐ). Surgical procedure of making an opening into the vas deferens.

vasothrombin (văs″ō-thrŏm′bǐn). Thrombin derived from the intima of blood vessels.   [deferens.

vasotomy (văs-ŏt′ō-mǐ). Incision of vas

vasotonic (văs″ō-tŏn′ǐk). Pert. to the tone of a vessel.

vasotribe (văs′ō-trīb). Pressure forceps used for controlling hemorrhages. SYN: *angiotribe.*

vasotripsy (văs-ō-trǐp′sǐ). Arrest of hemorrhages with a strong forceps by crushing an artery. SYN: *angiotripsy.*

vasotrophic (văs″ō-trof′ǐk). Affecting the nutrition by change in caliber of blood vessels.

vasovesiculectomy (văs″ō-vĕs-ǐk-ū-lĕk′tō-mǐ). Excision of the vas deferens and seminal vesicles.

vasovesiculitis (văs″ō-vĕs-ǐk-ū-lī′tǐs). Inflammation of the vas deferens and seminal vesicles.

Vater's ampullae (fäh′ter). Dilatation at junction of common bile duct and pancreatic duct, just before they empty into the duodenum.

   V.'s corpuscles. Ovoid end organs of nerves supplying the skin. SYN: *pacinian corpuscles.*

vection (vĕk′shŭn). Carrying of disease germ from the sick to well persons.

   v., circumferen'tial. Transference through an intermediate host.

   v., ra'dial. Direct transference of disease germs from one individual to another.

vectis (vĕk′tǐs). A curved lever for making traction on the presenting part of the fetus.

vector (vĕk′tor). A living carrier of disease germs from the sick to a well person. SEE: *vection.*

   v., circumferen'tial. One carrying infection from the sick to the well.

vectorial (vĕk-tō′rǐ-ăl). Relating to a vector.

vegetarian (vĕj-ĕ-tā′rǐ-ăn). One who eats no animal products, but who lives on vegetables.

vegetarianism (vĕj-ĕ-tā′rǐ-ăn-ǐzm). The belief and practice of eating vegetables and fruits only.

vegetation (vĕj-ĕ-tā′shŭn). A morbid luxurious outgrowth on any part, esp. wartlike projections made up of collections of fibrin in which are enmeshed white and red blood cells; sometimes seen on denuded areas of the endocardium covering the valves of the heart.

vegetative (vĕj′ĕ-tā″tǐv). 1. Having the power to grow, as plants. 2. Functioning involuntarily. 3. Quiescent, passive, noting a stage of development.

   v. nervous system. The sympathetic nervous system.

   v. pole. Area at end of ovum containing nutritive matter.

vehicle (vē′ǐ-kl). A substance used as a medium for the administration of medicine, as syrup in liquid preparations. SYN: *menstruum.*

veil (vāl). 1. Any veillike structure. 2. A piece of the amniotic sac occasionally covering the face of a newborn infant. SYN: *caul.* 3. Slight obscuration of the voice.

   v., acquired. Slight imperfection of the voice due to strain or exposure.

   v., uterine. Device for covering the cervix uteri to prevent impregnation.

vein (vān). Vessel carrying dark red (unaerated) blood to the heart, except for pulmonary vein.

velamen (vĕl-ā′mĕn) (pl. *velamina*). Any covering membrane.

   v. nativum. The skin covering the body.

   v. vul'vae. Abnormal elongation of the nymphae. SYN: *Hottentot apron.*

velamentous (vĕl-ă-mĕn′tŭs). Expanding like a veil, or sheet.

velamentum (vĕl-ă-mĕn′tŭm) (pl. *velamenta*). A membranous covering.

velar (vē'lar). Pert. to a veil or veillike structure.

vellication (vĕl-ĭk-ā'shŭn). Spasmodic twitching of muscular fibers.

velocity (vē-lŏs'ĭt-ĭ). Rate of speed of an object or process.

velosynthesis (vĕl-o-sĭn'thĕs-ĭs). Suture of a cleft palate, particularly the soft palate. SYN: *staphylorrhaphy.*

Velpeau's bandage (vĕl-pō'). A bandage for the shoulder. SEE: *bandage.*

V's deformity. Deformity seen in Colles'* fracture in which lower fragment is displaced backward.

velum (vē'lŭm). Any veil-like structure.

    v. palati'num. BNA. The soft palate.

vena (vē'nă) (pl. *venae*). A vein.

venenation (vĕn-ē-nā'shŭn). 1. Condition of being poisoned. 2. Act of poisoning.

venene (vē-nēn'). Toxic substance in snake venom.

veneniferous (vĕn-ē-nĭf'ĕr-ŭs). Transmitting or carrying poison.

venenific (vĕn-ē-nĭf'ĭk). Producing poison.

venenous (vĕn'ĕn-ŭs). Poisonous.

venepuncture (vĕn'ē-pŭnk''chūr). Puncture of a vein to withdraw blood or inject a remedy.

venereal (vē-nē'rē-ăl). Pert. to or resulting from sexual intercourse.

    v. bubo. Enlarged gland in the groin, the result of a venereal disease.

    v. collar. Mottled condition of the neck seen occasionally in syphilis.

    v. disease. One acquired ordinarily as a result of sexual intercourse with an individual who is afflicted.

    v. sore, or **v. ulcer.** Chancroid.

    v. wart. Moist reddish elevations on genitals and anus. SYN: *verruca acuminata, condyloma.*

venereologist (vē-nēr''ē-ŏl'ō-jĭst). A doctor who specilaizes in the treatment of venereal diseases.

venereology (vē-nēr''ē-ŏl'ō-jĭ). The scientific study and treatment of venereal diseases.

venereophobia (vē-nēr''ē-ō-fō'bĭ-ă). Abnormal fear of venereal disease. SYN: *cypridophobia.*

venery (vĕn'ĕr-ĭ). Sexual intercourse. SYN: *coitus.*

venesection (vĕn''ē-sĕk'shŭn). Opening of a vein for withdrawal of blood.

venin(e (vĕn'ĭn). Toxic substance in snake venom.

venin-antivenin (vĕn''ĭn-ăn''tĭ-vĕn'ĭn). Vaccine to counteract snake poison.

veniplex (vĕn'ĭ-plĕks). A plexus of veins.

venipuncture (vĕn''ĭ-pŭnk'chūr). Puncture of a vein for any purpose.

venisection (vĕn''ĭ-sĕk'shŭn). Opening of a vein for blood abstraction. SYN: *phlebotomy.*

venisuture (vĕn-ĭ-sū-chūr). Suture of a vein. SYN: *phleborrhaphy.*

venoauricular (vē''nō-aw-rĭk'ū-lar). Relating to the vena cava and the auricle.

venoclysis (vē-nŏk'lĭ-sĭs). The continuous injection of medicinal or nutrient fluid intravenously. SYN: *phleboclysis.*

venogram (vē'nō-grăm). 1. A roentgenogram of the veins. SYN: *phlebogram.* 2. A tracing of the venous pulse.

venography (vē-nŏg'ră-fĭ). 1. Roentgenography of veins. 2. The making of a tracing of the venous pulse.

venom (vĕn'ŏm). A poison excreted by some animals, such as insects or snakes, and transmitted by bites or stings.

venoperitoneostomy (vē''nō-pĕr''ĭ-tō-nē-ŏs'tō-mĭ). Attachment of the cut end of the saphenous vein into the cavity of the peritoneum.

venopressor (vē''nō-prĕs''or). Pert. to venous blood pressure and its supply to the right side of the heart.

venosclerosis (vē''nō-sklē-rō'sĭs). Sclerosis of veins. SYN: *phlebosclerosis.*

venosity (vē-nŏs'ĭ-tĭ). 1. Condition in which there is an excess of venous blood in a part causing venous congestion. 2. Deficient aeration of venous blood.

venostasis (vē-nŏs'tă-sĭs). Abstraction of blood from the circulation by compression of veins in an extremity. SYN: *phlebostasis.*

venostat (vē'nō-stăt). Appliance for performing venous compression.

venotomy (vē-nŏt'ō-mĭ). Incision of a vein.

venous (vē'nŭs). Pert. to the veins or blood passing through them.

    v. blood. The dark blood in the veins.

    v. hum. Murmur heard upon auscultation over larger veins of the neck.

    v. hypere'mia. Excess of venous blood in a part. SYN: *venosity.*

    v. sinus. Cerebral sinus.

venovenostomy (vē''nō-vē-nŏs'tō-mĭ). Formation of an anastomosis of a vein into a vein.

vent (vĕnt). An opening in any cavity, esp. one for excretion.

venter (vĕn'ter). 1. The abdomen. SYN: *belly.* 2. Any of the greater body cavities. 3. The uterus. 4. The hollowed part of a muscle or other structure.

ventilation (vĕn-tĭl-ā'shŭn). 1. Circulation of air or amt. of fresh air in a room and withdrawal of foul air. 2. Oxygenation of blood. 3. PHYS: The amt. of air inhaled per day.

    v., exhaustion. Forcible withdrawal of air from a room.

    v., ple'num. Forcible introduction of air into a room.

ventose (vĕn'tōs). Distended with gas. SYN: *flatulent.*

ventouse (vahn-tooz'). A glass for cupping.

ven'trad. Toward the ventral aspect, opp. to *dorsad.*

ventral (vĕn'trăl). Pert. to the ant. or front side of the body. Opp. of *dorsal.**

    v. aspect. Ant. or inf. view; toward the belly.

    v. hernia. One through the abdominal wall.

ventricle (vĕn'trĭk-l). 1. A small cavity. 2. One of 2 lower chambers of the heart, which propel blood into the arteries. The right ventricle forces it into the pulmonary artery and the lungs; the left, through the aorta. At each beat, each ventricle pumps more than 6 oz. of blood.

v., aortic. Left ventricle of the heart.

v. of the brain. Five cavities filled with cerebrospinal fluid.

v. of the larynx. The space bet. the true and false vocal cords.

v. of Morgagni. Space bet. true and false cords extending laterally to the thyroid cartilage.

v. of the myelon. Central canal of spinal cord. [and syphilis.

v., prolapse of. Seen in tuberculosis

ventricornu (věn-trĭ-kor'nŭ). The ant. ventral horn of gray matter of the spinal cord.

ventricornual (věn"trĭ-kor'nŭ-ăl). Relating to the ventricornu.

ventricose (věn'trĭ-kōs). 1. Inflated on 1 side. 2. Corpulent.

ventricular (věn-trĭk'ū-lar). Pert. to a ventricle.

v. aqueduct. Canal connecting 3rd and 4th cerebral ventricles. SYN: *aquaeductus Sylvii*.

v. bands. The false vocal cords or folds of mucous membrane parallel or above the vocal bands.

v. ligament. A false vocal band.

v. muscle. The thyreoepiglottideus.

v. septum. Septum between ventricles of the heart.

ventriculin (věn-trĭk'ū-lĭn). Dessicated, defatted hog stomach used in primary anemia.

DOSAGE: From 20-30 Gm. daily.

ventriculography (věn-trĭk-ū-lŏg'ră-fĭ). An x-ray process used for localization of cerebral tumors, following the injection of air into the cerebral ventricles.

ventriculometry (věn-trĭk"ū-lŏm'ě-trĭ). The measurement of the intraventricular cerebral pressure.

ventriculonector (věn-trĭk"ū-lō-něk'tor). Muscular band connecting auricles and ventricles of the heart. SYN: *atrioventricular bundle*.

ventriculoscopy (věn-trĭk"ū-lŏs'kō-pĭ). Examination of the ventricles of the brain with an endoscope.

ventriculus (věn-trĭk'ū-lŭs). BNA. 1. The stomach. 2. A ventricle of the brain or heart.

ventricumbent (věn-trĭ-kŭm'běnt). Lying on the belly. SYN: *prone*.

ventriduct (věn'trĭ-dŭkt). To draw toward the abdomen.

ventrimeson (věn-trĭ-měs'ŏn). The median line on the ventral surface of the body.

ventripyramid (věn"trĭ-pir'ă-mĭd). An ant. pyramid of the medulla oblongata.

ventrocystorrhaphy (věn-trō-sĭs-tor'ă-fĭ). Suture of a cyst to the abdominal wall to permit drainage.

ventrofixation (věn'trō-fĭks-ă-shŭn). The suture of a displaced viscus to the abdominal wall.

ventrohysteropexy (věn"trō-hĭs'těr-ō-pěks"ĭ). Attachment of the uterus to the abdominal wall.

ventroscopy (věn-trŏs'kō-pĭ). Examination of the abdominal cavity by illumination. SYN: *celioscopy*.

ventrose (věn'trōs). Having a belly or swelling like one.

ventrosuspension (věn"trō-sŭs-pěn'shŭn). Fixation of displaced uterus to abdominal wall.

ventrotomy (věn-trŏt'ō-mĭ). Incision into abdominal cavity. SYN: *celiotomy, laparotomy, q.v.*

ventrovesicofixation (věn"trō-věs-ĭ-kō-fĭks-ă'shŭn). Suture of uterus to abdominal wall and bladder. SYN: *hysterocystopexy*.

venula (věn'ū-lă). Venule.

venule (věn'ūl). A veinlet, a tiny vein continuous with a capillary.

venus (vē'nŭs). Sexual intercourse. SYN: *copulation*.

v.'s collar. Pigmentation around the neck in eruption due to syphilis.

verbigeration (věr-bĭj-ěr-ā'shŭn). Uncontrollable repetition of phrases, absence of coherent thought combined with voluble speech, seen in insanity.

verbomania (věr"bō-mā'nĭ-ă). The flow of talk in some forms of psychosis.

verdigris (věr'dĭg-rĭs). 1. Mixture of basic copper acetates. 2. Deposit of copper carbonate upon copper and bronze vessels.

Vergas' ventricle (věr'gă). Cleftlike space bet. the callosum and fornix of the brain.

vergency (věr'jěn-sĭ). 1. Any turning movement about the eyes. 2. The reciprocal of the focal distance of a lens taken as a measure of the divergence or convergence of rays.

Verheyen's stars (fěr-hī'ěn). Starlike venous plexuses on surface of the kidney below its capsule.

verjuice (věr'jūs). Acid juice from unripe fruit.

vermicidal (věr"mĭ-sĭ'dăl). Destroying worms parasitic in the intestines.

vermicide (věr'mĭ-sĭd). 1. Destroying worms. 2. An agent that will kill intestinal worms. Ex: *santonin, oil of chenopodium*.

vermicular (věr-mĭk'ū-lăr). Resembling a worm.

v. appendix. The vermiform appendix.

v. movements. The wormlike movements of peristalsis.

v. pulse. Small, rapid one resulting in wormlike feeling in the fingers.

vermiculation (věr-mĭk"ū-lā'shŭn). A wormlike motion, as in the intestines. SEE: *peristalsis*.

vermiculose, vermiculous (věr-mĭk'ū-lōs, věr-mĭk'ū-lŭs). 1. Infested with worms or larvae. 2. Wormlike.

vermiform (věr'mĭ-form). Contoured like a worm.

v. appendix. A small tube about the size of a goose quill opening into the cecum and closed at its other end.

Its inflammation is called *appendicitis.**

vermifugal (věr-mĭf'ū-găl). Expelling worms from the intestines.

vermifuge (vĕr'mĭ-fūj). 1. Expelling worms. 2. Agent for expelling intestinal worms. SYN: *vermicide.*

vermilion (vĕr-mĭl'yŭn). Red mercuric sulfide.

v. border. Junction of mucous membrane of the lips with the skin.

v. poisoning. Poisoning is slower and less marked, but resembles mercuric chloride, *q.v.*

vermin (vĕr'mĭn). Parasitic insects and animals, such as mice, lice, bedbugs.

v. killers. POISONING: SEE: *arsenic, strychnine, phosphorus* and *fluorides,* which are the principal poisonous ingredients.

vermination (vĕr-mĭn-ā'shŭn). Infestation with vermin or worms.

verminossi (vĕr-mĭn-ō'sĭs). Infestation with vermin.

verminous (vĕr'mĭn-ŭs). Pert. to or infested with worms.

vermiphobia (vĕr-mĭ-fō'bĭ-ă). An abnormal fear of being infestated with worms.

vermis (vĕr'mĭs). 1. A worm. 2. Median connecting lobe of the cerebellum.

v. cerebel'li. BNA. Same as vermis, 2.

vermography (vĕr-mŏg'ră-fĭ). Roentgenography of the vermiform appendix.

vernal (vĕr'năl). Occurring in or pert. to the spring.

v. catarrh. A chronic form of conjunctivitis occurring usually in spring and remaining until cool weather. SEE: *catarrh vernal.*

v. fever. Malarial fever.

Vernes' test (vārn). A blood test for syphilis.

vernix (vĕr'nĭks). Varnish.

v. caseo'sa. A sebaceous deposit covering the fetus due to secretion of skin glands.

After birth, rub the skin with olive oil and it will disappear. SEE: *sebum.*

verodigen (vē-rō'dĭj-ĕn). A purified digitalis principle.

DOSAGE: 1/80 gr. (0.0008 Gm.).

veronal (vĕr'ō-năl). USP. A brand of barbital, a white crystalline substance.

DOSAGE: 7-20 gr. (0.5-1.3 Gm.).

v. sodium. A brand of soluble barbital.

veronalism (vĕr'ō-năl-ĭzm). Addiction to the use of veronal and the resultant symptoms.

verruca (vĕr-rū'kă) (pl. *verrucae*). Elevation of the skin, small, circumscribed, formed by hypertrophy of the papillae and of various forms according to location. SYN: *wart.*

v. acuminata. A pointed reddish moist wart about the genitals and the anus, seen in gonorrhea. SYN: *venereal wart.*

v. digitata. Form seen on face and scalp, possibly serving as starting point of cutaneous horns, forming several filiform projections with horny caps closely grouped on a comparatively narrow base which in turn may be separated from skin surface by slightly contracted neck.

v. filiformis. Small threadlike growths on neck and eyelids covered with smooth and apparently normal epidermis.

v. plana. Flat oily wart, pigmented, on backs of old people.

v. plantaris. Warts on the soles of the feet.

v. senilis. SEE: *verruca plana.*

v. simplex. Verruca vulgaris, *q.v.*

v. vulgaris. Common warts, usually on backs of hands and fingers.

verruciform (vĕr-ū'sĭ-form). Wartlike.

verrucose, verrucous (vĕr'ū-kōs, vĕr-rū'kŭs). Wartlike, with raised portions.

versicolor (vĕr'sĭ-kŭl''er). 1. Having many shades or colors. 2. Changeable in color.

version (ver'shŭn). 1. Condition of uterus in which its axis is deflected from the normal position without being bent on itself. SEE: *anteversion, lateroversion, retroversion.* 2. Process of turning the fetus in the uterus to facilitate delivery.

v. cephalic. Turning of fetus so that the head presents.

v. pelvic. Manipulation of a cross presentation until it is changed to a pelvic presentation.

v. podalic. Manipulation of fetus by the feet so that the breech presents.

v. spontaneous. Version of fetus by uterine muscular contraction without artificial assistance.

vertebra (ver'tē-bră) (pl. *vertebrae*). Any one of the 33 bony segments of the spinal column. The vertebrae comprise 7 cervical, 12 thoracic dorsal, 5 lumbar, 5 sacral, and 4 coccygeal.

v. basilar. The lowest of the lumbar vertebrae.

v. cervical. The 7 vertebrae of the neck.

v. coccygeal. The rudimentary vertebrae of the coccyx.

v. cranial. The segments of the skull and facial bones, by some regarded as homologous with vertebrae.

v. dentata. The 2nd cervical vertebra. SYN: *axis.*

v. dorsal. The 12 vertebrae which connect the ribs and form part of the post. wall of the thorax. SYN: *thoracic vertebra.*

v. false. One of the segments of the sacrum and the coccyx.

v. lumbar. The 5 vertebrae bet. the dorsal vertebrae and the sacrum.

v. magnum. The sacrum.

v. odontoid. Same as *vertebra dentata.*

v. prominens. The 7th cervical vertebra.

v. sacral. The 5 fused segments forming the sacrum.

v. sternal. The segments of the sternum.

v. thoracic. SEE: *dorsal vertebra.*

v. true. The vertebrae which remain unfused through life.

vertebral (ver'tē-brăl). Pert. to a vertebra or the vertebral artery.

v. arch. Sup. loop of the vertebra enclosing the neural canal. SYN: *neural arch.*

v. canal. The spinal canal or cavity.

v. column. Spinal column.

v. foramen. 1. The hollow space enclosed by a vertebral arch. 2. A vertebrarterial foramen.

v. groove. The groove bet. the transverse and spinous processes of the spine.

v. ribs. The lower 2, or floating ribs.

vertebrarium (ver″tē-brā'rĭ-ŭm). The spinal column.

vertebrarterial (ver″tē-brar-tē'rĭ-ăl). Pert. to a vertebra and an artery.

v. foramen. A foramen in the transverse processes of the cervical vertebrae for passage of the vertebral artery.

vertebrate, vertebrated (ver′tē-brāt, ver′-tē-brā-tĕd). Having or resembling a vertebral column.

vertebrectomy (ver-tē-brĕk′tō-mĭ) Excision of a vertebra or part of one.

vertebrochondral (ver″tē-brō-kŏn′drăl). Denoting the false ribs (8th, 9th, 10th) connected with a vertebra at 1 end and the costal cartilages at the other.

vertebrocostal (ver″tē-brō-kŏs′tăl). Pert. to a vertebra and a rib. SYN: *costo-vertebral.*

vertebromammary (ver″tē-brō-măm′mă-rĭ). Pert. to the vertebral and mammary area.

v. diameter. The anteroposterior diameter of the thorax.

vertebrosternal (ver″tē-brō-ster′năl). Pert. to a vertebra and the sternum.

vertex (ver′tĕks). The top of the head. SYN: *crown.*

v. cordis. Apex of the heart.

v. presentation. Presentation in labor of vertex of the fetal skull.

vertical (ver′tĭk-ăl). 1. Pert. to or situated at the vertex. 2. Directed up or down at right angles to the plane of the body or part of the earth's surface.

verticillate (ver-tĭs′ĭl-āt, -tĭs-ĭl′āt). Arranged like the spokes of a wheel or a whorl.

vertiginous (ver-tĭj′ĭn-ŭs). Pert. to or afflicted with vertigo.

vertigo (ver′tĭg-ō, ver-tī′gō). Sensation of dizziness, a whirling motion of oneself or of ext. objects.

v., auditory, v., aural. Vertigo due to disease of the ear.

v., cerebral. Vertigo due to brain disease.

v., epileptic. Vertigo attending an epileptic attack or following it.

v., essential. Vertigo from an unknown cause.

v., gastric. Vertigo from gastric disturbance.

v., hysterical. Vertigo accompanying hysteria.

v., labyrinthine. Vertigo due to disease of labyrinth of the ear. SYN: *Ménière's disease.*

v., laryngeal. Vertigo accompanying laryngeal spasm.

v., lithemic. Vertigo experienced in gout or lithemia.

v., objective. Vertigo when objects seen appear to be moving when stationary.   [of the eye.

v., ocular. Vertigo caused by disease

v., organic. Vertigo from a brain lesion.

v., peripheral. Vertigo from disturbance distant from the brain.

v., subjective. Vertigo in which patient seems to be turning or rotating.

v., toxic. Vertigo from presence of a toxin in the body.

verumontanitis (ver″ū-mŏn-tăn-ī′tĭs). Inflammation of the verumontanum. SYN: *colliculitis.*

verumontanum (ver″ū-mŏn-tā′nŭm). An elevation on the floor of the prostatic portion of the urethra where the seminal ducts enter.

vesalianum (vĕs-a-lĭ-ā′nŭm). One of the sesamoid bones in the tendon of origin of the gastrocnemius muscle, and another on outer border of foot in the angle bet. the cuboid and fifth matatarsal.

Vesalius, foramen of (vĕs-ā′lĭ-ŭs). One in base of the skull transmitting an emissary vein.

v., vein of. Small vein giving from the cavernous sinus passing through Vesalius' foramen.

vesania (vē-sā′nĭ-ă). Mental derangement without coma or fever. SYN: *insanity.*

vesanic (vĕs-ăn′ĭk). Pert. to insanity.

vescette (vĕs-ĕt′). Commercial tablet made of compressed effervescent salts.

vesica (vĕs-ī′kă). A bladder.

v. fellea. BNA. The gallbladder.

v. prostat'ica. A minute pouch in the prostatic urethra, remnant of müllerian duct. SYN: *utriculus prostaticus.*

v. urinaria. BNA. The urinary bladder.

vesical (vĕs′ĭk-ăl). Pert. to or shaped like a bladder.

v. reflex. Inclination to urinate, caused by moderate bladder distention.

vesicant (vĕs′ĭk-ănt). 1. Blistering; causing or forming blisters. 2. Agent used to produce blisters. They are much less severe than escharotics. SYN: *epispastic.*

vesication (vĕs-ĭ-kā′shŭn). 1. Process of blistering. 2. A blister.

vesicatory (vĕs′ĭk-ă-tor′ĭ). 1. Causing or pert. to blisters. 2. Agent causing blisters. SYN: *vesicant.*

vesicle (vĕs′ĭ-kl). 1. A small sac or bladder containing fluid. 2. A blisterlike small elevation on the skin from the size of a pinhead to that of a split pea, containing serous fluid.

v., allantoic. Int. cavity of the allantois.

v., auditory. That portion of the cerebral vesicle from which the ext. ear is formed.

v., blastodermic. Sac developed from the blastoderm.

v., cerebral. Expansion of neural embryonic canal from which the brain develops.

v., compound. Vesicle with more than 1 cavity.

v., germinal. Nucleus of the ovum.

v., graafian. The ovarian structure containing the ovum.

v., seminal. One of the 2 membranous, sacculated tubes situated at the base of the bladder, bet. it and the rectum, serving as a reservoir for the semen and having a secretion of its own.

v., umbilical. Portion of embryonic yolk sac outside the body cavity.

vesico-. Combining form meaning *bladder*.

vesicocele (vĕs'ĭk-ō-sēl). Hernia of bladder. SYN: *cystocele*.

vesicocervical (vĕs″ĭk-ō-ser'vĭ-kăl). Relating to the urinary bladder and cervix uteri.

vesicoclysis (vĕs-ĭk-ŏk'lĭs-ĭs). Injection of fluid into the bladder.

vesicofixation (ves″ĭk-ō-fĭks-ā'shŭn). Attachment of the uterus to the bladder or the bladder to the abdominal wall.

vesicoprostatic (vĕs″ĭk-ō-prŏs-tăt'ĭk). Relating to the bladder and prostate.

vesicopubic (vĕs″ĭk-ō-pū'bĭk). Pert. to the bladder and the os pubis.

vesicospinal (vĕs″ĭk-ō-spī'năl). Relating to the urinary bladder and spinal cord.

vesicotomy (vĕs-ĭ-kŏt'ō-mĭ). Incision of the bladder.

vesicouterine (ves″ĭk-ō-ū'ter-ĭn). Pert. to the urinary bladder and the uterus.

vesicovaginal (vĕs″ĭk-ō-văj'ĭ-năl). Pert. to the urinary bladder and vagina.

vesicula (vĕs-ĭk'ū-lă) (pl. *vesiculae*). A small bladder, or vesicle.

v. seminalis. BNA. Tiny reservoir of semen at base of the bladder. SYN: *vesicle, seminal, q.v.*

vesicular (vĕs-ĭk'ū-lar). Pert. to vesicles or small blisters.

v. breathing. Murmur heard in normal breathing.

v. column, v. cylinder. Ganglion cells at base of post. horn of spinal cord.

v. eczema. Eczema accompanied by formation of vesicles.   [sema.

v. emphysema. Pulmonary emphy-

v. erysipelas. A form of erysipelas that develops vesicles on the inflamed surface.

v. fever. 1. Condition marked by vesicular eruption; rise in temperature, slight; localized pain. 2. Skin disease marked by formation of vesicles. SYN: *pemphigus.*

v. murmur. The normal sound of respiration heard on auscultation. Same as *vesicular breathing.*

v. râle. The crepitant râle, a crackling sound heard at end of inspiration.

v. resonance. Percussion sound heard over the normal lung.

vesiculase (vĕs-ĭk'ū-lās). An enzyme in prostatic fluid said to coagulate semen.

vesiculation (vĕs-ĭk-ū-lā'shŭn). Formation of vesicles or state of having or forming them.

vesiculectomy (vĕs-ĭk″ū-lĕk'tō-mĭ). Partial or complete excision of a vesicle, particularly a seminal vesicle.

vesiculiform (vĕs-ĭk'ū-lĭ-form). Having the shape of a vesicle.

vesiculitis (vĕs-ĭk″ū-lī'tĭs). Inflammation of a vesicle, particularly the seminal vesicle.

vesiculocavernous (vĕs-ĭk″ū-lō-kăv'ĕr-nŭs). Vesicular and cavernous.

vesiculogram (vĕs-ĭk'ū-lō-grăm). An x-ray picture of the seminal vesicles.

vesiculography (vĕs-ĭk″ū-lŏg'ră-fĭ). X-ray photography of the seminal vesicles.

vesiculopapular (vĕs-ĭk″ū-lō-păp'ū-lăr). Composed of vesicles and papules.

vesiculopustular (vĕs-ĭk″ū-lō-pŭs'tū-lăr). Having both vesicles and pustules.

vesiculotomy (vĕs-ĭk″ū-lŏt'ō-mĭ). Division of a vesicle, as a seminal vesicle.

vesiculotympanic (vĕs-ĭk″ū-lō-tĭm-păn'ĭk). Vesicular and tympanic.

vespajus (vĕs-pā'jŭs). Follicular, suppurative inflammation of the hairy part of the scalp.

vessel (vĕs'ĕl). A tube, duct, or canal to convey the fluids of the body. SYN: *vas.*

v.'s, absorbent. The lacteals, lymphatics and capillaries of the intestines.

v.'s, blood. Arteries, veins, and capillaries.

v.'s, chyliferous. Vessels arising in the villi of the intestinal walls carrying chyle and terminating in the thoracic duct.

v.'s, lymphatic. Vessels conveying lymph.

v.'s, nutrient. Those supplying interior of the bones.

v., radicular. Branch of a vertebral artery supplying cerebral nerve root.

vestibular (vĕs-tĭb'ū-lăr). Pert. to a vestibule.

v. bulbs. Two sacculated collections of veins, lying on either side of the vagina beneath the bulbocavernosus muscle, connected anteriorly by the *pars intermedia*, and through this strip of cavernous tissue communicating with the erectile tissue of the clitoris.

vestibule (vĕs'tĭb-ūl). A small space or cavity at the beginning of a canal, such as the aortic vessel.

v. of ear. The middle part of the inner ear, behind the cochlea, and in front of the semicircular canals; it contains the utriculus and sacculus.

v. of larynx. The portion of the larynx above the vocal cords.

v. of nose. The anterior part of the nostrils containing the vibrissae.

v. of pharynx. The fauces.

v. of vulva. An almond-shaped space bet. the lines of attachment of the labia minora. At the ant. angle the *clitoris* is situated; the post. boundary is the *fourchette.* The vestibule appears approximately 4 or 5 cm. long and 2 cm. in greatest width when the labia minora are separated. Four major structures open into vestibule: The *urethra anteriorly*, the *vagina posteriorly*, and the two *excretory ducts of the glands of Bartholin*, laterally. The covering membranes are pink in color and constructed of delicate stratified squamous epithelium. Collections of cavernous tissue are disposed beneath the integument. SEE: *vestibular bulbs, Bartholin's glands, vagina.*

vestibulotomy (věs-tĭb″ū-lŏt′ō-mĭ). Surgical incision into the vestibule of the inner ear.

vestibulourethral (věs-tĭb″ū-lŏ-ū-rē-thrăl). Relating to the vestibule of the vulva and the urethra.

vestibulum (věs-tĭb′ū-lŭm) (pl. *vestibula*). Vestibule.

   v. vagi′nae. BNA. Space behind glans clitoridis bet. the labia minora enveloping the vagina, urethra, and Bartholin's glands.

vestige (věs′tĭj). A small degenerate or incompletely developed structure which has been more fully developed in the embryo or in a past generation.

vestigial (věs-tĭj′ĭ-ăl). Of the nature of a vestige. SYN: *rudimentary.*

   v. fold. A fibrous band of the pericardium, a remnant of the obliterated left innominate vein.

vestigium (věs-tĭj′ĭ-ŭm). Vestige.

via (vī′ă) (pl. *viae*). Any passage in the body.

   v. prima. First channel for passage of food, the alimentary canal.

   v. secunda. The lacteals and blood vessels, the second path for entrance of nutriment into the body.

viability (vī-ă-bĭl′ĭ-tĭ). Ability to live, grow and develop.   [7 months' fetus.

viable (vī′ă-bl). Capable of living, as a

vial (vī′ăl). A small glass bottle for medicines or chemicals.

vibex (vī′běks) (pl. *vibices*). A linear subcutaneous extravasation of blood.

vibices (vĭb-ĭ′sēz). (sing. *vibex*). A form of macula, appearing as long narrow purple spots under the skin; hemorrhagic lesions.

vibratile (vī′bră-tĭl). Adapted to or used in vibratory motion; moving to and fro. SEE: *vibratory.*

vibration (vī-brā′shŭn). 1. A to and fro movement. SYN: *oscillation.* 2. Therapeutic shaking of the body, a form of massage.

vibrator (vī′brā-tor). Device for causing artificial vibration of body or its parts.

   v., mechanical. Machine driven by hand or motor to give general shake-up of part desired.

   v., ossicle. Instrument for breaking up aural adhesions.

vibratory (vī′bră-tō″rĭ). Having a vibrating or oscillatory movement.

Vibrio (vĭb′rĭ-ō). A genus of short, rigid, motile bacteria, shaped like an "S" or a comma.

   V. chol′erae asiat′icae, V. com′ma. The spirillum of Asiatic cholera.

   V. Fink′leri. Same as *Vibrio proteus.*

   V. pro′teus. A species in the feces of patients with cholera nostras and cholera infantum.

   V. sputig′enus. A species found in sputum septicemia.

vibrion septique (vē-brē-on′sěp-tēk). Bacillus causing malignant edema.

vibrissae (vī-brĭs′ē) (sing. *vibrissa*). Stiff hairs within the nostrils at the ant. nares.

vibrometer (vī-brŏm′ět-ěr). Device for the treatment of deafness which produces rapid vibrations of the membrana tympani.

vibrotherapeutics (vī″brō-thěr-ă-pū′tĭks). The therapeutic application of vibration.

vicarious (vī-kā′rĭ-ŭs). Taking the place of another; pert. to assumption of the function of 1 organ by another.

   v. menstruation. Menstruation through some other channel than the vagina, as hemorrhage from the nose, from the breast, or eyes, or in form of a leukorrhea at menstrual period.

   v. respiration. Increased respiration in 1 lung when the other is lessened or abolished.

vicious (vĭsh′ŭs). Faulty, defective.

   v. cicatrix. One causing a deformity.

   v. union. Deformity caused by improper uniting of ends of a fractured bone.

Vicq d'Azyr's bundle (vĭk-dă-zēr). Mass of nerve fibers from the optic thalamus to the corpus albicans.

vidian artery (vĭd′ĭ-ăn). Branch of int. maxillary artery passing through the vidian canal.

   v. canal. Sphenoidal foramen for vivian nerve and artery.

   v. nerve. A branch from the sphenopalatine ganglion.

vigil (vĭj′ĭl). Insomnia; wakefulness.

   v., coma. Condition of muttering delirium in which patient is partially conscious and not completely comatose. SEE: *vigilambulism.*

vigilambulism (vĭj-ĭl-ăm′bū-lĭzm). The secondary state of dual or multiple personality, occurring in a state resembling somnambulism, but not during sleep.

vigintinormal (vī-jĭn″tĭ-nor′măl). Consisting of one-twentieth of what is normal, as a solution.

Vigo plaster (vē′gō). A plaster containing mercury, turpentine, wax, lead plaster, and other materials.

Villate's solution (vē-lāt′). Preparation for injection into carious bones of zinc and copper sulfate, and lead subacetate.

villi (vĭl′ī) (sing. *villus*). Tiny projections from a surface. SEE: *villus.*

   v., chorionic. Tiny branching processes of surface of chorion which become vascular and help to form the placenta.

villiferous (vĭl-ĭf′ěr-ŭs). Having villi, or tufts of hair.

villikinin (vĭl-ĭk′ĭn-ĭn). A hormone supposed to stimulate the intestinal villi.

villoma (vĭl-lō′mă). A tumor of the papillae of the mucous surfaces. SYN: *papilloma.*

villose, villous (vĭl′ōs, vĭl′ŭs). Pert. to or furnished with villi or with fine hairlike extensions.

villositis (vĭl-ōs-ī′tĭs). A bacterial disease causing inflammation of the placental villi.

villosity (vĭl-ŏs-ĭ-tĭ). 1. Condition of being furnished with villi. 2. Proliferation of a membrane. SYN: *villus.*

villus (vĭl′ŭs) (pl. *villi*). One of the short

vascular hairlike processes found on certain membranous surfaces.

v., chorionic. Tiny vascular projections on the chorionic surface which help to form the placenta. SEE: *chorion.*

Vincent's angina (vĭn'sĕnts ăn-jī'nă). Painful ulceromembranous disease of the tonsils and pharynx. SYN: *trench mouth.* SEE: *Borrelia vincenti.*

vinculum (vĭn'kū-lŭm). A uniting band or bundle. SYN: *frenulum, frenum, ligament.*

v. ten'dinum. BNA. Tendinous, slender filaments connecting the phalanges with the flexor tendons. 2. The ringlike ligament of the ankle or wrist.

vinethene (vĭn'ĕth-ēn). Proprietary general anesthetic, acting rapidly, but of short duration.

vinous (vī'nŭs). Containing or of the nature of wine.

vinum (vī'nŭm). Wine.

The medicated wines are solutions of medicinal substances in wine. They are not often prescribed. None are official.

vioform (vī'ō-form). An almost odorless substitute for iodoform.

DOSAGE: Internally 4 gr. (0.25 Gm.).

violence (vī'ō-lĕns). The use of force or physical compulsion.

violet (vī'ō-lĕt). One of the colors of the spectrum resembling purple.

v. blindness. Inability to see violet tints.

viosterol (vī-ŏs'tĕr-ōl). A solution of irradiated ergosterol in vegetable oil.

AVERAGE INFANT DOSE: 8 to 10 drops.

viraginity (vĭr-ăj-ĭn'ĭ-tĭ). Presence in a woman of masculine qualities and sexual tendencies.

virgin (vĭr'jĭn). 1. A woman (or man) who has had no sexual contact. 2. Uncontaminated; fresh; new. SEE: *virginity.*

virginal (vĭr'jĭn-ăl). Relating to a virgin or to virginity.

v. membrane. The membrane occluding the ext. orifice of the vagina. SYN: *hymen.*

virginity (vĭr-jĭn'ĭt-ĭ). The state of being a virgin; not having sustained sexual relations with the opposite sex.

viricidal (vĭ-rĭ-sī'dăl). Destructive to or inhibiting a virus. SYN: *virucidal.*

virile (vĭr'ĭl). Having characteristics of a mature male. SYN: *masculine.*

v. reflex. 1. Sudden downward movement of penis when the prepuce or gland of a completely relaxed penis is pulled upward. 2. Contraction of bulbocavernous muscle on percussing dorsum of penis. 3. Contraction of bulbocavernous muscle resulting from compression of glans penis.

virilescence (vĭr-ĭl-ĕs'ĕns). The acquisition of masculine characteristics by an aged female. [organs.

virilia (vĭr-ĭl'ĭ-ă). The male generative

virilism (vĭr'ĭl-ĭzm). Presence or development of male secondary characteristics in a woman.

v., prosopopilary. Virilism with growth of hair on face of a woman.

virility (vĭr-ĭl'ĭ-tĭ). 1. The state of possessing masculine qualities. 2. Normal power of procreation in the male sex.

viripotent (vĭr-ĭp'ō-tĕnt). 1. Sexually mature, noting male sex. 2. Marriageable, applied only to a female. SYN: *nubile.*

virology (vī-rŏl'ō-jī). The phase of biology dealing with viruses and virus diseases.

virose, virous (vī'rōs, vī'rŭs). Having poisonous qualities or effects. SYN: *poisonous.*

virtual (vĭr'tū-ăl). Being in effect, but not in fact; potential.

v. cautery. Application of caustics to a part. [virus.

virucidal (vĭ-rū-sī'dăl). Destructive of a

virulence (vĭr'ū-lĕns). 1. Relative power possessed by organisms to produce disease. 2. Property of being virulent; venomousness, as of a disease. SEE: *attenuation, avirulent.*

virulent (vĭr'ū-lĕnt). 1. Very poisonous. 2. Infectious; able to overcome the host's defensive mechanism; distinguished from toxic and pathogenic.

viruliferous (vĭr-ū-lĭf'ĕr-ŭs). Conveying or producing a virus.

virulin (vĭr'ū-lĭn). A constituent of virulent bacteria making it possible for them to resist phagocytic action.

virus (vī'rŭs). 1. The specific living morbid principle by which an infectious disease is transmitted. 2. The fluid exudate from vesicles of vaccinia used for vaccination. SYN: *vaccine lymph.*

v., attenuated. A virus so treated that it is less pathogenic.

v., dehumanized. Vaccine obtained by the inoculation of a heifer with virus from a human being.

v., filtrable. A virus causing infectious disease, the essential elements of which are so tiny that they retain infectivity after passing through a filter of the Berkefield* type.

vis (vĭs) (pl. *vires*). Force, strength, energy, power.

v. afron'te. Force that attracts.

v. formati'va. Energy resulting in development of new tissue.

v. medica'trix natu'rae. The healing power of nature.

viscera (vĭs'ĕr-ă) (sing. *viscus*). Internal organs, esp. the abdominal.

viscerad (vĭs'ĕr-ăd). Toward the viscera.

visceral (vĭs'sĕr-ăl). Pert. to viscera.

v. arches. The 4 depressions of lateral walls of the embryonic cervical region.

v. cavity. Body cavity containing the viscera.

v. clefts. The fissures separating the visceral arches.

v. crisis. Severe paroxysmal pain in any of the viscera in tabes dorsalis.

v. skeleton. The pelvis, ribs and sternum enclosing the viscera.

visceralgia (vĭs-ĕr-ăl'jĭ-ă). Neuralgia of any of the viscera.

visceralism (vĭs'ĕr-ăl-ĭzm). The idea that disease originates in the viscera.

viscerimotor (vĭs-ĕr-ĭ-mō'tor). Conveying motor impulses to a viscus.

viscerogenic (vĭs″ĕr-ō-jĕn′ĭk). Originality in the viscera, noting reflexes.

visceroinhibitory (vĭs″ĕr-ō-ĭn-hĭb′ĭ-tō-rĭ). Checking the action of the viscera.

visceromotor (vĭs″ĕr-ō-mō′tor). Conveying motor impulses to the viscera. SYN: *viscerimotor*.

visceroparietal (vĭs″ĕr-ō-pă-rī′ĕ-tăl). Relating to the viscera and the abdominal wall.

visceroperitoneal (vĭs″ĕr-ō-pĕr″ĭ-tō-nē′ăl). Relating to the abdominal viscera and peritoneum.

visceropleural (vĭs″ĕr-ō-plū′răl). Relating to the thoracic viscera and the pleura. SYN: *pleurovisceral*.

visceroptosis (vĭs-ĕr-ōp-tō′sĭs). Downward displacement of a viscus. SEE: *Glénard's disease*.

viscerosensory (vĭs″ĕr-ō-sĕn′sō-rĭ). Noting sensation caused by visceral disorder.

visceroskeletal (vĭs″ĕr-ō-skĕl′ĕt-ăl). Relating to the visceral skeleton.

viscerosomatic (vĭs″ĕr-ō-sō-măt′ĭk). Relating to the viscera and the body.

viscid (vĭs′ĭd). Adhering, glutinous, sticky.

viscidity (vĭs-ĭd′ĭ-tĭ). The property of being viscid or sticky SYN: *viscosity*.

viscosimeter (vĭs-kōs-ĭm′ĕt-ĕr). Device for estimating the viscosity of a fluid, esp. of blood.

viscosity (vĭs-kŏs′ĭ-tĭ). State of being sticky or gummy.

   v., specific. The internal friction of a fluid, measured by comparing the rate of flow of the liquid through a tube with that of some standard liquid, or by measuring the resistance to rotating paddles.

viscous (vĭs′kŭs). Sticky, gummy, gelatinous.

viscus (vĭs′kŭs) (pl. *viscera*). Any internal organ enclosed within a cavity, such as the thorax or abdomen. SEE: *viscera*.

visile (vĭz′ĭl). 1. Pert. to vision. 2. Readily recalling what is seen, more than that which is audible or motile.

vision (vĭzh′ŭn). 1. Act of viewing external objects. SYN: *sight*. 2. Sense by which light and color are apprehended. 3. Imaginary sight. [ness.

   v., achromatic. Complete color blindness.

   v., binocular. Visual sensation which is produced when the images fall on symmetrical points of each retina.

   v., central, v., direct. Vision with the fovea centralis.

   v., day. Condition in which patient sees better during the day than at night, found in peripheral lesions of the retina, such as retinitis pigmentosa.

   v., double. Seeing of one object as two. SYN: *diplopia*.

   v., field of. The space within which an object can be seen while the eye remains fixed on some one point.

   v., half. Blindness in one or both eyes for half of the visual field. SYN: *hemianopia*.

   v., indirect, v., peripheral. Vision with the retina outside of the macular field.

   v., multiple. Seeing of one object as two or more. SYN: *polyopia*.

   v., night. Condition in which patient sees better after dusk, found in lesions of the macula.

visual (vĭzh′ū-ăl). 1. Pert. to vision. 2. One whose learning and memorizing processes are largely of a visual nature.

   v. angle. Angle bet. line of sight and the extremities of object seen.

   v. axis. The line of vision, from object seen through the pupil's center to macula lutea.

   v. cone. The cone whose vertex is at the eye and whose generating lines touch the boundary of a visible object.

   v. field. The area within which objects may be seen when the eye is fixed.

   v. line. The visual axis.

   v. plane. The plane in which both optic axes lie.

   v. point. Center of vision.

   v. purple. A purple pigment in retinal rods. SYN: *rhodopsin*.

visuoauditory (vĭzh″ū-ō-aw′dĭ-tor-ĭ). Relating to sight and hearing, as connecting nerve fibers bet. auditory and visual centers.

visuognosis (vĭzh-ū-ŏg-nō′sĭs). The recognition and appreciation of what is seen.

visuometer (vĭzh-ū-ŏm′ĕ-tĕr). Device for ascertaining the range of vision.

visuopsychic (vĭzh″ū-ō-sī′kĭk). Both visual and psychic noting cerebral area involved in apprehension of visual sensations.

visuosensory (vĭzh″ū-ō-sĕn′sō-rĭ). Relating to the recognition of visual impressions.

vitaglass (vī′tă-glăs). Window glass containing quartz for transmitting the ultraviolet antirachitic rays of sunlight.

vital (vī′tăl). Pert. to or characteristic of life.

   v. capacity. Volume of air that can be expelled following full inspiration.

   v. center. Respiratory center in medulla.

   v. principle. The energy upon which all life depends.

   v. signs. Respiration, pulse, and temperature.

   v. statistics. A record of births, marriages, disease, and deaths in a certain area.

vitalism (vī′tăl-ĭzm). The opinion that a vital force neither chemical nor mechanical is responsible for bodily functions.

vitalist (vī′tăl-ĭst). One who believes in vitalism.

vitalistic (vī-tăl-ĭs′tĭk). Relating to vitalism.

vitality (vī-tăl′ĭ-tĭ). 1. Principle of life. 2. Animation, action. SYN: *strength*. 3. State of being alive.

vitals (vī′tăls). Organs of the body, esp. the heart, liver, lungs, and brain, essential to life.

vitamin(e (vī′tă-mĭn, -mēn). Any of a group of accessory organic substances existing in most foods in minute amts. in their natural state, needed in the diet for metabolism, the absence of which results in malnutrition and specific deficiency diseases.

vitamin A (fat soluble). Evidently manufactured in the body from *carotin,** which is supposed to be responsible for this vitamin in green vegetables, carrots, egg yolk, and butter.

vitamin B (water soluble). An antineuritic and beriberi vitamin composed of 17 or 18 factors.

vitamin C. This vitamin is associated with vitamins A and D and calcium and phosphorous balance in development of bone.

vitamin D. Vitamin concerned with bone formation; derived from plants, food and from the sun and ultraviolet rays.

vitamin E (fat soluble). A vitamin concerned with sterility.

vitamin G (B_2) (water soluble). A vitamin needed for growth and a healthy nervous system.

vitamin H. A factor in the B group called biotin.* It is a powerful cellular stimulant found in animal tissues. It, with avertin,* a depressant found in white of eggs, acts as a gyroscope to maintain cellular, chemical equilibrium. Lack of this equilibrium may be the cause of disease. The two factors need to be balanced in the body.

vitamin K (K_1 and K_2). The antihemorrhagic vitamin complex which aids blood coagulation.

vitamin L. A vitamin found to be necessary for lactation in rats.

vitamin P (citron). Antiscorbutic.

vitamin T. Found in vegetable oils and in egg yolk, it increases blood platelet count in humans, and is effective in purpura.

vi′tamin diets. Those containing the vitamins necessary for health.

v. high diet. Emphasis placed on leafy vegetables, fresh fruits (esp. citrus), tomatoes, fresh or canned, whole-grain cereals, butter, glandular meats (esp. liver), eggs, milk, cream. Vitamin concentrates are given when ordered by physician.

vitaminoid (vī′tăm-ĭn-oyd). Of the nature of vitamin.

vitaminology (vī″tăm-ĭn-ŏl′ō-jĭ). The science dealing with vitamins.

vita sexualis (vī′tă sĕks-ū-ā′lĭs). The sex life.

vitellary (vĭt′ĕl-ă-rĭ). Pert. to the vitellus. SYN: *vitelline.*

vitellin (vī-tĕl′ĭn). A protein which can be extracted from egg yolk and contains lecithin. SEE: *nucleoprotein, ovovitellin.*

vitelline (vī-tĕl′ĕn). Pert. to the yolk of an egg or the ovum.

v. duct. The pedicle by which the umbilical vesicle is attached to the intestine of the embryo.

v. membrane. Membrane that surrounds the ovum.

v. veins. Veins from yolk sac to heart and portal vein in the embryo.

vitellus (vī-tĕl′ŭs). The protoplasmic contents of the ovum. The yolk of the egg with its germinal (*v. format′ivus*) and

nutritive portion (*v. nutriti′vus*). SEE: *cleavage nucleus.*

vitiation (vĭsh″ĭ-ā′shŭn). Injury, contamination, impairment of use.

vitiligo (vĭt-ĭl-ī′gō). An acquired cutaneous affection characterized by milk-white patches, surrounded by areas of normal pigmentation.

vitiligoidea (vĭt-ĭl-ĭg-oyd′ē-ă). Disease marked by formation of tiny yellow patches or nodules on the skin, as on the eyelids. SYN: *xanthoma.*

vitium (vĭsh′ĭ-ŭm) (pl. *vitia*). A fault, defect, or vice.

v. cordis. An organic heart lesion.

vitodynamic (vī″tō-dĭ-năm′ĭk). Relating to vital force.

vitreocapsulitis (vĭt″rē-ō-kăp-sū-lī′tĭs). Inflammation of the vitreous humor. SYN: *hyalitis.*

vitreous (vĭt′rē-ŭs). 1. Glassy. 2. Pert. to the vitreous body. SEE: *pseudoglioma.*

v. body. A transparent jellylike mass that fills the cavity of the eyeball, enclosed by the hyaloid membrane.

v. chamber. The portion of the cavity of the eyeball behind the lens.

v. degeneration. Retrogressive change of a part into a translucent shining substance, esp. of a blood vessel wall.

v. humor of the ear. The endolymph.

v. membrane. 1. Inner one of the choroid. 2. One of hair follicles bet. outer root sheath and internal layer.

v. table. The inner layer of compact tissue belonging to most of the bones of the cranium.

vitriol (vĭt′rē-ol). A sulfate of any of various metals.

v., blue. Copper sulfate, *q.v.*

v., green. Ferrous sulfate, *q.v.*

v., oil of. Sulfuric acid, *q.v.*

v., white. Zinc sulfate, *q.v.*

vitropression (vĭt″rō-prĕsh′ŭn). Method of temporarily eliminating redness of the skin cased by hyperemia by pressure with a glass slide on the skin for purpose of studying any lesions or discolorations.

vitrum (vĭt′rŭm). Glass. *In vitro* is an expression meaning, in a test tube or in glass.

Vitus dance, St. (vī′tŭs). A functional nervous disorder causing muscular spasms. SYN: *chorea, q.v.*

vivi-. Combining form meaning *alive.*

vividiffusion (vĭv-ĭ-dĭf-ū′zhŭn). Dialysis of the blood of a living animal by removing it from an artery, passing it through tubes and back into a vein, without exposure to air.

vivification (vĭv-ĭ-fĭ-kā′shŭn). 1. Trimming of the surface layer of a wound to aid union of tissues. 2. Transformation of protein food through assimilation into the living matter of cellular organisms.

viviparous (vĭv-ĭp′ăr-ŭs). Developing young within the body, the young being expelled and born alive, the opposite of *oviparous.*

vivipation (vĭv-ĭp-ā′shŭn). A form of generation in which the ovum matures in the womb.

viviperception (vĭv″ĭ-pĕr-sĕp′shŭn). The study of the vital processes of a living body without vivisection.

vivisect (vĭv′ĭ-sĕkt). To dissect a living animal for experimental purposes.

vivisection (vĭv″ĭ-sĕk′shŭn). Cutting of or operation upon a living animal for physiological investigation and the study of disease. SEE: *biotomy, callisection.*

vivisectionist (vĭv″ĭ-sĕk′shŭn-ĭst). One who practices or believes in vivisection.

vivisector (vĭv′-ĭs-ĕk′tor). One who practices vivisection.

vivisectorium (vĭv″-ĭs-ĕk-tō′rĭ-ŭm). A place where vivisection is performed.

Vleminckx's solution (flĕm′ĭnks). A solution of sulfurated lime.

DOSAGE: Externally diluted with 5 to 10 volumes of water.

vo′cal. Pert. to the voice.

v. area. That portion of glottis bet. the vocal cords.

v. cords. Four mucous membranous folds in int. of the larynx. SEE: *chorditis nodosa.*

v. frem′itus. Chest-wall vibration felt on palpation while patient is speaking.

v. ligaments. Agents producing voice. SYN: *thyroarytenoid ligaments.*

v. process. That of the arytenoid cartilage to which are attached the vocal cords.

v. res′onance. Sound heard in auscultation of lung while patient is speaking.

v. signs. Indication of disease by changes in the voice.

voice (voys). Sound uttered by human beings, produced by vibration of the vocal cords.

voices (voys′ĕs). Verbal, auditory hallucinations. SYN: *phoneme.*

void (voyd). To evacuate the bowels or bladder.   [the hand.

vola (vō′lă). The sole of foot or palm of

v. manus. Palm of hand.

v. pedis. Sole of foot.

volar (vō′lăr). Relating to the palm, or sole of foot.

volatile (vol′ă-tĭl). CHEM: Easily vaporized or evaporated.

volatillization (vŏl″ă-tĭl-ĭ-zā′shŭn). Conversion of a solid or liquid into a vapor.

volition (vō-lĭsh′ŭn). The act or power of willing or choosing.

Volkmann's contracture (fōlk′mahn). Degeneration, contracture, and atrophy of a muscle resulting from long-continued interference with normal circulation by bandage or elastics, or from exposure to cold or injury of an artery.

volley (vŏl′ĕ). A series of artificially induced rapid muscular contractions.

volsella (vŏl-sĕl′ă). Forceps with sharp pointed hooks at end of each blade.

volt (vōlt). An electrical unit of pressure, the electromotive force required to produce 1 ampere of current through a resistance of 1 ohm.

voltage (volt′āj). Electromotive force or difference in potential expressed in volts.

v., effective. Voltage of high frequency machine when patient is in the electrical circuit.

It is that voltage which is the driving force of the diathermy current.

v., load. Same as *effective voltage.*

v., no-load. Voltage produced by high frequency apparatus while the patient is not connected in the circuit.

v., peak. Two types of diathermy voltage: (1) Peak voltage, highest instantaneous value which it reaches in its course. (2) SEE: *effective voltage.*

v., roentgen ray. Quality of x-rays is a function of the voltage at which they are generated. The lower the voltage the larger the proportion of rays of long wave length (soft rays of low power of penetration) and the higher the voltage the greater the proportion of rays of short wave length (penetrating rays).

voltaic pile (vŏl-tā′ĭk). Alternate disks of 2 dissimilar metals, as copper and zinc separated by strips of cloth wet with acid for producing electrical current.

First means of generating a constant flow of current. Invented by Volta.

voltaism (vŏl′tă-ĭzm). Electricity produced by chemical decomposition in a battery. SYN: *galvanism.*

voltameter (vŏl-tăm′ĕt-ĕr). Device for measuring force of a current in volts.

voltmeter (vōlt′mē-tĕr). A meter calibrated to measure electromotive force in volts.

Voltmeters are connected in parallel with the circuit or resistance over which the potential drop is to be measured.

Voltolini's disease (vŏl-tō-lē′nē). Primary labyrinthitis in children with symptoms of meningitis, and subsequently a staggering gait and deaf-mutism.

volubil′ity. PSY: Excessive fluency of speech.

vol′ume in′dex. An expression of average size of individual red blood cells, normally about I; indices below this indicate abnormally small red cells; above, abnormally large ones. The volume index is found by dividing the percentage of red cells into the hematocrit* percentage. SEE: *color index.*

volumetric (vŏl″ū-mĕt′rĭk). Pert. to measurement of volume.

volumette (vŏl-ū-mĕt′). Device for administering predetermined dosages of fluid, repeatedly.

volumination (vŏl-ū″mĭn-ā′shŭn). Increase in size of bacteria produced by action of serum.

volumometer (vŏl″ū-mŏm′ĕ-tĕr). Apparatus for measuring volume or changes in volume.

voluntary (vŏl′ŭn-tă-rĭ). Pert. to or under control of the will.

v. muscles. Voluntary muscles are generally attached to the skeleton, are innervated by myelinated nerves coming directly from the brain or spinal cord, and under the microscope are seen to consist of long cylindrical fibers bearing crosswise striations.

v. nervous system. Brain and spinal cord and their nerves and end organs controlling voluntary movements. SYN: central nervous system, q.v.

voluntomotory (vŏl″ŭn-tō-mō′tō-rĭ). Relating to voluntary motor influence.

voluptuous (vō-lŭp′tū-ŭs). 1. Pert. to, arising from, or provoking consciously or otherwise, sensual desire, usually applied to the female sex. 2. Given to sensualism.

volupty (vŏl′ŭp-tĭ). Sexual pleasure.

volute (vō-lūt′). Spiral, rolled up. SYN: convoluted.

volvulosis (vŏl-vū-lō′sĭs). Disease characterized by cutaneous or subcutaneous elastic fibrous tumors due to infestation with the worm Oncocerca volvulus.

volvulus (vŏl′vū-lŭs). A twisting of the bowel upon itself causing obstruction.

vomer (vō′mer). The plow-shaped bone which forms the lower and post. portion of the nasal septum, articulating with the ethmoid, splenoid, the 2 palate bones, and 2 sup. maxillary bones.

vomerine (vō′mĕr-ĭn). Pert. to the vomer.

vomerobasilar (vō″mĕr-ō-băs′ĭl-ar). Concerning the vomer and the basilar region of the cranium.

v. canal. Canal occurring at junction of sphenoid bone and vomer.

vomica (vŏm′ĭk-ă). 1. A cavity in the lungs, as from suppuration. 2. Sudden and profuse expectoration of putrid, purulent matter.

vomicose (vŏm′ĭk-ōs). Marked by many ulcers; ulcerous; purulent.

vomit (vŏm′ĭt). 1. Matter ejected from stomach through the mouth. 2. To yield up gastric and intestinal contents through the mouth.

v., bilious. Bile forced back into the stomach and ejected with vomited matter.

v., black. Vomit containing blood acted on by the gastric juice. Seen in worst form of yellow fever.

v., coffee-ground. Bloody vomit of gastric malignancy.

vomiting (vŏm′ĭt-ing). Ejection through the mouth of the gastric contents. SYN: emesis.

v., cyclic. Recurring paroxysms of vomiting.

v., dry. Nausea without vomitus.

v., incoercible. Uncontrollable vomiting.

v., pernicious. Severe vomiting of pregnancy.

v. of pregnancy. That of morning sickness.

v., projectile. Ejection of vomitus with great force.

v., stercoraceous. Vomiting of fecal matter.

vomito negro (vŏm′ĭt-ō nā′grō). Vomit containing blood darkened by gastric secretion. SYN: black vomit.

vomitory (vŏm′ĭ-tō-rĭ). 1. Causing vomiting. 2. An agent inducing emesis. 3. A vessel to receive ejecta.

vomiturition (vŏm″ĭ-tū-rĭsh′ŭn). Repeated ineffective efforts to vomit. SYN: retching.

vomitus (vŏm′ĭt-ŭs). 1. Act of ejecting matter from the stomach through the mouth. 2. Material ejected from the stomach by vomiting.

v. mari′nus. Seasickness.

v. matuti′nus. Morning vomiting of chronic gastric catarrh.

von Graefe's sign (fŏn gra′fēz). Failure of lid to move downward promptly with eyeball, the lid moving tardily and jerkily; seen in exophthalmic goiter.

von Leube motor test meal (fŏn loy′be). Soup, 400 cc.; beef, 200 Gm.; water, 200 cc. If at end of 6 hours a gastric lavage fails to show a residue, the motility of the stomach is normal.

v. L.'s test meal. Clear soup, 200 cc.; beefsteak, 200 Gm.; bread, 50 Gm.; water, 200 cc. The stomach contents are expressed in 6 hours. This is a gastric test meal.

Von Pirquet's test (fŏn pēr′kā). A diagnostic test for tuberculosis, in which a little tuberculin is applied to a scarified area of the skin of the arm.

A positive reaction is seen if a red papillar eruption appears at the site of inoculation.

Von Recklinghausen's disease (fŏn rĕk′lĭng-how″zĕn). 1. Multiple neurofibromata occurring on the skin along the course of the nerves; associated with marked cutaneous pigmentation. 2. Generalized fibrocystic disease of the bones. SYN: molluscum fibrosum.

Voorhees' bag (voor′ēz). An inflatable rubber bag for dilating the cervix uteri to induce labor.

voracious (vō-rā′shŭs). Having an insatiable or ravenous appetite.

Voronoff's method (vo′rŏn-ŏf). Attempt to rejuvenate by transplantation of the testis of a young anthropoid ape into the male.

vortex (vor′tĕks) (pl. vortices). A spiral arrangement of the cardiac muscular fibers.

vorticose (vor′tĭk-ōs). Whirling.

vox (vŏks) (pl. voces). Voice.

v. choler′ica. The suppressed voice of last stages of cholera.

voyeur (voi-ŭr′). One whose erotic stimulus is derived from looking at sexual objects or situations, such as watching others during coitus.

vril (vrĭl). The initial energy with which man is supposed to be endowed from birth and which makes it possible for him to reach full maturity and to reproduce his kind; also applied to all living organisms.

vuerometer (vū″ĕr-ŏm′ĕt-ĕr). Apparatus for measuring distance bet. the eyes.

vulgaris (vŭl-gā′rĭs). Ordinary.

vulnerable (vŭl′nĕr-ă-bl). Easily injured or wounded.

vulnerary (vŭl′nĕr-ār-ĭ). 1. Pert. to wounds. 2. A remedy used to heal wounds.

vulnerate (vŭl′nĕr-āt). To wound.

vulnus (vŭl′nŭs) (pl. *vulnera*). A wound or injury.

vulsella, vulsellum (vŭl-sĕl′ă, vŭl-sĕl′ŭm). A forceps with a hook on each blade. SYN: *volsella*.

vulva (vŭl′vă) (pl. *vulvae*). The ext. female genitalia lying beneath the mons veneris consisting of the labia majora, labia minora, and clitoris.

    v. cerebri. A small opening leading from third ventricle of brain into the infundibulum.

    v., vestibule of. The portion of the vulva immediately behind the mouth of the vagina.

vulvar (vŭl′var). Relating to the vulva.

vulvectomy (vŭl-vĕk′tō-mĭ). Excision of the vulva.

vulvismus (vŭl-vĭz′mŭs). Painful spasm of the vagina. SYN: *vaginismus*.

vulvitis (vŭl-vī′tĭs). Inflammation of the vulva.

    v., leukoplakic. Atrophy and wrinkling of the vulva with discoloration.

vulvo-. Combining form meaning *a covering, the vulva.*

vulvocrural (vŭl″vō-krū′răl). Relating to the vulva and the thigh.

vulvopathy (vŭl-vŏp′ă-thĭ). Any disorder of the vulva.

vulvouterine (vŭl″vō-ū′tĕr-ĭn). Relating to the vulva and uterus.

vulvovaginal (vŭl″vō-văj′ĭn-ăl). Pert. to the vulva and vagina.

    v. glands. Small glands on either side of the vulvar orifice. SEE: *Bartholin's glands.*

vulvovaginitis (vŭl″vō-văj″ĭn-ī′tĭs). Inflammation of both the vulva and vagina at the same time, or of the vulvovaginal glands.

W

W. Chemical symbol for *tungsten*.

Wachendorf's membrane (vahk'ĕn-dōrf).
1. A thin vascular membrane occluding the pupil in the fetus. SYN: *membrana pupillaris*. 2. The outer membrane ensheathing a cell.

Wachsmuth's mixture (vahks'moot). Mixture of 5 parts of chloroform and 1 of oil of turpentine for general anesthesia.

wafer (wā'fer). 1. A thin sheet of flour paste used to enclose a medicinal dose of powder. 2. A flat vaginal suppository.

Wagner's corpuscles (vahg'ner). The oval-shaped end organs of certain nerve fibers. SYN: *tactile corpuscles*.

W.'s spot. Germinal spot in an ovum.

Wagstaffe's fracture (wăg'stăf). One with separation of the internal malleolus.

waist (wāst). Small part of body bet. thorax and hips. SEE: *cincture sensation*.

wakefulness (wāk'fŭl-nĕs). State marked by inability to sleep. SYN: *insomnia*.

Walcheren fever (vahl'kha-ren). A severe type of malarial fever found in Holland.

Walcher's position (vahl'ker). The patient assumes the dorsal-recumbent position with the legs hanging down over the end of the table from just above the knees, the legs fairly well separated.

walking (wauk'ing). Act or manner of movement on foot without running, as for exercise.

w. apparatus. Apparatus to aid walking of patients with weak or paralyzed leg muscles.

w. typhoid. Typhoid fever in which the symptoms are mild so that the patient is ambulatory.

wall (wawl). A limiting structure or partition often forming an enclosure, as the abdominal wall.

wallerian degeneration (wŏl-ē'rĭ-ăn). Degeneration of a nerve fiber severed from its trophic center.

walleye (wawl'ī). 1. Eye in which iris is light-colored or white. 2. Leukoma or dense opacity of cornea. 3. Squint in which both visual axes diverge. SYN: *divergent strabismus*.

wall-plate (wawl'plāt). Apparatus for furnishing low tension and low frequency current.

wan'dering. Moving about; not fixed.

w. abscess. One that burrows and comes to the surface at a point distant from its origin.

w. cell. A leukocyte which moves about the substance of an organ.

w. kidney, w. spleen. Dislocated floating kidney or spleen.

Wangensteen's method (wăng'ĕn-stēn). Technic for relieving postoperative distention, nausea and vomiting and certain cases of mechanical bowel obstruction.

ward (ward). A large room or hall in a hospital.

w., accident. One reserved for accident cases.

w., isolation. One for isolation of those suspected of being affected with an infectious disease.

w., psychopathic. One in a general hospital for temporary reception of mental cases.

Wardrop's disease (war'drŏp). Acute inflammation of matrix of the nail in scrofulous children. SYN: *onychia maligna*.

W.'s operation. Ligation of an artery for aneurysm at a distance beyond the sac.

warehousemen's itch (wār'hows-mēnz ĭtsh). Eczema of hands from touching irritating substances.

war gases. There are at least 4 classes of these gases: (1) Suffocating gases; (2) irritating gases; (3) vesicants, and (4) general poisons or toxic gases. Some of these are explosive.

warm-blooded. Having a high and constant body temperature. SYN: *homothermal*.

wart (wort). A circumscribed cutaneous elevation resulting from hypertrophy of the papillae and epidermis. SYN: *verruca, q.v.*

w., seborrheic. Patch of corneous hypertrophy on face of the aged.

w., senile. SEE: *seborrheic wart*.

w.'s venereal. Vegetating growths upon skin, esp. on the mucocutaneous juncture of the genitals, having an offensive discharge. SYN: *verruca acuminata*.

warty (war'tĭ). Relating to or covered with warts.

wash (wash). 1. To bathe with a fluid, as an injured part. 2. A lotion.

washerwomen's itch (wash'ĕr-wŭm"ăn). Eczema of the hands of laundry workers.

wash-leath'er skin. A trophic change in the skin in which silver drawn across it leaves a black mark.

wasp sting. Sting form a wasp, which causes a general urticaria. SEE: *hornet sting*.

Wassermann-fast (vas'ĕr-mahn). Indicating a positive reaction shown by a Wassermann test which continues after repeated antisyphilitic medication.

W. reaction. Serum complement fixation test as a diagnosis of syphilis.

The results are designated as 1, 2, 3, and 4 plus, the intensity of the reaction usually corresponding to the severity of the infection. The disease may still exist with a negative reaction. Several such reactions would indicate its absence. Several years after treatment and after last "negative" is obtained should pass before cure is definitely accepted.

waste (wăst). 1. To shrink in physical bulk or strength, as from disease. 2. Loss by breaking down of bodily tissue. 3. Refuse material no longer useful to an organism.

   w. products. Carbon dioxide, organic and inorganic salts, water, dead skin, hair, nails, undigested foods.

   w. p.'s, metabolic. Soluble salts in the form of nitrogenous salts (urea) and inorganic salts (sodium chloride); gas in form of carbon dioxide, and liquid in the form of water.

   They are excreta, removed by the process of elimination, q.v.

wasting (wăst'ĭng). Enfeebling; causing loss of strength or size; emaciating. SEE: *marasmus.*

   w. palsy or **paralysis.** Chronic disease marked by gradual atrophy of muscular tissue with paralysis. SYN: *progressive muscular atrophy.*

water (waw'tĕr). 1. A solution in water of a volatile substance. 2. The urine. 3. H_2O, hydrogen and oxygen, a tasteless, clear odorless fluid, constituting bet. 75% and 90% of all tissues.

   w.-bed. A rubber mattress, filled 3 parts full with warm water (temp. 100° F.); must not be too full or it will be hard. Fracture boards are placed across the wire mattress to produce a firm foundation and prevent sagging; it should be refilled every fortnight.

   w.-borne. Disease spread by germs in drinking water or bath water.

   w. on brain. Disease marked by abnormal increase in cerebral fluid. SYN: *hydrocephalus.*

   w. brash. Gastric burning pain with eructations. SYN: *heartburn.*

   w.-cure. Use of water in treatment. SYN: *hydrotherapy.*

   w.-hammer pulse. Pulse marked by quick powerful beat, collapsing suddenly. SYN: *Corrigan's pulse, q.v.*

   w., heavy. Water incapable of supporting life containing the mass 2 isotope of hydrogen.

   w.-pox. True chickenpox or varicella, q.v.

water balance diet. Water content of diet is calculated to individual prescription. The water content of foods as well as beverages is calculated as part of the fluid allowance given in the diet prescription.

waters (waw'tĕrs). Common term for the amniotic fluid surrounding the fetus.

   w., bag of. Sac enclosing liquor amnii surrounding the fetus. SYN: *amniotic sac.*

watt (wŏt). A unit of electric power equal to work done at rate of 1 joule per second or work represented by current of 1 ampere under a pressure of 1 volt.

   w.-hour. An electrical unit of work or energy. It is equal to the wattage multiplied by the time in hours. Its mechanical equivalent is 2655 foot-pounds.

wattage (wŏt'ăj). The consumption of electricity measured in watts.

wattmeter (wŏt'mē-tĕr). Device for measuring consumption of an electric current.

wave (wāv). 1. A disturbance of the equilibrium of a body or medium propagated from point to point with a continuous motion through a closed curve. 2. An undulating or vibrating motion.

   w., hertzian. Electromagnetic radiations used in radio and wireless transmission.

   w. length. The distance bet. corresponding points in 2 adjacent waves; e. g., bet. 2 crests.

   w., pulse. Elevation of the pulse noted by the finger or in curve graphically recorded by the sphygmograph.

   w.'s, Traube-Hering. Rhythmical fluctuations in arterial pressure due to disturbance of the respiratory center.

wax (wăks). 1. A substance secreted by bees. SYN: *cera.* 2. Anything having the physical properties of, or resembling beeswax. 3. Earwax. SYN: *cerumen.* SEE: *ceroplasty.*

waxing kernels (wăks'ĭng kĕr'nĕls). Enlarged lymph glands, forming small tumors, seen esp. in children.

waxy (wăks'ĭ). Resembling or pert. to wax.

   w. cast. Dense, highly refractile urinary cast.

   w. degeneration. Amyloid degeneration seen in wasting diseases.

weak (wĕk). Deficient in strength of body; infirm.

wean (wēn). To accustom to loss of breast milk by substitution of other nourishment.

weaning brash (wēn'ĭng brăsh). Severe diarrhea sometimes attacking infants just weaned.

weasand (wē'zănd). Esophagus or windpipe; loosely, the throat.

webbed (wĕbd). Having a membrane connecting adjacent structures, as the duck's feet.

   w. fingers, w. toes. Two or more toes or fingers connected by a membrane.

weber (wē'bĕr). 1. Ampere. 2. Coulomb. Both uses are obsolete.

Weber's syndrome (wĕb'er). Palsy of 3rd cranial nerve on 1 side and hemiplegia on the other side.

weeping (wēp'ĭng). 1. Shedding tears. 2. Moist; dripping.

   w. eczema. Dermatitis with eruption of vesicles exuding serum.

   w. sinew. Circumscribed cystic swelling of a tendon sheath.

Weidel's reaction (vī'dĕl). Test for presence of xanthine bodies or uric acid.

Weigert's law (vī'gĕrt). Loss or destruction of organic elements is usually followed by excessive production during reparative process.

weight (wāt). 1. The property of matter which causes it to fall to the earth by gravitation. 2. Amt. of such a tendency.

Weight and Height Ratio

Lbs.	H.	Lbs.	H.
115	5 ft. 0 in.	155	5 ft. 8 in.
120	5 " 1 "	160	5 " 9 "
125	5 " 2 "	165	5 " 10 "
130	5 " 3 "	170	5 " 11 "
135	5 " 4 "	175	6 " 0 "
140	5 " 5 "	180	6 " 1 "
145	5 " 6 "	185	6 " 2 "
150	5 " 7 "	190	6 " 3 "

w., atomic. Weight of an atom of elementary substances compared with that of oxygen, which is taken as 16.

w., molecular. Weight of a molecule of substance compared with hydrogen being equal to the sum of weights of its constituent atoms.

weights and measures. SEE: *apothecaries' measures, avoirdupois measures, metric system.*

Weil's disease (vīl, wīl). An acute infectious febrile disorder, caused by a spirochete.

Weir Mitchell's treatment (wēr mĭt'shĕl). Rest in bed, massage, nourishing diet and isolation for hysteria and neurasthenia.

Welch's bacillus (wĕlsh). Rod-shaped organism, nonmotile, encapsulated organism, frequently causing gas gangrene. SYN: *Bacillus aerogenes capsulatus.*

wen (wĕn). A cyst resulting from the retention of secretion in a sebaceous gland. SYN: *steatoma.*

Werlhof's disease (verl'hof). Form of progressive purpura marked by hemorrhages from the mucous membranes and severe prostration. SYN: *purpura haemorrhagica.*

Wernicke's syndrome (ver'nĭk-ē). Condition of old age frequently seen, marked by loss of memory and disorientation with confabulation. SYN: *presbyophrenia, q.v.*

Westphal's nucleus (vĕst'fahl). Small bulbar one post. to and above nucleus of the 4th cranial nerve.

W's. phenom'enon, W's. sign. Loss of the knee jerk, the patellar reflex.

wet (wĕt). Soaked with moisture.

w. brain. Increased amt. of cerebrospinal fluid with edema of the meninges, due to alcoholism.

w. cup. A cupping glass used after scarification.

w. dream. Nocturnal seminal emission during a sex dream.

w. nurse. A woman who gives suck to another's child.

w. pack. A form of bath, given by wrapping patient in hot or cold wet sheets, covered with a blanket, used esp. to reduce fever.

whartonitis (hwar"ton-ī'tĭs). Inflammation of Wharton's duct in the submaxillary gland.

Wharton's duct (hwar'ton). That of the sublingual gland (2 in. long) opening into the mouth at side of the *frenum linguae.*

W's. jelly. A gelatinous basic substance in the umbilical cord.

wheal (hwēl). More or less round and evanescent elevation of the skin, white in center with pale red periphery, accompanied by itching.

wheeze (hwēz). 1. A sound made by air as it passes with difficulty through the glottis and fauces in difficult respiration. 2. To breathe noisily or with effort.

wheezing (hwē'zĭng). Noisy and difficult breathing.

whelk (hwĕlk). A wheal; a protuberance on the face, as a nodule or tubercle.

whey (hwā). The liquid left after milk has been coagulated by the aid of rennet.

whipworm (hwĭp'worm). A round worm often parasitic in the human intestines. SEE: *Trichocephalus dispar.*

whirl (hwirl). To revolve rapidly; to feel giddiness.

whirlbone (hwirl'bōn). 1. The kneecap. SYN: *patella.* 2. The head of the femur.

whisky, whiskey (hwĭs'kē). A distilled alcoholic liquor made from grain. SYN: *spiritus frumenti.*

whisper (hwĭs'per). 1. Speech without voice; a low, sibilant sound. 2. To utter in a low, nonvocal sound.

w., cavernous. Direct transmission of a whisper through a cavity in auscultation.

white (hwīt). 1. The achromatic color of highest brilliance. 2. Of the color of milk.

w. cell, w. corpuscle. The leukocyte. SEE: *blood, corpuscle.*

w. gangrene. Gangrene due to local anemia.

w. leg. Phlebitis of femoral vein marked by white swelling of the leg. SYN: *phlegmasia alba dolens.*

w. line. White tendinous attachment of abdominal oblique and transverse muscles. SYN: *linea* alba.

w. matter, w. substance. Any nervous structure composed of white medullated nerve fibers.

w. precipitate. SEE: *ammoniated mercury.*

w. softening. Stage of softening of any substance in which the affected area has become white and anemic.

w. swelling. Tuberculous arthritis. SEE: *gonatocele.*

whites (hwīts). A thick, whitish vaginal discharge. SYN: *leukorrhea, q.v.*

White's operation (hwīt). Castration for relief of enlarged prostate.

whitlow (hwĭt'lō). Suppurative inflammation at the end of a finger or toe. SYN: *felon, panaris, paronychia, q.v.*

wholesome (hōl'sŭm). Promoting physical well-being.

whoop (hoop). The sonorous and convulsive inspiratory crow following a paroxysm of whooping cough.

whooping cough (hoop'ĭng kawf). An acute infectious disease with recurrent spasms of coughing ending in a whooping inspiration. SYN: *pertussis, q.v.*
SEE: *bex convulsiva, chin cough.*

whorl (hwurl). 1. Spiral arrangement of cardiac muscular fibers. SYN: *vortex.* 2.

A type of fingerprint in which the central papillary ridges turn through at least 1 complete circle.

Widal's reaction or **test** (vē-dal'). An agglutination test for typhoid fever.

wild cherry (*prunus virginiana*). USP. The dried bark of the plant, used principally in the form of the syrup as a vehicle for cough medicine.

DOSAGE: 2½ drams (10 cc.).

Wilde's cords (wīld). Fibrous bands which cross the callosum transversely.

W's. incision or **operation.** Incision behind the auricle for relief of mastoid abscess.

will (wĭl). Power of controlling one's actions or emotions.

Willis' bands (wĭl'ĭs). Those crossing the sup. longitudinal sinus, transversely.

W. circle. The intercommunications established at the base of the brain bet. the branches of the basilar and internal carotid arteries.

Wilson's disease (wĭl'sun). A rare disease of degeneration of corpus striatum and cirrhosis of the liver, characterized by tremulous distortion of the muscles (increased by activity), dysarthria, dysphagia, and emotionalism.

Wimshurst machine (wĭmz'hurst). A type of influence machine to produce static current.

Winckel's disease (vĭn'kĕl). A fatal disease of the newborn characterized by profuse hemorrhages, hematuria, jaundice, enlarged spleen, and punctiform hemorrhages upon the skin. SEE: *Buhl's disease.*

windage (wĭnd'ăj). Compression of air by passage of a missile near the body causing injury of an internal organ by the external concussion.

windpipe (wĭnd'pīp). Passage for breath from the larynx to the lungs. SYN: *trachea, q.v.*

wink (wĭnk). 1. To close and open the eyelids quickly. 2. Act of closing and opening the eyelids quickly. SEE: *mication, nictitation.*

win'ter itch. Itching occurring only in the winter. SYN: *pruritus hiemalis.*

Winternitz's ablutions (vĭn'ter-nĭts). Patient sits on edge of bathtub, back exposed. Cold water from hose is allowed to flow down back while the back is rubbed vigorously.

Wirsung, duct of (vēr'soong). Excretory duct of the pancreas. SYN: *pancreatic duct.*

wisdom tooth (wĭz'dŏm). The hindmost or last molar tooth on each side of the jaw, which may appear as late as the 25th year.

witches' milk (wĭtsh'es). Milk secreted by the newly born infant's breast, stimulated by the lactating hormone circulating in the mother.

witherings (wĭth'ĕr-ĭngs). Tumor due to fatty degeneration and absorption of epithelial cells. SYN: *scirrhus, atrophic.*

wolffian body (wool'fĭ-ăn). An embryonic organ on each side of the vertebral column. SYN: *mesonephros.* SEE: *archinephron, embryo, paroöphoron, parovarium.*

w. cyst. One of the broad ligaments of the uterus.

w. duct. The mesonephric canal that joins post. end of the intestine. SEE: *epoöphoron.*

w. tubules. Small tubes joining the wolffian duct at right angles.

wom'an. An adult female person. SEE: *misogyny.*

womb (woom). Female organ for protection and nourishment of the fetus. SYN: *uterus, q.v.*

wood alcohol (wud al'kō-hŏl). Alcohol obtained by distillation from wood.

It is a poisonous substance and frequently causes loss of sight. SEE: *methyl alcohol.*

Wood's filter. A screen that absorbs visible rays but allows a portion of the ultra-violet rays to be transmitted.

wood tick. Parasite which bites man and produces wheals with itching central punctures causing spotted or Rocky Mountain spotted* fever.

woolsorter's disease (wool'sor-ter). A pulmonary form of anthrax which develops in those who handle wool contaminated with *Bacillus anthrax.*

word blindness. Inability to comprehend written words; a form of aphasia, *q.v.*

w. salad. The use of words with no apparent meaning attached to them or to their relations one with another; usually found in schizophrenia.

work (wurk). For definition, SEE: *erg.* For comparison of various energy units, SEE: *calorie, unit.*

worm (werm). 1. An invertebrate, cylindrical animal of the group *Vermes.* 2. Any small, limbless, creeping animal. 3. Median portion of the cerebellum. 4. Any wormlike structure.

w. abscess. Abscess resulting from lodgment of a worm in the body.

w. fever. Fever due to irritation caused by worms in the intestinal canal.

worms (werms). Any disorder due to the presence of parasitic worms in the body.

wormian bones (wur'mĭ-ăn). Small, irregular bones in the course of the cranial sutures.

worsted test (wus'tĕd). Matching of the differently colored skeins of worsted yarn to detect color blindness. SYN: *Holmgren's test.*

wound (woond). Break in the continuity of soft parts from violence or trauma of tissues.

w., abdominal. Frequently sustained; ordinarily involves structure of abdominal wall.

w., bullet. A puncture wound from a bullet. Usually there is a small point of entrance; if the bullet left the body a larger point of exit; it is associated with injuries of bone, tendon, blood vessels, etc.

w., cellulitis of. When wounds have been closed without drainage, esp. ...

such cases as appendicitis, local inflammation of the wound may occur.

w., contused. A bruise. It may be caused by a blunt instrument.

w., crushing. If bleeding, apply cold cloths; if not, gently mold to proper shape, apply cloth dipped in warm water, and keep warm. If bone is fractured, apply splint.

w., fish-hook. Imbedded fish hooks are notably difficult to remove. Push the hook through, then cut off barb with an instrument. These injuries frequently become infected, so carefully saturate with an antiseptic and cover with a dressing, and observe for several days.

w., gunshot. Penetrating or perforating wound which may contain a foreign body, as a bullet.

w., incised. A clean-cut wound.

w., lacerated. A torn wound.

w., open. Contusion where skin is also broken, such as a gunshot wound, incised wound, or lacerated wound.

w., perforating. One in which the vulnerating body both enters and emerges from the cavity.

w., poisoned. This may be classed as a lacerated wound, or a punctured wound, depending on tearing of tissue.

w., punctured. One made by sharp-pointed instrument, such as a dagger, an ice pick, or needle. The chief danger is from thrombosis and possible release of emboli. A puncture wound never gives access to int. of wound. Tetanus germs thrive in such a wound, as they live in darkness and progress rapidly without air. Inspect instrument that caused the wound. The puncture should be found and, if possible, squeezed until the blood flows.

w., subcutaneous. Include all which are unaccompanied by break in skin. As contusions.

w. tearing off parts. If completely severed, treat same as lacerated wound. A few drops of carbolic acid should be used in water for washing wounds. Watch for shock. If parts are not completely severed, gently bring into position, apply splints where necessary, and bandage until surgical aid is obtainable. Watch for shock.

Wrisberg's ansa (vrĭz'berk). Loop made by anastomosis of right pneumogastric and great splanchnic nerves with right semilunar ganglion.   [of larynx.

W's. cartilage. Cuneiform cartilage

W's. ganglion. One often found in superficial cardiac plexus.

W's. nerve. 1. Small branch of the brachial plexus. 2. Small int. cutaneous nerve bet. facial and auditory nerves.

wrist (rĭst). The joint bet. hand and arm; the carpus, consisting of 8 bones.

w. clonus. Irregular convulsive movements of the hand due to inability to control the muscles that bend the wrist backward.

w. clonus reflex. Lateral clonic movements of hand occurring when hand is held down at arms length in extreme extension.

w.-drop. A dropping of the hand caused by paralysis of extensor muscles of fingers and wrist.

w. joint. Joint formed by the radius and the first row of carpal bones.

wri'ter's cramp. An occupational disability due to excessive writing.

writing hand. Position seen in paralysis agitans marked by contraction of muscle of the hand.

The fingers assume the position similar to holding a pen.

wryneck (rī'nĕk). Contracted state of 1 or more muscles of the neck, producing an abnormal position of the head. SYN: *loxia, torticollis.*

Wunderlich's curve (voon'dĕr-lĭk). The fever curve typical of typhoid fever.

X

X. 1. Chemical symb. for *xenon*. 2. Abbr. of *Kienböck's unit*. 3. Roman numeral 10. 4. Symb. of *reactance*.

xanthelasma (zăn-thĕl-ăz'mă). 1. Yellow. 2. Flat or slightly raised yellowish tumor occurring in elderly persons, found most frequently on the upper and lower lids, esp. near the inner canthus. SYN: *xanthoma*.

xanthelasmoidea (zăn-thel-ăz-moy'dē-ă). Chronic disease of childhood marked by wheals and followed by brownish-yellow patches. SYN: *urticaria pigmentosa*.

xanthematin (zăn-thĕm'ă-tĭn). A yellow substance derivable from hematin when treated with nitric acid.

xanthemia (zăn-thē'mĭ-ă). Yellow pigment in the blood. SYN: *carotinemia*.

xanthic (zăn'thĭk). 1. Yellow. 2. Pert. to xanthine.

    x. calculus. A urinary concretion containing xanthine.

xanthin(e (zăn'thĭn, -thēn). A nitrogenous extractive contained in muscle tissue, liver, spleen, pancreas, and other organs, and in the urine, formed during the metabolism of nucleoproteins.

    x. bases. Nitrogenous substances resulting from splitting up of nucleins. SEE: *purine bases*.

xanthinuria (zăn-thĭn-ū'rĭ-ă). Excretion of large amounts of xanthine in the urine.

xanthochromia (zăn"thō-krō'mĭ-ă). Yellow discoloration, as of the skin in patches or of the cerebrospinal fluid, resembling jaundice.

xanthochroous (zăn-thok'rō-ŭs). Having a yellowish or light complexion.

xanthocyanopia, xanthocyanopsia (zăn"thō-sĭ-ăn-ō'pĭ-ă, -ŏp'sĭ-ă). A form of color blindness in which yellow and blue are distinguishable, but not red and green.

xanthoderma (zăn"thō-der'mă). Yellowness of the skin.

xanthodont, xanthodontous (zăn'thō-dŏnt, zăn-thō-dŏn'tŭs). Having yellow teeth.

xanthokyanopy (zăn"thō-kĭ-ăn'ō-pĭ). Partial blindness for color, yellow and blue only being discerned. SYN: *xanthocyanopia*.

xanthoma (zăn-thō'mă). Flat, slightly elevated, soft, rounded, chamois-covered plaque or nodule, usually on the eyelids.

    x. diabeticorum. Cutaneous disease associated with diabetes mellitus.

    x. mul'tiplex. Xanthomas all over the body.   [the eyelids.

    x. palpebra'rum. Xanthoma affecting

    x. tuberosum. A form which may appear on the neck, shoulders, trunk, or extremities, consisting of small, elastic, and yellowish-colored nodules.

xanthomatosis (zăn-thō-mă-tō'sĭs). General eruption of xanthomas. SYN: *xanthoma multiplex*.

xanthomelanous (zăn"thō-mĕl'ăn-ŭs). Having black hair and an olive skin.

xanthopathy (zăn-thŏp'ă-thĭ). Yellowish pigmentation of the skin. SYN: *xanthochromia, xanthoderma*.

xanthophane (zăn'thō-fān). A yellow pigment in the retinal cones.

xanthoplasty (zăn-thō-plăs'tĭ). Yellow color of the skin. SYN: *xanthoderma*.

xanthoproteic (zăn"thō-prō-te'ĭk). Derived from or pertaining to xanthoprotein.

    x. reaction. Deep orange color produced by adding ammonia and heating proteids with nitric acid; a test for protein.

xanthoprotein (zăn"thō-prō'tē-ĭn). Yellowish substance produced by heating proteids with nitric acid.

xanthopsia (zăn-thŏp'sĭ-ă). Condition in which objects appear yellow.

xanthopsin (zăn-thŏp'sĭn). Visual yellow, the visual purple produced by light acting on rhodopsin.

xanthopsis (zăn-thŏp'sĭs). Yellow pigmentation seen in cancers.

xanthopsydracia (zăn"thŏp-sĭ-drā'shĭ-ă). Skin disease marked by the formation of yellow pustules or pimples on the skin.

xanthosarcoma (zăn"thō-sar-kō'mă). Giant cell sarcoma of tendon sheaths containing xanthoma cells.

xanthosis (zăn-thō'sĭs). A yellowish pigmentation, esp. seen in degenerating tissues and malignancies.

    x. diabet'ica. Yellowish skin seen in diabetics.

xanthous (zăn'thŭs). Yellow.

xanthuria (zăn-thū'rĭ-ă). Excretion of an excess of xanthine in the urine. SYN: *xanthinuria*.

x chromosome. A chromosome which probably carries sexual characteristics and passes whole into the daughter cell. SYN: *chromosome, accessory*.

x-disease. General malaise with disturbances of digestion, cardiac action, respiration, with extreme sensitiveness to cold.

x-element. Aggregate of accessory chromosomes, paired or unpaired with group of varying size or shape known as the y-element.

xenogenous (zĕn-ŏj'ĕn-ŭs). 1. Caused by a foreign body. 2. Originating in the host, as a toxin resulting from stimuli applied to cells of the host.

xenomenia (zĕn-ō-mē'nĭ-ă). Menstruation from a part of the body other than the normal one. SYN: *vicarious menstruation*.

xenon (zē'non). A gaseous element in the atmosphere. At. wt. 131.3. SYMB: Xe.

xenoparasite (zĕn"ō-păr'ă-sīt). One that may become pathogenic if the resistance of the host has been weakened.

xenophobia (zĕn″ō-fō'bĭ-ă). Abnormal reluctance to meeting strangers.

xenophonia (zĕn″ō-fō'nĭ-ă). Alteration in accent and intonation of a person's voice due to defect of speech.

xenophthalmia (zĕn-ŏf-thăl'mĭ-ă). Inflammation of the eye caused by a foreign body.

xeransis (zē-răn'sĭs). Loss of moisture in tissue or drugs brought about gradually. SYN: siccation.

xerantic (zē-răn'tĭk). Causing dryness. SYN: siccant, siccative.

xerasia (zē-rā'sĭ-ă). Disease of the hair in which there is abnormal dryness, followed by brittleness, and eventually loss.

xero- (zē″rō-). Prefix meaning dry.

xerocheilia (zē″rō-kī'lĭ-ă). Dryness of the lips; a type of cheilitis.

xeroderma (zē-rō-der'mă). Roughness and dryness of the skin; mild ichthyosis.

   x. pigmento'sum. A rare disease of the skin starting in childhood marked by disseminated pigment discolorations, ulcers, cutaneous and muscular atrophy and death. SYN: Kaposi's disease.

xerodermatic (zē″rō-der-măt'ĭk). Relating to xeroderma.

xeroma (zē-rō'mă). An abnormally dry state of the conjunctiva. SYN: xerophthalmia.

xeromenia (zē-rō-mē'nĭ-ă). The occurrence of the usual disturbances during menses without menstrual flow.

xeromycteria (zē-rō-mĭk-tē'rĭ-ă). Dryness of the nasal passages.

xeronosus (zē-rŏn'ō-sŭs). Dryness of the skin.

xerophagia (zē-rō-fā'jĭ-ă). The eating of dry food only.

xerophthalmia (zē-rŏf-thăl'mĭ-ă). Conjunctival dryness with keratinization of epithelium following chronic conjunctivitis and in disease due to deficency of Vitamin A.

xerosis (zē-rō'sĭs). 1. Abnormal dryness of skin, mucous membranes, or of the conjunctiva. 2. Normal sclerosis of tissues in the aged.

xerostomia (zē-rō-stō'mĭ-ă). Dryness of the mouth.

xerotes (zē'rō-tēz). Dryness of the body; dryness.

xerotocia (zē-rō-tō'shĭ-ă). Dry labor.

xerotic (zē-rŏt'ĭk). Dry; characterized by dryness.

xerotripsis (zē″rō-trĭp'sĭs). Dry friction.

xiphi-, **xipho-** (zif-i-, -o-). Prefixes pert. to the xiphoid cartilage.

xiphisternum (zĭf-ĭ-ster'nŭm). The pointed process of the lower end of the sternum. SYN: xiphoid cartilage.

xiphocostal (zĭf″ō-kŏs'tăl). Relating to the xiphoid cartilage and the ribs.

   x. ligament. One connecting the xiphoid cartilage to the cartilage of the 8th rib.

xiphodynia (zĭf-ō-dĭn'ĭ-ă). Pain in the ensiform cartilage.

xiphoid (zĭf'oyd). Sword-shaped, ensiform.

   x. process. The lowest portion of the sternum, a sword-shaped cartilaginous process supported by bone.

xiphoiditis (zĭf-oyd-ī'tĭs). Inflammation of the ensiform or xiphoid cartilage.

x-knee. Knock-knee.

xoanthropy (zō-ăn'thrō-pĭ). Monomania in which one believes himself to be an animal.

X-radiation unit. SYMB: r. Amt. of x-radiation which, when the secondary electrons are fully utilized, and wall effect of the chamber is avoided, produces in 1 cc. of atmospheric air at 0° C. and 76 cm. mercury pressure such degree of conductivity that 1 electrostatic unit of charge is measured at saturation current.

x-ray. 1. Any of the radiations of an extremely short wave length, emitted primarily as result of sudden change in velocity of a moving electric charge and as the result of atomic changes of target due to this impact. 2. A photograph obtained by use of x-rays.

   x. dermatitis. Cutaneous inflammation due to exposure to x-rays.

   x. unit. Unit of x-ray dosage equal to 1/10 the erythema dose.

xylenin (zī'lē-nĭn). A toxic substance extracted by xylene from tubercle bacilli.

xylo- (zī-lō-). Prefix pert. to or derived from wood.

xylol (zī'lŏl). A commercial mixture of the 3 xylenes (ortho, meta, and para dimethylbenzene).

xylose (zī'lōs). Wood sugar, a crystalline, nonfermentable pentose.

xylotherapy (zī″lō-ther'ă-pĭ). Therapeutic application of certain woods to the body.

xyrospasm (zī'rō-spăzm). Occupational neurosis of the fingers seen in barbers.

xysma (zĭz'mă). In diarrhea, flocculent pseudomembranous matter sometimes seen in stools.

xyster (zĭs'ter). A surgeon's rasp, used mainly for scraping bones. SYN: raspatory.

xystus (zĭs'tŭs). Scraped lint.

Y

Y. symb. of element *yttrium*.

yaghourt (yah-ghoort'). Milk curdled by a ferment possessing an active lactic acid bacillus, *B. bulgaricus*, used in Bulgaria.

Y-angle. Angle bet. line uniting lambda an inion and radius fixus.

yard. 1. A measure of 3 feet or 36 inches. 2. The penis.

yatren (yăt'rĕn). Commercial brand of chiniofon, *q.v.*

yava skin (yah'va skĭn). A form of elephantiasis due to the excessive use of kava. SEE: *elephantiasis*.

yawn. 1. To open the mouth involuntarily, as in drowsiness or fatigue. 2. Involuntary act of gaping, accompanied by attempts at inspiration, excited by drowsiness.

yawning (yawn'ĭng). Deep inspiration, gaping induced by drowsiness or fatigue. SYN: *oscitation*.

yaws (yawz). An infectious tropical disease. SYN: *frambesia*.

Yb. The symb. for *ytterbium*.

Y bacil'lus. A dysentery bacillus.

Y car'tilage. The cartilage uniting the 3 pelvic bones at bottom of the acetabulum early in life.

y chromosome. An accessory chromosome in male cells supposed to be the male determining principle in fertilization. SEE: *chromosome, heredity*.

yeast (yēst). 1. A substance composed of aggregated cells (Saccharomyces) of minute unicellular sac fungi. 2. A commercial product composed of meal impregnated with living yeast.

y. enema. One quart of warm water and ½ cake of yeast, thoroughly mixed and given very warm.

yelk (yelk). Variant of yolk.

yellow (yĕl'ō). 1. One of the primary colors resembling that of a ripe lemon. 2. Colored yellow, as the skin in disease.

y. fever. An acute infectious disease characterized by jaundice, epigastric tenderness, vomiting, hemorrhages, and a febrile course consisting of 2 paroxysms.

y. softening. A stage of softening of the brain marked by fatty degeneration and yellow discoloration.

y. spot. 1. Yellowish nodule at ant. end of vocal cord. 2. Center of the retina, the point of clearest vision. SYN: *macula lutea*.

y. vision. Condition in which objects seem yellow in color. SYN: *xanthopsia*.

yerba (yer'ba). An herb.

y. maté (mah'tā). Paraguay tea.

Yersin's serum (yer-san'). An antitoxic serum for the plague.

-yl. Suffix signifying, in chemistry, *a radical*.

-ylene. Suffix denoting, in chemistry, *a bivalent hydrocarbon radical*.

Y ligament. A y-shaped band covering the upper and front portions of the hip joint. SYN: *iliofemoral ligament*.

yoghurt (yŏg'hert). Curdled milk containing lactic acid.

Acts as intestinal antiseptic; lessens fermentation. Useful in arthritis and cecal obstructions. It contains only 2 lactic ferments, *i. e.*, a streptococcus bacillus and a streptobacillus. Much used in Bulgaria. SEE: *milk*.

yolk (yōk). The contents of the ovum; sometimes only the nutritive portion. SYN: *vitellus.* SEE: *zona pellucida, zona radiata*.

y. cavity. One within a yolk.

y. cells, y. granules. The granulations composing the yolk.

y. sac. Membranous sac surrounding food yolk in the embryo.

y. stalk. The umbilical duct connecting the yolk sac with the embryo.

y. of wool. Crude wool fat.

Young-Helmholtz theory (yŭng-hĕlm'hōlts). Belief that color vision depends on 3 different sets of retinal fibers responsible for perception of red, green, and violet.

The loss of either red, green, or violet as color perceptive elements in the retina causes an inability to perceive a primary color or any color of which it forms a part.

Young's rule (yŭng). A dose for children is arrived at by adding 12 to the age and dividing the result by the age, making the quotient the denominator of a fraction, the numerator of which is 1. The proportion of the adult dose to be given the child is represented by the fraction.

youth (yūth). Period bet. childhood and maturity.

y. s. Abbr. for *yellow spot* of the retina.

ytterbium (ĭ-tur'bĭ-ŭm). A rare metallic element. SYMB: Yb. At. wt. 173.5.

yttrium (ĭt'rĭ-ŭm). A metallic element. SYMB: Y. At. wt. 88.92.

Yvon's coefficient (ē'vŏn). The ratio bet. the amount of urea and phosphates in the urine.

Y's. tests. One for presence of acetanilide and the other for akaloids in urine.

Z

Zaglas' ligament (zah'glahz). The part of the post. sacroiliac ligament from post. sup. spinous process of ilium to side of sacrum.

Zahn's lines or ribs (zahn). Transverse whitish marks on the free surface of a thrombus made by the edges of the lamellae of blood platelets.

Zander apparatus (zan'der). Mechanical means for massage and exercise designed by Zander about 1857.

Zang's space (zang). One bet. the 2 lower tendons of the sternomastoid muscle in the supraclavicular fossa.

zaranthan (zar-an'than). Scirrhous hardening of the breast.

zein (zē'ĭn). A protein obtained from maize. It is deficient in tryptophane and lysine.

zeismus (zē-ĭz'mŭs). Pellagra believed to be due to excessive diet of corn or corn products.

Zeiss' gland (zīs). One of the sebaceous glands at free edges of eyelids.

zeist (zē'ĭst). A person who believes that pellagra is the result of a diet of maize.

zelotypia (zē-lō-tĭp'ĭ-ă). 1. Morbid or monomaniacal zeal in the interest of any project or cause. 2. Insane jealousy.

Zenker's degeneration, zenkerism (zĕng'-kĕr, -ĭzm). A glassy or waxy, hyaline degeneration of skeletal muscles in acute infectious diseases, esp. in typhoid.

zeoscope (zē'ō-skōp). Device for determining the alcoholic content of a liquid by means of its boiling point.

zero (zē'rō). 1. Figure corresponding to nothing. 2. The point from which the graduation of a scale commences.

zestocausis (zĕs''tō-kaw'sĭs). Cauterization with heated steam.

Ziehl-Neelsen method. One for staining *B. tuberculosis.*

zinc (zĭnk). A bluish-white, crystalline, metallic element. SYMB: Zn. At. wt. 65.38. Sp. gr. 7-7.2 It boils at 930° C. (1706° F.). It is found as a carbonate and silicate, known as *calamine,* as a sulfide, and as a blende.

   z. ac'etate. USP. White, pearly crystals.

   z. chlo'ride. USP. White granular powder.

   z. ointment. An ointment consisting of 20% of zinc oxide mixed with petrolatum or a lard base, used in treating skin diseases.

   z. ox'ide. USP. Very fine white powder.

   DOSAGE: 2-5 gr. (0.12-0.3 Gm.).

   z. stearate. USP. Very fine, smooth powder.

   z. sul'fate. USP. White, transparent crystals.

   DOSAGE: As an emetic, 15 gr. (1 Gm.).

Zinn's ligament (zĭn). Connective tissue giving attachment to the rectus muscles of the eyeball.

   Z., zonule of. Suspensory ligament of lens of the eye. SYN: *zonula ciliaris.*

zirconium (zĭr-kō'nĭ-ŭm). A metallic element found only in combination. SYMB: Zr. At. wt. 91.22.

Zn. Chemical symb. for *zinc.*

zoanthropy (zō-ăn'thrō-pĭ). Delusion that one is an animal.

zoetic (zō-ĕt'ĭk). Pert. to life. SYN: *vital.*

zoetrope (zō'e-trōp). Instrument in which pictures of objects viewed are apparently moving.

zomidin (zō'mĭd-ĭn). A component of meat extract.

zomotherapy (zō''mō-ther'ă-pĭ). Therapeutic administration of a meat diet or meat juice.

zona (zō'nă). 1. A band or girdle. 2. An acute inflammatory disease, characterized by groups of small vesicles mounted on inflammatory bases, associated with neuralgic pain and following the distribution of certain nerve trunks. SYN: *herpes zoster.*

   z. ciliaris. Ciliary processes taken together. SYN: *corona ciliaris.*

   z. facia'lis. Herpes zoster of the face.

   z. granulo'sa. A layer of cells lining the graafian follicle from which the corpus luteum develops.

   z. pellucida. Inner, thick, solid, membranous envelope of the ovum.

   It is pierced by many radiating canals, giving it a striated appearance.

   z. radiata. SEE: *zona pellucida.*

zonal (zō'năl). Pert. to a zone.

   z. stratum. A layer of white fibrous layers on the ventricular surface of the thalamus.

zonary (zō'nar-ĭ). Pert. to or shaped like a zone.

   z. placenta. One arranged in the form of a broad ring around the chorion.

Zondek-Aschheim test (zŏn'dĕk ahsh'hīm). A test for pregnancy. SEE: *test, Aschheim-Zondek.*

zone (zōn). A small zone or belt.

   z's., erotogenic. Areas of the body which when stimulated produce erotic desires.

   z. therapy. Therapeutic stimulation of a part, mechanically, in the same longitudinal zone as the diseased area.

   z. of Zinn. Suspensory ligament of crystalline lens of eye.

zonesthesia (zōn-ĕs-thē'zĭ-ă). A sensation, as of a cord constricting the body. SYN: *cincture sensation.*

zonifugal (zō-nĭf'ū-găl). Passing outward from within any zone or area.

zoning (zō'nĭng). The occurrence of a stronger fixation of complement in a lesser amount of suspected serum; a phenomenon occasionally observed in diagnosing syphilis by complement fixation method.

zonipetal (zō-nĭp'ĕt-ăl). Passing from without into a zone or area of the body.

zonula (zōn'ū-lă). A small zone. SYN: *zonule*.

   z. ciliaris. BNA. Suspensory ligament of the crystalline lens.

zonular (zōn'ū-lar). Pert. to a zonula.

   z. cataract. One with opacity limited to certain layers of the lens.

   z. fibers. Interlacing ones of the zonula ciliaris.

   z. spaces. Those bet. fibers of ligament of the lens.

zonule (zōn'ūl). A small band or area. SYN: *zonula*.

   z. of Zinn. Suspensory ligament of the crystalline lens. SYN: *zonula ciliaris*.

zonulitis (zōn-ū-lī'tĭs). Inflammation of Zinn's zonule.

zoöbiology (zō″ō-bī-ŏl'ō-jĭ). The study of animal life.

zoöchemistry (zō″ō-kĕm'ĭs-trĭ). Chemistry of solids and fluids in animal tissues.

zoödermic (zō″ō-der'mĭk). Performed with the skin of an animal, said of a method of skin grafting.

zoödynamics (zō″ō-dī-năm'ĭks). Science dealing with the vital powers of animals.

zoögenous (zō-ŏj'ĕn-ŭs). Derived or acquired from animals.

zoögeny, zoögony (zō-ŏj'ĕn-ĭ, -ŏn-ĭ). The generation of animals.

zoöglea (zō″ō-glē'ă). A stage in development of certain organisms in which colonies of microbes are embedded in a gelatinous matrix.

zoögraft (zō′ō-gräft). A graft of tissue obtained from an animal.

zoögrafting (zō″ō-gräft'ĭng). Use of animal tissue in grafting on a human body.

zoöid (zō-oyd). 1. Resembling an animal. 2. A form resembling an animal; an organism produced by fission. 3. An animal cell which can move or exist independently.

zoölogy (zō-ŏl'ō-jĭ). The science of animal life.

zoönomy (zō-ŏn'ō-mĭ). Laws of animal life. SYN: *zoöbiology*.

zoönosis (zō-ŏn'ō-sĭs). Any disease acquired from an animal or an animal parasite.

zoöparasite (zō″ō-par'ă-sīt). An animal parasite.

zoöpathology (zō″ō-păth-ŏl'ō-jĭ). Science of the diseases of animals.

zoöphagous (zō-ŏf'ăg-ŭs). Living upon animal food.

zoöphilism (zō-ŏf'ĭl-ĭzm). Abnormal love of animals.

zoöphobia (zō″ō-fō'bĭ-ă). Abnormal fear of animals.

zoöphyte (zō′ō-fīt). A plantlike animal; any of numerous invertebrate animals resembling plants in appearance or mode of growth.

zoöplasty (zō′ō-plăs-tĭ). Transplantation of animal tissue to man.

zoöprecipitin (zō″ō-prē-sĭp'ĭ-tĭn). A precipitin formed from repeated animal protein injections.

zoöpsychology (zō″ō-sī-kŏl'ō-jĭ). Psychology of animals.

zoösis (zō-ō'sĭs). Any disease caused by animal agents, as a parasite. SYN: *zoönosis*.

zoösmosis (zō″ŏz-mō'sĭs). Process of passage of living protoplasm into the tissues from blood vessels.

zoösperm (zō′ō-sperm). Mature male germ cell. SYN: *spermatozoon, q.v.*

zoöspore (zō′ō-spōr). Any spore moving by means of flagella.

zoötomy (zō-ŏt'ō-mĭ). Science dealing with the anatomy of the lower animals.

zoötoxin (zō″ō-tŏks'ĭn). Any toxin or poison produced by an animal, as *snake venom.*

zoster (zŏs'ter). Acute inflammatory disease with vesicles grouped in the course of cutaneous nerves. SYN: *herpes zoster, zona.*

   z. auricula'ris. Herpes zoster of the ear.

   z. ophthal'micus. Herpes affecting the ophthalmic nerve.

zosteriform (zŏs-ter'ĭ-form). Resembling herpes zoster. SYN: *zosteroid.*

zosteroid (zŏs'ter-oyd). Resembling herpes zoster. SYN: *zosteriform.*

zygal (zī'găl). Yoked.

   z. fissure. A cerebral fissure consisting of 2 pairs of branches connected by a stem.

zygapophysis (zī-găp-ŏf'ĭs-ĭs). One of the articular processes of the neural arch of a vertebra.

zygion (zĭj'ĭ-ŏn). Craniometrical point on the zygoma at either end of bizygomatic diameter.

zygocyte (zī'gō-sīt). A cell formed by the union of 2 gametes. SYN: *zygote.*

zygodactyly (zī″gō-dăk'tĭl-ĭ). Fusion of 2 or more fingers or toes. SYN: *syndactylism.*

zygolabialis (zī″gō-lā-bĭ-ā'lĭs). The zygomaticus minor muscle. :

zygoma (zī-gō'mă). 1. BNA. The long arch that joins zygomatic processes of the temporal and malar bones on the sides of the skull. 2. The malar bone.

zygomatic (zī″gō-măt'ĭk). Pert. to the zygoma.

   z. arch. The formation on each side of the cheeks of the zygomatic process of each malar bone articulating with the zygomatic process of the temporal bone.

   z. bone. Bone on either side of the face below the eye. SYN: *malar bone.*

   z. process. 1. A thin projection from the temporal bone bounding its squamous portion. 2. A part of the malar bone helping to form the zygoma.

   z. reflex. Movement of lower jaw toward percussed side when zygoma is percussed.

zygomaticoauricularis (zī″gō-măt″ĭk-ō-awrĭk″ū-lā'rĭs). Muscle which draws the pinna of the ear forward.

zygomaticum (zī″gō-măt′ĭk-ŭm). The zygomatic bone.

zygomaticus (zī-gō-mat′ĭk-ŭs). A muscle which draws the upper lip upward and outward.

zygomaxillary (zī″gō-măks′ĭl-ar-ĭ). Pert. to the cheekbone and upper jaw.

   z. point. A craniometrical point marked at the lower end of the zygomatic suture.

zygon (zī′gŏn). The bar connecting the 2 pairs of branches of a zygal fissure in the cerebrum.

zygoneure (zī′gō-nūr). A nerve cell connecting other nerve cells.

zygosis (zī-gō′sĭs). Fusion of the nuclei of 2 unicellular organisms in sexual union.

zygote (zī′gōt). Cell produced by union of 2 gametes. SYN: *zygocyte.*

zygotoblast (zī-gō′tō-blăst). Any germ originating within a zygote.

zymase (zī′mās). Any of a group of enzymes* which, in the presence of oxygen, convert certain carbohydrates into carbon dioxide and water or, in absence of oxygen, into alcohol and carbon dioxide or lactic acid.

zyme (zīm). A ferment; a disease-producing ferment, as the morbific principle of a zymotic disease.

zymic (zī′mĭk). 1. Pert. to or due to fermentation or a ferment. 2. Denoting an anaerobic microörganism.

zymin (zī′mĭn) . 1. A pancreatic preparation. 2. A ferment. SYN: *zyme.*

zymocyte (zī′mō-sīt). An organism causing fermentation.

zymogen (zī′mō-jĕn). 1. A substance that develops into a chemical ferment or enzyme.

zymogene (zī′mō-gēn). Microbe causing fermentation.

zymogenic (zī-mō-jĕn′ĭk). 1. Causing a fermentation. 2. Pert. to or producing a zymogen.

zymohydrolysis (zī″mō-hī-drŏl′ĭ-sĭs). Decomposition brought about by a ferment. SYN: *zymosis.*

zymoid (zī′moyd). 1. Resembling an enzyme or ferment. 2. An enzyme that can unite with the substratum, but not decompose it.

zymologic (zī-mō-lŏj′ĭk). Relating to zymology.

zymologist (zī-mŏl′ō-jĭst). One who specializes in study of ferments.

zymology (zī-mŏl′ō-jĭ). The science of fermentation.

zymolysis (zī-mŏl′ĭ-sĭs). Changes produced by an enzyme; action of enzymes. SYN: *fermentation, zymosis.**

zymolyte (zī′mō-līt). Substance upon which a ferment acts. SYN: *substrate.*

zymolytic (zī-mō-lĭt′ĭk). Causing fermentation; fermentative.

zymoma (zī-mō′mă). Any ferment.

zymometer (zī-mŏm′et-er). Device for measuring fermentation. SYN: *zymosimeter.* [fungi.

Zymonema (zī-mō-nē′mă). A genus of

zymonematosis (zī″mō-nē-măt-ō′sĭs). Infestation with Zymonema. SYN: *blastomycosis.*

zymophore (zī′mō-fōr). Noting the atomic group bearing the ferment.

zymophoric, zymophorous (zī-mō-for′ĭk, -mŏf′or-ŭs). Having fermentative properties.

zymophyte (zī′mō-fīt). A microörganism causing fermentation.

zymoplastic (zī-mō-plăs′tĭk). Producing a ferment.

zymoscope (zī′mō-skōp). Device for determining zymotic power of yeast.

zymose (zī′mōs). An enzyme that changes a disaccharide into a monosaccharide, such as cane sugar into invert sugar. SYN: *invertin.*

zymosimeter (zī-mōs-ĭm′ĕt-ĕr). Device for determining amount of fermentation.

zymosis (zī-mō′sĭs). 1. Fermentation. 2. Process by which an infectious disease is supposed to develop. 3. An infectious disease.

   z. gas′trica. Organic acid in the stomach.

zymosthenic (zī-mōs-thĕn′ĭk). Increasing the power and activity of an enzyme.

zymotic (zī-mŏt′ĭk). Relating to or produced by fermentation.

   z. disease. Any epidemic, endemic, or contagious disease capable of being induced or produced by some morbific agent or element incident to process or condition of fermentation.

   z. papilloma. Contagious skin disease characterized by reddish sores on the face and hands, feet and ext. genitals. SYN: *yaws.*

   z. principle. A specific matter or element that of itself propagates a zymotic disease, as the zymotic principle of smallpox or syphilis.

   z. theory. The hypothesis that a poisonous particle, either atmospheric or communicated by contact, acts as a ferment to produce certain diseases.